Sports physiotherapy

Applied science and practice

Sports physiotherapy

Applied science and practice

Edited by

Maria Zuluaga BAppSc(Phty) GradDipManipTher MAPA MMPAA
Consultant physiotherapist, Melbourne

Christopher Briggs BSc MSc PhD
Senior lecturer, Department of Anatomy and Cell Biology, University of Melbourne

John Carlisle BAppSc GradDipPhysio(Sports) MAPA
Private practitioner, physiotherapy, Melbourne

Virginia McDonald BAppSc(Phty) GradDipManipTher MAPA MMPAA
Private practitioner, physiotherapy, Melbourne

Joan McMeeken DipPhysio BSc(Hons) MSc MAPA
Professor and Head, School of Physiotherapy, University of Melbourne

Wendy Nickson DipPhys GradDipPhys(Sports) MAPA
Consultant physiotherapist, Melbourne

Pamela Oddy BA(Hons)
Public relations consultant, Australian Physiotherapy Association (Victorian Branch)

Dorothy Wilson BSc(Physio) MSc MAPA
Private practitioner, physiotherapy, Melbourne

Foreword by

Robert de Castella
Director, Australian Institute of Sport, Canberra

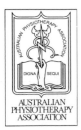

This book has been developed by the editors on behalf of the
Victorian Branch of the Australian Physiotherapy Association.

Churchill Livingstone

CHURCHILL LIVINGSTONE
An imprint of Harcourt Publishers Limited

© Harcourt Brace and Company Limited 1998
© Harcourt Publishers Limited 2000

◿ is a registered trademark of Harcourt Publishers Limited

First published 1995
Reprinted 1998
Reprinted 2000

National Library of Australia Cataloguing-in-Publication Data

Sports physiotherapy : applied science and practice.

  1st ed.
  Bibliography.
  Includes index.
  ISBN 0 443 04804 5.

1. Sports physical therapy. 2. Sports injuries – Treatment. I. Zuluaga,
Maria, 1957– .

615.82

A catalogue record for this book is available from the British Library
A Library of Congress Cataloging in Publication record is available for
this title

Note
Medical knowledge is constantly changing. As new
information becomes available, changes in treatment,
procedures, equipment and the use of drugs become
necessary. The editors / authors / contributors and the
publishers have, as far as it is possible, taken care to ensure
that the information given in this text is accurate and up to
date. However, readers are strongly advised to confirm that
information, especially with regard to drug usage, complies
with the latest legislation and standards of practice.

Neither the publishers nor the author will be liable for any
loss or damage of any nature occasioned to or suffered by any
person acting or refraining from acting as a result of reliance
on the material contained in this publication.

For Churchill Livingstone in Melbourne
Publisher: Judy Waters
Editorial: Pam Jonas
Copy Editing: Adrienne de Kretser
Desktop Preparation: Sandra Tolra
Typesetting: Friedo Ligthart, Designpoint
Indexing: Max McMaster
Production Control: Anke Liebmtz
Design: Churchill Livingstone
Printed in China
NPCC/04

The
publisher's
policy is to use
**paper manufactured
from sustainable forests**

Foreword

It is with great pleasure that I write this foreword. It is an opportunity to acknowledge the support I received from many sports science and medicine professionals who played a significant role in my successful athletic career, and who continue to support many of Australia's finest athletes. Physiotherapists are part of this vital group; they are individuals with specialized skills that assist athletes to maximize their athletic potential.

As Australia races towards the year 2000, expectations greater than ever before will be placed on our athletes to achieve in the international sporting arena. How we prepare our athletes and keep them fit, strong and able, has very much become the responsibility of our coaching, sports science and medicine experts.

Australia is now a recognized world leader in sporting performances, advanced technology, facilities, sports science and medicine. This infrastructure provides a much valued support system for our champion athletes. Today's athletes are required to train harder, for longer, and more often, than ever before. This gradual but continual increase in training and competition workload necessitates more exact injury prevention, diagnosis and recovery. As new training programs are developed to keep Australia ahead of the rest of the world, innovations in areas such as physiotherapy assist athletes in preventing and recovering from injuries that may otherwise adversely affect valuable training and competition opportunities.

Today national sporting bodies, recognizing the essential role of the physiotherapist and the masseur, regularly engage them to accompany teams performing both nationally and internationally. In this role they not only attend to the injured athletes, but also work extensively on recovery. The faster the body is able to recover from the stress of training and competition, the faster it is able to return to an optimal level of performance. This is extremely important in sports where athletes have to compete several times in one day, or several times over consecutive days.

I believe the greatest progress in sports medicine over the next few years will be in the area of recovery. For this reason, the Australian Institute of Sport and other state and national institutions are expanding their involvement from applied treatment into research to determine more precisely the benefits of different therapies and modalities in prevention and recovery.

In my own athletic career I extensively used the services of Australia's finest physiotherapists to keep me on the road. A number of these are contributors to this book. My career as a marathon runner spanned three decades and four Olympics. This was only possible with the help of these experts. In the past, a few individuals were able to succeed on their own. Today this is almost impossible. I often travelled with individuals from the field of sports science and medicine, accessing their knowledge and assistance to maximize my running performances.

When you have put your body through the trauma and stress mine has received over the years, you appreciate friends in the medical field who can help nurture it back to good health. I would not have been able to achieve all I accomplished in the marathon had it not been for such help. When I won the World Marathon Championship in 1993, I had sustained a lower back injury several weeks before the event that required intensive physiotherapy treatment. I was uncertain how it would respond under the stress of competition right up until the morning of the World Championships. Thanks to Craig Purdam and experts like him, my back remained strong and I won the World Championship. This was not the first or last time I relied on physiotherapy to get me through a major international competition, but perhaps, for me, it was the most important.

What is exciting about this book is that it is uniquely Australian: it relates to the Australian sporting experience and uses Australian expertise, which is comparable to any in the world. It draws on a cross-section of expert knowledge from nationally and internationally recognized sports medicine practitioners. Much of the sound advice and application of this book has been drawn from a strong scientific basis coupled with successful application. However, this is not just a book for managing the elite athlete.

Its directions and recommendations are appropriate for all those with a sporting involvement, from the recreational athlete to the Olympic champion.

Ultimately, all Australians can benefit from a lifestyle of sporting involvement. Sport is more productive and enjoyable if it is played without the trauma of injury. Good sports physiotherapy practice can lead to a reduction in the incidence of sports-related injuries. It can also speed recovery and repair.

Make use of the knowledge stored between these pages, and use this information to help the athletes in your care achieve everything they can in the sporting arena.

ROBERT DE CASTELLA

Preface

The stimulus for this book came from the Victorian Chapter of the Sports Physiotherapy Group (SPG) of the Australian Physiotherapy Association. The SPG was aware of the breadth of knowledge and expertise of the many talented Australians who work in the field of sports injury management, and the lack of—and need for—a comprehensive reference work bringing together this knowledge and expertise in a way that meets the specific needs of sports physiotherapists.

Sports Physiotherapy—Applied Science and Practice is the response to this expressed need. It gathers together the best theoretical and clinical knowledge of Australian sports physiotherapists, and integrates it with current information from related fields including applied anatomy, biochemistry, biomechanics, exercise physiology and psychology. Recognition is given to the primary contact status of physiotherapists in Australia and the vital role they play in managing the sports person. The information presented is relevant to the management of all those who participate in sport from the recreational to the elite athlete.

Deliberately written with a strong clinical bias, the book differs from clinical handbooks in that it attempts to reflect the scientific rationale for clinical assessment and management. Concepts are explained and some of the innovative techniques in the management of musculoskeletal injury are discussed. The book also focuses on management by region rather than by individual sport, which enables the reader to apply the information presented to a variety of situations. Further, the book is written specifically for the physiotherapist either actively engaged in working with athletes or aiming to do so, although it offers information valuable to any practitioner interested in the field of sport. These features distinguish the book from many others on sports medicine.

The book has been written by many authors, reflecting the multi-disciplinary team available for the management of athletes. They are drawn from a variety of backgrounds and include physiotherapists who have worked with Australian Olympic and Commonwealth Games teams, physiotherapists in private practice, and researchers and academics from a range of disciplines.

Their contributions reflect their diversity of experience and their individual approaches to management.

The book is divided into seven main sections. Section 1 presents fundamental background information on the biomechanical behaviour of bone, connective tissue, muscle and nerve as well as the ultrastructural properties of these basic tissues, with particular emphasis on their response to injury, training and de-training. It incorporates a review of the physiological mechanisms underlying the body's response to exercise and focuses on the responses which occur at the sub-cellular, cellular and whole body levels. The section concludes with an examination of current theories of pain, as well as the recent literature on the types and location of pain associated with joint and soft tissue injury.

Section 2 discusses the factors to be taken into account in trying to minimise sports injuries. Intrinsic as well as extrinsic factors are identified, including pre-season training, the selection and use of appropriate equipment, particularly footwear, and the need for balanced and progressive training. The research aspects of injury prevention are also highlighted.

Section 3 provides comprehensive information on the principles of assessment and of management. The components of assessment both on and off the field are identified, and presented in a useable format. The section highlights the important role of assessment in developing an appropriate management program.

Section 4 begins with a consideration of the role of fitness testing in the management of athletes of all levels of fitness, and offers advice on the selection of appropriate tests. A variety of management and treatment techniques is then discussed, ranging from manual therapy through isokinetic dynamometry to more recent additions to the fields of sports physiotherapy such as acupuncture.

Section 5 reinforces the team approach to treatment, and emphasises the importance of the athlete's mental state in achieving successful rehabilitation and return to sport or competition. Aptly titled 'Understanding and managing the injured athlete', the section is a reminder of the increasingly important role being played by sports psychology.

Section 6 presents a regional view of injuries and their management. The basic anatomy and biomechanics of each region are discussed, and authors' preferred protocols for assessment and management are presented, together with alternative approaches.

Section 7 recognises sports physiotherapists' need for knowledge beyond their own discipline if they are to play a fully effective role in athlete management. Nutrition, touring with teams, the role of drugs in sport and legal requirements are discussed by experienced practitioners in the relevant fields.

The development of *Sports Physiotherapy—Applied Science and Practice* was co-ordinated for the Australian Physiotherapy Association by a Committee that began as a collection of enthusiastic individuals keen to put their expertise and experience in sports physiotherapy at the project's disposal. These individuals gradually grew into a highly motivated team of scientific editors who acquired valuable editorial and project management skills along the way, as well as enjoying confirmation of the APA's—and their own—belief in the range and depth of local sports physiotherapy expertise.

The book is a reflection of their commitment to provide two things: a showcase for the talents of those involved in sports injury management in Australia; and a valuable resource that will enhance the quality of practice in sports physiotherapy both in Australia and overseas.

Acknowledgements

Any book that has been prepared by a Committee on behalf of an Association and involves over fifty authors is bound to have incurred quite a debt of gratitude.

In the first instance, the Australian Physiotherapy Association (Victorian Branch) would like to extend its thanks to those who served on in the Editorial Committee, in particular Maria Zuluaga, convenor at the project's end, and her colleagues Chris Briggs, John Carlisle, Virginia McDonald, Joan McMeeken, Wendy Nickson and Dorothy Wilson, assisted by Pamela Oddy of the APA Branch Office, who were also on board at publication date. Others who sat on the Committee for a time included Craig Allingham and Lisa Woolf, whose stint included a term as joint convenors, Graham Reid and Louise Jones (formerly of the Branch Office); their contributions were also invaluable.

Those who wrote for *Sports Physiotherapy—Applied Science and Practice* did so on a voluntary basis because they shared the APA's vision of the book's potential as an ambassador for Australian sports physiotherapy expertise. The APA extends its gratitude to these authors for investing many hours of their precious time and expertise in this project, in an outstanding demonstration of professional good will.

In overseeing the development of the book the Editorial Committee was fortunate enough to be able to call on a whole network of expert readers and advisers whose incisive comments helped shape the final form of each contribution. For their work in this capacity, the APA extends its thanks to Craig Allingham, Nick Ames, Frank Archer, Trish Ayers, John Bartlett, Kris Baskus, John Behrsin, Debbie Benger, Peter Bond, Elizabeth Burman, Sara Carroll, Peter Carson, Bev Dalziel, Rod Dalziel, Paula Davidson, Peter Duras, Diana Elton, Rosalie Freeman, Barry Gavin, Rob Hanna, John Hart, Philip Hart, Michael Hase, Robert Hutchinson, Trefor James, Elizabeth Kerr, Daisy Kong, Paul Lew, Wendy Lowe, Wayne MacCombie, Jenny McConnell, Julie Nitschke, Kath Philip, Bruce Reid, Graham Reid, Louisa Remedios, Steve Selig, Tracey Sjogren, Ross Smith, Peter Stanton, Nandor Steidler, Anthony Stewart, Patty Tam, Mary Taylor, Pat Trott, Elizabeth Tully, David Vivian, Harry Vontelas, Lyn Watson, Women's Health Physiotherapy Group (Victorian Chapter), David Young. To any whose names have inadvertently been omitted, apologies as well as thanks are extended.

The support and enthusiasm of the APA's Victorian Branch Council for 'the sports book' was always felt and appreciated by members of the Editorial Committee, who also benefited from the excellent secretarial services provided by the Branch throughout the project. Particular thanks are due to Sandra Rosenberg who set up many of the systems that made it possible.to keep track of so many contributors and manuscripts. Janet Christensen continued to keep things in excellent order during her brief stint at the book secretariat helm, whilst her successor Katie Paynter managed to keep track of myriad captions, illustrations, and authors' biographical details.

The unsung heroes of many a book are the families, partners and friends who remain loyal from the first to the last word, and this book is no exception. The Editorial Committee thanks its large team of supporters who themselves invested many hours in the book through tasks including child-minding, making not only dinner for the family but muffins for Committee meetings, soothing irritable editors, and finally even proofreading and checking references.

Contact with Churchill Livingstone has been a pleasure since the Editorial Committee's first timid efforts at a publication proposal. In addition to their professional expertise, the company's Melbourne publisher Judy Waters and editor Pam Jonas have provided much wise counsel and reassurance both to the Editorial Committee and to individual authors, for which the APA expresses its gratitude.

Last, but far from least, thanks are due to the Victorian Chapter of the Australian Physiotherapy Association's Sports Physiotherapy Group who set the ball rolling. The SPG convinced the APA that the time was ripe for Australian sports physiotherapy to make its mark in the professional literature, and this volume is the validation of their conviction.

Contributors

Jane Abbott BAppSc(Phty)
Hand therapist, Geelong Hand Clinic. Member of Australian Hand Therapy Association.

Jason Agosta BAppSci(Podiatry)
Podiatrist, Olympic Park Sports Medicine Centre and Lecturer (part time), Department of Podiatry, La Trobe University, Melbourne. Represented Australia in the World Cross Country Championships 1986.

Craig Allingham BAppSc(Phty) GradDipSportSc MAPA FASM
Australian team physiotherapist at the 1988 and 1992 Olympic Games. Consultant to the Australian Baseball Federation and guest lecturer on graduate sports medicine courses. Private practice, Healthfocus, specialising in sports physiotherapy, Albury, New South Wales.

Libby Austin BAppSc(Phty) GradDipAdvManipTher
Manipulative physiotherapist in private practice in Glen Osmond, South Australia. Physiotherapist to Garville Netball Team, State Netball League Premiers, 1994.

Wendy Braybon GradDipManipTher GradDipSportsPhys DipPhys(CSP) DipRemGym MAPA MCSP MMPAA
Physiotherapist to Australian Women's Softball Team. Private practitioner, Windsor Physiotherapy Centre, Melbourne.

Christopher Briggs DipPE DipEd BSc MSc PhD
Senior lecturer, Department of Anatomy and Cell Biology, University of Melbourne. Published in a number of areas including blood supply and development of the bone, and factors influencing exercise performance and metabolism.

Peter Brukner MB BS DRCOG FASMF FACSM FACSP
Medical Director, Olympic Park Sports Medicine Centre, Melbourne.

Louise Burke BSc(Nut) GradDip(Diet) PhD
Director, Sports Nutrition program, Australian Institute of Sport, Canberra. Published extensively in the area of sports nutrition.

David Butler BPhty GradDipAdvManipTher
Lecturer, University of South Australia and Neuro-orthopaedic Institute International. Principal of manipulative physiotherapist practice in Adelaide. Widely published in the area of adverse tension in the human nervous system.

John Carlisle BAppSc GradDipPhysio(Sports)
Private practitioner in Melbourne. Medical co-ordinator for umpires in Australian Football League. Lecturer in training courses for coaches in both Victorian Baseball and the Australian Football League. Physiotherapist for Victorian Baseball Team. Member of the AFL Fitness Advisory Committee.

Melinda M. Cooper B(Phty)(Qld) MAPA
Director of a physiotherapy practice specialising in women's health. Lectures and conducts workshops on a variety of women's health topics to physiotherapists, midwives and to public seminars. Writes for women's health publications.

Peter Duras BAppSc(Phty) FASMF
Private practitioner in Melbourne. Experience with over thirty sports at a national level. Has travelled extensively overseas with a range of track and field teams. Physiotherapist to Australian teams at the Commonwealth Games since 1982.

Diana Elton BA BAppSc DipPhysio PhD MAPsC MIASP MIHS LPIBA
Private practitioner who encompasses psychology and physiotherapy in the management of pain and stress. Academic Associate in Department of Psychology, University of Melbourne. Lectures on pain management and psychosomatic medicine.

Charles Flynn BAppSc(Phty) GradDipManipTher
Private practitioner in Ballarat, Victoria. Currently sitting on the Physiotherapy Registration Board of Victoria; member of the Advisory Committee for the Physiotherapy School, University of Melbourne.

Barry Gerrard MSc(Melb) BAppSc(Phty) GradDipManipTher HDDT
Private practitioner in Melbourne and Dandenong. Lecturer in postgraduate diploma courses in manipulative therapy and sports physiotherapy, La Trobe University, Melbourne. Main research interest and publications are in the area of the treatment of patellofemoral pain.

Margaret Grant BSc (Physio)
Lecturer in sport physiotherapy, Faculty of Health Sciences, La Trobe University, Melbourne. Physiotherapist, National Women's Road Cycling Team. Research interests in the biomechanics of lower limb sports injuries.

Rod Green BSc(Hons) DipEd MSc
Lecturer in the School of Human Biosciences, La Trobe University, Melbourne. Currently completing a PhD quantifying the benefits of health promotion in the workplace.

Peter Hamer DipPhys BPE(Hons) MEd FASMF
Private practitioner with a major focus on sports injuries. Currently completing a PhD in the area of muscle mechanics and physiology.

Christopher J. Handley BA(Hons) DipEd(Perth) DSc PhD
Reader, Department of Biochemistry and Molecular Biology, Monash University, Melbourne. Research interests and publications are in the areas of the basic molecular science of joint tissues, and changes that occur as a result of degenerative and inflammatory joint disease or mechanical trauma.

Mark Hargreaves BSc MA PhD
Lecturer, Department of Physiology, University of Melbourne. Current research interest and publications in the area of physiological and metabolic responses to exercise.

Dennis Hatcher BSc PhD
Consultant, exercise and sports management and practice.

Christopher Horsley BEd BSc MClinPsy
Psychologist at the Australian Institute of Sport in Canberra. Member of the 1992 Barcelona Olympic team. Has worked extensively with a number of Australian teams including Women's Hockey, Men's Water Polo and Women's Basketball teams. Consultant to professional rugby league and basketball teams. His particular research interest is the psychology of injury rehabilitation.

Peter Howley BAppSc GradDipManipTher
Private practitioner in Ballarat, Victoria. Specialist lecturer in sports physiotherapy courses; physiotherapist to various sporting clubs. Fellow of the Australian Sports Medicine Federation and joint winner of the BEIERSDORF Sports Medicine Award 1983.

Murray S. Hutchison BSc BAppSc(Phty) GradDipAdvManipTher

Private practitioner, Melbourne, and Associate Lecturer in orthopaedic physiotherapy at La Trobe University, Melbourne.

Jenny Keating BAppSc PostgradDipManipPhysio
Currently completing PhD full time in the Department of Behavioural Health Sciences, La Trobe University, Melbourne.

Michael A. R. Kenihan DipTechPhysio MAPA FASMF
Senior physiotherapist and Director of Sports Medicine Centres of Victoria.

Karim Khan MB BS BMedSci FACSP FASMF
Currently completing PhD in the Department of Medicine, University of Melbourne and Royal Melbourne Hospital. Sports Physician, Australian Goldmark Opals Basketball team.

Kay Knight BAppSc(Phty) GradDipHealthSc Acup(Beijing)
Principal physiotherapist at Rich River, Victoria. Specialises in acupuncture using Traditional Chinese Medicine principles. As a result of being awarded the RACV Sir Edmund Herring scholarship, studied at the Beijing College of Traditional Chinese Medicine in 1988.

John Lang BEd MHK PhD
New South Wales Manager of HBA Health Management. Research interests lie in the area of neuromuscular adaptation to exercise. His current work is in the area of corporate health management.

Colleen Liston MAppSc AUA GradDipHlthSc MCSP PhD
Senior lecturer and Director of the Centre for Applied Research in Exercise Science and Rehabilitation, School of Physiotherapy, Curtin University, Perth. Consultant on massage to Edith Cowan University and TAFE. Consultant on spinal deformity.

Paul C. Lew DipPhysio GradDipAdvManipTher MSc
Lecturer (part time), School of Physiotherapy, University of Melbourne. Private practitioner and physiotherapist to Essendon Football Club. Presented and published papers mainly in the area of neural stretching techniques in the treatment of lower back and leg pain.

Michael J. McKenna BSc(Hons) DipEd MSc PhD
Lecturer, Department of Physical Education and Recreation, Victoria University of Technology, Melbourne.

Joan McMeeken DipPhysio BSc(Hons) MSc
Professor and Head, School of Physiotherapy and Associate Dean, Faculty of Medicine, Dentistry and Health Sciences at the University of Melbourne. Extensive publications on various aspects of electrotherapy.

Mary Magarey DipTechPhysio GradDipAdvManipTher
Lecturer, graduate programs in manipulative, sports and orthopaedic physiotherapy, School of Physiotherapy,

University of South Australia, Adelaide. Co-ordinator, graduate programs in sports physiotherapy and is completing work towards a PhD. Current research interest and publications in the area of manipulative therapy and the musculoskeletal system.

G. D. Maitland MBE MAppSc(Phty)(Hon) FCSP FACP AVA
Visiting lecturer, School of Health and Biomedical Sciences, University of South Australia, Adelaide. Private consultant, manipulative physiotherapy.

Ken Niere BAppSc(Phty) GradDipManipTher
Private practitioner in Melbourne. Lecturer in manipulative therapy, School of Physiotherapy, La Trobe University, Melbourne.

Barry Oakes MB BS MD
Senior Lecturer, Department of Anatomy, Monash University, Melbourne. Director, Sports Medicine Centres of Victoria. Foundation Fellow of the Australian Sports Medicine Federation. Current research interests in the areas of ligament and articular cartilage repair and grafting. Clinical interests associated with soft tissue injuries. Associate editor, Australian Journal of Exercise Science and Sports Medicine.

Hayden Opie BComm LLB(Hons)(Melb) LLM(Tor)Barrister and Solicitor of the Supreme Court of Victoria.
Senior lecturer, Faculty of Law, University of Melbourne. President of the Australian and New Zealand Sports Law Association Inc. since its inception in 1990. Regular speaker at conferences; extensive publications on the relationship between sport and the law.

Jeffrey Oxley BAppSc(Phty) GradDip(Sport)
Private practitioner and Director, Corio Bay Sports Medicine Treatment Clinic in Geelong. Physiotherapist for the Geelong Football Club and the Geelong Basketball Club. President of the Australian Football League Physiotherapists Association. Current clinical interest in the rehabilitation of ACL reconstructions, massage as a therapeutic modality and TENS therapy.

Craig Purdam DipPhty GradDipSportsPhysio
Head, Department of Physiotherapy and Massage Services, Australian Institute of Sport, Canberra.

Margaret Reid Campion GradDipPhty(UK) MSCP MAPA
Hydrotherapy consultant. Extensive experience worldwide in lecturing undergraduate and postgraduate students in hydrotherapy. Numerous publications in this area for both adults and children.

Erica Rundle BAppSc(Phty) GradDipSpPhysio
GradDipManipPhysio
Private practitioner in Melbourne. Has been affiliated with variety of clubs whose sports include Australian Rules football, cricket and swimming.

Steven M. Sandor BAppSc(Physio)
Private practitioner and Director, Sports Medicine Centres of Victoria. Has lectured extensively in postgraduate sports medicine courses and published books and articles in the sports medicine area. Affiliated with the Richmond Football Club, Victorian Cricket Association and numerous local sporting clubs.

Peter J. Selvaratnam PhD BAppSc
GradDipManipTher DipAcup
Director of Melbourne Spinal and Sports Physiotherapy Clinic. Honorary lecturer, Department of Anatomy, Faculty of Medicine, Monash University, Melbourne. Visiting lecturer for the postgraduate diploma of manipulative therapy at La Trobe University, Melbourne. Formerly consultant physiotherapist for the Australian Men's and Women's Basketball teams.

Helen Slater MAppSc BAppSc(Phty) GradDipAdvManTher
Adjunct Lecturer, School of Physiotherapy, Faculty of Health and Biomedical Sciences, University of South Australia, Adelaide. Principal of manipulative physiotherapist practice in Adelaide.

James R. Taylor MB ChB DTM PhD FAFRM
Adjunct Professor, School of Health Sciences, Curtin University, Perth. Principal Research Fellow, Royal Perth Hospital. Private practice, Perth Pain Management Centre.

Mary Toomey BAppSc(Phty) GradDipExRehab
Senior Physiotherapist, Sports Medicine Centres of Victoria. Senior physiotherapist to Melbourne Football Club.

Elizabeth Tully BAppSc(Phty) DipEd
Lecturer, School of Physiotherapy, University of Melbourne. Co-ordinator of Applied Anatomy and Kinesiology for undergraduate and postgraduate courses.

Lance Twomey DipPhysio BAppSc BSc(Hons) PhD
Deputy Vice Chancellor at Curtin University of Technology, Perth. Consultant to a range of education committees, and private and government organisations. Published extensively on aspects of the anatomy of the vertebral column.

Bill Vicenzino BPhty GradDipSpPhysio(Dist) MSc
Associate Lecturer in sports and manipulative physiotherapy in the Department of Physiotherapy, University of Queensland.

Dorothy-Mary Vicenzino BPhty GradDipSpPhysio(Dist)
Staff physiotherapist, Prince Charles Hospital, Brisbane.

Henry Wajswelner BAppSc(Phty) GradDipManipTher
Lecturer in musculoskeletal physiotherapy and exercise prescription, School of Physiotherapy, University of Melbourne. Director, Olympic Park Sports Medicine Centre.

Gillian Webb DipPhysio GradDipExRehab
Lecturer, School of Physiotherapy, University of Melbourne.

Tim Wrigley BSc(Hons) MSc
Researcher, technologist and computer specialist in biomechanics and physiology in the Centre for Rehabilitation, Exercise and Sport Science and the Department of Physical Education and Recreation at Victoria University of Technology, Melbourne.

Guy Zito DipPhysio GradDipAdvManipTher
Course Co-ordinator and Lecturer, Masters programs and Graduate Diploma in Manipulative Physiotherapy, Faculty of Health Sciences, La Trobe University, Melbourne. Private practice, Carlton Physiotherapy Centre, Melbourne.

Contents

Introduction

Craig Purdam

Sports physiotherapy must surely rank as one of the most interesting, challenging and rewarding vocations available today. At a time when excellence in sport remains a national pursuit, opportunities abound for highly motivated and dedicated sports physiotherapists to fill a vital role in supporting the athlete in their quest.

The role of the sports physiotherapist has expanded markedly over the past few years, reflecting in part the information explosion that has occurred within sports medicine in general. Whilst the clinical setting remains the greatest source of contact with the athletic population, a greater emphasis is now being placed on preventive measures. These include areas such as coach and athlete education as well as pre-participation screening followed by appropriate generalized or specific remedial programs.

More team and individual sports are now utilizing physiotherapists as support staff at training and competition venues, where their role may vary greatly according to the sport, venue, country and availability of associated sports medicine practitioners such as doctors, trainers, masseurs, exercise physiologists.

Sports physiotherapists working closely with a sport may have much to offer the coach or physical educator in terms of performance enhancement of an individual or group by virtue of their unique combination of knowledge that includes kinesiology, biomechanics, physiology and pathology. This may be as a result of specific research pertaining to the particular athlete or sport, or through the application of pre-existing knowledge.

To increase the knowledge and awareness of the expertise available within the sports physiotherapy profession the education of peers and other members of the sports medicine support team on developments in sports physiotherapy remains very important.

Specialized knowledge

The sports physiotherapist requires specialized knowledge in many areas, and the keystone to a high level of expertise in sports physiotherapy is undoubtedly a thorough understanding of anatomy, functional anatomy and kinesiology, combined with a forte in clinical reasoning.

Investigations concerning the aetiology of many of the injuries managed by the physiotherapist demands a fundamental knowledge of sports biomechanics which is particularly pertinent when combined with kinesiology. This knowledge should include an understanding of the biomechanics of the foot/shoe interface, foot function in shock attenuation and propulsion, the storage and utilization of elastic energy within the musculo-tendinous unit, and a working knowledge of impact and translational forces encountered in different sporting activities. These would include running, throwing, swimming, jumping, cycling and rowing.

A working knowledge of sports psychology is of great advantage to the physiotherapist in terms of optimal management of the chronically injured athlete. Whilst it is not expected that the treating physiotherapist perform this role as such, an understanding of the functions of the sports psychologist helps to create the most favorable conditions for rehabilitation of long term injuries to take place.

Sports pharmacology is relevant in terms of understanding the effects of various medications on healing rates, alteration of pain perception or mood state, interactions with other substances, and physiological side effects. The physiotherapist also requires a comprehensive knowledge of banned substances, particularly when in the situation of sole medical support travelling with teams, as they may be required to assist or advise in drug screening and/or testing procedures.

Specialized knowledge is required in training physiology. This includes an awareness of the normal physiology and adaptive processes occurring in the various tissues of the cardiovascular, neuromuscular and musculoskeletal system in response to training loads. The physiotherapist must also recognise the potential for reversibility of these processes, because the level at which the athlete returns to sport following a prolonged lay-off requires integration of these principles into the training program set in collaboration with the coach.

The sports physiotherapist may often be involved in the later stages of rehabilitation in teaching skill acquisition or skill maintenance. Intrinsic or overuse injuries are frequently the result of poor movement patterns which must be addressed in order to prevent recurrence.

Understanding the particular sport, its biomechanics, anatomy and kinesiology gives the physiotherapist a basis for analysis of the causative factors in sports injuries. These will vary according to the nature of the injury (intrinsic, extrinsic or overuse) but form the basis of more complete management of sports injuries.

Specialized skills

As with all areas of special interest within our profession, sports physiotherapists require a number of specialized skills. These include:

- A high level of manual therapy skills, equipping the physiotherapist with the ability to treat effectively soft tissue and/or joint conditions with techniques that include massage, stretching, mobilisation, manipulation, trigger point or deep connective tissue therapy
- An ability to make a thorough postural analysis of athletes both in a static and dynamic sense as it relates to their sporting activities. This should be accompanied by the appropriate remedial skills for designing a variety of rehabilitation programs to suit
- The ability to apply appropriate strapping or bandaging to an injury or, where applicable, the ability to fabricate splints or temporary orthoses
- The ability to make accurate on-field diagnosis and follow this up with appropriate management of the acute injury, including the implementation of emergency procedures if required
- Utilizing previous experience and/or information from the sport and relevant literature, the sports physiotherapist must be capable of formulating and implementing injury preventive conditioning programs for that sport
- In preparation for championship or tournament competition individuals and teams often undertake a pre-participation examination. The sports physiotherapist should be capable of designing a meaningful method of screening participants and putting this into practice
- The sports physiotherapist must be capable of adapting his or her practice when touring with either individual or team sports, domestically or overseas. Variable factors such as venue, language, backup, equipment, travel, power supply and time constraints all add to the challenge of providing the best possible advice.

Inter-relationships

The sports physiotherapist working with an individual or team sport is in a unique situation in being part of the staff supporting the team. As with all teams it is imperative that for the best results each member of the support team have a respect and understanding of the role and expertise of the other members of that team. Each team member should also be aware of their own limitations and be constantly mindful of the person(s) best equipped for the task at hand. The relationships the sports physiotherapist develops with those other persons involved with the team can vary greatly.

The team doctor, physiotherapist, trainer and masseur must understand each other's roles in providing the most efficient and credible service to the sport. The importance of this cannot be over-emphasized as a breakdown in this unit will directly affect the management of injuries as well as the 'chemistry' and ultimately the performance of the athlete or team.

Likewise, it is important that the sports physiotherapist understands the role of the other sport health professionals, i.e. psychologists, nutritionists, physiologists and physical educators, and refers athletes or coaches to those professionals should the need arise. The physiotherapist is ideally situated to perform this task by virtue of regular contact with injured athletes.

It is important when dealing with the administration of any sport that the physiotherapist be scrupulously professional and apolitical. Politics abound within sport, often creating changing power bases.

The relationships that sports medicine personnel develop with the coach have the potential to be immensely satisfying. They become allied with the common goal of the athlete or team while they aim to remain objective for best results. Learning the sport and working with the coach in developing productive training sessions for the injured athlete can be rewarding; however, one should also remember the coach can become as frustrated as the athlete when injuries occur.

The relationship the sports physiotherapist develops with the athlete is generally a little more relaxed than that normally encountered in the consultation room. This generally works to the physiotherapist's advantage as he or she is accepted as 'one of the team'. However, this should be continually balanced against one's professionalism to achieve the ideal level of professional distance that ensures long term workability and mutual respect. The physiotherapist is also quite commonly the member of the medical team with the responsibility to ensure the athlete has a thorough understanding of his or her injury, its aetiology, expected conservative/operative management and estimated recovery time. The provision of this information at times will require sensitivity and tact whilst ensuring it is accurate and realistic.

In summary, sports physiotherapy can be an immensely satisfying field that demands of the practitioner a thirst for greater knowledge, accurate judgement in clinical and emergency situations, specialised physical skills, an awareness of responsibilities and the responsibilities of others associated with sport, and a full understanding of the aims and objectives of the coach and athletes in question.

Exercise and injury

1. Physiological responses to exercise

Michael J. McKenna, Mark Hargreaves

The integrated response to physical exercise involves the co-ordinated interplay between the physiological systems responsible for increased energy metabolism, supply of oxygen and substrates to contracting skeletal muscle, removal of metabolic waste products and heat, and the maintenance of fluid and electrolyte balance. This chapter will provide a brief overview of some aspects of exercise physiology, and for a more detailed discussion of the physiological responses to exercise readers are referred to the books and review articles listed at the end of the chapter.

Skeletal muscle

Skeletal muscle represents as much as 40–50% of the total body weight and is responsible for development of tension necessary for joint movement. The basic structure and function of skeletal muscle is well covered in recognized anatomy and physiology textbooks and will not be discussed further. Nevertheless, knowledge of the sequence of events involved in muscle contraction is crucial in understanding muscle function during exercise. (see box)

Sequence of events during muscle contraction and relaxation

1 Motor cortical activation and excitation of alpha motor neuron
2 Arrival of electrical impulse at neuromuscular junction
3 Propagation of muscle action potential across sarcolemma
4 Excitation-contraction coupling:
   —conduction of excitation in T-tubule system
   —release of calcium from sarcoplasmic reticulum
   —action of calcium on muscle myofibrils
5 Contraction of myofibrils ('sliding filament theory') and tension development
6 Re-uptake of calcium by sarcoplasmic reticulum and muscle relaxation

---

The immediate energy source for muscle contraction is adenosine 5' triphosphate (ATP). Activation of the myosin ATPase enzyme during excitation-contraction coupling results in the hydrolysis of ATP. ATP also is required for other energy-dependent processes within the muscle cell (e.g. ion exchange by the calcium pump in the sarcoplasmic reticulum and sodium-potassium pump in the sarcolemma). Since the intramuscular stores of ATP are relatively small (5 mmol/kg), other metabolic pathways must be rapidly activated to maintain ATP supply for continued contractile activity. Creatine phosphate (CP) is stored in larger amounts (approx. 20 mmol/kg) and serves as a reservoir of high-energy phosphate bonds for the rapid replenishment of ATP when broken down by creatine kinase. ATP also can be regenerated from ADP through the action of adenylate kinase. The majority of ATP, however, is produced from anaerobic glycolysis and oxidative metabolism. The major substrates for oxidation are carbohydrates and lipids, with a smaller contribution from amino acids. (Table 1.1)

The relative importance of these metabolic pathways is dependent upon the intensity and duration of exercise. During high-intensity short-duration exercise (sprint and power events), breakdown of the high energy phosphagens (ATP, CP) and the degradation of glycogen to lactate are the major energy-yielding processes. Static exercise, particularly above 30-40% of maximum voluntary contraction, is also primarily dependent upon ATP, CP and glycogen since blood flow, and therefore oxygen and

Table 1.1 Energy metabolism in skeletal muscle

ATP utilization
$$ATP \rightarrow ADP + Pi + H^+ + energy$$

ATP resynthesis
(1) Anaerobic
$$ATP + CP + H^+ \rightarrow ATP + creatine$$
$$2\ ADP \rightarrow ATP + AMP$$
$$Glucose\ (glycogen) + 2(3)\ ADP \rightarrow 2\ lactate + 2(3)\ ATP + 2H^+$$
(2) Aerobic
$$2\ pyruvate + 6\ O_2 + 36\ ADP \rightarrow 6\ CO_2 + 6\ H_2O + 36\ ATP$$
$$Palmitate + 23\ O_2 + 130\ ADP \rightarrow 16\ CO_2 + 16\ H_2O + 130\ ATP$$

substrate supply, is reduced. During prolonged submaximal exercise (endurance events), there is primary reliance on the oxidative metabolism of carbohydrates, lipids and, to a lesser extent, amino acids (Felig & Wahren 1975, Gollnick 1985).

One aspect of skeletal muscle physiology that has received considerable attention in the exercise sciences over the last 15-20 years has been the relationship between skeletal muscle fibre type composition and exercise performance. Skeletal muscle fibres can be classified into two main types on the basis of their contractile, metabolic and morphological characteristics: slow twitch (ST) and fast twitch (FT). The FT fibres have been further classified into FTa and FTb on the basis of differences in their oxidative and glycolytic potential (Table 1.2). An intermediate fibre type, with characteristics of both ST and FT fibres, has also been identified and is believed to represent a transitional stage in fibre transformation. The fibre types can be differentiated in human skeletal muscle using histochemical and biochemical techniques (Saltin & Gollnick, 1983). The most commonly used histochemical technique utilizes differences between ST and FT fibres in the acid/alkaline stability of myosin ATPase. (Table 1.2)

The ST fibres have a high oxidative capacity and capillary density and a low fatiguability, and are innervated by small motor neurons. Not surprisingly, they are well suited for prolonged low-intensity activity. In contrast, the FT fibres have a higher glycolytic capacity (FTb > FTa), with a lower oxidative capacity (FTa > FTb) and a greater fatiguability (FTb > FTa) and are innervated by large motor neurons. These fibres are well adapted for high-intensity exercise. The size principle (Henneman 1957) describes the muscle fibre recruitment pattern during exercise of varying intensity. Small motor neurons are activated first,

resulting in ST fibre involvement at low exercise intensities; at higher intensities, larger motor neurons, and therefore the FT fibres, are activated. This general pattern of fibre recruitment has been confirmed by studies utilizing histochemical visualization of glycogen staining intensity before and after exercise as an index of muscle fibre involvement. During prolonged submaximal exercise, the ST fibres are primarily involved (Vøllestad et al 1984), although in the latter stages there may be involvement of the FTa fibres. As exercise becomes more intense, there is progressive involvement of the FT fibres so that at exercise intensities approaching and above maximal oxygen uptake, all fibre types will be recruited (Vøllestad & Blom 1985, Vøllestad et al 1992). The differential involvement of muscle fibre types in activities of varying intensities has resulted in interest in the potential role of skeletal muscle fibre composition in specifically trained athletes as a determinant of exercise performance. Indeed, it has been observed that the muscles of elite endurance athletes are composed primarily of ST muscle fibres (70–90%), while the muscles of sprint and explosive athletes possess relatively more FT fibres (Bergh et al 1978, Costill et al 1975, Saltin & Gollnick 1983). This has generally been ascribed to genetic factors and natural selection, since skeletal muscle fibre composition is identical in monozygotic twins (Komi et al 1977). More recently, however, the observations that the increased percentage of ST muscle fibres in endurance athletes may be limited to the trained musculature (Tesch & Karlsson 1985) and evidence of intermediate fibres in muscle following training (Baumann et al 1987, Klitgaard et al 1990, Schantz 1986) raise the possibility that regular training can modify skeletal muscle fibre characteristics.

Exercise metabolism

During high-intensity dynamic exercise (e.g. sprint running and swimming, track cycling, interval training), the breakdown of the high energy phosphagens (ATP, CP) and the degradation of glycogen to lactate are the major energy-yielding pathways (Hermansen et al 1984). Muscle ATP levels may fall by as much as 30–50%, depending upon exercise intensity and duration, although they are never completely depleted. In contrast, muscle CP may be reduced almost to zero following maximal exercise. Muscle glycogen can be reduced by 50–60% following a single, maximal exercise bout, accompanied by a 10–20 fold increase in muscle lactate. Fatigue during such exercise is often associated with intramuscular acidosis and electrolyte disturbances, although CP depletion and glycogen depletion in FT fibres may also play a role. For exercise extending to a duration of minutes and hours, the oxidative metabolism of carbohydrates and lipids provides the vast majority of ATP. Although for many years protein was not thought to be utilized during prolonged exercise, recent reports have

Table 1.2 Characteristics of muscle fibre types in human skeletal muscle

Characteristics	ST	FTa	FTb
Contractile			
Ca^{2+} activated myosin ATPase (mmol/min.mg protein)	0.16	0.48*	0.48*
Time to peak tension (ms)	80	30*	30*
Substrate contents			
ATP	4.9	5.3	4.9
CP	12.6	14.5	14.8
Glycogen	78	83	89
Triglycerides	7.1	4.2*	4.2*
Enzyme activities			
Creatine kinase (mmol/min.g protein)	13.1	16.6*	16.6*
Phosphorylase	2.8	5.8	8.8
Phosphofructokinase	7.5	13.7	17.5
Citrate synthase	10.8	8.6	7.5
Hydroxyacyl-CoA dehydrogenase	14.8	11.6	7.1

Substrate contents are in mmol/kg; enzyme activities (unless otherwise stated) are in mmol/kg.min.
* determined on pools of FT fibres.
Source: Saltin & Gollnick (1983).

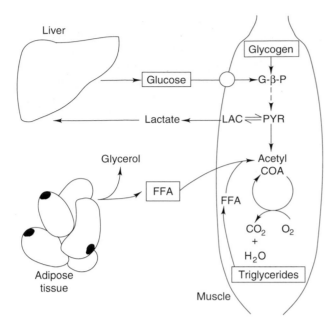

Fig. 1.1 Overview of carbohydrate and lipid metabolism during prolonged exercise. Source: Richter et al (1981)

indicated oxidation of amino acids during exercise (Hood & Terjung 1990). Despite these observations, carbohydrates and lipids remain the most important oxidative substrates. The relative mix of carbohydrate and lipid utilization during exercise is influenced by such factors as exercise intensity and duration, training status and diet (Fig. 1.1)(Felig & Wahren 1975, Gollnick 1985, Hargreaves 1991).

Muscle glycogen is the important substrate during both intense short-duration and prolonged exercise. Since fatigue during prolonged exercise is often associated with muscle glycogen depletion, glycogen loading prior to endurance exercise has become popular (see Ch. 35). The rate of muscle glycogen utilization is most rapid during the early stages of exercise and is exponentially related to exercise intensity (Vøllestad & Blom 1985). The regulation of muscle glycogenolysis during exercise involves the interplay between local and hormonal factors (Hargreaves & Richter 1988). Contraction-induced increases in intramuscular calcium and inorganic phosphate will stimulate glycogen breakdown, as will adrenaline released from the adrenal medulla during strenuous exercise. As the muscle glycogen level declines with exercise, and glucose delivery increases, blood glucose becomes more important as a carbohydrate substrate. Glucose uptake by contracting skeletal muscle can increase from 0.1 mmol.min^{-1} at rest to as high as 3-4 mmol.min^{-1}, depending upon the exercise intensity and duration (Katz et al 1986, Wahren 1977). The increase in glucose uptake is achieved by an increased muscle membrane glucose transport and activation of the glycolytic and oxidative enzymes responsible for glucose disposal (Hargreaves 1990). Liver glucose output also increases (Wahren 1977) so that blood glucose levels are maintained, or even

slightly increased during the early stages of exercise. This is initially due to increased liver glycogenolysis; however, as exercise continues, an increasing proportion of liver glucose output is due to the synthesis of new glucose (gluconeogenesis) from such precursors as lactate, pyruvate, glycerol and amino acids (Felig & Wahren 1975). During prolonged exercise lasting several hours, liver glucose output may fall behind muscle glucose uptake, resulting in hypoglycemia. Ingestion of carbohydrate during prolonged exercise will maintain blood glucose levels and a high rate of carbohydrate oxidation and improve endurance performance (Costill & Hargreaves 1992). In addition to being a gluconeogenic precursor, there is evidence that lactate is also a substrate for oxidative metabolism, particularly in ST fibres, during exercise (Brooks 1986). Contracting skeletal muscle also derives energy from the ß-oxidation of free fatty acids (FFA), mobilized from the adipose tissue triglyceride stores. The muscle uptake and utilization of FFA is determined by their arterial concentration and the ability of muscle to oxidize FFA. Peak plasma FFA levels are usually attained after 3–4 hours of exercise, at which time they have become the major fuel source (Felig & Wahren 1975). Muscle triglycerides can also contribute to exercise metabolism. It has been suggested that they are more important early in exercise and during exercise at higher intensity when adipose tissue lipolysis may be inhibited (Jones et al 1980, McCartney et al 1986). In contrast, plasma triglycerides are believed to make only a minor contribution to lipid metabolism during exercise.

OXYGEN TRANSPORT SYSTEM

The increase in oxidative metabolism that occurs during all intensities of exercise is critically dependent upon the delivery of oxygen to contracting skeletal muscle and, thus, upon the functional capacities of the cardiovascular and respiratory systems. Over the years there has been considerable interest in the physiological determinants of oxygen transport and utilization during exercise which contribute to maximal oxygen uptake (VO$_2$ max), the most widely accepted measure of aerobic (cardiorespiratory) fitness.

Cardiovascular system during exercise

During exercise, the cardiovascular system is regulated to perform a number of important functions: (1) to increase blood flow and oxygen delivery to contracting skeletal and cardiac muscle; (2) to maintain mean arterial blood pressure, thereby ensuring adequate cerebral blood flow; and (3) to minimize exercise-induced hyperthermia by transporting heat to the skin where it is used to evaporate sweat. With the onset of exercise, there is a marked and rapid vasodilation in active skeletal muscle due to the release of vasoactive metabolites from contracting muscle. These substances include potassium (K^+), hydrogen ion (H^+), and lactate ions and adenosine, together with development of local hypercapnia, hypoxia and hyperosmolality. Despite the large reduction in skeletal muscle vascular resistance, mean arterial pressure increases due to the increase in cardiac output and systolic blood pressure. Diastolic blood pressure is usually maintained at resting levels, due to vasoconstriction in the splanchnic, renal and inactive muscle vascular beds, although it may fall at higher exercise intensities as blood flow increases to contracting muscle. Cardiac output increases from about 5 l.min^{-1} at rest to as high as 20–25 l.min^{-1} during maximal exercise and can be even higher in endurance athletes. This is achieved by increases in both heart rate and stroke volume, mediated by withdrawal of vagal activity, activation of cardiac sympathetic nerves and increases in circulating adrenaline, released from the adrenal medulla. In addition, venous return is enhanced by the rhythmic action of the contracting muscles on peripheral veins ('muscle pump') and by alterations in intrathoracic pressure during the respiratory cycle. Regional vasoconstriction, mediated by the sympathetic nervous system, not only minimizes the fall in total peripheral resistance, but also causes displacement of blood into the large veins, thereby assisting in the maintenance of ventricular filling. As exercise continues, a rise in core temperature of $1–2°C$ results in vasodilation of the cutaneous circulation, which is greatly enhanced if the environmental temperature is high. While this is essential for heat loss, it has the unfortunate consequence of displacing blood to the periphery, resulting in reduced central venous pressure, a decline in stroke volume and an increase in heart rate. The cutaneous circulation, however, is a target of sympathetic vasoconstriction at higher exercise intensities when the need to maintain mean arterial pressure overrides thermoregulatory demands. The regulation of the cardiovascular response to exercise involves the coordination of a number of neurohumoral factors. Cardiovascular effector outflow ('central command'), generated in parallel with motor cortical activation of skeletal muscle, sets the pattern of cardiovascular activity (Mitchell 1990). This is then subject to feedback modulation by a number of reflex mechanisms including muscle chemoreflexes and the arterial baroreflexes (Rowell & O'Leary 1990). In addition, alterations in blood volume, body temperature and arterial O_2 content are likely to influence this activity. Some of these responses will be mediated by increases in the circulating levels of renin, angiotensin, vasopressin and adrenaline. For an excellent review of the cardiovascular responses to exercise, readers are referred to Rowell (1986).

Respiratory system during exercise

Accompanying the cardiovascular response to exercise is an increase in pulmonary ventilation, to ensure maintenance of arterial oxygenation and elimination of carbon dioxide. This is achieved by an increase in both tidal volume and breathing frequency. The success of the ventilation control systems in minimizing exercise-induced alterations in the chemical composition of the blood is demonstrated by the remarkable stability of arterial PO_2, PCO_2 and pH during mild to moderate exercise. During the early stages of incremental exercise, ventilation increases in proportion to the increases in oxygen consumption (VO_2) and carbon dioxide production (VCO_2). A point is reached, however, beyond which the increase in ventilation is larger than the increase in VO_2. This point is often referred to as the ventilatory or anaerobic threshold. It has been suggested that this abrupt increase in ventilation is due to increases in VCO_2, arising from bicarbonate buffering of lactic acid from contracting skeletal muscle (Wasserman et al 1986). There is considerable debate and controversy in the literature regarding the mechanisms of lactate production during exercise and the suggested causal link between blood lactate and ventilation, as summarized in a number of reviews (Brooks 1985, Davis 1985, Katz & Sahlin 1988, McLellan 1987, Walsh & Banister 1988, Wasserman et al 1986). Despite the controversy, the measurement of the ventilatory threshold has proved useful in the assessment of endurance athletes (Williams 1990), since it provides a measure of the maximal steady-state work rate during prolonged exercise and is a strong predictor of endurance exercise performance. The ventilatory responses to exercise involve the interaction between neural and humoral inputs to the respiratory centre. These include CO_2 flow to the lung, descending neural drive linked to motor cortical activation of skeletal muscle, feedback from chemoreceptors and proprioceptors in contracting muscle, increased body temperature, and alterations in the arterial levels of H^+, K^+ and adrenaline (Dempsey et al 1985, Forster & Pan 1991).

Maximal oxygen uptake

The transfer of oxygen from the atmosphere to the mitochondria within contracting muscle, where it is utilized during oxidative metabolism, involves a number of physiological systems and processes. While it is relatively difficult to assess the individual steps involved in oxygen transfer, it is possible to obtain an overall measure of the functional capacity of the aerobic energy system—maximal oxygen uptake or VO_2 max. Maximal oxygen uptake is a measure of the ability of the contracting muscle to consume oxygen in substrate metabolism and the combined abilities of the respiratory and cardiovascular systems to deliver oxygen to the muscle mitochondria. There has been considerable interest in the physiological factors that limit VO_2 max (Fig. 1.2). The argument usually divides into two views: that VO_2 max is limited by oxygen supply to the muscles or

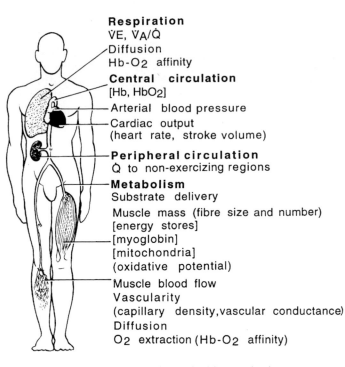

Respiration
$\dot{V}E$, $\dot{V}A/\dot{Q}$
Diffusion
Hb-O_2 affinity
Central circulation
[Hb, HbO$_2$]
Arterial blood pressure
Cardiac output
(heart rate, stroke volume)
Peripheral circulation
$\dot{Q}$ to non-exercizing regions
Metabolism
Substrate delivery
Muscle mass (fibre size and number)
[energy stores]
[myoglobin]
[mitochondria]
(oxidative potential)
Muscle blood flow
Vascularity
(capillary density, vascular conductance)
Diffusion
O_2 extraction (Hb-O_2 affinity)

Fig. 1.2 Potential physiological factors limiting maximal oxygen uptake. Source: Saltin & Rowell (1980)

by the ability of the muscles to consume oxygen (Wagner 1991). There seems to be reasonably general agreement that it is oxygen supply that limits VO_2 max (Saltin & Rowell 1980, Wagner 1991). The question arises of whether a single link in the oxygen transport system can be identified as the limiting factor. In the past, the respiratory system has been largely dismissed as a limiting factor on the basis of the observation that arterial oxygen saturation is well maintained during exercise at sea level.

Recent studies, however, have observed arterial desaturation during severe exercise in a number of highly trained athletes (Powers & Williams 1987). When arterial desaturation is prevented, VO_2 max is significantly increased (Powers et al 1989). The cause of this arterial desaturation appears to be a diffusion limitation, rather than inadequate hyperventilation. It has been suggested that in these athletes cardiovascular adaptations, resulting in increased cardiac output and reduced pulmonary transit times, expose the lung as the weak link (Dempsey 1986). Alternatively, it is possible that the athletes studied have a genetic predisposition to arterial desaturation. Nevertheless, in almost all healthy subjects, arterial desaturation usually does not occur and under these circumstances the respiratory system is not thought to be limiting. Other authors have suggested that there is a central cardiovascular limitation, due to an upper limit for maximal cardiac output and muscle blood flow when the amount of active muscle mass is large (Rowell 1988, Saltin 1985). In addition, elevated arterial hemoglobin levels, induced by 'blood doping', have been shown

to increase VO_2 max (Buick et al 1980). Finally, it has recently been suggested that oxygen supply to mitochondria is limited by the oxygen diffusion capacity of the tissues (Wagner 1991).

In view of the number of links in the oxygen transport system, it is unlikely that one single factor will limit VO_2 max in all situations. Rather, all components of the oxygen transport pathway, by influencing either oxygen delivery or tissue diffusion of oxygen, will play a role in determining VO_2 max (Wagner 1991). Thus, oxygen delivery will be determined by cardiac output, muscle blood flow and arterial oxygen content (influenced by inspired oxygen, pulmonary gas exchange and arterial hemoglobin), while tissue oxygen diffusion will be affected by hemoglobin oxygen dissociation, oxygen diffusion through the erythrocyte and plasma, capillary surface area and diffusion and myoglobin-facilitated transport of oxygen into the muscle mitochondria.

MUSCLE FATIGUE

Definitions and overview

Muscle fatigue is usually defined as a failure to maintain the required or expected force output (Edwards 1981), or as a loss of force generating capacity of muscle (Vøllestad & Sejersted 1988). However, these definitions are limited, since they omit several important manifestations of fatigue and do not adequately define fatigue during dynamic contractions. Since the muscular power output is substantially reduced with fatigue (McCartney et al 1986, de Haan et al 1989), fatigue may be more appropriately defined as an impairment in the force and power generating capacity of muscle. This definition covers the decline in maximal force and in the rate of force development with fatigue, as well as the marked slowing of muscular relaxation (Fig. 1.3).

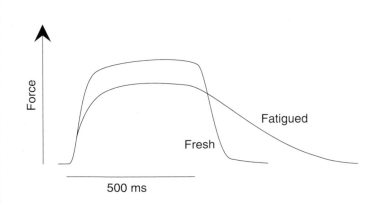

Fig. 1.3 Development and relaxation of force in the human first dorsal interosseous muscle when fresh and after 30 second fatiguing contraction. Source: Cady et al (1989a)

No single mechanism can account for all components of muscular fatigue; indeed, both the loss of force and slowing of relaxation appear to have a multi-factorial and possibly separate basis. Further, the mechanisms of muscular fatigue in prolonged submaximal contractions may well be different from those in short-duration intense exercise. This section outlines the possible sites and mechanisms of muscular fatigue during exercise. Recent reviews on muscle fatigue include those by Fitts and Metzger (1988), Vøllestad and Sejersted (1989), McClaren et al (1990), Westerblad et al (1991) and Fitts (1994).

Sites of fatigue: central vs peripheral

The exact site of fatigue remain controversial, but they may include central nervous and peripheral muscular processes (Asmussen 1978, Bigland-Ritchie 1981). Central nervous processes include the initiation of motor patterns in the motor cortex, propagation of impulses down descending motor pathways and the excitation of alpha motor neurons, ultimately resulting in the recruitment of the motor unit. Central fatigue has been demonstrated in some subjects by an inability to fully recruit all motor units during a fatiguing isometric contraction (Bigland-Ritchie et al 1978). However, this effect could be negated in most subjects by adequate familiarization, feedback and motivation. Recently, incomplete motor unit recruitment of the elbow flexor muscles (about 90% recruitment) has been demonstrated during fatiguing isometric contractions, indicating the presence of central fatigue (Gandevia 1992). However, central fatigue accounted for only a small proportion of the decline in force during isometric contractions.

Thus, while central fatigue may exist during isometric contractions, most of the fatigue originates at peripheral sites. Complete studies of the role of central fatigue during dynamic contractions remain to be undertaken, although a recent study has suggested that central fatigue may contribute (Newham et al 1991). Possible peripheral sites of fatigue include the sarcolemma, t-tubular system, sarcoplasmic reticulum (SR), and the actin-myosin cross-bridges. These reflect the processes of membrane excitation, excitation-contraction coupling and uncoupling and metabolic energy production.

Proposed mechanisms of muscular fatigue

Possible mechanisms of fatigue have traditionally been broadly categorized under the depletion of substrates, accumulation of metabolites, ionic disturbances and impairment of excitation-contraction coupling and uncoupling. Fatigue has been linked with each of these factors, but this link is clearly dependent upon such factors as exercise intensity and duration.

Substrate depletion

Both CP and glycogen may undergo substantial depletion during exercise. The early finding that CP was almost totally depleted with intense exercise lasting several minutes, suggested that CP depletion may be linked with fatigue through a deficiency in ATP generation (Hultman et al 1967). A more rapid and marked muscular fatigue is found during intense sprinting exercise lasting only 30 seconds in duration. Associated with this form of exercise are decreases in muscle CP by 70%, glycogen stores by up to 30% and ATP by up to 40-50% (Cheetham et al 1986, McCartney et al 1986). Although this reflects a greater rate of ATP utilization than ATP generation, it would appear from these results that sufficient CP and ATP stores remain for continued high-intensity exercise. More recently, investigations of changes in ATP and CP in single muscle fibres taken by muscle biopsy from the vastus lateralis after fatiguing electrical stimulation, demonstrated declines in ATP of up to 40–50%, with total depletion of CP in ST and FT fibres (Soderlund & Hultman 1991). This finding suggests that the rate of ATP resynthesis may indeed be limiting during very intense contractile activity. During prolonged exercise, muscle glycogen stores may become exhausted, particularly in ST fibres (Vøllestad et al 1984). Despite this dramatic metabolic substrate depletion, muscle ATP stores are reduced by only about 10–20% at the time of exhaustion (Broberg & Sahlin 1989). This relatively small decline in muscle ATP with prolonged exercise might suggest that an impairment in the rate of ATP resynthesis with glycogen depletion is not linked with fatigue. However, muscle glycogen loading has been shown to enhance prolonged exercise performance (Bergstrom et al 1967), indicating that glycogen depletion is linked with fatigue in some way during prolonged exercise. Recent hypotheses are that metabolite accumulation (e.g. ADP) may be responsible for fatigue.

Accumulation of metabolites

Vigorous muscular contraction is accompanied by the accumulation of many metabolites, including lactate and hydrogen ions (H^+), inorganic phosphate (Pi), adenosine diphosphate (ADP), inosine monophosphate (IMP) and glycolytic intermediates. Of these, the effects of the accumulation of lactate and H^+ on fatigue have been the most closely studied.

Acidosis

Intense short-duration exercise is characterized by a large rise in muscle lactate concentration, with the development of a marked intracellular acidosis (Hermansen & Osnes 1972, Wilson et al 1988). This acidosis has been linked to muscular fatigue through numerous mechanisms. These include a depression of the maximal Ca^{2+}-activated tension, an increase in the Ca^{2+}-activation threshold and a reduced Ca^{2+}-sensitivity in skinned single muscle fibres (Donaldson & Hermansen 1978, Fabiato & Fabiato 1978). Acidosis also causes a reduced maximal velocity of fibre shortening (Metzger & Moss 1987, Cooke et al 1988), which may contribute to the reduced power output particularly evident at higher velocities of contraction (de Haan et al 1989). Energy metabolism may also be impaired under acidotic conditions, with a reduction in the rates of glycogenolysis and glycolysis (Sutton et al 1981, Spriet et al 1989). Inhibition of cellular ATP production or energy charge may also impair the energy-dependent processes of muscle relaxation. Thus, elevations in intracellular H^+ may contribute directly to the slowing of muscle relaxation with fatigue (Cady et al. 1989b, Bergstrom & Hultman 1991). Hence, acidosis has been linked with both the decline in force and the slowing of relaxation. However, acidosis cannot account for all of the decline in force and slowing of relaxation with fatigue. In addition, acidosis is not an important factor in muscular fatigue with prolonged exercise, since muscle H^+ is only slightly elevated (Dawson et al 1978, Denis et al 1989).

Inorganic phosphate

Intramuscular Pi increases 4-5 fold during intense muscle contraction (Cady et al 1989b, Wilson et al 1988) and may directly reduce force development of the muscle fibre (Cooke et al 1988). This inhibitory effect is probably due to an increased concentration of the diprotonated inorganic phosphate ion ($H_2PO_4^-$), which will be exacerbated by acidosis (Cady et al 1989b, Nosek et al 1987, Wilson et al 1988). The rise in Pi is also closely related to the prolongation of muscle relaxation with fatigue (Bergstrom & Hultman 1991, Cady et al 1989a). The importance of elevations in Pi to fatigue induced by prolonged exercise has not been investigated.

Adenosine diphosphate

Muscle ADP concentration increases during contractile activity in proportion to the decline in force output (Dawson et al 1978). A rise in ADP and a decline in ATP will reduce the cellular energy charge, with a reduced energy yield from ATP hydrolysis (Sahlin et al 1978). Since ADP is rapidly removed in-vivo by creatine phosphokinase, adenylate kinase, glycolysis and oxidative metabolism, only small increases in ADP are found experimentally. This has made it difficult to determine the importance of ADP in the fatigue process. Removal of ADP by adenylate kinase produces adenosine monophosphate (AMP), which is subsequently deaminated to IMP and ammonia. Since IMP is removed only slowly from muscle, increases in IMP with exercise may reflect transient increases in AMP and ADP. Marked increases in muscle IMP have been reported at fatigue during both intense (Sahlin et al 1978) and prolonged exercise (Broberg & Sahlin 1989). These findings suggest that a transient rise in ADP occurs at exhaustion and may be an important factor in the development of fatigue. However, any causality of this link remains to be established.

Muscle ionic disturbances

Electrolytes are critical to normal muscle function, being intimately related to the processes of muscle membrane excitation, excitation-contraction coupling and relaxation. Disturbance of the normally tight regulation of electrolyte changes in muscle has been linked with fatigue (McKenna 1992, Sjøgaard 1991). Electrolyte fluxes across the muscle membrane have been implicated in muscular fatigue through two major mechanisms: (1) membrane depolarization and consequent reduced excitability (Sjøgaard et al 1985); and (2) via the development of intracellular acidosis (Lindinger et al 1987, Lindinger & Heigenhauser 1988, 1991). Potassium (K^+) efflux from the contracting muscle cell with each action potential leads to both an increased interstitial K^+ and a lower intracellular K^+ (Hnik et al 1986, Juel 1986, Sjøgaard et al 1985). These changes are marked during intense contraction (Juel 1986) and may depolarize the sarcolemmal and t-tubular membranes, causing a decline in action potential amplitude, Ca^{2+} release and consequently, muscle force development (Juel 1986, Sjøgaard et al 1985). It is likely that this effect is mediated at the t-tubular membrane, owing to the small volume and the low density of Na^+/K^+-pumps in the t-tubular system, as well as the inconsistent findings on muscle action potential changes with fatigue.

Disturbance to potassium homeostasis has also been implicated in fatigue during prolonged, submaximal and intermittent exercise, since intracellular K^+ may be substantially reduced under these conditions (Lindinger & Sjøgaard 1991). The decline in intracellular K^+ and increases in lactate and chloride ion concentrations also make a substantial contribution to the marked intracellular acidosis during intense contraction (Lindinger & Heigenhauser 1988, 1991).

Failure of excitation-contraction coupling

Due to the fundamental role of calcium (Ca^{2+}) in both muscle contraction and relaxation, disturbance to Ca^{2+} regulation may affect all aspects of muscle contractile function. A failure of skeletal muscle excitation-contraction coupling is now widely regarded as being intimately involved in the fatigue process (Vøllestad & Sejersted 1988, Westerblad et al 1991). Possible mechanisms include a reduced Ca^{2+} release from the SR (Allen et al 1989, Lannergren & Westerblad 1989) and impaired Ca^{2+} sensitivity (Allen et al 1989, Donaldson & Hermansen 1978), which are both closely linked with the reduction in force generating capacity with fatigue. Muscle relaxation is dependent upon the energy dependent processes of cross bridge detachment and Ca^{2+} removal by the SR.

It is apparent that the rate of Ca^{2+} removal by the SR is also reduced with muscular fatigue, in both single muscle fibres, muscle homogenate preparations and isolated SR fragments (Allen et al 1989, Byrd et al 1989, Gollnick et al 1991). Therefore, an impairment of SR function (Ca^{2+} transport) must also contribute to the slowed relaxation time with fatigue. This rate of Ca^{2+} removal in muscle homogenates may be reduced by about 50% with fatigue (Byrd et al 1989, Gollnick et al 1991) and is paralleled by a similar reduction in Ca^{2+}-ATPase activity (Byrd et al 1989). This slowing of relaxation is advantageous during an isometric contraction, allowing fusion of twitches at a lower motor neuron firing frequency, but it may interfere with muscle co-ordination during rapid ballistic contractions.

EFFECTS OF TRAINING

The effects of training on the mechanisms of adaptation have previously been thoroughly reviewed for the cardiovascular system (Blomqvist & Saltin 1983, Clausen 1977, Rowell 1986), the respiratory system (Dempsey et al 1985) and skeletal muscle (Booth & Thomason 1991, Saltin & Gollnick 1983). Physical training may be broadly classified into three categories—endurance, sprint and strength—which may be conceptualized as a continuum ranging from endurance to strength training. The intensity of contraction and the number of contractions performed with endurance training is inverse to strength training. The following section will focus on the effects of endurance training on cardiovascular, respiratory, skeletal muscle and metabolic adaptations and their relationship with exercise performance. Where possible, the effects of sprint and strength training will also be briefly described.

Muscle fibre types and ultrastructure

Although it has long been believed that skeletal muscle fibre composition is set by genetic factors, an increasing number of studies have documented fibre type transformation following intense and/or prolonged endurance training (Baumann et al 1987, Klitgaard et al 1990, Schantz 1986, Tesch & Karlsson 1985). Thus, the higher numbers of ST fibres in muscles of endurance athletes probably represent a combination of genetic endowment and a training-induced fibre type transition from FT to ST fibres. Table 1.3 summarizes some results which demonstrate the mutability of human skeletal muscle fibres.

Table 1.3 Histochemically determined vastus lateralis fibre type distribution before and after training in longitudinal training/detraining studies and in studies comparing trained and untrained subjects

Type of training		Fibre types		
		I	IIa	IIb
8 weeks high-intensity	Pre	41	37	19
endurance training (n = 12)	Post	43	42*	14*
24 weeks cross-country	Pre	58	26	9
running (n = 7)	Post	57	32*	3*
6 weeks high intensity	Pre	50	37	12
endurance training (n = 10)	Post	56*	34	10*
15 weeks high intensity	Pre	41	42	17
training (n = 24)	Post	47*	42	11*
11 weeks sprint training	Pre	69	20	10
after 4 weeks long distance	Post	52*	18	18*
running (n = 4)				
14 weeks detraining after	Pre	53	29	14
several years endurance	Post	52	30	13
training (n = 6)				
1–2 years detraining after	Pre	65	28	7
years of competitive rowing (n = 4)	Post	51*	37	11
6 weeks sprint training	Pre	57	32	8
(n = 15)	Post	48*	38*	12
Controls (n = 69)		54	32	13
Orienteers (n = 8)		68*	24	3*
Controls (n = 6)		51	41	7
Long distance runners (n = 9)		78*	19*	3*
Controls (n = 4)		38	31	26
Cross-country runners (n = 6)		52	35	12*

* denotes different from Pre or control.
Source: Adapted from Baumann et al (1987).

Strength training induces a marked muscular hypertrophy and even greater gains in muscular strength. Fibre type transformations are not evident in either upper or lower limb muscles after strength training (Luthi et al 1986, MacDougall 1986, Thorstensson et al 1976). Muscular hypertrophy results from increased FT and ST fibre areas, particularly in the FT fibres (MacDougall 1986). Since muscle (and individual fibre) cross-sectional area is well correlated with muscular strength, hypertrophy is an important factor in the gain in muscular strength evident with strength training (Fig. 1.4)(Saltin & Gollnick 1983). However, improvement in muscle strength with strength training also originates from neural factors (Sale 1988). This is indicated by the rapid gain in strength occurring early in a strength training program, without any muscular hypertrophy. It is also evidenced by the cross-training effect, where an improvement in muscular strength may be found not only in a trained limb, but also in a non-trained limb (Sale 1986). Further, muscle strength gains are highly specific to the mode of training; for example, with isometric strength training, isometric strength may be increased but dynamic strength may be unchanged, and vice versa (Sale 1986). Muscular strength does not appear to be greatly improved after endurance training or after short-term sprint training (McKenna 1991). However, long-term sprint training most likely induces considerable gains in muscular strength, although the pronouced hypertrophy evident in elite sprint athletes is most likely due to additional strength training. Sprint training may cause muscle fibre transformation within the FT pool of fibres, however, findings on ST to FT conversion remain inconclusive (Jansson et al 1990).

Cardiovascular system

Adaptations within the cardiovascular system with training may be considered as either central or peripheral in origin. Central adaptations include changes in cardiac output, blood volume and arterial oxygen-carrying capacity. Peripheral adaptations include skeletal muscle blood flow and capillarization. The functional significance of these changes may be assessed by examining their respective roles in the improvements in VO_2 max and endurance performance after endurance training. The Fick equation is useful in understanding the contributions of central and peripheral factors to VO_2 max: oxygen consumption is equal to the product of cardiac output and the arterio-mixed venous oxygen content difference ($VO_2 = Q \times Ca - \bar{v}O_2$). Physical training produces a number of central and peripheral cardiovascular adaptations, thereby enhancing oxygen delivery to skeletal muscle.

Cardiac output

During maximal exercise, cardiac output may reach 30 l.min^{-1} or more in elite athletes, compared with about 20 l.min^{-1} in sedentary control subjects. It may be reduced to only 15 l.min^{-1} following a period of bedrest (Blomqvist & Saltin 1983, Saltin et al 1968). These differences in maximal cardiac output are almost entirely due to differences in maximal stroke volume, with maximal heart rate being essentially unchanged (Saltin et al 1968). The time course of activity-induced changes in maximal cardiac output parallels that of VO_2 max (Saltin et al 1968), indicating the importance of central circulatory adaptations in determining VO_2 max. The increased maximal stroke volume reflects greater end diastolic volume, due to increased end diastolic dimensions (Keul et al 1982). During submaximal exercise, stroke volume is greater and heart rate reduced after endurance training (Saltin et al 1968).

The reduction in heart rate at rest and during submaximal exercise after training probably reflects a reduced sympathetic drive. In contrast to the enhanced cardiac performance with endurance training are the circulatory adaptations evident with strength or power training. In these subjects, VO_2 max is relatively low, end diastolic dimensions and volume are reduced, while ventricular wall thickness is greatly increased (Keul et al 1982). These changes represent an impaired cardiac performance in the power athlete. Little is known of the effect of sprint training on central cardiovascular function. Sprint training reduces the resting and submaximal heart rate in humans (McKenna 1991), and enhances maximal stroke volume and hence maximal cardiac output in rats (Hilty et al 1988).

Muscle blood flow

Almost all the increased cardiac output during exercise is directed to the contracting skeletal muscle, with peak muscle blood flow as high as 7 l.min^{-1} measured during single leg exercise. After endurance training, the blood flow to contracting skeletal muscle is reduced during submaximal exercise (Grimby et al 1967, Kiens & Saltin 1986). Although not yet demonstrated in humans, the maximal muscle perfusion must also be increased after endurance training, given the magnitude of increase in maximal cardiac output and the smaller increase in whole body oxygen extraction.

Blood volume

Blood volume is expanded by 6–10% after endurance training, primarily due to an increased plasma volume, with no change in red cell volume (Green et al 1991c, Oscai et al 1968). This hypervolemia causes the decline in blood hemoglobin concentration often found in athletes, known as a sports pseudoanemia, since red cell mass does not decline with training (Green et al 1991c). An expanded blood volume will increase maximal cardiac filling and output and thus contribute to the increase in VO_2 max after endurance training. Similarly, detraining caused a decline in blood volume and in VO_2 max (Coyle et al 1986). When blood volume was restored to normal levels, VO_2 max was also restored.

Muscle capillarization

Skeletal muscle capillarization increases dramatically with endurance training (Saltin & Gollnick 1983). When expressed as the number of capillaries per muscle fibre, capillarization increases by nearly 50% after 8 weeks of training (Fig. 1.4). The mechanisms underlying this adaptation remain undefined, but they may be linked with an increase in fibroblast growth factor in skeletal muscle (Booth & Thomason 1991). The functional significance of this adaptation lies in the increased cross-sectional area of the circulation-muscle interface. This reduces the mean capillary-fibre diffusion distance and increases the red blood cell mean transit time, effectively enabling a greater extraction of oxygen and metabolic fuels by skeletal muscle, as well as facilitating waste product removal (Saltin & Rowell 1980, Saltin 1984, Saltin & Gollnick 1983).

The increased oxygen extraction is, however, dependent upon an increased oxidative capacity of skeletal muscle. Despite the marked muscular hypertrophy following strength training, the muscle capillary-fibre ratio and capillary density remains unchanged (Luthi et al 1986). In contrast, sprint training in rats increased the muscle capillary-fibre ratio, as well as the number of capillaries (Dimauro et al 1992).

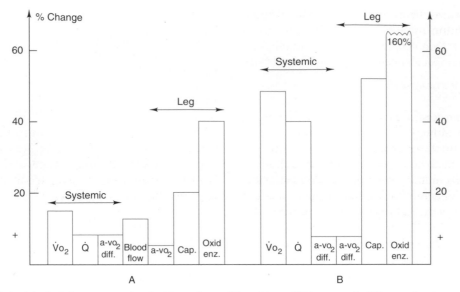

Fig. 1.4 Summary of physiological changes associated with moderate (A) and large (B) increases in VO_2 max in response to physical training. Source: Saltin & Gollnick (1983)

Respiratory system

Although organs such as skeletal muscle and the myocardium demonstrate marked adaptation to chronically increased physical activity, the extent of adaptation by the pulmonary system appears to be very limited. Although well trained athletes may have a greater vital capacity (VC) and forced expired volume (FEV) than untrained individuals, these differences are genetically determined. Resting pulmonary ventilation is unchanged after training, but endurance training lowers the ventilation at submaximal workrates, due principally to reductions in lactate and CO_2 production (Casaburi et al 1987). In the untrained person, arterial blood gases and pH are very well regulated during light to moderate exercise. With higher exercise intensities, arterial PO_2 is again well regulated, but PCO_2 declines markedly, possibly in response to the developing systemic acidosis.

In contrast, the very highly trained endurance athlete (VO_2 max > 65 ml.kg^{-1}.min^{-1}) may demonstrate imperfect arterial oxygenation during heavy exercise. This is evidenced by an increased widening of the alveolar to arterial PO_2 difference, with arterial PO_2 falling as low as 65 mmHg during heavy exercise. This hypoxemia is thought to be due to a combination of several factors, including the athletes' very high pulmonary blood flow (cardiac output > 25 l.min^{-1}) and a morphologically limited pulmonary capillary capacity, resulting in a reduced red blood cell transit time and inadequate gas equilibration during passage through the pulmonary capillary (Dempsey et al 1985, Powers & Williams 1987). Thus, the exercise performance of the very well trained athlete may be limited by the pulmonary system during heavy exercise (Dempsey 1986).

Skeletal muscle metabolic adaptations

Mitochondria and enzyme activities

One of the most striking peripheral adaptations with endurance training is the marked increase in mitochondrial enzyme activities, reflecting an increased mitochondrial volume (Saltin & Gollnick 1983). Enzymes involved in the Krebs cycle, electron transport chain and beta oxidation (fat metabolism) are all increased with endurance training (Fig. 1.4). These changes are reversible, demonstrating a sharp decline after only 1 week of detraining (Costill et al 1985, Henriksson & Reitman 1977). The molecular mechanisms underlying mitochondrial upregulation with training remain obscure, but may be associated with increases in 3'5'cyclic adenosine monophosphate (cAMP), or changes in CP stores in skeletal muscle with contractile activity (Booth & Thomason 1991).

The functional significance of these changes has been extensively discussed and probably confers: (1) increased control (sensitivity) over oxidative metabolic pathways; (2) more rapid increases in mitochondrial O_2 consumption; (3) diminished metabolic disturbances with exercise; and (4) enhanced lipid utilisation (Saltin 1984, Saltin & Rowell 1980, Saltin & Gollnick 1983). Myoglobin stores in human skeletal muscle are not increased with endurance training (Jansson et al 1982), but may in fact be elevated with immobilization (Jansson et al 1988). Sprint training is associated with elevations in phosphofructokinase (PFK) activity, but only small increases (if any) in oxidative enzyme activities (Jacobs et al 1987, Roberts et al 1982). The increased PFK activity may contribute to the greater glycolytic rate found after sprint training. Strength training is associated with a reduction in mitochondrial volume density, due to the large increase in myofibrillar volume

(Luthi et al 1986, MacDougall 1986). This may contribute to the poor aerobic performance of strength trained muscle.

Exercise metabolism

The metabolic adaptations to training have been extensively reviewed (Booth & Thomason 1991, Gollnick 1986, Gollnick & Hodgson 1986, Holloszy & Coyle 1984, Saltin & Gollnick 1983). Although endurance training does not modify the resting content of muscle ATP and CP, glycogen and lipid stores appear to be increased and there are marked differences in exercise-induced changes in these metabolites after endurance training. After endurance training, exercise at a given power output is characterized by a reduced decline in muscle phosphagen (ATP and CP) and glycogen stores and a smaller accumulation of lactate in both muscle and blood (Hurley et al 1986, Jansson & Kaijser 1987, Saltin & Karlsson 1971). These changes were originally suggested to result from the increased mitochondrial volume and capillarization evident with endurance training (Gollnick & Saltin 1982, Saltin & Rowell 1980); however, these metabolic changes are evident after only 5–12 days of training, when no increases in mitochondria or capillarization are apparent (Green et al 1991b, 1992). Thus, other mechanisms may also be responsible for these training-induced alterations in exercise metabolism.

These mechanisms have not been completely identified, but may include alterations in circulating catecholamines (Green et al 1991a). One of the most important metabolic adaptations after endurance training is the greater lipid utilization during exercise (Hurley et al 1986). There is debate on whether this increase in lipid oxidation is due entirely to enhanced muscle triglyceride breakdown (Hurley et al 1986, Jansson & Kaijser 1987) or also involves increased muscle uptake of circulating plasma FFA (Turcotte et al 1992). Increased fat utilization during exercise enables conservation of endogenous carbohydrate stores and confers an increased muscular endurance. However, due to the low metabolic power of lipid oxidation (i.e. rate of ATP production),

increased lipid oxidation does not contribute to the improvement in VO_2 max. Sprint training results in an unchanged decline in muscle ATP and CP, but an increased lactate accumulation in muscle and blood during intense exercise (Nevill et al 1989, Sharp et al 1986).

Electrolyte regulation during exercise

The effects of training on electrolyte regulation during exercise remain largely unexplored, despite the importance of electrolytes for normal muscle function and in fatigue. Potassium (K^+) regulation by skeletal muscle may be improved by both endurance and sprint training (McKenna 1991, Lindinger & Sjøgaard 1991). After endurance training, intracellular K^+ may be increased (Knochel et al 1985), K^+ release from contracting muscle reduced (Kiens & Saltin 1986), and plasma K^+ lower at a given power output (Fosha-Dolezal & Fedde 1989). The concentration of Na^+/K^+ pumps is increased in rat skeletal muscle after endurance training (Kjeldsen et al 1986), but not in human skeletal muscle after low-intensity endurance training (Kjeldsen et al 1990). The Na^+/K^+ pump concentration was higher in muscle of chronically trained elderly men compared with age matched controls (Klitgaard et al 1989). After sprint training, the concentration of Na^+/K^+ pumps in skeletal muscle was increased by 16%, with an attenuated rise in plasma K^+ during maximal intermittent exercise (McKenna et al 1993). Since K^+ loss from muscle is implicated in muscular fatigue, improved K^+ may be important in the improved exercise performance demonstrated after both endurance and sprint training. The marked rise in H^+ with intense sprint exercise was either reduced or unchanged after sprint training, despite a greater increase in muscle lactate (Nevill et al 1989, Sharp et al 1986). This improved muscle H^+ regulation may contribute to the reduced fatiguability after sprint training and is probably not due to increased muscle buffer capacity (in vitro), but rather to enhanced sarcolemmal ion exchange mechanisms (Nevill et al 1989, McKenna 1991, Sharp et al 1986).

REFERENCES

Allen D G, Lee J, Westerblad H 1989 Intracellular calcium and tension during fatigue in isolated single muscle fibres from Xenopus laevis. Journal of Physiology 415:433-458

Asmussen E 1978 Muscle fatigue. Medicine and Science in Sports 11:313-321

Baumann H, Jaggi M, Soland F, Howald H, Schaub M C 1987 Exercise training induces transitions of myosin isoform subunits within histochemically typed human muscle fibres. Pflugers Archives 40:349-360

Bergh U, Thorstensson A, Sjodin B, Hulten B, Piehl K, Karlsson J 1978 Maximal oxygen uptake and muscle fibre types in trained and untrained humans. Medicine and Science in Sports 10:151-154

Bergstrom J, Hermansen L, Hultman E, Saltin B 1967 Diet, muscle glycogen and physical performance. Acta Physiologica Scandinavica 71:140-150

Bergstrom M, Hultman E 1991 Relaxation and force during fatigue and recovery of the human quadriceps muscle: relations to metabolite changes. Pflugers Archives 418:153-160

Bigland-Ritchie B 1981 EMG and fatigue of human voluntary and stimulated contractions. In: Human muscle fatigue: physiological mechanisms. Pitman Medical, London (Ciba Foundation Symposium 82), pp. 130-156

Bigland-Ritchie B, Jones D A, Hosking G P, Edwards R H T 1978 Central and peripheral fatigue in sustained maximum voluntary contractions of human quadriceps muscle. Clinical Science 54:609-614

Blomqvist C G, Saltin B 1983 Cardiovascular adaptations to physical training. Annual Reviews of Physiology 45:169-189

Booth F W, Thomason D B 1991 Molecular and cellular adaptation of muscle in response to exercise: perspectives of various models. Physiological Reviews 71:541-585

Broberg S, Sahlin K 1989 Adenine nucleotide degradation in human skeletal muscle during prolonged exercise. Journal of Applied Physiology 67:116-122

Brooks G A 1985 Anaerobic threshold: review of the concept and directions for future research. Medicine and Science in Sports and Exercise 17:22-31

Brooks G A 1986 The lactate shuttle during exercise and recovery. Medicine and Science in Sports and Exercise 18:360-368

Buick F, Gledhill N, Spriet L L, Myers E 1980 Effects of induced erythrocythemia on aerobic work capacity. Journal of Applied Physiology 48:636-642

Byrd S K, McCutcheon L, Hodgson D, Gollnick P 1989 Altered sarcoplasmic function after high-intensity exercise. Journal of Applied Physiology 67:2072-2077

Cady E B, Elshove H Jones D A, Moll A 1989a The metabolic causes of slow relaxation in fatigued human skeletal muscle. Journal of Physiology 418:327-323

Cady E B, Jones D A, Lynn J, Newham D J 1989b Changes in force and intracellular metabolites during fatigue of human skeletal muscle. Journal of Physiology 418:311-325

Casaburi R, Storer T W, Wasserman K 1987 Mediation of reduced ventilatory response to exercise after endurance training. Journal of Applied Physiology 63:1533-1538

Cheetham M E, Boobis L H, Brooks S, Williams C 1988 Human muscle metabolism during sprint running. Journal of Applied Physiology 61:54-60

Clausen J P 1977 Effect of physical training on cardiovascular adjustments to exercise in man. Physiological Reviews 57:779-815

Cooke R, Franks K, Luciani G B, Pate E 1988 The inhibition of rabbit skeletal muscle by hydrogen ions and phosphate. Journal of Physiology 395:77-97

Costill D L, Daniels J, Evans W, Fink W J, Krahenbuhl G, Saltin B 1975 Skeletal muscle enzymes and fibre composition in male and female track athletes. Journal of Applied Physiology 40:149-154

Costill D L, Fink W J, Hargreaves M, King D S, Thomas R, Fielding R 1985 Metabolic characteristics of skeletal muscle during detraining from competitive swimming. Medicine and Science in Sports and Exercise 17:339-343

Costill D L, Hargreaves M 1992 Carbohydrate nutrition and fatigue. Sports Medicine 13:86-92

Coyle E F, Hemmert M K, Coggan A R 1986 Effects of detraining on cardiovascular responses to exercise: role of blood volume. Journal of Applied Physiology 60:95-99

Davis J A 1985 Anaerobic threshold: review of the concept and directions for future research. Medicine and Science in Sports and Exercise 17:6-18

Dawson M J, Gadian D, Wilkie D 1980 Mechanical relaxation rate and metabolism studied in fatiguing muscle by phosphorus nuclear magnetic resonance. Journal of Physiology 299:465-484

de Haan A, Jones D, Sargeant A 1989 Changes in velocity of shortening, power output and relaxation rate during fatigue of rat medial gastrocnemius muscle. Pflugers Archives 413:422-428

Dempsey J A 1986 Is the lung built for exercise? Medicine and Science in Sports and Exercise 18:143-155

Dempsey J A, Vidruk E, Mitchell G S 1985 Pulmonary control systems during exercise: update. Federation Proceedings 44:2260-2270

Denis C, Linossier M-T, Dormois D, Cottier-Perrin M, Geyssant A, Lacour J-R 1989 Effects of endurance training upon hyperammonaemia during a 45 minute constant exercise intensity. European Journal of Applied Physiology 59:268-272

Dimauro J, Balnave R J, Shorey C B 1992 Effects of anabolic steroids and high intensity exercise on rat skeletal muscle fibres and capillarisation: a morphometric study. European Journal of Applied Physiology 64:204-212

Donaldson S K B, Hermansen L 1978 Differential and direct effects of H^+ on Ca^{2+}-activated force of skinned fibres from the soleus, cardiac and adductor magnus muscles of rabbits. Pflugers Archives 376:55-65

Edwards R H 1981 Human muscle function and fatigue. In: Human muscle fatigue: physiological mechanisms. Pitman Medical, London (Ciba Foundation Symposium 82), pp. 1-18

Fabiato A, Fabiato F 1978 Effects of pH on the myofilaments and the sarcoplasmic reticulum of skinned cells from cardiac and skeletal muscles. Journal of Physiology 276:233-255

Felig P, Wahren J 1975 Fuel homeostasis during exercise. New England Journal of Medicine 293:1078-1084

Fitts R H 1994 Cellular mechanisms of muscle fatigue. Physiological Reviews 74: 49-94

Fitts R H, Metzger J M 1988 Mechanisms of muscular fatigue. In: Poortmans J R (ed) Principles of exercise biochemistry. Karger, Basel

Forster H V, Pan L G 1991 Exercise hyperpnoea: its characteristics and control. In: The lung: scientific foundations. Raven Press, New York

Fosha-Dolezal S R, Fedde M R 1988 Serum potassium during exercise in Hereford calves: influence of physical conditioning. Journal of Applied Physiology 65:1360-1366

Gandevia S C 1992 Some central and peripheral factors affecting human motoneuronal output in neuromuscular fatigue. Sports Medicine 13:93-98

Gollnick P D 1985 Metabolism of substrates: energy substrate metabolism during exercise and as modified by training. Federation Proceedings 44:353-357

Gollnick P D 1986 Metabolic regulation in skeletal muscle: influence of endurance training as exerted by mitochondrial protein concentration. Acta Physiologica Scandinavica 128 (Suppl. 556):53-66

Gollnick P D, Saltin B 1982 Significance of skeletal muscle oxidative enzyme enhancement with endurance training. Clinical Physiology 2:1-12

Gollnick P D, Hodgson D R 1986 Enzymatic adaptation and its significance for metabolic response to exercise. In: Saltin B (ed) Biochemistry of exercise VI. Human Kinetics, Champaign

Gollnick P D, Korge P, Karpakka J, Saltin B 1991 Elongation of skeletal muscle relaxation during exercise is linked to reduced calcium uptake by the sarcoplasmic reticulum in man. Acta Physiologica Scandinavica 142:135-136

Green H J, Jones S, Ball-Burnett M, Fraser I 1991a Early adaptations in blood substrates, metabolites, and hormones to prolonged exercise training in man. Canadian Journal of Physiology and Pharmacology 69:1222-1229

Green H J, Jones S, Ball-Burnett M E, Smith D, Livesey J, Farrance B W 1991b Early muscular and metabolic adaptations to prolonged exercise training in humans. Journal of Applied Physiology 70:2032-2038

Green H J, Sutton J R, Coates G, Ali M, Jones S 1991c Response of red cell and plasma volume to prolonged training in humans. Journal of Applied Physiology 70:1810-1815

Green H J, Helyar R, Ball-Burnett M, Kowalchuk N, Symon S, Farrance B W 1992 Metabolic adaptations to training precede changes in muscle mitochondrial capacity. Journal of Applied Physiology 72:484-491

Grimby G, Haggendal L, Saltin B 1967 Local xenon133 clearance from the quadriceps muscle during exercise in man. Journal of Applied Physiology 22:305-310

Hargreaves M 1990 Skeletal muscle carbohydrate metabolism during exercise. Australian Journal of Science and Medicine in Sport 22:35-38

Hargreaves M 1991 Carbohydrates and exercise. Journal of Sports Sciences (special issue) 9:17-28

Hargreaves M, Richter E A 1988 Regulation of skeletal muscle glycogenolysis during exercise. Canadian Journal of Sports Sciences 13:197-203

Henneman E 1957 Relation between size of neurons and their susceptibility to discharge. Science 126:1345-1347

Henriksson J, Reitman J S 1977 Time course of changes in human skeletal muscle succinate dehydrogenase and cytochrome oxidase activities and maximal oxygen uptake with physical activity and inactivity. Acta Physiologica Scandinavica 99:91-97

Hermansen L, Osnes J 1972 Blood and muscle pH after maximal exercise in man. Journal of Applied Physiology 32:304-308

Hermansen L, Orheim A, Sejersted O M 1984 Metabolic acidosis and changes in water and electrolyte balance in relation to fatigue during maximal exercise of short duration. International Journal of Sports Medicine 5:S110-S115

Hilty M R, Groth H, Moore R L, Musch T I 1989 Determinants of VO_2 max in rats after high-intensity sprint training. Journal of Applied Physiology 66:195-201

Hnik P, Vyskocil F, Ujec E, Vejsada R, Rehfeldt H 1986 Work-induced potassium loss from skeletal muscles and its implications. In: Saltin B (ed) Biochemistry of exercise VI. Human Kinetics, Champaign, pp. 345-364

Hodgkin A L, Horowicz P 1959 Movements of Na and K in single muscle fibres. Journal of Physiology 145:405-432

Holloszy J O, Coyle E F 1984 Adaptations of skeletal muscle to endurance exercise and their metabolic consequences. Journal of Applied Physiology 56:831-838

Hood D A, Terjung R L 1990 Amino acid metabolism during exercise and following endurance training. Sports Medicine 9:23-35

Hultman E, Bergstom J, McLennan-Anderson N 1967 Breakdown and resynthesis of phosphorylcreatine and adenosine triphosphate in connection with muscular work in man. Scandinavian Journal of Clinical and Laboratory Investigation 19:56-66

Hultman E, Sjoholm H 1983 Electromyogram, force and relaxation time during and after continuous electrical stimulation of human skeletal muscle in situ. Journal of Physiology 339:33-40

Hurley B F, Nemeth P M, Martin W H, Hagberg J M, Dalsky G P, Holloszy J O 1986 Muscle triglyceride utilisation during exercise: effect of training. Journal of Applied Physiology 60:562-567

Jacobs I, Esbjornsson M, Sylven C, Holm I, Jansson E 1987 Sprint training effects on muscle myoglobin, enzymes, fibre types and blood lactate. Medicine and Science in Sports and Exercise 19:368-374

Jansson E, Sylven C, Nordvang E 1982 Myoglobin in the quadriceps femoris muscle of competitive cyclists and untrained men. Acta Physiologica Scandinavica 114:627-629

Jansson E, Kiajser L 1987 Substrate utilization and enzymes in skeletal muscle of extremely endurance-trained men. Journal of Applied Physiology 62:999-1005

Jansson E, Sylven C, Arvidsson I, Eriksson E 1988 Increase in myoglobin content and decrease in oxidative enzyme activities by leg immobilisation in man. Acta Physiologica Scandinavica 132:515-517

Jansson E, Esbjornsson M, Holm I, Jacobs I 1990 Increase in the proportion of fast-twitch muscle fibres by sprint training in males. Acta Physiologica Scandinavica 140:359-363

Jones N L, Heigenhauser G J F, Kuksis A, Matsos C G, Sutton J R, Toews C J 1980 Fat metabolism in heavy exercise. Clinical Science 59:469-478

Juel C 1986 Potassium and sodium shifts during in-vitro isometric muscle contraction, and the time course of the ion-gradient recovery. Pflugers Archives 406:458-463

Juel C 1988 Intracellular pH recovery and lactate efflux in mouse soleus muscles stimulated in-vitro: the involvement of sodium/proton exchange and a lactate carrier. Acta Physiologica Scandinavica 132:363-371

Katz A, Broberg S, Sahlin K, Wahren J 1986 Leg glucose uptake during maximal dynamic exercise in humans. American Journal of Physiology 251:E65-E70

Katz A, Sahlin K 1988 Regulation of lactic acid production during exercise. Journal of Applied Physiology 65:509-518

Kiens B, Saltin B 1986 Endurance training of man decreases muscle potassium loss during exercise (abstract). Acta Physiologica Scandinavica 126:P5

Kjeldsen K, Richter E A, Galbo H, Lortie G, Clausen T 1986 Training increases the concentration of [3H]ouabain-binding sites in rat skeletal muscle. Biochimica Biophysica Acta 860:707-712

Kjeldsen K, Norgaard A, Hau C 1990 Human skeletal muscle Na,K-ATPase concentration quantified by 3H-ouabain binding to intact biopsies before and after moderate physical conditioning. International Journal of Sports Medicine 11:304-307

Klitgaard H, Clausen T 1989 Increased total concentrations of Na-K pumps in vastus lateralis muscle of old trained human subjects. Journal of Applied Physiology 67:2491-2492

Klitgaard H, Bergman O, Betto R, Salviati G, Schiaffino S, Clausen T, Saltin B 1990 Co-existence of myosin heavy chain I and IIa isoforms in human skeletal muscle fibres with endurance training. Pflugers Archives 416:470-472

Knochel J P, Blanchley J D, Johnson J H, Carter N W 1985 Muscle cell electrical hyperpolarisation and reduced exercise hyperkalaemia in physically conditioned dogs. Journal of Clinical Investigation 75:740-745

Komi P V, Viitasalo J H T, Havu M, Thorstensson A, Sjodin B, Karlsson J 1977 Skeletal muscle fibres and enzyme activities in monozygous and dizygous twins of both sexes. Acta Physiologica Scandinavica 100:385-392

Kuel J, Dickhuth H H, Lehmann M, Staiger J 1982 The athletes heart—haemodynamics and structure. International Journal of Sports Medicine 3:33-43

Lannergren J, Westerblad H 1989 Maximum tension and force-velocity properties of fatigued, single Xenopus muscle fibres studied by caffeine and high potassium. Journal of Physiology 409:473-490

Lindinger M I, Heigenhauser G J F, Spriet L L 1987 Effects of intense swimming and tetanic electrical stimulation on skeletal muscle ions and metabolites. Journal of Applied Physiology 63:2331-2339

Lindinger M I, Heigenhauser G J F 1988 Ion fluxes during tetanic stimulation in isolated perfused rat hindlimb. American Journal of Physiology 254: R117-R126

Lindinger M I, Heigenhauser G J F 1991 The role of ion fluxes in skeletal muscle fatigue. Canadian Journal of Physiology and Pharmacology 69:246-253

Lindinger M I, Sjøgaard G 1991 Potassium regulation during exercise and recovery. Sports Medicine 11:382-401

Luthi J M, Howald H, Classen H, Rosler K, Vock P, Hoppeler H 1986 Structural changes in skeletal muscle tissue with heavy resistance exercise. International Journal of Sports Medicine 7:123-127

MacDougall J D 1986 Morphological adaptations in human skeletal muscle following strength training and immobilisation. In: Jones N L, McCartney N, McComas A J (eds) Human muscle power. Human Kinetics, Champaign

McCartney N, Spriet L L, Heigenhauser G J F, Kowalchuk J M, Sutton J R, Jones N L 1986 Muscle power and metabolism in maximal intermittent exercise. Journal of Applied Physiology 60: 1164-1169

McClaren D P M, Gibson H, Parry-Billings M, Edwards R H T 1990 A review of metabolic and physiological factors in fatigue. Exercise and Sport Sciences Reviews 17:29-66

McKenna M J 1991 The effects of sprint training on electrolyte, acid-base regulation and fatigue during intense exercise in man. PhD thesis, University of Melbourne

McKenna M J 1992 The role of ionic processes in muscular fatigue during intense exercise. Sports Medicine 13:134-145

McKenna M J, Schmidt T A, Hargreaves M, Cameron L, Skinner S L, Kjeldsen K 1993 Sprint training increases human skeletal muscle Na$^+$K$^+$ATPase concentration and improves potassium regulation. Journal of Applied Physiology 75: 173-180

McLellan T M 1987 The anaerobic threshold: concept and controversy. Australian Journal of Science and Medicine in Sport 19:3-8

Metzger J M, Moss R L 1987 Greater hydrogen ion induced depression of tension and velocity in skinned single fibres of rat fast than slow muscles. Journal of Physiology 393:727-742

Mitchell J H 1990 Neural control of the circulation during exercise. Medicine and Science in Sports and Exercise 22:141-154

Nevill M E, Boobis L H, Brooks S, Williams C 1989 Effect of training on muscle metabolism during treadmill sprinting. Journal of Applied Physiology 67:2376-2382

Newham D J, McCarthy T, Turner J 1991 Voluntary activation of human quadriceps during and after isokinetic exercise. Journal of Applied Physiology 71:2122-2126

Nosek T M, Fender K Y, Godt R E 1987 It is diprotonated inorganic phosphate that depresses force in skinned skeletal muscle fibres. Science 236:191-193

Oscai L B, Williams B T, Hertig B A 1968 Effects of exercise on blood volume. Journal of Applied Physiology 24:622-624

Powers S K, Williams J 1987 Exercise-induced hypoxemia in highly trained athletes. Sports Medicine 4:46-53

Powers S K, Lawler J, Dempsey J A, Dodd S, Landry G 1989 Effects of incomplete pulmonary gas exchange on ¶O$_2$ max. Journal of Applied Physiology 66:2491-2495

Richter E A, Ruderman N B, Schneider S H 1981 Diabetes and exercise. American Journal of Medicine 70:201-209

Roberts A D, Billeter R, Howald H 1982 Anaerobic muscle enzyme changes after interval training. International Journal of Sports Medicine 3:18-21

Rowell L B 1988 Muscle blood flow in humans: how high can it go? Medicine and Science in Sports and Exercise 20:S97-S103

Rowell L B, O'Leary D S 1990 Reflex control of the circulation during exercise: chemoreflexes and mechanoreflexes. Journal of Applied Physiology 69:407-418

Sahlin K, Palmskog G, Hultman E 1978 Adenine nucleotide and IMP contents of the quadriceps muscle in man after exercise. Pflugers Archives 374:193-198

Sale D G 1986 Neural adaptation in strength and power training. In: Jones N L, McCartney N, McComas A J (eds) Human muscle power. Human Kinetics, Champaign

Sale D G 1988 Neural adaptation to resistance training. Medicine and Science in Sports and Exercise 20:S135-S145

Saltin B 1984 Physiological adaptation to physical conditioning: old problems revisited. Acta Medica Scandinavica 711:11-24

Saltin B 1985 Hemodynamic adaptations to exercise. American Journal of Cardiology 55:42D-47D

Saltin B, Blomqvist C G, Mitchell J H, Johnson R L, Wildenthal K, Chapman C B 1968 Response to exercise after bed rest and after training. Circulation 38 (Suppl. 7):1-78

Saltin B, Karlsson J 1971 Muscle ATP, CP and lactate during exercise after physical conditioning. In: Pernow B, Saltin B (eds) Muscle metabolism during exercise. Plenum Press, New York

Saltin B, Rowell L B 1980 Functional adaptations to physical activity and inactivity. Federation Proceedings 39:1506-1513

Saltin B, Gollnick P D 1983 Skeletal muscle adaptability: significance for metabolism and performance. In: Handbook of Physiology, Skeletal Muscle. American Physiological Society, Bethesda pp. 555-631

Schantz P 1986 Plasticity of human skeletal muscle. Acta Physiologica Scandinavica 128:Suppl 558

Sharp R L, Costill D L, Fink W J, King D S 1986 Effects of eight weeks of bicycle ergometer sprint training on human muscle buffer capacity. International Journal of Sports Medicine 7:13-17

Sjøgaard G 1991 Role of exercise induced potassium fluxes underlying muscle fatigue: a brief review. Canadian Journal of Physiology and Pharmacology 69:238-245

Sjøgaard G, Adams R, Saltin B 1985 Water and ion shifts in skeletal muscle of humans with intense dynamic knee extension American Journal of Physiology 248:R190-R196

Soderlund K, Hultman E 1991 ATP and phosphocreatine changes in single human skeletal muscle fibres after intense electrical stimulation. American Journal of Physiology 261:E737-E741

Spriet L L, Lindinger M I, McKelvie R S, Heigenhauser GJ F, Jones N L 1989 Muscle glycogenolysis and H+ concentration during maximal intermittent cycling. Journal of Applied Physiology 66:8-13

Sutton J R, Jones N L, Toews C J 1981 Effect of pH on muscle glycolysis during exercise. Clinical Science 61:331-338

Tesch P A, Karlsson J 1985 Muscle fibre types and size in trained and untrained muscles of elite athletes. Journal of Applied Physiology 59:1716-1720

Thorstensson A, Hulten B, von Dobeln W, Karlsson J 1976 Effect of strength training on enzyme activities and fibre characteristics in human skeletal muscle. Acta Physiologica Scandinavica 96:392-398

Turcotte L P, Richter E A, Kiens B 1992 Increased plasma FFA uptake and oxidation during prolonged exercise in trained vs untrained humans. American Journal of Physiology 262:E791-E799

Vøllestad N K, Vaage O, Hermansen L 1984 Muscle glycogen depletion patterns in type I and subgroups of type II fibres during prolonged severe exercise in man. Acta Physiologica Scandinavica 122:433-441

Vøllestad N K, Sejersted O M 1988 Biochemical correlates of fatigue. European Journal of Applied Physiology 57:336-347

Vøllestad N K, Blom P C S 1985 Effect of varying intensity on glycogen depletion in human muscle fibres. Acta Physiologica Scandinavica 125:395-405

Vøllestad N K, Tabata I, Medbø J I 1992 Glycogen breakdown in different human muscle fibre types during exhaustive exercise of short duration. Acta Physiologica Scandinavica 144:135-141

Wagner P D 1991 Central and peripheral aspects of oxygen transport and adaptations with exercise. Sports Medicine 11:133-142

Wahren J 1977 Glucose turnover during exercise in man. Annals of the New York Academy of Sciences 301:45-55

Walsh M L, Banister E W 1988 Possible mechanisms of the anaerobic threshold: a review. Sports Medicine 5:269-302

Wasserman K, Beaver W L, Whipp B J 1986 Mechanisms and patterns of blood lactate increase during exercise in man. Medicine and Science in Sports and Exercise 18:344-352

Westerblad H, Lee J A, Lannergren J, D G Allen 1991. Cellular mechanisms of fatigue in skeletal muscle. American Journal of Physiology 30:C195-C209

Williams C 1990 Value of physiological measurement in sport. Journal of the Royal College of Surgeons, Edinburgh 35:S7-S13

Wilson J R, McCully K K, Mancini D M, Boden B, Chance B 1988 Relationship of muscular fatigue to pH and diprotonated Pi in humans. Journal of Applied Physiology 64:2333-2339

2. Physiological responses to injury: muscle

Tim Wrigley

This chapter reviews the physiological challenges to muscle faced by the injured athlete. The importance of the pathophysiology of direct injury to muscle (e.g. muscle strain) is obvious; less commonly considered are the indirect consequences for muscle of injury to joints and long bones.

The injured athlete suffers in several ways: most obviously, there is the injury itself and its immediate consequences. The athlete also suffers as a result of the relative inactivity—detraining—imposed by the injury. Since the athlete's physiological fitness for their particular sport is reflected in the muscular adaptations that have been achieved as a result of training, it is imperative that consideration be given to minimizing the deleterious effects of relative inactivity on muscle and other organ systems.

While rest may have featured prominently in the treatment of injury in the past, it was justified mainly on the basis of ensuring adequate healing time. Rarely was consideration given to the physiological deterioration of other organ systems—including uninjured muscle—during the rest phase. These days, rest is no longer a universal prescription, and it is likely that muscle is less deleteriously affected as a result. However, it is important that the minimization of detraining of uninjured skeletal muscle is not simply a possible fortuitous side benefit of a more active approach to the rehabilitation of the injury site itself, but a primary aim of the overall rehabilitation program.

In this chapter, the physiological consequences of injury for muscle are considered in an approximately chronological sequence. Coverage progresses from the athlete's pre-injury physiological status, through the pathophysiology of the injury itself, to the response to surgery (if clinically necessary) and its sequelae, including pain, effusion, and immobilization, and the detraining adaptations that result from enforced inactivity.

Much of this material is equally relevant to both direct injury to muscle, and the indirect consequences for muscle of joint or long bone injury. Even the coverage of surgical considerations—although primarily concerned with the effect of *joint* surgery on surrounding muscle—will be important in the instances of muscle and tendon ruptures requiring surgical management.

This chapter is primarily a review of research. Although the primary intent of this book is to provide information for clinical practice, the research literature in several areas germane to this chapter does not lend itself to clearcut clinical recommendations. This may be due to a simple lack of sufficient research studies; the results of such few studies must be judged with caution until they have been replicated more widely. Alternatively, the experimental models employed (particularly animal models) may be of questionable relevance to the clinical context. In such instances, an attempt has been made to provide a summary of the existing research. Where relevant, some details of experimental protocols and other aspects are provided, so that the reader can appreciate the reasons for the lack of clear conclusions regarding clinical practice.

PHYSIOLOGICAL STATUS AT THE TIME OF INJURY

There has been considerable research interest in the deterioration in physiological performance indices when the trained athlete ceases training (see 'Detraining' p. 31). However, little of this work has been done in a clinical context. There is little information on whether or not the trained athlete is less subject to the physiological consequences of injury, either at the injury site itself or for uninjured organ systems, including skeletal muscle. There would appear to be several perspectives on this issue. On the one hand, the trained athlete has achieved a level of physiological conditioning which makes the extent of deconditioning that may be seen in other clinical settings highly unlikely. On the other hand, the athlete can ill afford to lose even the slightest amount of fitness. So, while the athlete has a greater reserve, it may be even more vital to maintain physiological fitness than for the sedentary individual. While athletes tend to over-estimate the physiologically deleterious effects of 1-2 days off training, longer term inactivity will result in rather rapid deterioration of physiological conditioning (see 'Detraining' p. 31).

Athletes may be at an advantage because the strength of their soft tissues will be greater as a result of long term training. Therefore, should they proceed to surgery, surgical procedures utilizing autogenous tissue grafts may be more likely to succeed. On the other hand, these tissues will be subjected to greater loads upon return to competition, as compared to the normal level of activity for the non-athlete.

So far only the pre-existing level of fitness has been considered. A related issue is that of deliberate *pre-training* to increase the existing level of fitness prior to surgery and/ or immobilization. In some instances this would not be feasible because of the need for immediate surgery, or where any exercise might exacerbate an injury. Where conservative management has been attempted before a decision regarding surgery is made, some pre-training will have occurred fortuitously. While no known clinical studies have investigated a possible benefit of pre-training in minimizing surgical and immobilization effects, there have been several non-clinical studies of the effect of pre-training on susceptibility to immobilization-induced changes in physiological function. Two animal studies have produced particularly encouraging results in this respect: Appell (1986b) studied atrophy of tibialis anterior after cast immobilization of female rat hindlimbs. Pre-immobilization training (treadmill running) of 7 days resulted in a substantial reduction in the atrophy seen after 7 days of subsequent immobilization (from 35% atrophy without pre-training to only 5% atrophy with pre-training). Notably, however, the treadmill training produced an hypertrophy of 16%; this would be unlikely in humans, and suggests that this experimental model may be not be appropriate for the human context. Karpakka et al (1990) have shown a beneficial effect of pre-immobilization swim training on the maintenance of normal muscle collagen biosynthesis, in tibialis anterior and soleus of adult rats.

Human studies of pre-immobilization training have produced somewhat more equivocal results. MacDougall et al (1977) initially strength trained the elbow flexors of healthy male volunteers for 5 months, resulting in 11% and 28% increases in arm circumference and strength respectively. The subjects were then cast immobilized for 5 weeks. In comparison a group who underwent the immobilization only, the pre-trained group actually showed greater losses of metabolic fuel stores (creatine phosphate and glycogen). In a subsequent study of muscle fibre atrophy subsequent to such immobilization, MacDougall et al (1980) found that pre-training did not alter the susceptibility to atrophy.

The effect of pre-training on strength loss was not reported in either of these studies. Appell (1990) reported an unpublished study where isokinetic strength was measured in healthy male subjects after 3 weeks of leg immobilization. With 2 weeks of isokinetic pre-training, the control strength losses—of up to 40%—were approximately halved. Sale et al (1982) also investigated the potential benefits of pre-training on ameliorating strength loss. They studied thenar muscles after 5 weeks of immobilization (thumb, wrist and elbow) with or without 18 weeks of prior thumb abduction strength training. The strength loss following immobilization was also approximately halved by pre-training.

Given the somewhat contradictory findings in relation to pre-training, it is clear that further studies are required. In particular, clinical studies that compare actual patient groups—managed with or without pre-training are necessary.

MUSCLE TRAUMA

This section concerns the pathological states of human skeletal muscle that result when muscle is exposed to forces that are beyond its capacity—in intensity or volume—to sustain, so that damage to the muscle occurs. Such muscle damage may occur at any point in the exercise intensity spectrum, from high intensity exercise where an acute force is beyond the tensile strength of individual fibres or connective tissue elements, to strenuous endurance exercise maintained beyond (poorly understood) limits for this type of exercise. Muscle damage also occurs in situations that are not directly related to the nature of the exercise itself, such as contusions that result from blunt trauma, muscle damage occurring when bone is fractured, and compartment syndromes. Muscle also suffers laceration-type injury when surgical incisions are necessary to gain access to other structures.

Another form of muscle damage, that associated with the phenomenon of delayed-onset muscle soreness (DOMS), has received much attention in the literature. However, its occurrence is essentially limited to unconditioned individuals undertaking unaccustomed exercise, usually with a significant eccentric component. It is not of great clinical significance, as it is only mildly disabling and transient, in that it resolves within days. It generally does not reoccur, as the individual becomes accustomed to the exercise intensity. The only possible exception to this concerns the post-competition soreness experienced by some highly trained athletes in some high intensity sports. The exact nature of such soreness has not been studied, but it would seem to resemble the DOMS of unaccustomed exercise. Why such trained athletes never become completely conditioned to the exercise stress of their sport is not known. In body contact sports, it may be difficult to differentiate such soreness from multiple small contusions that those athletes sustain. DOMS will not be covered further here; the reader wishing additional information is referred to the recent reviews of Armstrong et al (1991), Cleak and Eston (1992), Ebbeling and Clarkson (1989), and Evans and Cannon (1991).

Although there has been a reasonable amount of basic science research on the response of muscle to injury in several experimental models, the findings of such work have often failed to find their way into sports medicine textbooks and review articles. Instead, only the general pathological processes involved in the initial response and subsequent healing of soft tissue wounds (i.e. not specifically muscle) are often described. Even muscle pathology texts generally devote little coverage to the specific processes involved in the response to muscle trauma.

Various authors have employed different terminology to describe the phases of the general pathophysiologic response to soft tissue injury. These phases are briefly described below; the reader is referred to the sources cited for more detailed information.

Phase 1

Inflammatory phase (Oakes 1981, 1992, Prentice & Bell 1990)

Reaction phase (van der Meulin 1982)

This phase is characterized by the initial cellular and humoral responses to the tissue damage. Immediate haemorrhage occurs due to capillary rupture. Initial vasoconstriction is replaced by vasodilation within minutes. The blood borne elements of the humoral response are responsible for vasodilation, increased capillary permeability, clotting, chemotaxis, and phagocytosis. The systems involved are: the kinin system, the intrinsic coagulation system, the fibrinolytic system, and the complement system (van der Meulin 1982). The related cellular response involves mast cells (formation of histamine and serotonin, resulting in vasodilation), granulocytes (formation of prostaglandins, resulting in vasodilation and chemotaxis), and macrophages (chemotaxis and phagocytosis). Further details regarding the inflammatory response may be found in Zarro (1986).

Phase 2

Fibroplastic phase (Prentice & Bell 1990)

Repair phase (Oakes 1981)

Matrix and cellular proliferation phase (Oakes 1992)

Regeneration phase (van der Meulin 1982)

Macrophage and granulocyte activity results in the removal of cellular debris and the fibrin clot. Neovascularization occurs due to capillary endothelial budding from the existing capillary network. The clot is replaced by granulation tissue, which forms a vascularized, connective tissue mass. Fibroplasia results in the synthesis and deposition of connective tissue collagen 'scar'. Further details of this collagen deposition may be found in Chvapil and Koopmann (1984) and Forrest (1983).

Phase 3

Maturation phase (Prentice & Hall 1990, Oakes 1992)

Remodelling phase (Oakes 1981, 1992, van der Meulin 1982)

This phase involves the further strengthening of collagen scar tissue, and its contraction and alignment in the direction of tissue loading.

While some of the pathological responses of different types of soft tissue are similar (regardless of the type of tissue) there are important differences that are often overlooked when the above general schemes are presented. In relation to muscle, notably missing is the capacity of injured muscle to regenerate contractile material. While this was known as early as 1865 (Waldeyer 1865, cited in Caplan et al 1988), this capacity has not only often been ignored, but it has even been specifically denied (e.g. Glick 1980, Evans 1980). The current state of knowledge in this area has recently been summarized by Caplan et al (1988) in the excellent monograph from the American Academy of Orthopaedic Surgeons (see also the reviews of Allbrook 1981 and Carlson & Faulkner 1983).

Reid (1992) has provided one of the few schemes that is specific to muscle injury, including the regenerative capacity:

1. Peritrauma period: haemorrhage, myofibrillar retraction, cell disruption, oedema, chemotaxis.
2. Intense inflammation: inflammation fully established, mononuclear cell (macrophage) invasion, inflammatory triggers, oedema.
3. Phagocytosis: intense phagocytic activity, mechanical weakening of muscle, significant oedema.
4. Early healing: fibroblast proliferation, collagen formation, satellite cells and muscle regeneration.
5. Established healing: complete muscle fibre bridging, contractile ability returning (but still inhibited due to oedema and pain), tensile strength still low.
6. Restoration of function: collagen maturation, increased tensile strength.

The duration of each of these phases is dependent on the severity of injury. Furthermore, the above scheme notwithstanding, the pathophysiology of the various types of muscle trauma appears to be distinctively different in a number of ways. These differences reflect the particular way in which damage is caused, and are manifested in dissimilar rates and kinds of pathological responses. For example, externally observed swelling may represent different balances of haematoma versus inflammatory response in different types of muscle injury. Also, some types of damage are resolved by substantial regeneration of functional muscle fibres, while in other types, denervated fibres are common, or scar tissue may predominate.

Because of these distinctions, it is important that the clinical relevance of research is judged on the basis of appropriate experimental models, most of which are animal models. Among such models, complete muscle ruptures have been studied by Garrett and his colleagues (reviewed in Garrett & Duncan 1988), incomplete muscle strains by Nikolaou and associates (1987) and Almekinders and Gilbert (1986), laceration injury by Gay and Hunt (1954) and Garrett et al (1984), muscle trauma associated with bone fracture by Allbrook et al (1966) and Kakulas (1982), and muscle contusion injury by Jarvinen, Kvist and colleagues (Kvist et al 1974, Jarvinen 1975, 1976a, 1976b, Jarvinen & Sorvari 1978, Kvist & Jarvinen 1982). The following is a review of some of the pertinent aspects of the more common of these injury types. Considerable detail is included in this discussion, as such detail has rarely been covered in the past.

Muscle strain injury

Nikolaou et al (1987) studied rabbit tibialis anterior muscle stretched to approximately 80% of ultimate rupture force, producing strain injuries of the type commonly seen clinically. Disrupted muscle fibres and small haemorrhage were immediately evident, limited to the region of the muscle at the distal musculotendinous junction. In fact a large number of studies have now shown the musculotendinous junction to be the invariant location of damage in this experimental model, including when the muscle is pulled to rupture (see the studies of Garrett and colleagues, cited below). This would seem to be inconsistent with the more variable distribution of muscle strains along the length of muscle that are seen clinically. However, recent dissections of human hamstring muscles, for example, have shown that elements of musculotendinous junction extend through approximately 60% of each muscle's length (Garrett et al 1989b). Therefore, what may be commonly diagnosed as a muscle belly strain may in fact actually occur at musculotendinous junction. Alternatively, this experimental model may not be analogous to the type of muscle injury seen in the human context. This issue awaits further investigation.

In the above mentioned study of Nikolaou et al, the haemorrhage remained localized to the site of the disrupted muscle fibres. Clinically, the localization or spread of such bleeding is dependent on whether the muscle compartment fascia remains intact or is disrupted (Garrett 1990, Renstrom 1988). In the rabbit tibialis anterior tested in Nikolaou et al's study, an inflammatory response ensued over the subsequent few days. Oedema, muscle fibre necrosis, leukocyte invasion, granulation tissue with fibroblasts and inflammatory cells were evident.

After these injuries had been mechanically induced, the animals' muscles were reattached (the rabbits' limbs were not immobilized and normal cage activity was allowed). At 24 hours, although muscle contractile force had reached its lowest point (50% of control), no further ruptures of individual fibres were apparent, despite normal cage activity. By 48 hours, oedema was resolving and contractile force had recovered to approximately 75% of control, despite persistent inflammatory cell proliferation and fibroblast activity. The authors made the point that such apparent early recovery of contractile function does not match normal clinical experience, probably because they elicited contraction of the rabbit muscle by electrical stimulation under anaesthesia, whereas pain typically inhibits contraction following human muscle injury.

The early recovery of contractile capability which occurred in this study might be interpreted as providing support for early mobilization of human muscle injuries. However, it should be noted that maximum tensile strength (i.e. ultimate rupture strength) of muscle injured in this way does not appear to recover as quickly as contractile function. Almekinders and Gilbert (1986) advised against early post-injury loading, as they found that maximum failure load was still as low as 40% of control at 4 days. When these muscles failed, they usually did so just proximal to the original injury site near the musculotendinous junction. These authors suggested that the ongoing inflammatory reaction might be responsible for the continued decrease in tensile strength. If this is so, then it would seem that—as Nikolaou et al (1987) pointed out—contractile capacity may not be affected to the same extent as maximum tensile strength by the acute inflammatory response.

By 7 days, a large increase in fibrous tissue and fibroblasts was apparent. Few inflammatory cells remained. The entry of phagocytic cells (mostly macrophages) is dependent upon sufficient intact vasculature (Caplan et al 1988). Where the muscle sarcolemma is disrupted, calcium influx precipitates greater muscle fibre necrosis (Garrett et al 1989a). The extent of subsequent muscle fibre regeneration appears to be partly related to the integrity of the basal lamina (basement membrane); it has been suggested that it provides a 'scaffold' for regenerating fibres (Kakulas 1982, Vracko 1974).

Study of the same type of muscle strain injury in the tibialis anterior of rats has delineated some of the characteristics of the subsequent response (Almekinders & Gilbert 1986). Macrophage invasion removed necrotic muscle fibres, leaving the macrophage filled basal lamina intact. Many muscle fibres that did not appear to have been injured had in fact suffered damage, as evidenced by subsequent invasion by inflammatory cells.

At 4 days, muscle regeneration was evident, with numerous myotubes and well developed cytoplasm. Consequently, in contrast to the above mentioned study of Nikolaou et al (1987), extensive scar tissue was not often evident. The difference in the relative amounts of regenerated muscle fibres and scar tissue between these two studies may reflect interspecies differences in regenerative potential (i.e. rabbit vs rat). Clinicians currently aim towards the achievement of a flexible, functional scar (e.g. Dornan 1990). However, it is important that future studies attempt to determine the optimum post-injury course for maximizing regeneration of contractile muscle fibres, and minimizing the development of scar tissue.

Muscle rupture

Our knowledge of the pathophysiology of complete muscle rupture has considerably advanced in the last decade. This has been due largely to the work of Garrett and his colleagues at Duke University. A summary of relevant findings follows.

The point of muscle rupture in Garrett's experimental model (rabbit extensor digitorum longus) was almost invariably in the region of the distal musculotendinous junction (Garrett et al 1987, 1988). Although the region of failure was determined, the precise structural point of failure is still unknown. The fact that the avulsion of muscle from tendon often left a short length of muscle attached to the tendon suggests that it may actually have been muscle fibres that ruptured (Garrett & Tidball 1988). Again however, as with the muscle strain model described above, there is concern as to how closely this model mimics in vivo muscle rupture. First, not all in vivo ruptures occur in the region of the musculotendinous junction. Second, the degree of strain at failure in this experimental model indicates length changes of the order of 75-225%, which is much greater than that likely to occur during in vivo injuries (Tidball 1991).

Garrett and his colleagues have investigated various factors that may influence failure behaviour. The potential significance of muscle architecture in relation to failure behaviour was investigated by Garrett et al (1988). While the site of failure was again invariably in the region of the musculotendinous junction, muscles with more pennate architectures tended to elongate further before failing.

It is logical to expect that a muscle's pre-injury contraction history might influence failure behaviour. A single, electrically stimulated isometric contraction prior to stretching the muscle to failure resulted in a greater force required for failure (Safran et al 1988). Furthermore, failure occurred at a greater muscle length. These findings were interpreted by the authors as lending support to the notion of an injury reducing effect of warm-up. The effect of the contractile state of muscle during stretch to failure has also been examined: muscle that was electrically stimulated (maximally and submaximally) during stretch was found to require greater force to failure (but not greater length) than unstimulated muscle (Garrett et al 1987); the force at failure was about 15% greater when the muscle was stimulated (Garrett 1990).

Contusion injury

A series of papers by Jarvinen and colleagues (cited below) represents the major investigation into the pathophysiology of muscle contusion injury. Interestingly, these authors also examined the relative effects of immobilization versus early mobilization on the recovery from this type of injury. As with all animal studies, Kvist and Jarvinen (1982) cautioned against direct extrapolation of results to the human clinical context. In particular, the rate of repair in the rats used is considerably faster than in humans.

The experimental injury induced in these studies was a standardized contusion (crush) injury to the gastrocnemius of male rats. The injury and repair processes were studied over days 2-42 post-injury. The immobilized group had their injured limbs placed in a soft plaster cast. The mobilized group ran on a treadmill from day 1 post-injury for periods from 20 minutes progressing up to 60 minutes.

As described by Jarvinen (1975), the initial inflammatory reaction and haematoma formation were more pronounced in the mobilized group, but subsequently resolved more rapidly. Similarly, scar formation was initially greater in the mobilized group, but was no different from that of the immobilized group at 6 weeks. The amount of necrotic and degenerated muscle tissue was greater in the immobilized group. Regeneration of muscle fibres was substantial in both groups, but occurred to a greater extent and more rapidly in the mobilized group. The substantial extent of regeneration was possibly explained by the fact that the basal lamina generally remained intact. Penetration of regenerated fibres through the scar was more evident in the immobilized group, although the orientation of such fibres was more longitudinal in the mobilized group.

The recovery of tensile properties was described in Jarvinen (1976b). At day 2, breaking strength had decreased by 20-30%. Early mobilization was followed by a rapid increase in tensile properties. Mobilized muscle had generally recovered fully by 3 weeks, while immobilized muscle took up to 6 weeks (Kvist & Jarvinen 1982). The gain in tensile strength appeared to be related to the speed of collagen scar formation and muscle fibre regeneration.

As with other forms of muscle injury, restoration of the vascular supply to the injured area was important for early and optimal recovery. Jarvinen (1976a) found that the speed and intensity of tissue repair (connective tissue formation and muscle regeneration, especially myotube formation) were correlated with the extent of ingrowth of new capillaries, particularly in week 1. Sprouting of new capillaries was more rapid and extensive in the mobilized group.

More recently, the same experimental contusion model has been used to investigate the relative effects of mobilization and immobilization in more detail, especially the sequential appearance of connective tissue components and the optimal timing of mobilization (Lehto et al 1985b). For rat gastrocnemius muscle, an initial period of 5 days of immobilization appeared necessary for optimizing the early appearance of type I collagen. The expression of type I collagen at this stage is a sign of early progression; type III collagen often predominates at this stage, preceding the appearance of type I (Lehto et al 1985a). This early progression would have the effect of accelerating the recovery of tensile strength, thus perhaps allowing safe and effective mobilization to be commenced. Muscles mobilized after only 2 days showed signs of re-rupture, indicating a lack of sufficient tensile strength at this stage. A larger area of granulation tissue subsequently resulted in these muscles, and at 8 weeks this connective tissue was not as well resorbed compared to the group immobilized for 5 days before mobilization commenced. While regenerating muscle fibres can penetrate through such a connective tissue barrier (Hurme et al 1991a), the final extent of regeneration will be impaired, in comparison to injured muscle with less connective tissue proliferation.

The effect of ageing on the response to muscle contusion has been studied by Jarvinen et al (1983). In the same experimental model described above, older rats displayed a less vigorous inflammatory and fibroblastic response in injured gastrocnemius. The result was that the haematoma resolved more slowly, overall healing was delayed, and a less compact connective tissue scar—with less muscle regeneration—was formed. This would be expected to lead to a lower ultimate tensile strength in the aged muscle.

Finally, Hurme et al (1991b) have recently studied the potentially significant neurophysiological consequences of contusion injury. These authors identified denervation of muscle fibre regions adjacent to the injury site, principally due to the physical severing of muscle fibres; thus one half of a fibre became disconnected from its neuromuscular junction in the other half. Actual severing of intramuscular nerve fibres was a less common mechanism of denervation. While reinnervation may occur over several weeks, the lack of innervation in the initial post-injury period may retard the course of muscle regeneration, which appears to depend on an intact nerve supply (Carlson & Faulkner 1983).

Mobilization versus immobilization after muscle injury—further comments

We have obviously progressed since the early 1960s, when it was necessary for a Sydney doctor (George 1963) to write to the editor of the *Medical Journal of Australia* to rebuke the orthopaedic surgeon for a Victorian Football League team for his published opinion that muscle injuries should be treated in the same way as bone—with complete immobilization and rest.

Although such an approach is no longer common—at least not among those specializing in sports medicine—the optimal prescription for mobilization following muscle injury remains uncertain. Clearly, some degree of protection in the early post-injury phase is required (Reid 1992), as tensile strength is reduced and premature mobilization thus runs the risk of disrupting the healing of injured tissues (Almekinders & Gilbert 1986, van der Meulin 1982, Lehto et al 1985b).

As with most other aspects of muscle injury, there is a paucity of basic science and clinical studies on this issue. Of the former, the previously described contusion model of Jarvinen and colleagues is virtually alone. It is not clear whether their results can be broadly extrapolated to human injuries, contusion or otherwise. Likewise, the few clinical studies—although providing some support for mobilization—have not addressed the optimum prescription for a range of injury types and grades (e.g. Corrigan 1965, Millar 1975). New and even more aggressive approaches, such as Stanton's (1988) suggestion of immediate continuous passive motion (CPM) for 4-6 hours a day within the limits of pain, must be compared to more conservative mobilization regimes.

Furthermore, as treatment regimes for muscle injury are refined, so must treatment discharge criteria be improved, so that the athlete's return to competition is as early as possible, but with the minimum possible risk of reinjury. It is unlikely that such criteria will be developed until a better understanding of the pathomechanics and pathophysiology of many of the most common human muscle injuries is achieved. Only with reference to such knowledge can the ability of muscle to resist reinjury be judged.

CONSEQUENCES OF SURGERY FOR MUSCLE FUNCTION

The process of undergoing surgery, per se, has been shown to produce acute deficits in muscle strength at sites remote from the site of surgery (Maxwell 1980, Edwards et al 1982). The latter authors argued that the deficits persisted for too long to be attributed to the general anaesthetic. Eriksson (1981) and Arvidsson et al (1984) have noted the hormonally-mediated stress response to surgery, which may be an alternative explanation for such surgically-induced weakness. However, such general weakness is not a universal finding. Its absence was shown by Young and Stokes (1986). These researchers found after open meniscectomy that the unoperated leg showed normal EMG levels during attempted isometric knee extension in the days immediately following surgery. Thus the effect of the general anaesthetic, or other possible mediators of weakness, was not apparent.

In contrast to the issue of general weakness, the remainder of this section considers the potential deleterious consequences of the surgical tourniquet on the actual operated limb.

Effects of surgical tourniquet on muscle function

Most orthopaedic surgery of the extremities is performed in a bloodless field achieved by a pneumatic tourniquet. However, for some procedures the use of a tourniquet remains contentious (Thorblad et al 1985). Although post-tourniquet palsy is a recognized clinical syndrome, it is generally associated with tourniquet times much longer than those used for most common orthopaedic sports medicine procedures (see Saunders et al 1979 for a review). Potential deleterious consequences of the typically shorter tourniquet times for such orthopaedic procedures have not generally attracted much attention. However, where pain or effusion have not seemed sufficiently severe to account for profound post-surgical inhibition of muscle function, other explanations—such as the tourniquet—have been sought (e.g. Stokes et al 1985).

The study of tourniquet sequelae has focussed on direct effects of compression on underlying nerve and muscle, and indirect consequences of tourniquet-induced ischaemia for distal muscle. Effects on metabolism, muscle and nerve ultrastructure, muscle contractile properties, possible neuropathy, and integrated muscle function have all been investigated.

Animal studies

Animal studies have indicated various effects of the tourniquet on underlying and distal nerve, muscle, and vasculature. The acute metabolic effects of a tourniquet are evident in blood gas tensions and pH, which indicate anoxia and acidosis (Solonen et al 1968). While some acute effects such as these may resolve immediately upon release of the tourniquet, other effects may persist for some period of time, or may even be permanent. Mild mechanical pressure produces a physiological block to nerve conduction that is reversed as soon as the pressure is released; a greater level of pressure has been found to cause ultrastructural damage to nerves and localized myelin swelling which may persist after tourniquet release (Ochoa et al 1972).

It is not clear whether the deleterious effects of the tourniquet occur predominantly during the actual period of tourniquet application, or subsequent to its removal. Strock and Majno (1969a, 1969b) found evidence that some muscle remained ischaemic at 90 minutes following tourniquet release. Tissue oedema may also persist following release (Moore et al 1956). Post-tourniquet damage may be associated with the re-perfusion of previously occluded vasculature (Pedowitz et al 1992).

Patterson and Klenerman (1979) studied ultrastructural changes in soleus and extensor digitorum longus of adult rhesus monkeys following upper thigh tourniquet (1-5 hours duration, at a pressure of 300 mmHg). Distal muscles—that is, those subjected to ischaemia only—showed swollen mitochondria and, in fast twitch fibres, decreased glycogen immediately following a 3 hour tourniquet. These effects had resolved at 1 day post-tourniquet. For the 5 hour tourniquet, soleus showed a similar recovery time for a similar range of effects, however extensor digitorum longus took 3-7 days to recover from more severe signs of degeneration. The effect of direct tourniquet pressure on underlying muscle fibres was much more severe. Widespread disruption of sarcomere ultra-structure was seen (sufficient to render fibres non-contractile), becoming progressively more severe as fibres subsequently appeared to undergo degeneration prior to the initiation of regeneration. Such relatively severe deleterious effects in animal muscle have generally been found only for unusually long tourniquet times. However, Dahlback (1970) found muscle fibre degeneration of rabbit muscle at 1 day following tourniquets applied for only 30 minutes. The damage to mitochondria observed after only 1 hour indicate that these structures are particularly susceptible to ischaemia, although they also display substantial regenerative capacity.

Patterson and Klenerman followed-up their initial 1979 study with a study of muscle contractile properties following tourniquet application (Patterson et al 1981). Again monkeys were studied, with the quadriceps underlying the tourniquet and the distal gastrocnemius and soleus being examined. After a 3 hour tourniquet, changes in contraction and half-relaxation times were not consistent, but isometric tension was reduced by 80-98% and 40-60% in the distal and underlying muscles, respectively. At 6 days, isometric tension was still depressed by 20% in distal muscle, and by 0-36% in the underlying muscle.

The possibility that tourniquet application may have differential effects on slow and fast twitch muscle fibres received some support from the study of Patterson and Klenerman (1979) referred to above. Damage to sarcomere ultrastructure was found to be more severe in the fast extensor digitorum longus than in the slow soleus. A subsequent study provided weak evidence of a greater effect of a 2 hour tourniquet on contractile properties of fast guinea pig plantaris when compared to slow soleus (Gardner et al 1984). However, further study is required before the question of possible differential susceptibility of slow and fast twitch fibres to deleterious tourniquet effects can be definitively resolved.

Human studies

Among the human studies of tourniquet effects, the majority of studies have employed EMG techniques to investigate possible neuropathy. Open meniscectomy has been the most common surgical procedure studied in this context. Saunders et al (1979) evaluated 48 post-meniscectomy patients at 3-4 weeks for EMG indices of possible neuropathy (as well as nerve conduction velocity) in both the distal muscles and those underlying the tourniquet. Tourniquet pressures were 330-450 mmHg and tourniquet times ranged from less than 15 minutes to over 1 hour (depending mainly on whether a surgeon used a tourniquet only for the intra-capsular portion, or the whole procedure). EMG abnormalities were present in 62.5% of patients (most commonly in the distribution of the femoral nerve), with the likelihood of abnormalities increasing with tourniquet time. Abnormalities took from 27 days to 5 months to resolve. Peroneal nerve conduction velocity was unaffected.

Several of the surgeons whose patients were studied by Saunders et al had made particular attempts to minimize tourniquet time. The tourniquet was not inflated until the capsular incision was made; in some instances, it was not in fact inflated until haemostasis became absolutely necessary. Furthermore, the tourniquet was deflated as soon as possible, usually after closure of the capsule.

Krebs (1989) studied 32 patients by neurologic EMG and nerve conduction velocity measurements at 1 month following tourniquet-aided open meniscectomy. An 8.5 cm tourniquet, inflated to 350-450 mmHg, was applied for periods ranging 14-98 minutes (mean of 60.6 minutes). Of the patients 53% were found to have femoral neuropathies at 1 month. Although a complete follow-up was not completed, several patients showed a persistence of abnormal neurologic signs at 9 weeks. Importantly, the presence of neuropathic findings was associated with poorer results for other measures of muscle-joint function, such as isokinetic knee extensor torque, range of knee flexion, and qualitative assessment of gait on level surfaces and stairs.

As most of the human studies have involved patients actually undergoing joint surgery, it is difficult to differentiate the effects of the tourniquet, per se, from other possible deleterious peri-surgical stimuli. Therefore, Stokes et al (1985) examined the immediate post-tourniquet effects of a tourniquet alone, in terms of voluntary muscle activation (assessed by EMG), isometric quadriceps strength, height of a one-legged jump, and neurologic EMG evidence of partial denervation. A tourniquet was applied to the thigh of 4 normal awake subjects at 517 mmHg for the maximum tolerable duration (37-50 minutes). Such tourniquet times are relatively typical, but still shorter than for some common procedures. No evidence of deterioration in any of the indices of muscle function was found at any time from tourniquet release up to 4 weeks later. This finding suggests that the effects of a tourniquet of this type may be relatively benign.

Because of the difficulty in isolating the effects of the tourniquet from the effects of other peri-surgical factors, it is unfortunate that few studies have attempted to compare surgical sequelae with and without tourniquet application. Dobner and Nitz (1982) studied 48 military men after open meniscectomy; half of the patients had a tourniquet, the other half did not. The patients were evaluated at 6 weeks for neurologic EMG abnormalities, femoral nerve conduction, single-leg vertical leap, and isotonic strength. None of the 24 patients operated on without tourniquet showed EMG abnormalities; 71% of those who had a tourniquet exhibited abnormalities (signs of partial denervation). The muscles most affected were tibialis posterior and gastrocnemius (posterior tibial nerve); the next most affected were the quadriceps (femoral nerve). The peroneus longus and the hamstrings (peroneal and sciatic nerve branches) were the least often affected. No changes in nerve conduction velocity were observed.

Resolution of these abnormalities took 3-6 months (the latter for 3 patients). Among the tourniquet patients, there was no association of tourniquet time and pressure with EMG abnormalities, although the mode time for those with abnormalities was only 42 minutes. For the functional assessment of single-leg vertical leap, the performance of those patients with post-tourniquet EMG abnormalities was grossly worse than that of those with normal EMG findings. There were no functional differences between the tourniquet patients with normal EMG findings and those patients who did not have a tourniquet. The authors concluded that arthrotomy without a tourniquet was preferable in this instance for this procedure, despite the additional attention to haemostasis required, and slightly longer operative times.

The study of Thorblad et al (1985) differs from the others cited in several respects. First, as described earlier, the majority of human tourniquet studies have utilized neurologic EMG diagnostic techniques; Thorblad et al instead investigated muscle enzyme indices of direct muscle damage, as well as isokinetic strength of quadriceps and hamstrings. Second, arthroscopic meniscectomy was studied, in contrast to the open meniscectomies previously examined. Finally, the conclusion of this study was contrary to other studies' conclusions regarding the use of pneumatic tourniquets, as will be described. Nineteen patients were studied, 9 with tourniquets at 450 mmHg, and 10 with no tourniquet. Of the muscle enzymes, only creatine kinase rose significantly over 6 post-operative days, but equally for both groups. Furthermore, levels were less than those commonly found, for example, after heavy exercise in healthy subjects. At 4 weeks, isokinetic quadriceps torque had recovered from its 1 week deficit in the tourniquet group, but not in the no-tourniquet group. Hamstring torque was unaffected. The authors concluded that the persistent torque deficit was due to pain-and/or effusion-induced inhibition, probably due to the increased saline flow (used to manage in-surgery haemorrhage) and consequent fluid extravasation and increased pressure.

In summary, it would appear that some muscle damage and neuropathologic signs of partial denervation are not uncommon for typical tourniquet times and pressures. Most existing studies have investigated open surgical procedures. Now that arthroscopy is the procedure of choice in many instances, further study of functional outcomes of tourniquet-aided and no-tourniquet procedures is warranted.

INHIBITION OF VOLUNTARY MUSCLE ACTIVATION

Inhibition of muscle activation after injury and/or surgery is often assumed to reflect voluntary inhibition due to pain. However, other peri-articular afferents may mediate reflex inhibition via inhibition of spinal motoneuron pools (Young & Stokes 1986). Effusion is the factor most often implicated in such reflex inhibition (via pressure and/or volume afferents). Inhibition due to patient anxiety or lack of motivation should also be considered (Eriksson 1981).

It would seem that the presence of inhibition is often conceded in the early post-injury and/or post-surgery phase. However, the particular importance of such inhibition stems from the fact that the initiation of muscle atrophy occurs within hours of the cessation of normal voluntary muscle activation (see 'Immobilization'). Therefore, there should be an especially aggressive effort to minimize inhibition in this early phase, so that the restitution of normal voluntary muscle activation following injury is achieved as quickly as possible. In this way, there is the best chance that atrophy will be minimized.

The relative inhibitory contributions of all the factors normally present after injury and/or surgery is of more than purely academic interest. If it can be shown, for example, that effusion is the major cause of inhibition, then efforts can be primarily focussed on the minimization of effusion, with less attention given to other, less important, mediators of inhibition.

This section is written with the assumption that the inhibition of muscle activation in the early post-injury/post-surgical period is undesirable. That is, it is assumed that it is a desirable aim for patients to be able to activate their muscles to the greatest extent possible in this phase. Obviously, this may not always be true; muscle contraction (voluntary or otherwise) and even passive muscle tension,

may not be consistent with tissue healing constraints. If this is so, then inhibition, and the consequent accelerated atrophy, may have to be conceded.

Stokes and Young (1984) have characterized the extent of inhibition after open meniscectomy. They assessed inhibition by the decline in EMG during isometric knee extension, comparing it to pre-surgery level. Within 24 hours of surgery, inhibition reached 80% and lasted for 3-4 days. At 10-15 days, inhibition was still 35-45%, even though patients were fully weight-bearing. The inhibition was not associated with the general anaesthetic used during surgery, as the unoperated leg showed normal EMG levels in the post-surgical period (Young & Stokes 1986).

The reflex inhibition of muscle activation by afferent signals from articular receptors—independent of inhibition due to pain—was described as early as 1890 (Raymond 1890, cited by Stokes & Young 1984). Such a dissociation of inhibition of reflex origin from pain-induced inhibition has been reinforced by more recent findings (e.g. Shakespeare et al 1985).

Although it is clear that pain may lessen maximal voluntary contraction (e.g. Lysholm 1987), the relative roles of pain and reflex sources—such as effusion—in the overall extent of inhibition are somewhat uncertain. This uncertainty is mainly associated with the exact role of pain; in contrast, the fact that effusion exerts a potent (and generally underestimated) inhibitory action has been clearly demonstrated in the research literature in the past decade (see under 'Effusion' below). The inhibition resulting from effusion has been found to be dissociated from pain in several studies. Young et al (1983) found the lower of two doses of intra-articular anaesthetic in the early post-arthrotomy period ameliorated most of the patients' pain but little of the inhibition (a higher dose relieved both pain and inhibition).

Dissociation of inhibition from pain has also been demonstrated by their different time courses in certain circumstances. After open meniscectomy, Shakespeare et al (1985) found that inhibition at 3 days post-surgery remained near maximal, while contractions were near pain-free. These workers subsequently confirmed that when these results were recorded, an effusion was never clinically evident (Young & Stokes 1986). This suggested either a source of inhibition other than effusion or pain, or alternatively that effusions that were too slight to be clinically apparent were nevertheless capable of inducing severe inhibition. There is evidence to support the latter contention, as outlined below.

The extent of inhibition may be assessed in a number of ways. The above studies of Young and his colleagues have expressed inhibition in terms of the reduction in surface EMG (over rectus femoris) during attempted maximal isometric knee extension. Other studies have employed alternative criterion measures of the extent of inhibition:

Arvidsson (1987) assessed joint torque generation as the measure of inhibition; Spencer et al (1984) and others have assessed inhibition with the H-reflex measure of excitability of the spinal motoneuron pool.

Effusion

It has been known for some time that a large experimental saline infusion into normal knees—mimicking the joint distension of an effusion—produces significant inhibition (e.g. de Andrade et al 1965). Furthermore, aspiration of post-meniscectomy effusions (35-85 ml) have resulted in substantial restoration (although not complete) of previously inhibited maximal voluntary contraction (Stokes & Young 1984). Aspiration of chronically effused knees has also been shown to restore strength (Fahrer et al 1988).

Study of two normal subjects by Young et al (1987) found 60% inhibition (assessed by EMG) with subclinical, small volume experimental knee effusions of 20-30 ml. Young and Stokes (1986) have reported inhibition, as indicated by depressed reflex motoneuron excitability, with experimental saline infusions as low as 10 ml (in normal knees). Such small volume experimental effusions have also been shown to decrease dynamic (isokinetic) torque production by up to 40% in normal knees (Baxendale et al 1985); this study was unable to demonstrate a consistent effect on isometric torques. It is interesting to note that although the subjects did not generally experience pain with these small infusions, they did experience sensations of tightness or fullness. It was not reported whether the investigators attempted to discern clinical evidence of swelling, although similar small effusion volumes were not usually clinically apparent in other studies (Young & Stokes 1986). Therefore, if an effusion were not clinically apparent, a patient's subjective sensations might represent an alternative, clinically useful indicator of the need for an aggressive approach to a small effusion, given the apparent potent inhibitory affect.

Spencer et al (1984) examined reflex motoneuron excitability under experimental infusions of 10-60 ml in normal knees. Of particular interest was the separation of depressed excitability among vastus medialis, rectus femoris, and vastus lateralis. The threshold effusion volume that elicited inhibition of vastus medialis was 20-30 ml; for rectus femoris and vastus lateralis the threshold volume was 50-60 ml. The severity of inhibition between the respective quadriceps components exhibited the same difference trend, but did not achieve statistical significance. Additional studies are needed to replicate this result, and further investigate the notion of differential inhibition of different muscles in patients.

The extent of effusion induced inhibition seems to vary with joint angle, with less inhibition having been found at 30° of knee flexion than at full extension (Stratford 1981).

The fact that intra-articular pressure is less in flexion (Eyring & Murray 1964) is probably the explanation for this trend; alternatively, decreased tension in the posterior capsule of the knee may be significant. After meniscectomy, Shakespeare et al (1983) found greater EMG for a maximal isometric contraction in flexion (approximately 40°) than in extension, again indicative of less inhibition in flexion. The implication of such findings is that patients may be more effectively exercised in flexion than in extension.

Pain

The advent of arthroscopy as the procedure of choice in many instances has meant that significant pain is less widespread following surgical procedures in orthopaedic sports medicine. However, many procedures still require arthrotomy, with large incisions that are associated with significant post-operative pain.

The multidisciplinary research group of Eriksson, Arvidsson and colleagues in Sweden has been particularly concerned with the role of pain in post-surgical inhibition of voluntary muscle activation (Arvidsson 1987, Arvidsson & Eriksson 1988). Again, the concern stems from the apparent rapid onset of atrophy if muscle is inactive for any length of time. Their experimental model has generally been patients undergoing knee reconstruction (patellar tendon graft) for chronic anterior cruciate ligament (ACL) insufficiency.

Arvidsson et al (1986) compared EMG during attempted isometric knee extension before and after the epidural administration of dilute lidocaine. The subjects were 10 patients who were examined on the morning following open knee reconstruction. To verify that the epidural anaesthetic would not affect normal motor function, these investigators had previously administered the anaesthetic to two normal subjects. Concentric isokinetic torque, EMG, and H-reflex were essentially unchanged in these subjects. Prior to post-surgical injection, all of the reconstructed patients had significant pain and could only weakly contract their quadriceps. After injection, EMG during isometric contraction increased in comparison to pre-injection levels by 500%-10 000% over a 25 minute period; that is, the response was highly variable, but clearly beneficial. These findings have led this group to institute routine epidural anaesthesia (van Helder 1991) for 2-3 days after knee reconstruction (Eriksson & Arvidsson 1986).

However, Stokes and Young (1984) have questioned the interpretation of these findings, in particular the assumption that only pain fibres were blocked by the epidural anaesthetic. Although it had been demonstrated that the large motor fibres were not affected, Stokes and Young argued that other small afferents may have been blocked with the small pain fibres. If this were the case, then the inhibition observed may have been elicited by other factors—possibly more important than pain—and relieved when their afferents were blocked with the pain afferents. Stokes and Young's own studies—cited earlier—that showed substantial inhibition in open meniscectomy patients, independent of pain, certainly supports this suggestion. Effusion was identified as the most likely cause of inhibition in these studies; Arvidsson, Eriksson and their colleagues have not investigated the role of effusion in their patients.

Muscle fibre types

There is some evidence that muscle fibre types may be differentially affected by joint injury and its sequelae. The exact explanation for such differential effects remains uncertain. This possibility is also discussed later in the section devoted to 'Immobilization'. It is possible that pain or effusion may mediate such differential effects. For effusion, no known studies have investigated this question (Young & Stokes 1986). When the possible differential effects of pain on different fibre pools are discussed, the work of Gydikov (1976) is often cited. This study has been interpreted by Sherman et al (1982) as having shown that 'mild pain inhibits the monosynaptic reflexes to tonic motor units (slow twitch), while severe pain inhibits the monosynaptic reflexes to both tonic and phasic (fast twitch) units' (p 157). Haggmark et al (1981) concurred with this interpretation; however Rose and Rothstein (1982) interpreted Gydikov's study as follows: 'pain has a greater inhibitory effect on the motoneurons of type I fibres (slow twitch) than on the motoneurons of the type II fibres (fast twitch)' (p 1778). Not only are these slightly different interpretations, but they are both difficult to reconcile with Gydikov's methodology.

Gydikov's painful stimulus was electrical stimulation of the sural nerve, while motor unit activity was monitored with an EMG based technique in biceps femoris of healthy men and women. A transient decrease in motor unit activity was observed. Strength of the painful stimuli influenced only the duration of decreased motor unit activity. Furthermore, only tonic (slow twitch) motor units appear to have been investigated. In summary, Gydikov's methodology was such that extrapolation to injury or surgery induced pain is not justified. Therefore, there would currently appear to be no clear evidence to support differential effects of either pain or effusion on inhibition of different muscle fibre (motor unit) types.

Direct inhibition of muscle

Although the main subject of this section is muscle, inhibition—as it is usually considered—is in fact not a phenomenon that is mediated within muscle itself. It is in fact mediated via afferent pathways from various periarticular receptors that influence efferent command signals to muscle. There is, however, some evidence to suggest that with immobilization, for example, changes may occur in the electrolyte milieu of the muscle itself that change the extent of muscle activation for a given level of motor command (Wroblewski et al 1987). That is, the excitability of the muscle membrane itself may be altered—the muscle itself may be effectively 'inhibited'.

IMMOBILIZATION

In orthopaedic sports medicine, complete immobilization is less common following injury and surgery than it once was, except perhaps in the case of fractures. Early mobilization involving, for example, continuous passive motion (CPM) (Frank et al 1984, O'Donoghue et al 1991) and limited motion braces (Haggmark & Eriksson 1979a, Sandberg et al 1987) is widely employed. While the involved joint—rather than muscle—has generally been the focus of such early mobilization, deterioration of muscle has also probably been lessened by such efforts.

However, where immobilization is still employed, the deleterious consequences for many organ systems—including skeletal muscle—may be profound (Sandler & Vernikos 1986, Steinberg 1980). Furthermore, where atrophy and weakness have been identified long after injury, it is logical to consider whether immobilization at the time of injury and/or surgery may have contributed. A number of studies have found that large deficits in muscle *strength* persist long after knee ligament injury and/or surgery (Grimby et al 1980, Arvidsson et al 1981), femoral fractures (Damholt & Zdravkovic 1972, Danckwardt-Lilliestrom & Sjogren 1976, Rutherford et al 1990), and Achilles tendon injury (Sjostrom et al 1978). Whether such residual deficits were the result of atrophy, pain (leading to long standing relative disuse), instability, inadequate surgery or rehabilitation, or other factors, is not clear. However, persistent *atrophy* long after injury and/or surgery certainly has been identified (Edstrom 1970, Gerber et al 1985, Rutherford et al 1990). Again, however where pain and disability also remain it is not often possible to differentiate cause and effect. Thus it cannot be concluded from such studies whether persistent atrophy stems from an immobilization period at the time of injury/surgery.

The consideration of the deleterious effects of immobilization on skeletal muscle is complicated by a number of factors. Therefore, although there is a large body of literature available on this subject, neither the human nor animal studies allow a complete and unequivocal conclusion as to the obligatory effects of immobilization in a clinical context. The factors that are thought to possibly influence the effects of immobilization on muscle include (Appell 1990, Wills et al 1982):

1. Degree of immobilization (relative versus complete disuse)
2. Duration of immobilization
3. Age
4. Sex
5. Type of muscle
   Upper or lower limb muscle
   Anti-gravity muscle
   One or two joint muscle
6. Fibre composition of muscle
7. Muscle length during immobilization (degree of passive stretch)
8. Muscle activation during immobilization (voluntary or electrically stimulated)
9. Pre-immobilization physiological status
10. Accompanying joint or muscle pathology.

Changes in muscle morphology

The most readily recognizable muscle response to immobilization is atrophy. In humans, the extent of atrophy is difficult to determine accurately without imaging technology (Ingemann-Hansen & Halkjaer-Kristensen 1980), given the potentially confounding influences of unchanged or increased subcutaneous fat (Ingemann-Hansen & Halkjaer-Kristensen 1977, Lo Presti et al 1988), and interstitial fluid redistribution (Hargens et al 1983). Thus the apparent atrophy that is externally evident—e.g. by limb circumference measurement—underestimates the actual muscle atrophy.

A decrease in the rate of synthesis of myofibrillar protein is primarily responsible for muscle atrophy (Booth et al 1982), while protein degradation is relatively unchanged (Gibson et al 1987). Atrophy begins very early following immobilization and proceeds rapidly with an apparent exponential time course (Booth 1977, Rosemeyer & Sturz 1977, cited in Booth 1987). Lindboe & Platou (1984) studied men immobilized for 72 hours in a hip-to-ankle cast (15° knee flexion) and confined to bed, following medial ligament or meniscus injuries. Vastus medialis biopsy revealed atrophy of approximately 15% in both slow and fast twitch muscle fibres over this very short period of time. Changes in the function of immobilized muscle over periods as short as 1 week have also been observed (White et al 1984). These authors immobilized normal males in full leg casts for a total of 2 weeks, observing declines of 5% and 11% in calf area (muscle plus bone) and isometric plantar-flexion strength, respectively, after the first week. These values were approximately doubled at 2 weeks.

Therefore, clinicians should place an early emphasis on means of minimizing atrophy. These might include passive stretch (Goldspink & Goldspink 1986, Williams et al 1988, Williams 1988) via CPM or mobile brace (Haggmark & Eriksson 1979a, Sandberg et al 1987), voluntary con-

traction, and electrical stimulation (Duvoisin et al 1989, Gould et al 1983, Gibson et al 1989, Nitz & Dobner 1987). Surprisingly however, there appears to be little research evidence to support the common belief of clinicians that exercise of a *casted* limb (voluntary or electrically stimulated isometric contraction) has any beneficial effect (St Pierre & Gardner 1987). The studies of Halkjaer-Kristensen and Ingemann-Hansen (1985a, 1985b, 1985c, 1985d) represent the most extensive investigation of the potential ameliorating effects of such interventions while the limb is still immobilized. These authors studied almost 100 young male soccer players undergoing acute surgical or conservative (immobilization only) management of medial collateral ligament injury. The knees were immobilized in plaster casts for periods from 21-49 days, at 5-15° of knee flexion. Neither isometric contractions nor electrical stimulation had a preventative effect on muscle atrophy, aerobic/anaerobic enzyme activity, or static/dynamic muscle function. However, this may reflect to some extent the inhibitory influence of pain and/or effusion; these may have prevented a contraction of sufficient intensity being achieved (see 'Inhibition of voluntary muscle activation' p25). Clinicians should thus attempt to remove these potentially inhibitory influences, so that the chances of limiting muscle deterioration with traditional interventions are maximized.

When a muscle atrophies, the loss of muscle mass is the result of a decrease in size of individual muscle fibres; there is little evidence that an appreciable decrease in the actual number of muscle fibres occurs (Young et al 1982)—which would indicate an 'hypoplasia'—although some contrary results have been reported (e.g. Halkjaer-Kristensen & Ingemann-Hansen 1985b). Muscle atrophy is generally a combination of loss of sarcomeres in parallel and sarcomeres in series. The number of sarcomeres in parallel determines the cross-sectional area of muscle, which is the primary determinant of the intrinsic force generating capacity; the number of sarcomeres in series determines the length of the muscle, and thus its maximum contraction velocity (Wickiewicz et al 1983). In reviewing animal studies, it is important to bear in mind that atrophy reported in terms of muscle mass does not distinguish between loss of muscle length (sarcomeres in series) and muscle cross-sectional area (sarcomeres in parallel); their relative occurrence may not be the same.

There is considerable evidence to indicate that the length at which a muscle is immobilized will lead to adaptation in the number of sarcomeres in series, and thus muscle length. Muscles immobilized in a shortened position will tend to lose sarcomeres in series, thus shortening the overall muscle (Tabary et al 1972). This process involves actual degeneration of the central region of muscle fibres (Baker & Matsumoto 1988). Conversely, the opposite effect—addition of sarcomeres and lengthening of the muscle—is seen if muscle is immobilized in a lengthened position

(Tabary et al 1972). Animal studies have shown that muscles re-adapt to their previous length when immobilization is removed (Goldspink 1983), although this may take a number of weeks (Maxwell & Enwemeka 1992). The adaptation of sarcomere number to immobilized length is thought to be mediated by the passive tension that the muscle is exposed to and/or the degree of muscle activation (Hnik et al 1985).

Appell (1986a) has argued that these findings regarding the effect of immobilization length are of little practical clinical relevance. Appell's contention is based on the fact that joints are most often immobilized in relatively neutral positions, so that neither agonists nor antagonists are appreciably shortened or lengthened. While this may be so for some surgical procedures, it may not always be the case. Arvidsson and Eriksson (1988), in discussing their own studies and those of others, suggested that human knee extensor atrophy following open ACL reconstruction is less if immobilization is at 45° than if the knee is less flexed (Arvidsson et al 1986, Haggmark et al 1981, 1986, Halkjaer-Kristensen & Ingemann-Hansen 1985a). This possibility has not been fully studied, however Elmqvist et al (1988) compared immobilization angles of 30° and 70° for 6 weeks following ACL reconstruction; outcome was assessed in terms of knee stability, range of motion, isokinetic strength, and functional tests. The (incompletely reported) findings revealed no differences between knee flexion immobilization angles in terms of quadriceps atrophy or functional outcome.

While a particular joint immobilization position may result in an optimal length for a given muscle, that muscle's antagonist may be unavoidably shortened and, therefore, disadvantaged. While atrophy of the knee extensors is well recognized, the degree of atrophy experienced by the knee flexors following knee surgery and immobilization is not completely clear. This issue is particularly important in the case of ACL reconstruction, as these muscles have an important role as dynamic stabilizers against anterior translation of the tibia. Ingemann-Hansen and Halkjaer-Kristensen (1980) noted little atrophy of the knee flexors by computerized tomography. Likewise, in measuring isokinetic strength rather than actual atrophy, Vegso et al (1985) failed to find a statistically significant decline in strength at 5-22 weeks following extra-articular ACL reconstruction (4 weeks immobilization in full leg cast at 45° knee flexion) or open meniscectomy (7-10 days immobilization). However, the range of strength decline was quite large in Vegso et al's study, ranging from 20% superiority for the operated leg to 20% superiority for the uninvolved leg (this may have explained the failure to achieve significance). Thus some of their patients experienced large deficits in hamstring strength. In further support of the fact that the strength of the knee flexors can decline precipitously following knee surgery—most likely

due to atrophy—are the results of Morrissey and Brewster (1986) and Gould et al (1983), who found mean isometric strength decreases of 48% and 43% after 2 and 6 weeks of immobilization respectively.

No known human studies have compared knee flexor atrophy or strength loss following immobilization in different knee positions. In fact, there have been relatively few animal studies that have examined relative agonist-antagonist atrophy with immobilization of the involved joint in different positions. In one of the few such studies, Thomsen and Luco (1944) studied immobilization of the ankle joint in cats. They found that immobilization of up to 14 days in plantar-flexion resulted in decreased soleus weight and increased weight of tibialis anterior; conversely, immobilization in dorsi-flexion resulted in decreased weight of tibialis anterior and increased weight of soleus.

In summary, on the basis of animal studies and some evidence of differential human knee extensor atrophy with different immobilization lengths, it would seem that muscle length during immobilization should be considered if atrophy is to be minimised. This consideration must be weighed against the usual rationale for the choice of immobilization position, which is generally predicated upon biomechanical considerations in relation to the surgical procedure, and minimizing forces in repaired tissues during healing.

Muscle fibre types

A number of factors that may affect the nature of immobilization induced atrophy have been listed above.. Different combinations of these factors probably explain the conflicting results in the literature on some aspects of immobilization. For example, some studies have supported the suggestion that atrophy tends to predominate in certain muscle fibre types (see below); however, other studies have not agreed on which fibre type is more subject to immobilization induced atrophy, or indeed if there is a predominance at all.

Major emphasis is given here to clinical studies of human atrophy. Most of the human clinical studies have concerned knee ligament injuries. These have been acute or chronic injuries, usually managed surgically. Relative atrophy of muscle fibre types has generally been assessed by biopsy of vastus lateralis. A relatively large number of studies have suggested that the deleterious effects of such injury, surgery, and immobilization predominantly affect the slow twitch muscle fibres (Edstrom 1970, Gibson et al 1987, Haggmark & Eriksson 1979a, Haggmark et al 1981, 1986, Halkjaer-Kristensen & Ingemann-Hansen 1985b, Ingemann-Hansen & Halkjaer-Kristensen 1983, Karumo et al 1977, Young et al 1982, Wigerstad-Lossing et al 1988). Two studies of muscle atrophy following tendon rupture have also shown predominant slow twitch atrophy (Haggmark & Eriksson 1979b, Jozsa et al 1978). A small number of studies have shown a relatively equal atrophy of both fibre types (Gerber et al 1985, Lindboe & Platou 1982, 1984, Patel et al 1969, Sargeant et al 1977). Few studies have reported a predominant atrophy of fast twitch fibres (Baugher et al 1984, Lo Presti et al 1988).

Potential reasons for the different findings among these studies of relative fibre atrophy are difficult to discern; in some studies insufficient details were provided. In some cases, there was wide variation between individual patients in the balance of atrophy between fibre types. On the basis of the information available, there do not appear to be clear patterns that distinguish fibre type predominance between acute versus chronic injuries, surgical versus conservative management, ligament versus bone injuries, duration of immobilization, type of muscle biopsied, and so on. Some clinicians, however, are of the opinion that slow twitch fibres may be more susceptible to atrophy when the muscle has been immobilized in a shortened position (Arvidsson & Eriksson 1988, Haggmark et al 1986, Halkjaer-Kristensen & Ingemann-Hansen 1985b). Further review of the effects of immobilization on muscle fibre types—including animal studies—may be found in Appell (1986a, 1990).

It might be expected that immobilization of healthy subjects would perhaps allow the effects of immobilization, per se, on different muscle types to be separated from the many other potential influences that are present in the clinical context. Although several such studies have been made, they have involved elbow casting and biopsy of triceps brachii (MacDougall et al 1977, MacDougall et al 1980), in contrast to the clinical lower limb studies described above. To further complicate matters, these studies actually found predominant atrophy of fast twitch fibres over 5 weeks of immobilization (although both fibre types were significantly atrophied). It has been suggested that the discrepancy between these findings and those of most of the clinical studies may reflect functional differences between upper and lower limb muscles (MacDougall 1986a), or differences in the normal balance of fibre types in these muscles (MacDougall 1986b).

Notwithstanding the apparently conflicting research findings, Lieber et al (1988) have proposed a scheme to predict the relative susceptibility of different types of muscle (functional and fibre type differences) to immobilization induced atrophy. Under this scheme, the muscles most susceptible to atrophy are single joint, anti-gravity muscles that contain a high proportion of slow twitch fibres (e.g. soleus, vastus medialis); next most susceptible are muscles of similar function and fibre composition, but which cross 2 or more joints (e.g. erector spinae, rectus femoris, gastrocnemius); those muscles suggested to be least susceptible to atrophy are phasically activated and predominately fast twitch (e.g. tibialis anterior).

There is some evidence from animal studies that fibre type may also influence the rate of recovery following immobilization. Booth and Seider (1979) found that slow twitch rat muscle recovered more rapidly than fast muscle after 3 months of hind limb immobilization.

Muscle metabolic effects

Slow twitch fibres exhibit high activity of oxidative enzymes that favour aerobic energy metabolism. In contrast, fast twitch fibres possess high activities of the glycolytic enzymes associated with anaerobic metabolism (Saltin & Gollnick 1983). Although the findings reviewed above in relation to predominant fibre atrophy were variable, most studies showed that slow twitch fibres were the most subject to atrophy. Likewise, the enzymes of aerobic metabolism—that predominate in slow twitch fibres—decline more readily than those of anaerobic metabolism, which are relatively unaffected (Haggmark & Eriksson 1979a, Haggmark et al 1981, Halkjaer-Kristensen & Ingemann-Hansen 1985c, Jansson et al 1988, Wigerstad-Lossing et al 1988). The findings in relation to fibre atrophy and decline in enzyme activity would thus appear to indicate that the aerobic endurance capacity of muscle is likely to be most severely affected by immobilization. This is consistent with the faster decline in endurance indices found in detraining studies (see 'Detraining' p. 31).

Effects of bed rest (alone) on healthy muscle

Numerous studies have shown that bed rest alone—without limb immobilization—will cause a deterioration in various organ systems, including skeletal muscle (Greenleaf & Kozlowski 1982, Sandler & Vernikos 1986, Steinberg 1980). Le Blanc et al (1988) studied calf muscle area and isokinetic strength in 9 male subjects who underwent 5 weeks of complete horizontal bed rest. While plantar-flexor area decreased by 12% and strength by 26%, the area and strength of the dorsi-flexors did not change significantly. Differential effects on agonist-antagonist muscle groups was also shown in the study of Dudley et al (1989), who assessed isokinetic knee extensor and flexor strength (concentric and eccentric) after 30 days of bed rest. Knee extensor strength decreased by about 19%, while knee flexor strength did not decrease significantly (the actual decrease was about 6%). The changes were similar for both concentric and eccentric contractions, and all isokinetic test velocities. At 30 days post-bed rest, recovery of strength was almost complete. Finally, Gogia et al (1988) made similar findings following 5 weeks of bed rest: the muscle groups tested were plantar flexors, dorsi flexors, knee extensors, knee flexors, elbow flexors, and elbow extensors. The average strength of all muscle groups except the elbow extensors were reduced by 26%, 8%, 19%, 8%, and 7%, respectively, again suggesting differential susceptibility of agonist and antagonist.

Effects of crutch ambulation

Recently, several human experimental models that are similar to crutch ambulation have been described. In normal males, Berg et al (1991) found that 4 weeks of such unilateral lower limb unloading resulted in decreased isokinetic knee extensor strength of about 20%. Muscle cross-sectional area was reduced by about half this amount. At 4 days after return to normal ambulation, isokinetic strength was still down by about 10%. By the next measurements at 7 weeks, all indices had recovered to pre-unloading values. Hather et al (1992) employed a similar lower limb unloading method to study muscle morphology in 8 men and women, over 6 weeks. Knee extensor atrophy averaged 16%, although this was limited to the vasti; rectus femoris did not atrophy (the hip was not immobilized). Conversely, the knee flexors averaged only 7% atrophy. Atrophy of the triceps surae was similar to that of the vasti.

Those interested in further reading on the subject of the effects of immobilization on muscle should consult the reviews of Appell (1986a, 1990), Booth (1987), Booth & Gollnick (1983), Gossman et al (1982), St Pierre and Gardiner (1987), and Wills et al (1982).

DETRAINING

To say that an injured athlete has 'lost fitness' is as inadequate as a diagnostician stating that an athlete is simply 'injured'.

An important theme in the treatment of any injured athlete must be an understanding of the physiological requirements of a given athlete's sport. Only then can the clinician appreciate what it is that the athlete has lost—in terms of physiological fitness—due to an enforced layoff, and furthermore, what must be done to return the athlete to pre-injury physiological status as quickly as possible.

There is a substantial literature on the physiological consequences of the cessation of exercise training—detraining. However, many such studies of the regression of training induced improvements have been done following short term training programs of only moderately active or sedentary individuals. Relatively few studies have investigated the deterioration in physiological fitness that is experienced by athletes in long-term training who are forced to undergo a relative or complete layoff. Greatest emphasis is given here to those detraining studies that have been conducted with long term athletes. As clinicians who have attempted to prescribe rest for injured athletes will attest, such athletes are not easy to convince to stop training!

There is increasing evidence that many athletes (particularly endurance athletes) may be over-training. For such athletes, relative or even complete rest may result in improved performance (e.g. Koutedakis et al 1990). Furthermore, such over-training may be associated with the development of over-use injuries or illness, thus forcing

an athlete to reduce training, or cease completely. In such cases, athletes may be consoled to some extent by the fact that their loss of fitness may not be severe; short term rest or reduced training may in fact be physiologically beneficial.

Although the focus of this chapter is primarily on muscle, detraining affects both local muscular and central cardio-vascular adaptations to training; indeed such peripheral and central adaptations interact to determine an athlete's performance capability. It would be impossible to discuss one site of adaptation without the other, so both are covered here.

In order to understand the detraining response, one must understand the adaptive response to the initial exercise training. Readers who are unfamiliar with this area should refer to the earlier chapter on exercise physiology. A brief overview of endurance training adaptations is provided here, as most detraining studies have concerned endurance training. Among the adaptations to endurance training that occur locally in the trained muscles are increased activity of the enzymes of aerobic (oxidative) metabolism, increased mitochondria, increased energy substrate levels (e.g. glycogen) and muscle capillarization. Among the central adaptations to endurance-type training is an increase in maximal cardiac output (the product of stroke volume and heart rate). Alterations in stroke volume may be mediated by changes in blood volume and/or structural changes in cardiac dimensions. Endurance exercise performance is thus a function of all these adaptations, although some adaptations will be more important than others. Laboratory indices of aerobic fitness, such as the maximum oxygen consumption (VO_2 max), likewise reflect the combined effect of the underlying adaptations, local and central.

The results of the studies described below must be interpreted in the context of the level of inactivity imposed by various pathologies and interventions. Detraining studies have generally involved simply cessation of training; subjects have been able to maintain their 'normal' (albeit sedentary) activities of daily living. Certain pathologies, particularly those involving surgical intervention, will impose greater levels of inactivity. Such inactivity—including limb immobilization and bed rest—is specifically considered in the earlier section on Immobilization.

Detraining following aerobic endurance training

Most studies of detraining have investigated the phenomenon following aerobic, endurance-type training. Coyle et al (1984) followed endurance athletes (runners and cyclists, with mean training experience of 10 years) for 84 days after cessation of training. There was an average decline of 7% in maximum oxygen consumption (VO_2 max) after only 12 days of inactivity; this was almost half of the eventual decline seen at 84 days. Subjects who had the highest initial VO_2 max suffered the greatest loss. These researchers attempted to determine whether the decline in VO_2 max was due to a deterioration in local muscular or central factors. They found that the early decline in maximum oxygen consumption was due primarily to a decline in stroke volume. Despite the substantial deterioration in VO_2 max, sedentary levels were not reached, due primarily to stroke volume and arteriovenous oxygen difference remaining above that found in sedentary individuals. The latter was explained by the relative maintenance of local muscular factors such as muscle capillarization and oxidative enzyme activity (the latter declined, but did not approach sedentary levels). The findings of this study again emphasize the interaction of local muscular and central cardiorespiratory factors in the detraining response.

Rather than a decline in intrinsic heart function, which would seem unlikely over such a short period of time, the decline in stroke volume was attributed to the loss of the training induced plasma volume expansion; this loss would decrease venous return and thus limit left ventricular filling and stroke volume (Coyle et al 1986). A similar loss of plasma volume was also seen by Cullinane et al (1986) in their study of a 10 day training cessation in 15 male long distance runners. However, these researchers did not observe any decline in VO_2 max over this period (in contrast to Coyle et al 1984). Ehsani et al (1978) did find early regression (over 1-3 weeks detraining) of cardiac wall thickness, which had been modestly enlarged by 3 months training in college cross-country runners. An 11% decrease in VO_2 max was also found in this study.

In relation to physiological indices of *submaximal* endurance exercise performance, the athletes from Coyle et al's (1985) study still maintained a higher anaerobic threshold than untrained controls after 84 days of detraining. This would have allowed them to exercise for longer periods at higher intensity, with less lactic acid accumulation, than their untrained counterparts.

Costill et al (1985a) studied 8 male collegiate (short-distance) swimmers over 4 weeks of inactivity following 5 months of intense training (averaging 10 900 metres per week, training 6 days per week). In a standard 183 m swim at a speed equivalent to 90% of each swimmer's best time, the mean blood lactate accumulation during the swim almost doubled over the 4 weeks. A large decline of 50% in the respiratory capacity of the deltoid muscle was evident after only 1 week. While a swim of such a distance has a significant anaerobic component, the training of swimmers—even for such short-distance events—tends to involve large volumes of work, much of which is completed aerobically. These authors suggested that the physiological gains made over 5 months of training would be entirely lost within 6-8 weeks of ceasing training.

The pattern and extent of changes found in these studies are generally consistent throughout the literature on the cessation of long term training (see Coyle et al 1984 for a review); however, the detraining response following shorter periods of training may include more significant declines in physiological indices of aerobic function (Coyle 1988).

Although detraining-induced changes in indices of physiological function are interesting, actual effects on endurance performance are of much greater interest to the athlete. It cannot necessarily be assumed that declines in physiological function of the order indicated above will lead to similar relative declines in performance—performance could be affected to a greater, lesser, or similar extent. Among the detraining studies that have employed some form of test of endurance performance, there is a large variation in subject material, training history, and the nature of the endurance tests that have been employed; thus it is difficult to indicate the general extent of the decline in actual endurance performance that might be expected. Notably, the effect of detraining on endurance exercise performances of longer than 20 minutes duration does not seem to have been evaluated. These problems notwithstanding, a summary of relevant studies of actual exercise performance after detraining follows.

Houston et al (1979) followed 6 well trained distance runners over 15 days of detraining. Interestingly, these subjects' calf muscles were actually immobilized in a walking cast for the first 7 days. A decline of only 2.4-7.3% in VO_2 max was found, but there was an average decrease of 25% (range -2.5-50.5%) in run time to exhaustion at a speed equivalent to 90% of the athletes' VO_2 max. To put this in the context of race times, the duration of each athlete's run to exhaustion at this exercise intensity was in the range of about 10-20 minutes. Coyle et al (1986) noted a similar decline in VO_2 max among trained endurance cyclists and runners after 2-4 weeks detraining, but—in contrast to Houston et al's subjects—endurance time on a bicycle ergometer at 105-110% VO_2 max declined only about 8%. The difference may be due to the differences in test modes (running vs cycling), or in exercise intensity—and therefore duration—of the two studies' test bouts; Coyle et al's subjects lasted only in the order of 8-9 minutes before exhaustion. The work of Hickson et al (1985) provides further support for the notion of differential effects of detraining on endurance performances of different durations/intensities.

Reduced aerobic training

Maintenance of a reduced level of training—instead of total cessation—appears to lessen the extent of the decline in physiological function (Neufer 1989). Houmard (1991), in reviewing the growing literature on reduced training by endurance athletes, has concluded that periods of reduced training should not be longer than about 3 weeks if maximal aerobic endurance performance is to be maintained. Theoretically, total training load can be reduced by manipulating any combination of training frequency, volume, or intensity; however, it seems that aerobic endurance exercise performance is best maintained only under certain manipulations. Training frequency can be reduced, but probably only slightly (perhaps 20-50%); conversely, training volume can probably be reduced substantially, by perhaps 60-90%. Recent work has indicated that a failure to maintain training *intensity* will result in a decrement in running performance (McConnell et al 1992). In this study of male distance runners over 4 weeks, weekly training volume was reduced by 65%, and training frequency by 50% (which had been shown in previous work to produce minimal physiological deterioration). Intensity was reduced such that sessions were performed at a pace similar to, or slower than the athletes' easy running pace; this was well below their usual training intensity. While VO_2 max did not decline with this program, 5 km race performance time deteriorated significantly (by an average of 12 seconds). There was, however, no difference in times over the first 1600 m.

Note that the findings described above—of limited deleterious effects of short term reduced training—are contrary to the entrenched beliefs of most endurance athletes and coaches. Ironically, short term reductions in training loads are of course regularly practised by athletes in a number of sports in the lead-up to competition; this is commonly known as 'tapering'. The expectation underlying this practice is that performance will not only not decline, but will actually be improved by the reduction in training load. Although this phenomenon has not been widely studied, there is evidence to support the physiological and performance benefits of the practice (e.g. Costill et al 1985b). Where an athlete is required to reduce training load because of injury, it could be seen as analogous to tapering, and therefore potentially beneficial. However, it is not uncommon that the period of time involved with more serious injury will be longer than that generally associated with tapering.

Detraining following anaerobic training

There are fewer studies of detraining following anaerobic exercise training than those of detraining following aerobic training. Current evidence suggests that the deterioration of the physiological adaptations for high intensity anaerobic exercise is more modest than that seen for aerobic adaptations.

The study of Simoneau et al (1987) involved an initial 15 week high intensity, interval type bicycle ergometer training program, for 19 mixed sex sedentary subjects. Although such high intensity training is generally considered to be primarily anaerobic in nature, aerobic metabolism definitely contributes, so the categorization is somewhat blurred. Therefore, as is common with such training, improvements in both anaerobic and aerobic enzyme activities, as well as VO_2 max (increased by almost

20%) were observed in this study. The mechanical work done in 10 and 90 second 'all-out' efforts was also improved; the former task is considered to be predominantly anaerobic, while the latter has a significant additional aerobic component. Consistent with the discussion above, after 7 weeks of detraining, significant declines in those parameters associated with the aerobic component of the training adaptation were found. For example, half of the increase in VO_2 max had been lost, as had aerobic (oxidative) enzyme activities. Conversely, anaerobic (glycolytic) enzyme activities were unaffected. Work done in the 10 second test was unaffected, while 90 second work was decreased. This pattern is consistent with the relative contribution of anaerobic-aerobic metabolism to the respective work tests, and the changes in the physiological indices associated with these metabolic pathways.

Indices of anaerobic metabolism, such as glycolytic enzyme activities, do eventually decline with inactivity, but this takes much longer than is the case for the enzymes of aerobic metabolism (Green et al 1980—discussed under 'Sports with mixed physiological requirements' below). A decline in both aerobic and anaerobic enzyme activities after long term detraining (6 months) has been shown for late adolescent boys, following 3 months of either sprint or endurance training (Fournier et al 1982).

Although anaerobic (glycolytic) function may not decline appreciably in the short term, the sporting activities for which anaerobic metabolism is important typically also require a relatively high level of strength. Therefore, the loss of strength (discussed below)—with or without atrophy—may be particularly deleterious for these athletes, even though their relevant anaerobic metabolic pathways may not be greatly affected by detraining.

Detraining following strength training

Athletes in many sports utilize strength training to enhance their strength for performance. It is therefore of concern to know the extent of the loss of training-induced strength increases that might occur with enforced cessation of strength training. The physiological adaptations responsible for increases in strength resulting from strength training are both morphological (i.e. hypertrophy) and neural (Moritani & de Vries 1979). Both types of adaptations appear to regress with detraining (Hakkinen & Komi 1983).

Most studies of detraining following strength training have used relatively short periods of training, typically 6 months or less. Relatively few studies have been performed, and these studies have utilized various different types of subjects, ranging from sedentary to athletes experienced in strength training. Strength training equipment and protocols have also been different, as have the methods of strength assessment and the muscle groups studied.

Hakkinen and his colleagues have performed most of the studies on this subject, using heavy resistance training (including different combinations of concentric and eccentric muscle actions) and explosive, stretch-shortening cycle (plyometric) exercises (Hakkinen et al 1981, 1985; Hakkinen & Komi 1983, 1985a, 1985b; Tesch et al 1987), focussing on the knee extensors. The effects of the actual strength training in these types of studies have generally included hypertrophy (predominantly of fast-twitch fibres) of the order of 20-30% (Hakkinen et al 1981, 1985; Houston et al 1983). In studies of male detraining following strength training lasting 2.5-6 months, approximately half of the increase in fast twitch fibre area was lost after detraining periods of 2 (Hakkinen et al 1981) to 3 months (Hakkinen et al 1985, Houston et al 1983). Although these particular studies have involved male subjects only, it is now clear that women are capable of achieving significant hypertrophy if the training intensity is sufficient (Cureton et al 1988, Staron et al 1990). Staron et al's (1991) study of college females, who detrained for 8 months after 5 months heavy resistance training, found minimal regression of hypertrophy but significant strength loss (although not to pre-training levels).

Loss of strength training-induced hypertrophy has recently been studied over shorter periods by Dudley and his colleagues (Dudley et al 1991, Hather et al 1991). The subjects were recreationally active males, rather than athletes. After 1 month of familiarization, they underwent lower body heavy resistance training twice a week for 19 weeks. After 4 weeks of detraining, approximately half of the hypertrophy and strength gains had been lost.

As with the studies of aerobic and anaerobic detraining discussed above, the athlete who must cease strength training is most concerned about the loss of performance (i.e. strength), rather than laboratory physiological measures. Some details of substantial strength loss were mentioned among the details of loss of hypertrophy reviewed above. Conversely, Berger (1965) found little loss of leg squat strength with 6 weeks of detraining in male college physical education students. However, these results followed only 3 weeks of initial strength training. Although it was reported that strength had increased over this training period, the actual magnitude was not reported. Therefore, it is possible that the lack of a significant decline in strength with detraining may have been due to a limited training induced strength increase. However, an alternative explanation is also tenable. Increases in strength over such short training periods are generally attributed to neural changes (Moritani & DeVries 1979). Therefore, it is likely that any training-induced strength increases in Berger's study were largely due to such adaptations. Given Berger's finding of minimal strength loss with detraining, it is thus possible that neurally mediated strength increases may be relatively insensitive to detraining. Definitive support for this hypothesis awaits detraining studies that assess the time course of strength loss more closely.

Staron et al's (1981) case study of a 7 month detraining period by a single elite power lifter is also worth consideration. This athlete had been in heavy training for several years. After 7 months of inactivity, muscle biopsy of vastus lateralis demonstrated an atrophy of 41% in fast twitch fibres, and 31% in slow twitch fibres. Body mass decreased from 121.5 to 94.0 kg over the same period. Interestingly, the oxidative capacity of the muscle actually increased. This was possibly due to a relative maintenance of the number of mitochondria while muscle mass decreased, effectively increasing mitochondrial volume density. This adaptation was reflected in an increase in VO_2 max from 32.6 to 49.1 ml/kg/min (only partially explained by the change in body mass). Although probably of little interest to a power lifter, it is startling to note this degree of improvement in aerobic capacity resulting from no training whatsoever. It is in fact indicative of the extent to which high levels of strength and aerobic endurance capacity in muscle are largely mutually exclusive. Paradoxical increases in the speed of muscle tension development have also been observed with detraining following short term strength training (Ishida et al 1990).

Finally, it is worth considering the possibly different response to detraining after 'explosive', stretch-shortening cycle, strength training (e.g. plyometrics). Hakkinen and Komi (1985b) have studied detraining of 12 weeks following 24 weeks of such training of the lower limbs. Emphasizing the difference between this type of training and conventional strength training, maximal squat lift did not increase with this type of training to the same extent as that seen for these authors' heavy resistance training studies (referred to above). Furthermore, almost all of the 6.9% increase in squat lift was lost with detraining. However, most importantly, the decline in parameters related to explosive force production were relatively slight, suggesting that such training adaptations may be relatively resistant to detraining.

Readers may also wish to refer again to the several human studies of immobilization following strength training that were discussed at the start of this chapter in 'Physiological status at the time of injury'.

Sports with mixed physiological requirements (aerobic and anaerobic)

The physiological requirements of some sports (e.g. court sports, many team sports) are a mixture of aerobic and anaerobic capacities. Such sports do not generally attract as much research interest among physiologists as those sports that involve only single exercise forms and intensities. Given the mixed physiological requirements of such sports, the likely loss of the different components of athletes' physiological fitness with detraining can probably be inferred from the research on detraining after pure aerobic and anaerobic training. However, several studies have looked specifically at detraining from such sports. Allen (1989) followed 6 elite Rugby League players for 6 weeks following a competitive season. VO_2 max was initially only moderately high in these athletes (55.8 ml/kg/min), but it remained relatively stable for the first 4 weeks of detraining; by 6 weeks it had approached sedentary levels. Consistent with other studies, oxidative (aerobic) enzyme activity decreased by 25% over this period. Glycolytic (anaerobic) enzyme activity also decreased, but only by 16%.

In a study of college ice hockey players, Green et al (1980) monitored the detraining response during the off-season following a 5-month competitive season. VO_2 max and enzymes of aerobic and anaerobic metabolism were assessed at 6 and 18 weeks after cessation of training. VO_2 max decreased by an average of 5.2% over the first 6 weeks. This is somewhat less than that found in studies of detraining following endurance type training. Following the season's training, the VO_2 max of these athletes had reached moderately high levels (mean of 60 ml/kg/min), not dissimilar to those of the athletes in Coyle et al's (1984) endurance detraining study (discussed above), for example. Among the enzymes of muscle metabolism studied by Green et al (1980), aerobic enzyme activities declined most rapidly, reaching a plateau by 6 weeks. A significant decline in the activity of the important anaerobic enzyme, phospho-fructokinase (PFK), was not apparent at 6 weeks, but had occurred by 18 weeks.

Cross-training

This section would be incomplete without some discussion of the relatively common practice of 'cross-training' by injured athletes, that is, attempting to maintain fitness by exercising with uninjured limbs. However, despite its wide use (e.g. Croce & Gregg 1991), it may surprise clinicians to learn that the evidence to support the assumed benefits of this practice is far from definitive (Franklin 1989).

As indicated earlier, adaptations to normal endurance training involve enhancements to both local muscle metabolism and central cardiovascular function. Of these, it might seem reasonable to expect central cardiovascular fitness to be maintained, as long as this system were stressed with any form of exercise of sufficient intensity, regardless of which limbs were used. Conversely, maintenance of local muscle metabolic adaptations would logically seem to require exercise of the specific muscles. By this reasoning, cross-training might be expected to maintain central cardiovascular adaptations, but not local muscular adaptations. Does the existing research support these hypotheses? Despite this hypothesized 'generality' of central adaptations, studies have generally shown that the central enhancements that result from training are only apparent when exercise is performed with the same limbs as performed the actual training (e.g. Clausen et al 1973). The exact mechanisms whereby the heart only functions in a trained fashion when the limbs that performed the training are used are not fully understood (Saltin 1987, Kanstrup et al 1991). It is clear, though, that both central and peripheral factors govern the cardiovascular response to exercise (Rowell & O'Leary 1990). Conversely, as far as the local muscular adaptations are concerned, research does indeed support the hypothesis that enhancements in physiological markers of local muscle metabolism are limited to the trained limbs (Saltin et al 1976).

Although the weight of evidence supports the restriction of training enhancements to the trained limbs, some studies have found slight improvements in the performance of untrained limbs. The explanation for this effect has generally been a slight carry-over of central cardiovascular adaptations to exercise with the untrained limb, as local metabolic changes have not been detected in the untrained limb (Hardman et al 1987).

The studies referred to thus far in this discussion have trained their subjects with one set of limbs, and then tested the subjects' performance after training, but with the exercise being performed with another set of limbs. A small number of studies have also been performed where subjects who have trained with one set of limbs (or one form of exercise) are switched to another set of limbs (or exercise form) for a new training period, and then their performance in the original form of exercise is subsequently re-tested. Few such studies have been done with athletes; studies have generally involved previously untrained individuals. Among the factors that differ between the existing studies—and tend to confound definitive conclusions on the issue—are the duration of cross-training and the criterion variables on which the outcome was judged. In relation to the latter, studies have been variously judged on maximum oxygen uptake, anaerobic threshold, and submaximal exercise performance.

Pate et al (1978) studied 13 males (college physical education students) who initially trained their legs on a bicycle ergometer for 8 weeks (30 minutes/day, 5 days/week, at about 85% of maximum heart rate). For the subsequent 4 weeks, one group changed to arm training using an arm crank ergometer (at about 75% of maximum heart rate), while another group ceased training. Upon post-training assessment of VO_2 max during leg work on the bicycle ergometer, the arm training group did not perform any better than the group who stopped training. That is, arm training did not prevent the normal detraining response for leg exercise performance that occurred with no further training at all.

The study of Moroz and Houston (1987) employed a different design: the subjects were female runners in training for at least 6 weeks. One group continued to train in running for 4 weeks (30 minutes/day, 4 days/week, 80-85% of maximum heart rate), while another group undertook the same regime on a bicycle ergometer. VO_2 max and treadmill run time to exhaustion (at a speed and grade equivalent to 90% VO_2 max) were assessed. The results showed no decrement in either index of running performance as a result of the switch to cycling training. Thus cycling training was able to maintain running performance. Similarly, Maw (1991) found that female recreational runners could maintain their performance level by arm ergometer training (30 minutes/day, 3 days/week) when run training was stopped for 5 weeks.

The findings of these last two studies—showing a maintenance of performance with a dissimilar training mode—are somewhat unique. Further research is needed before definitive conclusions can be drawn regarding the possible clinical utility of cross-training by injured athletes. There is an almost complete lack of clinical studies on any aspect of this phenomenon. A small element of the study of Halkjaer-Kristensen and Ingemann-Hansen (1985a) investigated the effect of contralateral limb bicycle ergometer training on atrophy of knee injured soccer players. These authors found no ameliorating affect of this healthy-limb training on injured limb atrophy, but one hesitates to draw any conclusions until further studies have been done.

Interestingly, the apparent need to exercise the specific muscles in which maximal local metabolic adaptations are desired, does not necessarily apply to adaptations in muscle strength. There appears to be a 'cross-transfer' of muscle strength training effects—achieved by training one limb—to the other limb (see Enoka (1988) for a review of studies of this phenomenon; see also the comments of Kannus et al (1992) regarding such studies). No known studies have investigated the use of this phenomenon in a clinical context to ameliorate the strength loss in an injured limb. This context is obviously somewhat different to the enhancement of strength in healthy limbs, which is the paradigm that has been investigated in cross-transfer studies to date. Given that the cross-transfer effect is most likely neurally mediated, the prevention of strength loss—if it occurs—may be unlikely to extend to the reduction of morphological changes, such as muscle atrophy. However, the loss of the neural adaptations to strength training might possibly be lessened. These suggestions await further investigation.

Notwithstanding the questionable physiological benefits of cross-training, it is however worth considering the possible psychological benefit of allowing an injured athlete to maintain at least some type of exercise while recovering from injury. Furthermore, it is sometimes difficult to restrain over-zealous athletes from doing 'too much, too soon' when exercising injured limbs; if allowing them to exercise other limbs is helpful in restraining them in this regard, then it should be considered.

If one were to suggest recommendations for clinical practice on the basis of the existing research, one would suggest that some attempt should be made to reduce the detraining response in the injured athlete. If possible, this should involve the same type of exercise in which the athlete is usually engaged. While joint, bone, and/or muscle loading usually have to be reduced, exercise intensity should be maintained if possible, as should training frequency. One way in which this might be achieved for land based athletes is water training (e.g. Gatti et al 1979).

One of the most important areas of investigation in the last decade in relation to the physiology of exercise training has been that of the genetics of training. It is now clear that the susceptibility to improved performance with training—'trainability'—varies considerably between individuals, and appears to be strongly inherited (Bouchard et al 1988, 1992). The converse of this phenomenon—'detrainability'—has not been specifically studied. However, it is highly likely that there is a similar variability among individuals in the response to the removal of a training stimulus, as there is for the application of a training stimulus. This reinforces the clinical wisdom of individualization of rehabilitation programs, in contrast to 'cookbook' approaches based on fixed rates of progression.

Finally, the possibility of a detraining response following the formal rehabilitation phase should not be ignored. It is perhaps simplistic to assume that improvements in functional status—achieved by the time a patient is discharged from rehabilitation—will be maintained indefinitely after discharge. Typically, athletes will return to their sport, including their previous level of training, but often will not continue to perform any exercises specific to their previous injury. Especially where potentially-inhibitory influences persist (see earlier 'Inhibition of voluntary muscle activation', p25)—such as effusion, pain, or instability—it is likely that a decline in function will re-occur. Follow-up studies of patients following ACL injury (with or without reconstruction) have found persistent atrophy and strength deficits (Arvidsson et al 1981, Edstrom 1970, Grimby et al 1980). It is not certain from these studies whether the initial rehabilitation program redressed the acute responses to the injury, but then a regression of the gains occurred when rehabilitation ceased. No known studies have assessed patients throughout their initial rehabilitation, and then re-assessed them regularly for a number of years to investigate this possibility.

Some clinical conditions may be particularly prone to regress following the end of formal rehabilitation. For example, such conditions might include those that have been rehabilitated by emphasizing the strengthening of a particular muscle group in an agonist-antagonist pair. That is, rehabilitation has attempted to alter the normal strength ratio of the agonist to the antagonist. For example, this is often attempted for ACL insufficiency, where relative hamstring strength is increased in order to increase dynamic stabilization. It would seem unlikely that such an alteration in reciprocal muscle balance achieved by preferential strengthening of one muscle group—although beneficial—would persist once the rehabilitative exercise is terminated.

VARIABILITY OF PATIENT RESPONSE AND PROGRESS

Surgeons, physicians, and physiotherapists attribute failure, success, or variable rate of progression following injury to many factors, such as injury severity, surgical procedure and technique, patient access to and compliance with appropriate rehabilitation, and so on. Less often considered is variability in many of the factors mentioned so far in this chapter. For example, variable responses might also be due to:

1. The degree of inhibition of voluntary muscle activation. This might vary due to variable pain sensitivity, mechanoreceptor sensitivity (e.g. sensitivity to effusion volume and pressure), or in-surgery severing of articular mechanoreceptors, pain, or proprioceptive afferents.

2. Variable tourniquet time and responses.
3. Variable muscle protein turnover rates, thus affecting atrophy initiation and recovery.
4. Genetic variability in sensitivity to atrophy, detraining, and retraining adaptations.

FINAL NOTE

While all of the material covered in the preceding discussions is of varying degrees of clinical relevance, not all of it has been derived from clinical research. Some of the material comes from animal studies, some of it comes from studies of healthy humans; even among the coverage of clinical studies, not all are studies of injured athletes. Because of this state of affairs, one hesitates in many cases to draw definitive conclusions for clinical practice. Hopefully this state of affairs will encourage clinical researchers to take the implications of the animal and non-clinical human literature and test their extrapolation to the sports medicine context.

REFERENCES

Allbrook D 1981 Skeletal muscle regeneration. Muscle and Nerve 4:234-245
Allbrook D, Baker W de C, Kirkaldy-Willis W H 1966 Muscle regeneration in experimental animals and in man. The cycle of tissue changes that follows trauma in the injured limb syndrome. Journal of Bone and Joint Surgery 48-B(1):153-169
Allen G D 1989 Physiological and metabolic changes with six weeks detraining. Australian Journal of Science and Medicine in Sport 21(1):4-9
Almekinders L C, Gilbert J A 1986 Healing of experimental muscle strains and the effects of nonsteroidal antiinflammatory medication. American Journal of Sports Medicine 14(4):303-308
Appell H-J 1986a Skeletal muscle atrophy during immobilization. International Journal of Sports Medicine 7:1-5
Appell H-J 1986b Morphology of immobilized skeletal muscle and the effects of a pre- and postimmobilization training program. International Journal of Sports Medicine 7:6-12
Appell H-J 1990 Muscular atrophy following immobilization. A review. Sports Medicine 10(1):42-58
Armstrong R B, Warren G L, Warren J A 1991 Mechanisms of exercise-induced muscle fibre injury. Sports Medicine 12(3):184-207
Arvidsson I 1987 Rehabilitation of athlete's knee. A methodological approach. In: Marconnet P, Komi P V (eds) Muscular function in exercise and training. Karger, Basel, p 238-246
Arvidsson I, Eriksson E 1988 Counteracting muscle atrophy after ACL injury: scientific bases for a rehabilitation program. In: Feagin J A (ed) The crucial ligaments. Churchill Livingstone, New York, ch 25, p 451-459
Arvidsson I, Eriksson E, Haggmark T, Johnson R J 1981 Isokinetic muscle strength after ligament reconstruction in the knee joint: results from a 5-10 year follow-up after reconstruction of the anterior cruciate ligament in the knee joint. International Journal of Sports Medicine 2(1):7-11
Arvidsson I, Eriksson E, Pitman M I 1984 Neuromuscular basis of rehabilitation: muscle physiology and special techniques of evaluation. In: Hunter L Y, Funk F J (eds) Rehabilitation of the injured knee. C V Mosby, St Louis, p 210-234
Arvidsson I, Eriksson E, Knutsson E, Arner S 1986 Reduction of pain inhibition on voluntary muscle activation by epidural analgesia. Orthopedics 9(10):1415-1419

Baker J H, Matsumoto D E 1988 Adaptation of skeletal muscle to immobilization in a shortened position. Muscle and Nerve 11:231-244
Baugher W H, Warren R F, Marshall J L, Joseph A 1984 Quadriceps atrophy in the anterior cruciate insufficient knee. American Journal of Sports Medicine 12(3):192-195
Baxendale R H, Ferrell W R, Wood L 1985 Knee-joint distension and quadriceps maximal voluntary contraction in man. Journal of Physiology 367:100P
Berg H E, Dudley G A, Haggmark T, Ohlsen H, Tesch P A 1991 Effects of lower limb unloading on skeletal muscle mass and function in humans. Journal of Applied Physiology 70(4): 1882-1885
Berger R A 1965 Comparison of the effect of various weight training loads on strength. Research Quarterly 36(2):141-146
Booth F W 1977 Time course of muscular atrophy during immobilization of hindlimbs in rats. Journal of Applied Physiology 43:656-661
Booth F W 1987 Physiologic and biochemical effects of immobilization on muscle. Clinical Orthopaedics and Related Research 219:15-20
Booth F W, Gollnick P D 1983 Effects of disuse on the structure and function of skeletal muscle. Medicine and Science in Sports and Exercise 15(5):415-420
Booth F W, Nicholson W F, Watson P A 1982 Influence of muscle use on protein synthesis and degradation. In: Terjung R L (ed) Exercise and sport sciences reviews, vol 10. Franklin Institute Press, Philadelphia, p 27-48
Booth F W, Seider M J 1979 Recovery of skeletal muscle after 3 months of hindlimb immobilization in rats. Journal of Applied Physiology 47:435-439
Bouchard C, Boulay M R, Simoneau J-A, Lortie G, Perusse L 1988 Heredity and trainability of aerobic and anaerobic performances. An update. Sports Medicine 5:69-73
Bouchard C, Dionne F T, Simoneau J-A, Boulay M R 1992 Genetics of aerobic and anaerobic performances. In: Holloszy J O (ed) Exercise and sport sciences reviews, vol 20. Williams & Wilkins, Baltimore, p 27-58
Caplan A, Carlson B, Faulkner J, Fischman D, Garrett W 1988 Skeletal muscle. In: Woo S L-Y, Buckwalter J A (eds) Injury and repair of musculoskeletal soft tissues. American Academy of Orthopaedic Surgeons, Park Ridge, Illinois, ch 6, p 213-291
Carlson B M, Faulkner J A 1983 The regeneration of skeletal muscle fibers following injury: a review. Medicine and Science in Sports and Exercise 15(3):187-198

Chvapil M, Koopmann C F 1984 Scar formation: Physiology and pathological states. Otolaryngologic Clinics of North America 17(2):265-272

Clausen J P, Klausen K, Rasmussen B, Trap-Jensen J 1973 Central and peripheral circulatory changes after training of the arm and legs. American Journal of Physiology 225(3):675-682

Cleak M J, Eston R G 1992 Delayed onset muscle soreness: mechanisms and management. Journal of Sports Sciences 10:325-341

Corrigan A B 1965 The immediate treatment of muscle injuries in sportsmen: a trial involving direct contusion injuries. Medical Journal of Australia I(25):926-928

Costill D L, Fink W J, Hargreaves M, King D S, Thomas R, Fielding R 1985a Metabolic characteristics of skeletal muscle during detraining from competitive swimming. Medicine and Science in Sports and Exercise 17(3):339-343

Costill D L, King D S, Thomas R, Hargreaves M 1985b Effects of reduced training on muscular power in swimmers. Physician and Sports Medicine 13(2):94-101

Coyle E F 1988 Detraining and retention of training-induced adaptations. In: Blair S N, Painter P, Pate R R, Smith L K, Taylor C B (eds) Resource manual for Guidelines for exercise testing and prescription. Lea & Febiger, Philadelphia, ch 12, p 83-89

Coyle E F, Martin W H, Sinacore D R, Joyner M J, Hagberg J M, Holloszy J O 1984 Time course of loss of adaptations after stopping prolonged intense endurance training. Journal of Applied Physiology 57(6):1857-1864

Coyle E F, Martin W H, Bloomfield S A, Lowry O H, Holloszy J O 1985 Effects of detraining on responses to submaximal exercise. Journal of Applied Physiology 59(3):853-859

Coyle E F, Hemmert M K, Coggan A R 1986 Effects of detraining on cardiovascular responses to exercise: role of blood volume. Journal of Applied Physiology 60(1):95-99

Croce P, Gregg J R 1991 Keeping fit when injured. Clinics in Sports Medicine 10(1):181-195

Cullinane E M, Sady S P, Vadeboncoeur L, Burke M, Thompson P D 1986 Cardiac size and VO$_2$ max do not decrease after short term exercise cessation. Medicine and Science in Sports and Exercise 18(4):420-424

Cureton K J, Collins M A, Hill D W, McElhannon F M 1988 Muscle hypertrophy in men and women. Medicine and Science in Sports and Exercise 20(4):338-344

Dahlback L O 1970 Effects of temporary tourniquet ischemia on striated muscle fibers and motor end-plates. Morphological and histochemical studies in the rabbit and electromyographical studies in man. Scandinavian Journal of Plastic and Reconstructive Surgery (suppl 7):1-91

Damholt V, Zdravkovic D 1972 Quadriceps function following fractures of the femoral shaft. Acta Orthopaedica Scandinavica 43:148-156

Danckwardt-Lilliestrom G, Sjogren S 1976 Postoperative restoration of muscle strength after intramedullary nailing of fractures of the femoral shaft. Acta Orthopaedica Scandinavica 47:101-107

de Andrade J R, Grant C, Dixon A St J 1965 Joint distension and reflex muscle inhibition in the knee. Journal of Bone and Joint Surgery 47-A:313-322

Dobner J J, Nitz A J 1982 Postmeniscectomy tourniquet palsy and functional sequelae. American Journal of Sports Medicine 10(4):211-214

Dornan P 1990 The significance of scar tissue in rehabilitation of the athlete. Sport Health 8(4):17-19

Dudley G A, Duvoisin M R, Convertino V A, Buchanan P 1989 Alterations in the in vivo torque-velocity relationship of human skeletal muscle following 30 days exposure to simulated microgravity. Aviation, Space, and Environmental Medicine 60:659-663

Dudley G A, Tesch P A, Miller M A, Buchanan P 1991 Importance of eccentric actions in performance adaptations to resistance training. Aviation, Space, and Environmental Medicine 62:543-550

Duvoisin M R, Convertino V A, Buchanan P, Gollnick P D, Dudley G A 1989 Characteristics and preliminary observations of the influence of electromyostimulation on the size and function of human skeletal muscle during 30 days of simulated microgravity. Aviation, Space, and Environmental Medicine 60:671-678

Ebbeling C B, Clarkson P M 1989 Exercise-induced muscle damage and adaptation. Sports Medicine 7:207-234

Edstrom L 1970 Selective atrophy of red muscle fibres in the quadriceps in long-standing knee-joint dysfunction. Injuries to the anterior cruciate ligament. Journal of the Neurological Sciences 11:551-559

Edwards H, Rose E A, King T C 1982 Postoperative deterioration in muscular function. Archives of Surgery 117:899-901

Ehsani A A, Hagberg J M, Hickson R C 1978 Rapid changes in left vetricular dimensions and mass in response to physical conditioning and deconditioning. American Journal of Cardiology 42:52-56

Elmqvist L-G, Lorentzon R, Langstrom M, Fugl-Meyer A R 1988 Reconstruction of the anterior cruciate ligament. Long term effects of different knee angles at primary immobilization and different modes of early training. American Journal of Sports Medicine 16(5):455-462

Enoka R M 1988 Muscle strength and its development: New perspectives. Sports Medicine 6:146-168

Eriksson E 1981 Rehabilitation of muscle function after sport injury—major problem in sports medicine. International Journal of Sports Medicine 2(1):1-6

Eriksson E, Arvidsson I 1986 Rehabilitation after knee surgery. In: XXIII FIMS World Congress of Sports Medicine Abstracts. Brisbane, p 57-57a

Evans P 1980 The healing process at cellular level. A review. Physiotherapy 66(8):256-259

Evans W J, Cannon J G 1991 The metabolic effects of exercise-induced muscle damage. In: Holloszy J O (ed) Exercise and sport sciences reviews, vol 19. Williams & Wilkins, Baltimore, p 99-125

Eyring E J, Murray W R 1964 The effect of joint position on the pressure of intra-articular effusion. Journal of Bone and Joint Surgery 46-A:1235-1241

Fahrer H, Rentsch H U, Gerber N J, Beyeler Ch, Hess Ch W, Grunig B 1988 Knee effusion and reflex inhibition of the quadriceps. A bar to effective retraining. Journal of Bone and Joint Surgery 70-B(4):635-638

Forrest L 1983 Current concepts in soft connective tissue wound healing. British Journal of Surgery 70:133-140

Fournier M, Ricci J, Taylor A W, Ferguson R J, Montpetit R R, Chaitman B R 1982 Skeletal muscle adaptation in adolescent boys: sprint and endurance training and detraining. Medicine and Science in Sports and Exercise 14(6):453-456

Frank C, Akeson W H, Woo S L-Y, Amiel D, Coutts R D 1984 Physiology and therapeutic value of passive joint motion. Clinical Orthopaedics and Related Research 185:113-125

Franklin B A 1989 Aerobic exercise training programs for the upper body. Medicine and Science in Sports 21(suppl 5):S141-S148

Gardner V O, Caiozzo V J, Long S T, Stoffel J, McMaster W C, Prietto C A 1984 Contractile properties of slow and fast muscle following tourniquet ischemia. American Journal of Sports Medicine 12(6):417-423

Garrett W E 1990 Muscle strain injuries: clinical and basic aspects. Medicine and Science in Sports and Exercise 22(4):436-443

Garrett W E, Duncan P W 1988 Muscle injury and rehabilitation. Sports Injury Management 1(3):1-76

Garrett W E, Tidball J 1988 Myotendinous junction: structure, function, and failure. In: Woo S L-Y, Buckwalter J A (eds) Injury and repair of musculoskeletal soft tissues. American Academy of Orthopaedic Surgeons, Park Ridge, Illinois, ch 5, p 171-207

Garrett W E, Seaber A V, Boswick J, Urbaniak J R, Goldner J L 1984 Recovery and repair of skeletal muscle after laceration and repair. Journal of Hand Surgery 9A(5):683-692

Garrett W E, Safran M R, Seaber A V, Glisson R R, Ribbeck B M 1987 Biomechanical comparison of stimulated and nonstimulated skeletal muscle pulled to failure. American Journal of Sports Medicine 15(5):448-454

Garrett W E, Nikolaou P K, Ribbeck B M, Glisson R R, Seaber A V 1988 The effect of muscle architecture on the biomechanical failure properties of skeletal muscle under passive extension. American Journal of Sports Medicine 16(1):7-12

Garrett W, Bradley W, Byrd S, Edgerton V R, Gollnick P 1989a Muscle. Part B. Basic science perspectives. In: Frymoyer J W, Gordon S L (eds) New perspectives on low back pain. American Academy of Orthopaedic Surgeons, Park Ridge, Illinois, p 335-379

Garrett W E, Rich F R, Nikolaou P K, Vogler J B 1989b Computed tomography of hamstring muscle strains. Medicine and Science in Sports and Exercise 21(5):506-514

Gatti C J, Young R J, Glad H L 1979 Effect of water-training in the maintenance of cardiorespiratory endurance of athletes. British Journal of Sports Medicine 13:161-164

Gay A J, Hunt T E 1954 Reuniting of skeletal muscle fibres after transection. Anatomical Record 120:853-871

George J F 1963 Medical aspects of football. Medical Journal of Australia I:870-871

Gerber C, Hoppeler H, Claassen H, Robotti G, Zehnder R, Jakob R 1985 The lower-extremity musculature in chronic symptomatic instability of the anterior cruciate ligament. Journal of Bone and Joint Surgery 67-A(7):1034-1043

Gibson J N A, Halliday D, Morrison W L, Stoward P J, Hornsby G A, Watt P W, Murdoch G, Rennie M J 1987 Decrease in human quadriceps muscle protein turnover consequent upon leg immobilization. Clinical Science 72:503-509

Gibson J N A, Morrison W L, Scrimgeour C M, Smith K, Stoward P J, Rennie M J 1989 Effects of therapeutic percutaneous electrical stimulation of atrophic human quadriceps on muscle composition, protein synthesis and contractile properties. European Journal of Clinical Investigation 19:206-212

Glick J M 1980 Muscle strains: prevention and treatment. Physician and Sports Medicine 8(11):73-77

Gogia P P, Schneider V S, Le Blanc A D, Krebs J, Kasson C, Pientok C 1988 Bed rest effect on extremity muscle torque in healthy men. Archives of Physical Medicine and Rehabilitation 69:1030-1032

Goldspink D F, Goldspink G 1986 The role of passive stretch in retarding muscle atrophy. In: Nix W A, Vrbova G (eds) Electrical stimulation and neuromuscular disorders. Springer-Verlag, Berlin, p 91-100

Goldspink G 1983 Alterations in myofibril size and structure during growth, exercise, and changes in environmental temperature. In: Peachey L D (ed) Handbook of physiology. Section 10: Skeletal muscle. American Physiological Society, Bethesda, Maryland, p 539-554

Gossman M R, Sahrmann S A, Rose S J 1982 Review of length-associated changes in muscle. Experimental evidence and clinical implications. Physical Therapy 62(12):1799-1808

Gould N, Donnermeyer D, Gammon G G, Pope M, Ashikaga T 1983 Transcutaneous muscle stimulation to retard disuse atrophy after open meniscectomy. Clinical Orthopaedics and Related Research 178:190-197

Green H J, Thomson J A, Daub B D, Ranney D A 1980 Biochemical and histochemical alterations in skeletal muscle in man during a period of reduced activity. Canadian Journal of Physiology and Pharmacology 58:1311-1316

Greenleaf J E, Kozlowski S 1982 Physiological consequences of reduced physical activity during bed rest. In: Terjung R L (ed) Exercise and sport sciences reviews, vol 10. Franklin Institute, Philadelphia, p 84-119

Grimby G, Gustafsson E, Peterson L, Renstrom P 1980 Quadriceps function and training after knee ligament surgery. Medicine and Science in Sports and Exercise 12(1):70-75

Gydikov A A 1976 Pattern of discharge of different types of alpha motoneurones and motor units during voluntary and reflex activities under normal physiological conditions. In: Komi P V (ed) Biomechanics V-A. University Park Press, Baltimore, p 45-57

Haggmark T, Eriksson E 1979a Cylinder or mobile cast brace after knee ligament surgery. A clinical analysis and morphologic and enzymatic studies of changes in the quadriceps muscle. American Journal of Sports Medicine 7(1):48-56

Haggmark T, Eriksson E 1979b Hypotrophy of the soleus muscle in man after Achilles tendon rupture. Discussion of findings obtained by computed tomography and morphologic studies. American Journal of Sports Medicine 7(2):121-126

Haggmark T, Jansson E, Eriksson E 1981 Fibre type area and metabolic potential of the thigh muscle in man after knee surgery and immobilization. International Journal of Sports Medicine 2(1):12-17

Haggmark T, Eriksson E, Jansson E 1986 Muscle fibre type changes in human skeletal muscle after injuries and immobilization. Orthopedics 9(2):181-185

Hakkinen K, Komi P V 1983 Electromyographic changes during strength training and detraining. Medicine and Science in Sports and Exercise 15(6):455-460

Hakkinen K, Komi P V 1985a Changes in electrical and mechanical behavior of leg extensor muscles during heavy resistance strength training. Scandinavian Journal of Sports Science 7(2):55-64

Hakkinen K, Komi P V 1985b Effect of explosive type strength training on electromyographic and force production characteristics of leg extensor muscles during concentric and various stretch-shortening cycle exercises. Scandinavian Journal of Sports Science 7(2):65-76.

Hakkinen K, Alen M, Komi P V 1985 Changes in isometric force- and relaxation-time, electromyographic and muscle fibre characteristics of human skeletal muscle during strength training and detraining. Acta Physiologica Scandinavica 125:573-585

Hakkinen K, Komi P V, Tesch P A 1981 Effect of combined concentric and eccentric strength training and detraining on force-time, muscle fibre and metabolic characteristics of leg extensor muscles. Scandinavian Journal of Sports Science 3(2):50-58

Halkjaer-Kristensen J, Ingemann-Hansen T 1985a Wasting of human quadriceps muscle after knee ligament injuries. I Anthropometrical consequences. Scandinavian Journal of Rehabilitation Medicine (Suppl 13):5-11

Halkjaer-Kristensen J, Ingemann-Hansen T 1985b Wasting of human quadriceps muscle after knee ligament injuries. II Muscle fibre morphology. Scandinavian Journal of Rehabilitation Medicine (Suppl 13):12-20

Halkjaer-Kristensen J, Ingemann-Hansen T 1985c Wasting of human quadriceps muscle after knee ligament injuries. III Oxidative and glycolytic enzyme activities. Scandinavian Journal of Rehabilitation Medicine (Suppl 13):21-28

Halkjaer-Kristensen J, Ingemann-Hansen T 1985d Wasting of human quadriceps muscle after knee ligament injuries. IV Dynamic and static muscle function. Scandinavian Journal of Rehabilitation Medicine (Suppl 13):29-37

Hardman A E, Williams C, Boobis L H 1987 Influence of single-leg training on muscle metabolism and endurance during exercise with the trained limb and the untrained limb. Journal of Sports Sciences 5:105-116

Hargens A R, Tipton C M, Gollnick P D, Mubarek S J, Tucker B J, Akeson W H 1983 Fluid shifts and muscle function in humans during acute simulated weightlessness. Journal of Applied Physiology 54(4):1003-1009

Hather B M, Tesch P A, Buchanan P, Dudley G A 1991 Influence of eccentric actions on skeletal muscle adaptations to resistance training. Acta Physiologica Scandinavica 143:177-185

Hather B M, Adams G R, Tesch P A, Dudley G A 1992 Skeletal muscle responses to lower limb suspension in humans. Journal of Applied Physiology 72(4):1493-1498

Hickson R C, Foster C, Pollock M L, Galassi T M, Rich S 1985 Reduced training intensities and loss of aerobic power, endurance, and cardiac growth. Journal of Applied Physiology 58(2):492-499

Hnik P, Vejsada R, Goldspink D F, Kasicki S, Krekule I 1985 Quantitative evaluation of electromyogram activity in rat extensor and flexor muscles immobilized at different lengths. Experimental Neurology 88:515-528

Houmard J A 1991 Impact of reduced training on performance in endurance athletes. Sports Medicine 12(6):380-393

Houston M E, Bentzen H, Larsen H 1979 Interrelationships between skeletal muscle adaptations and performance as studied by detraining and retraining. Acta Physiologica Scandinavica 105:163-170

Houston M E, Froese E A, Valeriote St P, Green H J, Ranney D A 1983 Muscle performance, morphology amd metabolic capacity during strength training and detraining: a one leg model. European Journal of Applied Physiology 51:25-35

Hurme T, Kalimo H, Lehto M, Jarvinen M 1991a Healing of skeletal muscle injury: an ultrastructural and immunohistochemical study. Medicine and Science in Sports and Exercise 23(7):801-810

Hurme T, Lehto M, Falck B, Tainio H, Kalimo H 1991b Electromyography and morphology during regeneration of muscle injury in rats. Acta Physiologica Scandinavica 142:443-456

Ingemann-Hansen T, Halkjaer-Kristensen J 1977 Lean and fat component of the human thigh. The effects of immobilization in plaster and subsequent physical training. Scandinavian Journal of Rehabilitation Medicine 9:67-72

Ingemann-Hansen T, Halkjaer-Kristensen J 1980 Computerized tomographic determination of human thigh components. The effects of immobilization in plaster and subsequent physical training. Scandinavian Journal of Rehabilitation Medicine 12:27-31

Ingemann-Hansen T, Halkjaer-Kristensen J 1983 Progressive resistance exercise training of the hypotrophic quadriceps muscle in man. Scandinavian Journal of Rehabilitation Medicine 15:29-35

Ishida K, Moritani T, Itoh K 1990 Changes in voluntary and electrically induced contractions during strength training and detraining. European Journal of Applied Physiology 60:244-248

Jansson E, Sylven C, Arvidsson I, Eriksson E 1988 Increase in myoglobin content and decrease in oxydative enzyme activities by leg muscle immobilization in man. Acta Physiology Scandinavica 132:515-517

Jarvinen M 1975 Healing of a crush injury. 2. A histological study of the effect of early mobilization and immobilization on the repair process. Acta Pathologica Microbiologica Scandinavica (Sect A) 83:269-282

Jarvinen M 1976a Healing of a crush injury in rat striated muscle. 3. A micro-angiographical study of the effect of early mobilization and immobilization on capillary ingrowth. Acta Pathologica Microbiologica Scandinavica (Sect A) 84:85-94

Jarvinen M 1976b Healing of a crush injury in rat striated muscle. 4. Effect of early mobilization and immobilization on the tensile properties of gastrocnemius muscle. Acta Chirugica Scandinavica 142:47-56

Jarvinen M, Aho A J, Toivonen H 1983 Age dependent repair of muscle rupture. A histological and microangiographical study in rats. Acta Orthopaedica Scandinavica 54:64-74

Jarvinen M, Sorvari T 1978 A histochemical study of the effect of immobilization on the metabolism of healing muscle injury. In: Landry F, Orban W A R (eds) Sports medicine. Symposia Specialists, Miami, p 177-181

Josza L, Balint J B, Demel S 1978 Histochemical and ultrastructural study of human muscles after spontaneous rupture of the tendon. Acta Histochemica Budapest 63 S:61-73

Kakulas B A 1982 Muscle trauma. In: Mastaglia F L, Walton J (eds) Skeletal muscle pathology. Churchill Livingstone, Edinburgh, ch 21, p 592-604

Kannus P, Alosa D, Cook L, Johnson R J, Renstrom P, Pope M, Beynnon B, Yasuda K, Nichols C, Kaplan M 1992 Effect of one-legged exercise on the strength, power and endurance of the contralateral leg. A randomized, controlled study using isometric and concentric isokinetic training. European Journal of Applied Physiology 64:117-126

Kanstrup I-L, Marving J, Hoilund-Carlsen P F, Saltin B 1991 Left ventricular response upon exercise with the trained and detrained leg muscles. Scandinavian Journal of Medicine and Science in Sports 1:112-118

Karpakka J, Vaananen K, Orava S, Takala T E S 1990 The effects of preimmobilization training and immobilization on collagen synthesis in rat skeletal muscle. International Journal of Sports Medicine 11(6):484-488

Karumo I, Rehunen S, Naveri H, Alho A 1977 Red and white muscle fibres in meniscectomy patients. Effects of postoperative physiotherapy. Annales Chirurgiae et Gynaecologiae 66:164-169

Koutedakis Y, Budgett R, Faulman L 1990 Rest in underperforming elite competitors. British Journal of Sports Medicine 24(4):248-252

Krebs D E 1989 Isokinetic, electrophysiologic, and clinical function relationships following tourniquet-aided knee arthrotomy. Physical Therapy 69(10):803-815

Kvist M, Jarvinen M 1982 Clinical, histochemical and biomechanical features in repair of muscle and tendon injuries. International Journal of Sports Medicine 3 (suppl 1):12-14

Kvist H, Jarvinen M, Sorvari T 1974 Effect of immobilization on the healing of contusion injury in muscle. A preliminary report of a histological study in rats. Scandinavian Journal of Rehabilitation Medicine 6:134-140

Le Blanc A, Gogia P, Schneider V, Krebs J, Schonfeld E, Evans H 1988 Calf muscle area and strength changes after five weeks of horizontal bed rest. American Journal of Sports Medicine 16(6):624-629

Lehto M, Sims T J, Bailey A J 1985a Skeletal muscle injury—molecular changes in the collagen during healing. Research in Experimental Medicine 185:95-106

Lehto M, Duance V C, Restall D 1985b Collagen and fibronectin in a healing skeletal muscle injury. An immunohistological study of the effects of physical activity on the repair of injured gastrocnemius muscle in the rat. Journal of Bone and Joint Surgery 67-B(5):820-828

Lieber R L, Friden J O, Hargens A R, Danzig L A, Gershuni D H 1988 Differential response of the dog quadriceps muscle to external fixation of the knee. Muscle and Nerve 11:193-201

Lindboe C F, Platou C S 1982 Disuse atrophy of human skeletal muscle. An enzyme histochemical study. Acta Neuropathologica 56:241-244

Lindboe C F, Platou C S 1984 Effect of immobilization of short duration on muscle fibre size. Clinical Physiology 4:183-188

Lo Presti C, Kirkendall D T, Street G M, Dudley A W 1988 Quadriceps insufficency following repair of the anterior cruciate ligament. Journal of Orthopaedic and Sports Physical Therapy 9(7):245-249

Lysholm J 1987 The relation between pain and torque in an isokinetic strength test of knee extension. Arthroscopy 3(3):182-184

McConnell G K, Costill D L, Widrick J J, Hickey M S, Tanaka H, Gastin P B 1992 Reduced training volume and intensity maintain VO$_2$ max but not performance in distance runners. International Journal of Sports Medicine

MacDougall J D 1986a Morphological changes in human skeletal muscle following strength training and immobilization. In: Jones N L, McCartney N, McComas A J (eds) Human muscle power. Human Kinetics, Champaign, Illinois, p 269-288

MacDougall J D 1986b Discussion from the session. Halkjaer-Kristensen U, Ingemann-Hansen T Wasting and growth of skeletal muscle. In: Saltin B (ed) Biochemistry of exercise VI. Human Kinetics, Champaign, Illinois, p 563-566

MacDougall J D, Ward G R, Sale D G, Sutton J R 1977 Biochemical adaptation of human skeletal muscle to heavy resistance training and immobilization. Journal of Applied Physiology 43(4):700-703

MacDougall J D, Elder G C B, Sale D G, Moroz J R, Sutton J R 1980 Effects of strength training and immobilization on human muscle fibres. European Journal of Applied Physiology 43(1):25-34

Maw G 1991 The role of arm ergometry during lower body injury. In: Abstracts of the Annual Scientific Conference of the Australian Sports Medicine Federation. Australian Sports Medicine Federation, Canberra

Maxwell A 1980 Muscle power after surgery. Lancet i:420-421

Maxwell L C, Enwemeka C S 1992 Immobilization-induced muscle atrophy is not reversed by lengthening the muscle. Anatomical Record 234:55-61

Millar A P 1975 An early stretching routine in hamstring strains. Australian Journal of Sports Medicine 7(5):107-109

Moore D H, Ruska H, Copenhaver W M 1956 Electron microscopic and histochemical observations of muscle degeneration after tourniquet. Journal of Biophysics and Biochemical Cytology 2(6):755-763

Moritani T, de Vries H A 1979 Neural factors versus hypertrophy in the time course of muscle strength gain. American Journal of Physical Medicine 58:115-130

Moroz D E, Houston M E 1987 The effects of replacing endurance running training with cycling in female runners. Canadian Journal of Sports Science 12:131-135

Morrissey M C, Brewster C E 1986 Hamstring muscle weakness after surgery for anterior cruciate injury. Journal of Orthopaedic and Sports Physical Therapy 7(6):310-313

Neufer P D 1989 The effect of detraining and reduced training on the physiological adaptations to aerobic exercise training. Sports Medicine 8(5):302-321

Nikolaou P K, MacDonald B L, Glisson R R, Seaber A V, Garrett W E 1987 Biomechanical and histological evaluation of muscle after controlled strain injury. American Journal of Sports Medicine 15(1):9-14

Nitz A J, Dobner J J 1987 High intensity electrical stimulation effect on thigh musculature during immobilization for knee sprain. A case report. Physical Therapy 67(2):219-222

Oakes B W 1981 Acute soft tissue injuries. Nature and management. Australian Family Physician 10(7, suppl):3-16.

Oakes B W 1992 The classification of injuries and mechanisms of injury, repair and healing. In: Bloomfield J, Fricker P A, Fitch K D (eds) Textbook of science and medicine in sport. Blackwell Scientific, Melbourne, p 200-217

Ochoa J, Fowler T J, Gilliatt R W 1972 Anatomical changes in peripheral nerves compressed by a pneumatic tourniquet. Journal of Anatomy 113(3):433-455

O'Donoghue P C, McCarthy M R, Gieck J H, Yates C K 1991 Clinical use of continuous passive motion in athletic training. Athletic Training 26:200-208

Pate R R, Hughes R D, Chandler J V, Ratliffe J L 1978 Effects of arm training on retention of training effects derived from leg training. Medicine and Science in Sports and Exercise 10:71-74

Patel A N, Razzak Z A, Dastur D K 1969 Disuse atrophy of human skeletal muscles. Archives of Neurology 20:413-421

Patterson S, Klenerman L 1979 The effect of pneumatic tourniquets on the ultrastructure of skeletal muscle. Journal of Bone and Joint Surgery 61-B(2):178-183

Patterson S, Klenerman L, Biswas M, Rhodes A 1981 The effect of pneumatic tourniquets on skeletal muscle physiology. Acta Orthopaedica Scandinavica 52:171-175

Pedowitz R A, Friden J, Thornell L-E 1992 Skeletal muscle injury induced by a pneumatic tourniquet: An enzyme- and immunohistochemical study in rabbits. Journal of Surgical Research 52:243-250

Prentice W E, Bell G W 1990 Pathophysiology of musculoskeletal injuries and the healing process. In: Prentice W E (ed) Rehabilitation techniques in sports medicine. Times Mirror / Mosby, St Louis

Raymond 1890 Recherches experimentales sur la pathogenie des atrophies musculaires consecutives aux arthrites traumatiques. Revue de Medicine 10:374-392

Reid D C 1992 Muscle injury: classification and healing. In: Reid D C Sports injury assessment and rehabilitation. Churchill Livingstone, New York, p 85-101

Renstrom P 1988 Muscle injuries. In: Dirix A, Knuttgen H G, Tittel K (eds) Olympic book of sports medicine. Blackwell Scientific, Oxford, p 413-427

Rose S J, Rothstein J M 1982 Muscle mutability. Part 1. General concepts and adaptations to altered patterns of use. Physical Therapy 62(12):1773-1787

Rosemeyer B, Sturz H 1977 Musculus quadriceps femoris bei immobilization und remobilisation. Z Orthop 115:182

Rowell L B, O'Leary D S 1990 Reflex control of the circulation during exercise: chemoreflexes and mechanoreflexes. Journal of Applied Physiology 69(2):407-418

Rutherford O M, Jones D A, Round J M 1990 Long-lasting unilateral muscle wasting and weakness following injury and immobilization. Scandinavian Journal of Rehabilitation Medicine 22:33-37

Safran M R, Garrett W E, Seaber A V, Glisson R R, Ribbeck B M 1988 The role of warmup in muscular injury prevention. American Journal of Sports Medicine 16(2):123-129

St Pierre D, Gardiner P F 1987 The effect of immobilization and exercise on muscle function: a review. Physiotherapy Canada 39(1):24-36

Sale D G, McComas A J, MacDougall J D, Upton A R M 1982 Neuromuscular adaptation in human thenar muscles following strength training and immobilization. Journal of Applied Physiology 53(2):419-424

Saltin B 1987 Discussion following: Savard G, Kiens B, Saltin B Central cardiovascular factors as limits to endurance; with a note on the distinction between maximal oxygen uptake and endurance fitness. In: MacLeod D, Maughan R, Nimmo M, Reilly T, Williams C (eds) Exercise. Benefits, limits and adaptations. Spon, London, p 162-180

Saltin B, Gollnick P D 1983 Skeletal muscle adaptability: significance for metabolism and performance. In: Peachey L D (ed) Handbook of physiology. Section 10: Skeletal muscle. American Physiological Society, Bethesda, Maryland, p 555-631

Saltin B, Nazar K, Costill D L, Stein E, Jansson E, Essen B, Gollnick P D 1976 The nature of the training response; peripheral and central adaptations to one-legged exercise. Acta Physiologica Scandinavica 96:289-305

Sandberg R, Nilsson B, Westlin N 1987 Hinged cast after knee ligament surgery. American Journal of Sports Medicine 15(3):270-274

Sandler H, Vernikos J (eds) 1986 Inactivity: physiological effects. Academic Press, Orlando, Florida

Sargeant A J, Davies C T M, Edwards R H T, Maunder C, Young A 1977 Functional and structural changes after disuse of human muscle. Clinical Science and Molecular Medicine 52:337-342

Saunders K C, Louis D L, Weingarten S I, Waylonis G W 1979 Effect of tourniquet time on postoperative quadriceps function. Clinical Orthopaedics and Related Research 143:194-199

Shakespeare D T, Stokes M, Sherman K P, Young A 1983 The effect of knee flexion on quadriceps inhibition after meniscectomy. Clinical Science 65:64-65P

Shakespeare D T, Stokes M, Sherman K P, Young A 1985 Reflex inhibition of the quadriceps after meniscectomy: lack of association with pain. Clinical Physiology 5:137-144

Sherman W M, Pearson D R, Plyley M J, Costill D L, Habansky A J, Vogelgesang D A 1982 Isokinetic rehabilitation after surgery. A review of factors which are important for developing physiotherapeutic techniques after knee surgery. American Journal of Sports Medicine 10(3):155-161

Simoneau J-A, Lortie G, Boulay M R, Marcotte M, Thibault M-C, Bouchard C 1987 Effects of two high-intensity intermittent training programs interspaced by detraining on human skeletal muscle and performance. European Journal of Applied Physiology 56:516-521

Sjostrom M, Fugl-Meyer A R, Wahlby L 1978 Achilles tendon injury. Plantar flexion strength and structure of the soleus muscle after surgical repair. Acta Chirugica Scandinavica 144:219-226

Solonen K A, Tarkkanen L, Narvanen S 1968 Metabolic changes in the upper limb during tourniquet ischemia. Acta Orthopaedica Scandinavica 39:20-32

Spencer J D, Hayes K C, Alexander I J 1984 Knee joint effusion and quadriceps reflex inhibition in man. Archives of Physical Medicine and Rehabilitation 65:171-177

Stanton P 1988 CPM for muscle injuries. In: Torode M (ed) Proceedings of 25th Australian Sports Medicine Federation Conference. Cumberland College of Health Sciences, Sydney, p 95-102

Staron R S, Hagerman FC, Hikida RS 1981 The effects of detraining on an elite power lifter. A case study. Journal of the Neurological Sciences 51:247-257

Staron R S, Malicky E S, Leonardi M J, Falkel J E, Hagerman F C, Dudley G A 1990 Muscle hypertrophy and fast fibre type conversions in heavy resistance-trained women. European Journal of Applied Physiology 60:71-79

Staron RS, Leonardi MJ, Karapondo DL, Malicky ES, Falkel JE, Hagerman FC, Hikida RS 1991 Strength and skeletal muscle adaptations in heavy resistance-trained women after detraining and retraining. Journal of Applied Physiology 70(2):631-640

Steinberg F U 1980 The immobilized patient. Plenum, New York

Stokes M, Mills K, Shakespeare D, Sherman K, Whittle M, Young A 1985 'Post-meniscectomy inhibition': voluntary ischaemia does not alter quadriceps function in normal subjects. In: Whittle M, Harris D (eds) Biomechanical measurement in orthopaedic practice. Clarendon Press, Oxford, p 188-193

Stokes M, Young A 1984 The contribution of reflex inhibition to arthrogenous muscle weakness. Clinical Science 67:7-14

Stratford P 1981 Electromyography of the quadriceps femoris muscles in subjects with normal knees and acutely effused knees. Physical Therapy 62:279-283

Strock P E, Majno G 1969a Vascular responses to experimental tourniquet ischemia. Surgery, Gynecology and Obstetrics 129:309-318

Strock P E, Majno G 1969b Microvascular changes in acutely ischemic rat muscle. Surgery, Gynecology and Obstetrics 129:1213-1224

Tabary J C, Tabary C, Tardieu C, Tardieu G, Goldspink G 1972 Physiological and structural changes in the cat's soleus muscle due to immobilization at different lengths. Journal of Physiology 224:231-244

Tesch P A, Komi P V, Hakkinen K 1987 Enzymatic adaptations consequent to long term strength training. International Journal of Sports Medicine 8(Suppl 1):66-69

Thomsen P, Luco J V 1944 Changes in weight and neuromuscular transmission of muscles of immobilized joints. Journal of Neurophysiology 7:245-251

Thorblad J, Ekstrand J, Hamberg P, Gillquist J 1985 Muscle rehabilitation after arthroscopic meniscectomy with or without tourniquet control. A preliminary randomized study. American Journal of Sports Medicine 13(2):133-135

Tidball J G 1991 Myotendinous junction injury in relation to junction structure and molecular composition. In: Holloszy J O (ed) Exercise and sport sciences reviews, vol 19. Williams and Wilkins, Baltimore, p 419-445

van der Meulen J C H 1982 Present state of knowledge on processes of healing in collagen structures. International Journal of Sports Medicine 3 (suppl. 1):4-8

van Helder W 1991 Spinal anaesthesia and its common side effects. Canadian Journal of Sport Sciences 16(3):167

Vegso J J, Genuario S E, Torg J S 1985 Maintenance of hamstring strength following knee surgery. Medicine and Science in Sports and Exercise 17(3):376-379

Vracko R 1974 Basal lamina scaffold—anatomy and significance for maintenance of orderly tissue structure. American Journal of Pathology 77(2):314-335

Waldeyer W 1865 Ueber die Veranderungen der quergestreiften Muskeln bei der Entzundung und dem Typhusprozess, sowie uber die Regeneration derselben nach Substanz-defekten. Arch Path Anat Physiol Klin Med 34:473-514

White M J, Davies C T M, Brooksby P 1984 The effects of short term voluntary immobilization on the contractile properties of the human triceps surae. Quarterly Journal of Experimental Physiology 69:685-691

Wickiewicz T L, Roy R R, Powell P L, Edgerton V R 1983 Muscle architecture of the human lower limb. Clinical Orthopaedics and Related Research 179:275-283

Wigerstad-Lossing I, Grimby G, Jonsson T, Morelli B, Peterson L, Renstrom P 1988 Effects of electrical muscle stimulation combined with voluntary contractions after knee ligament surgery. Medicine and Science in Sports and Exercise 20(1):93-98

Williams P E 1988 Effect of intermittent stretch on immobilised muscle. Annals of the Rheumatic Diseases 47:1014-1016

Williams P E, Catanese T, Lucey E G, Goldspink G 1988 The importance of stretch and contractile activity in the prevention of connective tissue accumulation in muscle. Journal of Anatomy 158:109-114

Wills C A, Caiozzo, V J, Yasukawa D I, Prietto C A, McMaster W C 1982 Effects of immobilization on muscle. Orthopaedic Review 11(11):57-64

Wroblewski R, Arvidsson I, Eriksson E, Jansson E 1987 Changes in elemental composition of human muscle fibres following surgery and immobilization. An X-ray microanalytical study. Acta Physiologica Scandinavica 130:491-494

Young A, Stokes M 1986 Reflex inhibition of muscle activity and the morphological consequences of inactivity. In: Saltin B (ed) Biochemistry of exercise VI. Human Kinetics, Champaign, Illinois, pp 531-544

Young A, Hughes I, Round J M, Edwards R H T 1982 The effect of knee injury on the number of muscle fibres in the human quadriceps femoris. Clinical Science 62:227-234

Young A, Stokes M, Shakespeare D T, Sherman K P 1983 The effect of intra-articular bupivacaine on quadriceps inhibition after meniscectomy. Medicine and Science in Sports and Exercise 15:154

Young A, Stokes M, Iles J F 1987 Effects of joint pathology on muscle. Clinical Orthopaedics and Related Research 219:21-27

Zarro V 1986 Mechanisms of inflammation and repair. In: Michlovitz S L (ed) Thermal agents in rehabilitation. F A Davis, Philadephia, pp 3-17

3. Physiological responses to injury: ligament, tendon and bone

Barry W. Oakes

In musculoskeletal practice it is important to develop clinical skills and to establish a diagnosis with anatomical precision to manage a patient optimally. Management regimes are based on both previous practical experience of the clinician and of others as well as information based on experimentation be it animal or human. This chapter will review briefly recent basic science information in relation to bone and ligament/tendon and the response of these unique tissues to mechanical perturbations including exercise, and attempt to relate this to practical clinical patient management.

BONE

The measurement of bone mineral content to assess the long-term effects of physical activity or inactivity on bone composition has been possible using quantitative single or dual photon absorptiometry (Fig. 3.1) and, more recently, quantitative CT scanning and dual energy X-ray densitometry (DEXA) to localize changes within bones. For a comprehensive review of osteoporosis see Riggs and Melton (1986). The use of ultrasound to monitor changes in bone with loading has also been used but its interpretation requires more clarification. The combination of the above with biochemical parameters such as urine and serum hydroxyproline determinations may be useful for predicting individuals who may develop problems when subjecting themselves to musculoskeletal stress (Marguia et al 1988). The relationship between the relative contribution of the genome, the mechanical and hormonal environments to bone remodelling and maintenance of bone mass is still not well understood. The concept of an 'optimal strain environment' genetically programed but specific to the region of bone and its functional loading has been supported by recent work. The approximate type and magnitude of strain required to maintain bone mass and to induce fatigue fractures is now appreciated. As of writing this knowledge has not been successfully applied to patients, in that bone loss cannot be totally prevented with prolonged recumbency

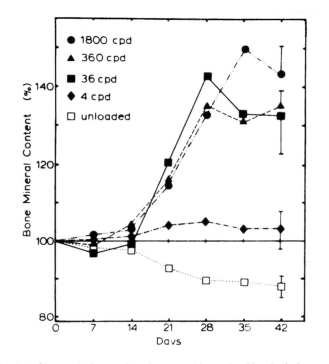

Fig. 3.1 Changes in bone mineral content (determined by single-beam photon absorption densitometry) that occurred over the 6 week experimental period. The rooster ulnae were subjected to zero (o), 4 (u), 36 (n), 360 (s), or 1800 (l), consecutive loading reversal cycles per day of an identically applied load regime. The vertical lines at 6 weeks indicate one standard deviation. Source: Rubin & Lanyon (1987)

or weightlessness (space flight). More longitudinal studies are required to determine the rate of change of bone remodelling and mechanisms to prevent bone resorption with prolonged bed rest and space flight. Similar studies are required to be done to predict which patients and which bones in these patients are at risk from stress fractures. The use of pulsed electromagnetic fields to minimize bone loss in experimental animal models is encouraging. Its usefulness as a clinical tool will soon begin to be evaluated. More longitudinal studies are also required to determine the relative contribution of various activities to bone growth in children.

Bone response to loading and unloading

Numerous animal experiments (reviewed by Tipton & Vailas 1988) have shown that exercise and the opposite unloading will positively and negatively influence the composition and hence mechanical properties of bone. Muscle mass and bone mass are directly related (Cohn et al 1977). Studies by Leichter et al (1989) demonstrated 7.5% increase in bone mineral density in male army recruits subjected to a 14-week intensive physical training period. Excessive exercise may also have deleterious effects such as stress fractures (Clement et al 1984) and may retard bone growth, particularly high intensity exercise (Forwood 1987). Also, stress fractures may develop because of loss of bone mass. There appears to be an empirical critical threshold level of bone density of about 1 g per square centimetre for the femur and the vertebrae. With bone densities below this critical fracture threshold level the incidence of hip and vertebral fractures increases (Riggs & Melton 1986).

Definitions of terms

Load

Applied force (Newton:N)

Deformation

Amount object stretches or elongates (millimetres:mm)

Stress

Deformation divided by area over which it is applied (megapascals: MPa)

Strain

Deformation divided by the initial length (microstrain = .001 strain)

Stiffness

Amount of applied load necessary to produce a given deformation (N/mm)

Ultimate strength

Measure of how much load a structure can bear prior to failure (also maximal load)

Load-deformation curve

A graph of the relationship between the load applied to an object and its resulting change in dimension (depends upon the structural properties of the specimen)

Stress-strain curve

A graph of the relationship between the stress applied to a material and its resulting strain (similar to load-deformation curve, but does not depend upon the specimen physical dimensions; measurement of material properties)

Creep

Progressive material deformation over time under constant load.

Experimental exercise studies are limited because of the difficulty in controlling and quantifying the precise level of mechanical loading, especially in relation to the strains imposed. Lanyon, Rubin and coworkers have addressed some of these problems by using quantitative methodology (Rubin & Lanyon 1987). This was the first work in vivo using direct mechanical loading of bone which determined the actual strains and the frequency of their application which would prevent bone loss or encourage new periosteal bone formation.

Functionally isolated avian ulnar model of bone adaptation to loading

The avian bone response to loading and unloading was examined (Rubin & Lanyon 1987b) using the 'functionally isolated avian ulnar model'. They determined with an applied physiological strain of 2050 microstrain at 4, 36, 360 and 1800 consecutive 0.5 Hz load reversals (cycles) that 4 cycles or only 8 s of loading per day was sufficient to prevent disuse osteoporosis. 36 cycles per day or only 72 s of loading was sufficient to trigger and maximize the osteogenic response. Loading times greater than 36 cycles (72 s) did not increase the osteogenic response (Fig. 3.1.) They also determined from a similar series of experiments but using increasing microstrains from -500 to -4000 microstrain at 100 consecutive 1 Hz reversals that there was a distinct 'dose response' curve for the deposition of new endosteal and periosteal bone. Strains less than 500 microstrain were associated with bone loss and strains greater than 1000 were associated with increase in osteogenic activity. Loading the functionally isolated ulna statically with springs to induce -2000 microstrain over 8 weeks induced no new bone formation and in fact intracortical porosis was observed. From these observations they concluded that cyclical dynamic loading rather than static loading was more effective in the transduction of the experimentally imposed mechanical strain via an unknown biochemical effector to surface osteoblasts. Lanyon coined the use of the term 'minimum effective strain' which is the strain magnitude required to maintain balanced remodelling and hence retain bone mass at its 'normal physiological' level.

Rubin and Lanyon also determined that normal peak physiological strains in adult bones which were weight-bearing were in the range of 0.002-0.003. From these observations Rubin and Lanyon (1987b) and Lanyon (1987) have suggested that osteocytes are very sensitive to the distribution, rate of change and magnitude of strain within the bone matrix. Osteoblasts entombed in bone matrix seem to be able to monitor dynamic strain matrix deformation within 6 s (probably by a biochemical message) and transmit this 'mechanical information' via gap junctions of their long cytoplasmic extensions to the surface osteoblasts and osteoclasts to remodel the bone appropriately. Hence the functional syncytium or network of bone cells responding to mechanical influences is critical to this concept of bone architectural adaption to loading.

Skerry et al (1988) have reported with bone loading that bone matrix proteoglycans may in fact be the biochemical transducer monitoring matrix strain. This was further suggested by the use of cuprolinium blue to demonstrate proteoglycans at the ultrastructural level. With bone loading proteoglycans were seen to reorient themselves in relation to the collagen fibrils of the bone matrix. Proteoglycans would be a strong contender as a biochemical transducer of matrix strain because of their strong negative charge profile which could inform the osteocytes by a change in charge relationships with the cell membrane. This has led to the attractive concept of the reorientation of proteoglycans being a matrix 'strain memory' and could explain the observation that in a single period of loading the remodelling response appears to saturate after a few loading cycles; although such a concept awaits further experimental validation. Recent results from the same group indicate that osteocytes can respond to a single loading cycle by the uptake of ^{3}H-uridine 24 hours after loading and that direct transformation from quiescence to bone formation appears to occur after this single loading cycle within five days of loading (Pead et al 1988).

Of even greater practical clinical importance is the report by Rubin et al (1989) of the prevention of osteoporosis in the functionally isolated avian ulnar model by the application of a pulsed electromagnetic field. Brighton et al (1988) have also shown that a capacitively coupled electrical field applied to osteoporotic rats could enhance bone deposition.

Greater understanding of bone performance in relation to fatigue failure or stress fractures has occurred since the start of the 1980s. Bone fatigue failure is currently topical because of the large numbers of individuals involved in distance running or jogging for lifestyle benefits, who sustain stress fractures.

The threshold level of physical activity or mechanical loading at which bone remodels positively or accumulates microdamage has not been defined. In fact the concept of microdamage is poorly defined except in terms of the status or integrity of the bone prior to a clearly diagnosable problem such as a stress fracture. Carter et al (1977, 1981) have demonstrated that repetitive cyclical physiological loading in vitro can cause a progressive gradual loss of stiffness and ultimate strength due to microcracks. The total number of cycles to fatigue failure was influenced only by

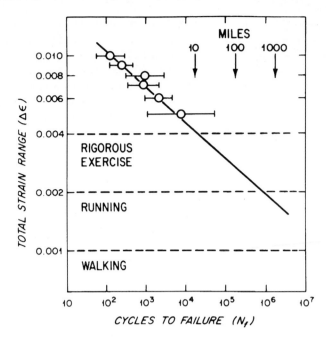

Fig. 3.2 The in vitro strain-related fatigue behaviour of cortical bone compared to the levels of cyclical strain range that are expected during various in vivo activities. Note prolonged rigorous exercise may lead to cortical fatigue or 'stress' failure as may prolonged running. Source: Carter et al (1981)

the total strain range and was not affected by mean strain. Bone was shown to have extremely poor fatigue resistance and fully reversed cyclic loading to half of the yield strain caused fatigue fracture in 1000 cycles. Carter et al (1981) compared their strain ranges (0.005–0.010) and fatigue results and extrapolated this data to that which may occur in bone in vivo with the clinical experience with fatigue fractures in military recruits and athletes. They concluded that military recruits would within 6 weeks (the earliest appearance of stress fractures) accumulate a loading history equivalent to 100–1000 miles (160–1600 km) of very rigorous exercise, which was according to them equivalent to 100 000 to 1 000 000 loading cycles. From their data extrapolation they predicted cyclic strain ranges of 0.0029 and 0.0019 respectively for these fatigue fractures in these recruits (Fig. 3.2).

They also determined that tensile fatigue caused failure at the cement lines which resulted in debonding of the osteons from surrounding interstitial bone, whereas compressive fatigue resulted in the formation of 'diffuse shear microcracks throughout bone which are oblique to the loading direction'. Carter also estimated the fatigue strength of bone as being about 7 MPa at 10^7 cycles and suggested that this extremely low value for fatigue strength of human cortical bone would require that our bones are constantly accumulating fatigue damage during everyday activities and that the processes of normal bone remodelling and repair are necessary for long term structural integrity of bone. The use of plasma hydroxproline levels may be a useful marker for predicting the onset of stress fractures of bone in those vigorously exercising (Marguia et al 1988).

Similar observations were made by Burr et al (1985) using physiological loads applied to the dog radius and by Forwood and Parker (1989) using in vitro torsional testing of the rat tibia. Burr et al (1985) observed crack fractures across osteons which were 40 times more frequent than in the control radius. For further detail reading on the mechanical adaptation of bone the monograph by Bruce Martin and Burr (1989) should be consulted.

In a fascinating study Rubin et al (1987) measured the velocity of ultrasound across the patella and tibia in 98 volunteers before and after running the Boston Marathon. They found that absolute sound velocities were 2.9% higher in those runners finishing in less than 3 hours compared to those finishing after 3 hours. Tibial velocities in males were 8.8% higher than in female runners. The mean velocity across the patella of three wheelchair racers was 28% lower than the mean combined patellar velocity measures in all runners. They suggested that faster velocities were associated with bone more suited to greater functional demands. It was also shown that there was a 1.6% increase in ultrasonic velocity across the tibia, and a 3.5% increase across the patella between pre and post race velocities, indicating change had occurred within the bone during the race. The nature of this change is speculative but it is tempting to suggest it could be due to fatigue fracture damage as has been postulated by Carter et al. However, with fatigue fractures we would expect a marked decrease in sound velocity. Rubin et al suggested that the increase in sound transmission observed post-race may be due to other organic mechanisms such as proteoglycan orientation. Unfortunately, individual biomechanical profiles which may have identified structural abnormalities likely to promote a damaging overload situation were not reported.

Work by Forwood and Parker (1986, 1987, 1989) using pubescent rats has shown that after an intensive month of exercise, the tibia showed an increased number of Haversian canals in the middle one third of the cortex, significant reductions in energy to failure, bone length and width of the proximal epiphyseal plate. No change was observed in the mechanical properties of the femur, but significant reductions occurred in bone length and weight. This suggests that intensive exercise in young rats is not beneficial for their normal growth and development. This is similar to the findings of others.

Carter et al (1987) and Wong and Carter (1988) have demonstrated both continuous and intermittent compressive force increased cartilage calcification in vitro. Carter et al have demonstrated that calcification in vivo can be accurately predicted by determining strain energy density in the developing cartilage anlagen of the femur and the more complex sternum. This is the first step in the proof of Wolff's Law, in that Julian Wolff predicted in 1892 that the 'internal architecture and external conformation' of bone is in accordance with mathematical laws. His prediction is now realized in part by Carter et al's mathematical analyses.

Hence at both the micro and macro levels it has been demonstrated that both the cells and the matrix respond to loading in such a manner that adaption including calcification during development are determined by mechanical forces. There is now strong evidence from Carter et al's observations that stress histories play a major role in regulating gene expression, especially during development.

LIGAMENT AND TENDON

In this section the following will be discussed:

- The development, normal structure and biomechanics of ligaments and tendons
- The time frame for adequate ligament collagen fibril biosynthesis and deposition in sufficient quantity, diameter and orientation to allow a patient to weight bear without compromising the repair
- Correlation of collagen fibril diameter and the mechanical properties of ligaments/tendons

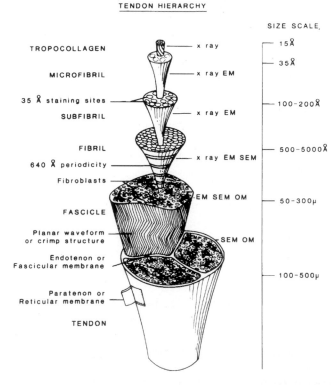

Fig. 3.3 Ligament/tendon structural hierarchy with size scale on the right. Note the planar crimp which can be seen at the level of light microscopy within each fascicle. Source: adapted from Kastelic et al (1978)

- The recent literature with reference to the effects of immobilization on ligament tensile strength, and the effects of mobilization (exercise) on ligament tensile strength and repair
- Ultrastructural and clinical observations on patients with anterior cruciate ligament autografts and allografts, and acute and chronic achilles tendon injury.

Structure and biomechanics

Mature adult ligament and tendon are composed of large diameter type I collagen fibrils (>1500 Å diam.) tightly packed together with a small amount of type III collagen dispersed in an aqueous gel containing small amounts of proteoglycan and elastic fibres. The outstanding feature of both these unique load-bearing tissues is the collagen 'crimp' which is a planar wave pattern found extending in phase across the width of all tendons and ligaments (Fig. 3.3). This collagen crimp appears to be built into the tertiary stucture of the collagen molecule and is probably maintained in vivo by inter- and intramolecular collagen cross-links as well as a strategically placed elastic fibre network. The crimp may help to attenuate muscle loading forces at the tendoperiosteal junction as well as the musculotendinous junction.

Ligament and tendon injury can be closely correlated with the load-deformation curve (Viidik 1973, Butler et al 1979, Oakes 1981). The load-strain curve can be divided into three regions (Fig. 3.4).

The 'toe' region or initial concave region represents the normal physiological range of ligament/tendon strain up to about 3–4 % of initial length and is due to the flattening of the collagen 'crimp'. Repeated cycling within this 'toe region' or 'physiological strain range' of 3–4 % (may be up to near 10% in cruciate ligaments, due to intrinsic macrospiral of collagen cruciate fibre bundles) can normally occur without irreversible macroscopic or molecular damage to the tissue.

The second part of the load-deformation curve is the linear region, where pathological irreversible ligament/tendon elongation occurs due to partial rupture of intermolecular cross-links (Rigby et al 1959). As the load is increased further intra- and intermolecular cross-links are disrupted until macroscopic falure is evident clinically. The early part of the linear region corresponds to mild ligament tears or grade 1, 0–50% fibre disruption and the latter part to grade 2, 50–80% fibre disruption where there is obvious clinical laxity on stress testing.

Grade 1 and 2 injuries always have some pain after the initial trauma and usually with a grade 2 injury the athlete cannot continue. This is a rough guide to the clinical severity of the injury.

In the third region, if continued loading occurs the linear part of the curve flattens and the yield or failure point is

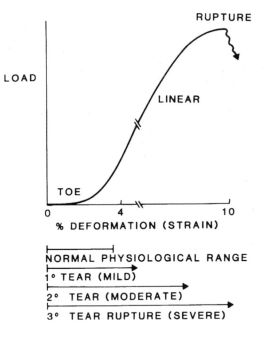

Fig. 3.4 Load-deformation (strain) curve for ligament/tendon and the clinical correlation with the grading of the injury. Note the 'toe' region of the curve (probably a function of the collagen crimp) is entirely within the normal physiological range and that greater than about 4% strain causes tissue damage

reached at 10–20% strain dependent upon ligament/tendon fibre bundle macro-organization.

In this region complete ligament tendon rupture occurs at 'maximal breaking load'. This is the dangerous grade 3 ligament rupture on clinical testing. It is dangerous because the athlete has severe momentary pain when the trauma is applied and then little pain, and the athlete (and often inexperienced examiners) believe the injury is trivial and treat it as such, with disastrous consequences.

Collagen biosynthesis and development of the rat anterior cruciate ligament

The morphology of the developing rat anterior cruciate ligament (ACL) has been studied in detail using both light and electron microscopy from the 14-day-old fetus through to senile 2-year-old adult rats (Oakes 1988). The observations made by Amiel (1983) with light microscopy on the rabbit ACL confirmed earlier observations made by the author on the cell types present in both the developing and adult rat ACL which are similar to cells in the adult human ACL. Fibroblasts in the developing foetal rat ACL align themselves via junctional complexes in the direction of the future ACL between the femoral and tibial condyles. Collagen fibrils appear to be deposited in long grooves or furrows of the cell membrane, and hence the cell directs collagen fibril orientation similar to that described for the developing tendon. As collagen fibrils are deposited between

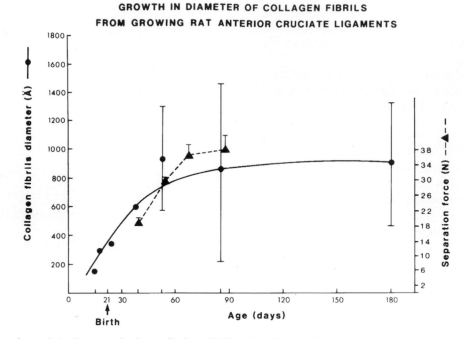

GROWTH IN DIAMETER OF COLLAGEN FIBRILS FROM GROWING RAT ANTERIOR CRUCIATE LIGAMENTS

Fig. 3.5 Comparison of growth in diameter of collagen fibrils (solid line through mean diameters with bar representing the largest and smallest fibrils) and tensile strength (dotted line with triangles) with age in the growing rat anterior cruciate ligament. Note both curves plateau at about 90 days post-conception or about 70 days after birth

the rows of cells they become pushed apart, eventually losing their junctional complex association with one another. This occurs in the rat just before birth and after the collagen crimp is established. It may be via these junctional complexes that the coordination of the collagen 'crimp' is achieved in register across the width of developing ligaments and tendons. Danhers et al (1986) have demonstrated that ligament fibroblasts contain actin filaments which could be involved in crimp formation via fibronectin. By 2 weeks postnatal the fibroblasts become collected into groups of 2–4 cells aligned in rows between the collagen bundles. In the adult rat ACL the fibroblasts lose their long cytoplasmic extensions and become rounded and 'chondrocyte' in shape, and often have a pericellular matrix not unlike that of articular cartilage. Survival by diffusion as a primary nutrient pathway is likely. Effete cells were common amongst viable cells in senile rats of 2 years, as were large masses of electron dense material some of which resembled fibrin. Similar observations in the ageing dog cruciate have been described. In comparison with the ACL, patellar tendon fibroblasts remain elongated with flattened nucleii. Presumably this is due to the continual loading that the parent muscle exerts on tendon collagen which tends to 'squeeze' these tendon fibroblasts. Amiel et al (1984) have shown that ligaments are different biochemically as well as morphologically compared to tendons. Indeed there are distinct differences between the collateral ligaments and the cruciate ligaments. The cruciate ligaments were shown to have larger cells with more DNA, more total collagen and a larger glycosaminoglycan (GAG) content than the patellar or the achilles tendon. Work by Hey et al (1990)

demonstrates there are two types of proteoglycan in bovine collateral ligament similar to that found in tendons.

Collagen fibril diameter quantification with age and correlation with ACL tensile strength

Some 50 collagen fibrils were measured at various ages of the rat from 14 days fetal to 2-year-old senile adult rats. The mean diameter and the range of fibrils from the largest to the smallest for each time interval were plotted against age (Fig. 3.5.) The mean fibril diameter begins to plateau at about 7 weeks postnatal. Also plotted on this figure is the separation force required to rupture the ACL in the rat with age. Special grips were used in this study to obviate epiphyseal separation and 70% of the failures occured within the ACL (Parker & Larsen 1981). It can be seen that the two curves closely coincide, indicating a correlation between the size of the collagen fibrils and the ultimate tensile strength of the ACL, as has been suggested by Parry et al (1978).

Correlation of collagen fibril size with mechanical properties of tissues

Parry et al (1978) also have completed detailed quantitative morphometric ultrastructural analyses of collagen fibrils from a large number of collagen containing tissues in various species. They came to a number of conclusions. Those that are pertinent for this discussion can be summarized:

- Type 1 oriented tissues such as ligament and tendon have a bimodal distribution of collagen fibril diameters at maturity.

- The ultimate tensile strength and mechanical properties of connective tissues are positively correlated with the 'mass average diameter' of collagen fibrils (Fig. 3.6). In the context of response of ligaments to exercise they also concluded that the collagen fibril diameter distribution is closely correlated with the magnitude and duration of loading of tissues.

Shadwick (1986) has also demonstrated a clear correlation between collagen fibril diameter and the tensile strength of tendons. He showed the tensile strength of pig flexor tendons was greater than that of extensor tendons and that this greater flexor tendon tensile strength was correlated with a population of larger diameter collagen fibrils not present in the weaker extensor tendons.

Effect of immobilization on ligament tensile strength

The most important study in this context is that by Noyes et al (1974). This study used the anterior cruciate ligament in monkeys as a part of a NASA study to examine the effects of prolonged unloading of ligaments in astronauts. They demonstrated clearly that 8 weeks lower limb cast immobilization led to a substantial loss of ligament tensile strength which took over 9 months to recover, even with a reconditioning program. The predominant mode of failure in these experiments was ligament failure, not avulsion fracture failure. The latter mode of failure was more predominant in the immobilized group due to resorption of Haversian bone at the ligament attachment but after 5 months of recon-

ditioning femoral avulsion fractures did not occur. This was without surgery, just simple immobilization.

Another important study that has direct implications for clinical practice is that by Amiel et al (1983). Although this work was done in rabbits, in the context of the previous work of Noyes it is very relevant. The time frames for the changes in ligament tensile strength are similar and hence are probably relevant to clinical orthopaedics. Amiel et al showed that 12 weeks immobilization of the medial collateral ligament (MCL) in the growing rabbit led to profound atrophy of the MCL such that there was an approximate 30% decrease in collagen mass due to increased collagen degradation in the immobilized MCL. Most of this atrophy occured during weeks 9–12 of immobilization. Again in this study there was no trauma or surgery to the MCL.

Hence it appears from the above two studies that prolonged immobilization, i.e. 6–12 weeks without trauma can itself lead to profound atrophy of both collateral and cruciate ligaments of the knee joint and recovery may require many months. This time frame must be kept in mind when managing patients after prolonged knee immobilization and advising them when they can return optimally to full competitive sport.

Amiel et al (1985) have also shown there is a close relationship between joint stiffness induced by immobilization and a decrease of total glycosaminoglycan and particularly hyaluronan in the periarticular connective tissues. They demonstrated alleviation of this joint stiffness in a rabbit model using intra-articular hyaluronate.

Apart from the original work of Noyes et al (1974) in which the effects of immobilization on the anterior cruciate ligament (ACL) of the primate were examined, there have been few studies to examine the cause of the decreased strength and elastic stiffness of the ACL in response to immobilization. Tipton et al (1970) reported that collagen fibre bundles with light microscopy were decreased in number and size (in dogs), suggesting that this was the cause of the decreased cross-sectional area seen in immobilized medial collateral rabbit ligaments (Woo et al 1987). The explanation for the decreased strength and elastic stiffness in these immobilized ligaments may be found at the collagen fibril level. Binkley and Peat (1986) showed a decrease in the number of small diameter fibrils with 6 weeks of immobilization of the rat medial collateral ligament. Tipton et al (1975), Cabaud et al (1980), Parker and Larsen (1981) and others observed that ligament strength was dependent on physical activity. Increased collagen content was found in the ligaments of exercised dogs and this correlated with increased cross-sectional area and larger fibre bundles. This accounts for the increased ligament tensile strength but whether this increased collagen was due to deposition of collagen on existing fibrils or due to the synthesis of new fibrils has not been investigated. Larsen and Parker (1982) have shown that with a 4-week intensive exercise program in young male Wistar

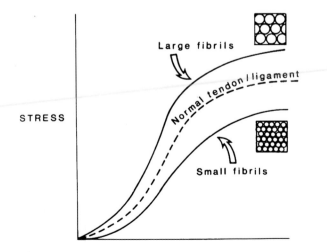

POSTULATED FORM OF STRESS/STRAIN CURVES FOR TENDONS COMPOSED SOLELY OF LARGE OR SMALL DIAMETER FIBRILS

Large fibrils

Normal tendon/ligament

STRESS

Small fibrils

STRAIN

Fig. 3.6 Load-strain curves with large and small fibrils and the intermediate curve representing the normal mix of small and large fibrils seen in ligaments and tendons in vivo. Source: adapted from Parry et al (1978).

rats both the anterior and posterior cruciate ligaments showed a significant strength increase (p < 0.05).

The above observations prompted an ultrastructural investigation of the mechanism of this increase in tensile strength within ligaments. Oakes et al (1981) quantified the collagen fibril populations in young rat anterior and posterior cruciate ligaments subjected to an intensive 1 month exercise program in an attempt to explain the increased tensile strength found in these ligaments with the intensive endurance exercise program.

Effect of mobilization on ligament tensile strength

There have been a large number of studies investigating this very question. The literature has been reviewed by Tipton et al (1986), Butler et al (1979), Parker and Larsen (1981).

Normal ligaments

The results in experimental animals generally indicate an increase in bone-ligament-bone preparation strength as a response to endurance type exercise. However, no change

in ligament or tendon strength has been recorded by some workers and this may reflect different exercise regimens and methods of testing as well as species differences.

Oakes et al (1981) and Oakes (1988) investigated collagen fibril changes within exercised rat cruciate ligaments. Five 30-day old pubescent rats were placed on a progressive 4-week exercise program of alternating days of swimming and treadmill running. At the conclusion of the exercise program the rats were running 60–80 minutes at 26 m/min on a 10% treadmill gradient and on alternate days swimming 60 minutes with a 3% body weight attached to their tails. Five caged rats of similar age and commencing body weights were controls. After 30 days the exercise and control rats underwent total body perfusion fixation and the anterior cruciate ligaments (ACL) and posterior cruciate ligaments (PCL) were removed and prepared for electron microscopy. Analysis of ultrathin transverse sections cut through collagen fibrils of the exercised ACLs revealed:

- a larger number of fibrils per unit area examined (29% increase, p < 0.05) compared to the non-exercised caged control ACLs

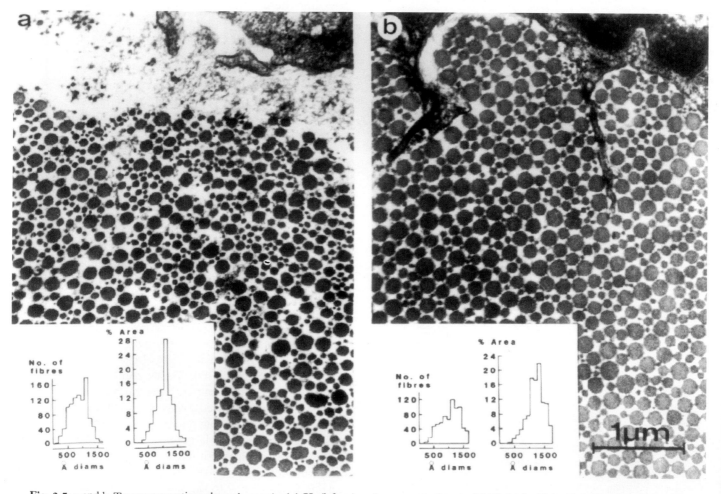

Fig. 3.7: a and b Transverse sections through exercised ACL (left, a) and nonexercised control ACL (right, b) (x 21 600). Insets: Histogram profiles of mean data for number of fibrils and percentage area occupied for each diameter group

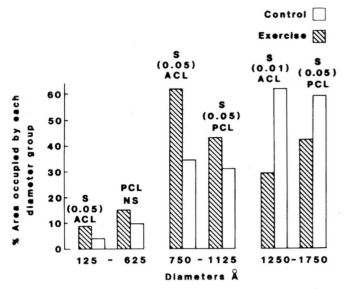

Fig. 3.8 Comparison of % area occupied by three diameter groupings used for statistical analysis for exercised and control ACL and PCL. Note increase in intermediate sized fibrils in the exercised rats

- a fall in mean fibril diameter from 966 +/- 30 Å in the control ACL's to 830 +/- 30 Å in the exercised ACLs, p < 0.05
- the major cross-sectional area of collagen fibrils was found in the 1125 Å diameter group in the exercised ACLs and in the 1500 Å diameter group in the control ACLs. However, total collagen fibril cross-section per unit area examined was approximately the same in both the exercised and the non-exercised control ACLs. Similar changes occurred in the exercised and control PCLs (Figs 3.7, 3.8 and 3.9). In the exercised PCL, collagen/ug DNA was almost double that of the control, suggesting that the PCL was more loaded with this exercise regime than the ACL.

The conclusion from this study is that ACL and PCL 'fibroblasts' deposit tropocollagen as smaller diameter fibrils when subjected to an intense month intermittent loading (exercise) rather than the expected accretion and increase in size of the pre-existing larger diameter collagen fibrils. Very similar ultrastructural observations to this study have been made for collagen fibrils of exercised mice flexor tendons (Michna 1984).

The mechanism of the change to a smaller diameter collagen fibril population is of interest and may be related to a change in the type of glycosaminoglycans and hence proteoglycans synthesized by ligament fibroblasts in response to the intermittent loading of exercise. It is well recognized since the original work of Toole and Lowther (1968) that glycosaminoglycans have an effect on determining collagen fibril size in vitro. This has been recently confirmed in vivo by Parry et al (1982). Merrilees and Flint (1980) demonstrated a change in collagen fibril diameters between the compression and tension regions of the flexor

digitorum profundus tendon as it turns 90° around the talus. Amiel et al (1984) have shown that the rabbit cruciate ligaments have more glycosaminoglycans than the patellar tendon and hence it is likely that glycosaminoglycans also play an important role in determining collagen fibril populations in cruciate ligaments.

Surgically repaired ligaments

Tipton et al (1970) demonstrated a significant increase in the strength of surgically repaired medial collateral ligaments (MCL) of dogs which were exercised for 6 weeks after 6 weeks cast immobilization. However, Tipton et al (1970) emphasized that at 12 weeks post-surgery (6 weeks immobilization and 6 weeks exercise training) the repair was only approximately 60% of that for the normal dogs and results suggested that at least 15–18 weeks of exercise training may be required before return to 'normal' tensile strength is achieved. Similar observations have been made by Piper and Whiteside (1980), using the MCL of dogs. They observed that mobilized MCL repairs were stronger and stretched out less, i.e. less valgus laxity than MCL repairs managed by casting and delayed mobilization. This conclusion is supported by the work of Woo et al (1987).

Some insight into the biological mechanisms involved in the repair response with exercise has come from Vailas et al (1981). By using ^{3}H-proline pulse labelling to measure collagen synthesis in rat MCL surgical repairs and coupling this with DNA analyses and tensile testing of repaired ligaments subjected to exercise and non-exercise regimens, they were able to document that exercise commencing 2 weeks post-surgical repair enhanced the repair and re-modelling phase by inducing a more rapid return of cellularity, collagen synthesis and ligament tensile strength to within normal limits. Further, Woo et al (1987) demonstrated almost complete return (98%) of structural properties of the transected canine femoral-medial collateral ligament-tibial (FMT) complex at 12 weeks post-transection without immobilization. Canines immobilized for 6 weeks and the FMT complex tested at 12 weeks had

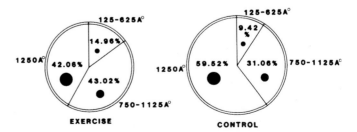

Fig. 3.9 Comparison of % area occupied by the three diameter groupings used for statistical analysis in the exercised and control PCL. Note increase in intermediate sized fibrils in the exercised rats

NORMAL LIGAMENT

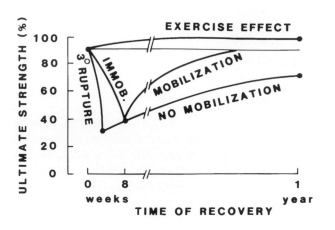

Fig. 3.10 Effects of immobilization, mobilization and exercise on ligament ultimate tensile strength (UTS) recovery. After a relatively short period of immobilization of about 8 weeks, ligament tensile strength takes many months to recover. Note the effect of exercise on ligament UTS is small. Source: adapted from Woo et al (1987)

mean loads to failure 54% that of the control. However, the tensile strength of the medial collateral ligament (MCL) was only 62% of controls at 48 weeks. This apparent paradox was explained by the doubling in cross-sectional area of the healing MCL (and hence increased collagen deposition) during the early phases of healing.

Woo et al (1987) examined the effects of prolonged immobilization and then mobilization on the rabbit MCL. Both the structural properties of the FMT complex and the material properties of the MCL were examined. After immobilization, there were significant reductions in the ultimate load and energy-absorbing capabilities of the bone-ligament-bone complex. The MCL became less stiff with immobilization and the femoral and tibial insertion sites showed increased osteoclastic activity, bone resorption and disruption of the normal bone attachment to the MCL. With mobilization, the ultimate load and energy absorbing capabilities ot the FMT complex improved but did not return to normal. The stress-strain characteristics of the MCL returned to normal, indicating the material properties of the collagen of the MCL in the rabbit return relatively quickly after remobilization but the delayed ligament bone-junction strength return to normal may take many months (Fig. 3.10.)

The detailed biological cellular mechanisms involved in this enhancement and remodelling of the repair are not understood, but they may involve prostaglandin and cyclic-AMP synthesis by fibroblasts subjected to repeated mechanical deformation by exercise.

Amiel et al (1987) have shown that maximal collagen deposition and turnover occurs during the first 3–6 weeks post-injury in the rabbit. Chaudhuri et al (1987) used a Fourier domain directional filtering technique to quantify collagen fibril orientation in repairing ligaments. Results indicated ligament collagen fibril reorientation does occur in the longitudinal axis of the ligament during remodelling. MacFarlane et al (1989) further showed that collagen remodelling of the repairing rabbit MCL appears to be encouraged by early immobilization but after 3 weeks collagen alignment and remodelling appears to be favoured by mobilization.

With this basic biological knowledge there is now a rationale for the use of early controlled mobilization of patients with ligament trauma. The use of a limited motion cast with an adjustable double action hinge for the knee joint is now accepted. It enhances more rapid repair and remodelling as well as preserving quadriceps muscle bulk. Patients are now usually mobilized in a limited motion cast at 3 weeks rather than the previously empirical time of 6 weeks.

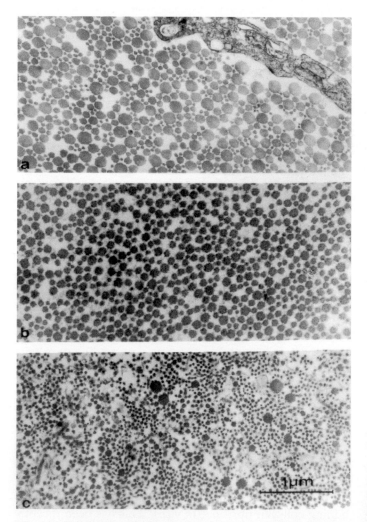

Fig. 3.11 Electronmicrographs of transverse sections through collagen fibrils of: (a) the normal young adult patellar tendon (PT) (mean of 6 biopsies), (b) normal young adult ACL (mean of 6 biopsies), (c) Jones' free graft (mean of 9 biopsies). All x 34 100

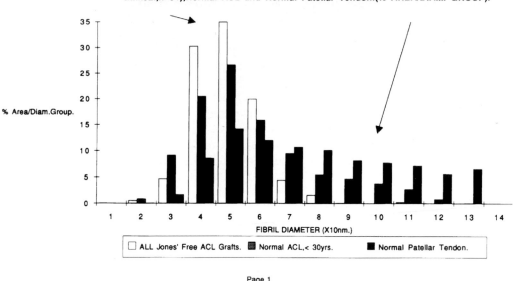

Comparison SUMMARY of ALL Jones' FREE ACL Grafts,IRRESPECTIVE OF GRAFT AGE,(O.D. &I.McL.,n=51),Normal ACL and Normal Patellar Tendon.(% AREA/DIAM. GROUP).

Page 1

Fig. 3.12 Histogram analyses of 51 Jones' free grafts compared with the normal ACL and the normal patellar tendon expressed as % area/diameter group vs fibril diameter (nm.) Note the Jones' free grafts have their major cross-sectional area in the small fibril region whereas the patellar tendon from which the grafts were derived are composed predominantly of large fibrils. The normal human ACL is composed of intermediate sized fibrils

Collagen fibre populations in human knee ligaments and grafts

In order to gain some biological insight into collagen repair mechanisms within human cruciate ligament grafts, biopsies were obtained from autogenous ACL grafts from patients subsequently requiring arthroscopic intervention because of stiffness, meniscal and/or articular cartilage problems or removal of prominent staples used for fixation. Most of the the ACL grafts were from the central one-third of the patellar tendon as a free graft (N = 51), or in some left attached distally (N = 8) and in others the hamstrings or the iliotibial tract was used (N = 7). These biopsies represented approximately 20% of the total free grafts performed over the 3 years of this study. The clinical ACL stability of the biopsy group differed little from the remainder. All had a grade II–III pivot shift (jerk) pre-operatively (10–15 mm anterior drawer neutral, ADN), eliminated post-operatively in 87% of patients (0.5 mm ADN). Subsequent clinical review at 3 years showed an increase in ADN with a return in 20% of a grade I pivot shift.

A total of 51 biopsies have been quantitatively analyzed for collagen fibril diameter populations in patients aged 19–42 years. This data was compared with collagen fibril populations obtained from biopsies of cadaver ACL's (N = 5) and biopsies of ACLs from young (< 30 years, N = 10) and old patients (> 30 years, N = 6) who had sustained a recent tear. Biopsies were also obtained from normal patellar tendons at operation (N = 7) and cadavers (N = 3).

The results (Fig. 3.11) from the collagen fibril diameter morphometric analysis in all the ACL grafts clearly indicated a predominance of small diameter collagen fibrils. Absence of a regular crimping of collagen fibrils was observed by both light and electron microscopy, as was a less ordered parallel arrangement of fibrils. In most biopsies capillaries were present and most fibroblasts appeared viable.

- Large diameter collagen fibrils (>1000 Å diam.) form a large proportion (approx. 45%) of the percentage cross-sectional area in the normal human patellar tendon.
- Collagen fibrils <1000 Å diam. form a large proportion (approx. 85%) of the percentage cross-sectional area in the normal human ACL.
- In all the ACL grafts, collagen fibrils < 1000Å diameter (majority 250–750 Å diam.) are the major contributor to the collagen fibril cross-sectional area, be they young (9 month) or old grafts (6 years) (Fig. 3.12).

Recent biochemical analysis of human patellar tendon autografts in situ for 2 years has shown about 70% type I and 30% type III collagen. Similar amounts of these types of collagen are also found in the normal human ACL. This large amount of type III collagen in the normal human ACL and the autografts is of great interest and is much larger than that found in the collaterals and other conventional ligaments and tendons. The usual collagen composition of ligaments and tendon is that 95% of the collagen is type I and the other 5% is composed of type III and V collagen. The significance of the large amount of type III in the normal human ACL and the ACL autografts is still to be determined.

Recent further studies of biopsies obtained from ACL human allografts utilizing fresh frozen achilles or tibialis anterior tendons ranging in age from 3–54 months indicated a similar predominance of small diameter collagen fibrils (Shino et al 1990).

Before discussing the biopsy data it is of interest to compare the collagen fibril profiles of the normal human patellar tendon with the normal human ACL. It can be seen the profiles are different in that the distribution in the patellar tendon is skewed to the right, with a small number of large fibrils not present in the normal ACL. Butler et al (1985) have shown that the patellar tendon is significantly stronger than the human ACL, PCL and LCL from the same knee in terms of maximum stress, linear modulus and energy density to maximum strength. The larger fibrils observed in the patellar tendon and not found in the ACL are an obvious explanation for the stronger biomechanical properties.

The biopsies from the grafts were obtained from patients with a good to fair rating in terms of a moderate anterior drawer (0–5 mm, ADN) and correction of the pivot shift, but both these tests of ACL integrity showed an increasing laxity of the ACL at the 3 year clinical review. The length of time the grafts were in vivo prior to biopsy varied from 6 months to 6 years. The collagen fibril population did not alter that much for the older grafts (> 3 years) which is in keeping with the observation clinically that the ACL grafts 'stretched out' post-operatively.

The most striking feature of all the biopsies from the grafts irrespective of whether they were free grafts, Jones' grafts, fascia lata or hamstring grafts was the invariable prevalence of small diameter fibrils among a few larger fibrils which probably were the original large diameter patellar fibrils. The packing of the small fibrils in the grafts was not as tight as is usually observed in the normal patellar tendon (compare Figs 3.2a & c). The Jones' free grafts had more large diameter fibrils than the Jones' grafts.

It appears from the quantitative collagen fibril observations in this study using a non-isometric surgical procedure that the large diameter fibrils of the original graft are removed and almost entirely replaced by smaller, less well packed and oriented than the larger diameter fibrils found in the normal patellar tendon. The smaller diameter fibrils are probably recently synthesized because they are of smaller diameter than those found in the original patellar tendon.

Is gentle mechanical loading in the ACL grafts an important stimulus to fibroblast proliferation and collagen deposition? Inadequate mechanical stimulus may occur especially if grafts are non-isometric and are 'stretched out' by the patient before they have adequate tensile strength. A lax ACL graft may not induce sufficient mechanical loading on graft fibroblasts to alter the glycosaminoglycans/ collagen biosynthesis ratios to favour large diameter fibril formation. Certainly in this study there was ACL graft laxity which increased post-operatively. This would lend credence

to the above notion. However, use of continuous passive motion in grafted primates does not increase the strength of grafts.

Another more likely possibility is that the replacement fibroblasts in the ACL grafts are derived from stem cells from the synovium (and synovial perivascular cells) which are known to synthesize hyaluronate which in turn favours small diameter fibril formation (Parry et al, 1982).

The strong correlation of small diameter fibrils with a lower tensile strength has been observed by Parry et al (1978) and the observations in that study would confirm this and correlates with the observations of Clancy et al C1981) and Arnoczky et al (1986).

The observations by Amiel et al (1989) indicates that collagenase may play a role in the remodelling of ACL tears/ grafts.

The conclusion from this study is that the predominance of the small diameter collagen fibrils (< 750 Å diameter) and their poor packing and alignment in all the ACL grafts irrespective of the type of graft, their age and the surgeon may explain the clinical and experimental evidence of a decreased tensile strength in such grafts compared to the normal ACL. It appears that in the adult, the replacement fibroblasts in the remodelled ACL graft cannot reform the large diameter, regularly crimped and tightly packed fibrils seen in the normal ACL even after 6 years (which was the oldest graft analyzed).

The origin of the replacement fibroblasts which remodel the ACL grafts is not known. It is the author's idea that they will not come from the actual graft itself although some of these cells may survive due to diffusion. However, the bulk of the stem cells involved in the remodelling process is probably derived from the surrounding synovium and its vasculature.

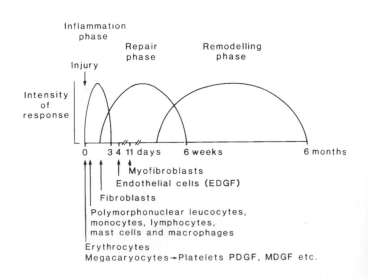

Fig. 3.13 The three phases of ligament/tendon healing and the cells involved.

Pathophysiology of repair of ligaments and tendons

Acute inflammatory phase

The gap in the ligament/tendon is filled with immediately with erthrocytes and inflammatory cells, especially polymorphonuclear leukocytes (Fig. 3.13). Within 24 hours monocytes and macrophages are the predominant cell and actively engage in phagocytosis of debris and necrotic cells. These are gradually replaced by fibroblasts from intrinsic or extrinsic sources and commence the initial deposition of the type III collagen scar. At this stage collagen concentration may be normal or slightly decreased but the total mass of ligament collagen scar is increased. Glycosaminoglycan (GAG) content, water, fibronectin and DNA content are increased.

Proliferation

Fibroblasts predominate. Water content remains increased and collagen content increases and peaks during this phase (3–6 weeks). Type I collagen now begins to predominate and GAG concentration remains high. The increasing amount of scar collagen and reducible cross-link profile has been correlated with the increasing tensile strength of the ligament matrix. Recent quantitative collagen fibril orientation studies indicates that early mobilization of a ligament at this stage (within first 3 weeks) may be detrimental to collagen orientation. After this time frame there is experimental evidence that mobilization increases the tensile strength of the repair and probably enhances this phase and the next phase of remodelling and maturation (Vailas et al 1981, Woo et al 1987, Hart & Danhers 1987).

Remodelling and maturation (6 weeks–12 months)

There is a decreasing cell number and hence decreased collagen and GAG synthesis. Water content returns to normal and collagen concentration returns to slightly below normal but total collagen content remains slightly increased. With further remodelling there is a trend for scar parameters to return to normal but the matrix in ligament scar region continues to mature slowly over months and even years. Collagen fibril alignment in the longitudinal axis of the ligament occurs even though it is small diameter collagen fibrils (Fig. 3.14).

Occasionally calcium apatite crystals will be deposited in the damaged tissues. The classic site for this to occur is in the rotator cuff supraspinatus tendoperiosteal attachment to the greater tubercle of the humerus.

Achilles tendon injuries, especially partial tears, present a dilemma for the clinician in that they are often intractable to management, although Stanish et al (1986) claim good clinical results from graded eccentric loading regimes. The author has examined achilles tendon biopsies of patients with chronic localized tears and more generalized thickened

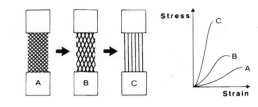

COLLAGEN REPAIR WITH IDENTICAL FIBRILS BUT DIFFERENT GEOMETRY

Modified from Viidik, 1979b

Fig. 3.14 The effect of collagen repair with identical fibrils but different geometry and their corresponding load-strain response to tensile testing. Source: adapted from Viidik (1980)

tender chronic achilles tendons. The feature which characterized the pathology ultrastructurally was the persistence of small diameter collagen fibrils. The large fibrils of the original tendon do not appear to be replaced in either a repairing tendon or ligament (Fig. 3.15).

ACL injuries appear to be unique in that the chondrocyte-like cells in this special ligament apparently have a limited capacity to proliferate and synthesize a new collagen matrix and hence repair appears to be limited. Collagenase release may also affect the effectiveness of the ACL repair process.

Clinical and ultrastructural observations on achilles tendon injuries

This section relates the three phases of healing of soft tissues as just described with that seen in achilles tendon injuries. Achilles tendon injuries can be classified as described for

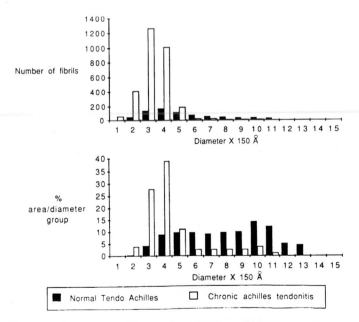

Fig. 3.15 Comparison of the number of fibrils vs. fibril diameter in patients with chronic achilles tendonitis. Also expressed as % area occupied for each diameter group vs diameter. Note the preponderance of small diameter fibrils in repairing chronic achilles tendonitis. The large normal fibrils are not replaced

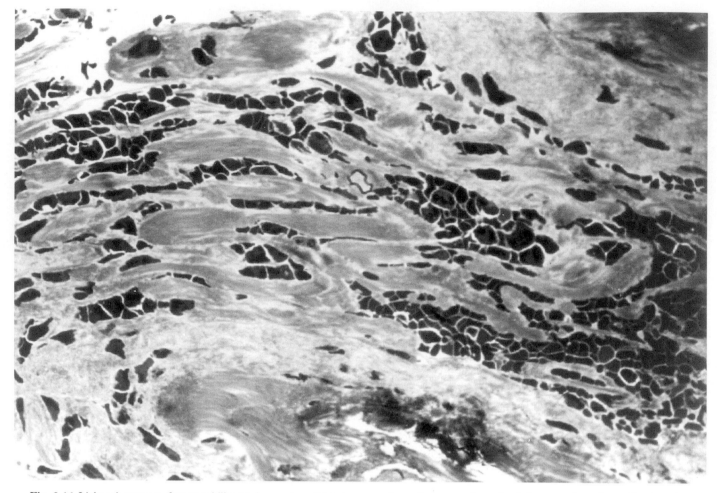

Fig. 3.16 Light microscopy of acute achilles tendon rupture. Note large numbers of extravascular red cells between the collagen fibre bundles

ligament injury, i.e. grades 1–3, with the last being complete rupture. Several patient histories will be used to illustrate these three phases of healing and attempted repair.

Grade 3: complete rupture

Patient profile: Australian Rules footballer, aged 26, powering off to avoid an opponent. Biopsy taken during surgical repair. Clinical signs were a palpable defect in the tendoachilles as well as a positive Thompson's sign.

With this disastrous injury there is both collagen bundle failure as well as vascular disruption. Hence, bleeding is a feature of these injuries when seen at an early surgical repair. This trauma to the tendon initiates the acute inflammatory phase and hence microscopically there is massive red cell extravasation and fibrin clot formation as well as collagen fibril disruption. The damaged tendon becomes oedematous and polymorphonuclear monocytes migrate into this area and release their lysosomal contents as well as actively phagocytosing cellular and other debris. Macrophages also move into the rupture site and commence phagocytosis of damaged cells and tissue. This phase lasts up to 72 hrs and is followed by the repair phase (Fig. 3.16).

Grade 2: tear

Patient profile: Australian Rules footballer with 6 months painful thickened tendoachilles. Operation: Excision of paratenon and tendon incision to remove damaged, haemorrhagic and necrotic regions. Biopsy taken for light and electronmicroscopy.

Light microscopy demonstrated a thickened paratenon and an oedematous thickened tendon. Ultrastructurally many fibroblasts have dilated rough endoplasmic reticulum and prominent nucleoli indicative of increased collagen synthesis. Apart from the many free red cells the other feature was the prevalence of many small diameter collagen fibrils not aligned or closely packed (180–200Å diameter) among the older larger pre-existing fibrils ranging from 800–1500Å diameter. Polymorphonuclear monocytes and macrophages were not common at this stage and perhaps reflects the slowness of repair in this unique tissue (Fig. 3.17).

This biopsy demonstated the features of the repair phase which follows the acute inflammatory phase and lasts from 72 hours to 4–6 weeks, but in this patient the repair phase had been perpetuated because of continued activity by the athlete. This is a common problem with these athletes because when they run the achilles tendon pain usually subsides, returning on cool-down often with a vengeance. In other patients where there is less florid tendonitis the tendon was clinically painful but not obviously enlarged, discrete areas of increased cellularity were seen in the tendon in the form of free red cells, cell debris and viable fibroblasts which were surrounded by both large and many small diameter collagen fibres. These areas were almost walled-off from the densely packed collagen of the rest of the tendon by a fibrin precipitate . These discrete areas are probably due to collagen fibre ruptures or microtears corresponding to the early part of region 2 of the load-deformation curve.

There is as yet no evidence that the use of massage or deep friction enhances this repair phase (Walker 1984).

Grade 1: injury

Patient profile: Runner, aged 25, with a painful tender lump in the achilles tendon for 18 months. Biopsy obtained at open operation.

The lump at operation was firmer than the rest of the tendon and was slightly darker in colour. On light microscopy of the biopsy taken from the nodule the changes in the collagen bundles were very subtle. There was less regular 'crimping' of the collagen bundles and they were not as tightly packed. However, ultrastructurally the cause of this less regular collagen crimp was obvious in that between large diameter fibrils were many small diameter fibrils less well oriented longitudinally. These tendons were interpreted as being in the remodelling phase as there was no increased fibroblast numbers in the nodules and no inflammatory cells were observed.

The mechanism of acute complete rupture in young athletes 'powering-off' during sprinting indicates that the gastrocnemius-soleus complex can generate sufficient force to rupture the tendon. However, tendon strength usually exceeds that of its muscle by a factor of two and hence rupture is unusual. The mechanisms involved in partial grade 1 and 2 tears in the achilles tendon are not as obvious. Viidik (1973) has shown that rat tendons in vitro undergo increasing deformation or 'plasticity' if cycled to loads less

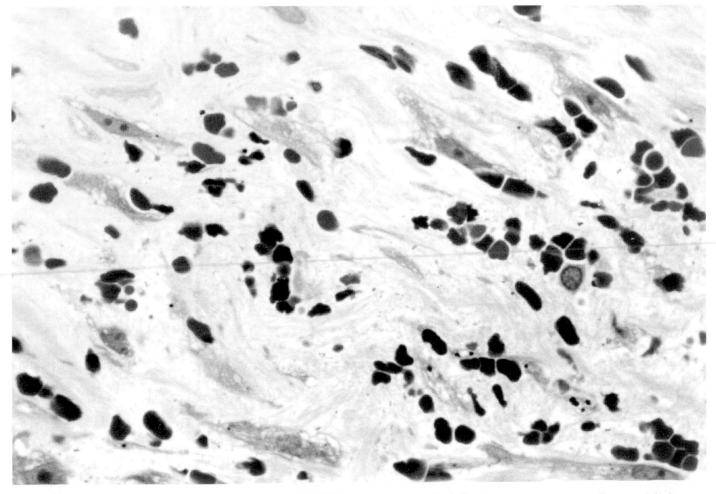

Fig. 3.17 Light micrograph of chronic repair response in the achilles tendon. Note the large fibroblasts synthesizing new collagen and the large number of extravasated red cells in this oedematous thickened tendon

than one-tenth of its failure load and the strain or deformation is well before region two or the linear part of the load-strain curve begins . Similar observations have been made both in vivo and in vitro for rat knee joint ligaments by Weisman et al (1980). It is possible that in distance runners a similar fatigue plasticity and elongation occurs in the tendon and this causes the microruptures and repair nodules already described.

The notion that some running athletes may not have an achilles tendon of sufficient cross-sectional area to sustain the repetitive tendon loading of distance without injury has been investigated by Engstrom et al (1985). They used ultrasound to measure the cross-sectional area of the human achilles tendon in vivo and validated this technique as a reliable method to measure the achilles tendon cross-sectional area using cadaver achilles tendons. Two groups of distance athletes with and without grade I achilles tendonitis who were age, weight and distance matched had their achilles tendon cross-sectional area measured using the previously validated ultrasound technique. Engstrom et al demonstrated that athletes with grade 1 type achilles tendonitis had about a 30% decrease in the cross-sectional areas of their achilles tendons (p < 0.05). This indicates that a major mechanism in this type of common injury may simply be fatigue creep failure of achilles tendon collagen (Fig. 3.18). Komi et al (1987) have recently developed an in vivo buckle tranducer which they located around the achilles tendon in a number of subjects. Direct force measurements were made on several subjects who were involved in slow walking, sprinting, jumping and hopping after calibration of the transducer. During running and jumping forces close to the previous estimated ultimate

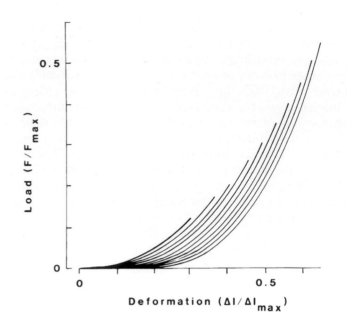

Fig. 3.18 Fatigue elongation curves postulated to occur in those athletes with chronic achilles tendonitis. These curves are from a rat hind limb tendon subjected to repeated loadings to successively higher load values to demonstrate that plasticity (the curve for the next loading is shifted to the right) before and within the linear part of the load-deformation curve. Load values are expressed i n units of maximal load and deformation values in units of the deformation at maximal load. Source: adapted from Viidik (1973)

tensile strength of the tendon were recorded, indicating that fatigue creep in a small cross-sectional tendon is a possible mechanism of injury without the need to invoke other lower limb biomechanical pathology, as has been suggested by Clement et al (1984) and Williams (1986).

REFERENCES

Amiel D, Akeson W H, Harwood F L, Frank C B 1983 Stress deprivation effect on the metabolic turnover of the medial collateral ligament collagen: a comparison between nine and 12 week immobilization. Clinical Orthopaedics and Related Research 172:265–270

Amiel D, Frank C B, Harwood F, Fronek J, Akeson W H 1984 Tendon and ligaments: a morphological and biochemical comparison. Journal of Orthopedic Research 1:257–265

Amiel D, Frey C, Woo S L-Y, Harwood F, Akeson W H 1985 Value of hyaluronic acid in the prevention of contracture formation. Clinical Orthopaedics and Related Research 196:306–311

Amiel D, Frank C B, Harwood F L, Akeson W H, Kleiner J B 1987 Collagen alteration in medial collateral ligament healing in a rabbit model. Connective Tissue Research 16:357–366

Amiel D, Ishizue K K, Harwood F L, Kitayashi L, Akeson W H 1989 Injury of the anterior cruciate ligament: the role of collagenase in ligament degeneration. Journal of Orthopedic Research 7:486–493

Arnoczky S P, Warren R F, Ashlock M A 1986 Replacement of the anterior cruciate ligament by an allograft. Journal of Bone and Joint Surgery 63A:376–385

Binkley J M, Peat M 1986 The effects of immobilization on the ultrastructure and mechanical properties of the medial collateral ligament of rats. Clinical Orthopaedics and Related Research 203:301–308

Brighton C T, Tadduni G T, Goll S R, Pollack S R 1988 Treatment of denervation/disuse osteoporosis in the rat with a capacitively coupled electrical signal: effects on bone formation and bone resorption. Journal of Orthopedic Research 6:676–684

Bruce Martin R, Burr D B 1989 Mechanical adaptation. In: Bruce Martin R, Burr D B Structure, function and adaptation of compact bone. Raven Press, New York. Ch. 6:, pp 143–185

Burr D B, Martin R B, Schaeffer M B, Radin E L 1985 Bone remodelling in response to in vivo fatigue microdamage. Journal of Biomechanics 18:189–200

Butler D L, Grood E S, Noyes F R, Zernicke R F 1979 In: Hutton R S (ed) Exercise and sports science reviews. Franklin Institute Press 6:125–181

Butler D L, Kay M D, Stouffer D C 1985 Comparison of material properties in fascicle-bone units from human patellar tendon and knee ligaments. Journal of Biomechanics 18:1-8

Cabaud H.E, Feagin J F, Rodkey W G 1980 Acute anterior cruciate ligament injury and augmented repair: experimental studies. American Journal of Sports Medicine 8:79–86

Carter D R, Hayes.W C 1977 Compact bone fatigue damage: a microscopic examination. Clinical Orthopaedics and Related Research 127:265–274

Carter D R, Caler W E, Spengler D M, Frankel V H 1981 Fatigue behaviour of adult cortical bone: the influence of mean strain and strain range. Acta Othopedica Scandinavica 52:481–490

Carter D C T, Orr E, Fyhrie D P, Schurman D J 1987 Influences of mechanical stress on prenatal and postnatal skeletal development. Clinical Orthopaedics and Related Research 219:237–250

Chaudhuri S, Nguyen H, Rangayyan R M, Walsh S, Frank C B 1987 A Fourier domain directional filtering method for analysis of collagen alignment in ligaments. IEEE Trans. Biomed. Eng. 34:509–518

Clancy W G, Narechania R G, Rosenberg T D, Gmeiner J G, Wisnefske D D, Lange T A 1981 Anterior and posterior cruciate reconstruction in Rhesus monkeys: a histological microangiographic and biochemical analysis. Journal of Bone and Joint Surgery 63A:1270–1284

Clement D B, Taunton J E, Smart G W 1984 Achilles tendinitis and peritendinitis: aetiology and treatment. American Journal of Sports Medicine12:179–184

Cohn S H, Abesemis C, Yasumura S, Aloia J, Zanzi L F, Ellis K J 1977 Comparative skeletal mass and radial bone mineral content in black and white women. Metabolism 26:171–178

Danhers L. E, Barnes A J, Burridge K W 1986 The relationship of actin to ligament contraction. Clinical Orthopaedics and Related Research 210:246–251

Engstrom C M, Hampson B.A, Williams J, Parker A W 1985 Muscle-tendon relations in runners. Abstract Proceedings of the Australian Sports Medicine Federation National Conference, Ballarat, p 56

Forwood M R, Parker D A W 1986 Effects of exercise on bone morphology. Acta Orthopedica Scandinavica 57:204–208

Forwood M R, Parker A W 1987 Effects of exercise on bone growth: mechanical and physical properties studied in the rat. Clinical Biomechanics 2:185–190

Forwood M R, Parker A W 1989 Microdamage in response to repetitive torsional loading in the rat tibia. Calcified Tissue International 45:47–53

Hart D P, Danhers L E 1987 Healing of the medial collateral ligament in rats. Journal of Bone and Joint Surgery 69A:1194–1199

Handley C J, Bateman J F, Oakes B W, Lowther D A 1975 Characterization of the collagen synthesized by cultured cartilage cells. Biochim.Biophys.Acta 386:444–450

Hey N J, Handley C J, Ng C K, Oakes B W 1990 Characterization and synthesis of macromolecules by adult collateral ligament. Biochemica et Biophysica Acta 1034:73–80

Kastelic J, Galeski A, Baer E 1978 The multicomposite structure of tendon. Connective Tissue Research 6:11-23

Komi P V, Salonen M, Jarvinen M, Kokko O 1987 In vivo registration of achilles tendon forces in man. Methodological development. International Journal of Sports Medicine 8:3–8

Lanyon L E 1987 Functional strain in bone as an objective, and controlling stimulus for adaptive bone remodelling. Journal of Biomechanics 20(11/12):1083–1093

Larsen N, Parker A W 1982 In: Sports medicine: medical and scientific aspects of elitism in sport, vol. 8. Howell M L, Parker A W (eds) Proceedings of the Australian Sports Medicine Federation. pp 63–73

Leichter I, Simkin A, Margulies J Y, Bivas A, Steinberg R, Giladi M, Milgrom C 1989 Gain in mass density of bone following strenous activity. Journal of Orthopaedic Research7:86–90

MacFarlane B J, Edwards P, Frank C, Rangayyan B, Liu Z-Q 1989 Quantification of collagen remodelling in healing nonimmobilized and immobilized ligaments. Transactions of Orthopaedic Research Society 14:300

Marguia M J, Vailas A, Mandelbaum B, Norton Hodgdon J, Goforth H, Riedy M 1988 Elevated plasma hydroxyproline: a possible risk factor associated with connective tissue injuries during overuse. American Journal of Sports Medicine16:660–664

Merrilles M J, Flint M H 1980 Ultrastructural study of the tension and pressure zones in a rabbit flexor tendon. American Journal of Anatomy 157:87–106

Michna M 1984 Morphometric analysis of loading-induced changes in collagen-fibril populations in young tendons. Cell Tissue Research 236:465–470

Noyes F R, Torvic P J, Hyde W B, De Lucas J L 1974 Biomechanics of ligament failure. 2. An analysis of immobilization, exercise and reconditioning effects in primates. Journal of Bone and Joint Surgery 56A:1406–1418

Oakes B W 1981 Acute soft tissue injuries-nature and Management. Australian Family Physician 10:Supplement 1–16

Oakes B W 1988 Ultrastructural studies on knee joint ligaments: quantitation of collagen fibre populations in exercised and control rat cruciate ligaments and in human anterior cruciate ligament grafts. In: Buckwalter J, Woo S L-Y (eds) Injury and repair of the musculoskeletal tissues. American Academy of Orthopaedic Surgeons, Illinois, Section 2, pp 66–82

Oakes B W, Parker A W, Norman J 1981 Changes in collagen fibre populations in young rat cruciate ligaments in response to an intensive one month's exercise program. In: Russo P, Gass G (eds) Human adaption. Department of Biological Sciences, Cumberland College of Health Sciences, pp 223–230

Parker A W, Larsen N 1981 Changes in the strength of bone and ligament in response to training. In: Russo P, Gass G (eds) Human adaption. Department of Biological Sciences, Cumberland College of Health Sciences pp 209–221

Parry D A D, Flint M H, Gillard G C, Craig A S 1982 A role for glycosaminoglycans in the development of collagen fibrils. FEBS Letters 149:1–7

Parry D A D, Barnes G R G, Craig A S 1978 A comparison of the size distribution of collagen fibrils in connective tissues as a function of age and a possible relation between fibril size and distribution and mechanical properties. Proceedings of Royal Society London B, 203:305–321

Pead M, Skerry T M, Lanyon L E 1988 Direct transformation from quiescence to bone formation in the adult periosteum following a single brief period of bone loading. Journal of Bone and Mineral Research 3:647–656

Piper T L, Whiteside L A 1980 Early mobilization after knee ligament repair in dogs: an experimental study. Clinical Orthopaedics and Related Research 150:277–282

Riggs B L, Melton J L 1986 Involutional osteoporosis. New England Journal of Medicine 314:1676–1686

Rubin C T, McLeod K J, Lanyon L E 1989 Prevention of osteoporosis by pulsed electromagnetic fields. Journal of Bone and Joint Surgery 71-A:411–416

Rubin C T, Pratt G W, Porter A L, Lanyon L E, Poss R 1987 The use of ultrasound in vivo to determine acute change in the mechanical properties of bone following intense physical activity. Journal of Biomechanics 20(7):723–72

Rubin C T, Lanyon L E 1987 Osteoregulatory nature of mechanical stimuli: function as a determinant for adaptive remodelling in bone. Journal of Orthopedic Research 5:300–310

Shadwick R E 1986 The role of collagen crosslinks in the age related changes in mechanical properties of digital tendons. Proceedings of North American Congress on Biomechanics 1:137–138

Shino K, Oakes B.W, Inoue M, Horibe S, Nakata K, Ono K 1990 Human ACL allograft: collagen fibril populations studied as a function of age of the graft. Transactions of 36th Annual Meeting of Orthopaedic Research Society

Skerry T M, Bitensky L, Chayen J, Lanyon L 1988 Loading-related reorientation of bone proteoglycan in vivo. Strain memory in bone tissue? Journal of Orthopaedic Research 6:547–551

Stanish W, Rubinovich R M, Curwin S 1986 Eccentric exercise in chronic tendonitis. Clinical Orthopaedics and Related Research 208:65–68

Tipton C M, James S L Mergner W, Tcheng T K 1970 Influence of exercise on the strength of the medial collateral knee ligament of dogs. American Journal of Physiology 218:894–902

Tipton C M, Matthes R D, Maynard J A, Carey R A 1975 The influence of physical activity on ligaments and tendons. Medicine and Science in Sports 7:165–175

Tipton C M, Vailas A C, Matthes R.D 1986 Experimental studies on the influences of physical activity on ligaments, tendons and joints: a brief review. Acta Medica Scandinavica Supplement 711:157–168

Tipton C M, Vailas A C 1989 Bone and connective tissue adaptions to physical activity. In: Bouchard C, Shephard R J, Stephens T, Sutton J R, McPherson B D (eds) Exercise, fitness and health. A consensus of current knowledge. Proceedings of International Conference on Exercise Fitness and Health, Toronto 1988. Human Kinetics, Champaign, Ilinois pp 331–344

Toole B P, Lowther D A 1968 The effect of chondroitin sulphate-protein on the formation of collagen fibrils in vitro . Biochemical Journal 109:857–866

Vailas A C, Tipton C M, Matthes R D, Gart M 1981 Physical activity and its influence on the repair process of medial collateral ligaments. Connective Tissue Research 9:25–31

Viidik A 1973 Functional properties of connective tissues. International Review of Connective Tissue Research 6:127–215

Viidik A 1980 Interdependence between structure and function. In: Viidik A, Vuust J eds Biology of collagen. Academic Press, London

Walker J 1984 Deep transverse frictions in ligament healing. Journal of Orthopaedic Sports Physical Therapy 6:89–94

Wong M, Carter D R 1988 Mechanical stresses and morphogenic enchondral ossification in the sternum. Transactions of Orthopaedic Research Society 13:241

Woo L-Y, Gomez M A T, Sites J, Newton P O, Orlando C A, Akeson W H 1987 The biomechanical and morphological changes in the medial collateral ligament of the rabbit after immobilization and remobilization. Journal of Bone and Joint Surgery 69A:1200–1211

Weisman G, Pope M H, Johnson R J 1980 Cyclical loading in knee ligament injuries. American Journal of Sports Medicine 8:24–30

Williams J G P 1986 Achilles tendon lesions in sport. Sports Medicine 3:114–135

4. Physiological responses to injury: synovial joint structures

Christopher J. Handley

This chapter reviews the structure and function of two important tissues of the diarthrodial joint, namely articular cartilage and synovial membrane. Articular cartilage covers the ends of bones and allows the distribution of compressive loads over the cross-section of bones as well as providing a near-frictionless and wear-resistant surface for joint movement. The synovial membrane covers all the internal surfaces of the synovial joint other than those made up of articular cartilage or meniscal cartilage if present. The cells of the synovial membrane are responsible for the synthesis of some macromolecular components of synovial fluid. The other components of synovial fluid originate from blood plasma. Both articular cartilage and synovial membrane are exposed in vivo to varying mechanical forces as a consequence of movement of the diarthrodial joint. This chapter will also review the role of mechanical force on the function and rehabilitation of these two tissues.

ARTICULAR CARTILAGE

Structure of articular cartilage

Adult articular cartilage is an avascular and aneural tissue made up of cells, known as chondrocytes, that are embedded in an extracellular matrix consisting of an insoluble network of mainly type II collagen fibres (Hascall & Hascall 1981). Trapped within the pores of the collagen network is a highly hydrated gel made up of proteoglycan aggregate (Fig. 4.1A). It is the extracellular matrix of the articular cartilage that gives this tissue its unique biomechanical properties. In both adult and developing articular cartilage, chondrocytes are responsible for the synthesis and maintenance of the extracellular matrix. If the metabolism of chondrocytes is altered or components of the extracellular matrix of articular cartilage are lost as a consequence of disease or injury, there will be a change in the mechanical function of the tissue (Kempson 1975).

Type II collagen molecules exist in the extracellular matrix of articular cartilage as covalently cross-linked fibres (Fig. 4.1A). It is these fibres that give articular cartilage its

tensile mechanical properties (Eyre 1980). If the formation of inter- and intra-molecular cross-links are interfered with, the tensile properties of the collagen network will be reduced. Also present in the extracellular matrix of cartilage is type IX collagen, which can make up to 20% of the total collagen present in this tissue. Type IX collagen belongs to the group of collagen molecules that do not form fibres and has been shown to contain one chondroitin sulphate chain (Vaughan et al 1985). Immunolocalization experiments have shown that type IX collagen is located throughout the extracellular matrix of articular cartilage and appears to be closely associated with the type II collagen fibres. Indeed, it has recently been shown that covalent cross-links exist between type II and type IX collagen (Eyre

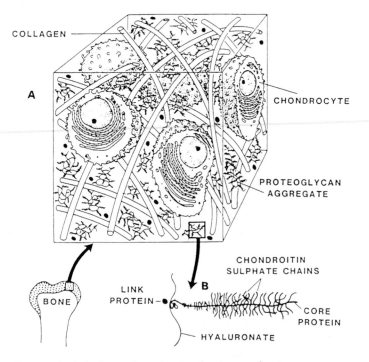

Fig. 4.1 A. Articular cartilage showing the macromolecular components of the extracellular matrix of the tissue; B. detailed structure of the proteoglycan aggregate

et al 1990). This has led to the suggestion that type IX collagen may be involved in the cross-linking of type II collagen fibres, thereby increasing the stability and strength of the collagen network. It has been further suggested that in early stages of osteoarthritis the cross-links formed between type II and IX collagen may be broken, resulting in larger pores within the collagen fibre network.

The major proteoglycan species present in cartilage is the cartilage specific aggregating proteoglycan (aggrecan). This macromolecule is very large ($\sim 3 \times 10^6$ daltons). It comprises a protein core to which approximately 80 keratan sulphate and 120 chondroitin sulphate glycosaminoglycan chains are attached (Fig. 4.1B) (Hascall & Hascall 1981, Handley et al 1985). These glycosaminoglycan chains contain on average one sulphate and one carboxyl group per disaccharide, which results in the aggregating proteoglycan having an extremely high negative fixed charge. The N-terminal region of the core protein of the aggregating proteoglycan contains a domain that binds to hyaluronate, a linear non-sulphated glycosaminoglycan present in cartilage. The binding between these two macromolecules is stabilized by a third component, the link protein. Many aggregating proteoglycans can bind to a molecule of hyaluronate to give an enormous structure referred to as the proteoglycan aggregate (Fig. 4.1B). The size of the proteoglycan aggregate is believed to be important in holding it within the collagen network. Other proteoglycan types have been reported to be present in the extracellular matrix of articular cartilage; they belong to the group of small proteoglycans (decorin and biglycan) which contain one or two glycosaminoglycan chains (Handley & Ng 1992). These proteoglycans appear to be associated with type II collagen fibres and there is evidence they may be involved in the regulation of the formation and maintenance of the collagen fibre network (Scott & Orford 1981).

Other non-collagenous macromolecular components of the extracellular matrix of articular cartilage have been isolated and characterized (Heinegärd & Oldberg 1989). Because little is known about the exact function of these macromolecules it is difficult to comment on their role in the maintenance and organization of the extracellular matrix of articular cartilage. Indeed, their physiological role is likely to be subtle and perturbations in the concentrations of these components in the extracellular matrix of cartilage as the result of disease and injury may be reflected in the physical properties of the tissue.

Articular cartilage is not a homogeneous tissue. This tissue, in mature animals, can be divided into three distinct regions, the superficial, middle and deep regions (Schenk et al 1986). Within each region there are differences among the size, distribution and metabolism of chondrocytes as well as in the organization, concentration and species of macromolecular components that make up the extracellular matrix of the tissue. The surface layer has greater cellularity but the cells are small, flattened and arranged so that their longitudinal axis is parallel to the surface. The collagen fibres within this region are so organized that they run parallel to the surface and the proteoglycan content of this layer is low. There have been reports that at the extreme superficial surface of this region there is an amorphous layer which appears to contain negatively charged macromolecules (Stanescu 1990). Proteoglycans do not appear to be present in this structure and it has been suggested that this region is made up of glycoproteins which act to lubricate the movement of the two opposing cartilage surfaces.

The middle region consists of chondrocytes randomly distributed in an extracellular matrix of type II collagen fibres rich in proteoglycan aggregate. The deep region contains chondrocytes arranged in columns in an extracellular matrix with a composition similar to that of the middle region of articular cartilage. The cells in this region undergo division and are morphologically distinct from the chondrocytes in the middle region. In the deeper zones of this region the columns of chondrocytes are surrounded by a non-mineralized matrix which subsequently calcifies next to the subchondral bone. Chondrocytes from these different regions of articular cartilage synthesize macromolecular components of the extracellular matrix at different rates. The chondrocytes in the hypertrophic region have the highest rate of metabolism. As well as regional differences through articular cartilage, there are reports that differences occur both in the composition and metabolism of articular cartilage from the same regions in low and high weight-bearing regions of the tissue (Maroudas et al 1990).

Regardless of the region of articular cartilage, the macromolecular components present in the extracellular matrix of cartilage are constantly being turned over: they are synthesized, incorporated into the extracellular matrix and selectively degraded, resulting in the loss of the macromolecules from the tissue (Handley et al 1990). These processes are dependent on the metabolic activity of the chondrocytes and in mature articular cartilage are so regulated that the rate of synthesis and incorporation into the extracellular matrix equals the rate of degradation of the molecule. This steady state metabolism results in the maintenance of constant levels of macromolecular components of the extracellular matrix of articular cartilage.

The avascularity of articular cartilage in mature animals raises the question of how chondrocytes obtain metabolites necessary for their metabolic activities. All metabolites and growth factors appear to reach the chondrocytes by passive diffusion from the synovial membrane through the extracellular matrix of cartilage. The thickness of articular cartilage increases with the size of animal. In the humans the articular cartilage present on the femur can be as much as 2.3 mm thick (Stockwell 1971). Since the overall cellularity of cartilage does not differ significantly among species, this means that individual chondrocytes are

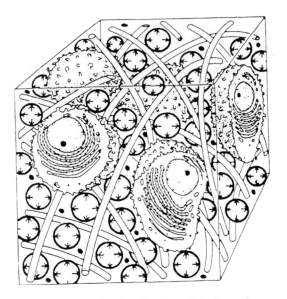

Fig. 4.2 Articular cartilage showing the effect of the internal pressure created by the affinity of the proteoglycan aggregate for water; circles and arrows depict the direction of the pressure

separated by more extracellular matrix. Therefore, in larger animals, metabolites and growth factors must travel greater distances in order to reach the chondrocytes. This limitation on the availability of nutrients and growth factors means that chondrocytes exist in vivo under conditions of limiting oxygen and metabolite concentrations. In terms of the generation of energy necessary for cellular activity, chondrocytes generate energy by substrate level phosphorylation via the conversion of glucose to lactate.

Mechanical properties of articular cartilage

Movement of the diarthrodial joint results in articular cartilage being exposed to both compressive and shear loads. The molecular composition of the extracellular matrix of articular cartilage allows for the absorption of

such mechanical loads as well as the distribution of compressive loads over the entire cross-section of the underlying bone. The tensile properties of articular cartilage come from the collagen network: the intra- and intermolecular cross-links give an insoluble network that will resist tensile forces originating from both shear and compressive loads experienced by this tissue. The collagen network may be further stabilized by interactions with minor collagens and proteoglycans, as well as with non-collagenous macromolecules. Within the pores of the collagen network, which have been estimated to be approximately 4 nm in diameter, proteoglycan aggregate is trapped mainly because of its very large size (Maroudas et al 1986). There may be specific interactions between components of the proteoglycan aggregate and other macromolecular components of the extracellular matrix.

The high fixed charge density associated with the proteoglycan aggregate results in the macromolecule being able to attract and bind water. Since proteoglycan aggregate is confined within the pores of the collagen network, it is unable to swell because of the tensile constraints exerted by the collagen network. This results in the generation of an internal pressure within the extracellular matrix of cartilage (Maroudas et al 1986). This internal pressure results in the extracellular matrix of articular cartilage being stiff and able to resist both compressive and shear forces (Fig. 4.2). When cartilage is compressed, water is displaced from the proteoglycan aggregate. After some time, an equilibrium is reached where no more movement of water occurs. On release of the compressive load, water will re-enter the tissue, driven by the affinity of the proteoglycan aggregate for water (Fig. 4.3). This movement of water is critical for a number of reasons. Fluid that is displaced from the surface of articular cartilage is believed to enhance the lubricating properties of the surface of articular cartilage. Since water is incompressible, the movement of fluid within the extracellular matrix of articular cartilage brought about

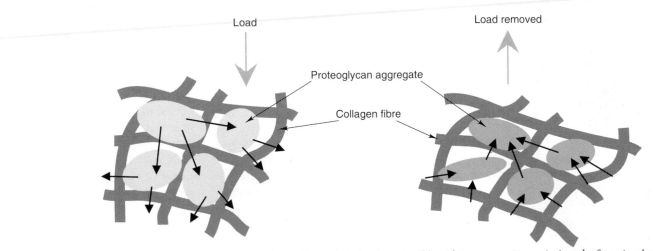

Fig. 4.3 Movement of water in and out of articular cartilage when the tissue is subjected to compression and when the force is relaxed

by a compressive load will result in the further displacement of fluid on either side of the point of compression. This results in the articular cartilage being able to spread compressive loads over a considerable surface area, which is important in protecting the underlying bone from excess loading. As pointed out previously since articular cartilage is avascular, nutrients and growth factors can only reach the cells from the synovial fluid by diffusion, which is a very slow process. Therefore, movement of fluid within and into and out of the extracellular matrix of articular cartilage, as the result of compressive loading and unloading the tissue, will enhance the rate at which these molecules reach the chondrocytes in the extracellular matrix.

A net loss of proteoglycans from the extracellular matrix of cartilage, such as that observed in diseased cartilage, will result in changes in the biomechanical properties of the tissue. The tissue will become less resistant to both compressive and shear forces (Kempson 1975). This will result in wear and damage of the collagen network, leading to fibrillation of the articular surface. The loss of proteoglycan aggregate will also result in a decreased ability of articular cartilage to distribute mechanical loads over the underlying bone, leading to degenerative changes in this tissue. These changes in the mechanical properties of the extracellular matrix of cartilage will ultimately result in changes to the metabolism of the chondrocytes and further exacerbate the already degenerative condition of the tissue.

Proteoglycan aggregate loss from articular cartilage is observed in a number of pathological conditions, including mechanical trauma, inflammation (inflammatory arthritis) and degenerative changes (osteoarthritis).

In contrast to articular cartilage, the meniscal cartilage of the knee joint is an example of fibrocartilage being made up of thick fibres of type I collagen arranged in a radial manner. Trapped within this collagen network are proteoglycan aggregates similar to those observed in articular cartilage. When the knee joint is compressed the meniscus, being wedge-shaped, is forced towards the outside of the joint, resulting in the generation of radial tensile stresses within the meniscus. These are counteracted by the orientation of the collagen fibres within this tissue (Mow et al 1990). In the knee joint, the meniscal cartilage has been reported as enhancing the distribution of loads across the tibial and femoral surfaces as well as assisting in the lubrication of these two articular surfaces (Dettaven 1990). The meniscal cartilage has also been implicated in maintaining the mechanical stability of the knee joint. Removal of the meniscus has been shown to decrease the contact area between the two articular surfaces of the knee joint, resulting in greater stresses being applied to areas of articular cartilage in this joint (Dettaven 1990). Meniscetomy has been shown to induce degenerative changes in the articular cartilage of the knee joint of experimental animals and it has been suggested that similar degenerative changes occur in humans on removal of the meniscus (DeHaven et al 1990). It is now common for partial meniscetomy to be performed to correct torn menisci, and suturing the torn meniscus is often attempted in order to maximize its contribution to the function of the knee joint.

Response of articular cartilage to injury

Buckwalter et al (1990) have separated articular cartilage injuries into three categories: conditions involving (1) the loss of macromolecules from the extracellular matrix of the tissue; (2) the mechanical disruption of the extracellular matrix and cells of cartilage; and (3) the disruption of both cartilage and the underlying bone.

Injuries that result in the loss of macromolecules from the extracellular matrix of articular cartilage are the consequence of infection or inflammation within the synovial capsule, prolonged immobilization of a joint over a week and mild blunt trauma such as falling on a joint. In all these conditions, loss of proteoglycan aggregate from the extracellular matrix of articular cartilage is a common feature. In inflammation and infection of the synovial joint, this loss of proteoglycan aggregate from cartilage can be brought about by factors such as proteolytic enzymes and free radicals entering the matrix of the tissue and directly degrading the proteoglycan aggregate. Furthermore these factors, with cytokines from inflammatory cells and toxins from bacteria if present, interact with the chondrocytes and change their metabolism, resulting in elevated rates of breakdown of proteoglycan aggregate and inhibition in the synthesis of proteoglycan (Handley et al 1990). In the early stages of these injuries the loss of proteoglycan aggregate is usually reversible if the damaging stimulus is stopped. However, if the situation is allowed to continue, the loss of proteoglycan is irreversible and the permanent depletion of proteoglycan from the cartilage matrix will lead to further degenerative changes in the tissue, including the loss of the collagen network.

For example, when a single inflammatory reaction occurs in a synovial joint, there is an immediate loss of proteoglycan aggregate from the tissue and a decrease in the ability of the chondrocytes to replace the lost proteoglycan (Lowther & Gillard 1976, Gillard & Lowther 1976). This situation remains for 5–6 days, after which the chondrocytes regain the ability to synthesize and replace proteoglycans. After 3–4 weeks, the proteoglycan content of the tissue is returned to normal and the extracellular matrix regains its normal biomechanical properties. If the joint is exposed to a number of inflammatory attacks, as in inflammatory arthritis, the ability of the chondrocytes to replace the proteoglycan is lost and the chronic situation results in the severe damage of the collagen network and ultimately the loss of cartilage from the bone.

Mechanical disruption of articular cartilage can result from blunt trauma of the tissue which may not result in fractures to the matrix. Little is known about the response of articular cartilage to blunt trauma, except that changes in the water content and collagen fibre structure have been observed (Donohue et al 1983). Buckwalter et al (1990) suggested that the response of cartilage to this type of injury probably depends on the degree of injury. Penetrating injuries of articular cartilage will result in fractures through the matrix of the tissue. A similar situation is observed in osteoarthritis where fibrillation of the matrix of articular cartilage occurs. This fibrillation begins at the articular surface and, with time, proceeds into the deeper regions of the tissue. In both situations there is poor repair of the extracellular matrix since this type of injury does not elicit an inflammatory response or migration of chondrocytes to the site of injury. Inflammation is an important process in the repair of other connective tissues, such as skin and bone, where cells (fibroblasts) which are responsible for repair, can migrate into the injury and secrete collagen, thus creating an area of repair. In cartilage, chondrocytes near the fracture site divide and form clusters of cells in an attempt to synthesize matrix components. However, the repaired matrix is weak and breaks down easily when subjected to normal mechanical loads over 6 months (Buckwalter et al 1990).

When the injury to articular cartilage involves the underlying bone, an inflammatory response occurs, a fibrin clot is formed and fibroblasts migrate into the wound from the bone and secrete an extracellular matrix which is initially indistinguishable from the normal cartilage. However, with time fibrillation and degeneration of the repaired matrix occur within the repair site, whic suggests that there are differences in both the composition and the biomechanical properties of the normal and the repaired area.

Response of articular cartilage to immobilization and mechanical stimulation

Articular cartilage has been shown to be sensitive to both immobilization and mechanical stimulation. Caterson & Lowther (1978) showed changes in the metabolism and composition of articular cartilage of the metacarpal-phalangeal joint, when the forelimb of a sheep was placed in a cast so that the whole limb was immobilized and did not bear weight. After 4 weeks' immobilization there was an observed decrease in both the rate of synthesis and in the tissue levels of proteoglycan of articular cartilage from the immobilized joint compared to similar tissue from the metatarsalphalangeal joints of the rear limbs. The contralateral joint of the forelimb of the experimental animal was subjected to increased compressive loads. Analysis of the articular cartilage from the limb revealed elevated tissue levels and rates of synthesis of proteoglycan. Palmoski et al (1979) described similar results for dogs that had one hind limb immobilized for 1 week. They further demonstrated

that the removal of the cast stimulated the synthesis of proteoglycan by the tissue and, 2 weeks later, the tissue proteoglycan levels had returned to normal. In a later series of experiments it was shown that if the animals were subjected to vigorous exercise after removal of the cast there was no reversal in either the synthesis or tissue levels of proteoglycan (Palmoski & Brandt 1981).

It has been suggested that the above effects on articular cartilage from immobilized joints may partly be due to the lack of nutrients or growth factors reaching the chondrocytes since there is neither mixing of the synovial fluid or movement of fluid within the extracellular matrix of the tissue (Caterson & Lowther 1978). Investigations using chondrocyte cultures or explant cultures of articular cartilage, where gradients of nutrients or growth factors were minimized, showed that the chondrocytes themselves appear to be sensitive to compressive forces of frequencies greater than 0.01 Hz (De Witt et al 1984). These observations point to a direct sensing of mechanical loads by chondrocytes and thereby suggests that mechanical stimulus and joint movement must be considered in the therapy of articular cartilage. Regular running of moderation duration has been shown in a number of animal models to increase the amount of proteoglycan present in the matrix of the tissue (Säämänen et al 1989). This suggests that, in training, a moderate running regime will increase the compressive strength of articular cartilage over time.

Response of articular cartilage to rehabilitation

A number of approaches have been taken to repair articular cartilage after injury. Invasive procedures include shaving the surface of articular cartilage, exposing cartilage to the subchondral bone in order to induce cell invasion and repair, grafting articular cartilage, implantating synthetic matrices and implantating chondrocytes. It has been suggested that the use of various growth factors, either specific to cartilage or capable of inducing chondrogenesis, may be of future use with the above surgical procedures or on their own (Handley et al 1986). With the exception of the shaving of cartilage, these approaches are largely experimental and there is little data on the long-term outcome on articular cartilage structure and biomechanics.

Non-invasive therapies, including passive movement of joints, have been investigated as possible ways to induce repair of articular cartilage. As previously pointed out, articular cartilage will respond to movement and mechanical force since immobilization of joints leads to degradation of the tissue. There have been a number of studies investigating the potential of the application of mechanical stimulus to joints to enhance the rate and quality of repair by articular cartilage. Salter, one of the original researchers in the area, and others have investigated the effect of continuous passive motion on the ability of cartilage to repair itself (for review see Salter 1990). Using young rabbits, they showed that continual passive motion enhances articular cartilage repair after full-thickness injury or septic inflammation to the tissue. The use of continuous passive motion to enhance repair by cartilage is still to be assessed in humans.

SYNOVIAL MEMBRANE

Structure and function of the synovial membrane

The synovium can be divided into three regions; the synovial lining or membrane, the subsynovial tissue and the joint capsule. The synovial membrane in normal tissue is three or four cell layers thick and is attached to the subsynovial tissue. The role of the synovial membrane is to synthesize components of synovial fluid and to remove particulate matter by phagocytosis. To this end, the cells that make up the synovial membrane can be divided into two populations, type A and type B cells (Barland et al 1962). The morphology of the type A cells suggests they are involved in the uptake of material from synovial fluid and it has been suggested that they are involved in the phagocytotic activity of the synovial membrane. Similarly, the synthetic activity of the synovial membrane is attributed to the type B cells (Barland et al 1962).

The synovial lining cells are attached to the subsynovial tissue that contains connective tissue cells surrounded by an extracellular matrix, fat cells, a fine blood capillary network, lymph vessels and a few nerve endings. The subsynovial tissue is associated with the joint capsule which is a fibrous connective tissue of similar composition to the collateral ligament which gives the synovium its mechanical strength. The joint capsule contains most of the nerve endings present in the synovium.

The synovial fluid is made up of components originating from blood plasma and from type B synovial cells. Electrolytes and low molecular weight nutrients present in the synovial fluid originate from plasma and reach the synovial space from the capillary bed in the subsynovial tissue by diffusion. The transport of glucose into the synovial fluid appears to be through a specific transport system. The transport of large molecules from the plasma into the synovial fluid is a selective process which is dependent on the molecular size of the macromolecules and is regulated by the exclusion effect of the extracellular matrix of the subsynovial tissue. In normal synovial fluid, large molecules such as immunoglobulin M and fibrinogen are present in small amounts. Other macromolecular components of the synovial fluid are synthesized by the cells of the synovial membrane. These include hyaluronate and a glycoprotein involved in lubrication of the articular surfaces. The synovial lining cells remove debris present in the synovial fluid and some macromolecules by phagocytosis. Other macromolecules exit from the synovial fluid via the lymphatic system present in the synovium. The dynamics of loss of these macromolecules suggest that there is an active process of removal which is not dependent on the molecular size of the exiting molecules.

Response of synovial membrane to injury, immobilization and rehabilitation

Inflammation within the synovial space leads to dramatic changes in not only the structure but also the function of the synovial membrane. Cell division results in the thickening of the synovial membrane as well as the subsynovial tissue. Associated with this is pain and discomfort when joint movement occurs (Fassbender 1986). With time, the synovium will invade the joint space and form a pannus which covers the surface of articular cartilage. The metabolism of the synovial cells is altered, proteolytic enzymes are secreted into the synovial fluid and onto the surface of articular cartilage. These proteolytic enzymes are responsible for the loss of components of the extracellular matrix of cartilage (Harris 1981). The permeability of the synovium also changes as a consequence of inflammation, resulting in more larger macromolecules appearing in the synovial fluid from the plasma. The inflammation of the synovium may be severe enough to change the mechanical properties of the joint capsule and associated ligaments, thus leading to joint destabilization. The immobilization of human joints over various periods of time has been reported to lead to the proliferation of the synovium and a pannus type of structure similar to that observed in inflammatory arthritis (Enneking & Horowitz 1972).

Surgical removal of the inflamed synovium is a common procedure in a number of inflammatory joint disorders (Gschwend 1985). Removal of the tissue reduces the symptoms and slows the progression of the inflammation. However, with time, the synovium will grow back. A number of approaches to control this regrowth have been used. These include chemical and radiation therapy. Continuous passive motion is used in the post-operative management of the joint to enhance motion of the affected joint (Salter 1990).

SUMMARY

Without mechanical stimulation, both articular cartilage and synovial membrane undergo degenerative changes that result in these tissues losing their biological function. In the case of articular cartilage there is a loss of proteoglycan which results in the tissue being unable to support compressive and shear loads. Gentle mechanical loading of the immobilized joint will result in increasing the rate of proteoglycan synthesis and, after 2–3 weeks, normal proteoglycan levels are observed in the extracellular matrix of the tissue. A similar reversal of tissue proteoglycan levels is seen in articular cartilage from joints in which a single acute inflammatory reaction has occurred. However, when the collagen network of articular cartilage has been damaged, as occurs in long-term immobilization of joints, excessive load-bearing or multiple inflammatory attacks, it is apparent that the chondrocytes are unable to repair this structural component. This inability of articular cartilage to repair the collagen network also restricts the capacity of the tissue to respond to surgical procedures. There is still no clear method of how to induce articular cartilage to heal, especially to repair damage to the collagen network so as to give a biomechanically functional tissue.

REFERENCES

Barland P, Novikoff A B, Hamermond 1962 1962 Electron microscopy of the human synovial membrane. Journal of Cell Biology 14:207-220

Buckwalter J A, Rosenberg L C, Hunziker 1990 Articular cartilage: composition, structure, response to injury, and methods of facilitating repair. In: Ewing J W (ed) Articular cartilage and knee joint function: basic science and arthroscopy. Raven Press, New York

Caterson B, Lowther D A 1978 Changes in the metabolism of the proteoglycans from sheep articular cartilage in response to mechanical stress. Biochimica et Biophysica Acta 540:412-422

DeHaven K E 1990 Articular cartilage: composition, structure, response to injury, and methods of facilitating repair. In: Ewing J W (ed) Articular cartilage and knee joint function: basic science and arthroscopy. Raven Press, New York

De Witt M T, Handley C J, Oakes B W, Lowther D A 1984 In vitro response of chondrocytes to mechanical loading. The effect of short term mechanical tension. Connective Tissue Research 12:97-109

Donohue J M, Buss D, Oegema T R, Thompson R C 1983 The effects of indirect blunt trauma on adult canine articular cartilage. Journal of Bone and Joint Surgery 65A:948-957

Enneking W F, Horowitz M 1972 The intra-articular effects of immobilization on the human knee. Journal of Bone and Joint Surgery 54A:973-985

Eyre D R 1980 Collagen: molecular diversity in the body's protein scaffold. Science 207:1315-1322

Eyre D R, Wu J J, Niyibizi C, Chun L 1990 The cartilage collagens—analysis of their cross-linking interactions and matrix organization. In: Maroudas A, Kuettner J (eds) Methods in cartilage research. Academic Press, London

Fassbender H G 1986 Joint destruction in various arthritic diseases. In: Kuettner K E, Schleyerbach R, Hascall V C (eds) Articular cartilage biochemistry. Raven Press, New York

Gillard G C, Lowther D A 1976 Carrageenin-induced arthritis. II. Effect of intraarticular injection of carrageenin on the synthesis of proteoglycan in articular cartilage. Arthritis and Rheumatism 19:918-922

Gschwend N 1985 Synovectomy. In: Kelley W N, Harris E D, Ruddy S, Sledge C B (eds) Textbook of rheumatology. W B Saunders, Philadelphia

Handley C J, Lowther D A, McQuillan D J 1985 The structure and synthesis of proteoglycens of articular cartilage. Cell Biology International Reports 9:753-782

Handley C J, McQuillan D J, Campbell M A, Bolis S 1986 Steady-state metabolism in cartilage explants. In: Kuettner K E, Schleyerbach R, Hascall V C (eds) Articular cartilage biochemistry. Raven Press, New York

Handley C J, Ng C K, Curtis A J 1990 Short- and long-term explant culture of cartilage. In: Maroudas A, Kuettner J (eds) Methods in cartilage research. Academic Press, London

Handley C J, Ng C K 1992 Proteoglycan, hyaluronan and non collagenons matrix protein metabolism by chardrocytes. In: Adolphe m (ed) Biological regulation of the chondrocytes. CRC Press, Boca Raton

Harris E D 1981 Pathogenesis of rheumatoid arthritis. In: Kelley W N, Harris E D, Ruddy S, Sledge B (eds) Textbook of rheumatology. W B Saunders, Philadelphia

Hascall V C, Hascall G K 1981 Proteoglycans. In: Hay E (ed) Cell biology of the extracellular matrix. Plenum, New York

Heinegärd D, Oldberg Å 1989 Structure and biology of cartilage and bone matrix non-collagenous macromolecules. Federation of American Societies for Experimental Biology Journal 3:2042-2051

Kempson G E 1975 The effects of proteoglycan and collagen degradation on the mechanical properties of adult human articular cartilage. In: Burleigh P M C, Poole A R (eds) Dynamics of connective tissue macromolecules. North-Holland, Amsterdam

Lowther D A, Gillard G C 1976 Carrageenin-induced arthritis. I. The effect of intraarticular carrageenin on the chemical composition of articular cartilage. Arthritis and Rheumatism 19:769-776

Maroudas A, Katz E P, Wachtel E J, Soudry M 1986 Physiochemical properties and functional behavior of normal and osteoarthritic human cartilage. In: Kuettner K E, Schleyerbach R, Hascall V C (eds) Articular cartilage biochemistry. Raven Press, New York

Maroudas A, Schneirderman R, Weineberg C, Grushko G 1990 Choice of specimens in comparative studies involving human femoral head cartilage. In: Maroudas A, Kuettner K (eds) Methods in cartilage research. Academic Press, London

Palmoski M J, Brandt K D 1981 Running inhibits the reversal of atrophic changes in canine knee cartilage after removal of a leg cast. Arthritis and Rheumatism 24:1329-1337

Palmoski M J, Perricone, E, Brandt K D 1979 Development and reversal of a proteoglycan aggregation defect in normal canine knee cartilage after immobilization. Arthritis and Rheumatism 22:508-517

Säämänen A-M, Tammi M, Kiviranta I, Jurvellin J, Helminen H J 1989 Levels of chondroitin-6-sulphate and nonaggregating proteoglycans at articular cartilage contact sites in the knees of young dogs subjected to moderate running exercise. Arthritis and Rheumatism 32:1282-1292

Salter R B 1990 The biological concept of continuous passive motion of synovial joints: the first 18 years of basic research and its clinical application. In: Ewing J W (ed) Articular cartilage and knee joint function: basic science and arthroscopy. Raven Press, New York

Schenk R K, Eggli P S, Hunziker E B 1986 Articular cartilage morphology. In: Kuettner K E, Schleyerbach R, Hascall V C (eds) Articular cartilage biochemistry. Raven Press, New York

Scott J E, Orford C R 1981 Dermatan sulphate rich proteoglycan associates with rat tail tendon collagen at the d band in the gap region. Biochemical Journal 197:213-216

Stanescu R 1990 Electron-microscopic study of the articular surface using cationized ferritin labeling. In: Maroudas A, Kuettner K E (eds) Methods in cartilage research. Academic Press, London

Stockwell R A 1971 The interrelationship of cell density and cartilage thickness in mammalian articular cartilage. Journal of Anatomy 109:411-21

Vaughan L, Winterhalter K M, Bruckner P 1985 Proteoglycan Lt from chicken embryo sternum identified as type IX collagen. Journal of Biological Chemistry 260:4758-4763

5. Physiological responses to injury: nervous system

David Butler, Helen Slater

The nervous system is a mechanically and physiologically continuous organ. Mechanical continuity is observed throughout connective tissue coverings and physiological continuity via the action potential and the flow of cytoplasm (axoplasm) that occurs within all neurones. Such continuity means that the consequences of neural injury cannot be purely local.

This continuous tract is a dynamic system. It possesses mechanical features that protect the conducting elements while allowing the body to perform a symphony of motions. For example, when the vertebral column is flexed, the neuraxis and meninges must adapt to a spinal canal that is 7-9 cm longer than in extension (Breig 1978, Louis 1981). From a starting position of wrist and elbow flexion, to full wrist and elbow extension, the median nerve in the arm adapts to a 20% change in the length of the nerve bed (Millesi 1986). It should be apparent that the nervous system requires specialised mechanics to cater for such responses to movement.

A state of normal biomechanics of the nervous system is equally important as in other musculoskeletal structures, perhaps more so because the nervous system innervates these other structures. Unlike muscle, joint and fascia, the concept of the nervous system as a dynamic structure, in particular mechanically dynamic, is being accepted slowly.

Sport places particular mechanical and physiological demands upon the nervous system. Rowing requires repetitive movement and forces. Rugby players are subjected to traction and compression forces, gymnastics demands soft tissue stretch, and athletics and martial arts demand ballistic forces. In sport, neural injury and its consequences are frequently masked by injuries to soft tissues and joints. Signs and symptoms of neural involvement may go unrecognized, with repercussions for prognosis and performance based on inadequate or inappropriate treatment.

This chapter discusses basic neuroanatomy and neurobiomechanics. For a more detailed understanding of the potential of the nervous system to contribute to injury states, refer to the reference list.

ESSENTIAL ANATOMY AND PHYSIOLOGY

Although the system is a continuum, there is diversity of structure and function. An understanding of basic neuroanatomy and neurophysiology helps give a clear perspective of the potential responses of the nervous system to injury.

The neurone

The neurone is the basic functional unit of the nervous system. The axon is its main outgrowth and an individual axon can extend the length of a limb. Functionally, the axon is dependent on the cell body, a biological fact of particular relevance in neural injury. Action potential mechanisms associated with injury are well understood, but perhaps the non-impulse mechanisms are not.

Within the axon lies the cytoplasm of the neurone—the axoplasm. Axoplasm is moving continually within the axon. Axoplasmic flow provides material synthesized by the cell body to meet the physiological requirements of the cell body, the axon and the target tissues. Within a single axon, there is a bidirectional axoplasmic flow of varying rates. Antegrade flow (from cell body to target tissues) occurs differentially. Slow antegrade flow travels at approximately 6 mm per day, transporting material which includes subunit proteins of neurofilaments and microtubules—essential components for maintenance of the axon structure. Fast antegrade transport, at a rate of approximately 400 mm per day, carries materials essential for impulse transmission (Lundborg 1988). This includes membrane material for the axolemma, neurotransmitters and neurotransmitter storage vesicles.

There is also a constant retrograde stream moving at 200 mm per day towards the cell body, comprising recycled materials carried in the antegrade flow, and chemical 'messages' from the target tissues and axon (Varon & Adler 1980). These chemical messages 'inform' the cell body of activities involving the neurone and its environment, inviting the cell body to react accordingly. Together with an uncompromised blood supply, we propose that a mechanically patent nervous system is necessary for the optimal flow of axoplasm. The consequences of impairment of axoplasmic flow are discussed below.

Protection of neuronal function during movement

Complex protective mechanisms exist to ensure optimal neuronal function during the demands of any physical activity.

The conducting tissues

The conducting tissues have their own protection. Neurones will stretch, and axon cylinders are quite flexible with layers of myelin which slide on each other. Neurones run a wavy course in the endoneurial tubes. The fascicles in peripheral nerve and spinal cord tracts also do not run a straight course. They are therefore equipped to respond to movement.

The connective tissues

The connective tissue coverings give the nervous system mechanical protection and help to maintain a balanced neuronal environment. A number of connective tissues are represented in the nervous system.

The outermost and strongest of the meninges, the dura mater, has limited elasticity due to a low concentration of elastic fibres (Tunturi 1977). In a relaxed state the collagen fibres of the dura assume a wavy appearance, but under tension the collagen fibres elongate (Breig 1978).

In the dura lie the leptomeninges; the arachnoid and pia are both mechanically weaker than the dura. The arachnoid contains the cerebrospinal fluid (CSF). Besides acting as a protective cushion, the CSF provides part of the nutritional requirements of the cord and nerve roots.

Peripheral nerves possess considerable tensile strength and gain protection from compression due to their connective tissue coverings. The outer epineurium surrounds, protects and cushions the fascicles. Each fascicle is surrounded by the perineurium which acts as a mechanical and physiological barrier and protects the contents of the endoneurial tubes. The endoneurium forms a sheath around individual myelinated nerve fibres, and groups of unmyelinated nerve fibres and helps to maintain a constant internal environment for the nerve fibre (Fig. 5.1).

Approximately half of a peripheral nerve is connective tissue although this varies greatly. There is more connective tissue where nerves cross joints, and where nerves are exposed to compressive forces (for example, the common peroneal nerve at the head of the fibula).

Diffusion barriers

In addition to protection by physical means, the continuity of the connective tissues assists in regulating and maintaining a constant osmotic and ionic environment for the

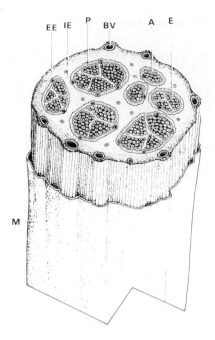

Fig. 5.1 The connective tissue sheath of a multifascicular segment of peripheral nerve. A = axon, BV = blood vessel, E = endoneurium, EE = external epineurium, IE = internal epineurium, M = mesoneurium, P = perineurium
Source: Butler (1991)

neurone. Diffusion barriers between the arachnoid and the CSF and between the CSF and the pia. In peripheral nerve, the perineurium has 'tight junctions' between cells which allow only small blood vessels to cross (Lundborg 1988). Significantly, lymphatics do not cross these tight junctions. Another barrier exists at the endothelium of the endoneurial capillaries. The internal neuronal environment, and therefore the conducting elements, are well protected. A clear example is seen where peripheral nerve passes through an infected body part. While the perineurium remains intact, neuronal function is unaffected.

If these protective barriers are breached by mechanical, viral or infective means there can be serious consequences for the nervous system. The maintenance of an increased endoneurial fluid pressure and the proliferation of intraneural connective tissue can ultimately result in intraneural fibrosis.

Neurovascular dynamics

Neurones are 'bloodthirsty' cells. The vasa nervorum possesses mechanical and structural features that ensure an adequate supply of blood to nerves while the body moves. The nervous system has extraneural and intraneural supplies. Because the nervous system is dynamic, extraneural or feeder vessels are functionally adapted for movement. For example, the vessels are often highly coiled, especially those supplying nerve roots and peripheral nerves (Parke & Watanabe 1985). In peripheral vessels, blood flow in arteries and in valveless veins is reversible, allowing for rapid shunting of blood in the event of blockage or pressure alterations (Lundborg 1988). Vessels enter the nervous system at the least vulnerable sites. These may occur near joints where minimal nervous system movement occurs in relation to surrounding structures. Similarly, the supply to the cord is derived from between 2 and 17 medullary feeder vessels (Dommisse 1986). These arise predominately in the cervical and lumbar plexuses where the nervous system migrates little during body movements in relation to interfacing structures (Louis 1981).

Innervation of the nervous system

The connective tissues of the nervous system are innervated. They are potential sources of pain and can therefore provide the nervous system with an early warning mechanism against overstretching, compression or irritation. Segmental sinuvertebral nerves innervate the dura mater, dural connections to the anterior aspect of the spinal canal, dural sleeves and blood vessels. These nerves are mixed with fibres from the ventral rami and sympathetic fibres via grey rami communicantes. On entering the canal each nerve joins a neural mesh in the dura and may innervate dural segments four or five levels above and below the entry site (Cuatico et al 1988, Groen et al 1988).

Connective tissue coverings of peripheral nerve are innervated via axonal branches within the nerve, the nervi nervorum. There is also sympathetic innervation from the perisvascular plexuses (Hromada 1963). This dense innervation, coupled with rich vascularization, means that nerve trunks are potentially reactive tissues.

VULNERABLE SITES OF THE NERVOUS SYSTEM

There are areas within the nervous system where the neuroanatomy or adjacent interfacing tissues predispose the system to injury:

1 areas of impulse generation—in particular, the dorsal root ganglion, neuronal pools in the spinal cord and terminal buttons (Devor 1991);
2 where the system passes through a tunnel, especially if the tunnel boundaries are unyielding. Examples of this are the carpal and tarsal tunnels and the intervertebral foramen;
3 where the system branches, for example the radial nerve at the elbow or the interdigital nerve to the web space between the third and fourth toes;
4 where there is a hard interfacing surface such as bone, fascia (small branches of the plantar nerves in the plantar fascia), or tendon (radial sensory nerve between the tendons of brachioradialis and extensor carpi radialis longus);
5 where nerves by virtue of their morphology (e.g. less fascicles, less connective tissue coverings) are more

vulnerable to injury. The common peroneal and ulnar nerves are significant examples.

RANGE OF INJURIES

The diverse dynamic demands of sport lead to a wide spectrum of neural injury, from a subclinical injury affecting performance, to the far more uncommon peripheral nerve severance and cord injury leading to quadriplegia. Injury to the nervous system may be direct or indirect. A direct injury can occur from overstretching or an irritation from repetitious activity. Indirect injury can result from bleeding due to a hamstring tear. The mechanics of the sciatic nerve may be affected by altering the pressure around the nerve, or at a later stage by scarring. Inflammatory irritation or mechanical compression of nerve roots caused by disc lesions are other examples. External forces resulting from ill-fitting footwear or bicycle seats could irritate or compress the peroneal and pudendal nerves respectively.

Certain diseases predispose the nervous system to injury. The most common is diabetes mellitus, present in approximately 5% of the population, and surely represented in the sporting population.

PATHOLOGY

Because of the continuum, the nervous system's direct or indirect involvement almost inevitably occurs after trauma. Its significance is often masked by injury to bones, joints and soft tissues. The spectrum of clinically overt peripheral nerve injuries and their consequences have been well described and classified by Seddon (1975) and Sunderland (1991). Although a similar spectrum exists in the central nervous system, it has perhaps received less attention. The more minor changes in nerve function are probably underestimated. They can be linked to alterations in neuronal processing in the dorsal horn and in some cases to the maintenance of pain (Wells & Woolf 1991).

Neural tissue also exhibits an inflammatory response similar to that of other tissues following trauma, typified by haemorrhage, oedema, increased vascular permeability, elevated intrafascicular pressures and the possibility of intraneural fibrosis (Sunderland 1976). If chronic, these pathological processes may be linked not only to local symptoms, but to symptoms remote from the site of the primary insult (Mackinnon 1992).

PATHOLOGICAL PROCESSES

Altered microcirculation and axonal transport

The ability of the nervous system to withstand temporary, mechanically induced vascular insufficiency is dependent on the magnitude and duration of the mechanical forces. At low compression forces there may be temporary and partial compromise of intraneural microcirculation resulting in impaired oxygenation and slowed axonal transport. If the compression persists, eventually the target tissue–cell body relationship will deteriorate, and in simple terms, the neurone becomes 'sick'. The entire axon becomes more susceptible to compressive forces (Dahlin & McLean 1986, Dahlin et al 1986).

The well developed peripheral vascular networks tolerate a considerable amount of stretching before blood flow is altered. Circulation begins to decrease at 6% elongation and ceases at 15%. (Elongation is only part of the adaptive measures to movement—the nervous system also slides with respect to interfacing structures: Lundborg & Rydevik 1973, Ogata & Naito 1986). The demands of some sports, especially those involving ballistic movements, must at times approach this threshold. There is no harm to the system provided the forces are not sustained.

Pressure gradients

Pressure gradients exist within the fluids and tissues of the nervous system and its surrounds. Minor alterations in these pressure gradients may be sufficient to effect changes in blood flow and axoplasmic flow. Sites that are particularly sensitive to changes in pressure gradients include the vulnerable sites listed above.

Sunderland (1976) has documented a model for carpal tunnel syndrome which relates to altered pressure gradients within the carpal tunnel and is applicable elsewhere in and around the nervous system. For adequate neuronal nutrition blood must flow into the tunnel, into the nerve, into the fascicle then out of the nerve and tunnel (Fig. 5.2A). Veins may collapse at pressure of approximately 20–30 mm Hg (Rydevik et al 1981). These pressures are much less than those present in patients with early symptoms of carpal tunnel syndrome (Gelberman et al 1981).

Sunderland (1976) describes three distinct stages (Fig. 5.2B, C, D) that may follow an elevated tunnel pressure:

1 hypoxia from venous stasis. This may be the basis of neuroischaemic pain;
2 oedema. Damaged capillary endothelium results in leakage of protein-rich oedema which is trapped within the endoneurium. The resultant increase in intrafascicular pressure swells the fascicle;
3 fibrosis. Fibroblasts proliferate in this environment, and the outcome is intraneural fibrosis.

Crush syndrome

Axoplasmic flow relies on a mechanically unimpeded nervous system and an uninterrupted blood flow. Alterations in the flow of axoplasm or quality of the flow may cause insidious attrition to both target tissues and neurones (Mackinnon & Dellon 1988). Double crush is serial impingement of a nerve tract. An initial injury predisposes

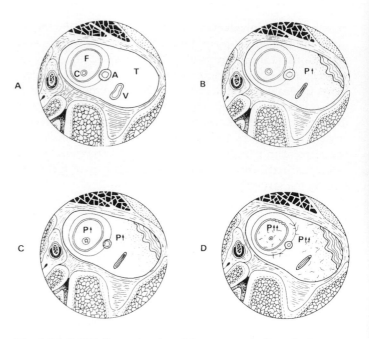

Fig. 5.2 A,B,C,D Representation of the pressure gradients in the carpal tunnel and the stages that follow alteration of the pressure gradients. For simplicity, one nerve fibre in a fascicle is represented. A = arteriole, C = capillary, F = fascicle, P = pressure, T = tunnel, V = venule
Source: Butler (1991)

neurones to injury elsewhere along the tract. For example, patients with carpal tunnel syndrome (CTS) are more likely to develop a compression lesion of the ulnar nerve in Guyon's canal (Cassvan et al 1986), and those suffering CTS frequently have bilateral symptoms (Hurst et al 1985).

The original double crush syndrome described neural injuries at the neck predisposing to carpal tunnel syndrome (Upton & McComas 1973). Reversed double crush occurs where a distal neural injury (e.g at the wrist) predisposes to a proximal injury, perhaps at the shoulder (Lundborg 1988). Mackinnon and Dellon (1988) and Mackinnon (1992) also describe multiple crush syndromes, where following initial neural injuries patients experience multiple and related areas of symptoms.

Clinical presentations of crush syndromes may be widespread and unfamiliar in nature. Athletes complaining of a 'string of injuries' or 'multiple areas of spot pains' may have a common pathophysiology that represents a minor form of the crush syndromes. Abnormal responses to tension tests such as the straight leg raise, the slump and the upper limb tension tests, may be clues to altered nervous system mechanics and physiology.

An athlete with diabetes or a pretensioned nervous system will be particularly susceptible to multiple sites of injury (Mackinnon 1992). We believe that the use of supports in sport, such as patella bands or tennis elbow straps, may mechanically and physiologically compromise the nervous system. This should be considered when advising athletes to use external supports for sport.

Autonomic nervous system influences

The concept of the nervous system as a mechanical and physiological continuum must extend to the autonomic nervous system, particularly the trunks, rami and ganglia of the sympathetic nervous system. These neurones are as much at risk from deformation, unphysiologic postures and entrapment as are somatic neurones. While not proven, we suggest that the location of the cervical sympathetic ganglia in a highly mobile part of the body may particularly predispose these ganglia to microtrauma. An example is hyperextension injuries of the neck commonly seen in contact sports such as rugby.

Thoracic and lumbar ganglia are vulnerable to distortion and compression due to their close proximity to bony structures (ribs, costovertebral joints) and by adhesion to periosteum and parietal pleura (Nathan 1986). We believe that abnormal autonomic activity associated with sports injuries is probably underestimated, and often goes unrecognized. Examination of the nervous system through tension tests such as the prone knee bend, upper limb tension tests and the obturator slump, and through interfacing tissues, should help the clinician to locate possible sources of the symptoms.

Abnormal impulse generating sites

Impulses are usually generated from sites such as neuronal pools in the cord, dorsal root ganglia and terminal buttons. With neural injury, an abnormal or ectopic impulse generating site may develop. A normal impulse passing this deformed locus may initiate a train of impulses in the nerve fibre or trigger impulses in neighbouring fibres. Common examples of abnormal impulse generating sites are neuromas, ephaptic synapses, immature axons, dysmyelination, demyelination and combinations of these neuropathologies. These sites may become mechanosensitive and/or chemosensitive and are potential sources of pain (Devor 1991).

Mechanical influences

It is important to emphasize that continuity of the neuraxis, meninges and peripheral nervous system dictates that movement in one part of the body will have implications all the way along the tract. For example, the upper limb tension test is likely to move and tension the nervous system from terminal fibres in the fingertips, along the upper limb peripheral nerve trunks to the cord, meninges, sympathetic trunk and neural tissue in the other arm (Butler 1991).

It follows that altered mechanics of the nervous system in one region may affect the mechanics of the system at other sites. Adverse tension in the nervous system has been defined by Butler (1991) as 'abnormal mechanical and physiological responses produced from the nervous system when its range of movement and stretch capabilities are tested'. Body movements not only produce an increase in tension within the nervous system but also move it in relation to adjacent or 'interfacing structures' (Butler 1991).

Pathology may affect nervous system mechanics from outside the system, termed 'extraneural', or from within the system, termed 'intraneural'. The two sources often co-exist, although one will usually dominate. Examples of vertebral extraneural pathologies are spinal canal stenosis, narrowing of the intervertebral foramen, adhesions between the dura and spinal canal, and lumbar disc protrusions irritating a nerve root. In the peripheral nervous system, examples include the sciatic nerve lying in a bed of blood from a hamstring tear, tight fascial bands across nerve and the tibial nerve as it passes through an oedematous posterior tarsal tunnel.

Intraneural pathology affects the elasticity of the nervous system. Sunderland (1991) refers to fibrosed nerve setting a 'friction fibrosis' elsewhere in the system. In this instance, tension has been taken up at one site in the nervous system, thereby compromising the amount of available slack elsewhere in the system. We propose that, as a consequence, the nervous system/mechanical interface relationship has been altered with the potential for symptoms. An example is a fibrotic length of common peroneal nerve at the head of the fibula that may lead to abnormal deep peroneal nerve/ interface relationships at the ankle. We suggest that this may contribute to altered proprioceptive input from the ankle and, in combination with less slack in the nervous system, influence the neurological functioning of the ankle joint, perhaps predisposing to recurrent ankle sprains.

The C6, T6 and L4 intervertebral levels are frequently implicated in injuries that lead to physical signs of adverse neural tension (Butler 1991). At these levels the spinal canal is typically smaller and the nervous system more bulky than other areas. They are well worth examining as sites remote from the initial injury when there are abnormal responses to tension testing.

Anomalies

Anomalies in the nervous system and its interfacing structures may result in bizarre symptomatology and difficulties in interpretation of the origin of symptoms. An example is the furcal nerve (arising from the L4 and L5 roots) which, by contributing to the femoral and obturator nerves and the lumbosacral trunk, may explain some of the atypical sensory deficits and the unusual areas of symptom response reported by patients (Kikuchi et al 1984). Other examples include split emerging nerve roots, tethering associated with dysraphisms such as spina bifida, and the Martin Gruber anastamosis where the median and ulnar nerves are connected in the forearm. Torg et al (1986) reported transient quadriplegia in 32 athletes (football, hockey, basketball, boxing) as a result of hyperextension and hyperflexion forces. Radiographs showed a decrease in the anteroposterior diameter of the cervical spine in all the tested athletes from causes such as congenital stenosis and fusion, cervical instability and disc protrusion. They postulated a direct compression of the spinal cord causing transient (10–15 min) motor and sensory manifestations. The 'at risk' athlete may not be aware of the potential for injury. The treating clinician may not appreciate the significance of a spond-xylolisthesis to the slow recovery of a hamstring tear.

In summary, the consequences of neural injury are:

1 symptoms from the nervous system (either conducting or connective tissues or both);
2 alteration of impulses to and from non-neural target tissues;
3 non-neural tissue injury from gross denervation leading to muscle weakness, loss of proprioception, or a more insidious alteration via changes in the quality and quantity of axoplasmic flow.

Immobilization and mobilization

There is little research on the effects of immobilization of the nervous system although, with a severe injury involving neuronal severance, a relatively tension free environment is widely regarded as optimal for healing. This allows the greatest proportion of regenerating axons to neuroticize the scar. However, the nervous system is a difficult structure to immobilize completely. Its continuity dictates that if the fingers, wrist and elbow of one arm were to be immobilized, movements of the neck and shoulder and the other arm would still have mechanical influences on the system along the affected arm to the finger tips. The cadaver work of McLellan and Swash (1976), Breig (1978), Millesi (1986), and Wilgis and Murphy (1986) supports this.

In common with all musculoskeletal structures, movement is essential for health. The 'use it or lose it' doctrine is as applicable to the nervous system as it is to joint, muscle and fascial tissues. Mechanically compromised neural tissue may scar, adhere to, or be irritated by surrounding structures. Those features of the nervous system that are essential to allow it to respond to movement, need movement to function optimally. To some degree circulation and CSF flow are dependent on movement. Movement probably helps the flow of axoplasm and will certainly affect the pressures in fluids and tissues.

The nervous system can be mobilized just like joint and soft tissues. Some techniques of examination are described in this text. Others, including treatment rationales, are detailed in Elvey (1986), Maitland (1986), Butler and Gifford (1989) and Butler (1991).

Possible effects of mobilization

Mobilization of the nervous system has a mechanical effect on neural structures that in turn influence vascular dynamics and axoplasmic flow. Possible influences on some of the neuropathologies commonly encountered by sports physiotherapists are discussed below.

It is easy to envisage that both the 'stuck' peripheral nerve, and dura mater surrounded by fresh blood and oedema, would benefit from gentle movement. Kornberg & Lew (1989) demonstrated the beneficial effect of neural mobilization in the treatment of hamstring injuries.

Dispersion of an intraneural oedema could be enhanced by alteration of the pressures in the nervous system during movement. This may in part explain the relief experienced by some sufferers of carpal tunnel syndrome when they mobilize their wrist.

It is not inconceivable that dysmyelination could be beneficially influenced by mobilizing the nervous system.

Restoration of normal mechanics of the connective tissues after injury lessens the possibility of the nerves being entrapped in surrounding connective tissues. The sinu-vertebral nerve could be caught in dural scar. Other examples include the nervi nervorum caught in the connective tissue sheath, and injured or regenerating nerve fibres caught in endoneurial scar.

It is possible that the nervous system can be 'trained' to lengthen. While a degree of pure stretch is possible, more complex mechanisms probably occur. Bora et al (1980) showed that sutured rats' nerves could become more compliant and suggested that this feature allowed repaired nerves to adjust to mobilization. While not proven, we suggest that the cell body may be signalled from an injury site (presumably by the neurotransmitters carried in the retrograde axoplasmic flow) and 'requested' to alter the compliance of the nerve.

Similar signalling could occur from target tissues. For example, stretch of the hamstring muscle may result in neurotropic messages 'requesting' that the compliance of the sciatic nerve be altered. There is an interesting clinical study that would provide support for this hypothesis. Ramamurthi (1980) noted that tension signs in patients with surgically proven disc lesions were more significant in Westernised Indian women and men, compared with those who followed a more traditional way of life where squatting and bending were more commonly adopted postures. The common stretches performed in sport must not be seen solely as musculoskeletal stretches. The nervous system is inevitably affected. Benefits from stretching may be attributed to a combination of effects on neural and non-neural tissues and structures.

Where a rapid improvement occurs following mobilization, this could in part be due to enhanced blood supply to hypoxic nerve fibres. The pressure gradients around the nervous system are in delicate balance. Treatment of interfacing tissues and mobilization of the nervous system may normalize the gradients and normalize the blood supply. In this regard, the effect of mobilization of the sympathetic trunk, either directly or via the ribs, cannot be underestimated. Distortion and angulation of the sympathetic trunk have not been associated with sympathetically maintained pain syndromes and altered microcirculation, although clear pathological evidence of alterations in the sympathetic trunk and ganglia has been provided by Nathan (1986). Marked neuroischaemia in rabbits' sciatic nerves following stimulation of the lumbar sympathetic chain has been shown (Selander et at 1985).

The circulation and percolation of CSF would be assisted by normal movement. At least half of a nerve root's metabolic requirements come from the CSF (Parke & Watanabe 1985). It is therefore reasonable to propose that normal movement will optimize the axonal transport systems. This may be achieved by altering mechanical restraints and/or improving blood flow, and thus increasing the energy available for axonal transport. It is probable that normal movement is part of the energetics of axoplasmic flow.

Surgery

There are two aspects to consider: first, the effects of surgery on neural structures, and second the effect on the nervous system of surgery to non-neural structures.

Surgical release or removal of structures that may be compressing neural tissue and thereby altering neurobiomechanics is the most common procedure, for example, external neurolysis to free a constricting band across a peripheral nerve or a laminectomy to remove a protruding disc fragment. With this form of surgery the nervous system has not been breached and early gentle mobilization is recommended. The continuity of the nervous system means that neural tissues may be mobilized without compromising the operated structures. For example, passive cervical flexion will mobilize the nervous system through the lumbar spinal canal with minimal movement of interfacing canal structures.

Surgery that requires entering the nervous system carries greater potential for intraneural scarring, slower recovery and a poorer prognosis. Examples of this type of surgery include durotomy and internal neurolysis. Where the nervous system is damaged severely from nerve laceration or severance, while good recovery may follow surgery some functional irreversibility is almost inevitable as diffusion barriers and connective tissue strength and elasticity have been altered.

Surgery not directed at the nervous system also has its neurological consequences; either purely from the mechanical trauma of the surgery or from post-surgical swelling and immobilization. In a knee reconstruction, the peroneal, saphenous and tibial nerves could be inadvertently traumatized during surgery or affected by post-operative swelling. Post surgical swelling may organize and irritate or compress nerves, particularly in the extremities. Where possible, and with agreement from the surgeon, the authors suggest that *careful* early nervous system mobilization is indicated. We believe that continuous passive motion is frequently overlooked as a beneficial way to mobilize neural tissue. Precautions and contraindications are detailed in Butler (1991).

SUMMARY

The nervous system is a complex continuum of multiple tissues that has the potential to be injured. In some cases the injury need only be minor to cause symptoms. The pathophysiology of neural injury deserves to be considered in conjunction with the wealth of knowledge on the pathophysiology of the musculoskeletal system in sports medicine. The significance of neural injury is:

1 the nervous system could be a source of symptoms itself;
2 it may affect other sites of both neural and non-neural injury;
3 it may alter impulses to and from non-neural structures.

An understanding of the pathophysiology and pathomechanics of the nervous system and its integration with the musculoskeletal system offers the clinician a new direction in assessment, treatment and prevention of sporting injuries.

REFERENCES

Bora F W, Richardson S, Black J 1980 The biomechanical responses to tension in a peripheral nerve. Journal of Hand Surgery 5:21–25

Breig A 1978 Adverse mechanical tension in the central nervous system. Almquist and Wiksell, Stockholm

Butler D S 1991 Mobilisation of the nervous system. Churchill Livingstone, Melbourne

Cassvan A, Rosenberg A, Rivers L F 1986 Ulnar nerve involvement in carpal tunnel syndrome. Archives of Physical Medicine and Rehabilitation 67:290-292

Cuatico W, Parker J C, Pappert E, Pilsl S 1988 An anatomical and clinical investigation of spinal meningeal nerves. Acta Neurochirurgica 90:139–143

Dahlin L B, Rydevik B, McLean W G et al 1986 Changes in fast axonal transport during experimental nerve compression at low pressures. Experimental Neurology 84:29–36

Dahlin L B, McLean W G 1986 Effects of graded experimental compression on slow and fast axonal transport in rabbit vagus nerve. Journal of the Neurological Sciences 76:221–230

Devor M 1991 Neuropathic pain and injured nerve: peripheral mechanisms. In: Wells J C D, Woolf C J 1991 Pain mechanisms and management. British Medical Bulletin. Churchill Livingstone, Edinburgh

Dommisse G F 1986 The blood supply of the spinal cord. In: Grieve G P (ed) Modern manual therapy of the vertebral column. Churchill Livingstone, Edinburgh

Elvey R L 1986 Treatment of arm pain associated with abnormal brachial plexus tension. Australian Journal of Physiotherapy 32:224–229

Groen G J, Balget B, Drukker J 1988 The innervation of the spinal dura mater: anatomy and clinical considerations. Acta Neurochirurgica 92:39–46

Gelberman R H, Hergenroeder P T, Hargens A R et al 1981 The carpal tunnel syndrome—a study of carpal canal pressures. The Journal of Bone and Joint Surgery 63A:380–383

Hromada J 1963 On the nerve supply of the connective tissue of some peripheral nervous system components. Acta Anatomica 55:343–351

Hurst L C, Weissberg D, Carroll R E 1985 The relationship of double crush to carpal tunnel syndrome (an analysis of 1000 cases of carpal tunnel syndrome). Journal of Hand Surgery 10B:202–204

Kornberg C, Lew P 1989 The effect of stretching neural structures on grade I hamstring injuries. The Journal of Orthopaedic and Sports Physical Therapy June:481-487

Kikuchi S, Hasue M, Nishiyama K, Tsukasa I 1984 Anatomic and clinical studies of radicular symptoms. Spine 9:23-30

Louis R 1981 Vertebroradicular and vertebromedullar dynamics. Anatomica Clinica 3:1–11

Lundborg G, Rydevik B 1973 Effects of stretching the tibial nerve of the rabbit. A preliminary study of the intraneural circulation and barrier function of the perineurium. Journal of Bone and Joint Surgery 55B:390–401

Lundborg G 1988 Nerve injury and repair. Churchill Livingstone, Edinburgh

Maitland G D 1986 Vertebral manipulation, 5th edn. Butterworths, London

Mackinnon S E , Dellon A L 1988 Surgery of the peripheral nerve. Thieme, New York

Mackinnon S E 1992 Double and multiple 'crush' syndromes. Hand Clinics 8:369-390

McLellan D C, Swash M 1976 Longitudinal sliding of the median nerve during movements of the upper limb. Journal of Neurology, Neurosurgery and Psychiatry 39:566–570

Millesi H 1986 The nerve gap: theory and clinical practice. Hand Clinics 4:651–663

Nathan H 1986 Osteophytes of the spine compressing the sympathetic trunk and splanchnic nerves in the thorax. Spine 12:527–532

Ogata K, Naito M 1986 Blood flow of peripheral nerve. Effects of dissection, compression and stretching. Journal of Hand Surgery 11B:11–14

Parke W W, Watanabe R 1985 The intrinsic vasculature of the lumbosacral spinal nerve roots. Spine 10:508–515

Ramamurthi B 1980 Absence of limitation of straight leg raising in proved lumbar disc lesion. Journal of Neurosurgery 52:852–853

Rydevik B, Lundborg G, Bagge U 1981 Effects of graded compression on intraneural blood flow. Journal of Hand Surgery 6:3-12

Seddon H 1975 Surgical disorders of the peripheral nerves, 2nd edn. Churchill Livingstone, Edinburgh

Selander D, Mansson L G, Karlsson L et al 1985 Adrenergic vasoconstriction in peripheral nerves in the rabbit. Anesthesiology 62: 6-10

Sunderland S 1976 The nerve lesion in carpal tunnel syndrome. Journal of Neurology, Neurosurgery and Psychiatry 39:615-616

Sunderland S 1991 Nerve and nerve injuries: a critical appraisal Churchill Livingstone, Edinburgh

Torg J S, Pavlov H, Genuario S E et al 1986 Neuropraxia of the cervical spinal cord with transient quadriplegia. The Journal of Bone and Joint Surgery 68A:1354-1370

Tunturi A R 1977 Elasticity of the spinal cord dura in the dog. Journal of Neurosurgery 47:391-396

Varon S, Adler R 1980 Nerve growth factor and control of nerve growth. Current Topics in Developmental Biology 16:207-252

Upton A R M, McComas A J 1973 The double crush in nerve entrapment syndromes. Lancet 2:359-362

Wells J C D, Woolf C J 1991 Pain mechanisms and management. British Medical Bulletin. Churchill Livingstone, Edinburgh

Wilgis E F S, Murphy R 1986 The significance of longitudinal excursion in peripheral nerves. Hand Clinics 2:761-766

6. Injury and pain

Diana Elton

Pain and disability require a multidimensional approach, as many functions of the central nervous system (CNS) are sensitive to stress and psychological dysfunction. Psychological events can change biochemical activity of the body, and the biochemistry of the body can have an impact on the psychological state of the individual. Therefore, pain needs to be considered as a psycho-neuro-endocrine phenomenon. Furthermore, a distinction needs to be made between pain and suffering. Pain may be considered a sensory event, while suffering includes all the psychological processing involved in the pain experience, such as worry, anxiety, concern about the meaning of pain, and the context of the situation.

A physiotherapist should not only excel in the physical treatment of pain and injury, but also understand complex biochemical and neurophysiological processes which may aid or hinder recovery. This knowledge can lead to the design of more effective physical programs. Ultimately, effective treatment must be aimed at stimulation of the body's own endogenous systems as well as administration of external interventions. Furthermore, a patient's motivation to follow the prescribed self-help of exercises and life style changes frequently depends on his or her mood state at the time. A depressed, over-anxious individual may be more difficult to motivate than someone who feels positive about the treatment outcome. Since mood states are related to the biochemistry and neurophysiology of the body, they affect all behavioural and psychological dimensions. They have an impact on both the frequency of sport injuries and on recovery from injury (Elton 1992).

There are increasing numbers of participants in recreational amateur and professional sport every year. There are also increasing numbers of sport injuries, notwithstanding better training and conditioning programmes and safer equipment. Australians suffer around 1 000 000 sporting injuries a year. Some of them are severe and 40 000 per year require hospitalization or surgery. The severity of injury varies from cuts and bruises to permanent spinal-cord injury. The cost of sports injuries in 1990 was estimated at between $2–4 billion dollars per year (Quinn 1992).

Many injured athletes show profound emotional disturbance if injured (Smith et al 1990). Understanding psychophysiological variables is required for an adequate program for rehabilitation of injured athletes. Psychological effects of sports injury include the emotional trauma of being injured, the psychological factors influencing the recovery process and the psychological impact of an injury on the athlete's future performance. These states can inhibit the recovery processes. For some athletes, an injury may result in a severe disturbance in their overall lifestyle and, in some cases, in the end of their athletic career (Feltz 1986). The psychological problems may include a loss of self-esteem, feelings of helplessness, anger and depression, irrational thoughts and beliefs and uncertainty about the future (Rotella & Heyman 1988).

Recently, there has been much interest in sports injury in the relevant literature (Crossman 1985); however the research has mainly focused on the psychological antecedents and on the effects of injury rather than on psychological intervention.

Just as negative emotions produce negative biochemical and neurophysiological changes, positive emotions can reverse this trend, and facilitate recovery. This is important in designing treatment programs.

This chapter will discuss on the neurophysiology and biochemistry of pain, and emphasize the body-mind interaction and the body's inner resources to heal itself. Attention will be focused on concomitant psychological variables.

BIOCHEMISTRY OF PAIN

The history of treatment of pain and disability presents various dilemmas. We still lack adequate understanding of treatment failures, that is the persistence of a condition, in spite of the best efforts to alleviate it . Equally puzzling are the 'miracle cures', where as a result of a non-medical intervention the symptoms abate or disappear. Placebo effects indicate that 33% of individuals are capable of controlling their pain as a result of administration of a chemically inert substance (e.g. a sugar pill), presented with a suggestion of analgesia. To add to this confusion, there is no clear knowledge of why some of the drugs administered for pain relief produce positive results. An exogenous substance can only be effective if it combines with a receptor in the human body (Elton et al 1983). It seems obvious that such receptors are there in order to combine with endogenous substances. This indicates an inherent capacity of the human body to produce substances to heal itself. This knowledge is still inadequately understood, and it is not well utilized in the treatment of pain.

Understanding placebo effects is important to the physiotherapist, as placebo effects include more than drug administration. Any situation where a person receives attention and care is potentially a placebo situation. Physiotherapy, offering hands-on intervention, contains powerful placebo elements. It is sometimes difficult to ascertain how much improvement is due to treatment, and how much to the placebo effects. While this chapter will confine itself to discussing placebo effects in drug and psychological interventions, the findings can include all therapy.

Dilemmas in the drug treatment of pain

Some information about the healing processes comes from the study of the effectiveness of drugs, and much research is available about the role of opiates in the treatment of pain. The study of morphine may be used to illustrate the point.

Morphine, like many other interventions, is not uniformly effective. Many researchers studying the effects of morphine are puzzled by conflicting results: in some studies morphine seemed to be effective in the control of pain while in others it showed only placebo-like effects. Arner and Meyerson (1988) showed that morphine was effective in the control of suffering but not in the control of pain sensation. Kupers et al (1991) further isolated differences in response between people suffering from neurogenic pain (pain of defined physiological origin) and idiopathic pain, such as pain without well defined physiological correlates (Wall 1990, Portenoy et al 1990). Morphine was effective in relieving suffering in patients with defined neurogenic pain, but did not produce relief in patients with psychologically based pain. This is an interesting finding, as it explains some of the reasons for non-improvement.

Research into the role of anti-depressants, which are being used to control pain, throws light on the relationship between mood and pain. While it is understandable that pain can depress an individual, it is harder to explain depression resulting in physical pain (Melzack 1990, Zitman et al 1991).

There is a common belief that individuals in pain are totally committed to attaining pain relief. Regrettably, this is only partially accurate. There are individuals who escape into pain as a way of giving up coping with the world, where they perceive their efforts as futile. Primary and secondary gains may operate on the situation (Elton 1983). These individuals usually have a low self esteem, and they may form the hard core of the 'pain prone' group, described by Sternbach (1975). While most people suffering from sport injuries suffer from acute rather than chronic pain, their trauma is more clearly defined, and they often have a high motivation to resume their normal lives. However, they are also subject to doubts and misgivings, and may fear the renewed strain of competitive sport.

This implies that while treatment of sports injuries may generally show better results than the treatment of chronic pain in general practice, this cannot be taken for granted.

Studies looking at the interaction between exogenous and endogenous opiates (Lipman et al 1990) indicate that to act on the body an exogenous substance may need not only the receptors, but also the presence of other facilitating substances in the body. It has been shown that the effectiveness of morphine varies, depending on the presence in the plasma of a metabolite *morphine-6-glucuronide* (Portenoy et al 1990). This is in line with the earlier research of Pasternak et al (1987).

History of endorphins

The search for endogenous biochemical substances implicated in the alleviation of pain started with drug research. Scientists attempted to find receptors in the human body for drugs of addiction such as morphine and pethidine. It seemed obvious that these substances could not act upon the human body unless they combined with an appropriate inner ligant. In 1973 three independent research teams (Pert & Snyder 1973, Simon et al 1973, Terenius 1973) found many such receptors in the central nervous system. This suggested that some normally occurring substance such as a neurotransmitter of pain pathways may be the endogenous connection for the opiate receptors. As the research continued, Hughes et al (1975) discovered enkephalins and Teschemacher et al (1975) discovered endorphins. Both are endogenous polypeptides which have analgesic effects. Hughes, demonstrated that met-enkephalin and leu-enkephalin had properties similar to morphine. Teschemacher showed that alpha and beta endorphins in the original research have opioid qualities and analgesic effects and are more powerful than the enkephalins.

It is interesting that both substances were quite different from morphine in chemical structure, although they were bound by the same receptors and produced the same pharmacological response. Furthermore, in the early studies, the effects of the endogenous polypeptides could be reversed by naloxone, which is a known morphine inhibitor. This finding resulted in research which used naloxone to demonstrate the presence of endorphins. At present about 30 endorphins have been isolated. Some are more stable or effective than others (Terenius 1987). They are now considered as links in pain modulatory neuronal systems as well as modulators at the endocrine level. Some receptors have generalised functions, while others are more selective for peptides which mediate pain relief (Terenius, 1987).There is ever-increasing data for multiple opioid analgesic systems.

Endorphins and stress

The relationship between endorphins and stress response is interesting. Pain generates stress and stress in turn aggravates pain. Endorphins seem to be produced in response to body stress. Very little is known about the physiological mechanisms activating the various endorphin systems. Mild stimulation, such as jogging, may induce a sense of well being. Physical exhaustion, pain or psychological stress may trigger intense activation leading to anaesthesia and inactivity. Both hypo- and hyper-activation of the endorphin system may lead to psychosomatic or psychiatric problems.

It is significant that the production of endorphins in the human body occurs naturally and has no adverse side effects such as addiction or physical dependence[1]. One of the explanations offered is that the last molecule in the endogenous polypeptide chain is unstable. However, when endorphins have been extracted from the human body, artificially stabilised in a laboratory, and given to an individual in the form of an injection, addiction and dependence have been produced (Inversen & Dingledine 1976). Endorphins play a role in a number of physiological processes, including pain threshold and tolerance, thermoregulation, eating, learning, sexual behaviour, and the regulation of central cardiovascular control and respiration. They are capable of diminishing both pain and suffering.

While exercise has a beneficial effect on the function of the human body, there is a puzzling connection between the level of exercise and stress. Research has been done on Olympic events, where high levels of ill health and injuries have been noted in some athletes (Quinn 1992).

It is an established fact that moderate exercise not only increases fitness, but improves general physical health and resistance to sickness. This implies that it is beneficial to the immune system. This is less evident in athletes competing at a national or international level. In fact Weidemann et al (1992) indicate that intensive exercise lowers the levels of immunoglobulins in the bloodstream. Weidemann et al suggested that immunoglobulins are implicated in neutralising antibodies secreted by the immune system's secondary line of defence (B-cells), and

their diminution increases susceptibility to infection. The authors also indicated that many athletes involved in competitive sports suffer from sports anaemia. Weidemann et al (1992) suggested that during intensive exercise red blood cells tend to produce high levels of free oxygen radicals, which may have a negative effect upon those cells.

There is new research investigating the effect of strenuous exercise upon leucocytes. Some of the results indicate that while moderate exercise increases the number of leucocytes, severe and prolonged exercise may reverse the trend. It seems that overall the degree of immunosuppression evidenced by the athletes is similar to that seen in individuals suffering from a high degree of prolonged situational stress.

There is a highly complex system of interaction between the immune system and the neuro-endocrine system, as the neurotransmitters and hormones regulate all cell functions, including the activity of the immune system. During exercise, the neuro-endocrine system secretes endorphins. This results in an abatement of pain and a mild euphoria. There is also a release of growth hormones and a release of beta-oestradiol in females and testosterone in males. Both of these hormones can produce a higher sex drive. The other substance released is adrenocorticotrophic hormone (ACTH), which signals to the adrenal glands the need to produce cortisone.

The Institute of Sports Research (Weidemann et al 1992) found that after several hours of moderate exercise, there is up to a 10-fold increase of growth hormone levels. However, these changes are transient and there is a return to homeostasis within six hours. Moderate exercise causes the pituitary gland to secrete the growth hormone which boosts the immune system. However, when the exercise reaches a stressful level, the adrenals release ACTH, which neutralizes the positive effects of exercise and suppresses the immune system.

Physiological stress produces only transient increases in cortisone. If, however, an athlete competes in a major event and a psychological stress is added to the physiological stress, there is more ACTH released, thereby decreasing the immune response.

These studies are relatively new and require further validation. However, their implication is that too much competitive sport creates physical and psychological states which may be detrimental to the individual's well being. As a corollary, we may face a possibility that dealing with some injured athletes may require skills not too different from those dealing with the 'pain prone' group of chronic pain patients.

Endorphins and naloxone studies

At this point the exact mechanism of effectiveness of endorphins is still unknown, although their effects are well established and their physiology is evident. Study of

---

[1] Note: Physical dependence can be differentiated from psychological dependence, i.e. withdrawal of exercise or jogging may produce a negative effect on the mood state.

naloxone inhibition still produces controversial results (Grevert & Goldstein 1978, Levine et al 1978a).

Endorphins and placebo response

Hilgard (1980) showed that some placebo responsiveness is due to increased production of endorphins in the body as a result of self-suggestion of pain relief. An important study of pain (Levine et al 1978b) examined the relationship between placebo and endorphins in a clinical situation. Patients listed for surgery for dental pain were assessed for placebo responsiveness. When the whole group was given placebo with a suggestion of pain relief, the positive placebo respondents reported less pain, while negative placebo respondents did not. Four hours after surgery, in a double-blind trial, some patients received placebo, while others received naloxone. Naloxone did not increase the pain of the negative responders to placebo, but it increased the pain in positive placebo responders. Furthermore, if naloxone was given prior to placebo, it decreased the number of positive placebo responders. This suggests that endorphins release mediated placebo-induced analgesia for post-operative dental pain. This study confirms other findings which show that positive placebo respondents produce endogenous analgesics to control their pain if they believe that the treatment of pain is effective.

An interesting link between pain, placebo and side effects of medication comes from the study of Elton et al (1983). Pain-prone patients suffering from prolonged pain lasting up to 25 years were divided into four experimental groups: hypnosis, biofeedback, placebo and interaction. In the placebo group the patients were divided into two subgroups, and were offered 'medication' in a double-blind trial. Some received small blue tablets, which looked like Stellazine, a powerful relaxant. The others were presented with white and yellow capsules, which looked like a tricyclic drug Amytriptiline. All patients were told that the medication may be a powerful pain reliever to be taken for a period of 12 weeks. While the experimenter was less familiar with the two substances, the patients had prior experience of them.

While relief from pain was negligible, both subgroups complained of unfortunate side effects. The group on blue tablets reported feeling drowsy all the time, having difficulty driving, falling asleep at parties, etc. The patients taking the capsules complained of double vision, dryness of mouth, disorientation, etc. Each report was consistent with the side effects of Stellazine and Amytriptiline. After termination of the research the experimenter was informed that in fact all the patients were given only sugar pills.

It seems that as a result of their belief in side effects of the 'drugs' and a scepticism regarding their effects on pain, the patients produced 'side effects' rather than pain relief.

All patients were re-assigned to other treatment modalities, where they have shown better gains.

Relationship between endorphins and substance P

Various researchers have focused on the relationship between the enkephalins and neurotransmitters such as substance P, which exists in high quantities in the substantia gelatinosa and the central amygdala (Uhl et al, 1977). This led Snyder (1978) to postulate a model of analgesia functioning at the level of the spinal cord. While some initial research suggested that the analgesic effects of substance P were short-term, work by Nakamura-Craig and Smith (1989) presented evidence that substance P is an important modulator in peripheral inflammatory pain, sensitising nociceptors to its own action and to the action of other mediators. This sensitising process can be associated with chronic inflammatory pain.

Endorphins and hypnosis

Initially there was insufficient evidence for a link between endorphins and hypnotic analgesia, however in 1978 Carli reported that morphine-like mechanisms may be responsible for the suppression of the behavioural and EEG manifestations of pain during animal hypnosis. Since in many experimental studies the effects of hypnotic analgesia cannot be reversed by naloxone, this suggests that either there are still undiscovered endorphins whose effectiveness cannot be reversed by naloxone, or that hypnotic analgesia occurs as a result of a release of still unknown non-opioid mechanisms. Hypnotic analgesia seems to occur too quickly and strongly to be mediated by the slow acting endorphin chain (Elton 1992). Both possibilities provide exciting scope for research.

Hypnosis can produce powerful positive changes to the body's healing processes. There is extensive literature describing the effects of hypnosis on the treatment of pain, psychosomatic conditions and results of injury (Elton 1992). While at present physiotherapists are not permitted to practise hypnosis on their patients, knowledge of the benefits offered by using hypnosis as an adjunct to standard physiotherapy treatment has merit. In the author's, opinion all physiotherapists would benefit from gaining a reasonable awareness of hypnotic phenomena.

Hypnosis has been used in the treatment of acute and chronic conditions. Many sports clubs employ a psychologist (Quinn 1992) versed in hypnotic training, to treat injured athletes. While we do not know the exact nature of the biochemical mechanisms of hypnosis, the empirical evidence of positive changes is compelling. Elton et al (1978c) report a study where pain sufferers who were treated by hypnosis lost most or all of their chronic pain. Hypnosis has been used in acute injuries to stop pain, reduce swelling and heal skin. While relief of pain can be measured mainly by self report of the individual, it is easier to measure reduction of swelling of the affected part.

Interactions between endorphins and other substances

The hypothalamus-pituitary-adrenal axis can indirectly affect endocrine and endorphin biosynthesis; cortisol seems to suppress their production. Stress may also induce analgesia via opioid or non-opioid mechanisms. The relationship between cortisol and endorphins is very important. A study by Lascelles et al (1974) indicated that chronic pain patients seemed to have higher than normal cortisol plasma levels. Furthermore, Terenius (1981) produced evidence that patients with pain of neurogenic origin had very low cerebral spinal fluid (CSF) endorphin levels, although there were higher levels of endorphins in some patients with psychologically-based pain. There was also evidence of a relationship between the presence of high levels of serotonin and low levels of endorphin activity.

Iggo (1987) pointed out a relationship between prostaglandin and pain: the higher the level of prostaglandin, the higher the pain. Peripheral analgesics do not seem to modify the sensitivity of the receptors in the absence of hyperalgesia, an effect in the case of non-steroidal anti-inflammatory drugs which act by diminishing production of prostaglandin.

Endorphins and acupuncture

Acupuncture has been known to stimulate endorphin and other pain modulator systems in the CNS (Han & Terenius 1982). Terenius (1987) found that the higher the level of endorphins in CSF the higher the tolerance to postoperative pain. High levels of beta-endorphin in plasma have been found in patients with chronic pain and major depressive disorders. Mayer et al (1977) demonstrated that endorphins are associated with acupuncture-induced analgesia.

The research into acupuncture-induced analgesia by Lianfang He & Xiaoding Cao (1987) has particular relevance to the physiotherapists, some of whom are using acupuncture in the treatment of pain. Recently, laser acupuncture and electro-acupuncture have become useful adjuncts to the physiotherapy treatment (Richards 1989). Traditionally, the effectiveness of acupuncture was explained by the Gate Control theory of pain (Melzack & Wall 1965). Linking this theory to the biochemical elements can produce an important breakthrough in the understanding of the theory behind the practice.

Non-opioid neurotransmitters

Further study is needed to understand non-opioid neurotransmitters in pain perception and analgesia (Messing & Wilcox 1987). Messing suggests that serotonin mediates endogenous opioid and non-opioid pain control systems. The role of non-opioid neurotransmitters may explain why naloxone does not reverse the analgesic effects of hypnosis.

Messing presents a strong case that drugs which enhance serotogenic neurotransmission may have potential therapeutic use, either by themselves or in conjunction with opioids. The biochemical markers of pain and stress and their modulation present important new fields for research in the laboratory and in the clinic.

In summary, the field of biochemistry of the body is a relatively new science with an unlimited scope for development. Each year there are new breakthroughs and new findings. This exciting field will eventually lead to a reformulation of much of our understanding of the therapeutic effectiveness of all treatment modalities.

NEUROPHYSIOLOGY AND PAIN: SPINAL MECHANISMS OF NOCICEPTION

Pain cannot be considered simply as a sensation, as there are no specific pain receptors in body tissues, nor is there a pain centre in the cortex. Melzack (1973) argued that although pain fibres terminate in the thalamus, there is no clear definition of where they end. The brain stem, particularly the mid-brain periaqueductal grey in its ventrolateral aspects, and periventicular thalamic sites, are involved in the transmission of pain (Fields & Basbaum 1978).

Early theories

The early theory of Specificity (Muller 1842) assumed that there were pain endings the same as there are sensory spots for other sensations. On the other hand, the Pattern theory of pain (Goldscheider 1894) assumed that pain was evoked by a summation of sensory inputs at the dorsal horn cells.

Nociceptors

In a recent description of the system, Iggo (1987) stated that the primary detectors of noxious or potentially noxious stimuli applied to the peripheral tissues are the nociceptors. These sensory receptors transmit stimuli which exceed the threshold magnitude of intensity. They have a much higher excitatory threshold than the thresholds for other sensations such as cold, heat, pressure, etc. Some nociceptors are generalised and transmit information via non-myelinated (C) afferent fibres. Others have greater selectivity. These include the mechanical nociceptors with small myelinated (A delta) afferent fibres. The transmission of impulses varies between the two fibres, giving rise to two sensory responses such as first and second pain (Iggo 1987).

Gate Control theory of pain

A breakthrough in neurophysiological approaches occurred with the advent of the Gate Control theory of pain (Melzack & Wall 1965, Melzack 1973, 1990). This influential theory has provided a useful framework for understanding the mechanisms of pain. Nearly 30 years later, the theory has not been invalidated. The basic assumption of the Gate Control theory is that there is, within the substantia gelatinosa of the dorsal horns of the spinal columns, a neural mechanism which acts as a pain gate. This gate can increase or decrease the flow of nerve impulses from peripheral fibres to the central nervous system, because of the reciprocal activity of the large-diameter A-beta and the small-diameter A-delta and C fibres, and the influence from the cortex via the descending pyramidal and extrapyramidal tracts. When the amount of information that passes through the gate exceeds a critical level, it activates the neural mechanisms responsible for pain experience and control. The large, fast-conducting A-beta fibres can depolarise the intramedullary afferent terminals, close the gate, and thereby decrease the effectiveness of the excitatory synapses and lower the experience of pain. Although these effects occur mainly at the pre-synaptic level, they are coupled with a simultaneous change in the post-synaptic transmission cells (see Fig. 6.1).

Melzack (1973) suggested that there are three features of the afferent input which are significant for the pain experience: the ongoing activity which precedes the stimulus, the stimulus-evoked activity, and the relative balance of the activity in large versus small fibres. He argued that when pain stimulus occurs and activates the receptor system, it enters an active nervous system which is already the substrate of past experience, cultural learning, anxiety, the present meaning of pain and so on. These cerebral processes participate actively in the selection, abstraction and synthesis of the information on pain received from the total afferent sensory input. Pain is not simply the end product of a linear sensory transmission; it is a dynamic process which involves continuous interactions between complex ascending and descending systems. Therefore the specificity theory cannot be applied to pain. General anxiety, worry over the consequences of the pain, the meaning of pain, and attention to pain may all stimulate the small-diameter fibres and potentiate the pain experience. Relaxation, focusing attention on something else and general mental calmness can stimulate the large-diameter fibres and thus decrease the experience of pain. Somatic input is therefore subject to the modulating influence of the gate before it evokes pain perception and response.

Modifications of the Gate Control theory

Further findings suggested that there is more than one gate (Melzack & Dennis, 1978); in fact, there may be successive synapses which act as pain gates throughout the pathways of pain, from the spinal cord to the brain area responsible for pain experience and response. Indeed, Melzack and Dennis (1978) have shown that laminae 1, 2, 3, 4 and 5 are concerned with conduction of nociceptive information. Virtually all dorsal horn cells have extensive projections to the brain and project through the spinothalamic tract, and the dorsolateral and dorsal column systems. All are under the control of the descending fibres. The presynaptic and post-synaptic effects are believed to be produced by the cells in laminae 2 and 3.

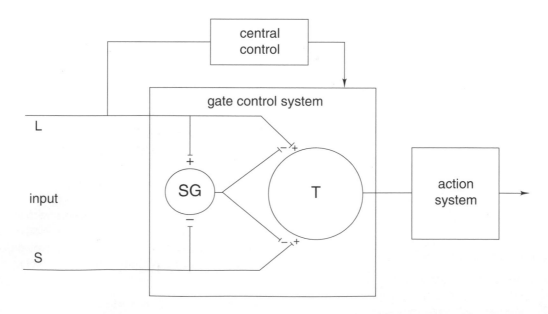

Fig. 6.1 Schematic diagram of the gate-control theory of pain mechanisms: L = the large-diameter fibres; S = the small-diameter fibres; + = excitation; - = inhibition. The fibres project to the substantia gelatinosa (SG) and first central transmission (T) cells. The inhibitory effect exerted by SG on the afferent fibre terminals is increased by activity in L fibres and decreased by activity in S fibres. The central control trigger is represented by a line running from the large fibre system to the central control mechanisms; these mechanisms, in turn, project back to the gate-control system. The T cells project to the entry cells of the action system. Source: Melzack and Wall (1965) ©1965 American Association for the Advancement of Science

The Gate Control theory of pain has remained an important explanatory system in understanding pain. According to Wall (1978) some modifications were necessary in view of ongoing neurological discoveries. They included redefinition of the role of the substantia gelatinosa, the role of large-diameter cells, and the various post-synaptic mechanisms which may facilitate or inhibit the pain experience.

Neurophysiological basis of the Gate Control theory

Melzack and Dennis (1978) argued that the sensory-discriminative information is directly associated with the neurons in the ventrobasal thalamus, and that transmission to reticular and limbic structures involving the motivational affective dimension may be indirect.

The reticular formation medulla and central grey in adjacent areas of the mid-brain produce pain behaviour (Elton Stanley and Burrows 1983). The limbic system, because of its reciprocal interconnection with the reticular formation, plays an important role in the transmission of pain. Its major pathway is the central grey which projects to the medial thalamus, hypothalamus and the limbic fore-brain structures. This pathway interacts with the frontal cortex. Surgical relief of pain has been achieved by a section of the singulum bundle or via a lesion of the medial thalamus and intralaminar nuclei. This points to the role of these structures in the experience of pain.

Frontal lobes seem to be associated with the motivational-affective dimension of pain. The cognito-evaluative dimension of pain is associated with the dorsal column and the dorsolateral projection pathway. This association, by involving the descending pyramidal and other central control threads, may modulate the incoming information and inhibit the firing in the dorsal horn cells in the spinal cord. Melzack and Dennis (1978) have suggested that neuron pools at many levels of the spinal cord and brain can act as pattern-generating mechanisms.

The Gate Control theory of pain (1965) has been used for years to explain the effectiveness of various therapeutic interventions. It led to development of TENS machines, which are believed to stimulate the large diameter fibres, providing alternative sources of information to the brain , closing the pain gate and thereby decreasing the pain experience. There is less clear evidence of the use of interferential current, however all use of current could be interpreted as affecting the closing of the pain gate.

Acute and chronic pain

While discussing the neurophysiology of pain, a distinction needs to be made between acute and chronic pain (Bonica 1977). Acute pain is usually associated with a well-defined cause, has a characteristic time course and usually terminates when healing has occurred. It has a rapid onset, a phasic component, and a subsequent tonic component, persisting for various periods of time. Biochemically, acute pain is similar to an anxiety state. It involves a fight or flight reaction, an excessive activity of the sympathetic system and feelings of anxiety and fear.

In chronic pain, the tonic component, which begins when the phasic component is over, may persist long after the healing of the initial injury. The neural mechanisms in chronic pain are more complex. The pain may also spread to other parts of the body and be resistant to standard forms of pain control. On a biochemical level chronic pain has effects similar to depression. There is a habituation of responses, lower sympathetic activity, depression, feelings of helplessness and somatic preoccupation. There is also narrowing of interests, sleep disturbance and changes in eating habits (Elton, Stanley and Burrows 1983). There are changes in the levels of serotonin and brain amines.

The neural pathways conducting the message of acute pain are the fast-conducting, dorsal column, post-synaptic system, the spino-cervical tract, and the neospinothalamic tract. The neural pathways conducting the message of chronic pain carry tonic information. The slow-conducting fibres associated with this experience are the spino-reticular tract and the paleo-spinothalamic tract. These pathways determine the level of arousal and general behavioural state necessary to protect the body from further damage, and to foster rest, protection and care of the damaged areas. As the healing progresses, their activity decreases.

It is of interest that while morphine generally diminishes tonic post-surgical pain, it is less effective in alleviating the phasic pain.

Melzack (1973) suggested that long-lasting chronic pain without well-defined physiological antecedents may be due to reverberatory or other self-sustaining neural activities that subserve memory-like processes related to pain. It is not clear which neural mechanisms subserve the long-term memory of sensory experiences. We can speculate about reverberatory neuron loops (Livingstone 1943) or a simpler two-neuron circuit (Anderson & Eccles 1962) which can produce rhythmic, sustained activity.

While physiotherapists working in the area of sports physiotherapy deal mainly with acute pain, the symptoms of chronic pain and its associated mood states may occur earlier than suggested in the literature (Weidemann et al 1992). If an athlete is depressed due to injury, the hormonal changes within the body will be similar to those in chronic pain, and the healing processes will be similarly affected. When anxiety turns into depression, it is useful to consider the psychological strategies used in control of chronic pain even if this occurs within weeks of the injury.

Endorphins and neural pathways

Some neural circuits may play a role in prolonged pathological pain. Immuno-histo-chemical studies show that

Goal setting

The Self-efficacy theory (Kelley 1990) implies a conviction that a person can successfully attain certain outcomes by an appropriate behaviour. These views are shared by Yukelson (1986), who suggested that an individual's performance may be predicted by his or her feelings of competence or expectations of personal effectiveness. This has an implication for setting therapeutic goals.

If the injured athlete can set a series of specific measurable and attainable goals which require continuous effort but which can lead to gradual improvement, the corresponding success will increase the athlete's belief in his or her capability to be in control. Attaining goals is important to athletes as they are involved in setting goals for themselves with every competition and are therefore in touch with these needs. Therefore goal-setting techniques and positive expectations can increase motivation to improve and can improve athlete's self-esteem when it is eroded by injury.

Orlick and Partington (1988) considered goal-setting an important first step in the initiation of positive action towards a speedy recovery. The research indicated that the sports psychologist may have an important role to play as a team member in the process of rehabilitating an injured athlete (see Ch. 19).

Recovery enhancement skills

These include goal-setting, positive self-taught imagery, relaxation, etc. which seem critical in attaining maximal physical rehabilitation (Orlick & Partington 1988). The authors surveyed 39 injured athletes, post-recovery, and divided them into 3 groups: fast, average and slow healers. All three groups were examined on cognitive skills. It was found that the group who scored high on goal-setting, positive thought and positive healing imagery, were the fastest healers.

There is a possibility that studying recovery after completion may yield biased results, since the fast-healing athletes may show selective memories of their attitudes to healing and view them as more positive whereas the slow healers might show negative selected memories, but the study indicates that the human mind may be a powerful agent in achieving positive change.

Relaxation techniques

Imagery, visualization and relaxation have not been researched adequately as they are mainly used in combination with other treatments.

For instance, athletes may be trained to use imagery in conjunction with relaxation to cope with stress of injury (Rotella & Heyman 1986). They may be used to reduce pain and improve healing, and later they may be used as a motive rehearsal to deal with the fear of returning to competition. Finally, mastery rehearsal may be used to improve performance skills (Feltz 1986). When athletes realize that their performance will be enhanced by mental rehearsal even if they are not able to rehearse physically, this may augment their motivation for the task.

Elton and Stanley (1976) provided an interesting demonstration of usefulness of relaxation and visualization in control of acute pain. 150 physiotherapy students were divided into two groups. Each group received initially painful stimulation by inflating a sphygmanometer cuff with plastic projections inside it. This pressure was applied to the long head of the biceps, and produced rapid pain. There was no significant difference in pain scores for both groups. Subsequently one group received training in relaxation and visualization. It was suggested that people can move away from pain by going to a favourite place away from the body. Both groups were then re-tested. The group trained in relaxation and visualization showed significantly better pain control. One subject reported that she could not go to another place (i.e. the beach) because the pain in her arm held her there. Instead, she stood mentally at the foot of the bed, leaving her arm behind, and the pain diminished anyway.

Affirmation imagery

The idea of affirmation imagery was suggested by Porter and Foster (1986). Repeating positive affirmations throughout the day may alter the negative thoughts related to the injury and improve belief in self-control. Positive images of healing as well as images of being fully recovered may mobilize a person's healing powers (Rotella & Heyman 1986). These techniques are particularly useful with hypnosis (Elton 1982) but they can also be used by physiotherapists with other relaxation techniques.

While athletes cannot change the fact that they have been injured, they can control their attitude towards the injury and recovery by a positive dialogue with their bodies (Porter & Foster 1986). This is easier to attain if the treatment is providing them with evidence of success, and if it is interesting and enjoyable.

Sometimes it is useful to provide the athletes with literature related to the treatment used, even if it is not entirely comprehensible. There is power in the written word, and people believe the efficacy of treatment more, particularly if relaxation and visualization (which may be assessed wrongly as 'soft' techniques) are used in conjunction with standard physiotherapy treatment.

Biofeedback training

Biofeedback can be used in conjunction with hypnosis, relaxation, visualization and other methods of rehabilitation. It provides instant evidence of change by 'a machine that does not lie' and helps enhance the patient's motivation by giving them a renewed feeling of personal control. The actual mechanisms of change in biofeedback therapy are more obscure than its effects. It shows changes in the physiological processes of the body and, by implication, in biochemical processes with which they are connected. This can affect the psychological state of the individual and may, in turn, be affected by it.

Return to competition

Often, when athletes return to competition, it is assumed that they are totally rehabilitated. This is not always valid (Weiss & Troxel 1986). Some athletes may experience anxiety and lack of confidence upon returning to competition and, in the process, find it extremely difficult to adjust to the demands of full training. Some are not ready physically although they are emotionally prepared to assume their tasks. Others, although physically ready, may not be psychologically ready to return to the rigours of competition. In such cases even a suggestion of return may produce negative feelings of doubts, fears and anxieties (Quinn 1992). Such anxiety may result in re-injury or in temporary or permanent performance decrease. Rotella and Heyman (1986) suggested that attention to both the physical and psychological components of rehabilitation is crucial in the recovery of an athlete. Sometimes, when the physiotherapy treatment is over, it may be useful to re-examine the psychological state of an individual prior to returning him or her to competitive sport.

SUMMARY

Biochemical and neurophysiological events have an impact on the experience of pain , and on the response to pain and injury. This chapter has illustrated the difficulty in isolating each variable, since they interact in a complex way. The human body has the capacity to heal itself even without treatment, but with treatment this capacity is greatly enhanced.

The physiotherapist in the area of sports medicine needs a thorough knowledge of all aspects of pain and injury. While the predominant method of treatment is physical, other knowledge is important to explain some patients' failure to improve, even with the best of physiotherapy approaches. It is equally useful to understand placebo effects in improvement. A physiotherapist has a great potential for generating the placebo response, by providing a caring atmosphere, visible methods of treatment and a tangible evidence that change is occurring.

Effective physiotherapy needs a committed and motivated patient. Fortunately, in the area of sports physiotherapy most patients have greater commitment to getting well quickly than in other areas of physiotherapy practice. They are generally younger and healthier, and they are less likely to submit to chronic pain. Nevertheless, not all of them have a positive approach to injury Their improvement can be enhanced by a thorough knowledge of all the variables involved in pain and injury. These include an understanding of biochemistry, neurophysiology and the psychology of injury and pain.

REFERENCES

Anderson P, Eccles J C 1962 Inhibitory phasing of neuronal discharge. Nature 196:645–647

Andersson S A, Rydenhag B 1985 Cortical nociceptive systems. Philos. Trans. R. Soc. London Ser B 308:347–355

Arner S, Meyerson B 1988 Lack of analgesic effect of opioids on neuropathic and idiopathic forms of pain. Pain 31(1):11–23

Beecher H K 1959 Measurement of subjective response. Oxford University Press, New York

Beecher H K 1968 The measurements of pain in man. In: Soulairac A, Cahn J, Charpentier J (eds) Pain. Academic Press, London

Blackwell B, McCullagh P 1990 The relationship of athletic injury to life stress, competitive anxiety and coping resources. Athletic training 25:23–27

Bonica J J (ed) 1977 Advances in pain research and therapy. Raven Press, New York, vol 2

Brock T C, Buss A H 1962 Dissonance, aggression, and evaluation of pain. Journal of Abnormal and Social Psychology 65:197-202

Burrows G D, Elton D, Stanley G V (eds) Handbook of chronic pain management. Elsevier, Science Publishers B.V. (Biomedical Division), Amsterdam pp 33–39

Carli G, Farabollini F, Fontani G 1978 Pain and animal hyposis: further studies on the effects of morphine and naloxone. In: Second world congress on pain VI (pain abstracts). Association for the Study of Pain, Seattle

Cavangah M E 1985 An investigation of the relationship between selected personality traits and the injury frequency of intercollegiate athletes. Unpublished master's thesis, University of North Carolina, Chapel Hill

Cervero F, Iggo A 1980 Substantia gelatinosa of the spinal cord column: a critical review. Brain 103:717–772

Crossman J 1985 Psychosocial factors and athletic injury. Journal of Sports Medicine and Physical Fitness 25:151–154

Cryan P O, Alles E F 1983 The relationship between stress and football injuries. Journal of Sports Medicine and Physical Fitness 23:52–58

Davidson P O, Bobey M J 1970 Repressor-sensitizer differences on repeated exposures to pain. Perceptual and Motor Skills 31:711–714

Duda J L, Smart A E, Tappe M K 1989 Predictors of adherence in the rehabilitation of athletic injuries: an application of personal investment theory. Journal of Sport and Exercise Psychology ll:367–381

Elton D 1980 Stress, anxiety and coping. Mental health in the 80s. Public Lecture Series. Victorian Association of Mental Health, Melbourne, October pp 20–24

Elton D 1982 Hypnosis and hypnotherapy. Australian Rationalist Quarterly Jan–Feb–March:11–14

Elton D 1992 Combined use of hypnosis and biofeedback in the treatment of stress induced conditions. Stress Medicine 9:25-35

Elton D, Stanley G V 1976 Relaxation as a method of pain control. Australian Journal of Physiotherapy 22:121–123

Elton D, Burrows G D, Stanley G V 1978a Relaxation: theory and practice. Australian Journal of Physiotherapy 24–183–186

Elton D, Quary P R, Burrows G D, Stanley G V 1978 A study of perceptual and psychophysical correlates of pain. Perceptual and Motor Skills 47:125–126

Elton D, Stanley, G V, Burrows G D 1978 Self esteem and chronic pain. Journal of Psychosomatic Research 22:25–30

Elton D, Stanley G, Burrows G 1983 Psychological control of pain. Grune & Stratton, Sydney

Eysenck H J 1957 The dynamics of anxiety and hysteria. Routledge & Kegan Paul, London

Feltz D L 1986 The psychologic aspects of sports injuries. In: Vinger P F, Hoerner E F (eds) Sports injuries: the unthwarted epidemic, 2nd edn. PSG Publishing, Littleton, Massachusetts pp 336–344

Ferreira S H 1986 Control of inflammatory pain. In: Advances in inflammation research. Raven Press, New York

Fields H L, Basbaum A I 1978 Brainstem control of spinal pain–transmission neurons. Annual Revue of Physiology 40:217–248

Fleetwood–Walker S M, Mitchell R, Hope P J, Molony V 1985 Effects of opioid peptide agonists selective for xx and x receptors on identified dorsal horn neurons. In: Iggo A, Iversen L L, Cervero F (eds) Nociception and pain. Royal Society, London, p 427

Fordyce W E 1978 Learning process in pain. In: Sternbach R A (ed) The psychology of pain. Raven Press, New York

Goldscheider A 1894 Ueber den schmerz in physiologischer and klinischer hinsicht. Hirschwald, Berlin

Goldstein A 1976 Opioid peptides (endorphins) in pituitary and brain. Science 193:1081–1086

Gordon N C, Heller P H, Levine J D 1991 Lack of effect of ephedrine on opiate analgesia. Pain 47:21–23

Grevert P, Goldstein A 1978 Endorphins: naloxone fails to alter experimental pain or mood in humans. Science 199:1093–1095

Han J S, Terenius L 1982 Neurochemical basis of acupuncture analgesia. Annual Review of Pharmacological Toxicology 22:193–220

Hilgard E R 1980 Hypnosis in the treatment of pain. In: Burrows G D, Dennerstein L (eds) Handbook of hypnosis and psychosomatic medicine. Excerpta Medica, Elsevier/North Holland Biomedical Press, Amsterdam

Hokfelt T, Ljungdahl A, Terenius L, Elde R, Nilsson G 1977 Immunohistochemical analysis of peptide pathways possibly related to pain and analgesia: enkephalin and substance P. Proceedings of the National Academy of Sciences of the United Sstates of America 74:3081–3085

Hughes J, Smith T W, Kosterlitz H W 1975 Identification of two related pentapeptides from brain with potent opiate agonist activity. Nature 258:577–579

Iggo A 1985 Sensory receptors in the skin of mammals and their sensory functions. Rev. Neurol., Paris 141:599–613

Iggo A 1987 Physiology of pain. In: Burrows G D, Elton D, Stanley G V (eds) Handbook of chronic pain management. Elsevier Science Publishers B.V. (Biomedical Division), Amsterdam, pp 7–18

Irvin R F 1975 Relationship between personality and the incidence of injuries to high school football participants. Dissertation abstracts. University of Oregon 36(7):4328–A

Iversen L, Dingledine R 1976 Enkephalin: the latest instalment. Nature 262:738–739

Kelley M J 1990 Psychological risk factors and sports injuries. Journal of Sports Medicine and Physical Fitness 30(2):202–221

Kerns J M, Braverman B, Mathew A, Lucchinetti C, Ivankovich A D 1991 A comparison of cryoprobe and crush lesions in the rat sciatic nerve. Pain 47:31–39

Kerr G, Minden H 1988 Psychological factors related to the occurrence of athletic injuries. Journal of Sport and Exercise Psychology 10:167–173

Kubler–Ross E 1969 On death and dying. Tavistock, London

Kupers R C, Konings H, Adriaensen H, Gybels J M 1991 Morphine differentially affects the sensory and affective pain ratings in neurogenic and idiopathic forms of pain. Pain 47:5–12

Lascelles P T, Evans P R, Merskey H, Sabur M A 1974 Plasma cortisol in psychiatric and neurologic patients with pain. Brain 97:533–538

Lazarus R S, Folkman S 1984 Stress, appraisal and coping. Springer, New York

Lianfang He, Xiaoding Cao 1987 Endogenous opioid peptides and acupuncture analgesia. In: Burrows G D, Elton D, Stanley G V (eds) Handbook of chronic pain management. Elsevier Science Publishers B.V. (Biomedical Division) Amsterdam pp 47–52

Levine J D, Gordon N C, Fields H L 1978 Evidence that the analgesic effect of placebo is mediated by endorphins. In: Second world congress on pain. International Association for the Study of Pain, vol 1, Pain abstracts

Levine J D, Gordon N C, Fields H L 1978 The mechanism of placebo analgesia. Lancet 2:654–657

Liebeskind J C, Paul L A 1977 Psychological and physiological mechanisms of pain. Annual Review of Psychology 28:41–60

Lipman J J, Miller B E, Mays K S, Miller M N, North W C, Byrne W L 1990 Peak B endorphin concentration in cerebrospinal fluid: reduced in chronic pain patients and increased during the placebo response. Psychopharmacology 102:112–116

Livingstone W K 1943 Pain mechanisms. Macmillan, New York

May J R 1990 Psychological sequelae and rehabilitation of the injured athlete. Sports Medicine Digest 12(11):1–2, 85

May J R, Sieb G E 1987 Athletic injuries: psychosocial factors in the onset, sequelae, rehabilitation and prevention. In: May J R, Asken M J (eds) Sports psychology. PMA Publishing, New York, p 157-185

Mayer D J, Price D D, Rafii 1977 Antagonism of acupuncture analgesia in man by the narcotic antagonist naloxone. Brain Research 121:368–372

Melzack R 1973 The puzzle of pain. Penguin, Harmondsworth, Middlesex

Melzack R 1990 The tragedy of needless pain. In: Scientific American 262:19–25

Melzack R, Dennis S G 1978 Neurophysiological foundations of pain. In: Sternbach R A (ed) The psychology of pain. Raven Press, New York

Melzack R, Wall P D 1965 Pain mechanisms: a new theory. Science 150:971–979

Merskey H, Spear E G1967 Pain: psychological and psychiatric aspects. Bailleiere, Tindall and Cassell, London

Messing R B, Wilcox G L 1987 Non-opioid neurotransmitters in pain perception and analgesia. In: Burrows G D, Elton D, Stanley G V (eds) Handbook of chronic pain management. Elsevier Science Publishers B.V. (Biomedical Division), Amsterdam, pp 7–18

Muller J 1842 Elements of physiology. Taylor, London

Nakamura–Craig M, Smith T W 1989 Substance P and peripheral inflammatory hyperalgesia. Pain 38(1):91–98

Orlick T, Partington J 1988 Mental links to excellence. The Sport Psychologist 2:105–130

Otis C 1992 Problems of female athletes. Lecture, The American College of Sports Medicine Conference, Washington, June

Pasternak G W, Bodnar R J, Clark J A, Inturrisi C E 1987 Morphine–6–glucuronide, a potent mu agonist. Life Science 41:2845–2849

Pert C B, Snyder S H 1973 Opiate receptor: demonstration in nervous tissue. Science 179:1011–1014

Portenoy R K, Foley K M, Inturissi C E 1990 The nature of opioid responsiveness and its implications for neuropathic pain: new hypotheses derived from studies of opioid infusions. Pain 43:273–286

Porter K, Foster J 1986 The mental athlete: inner training for peak performance. Ballantine, New York

Quinn A 1992 Psychological factors which predispose athletes to injury. Unpublished Doctoral thesis. Psychology Department, University of Melbourne

Richards D 1989 Your health is in your hands. Superior Health Products, Rose Park SA

Rotella R J, Heyman S R 1986 Stress, injury and the psychological rehabilitation of athletes. In: Williams J M (ed) Applied sport psychology: personal growth to peak performance. Mayfield. Palo Alto Ca, pp 343–364

Sanderson FH 1981 The psychology of the injury-prone athlete. In: Reilly T (ed) Sports fitness and sports injuries. Faber & Faber, London pp 31–36

Sauerbruch F, Wenke H 1963 Pain: its meaning and significance. Allen & Unwin, London

Schmidt P, Poulsen S S, Rasmussen T N, Bersani M, Holst J J 1991 Substance P and neurokinin A are codistributed and colocalized in the porcine gastrointestinal tract. Peptides, Pergamon Press, New York

Silva J M, Hardy C J 1991 The sport psychologist. In: Mueller F O, Ryan A J (eds) Prevention of athletic injuries: the role of the sports medicine team. Contemporary exercise and sports medicine. F A Davis, Philadelphia, pp 114–132

Simon E J, Hiller J M, Edelman I 1973 Stereospecific binding of the potent narcotic analgesic [3H]-etorphine to rat brain homogenate. Proceedings of the National Academy of Sciences 70:1947–1949

Smith A M, Scott S G, Wiese D M 1990 The psychological effects of sports injuries. Coping. Sports Medicine 9(6):352–369

Snyder S H 1978 The opiate receptor and morphine–like peptides in the brain. American Journal of Psychiatry 135:645–652

Sternbach R A 1968 Pain: a psychophysiological analysis. Academic Press, New York

Sternbach R A 1974 Pain patients: traits and treatments. Academic Press, New York

Terenius L 1973 Stereospecific interaction between narcotic analgesics and a synaptic plasma membrane fraction of rat cerebral cortex. Acta Pharmacologica et Toxicologica 32:317–320

Terenius L 1981 Endorphins and pain. Hormonal Research 8:162–177

Terenius L 1987 Endorphins and cortisol in chronic pain. In: Burrows G D, Elton D, Stanley G V (eds) Handbook of chronic pain management. Elsevier, Science Publishers B.V. (Biomedical Division), Amsterdam, pp 33–39

Teschemacher H, Opheim K G, Cox B M, Goldstein A 1975 A peptide-like substance from pituitary that acts like morphine. Isolation. Life Sciences 16:1771–1775

Uhl G R, Kuhar J J, Snyder S H 1977 Neurotensin: immunohistochemical localisation in rat central nervous system. Proceedings of the National Academy of Sciences 74:4059–4063

Vallient P M 1980 Injury and personality traits in non-competitive runners. Journal of Sports Medicine and Physical Fitness 20(3):341–346

Vargas M L, Bansinath M, Turndorf H, Puig M M 1989 Antinociceptive effects of azepexole (BHT 933) in mice. Pain 36(1):117–123

Voudouris N J, Peck C L, Coleman G 1989 Conditional response models of placebo phenomena: further support. Pain 38(1):109–116

Wall P 1978 The gate control theory of pain mechanisms: a re-examination and re-statement. Brain 101:1–18

Wall P D 1990 Neuropathic pain (editorial). Pain. 43:267–268

Weidemann M K, Smith J A, Grey A B, McKenzie S J, Pine D D, Kolbech-Braddon M E, Telford R D 1992 Exercise and the immune system. Today's Life Science July:24–33

Weiss M R, Troxel R K 1986 Psychology of the injured athlete. Athletic Training 21:104

Willer J C, Roby A, Gerard A, Maulet C 1982 Electrophysiological evidence for a possible serotoninergic involvement in some endogenous opiate activity in humans. European Journal of Pharmacology 78:117–120

Willer J, De Broucker T, Bussel B, Roby-Brami A, Harrewyn J 1989 Central analgesic effect of ketoprofen in humans: electrophysiological evidence for a supraspinal mechanism in a double-blind and cross-over study. Pain 38(1):1–7

Williams J M, Tonymon P, Wadsworth W A 1986 Relationship of life stress to injury in intercollegiate volleyball. Journal of Human Stress 12:38–43

Witkin H A, Dyk R B, Faterson H F, Goodenough D R, Karp S A 1962 Psychological Differentiation. Wiley, New York

Yukelson D 1986 Psychology of sports and the injured athlete. In: Bernhardt D B (ed) Clinics in physical therapy. Churchill Livingstone, New York, vol 10 Sports physical therapy

Zitman F G, Linssen A C G, Edelbroek P M, Van Kempen G M J 1991 Does addition of low-dose flupentixol enhance the analgesic effects of low-dose amitriptyline in somatoform pain disorder? Pain 47:25–30

Prevention of injury

7. Considerations in injury prevention

Bill Vicenzino, Dorothy Vicenzino

Participation in sport is encouraged as a way of preventing diseases of many of the body's systems, especially the cardiovascular system. Recently it has become evident that participation in sport also constitutes an increased risk of injury (Van Mechelen et al 1992). In Australia, approximately 1 000 000 people suffer a sports injury every year (Australian Sports Medicine Federation 1990). At an estimated total cost to the community of approximately $A1 billion (Australian Sports Medicine Federation 1990), there is considerable motivation for promoting the prevention of sports injuries. For this reason and for other sociological and ideological reasons the contemporary approach to health care is one of prevention (Meeuwisse 1991, Ritchie 1989, Van Mechelen et al 1992).

The musculoskeletal system is most at risk of injury in sports participation (Durant et al 1985). Since physiotherapy is the health care profession that is recognized for its role in the management of musculoskeletal dysfunction, physiotherapists have an important role to play in the prevention of sports injury.

A survey of American physical therapists by the Sports Physical Therapy section of the American Physical Therapy Association highlighted this importance (Skovly 1980). Some of the competencies that the survey identified were the development of preventative conditioning programs; the provision of health care status information and recommendations to coaches, parents and physicians; administration preparticipation physical evaluations; the recommendations for safer playing environments; the selection, fitting and maintenance of athletic equipment and counselling on ergogenic[1] aids (Malone 1986).

The prevention of injury can be classified into primary, secondary and tertiary levels (Lysens et al 1991).

The primary level of prevention refers to specific strategies that are used to prevent injury or illness occurring,

[1] Note: Ergogenic means to increase work output. It is used in reference to performance enhancing drugs, doping and other strategies (legal or illegal) that are implemented in order to increase work output or performance.

e.g. the advertising campaigns that focused on the harmful effects of smoking and excessive alcohol consumption. The implementation of rules to outlaw spear tackles in rugby football and the compulsory wearing of shin guards for all soccer players are some other examples of sport-specific strategies. This chapter focuses on the primary level of prevention.

The secondary level of prevention refers to the early detection of injury, the prevention of the progression of the extent or severity of injury, the prevention of the development of any complications, the prevention of the severity and amount of disability, and the prompt administration of appropriate therapy.

The tertiary level of prevention refers to the restoration of function and the prevention of recurrence by the administration of appropriate rehabilitation programs and implementation of specific preventative measures, most of which are used as strategies in the primary level of prevention.

At the primary level of prevention, an epidemiological investigation of a sport and the identification of injury risk factors are precursors to the implementation of preventative strategies (Van Mechelen et al 1987). Following the implementation of these strategies, further investigations are required to ascertain the effectiveness of the preventative strategies (Van Mechelen et al 1987). This model is similar to that which is used in clinical practice. The clinical assessment of the client is similar to the initial epidemiological investigation and the identification of the risk factors; the implementation of a clinical intervention is similar to the implementation of a preventative strategy and the reassessment following a clinical intervention is similar to follow-up epidemiological investigations.

This chapter reflects the basis of this model in that it is divided into three sections:

- the risk factors predisposing to sports injuries,
- the preparticipation evaluation that is used for the identification of the risk factors, and
- the strategies that are used to prevent sports injury.

RISK FACTORS IN SPORTS INJURIES

Risk factors are usually classified as intrinsic or extrinsic to the participant (Lysens et al 1984). The intrinsic risk factors listed by Lysens et al (1984) are the individual physical and psychological characteristics of the participant; the extrinsic risk factors are the exposure to the sporting activity, the manner in which preparation for the activity is undertaken, the equipment used and the prevailing environmental conditions. To date, the extrinsic factors have received most attention.

The study of the predisposing factors of sports injury is multifaceted and complex (Van Mechelen et al 1992). Unfortunately, many of the studies that have been conducted have methodological errors that detract from their results (Hoeberigs 1992, Taerk 1977). A common type of study that is used seeks to determine correlations between risk factors and injury even though a correlation between two factors does not infer causation (Meeuwisse 1991). Thus a correlation between risk factor and injury does not indicate that the risk factor causes the injury. Consequently, the evidence for many risk factors, especially the intrinsic risk factors, is still conjectural at this stage (Lorenzton 1988, Van Mechelen et al 1992).

Intrinsic factors

The intrinsic risk factors that may be important in the prevention of sports injuries are the existence of any mechanical imbalances; a history of previous injury; the physical fitness level of the participant; and psychological/psychosocial factors.

Mechanical imbalances

Mechanical imbalance can be defined as an alteration of structure and function which is reflected in a variety of combinations of muscle tightness and weakness, ligamentous laxity and/or poor alignment of body segments. Physiotherapists are acutely aware of the importance of accurately identifying these components of mechanical imbalance because they form the basis of any preventative strategies (Sahrmann 1988).

The obvious role of muscles is in the production and control of movements or sustained positions between two or more body segments. The length of a muscle determines many of its structural and functional characteristics of strength, endurance, power and fatigue (Fitch 1984, Gossman et al 1982, Soderberg 1983), and probably plays a role in the control of motor activity (DeDomenico 1984, McCloskey 1982). This is clinically significant because the length of muscles are reported to play a large role in dysfunction of the musculoskeletal system (Janda 1978, Sahrmann 1983).

An alteration in muscle length due to a multitude of biological and environmental factors may alter the joint function through at least two possible avenues, neurological and mechanical. Neurologically, the altered muscle length will affect the fusimotor activity and the feedback to the central regulating mechanisms with a resulting alteration in the level of facilitation of the muscles locally, and at a distance from the muscle with the altered muscle length. (Bullock-Saxton 1991, Cameron-Tucker 1983, Janda 1980). The other avenue is mechanically based, in that the decreased extensibility of connective tissue will alter the muscle's ability to function (Garrett 1990, Herbert 1988). It will also alter the amount of joint excursion that the muscle controls (Janda 1980, Sahrmann 1983, Steindler 1983). A differential in length and strength of agonistic to antagonistic muscles that deviates from an accepted ideal value is referred to as a muscle imbalance.

Muscle tightness. Physiotherapists are very diligent in encouraging athletes to maintain or improve muscle flexibility in order to prevent injury. Surprisingly, few studies have documented a direct causal relationship between muscle tightness and injury (Lorenzton 1988).

Ekstrand and Gillquist (1982) found that soccer players with tight muscles were more likely to injure the tight muscles. However, this was not statistically significant. In a prospective study, Ekstrand and Gillquist (1983a), found a statistically significant relationship between muscle tightness and muscle strain injury and tendonitis. As Keller et al (1987) state, 'This association does not prove causality, but it does suggest that soccer players may benefit from programs designed to increase their flexibility' (p 235).

Lysens et al (1984, cited in Lysens et al 1991) in a prospective study found that athletes with reduced extensibility of the calf muscles were more likely to sustain ankle sprains (lateral ligament). This substantiates the claims made by McCluskey et al (1976) that maintenance of appropriate calf length is important as a preventative measure against injury and reinjury of the ankle. It also validates the authors' clinical observations that clients who returned with recurrent ankle injuries are those who were unable to achieve 10° of talocrural dorsiflexion (with subtalar joint in neutral), either because of muscular or joint restrictions. It is postulated this is because of an inability of the ankle to gain optimum bony stability that is afforded in dorsiflexion (Donatelli 1990).

There are some instances when a high degree of flexibility may result in a lack of protection of the associated joint(s) and culminate in injury. Lysens et al (1989) found evidence for this in a prospective longitudinal study of physical education students. Kirby et al (1981) found that gymnasts who had greater toe touching ability also experienced low back discomfort. Hamilton et al (1992) found that the more flexible male dancers developed more injuries. The deleterious effect of a lengthened muscle on a joint may well be via an interruption in the fine balance of the synergistic contractions required to produce appropriate movement patterns (Richardson 1992), and may predispose the athlete to excessive stresses of the capsulo-ligamentous and cartilaginous structures. It would seem that a fine balance between flexibility, tightness and synergistic co-activation of muscles is essential for the prevention of sports injuries.

Muscle weakness. It seems that muscle weakness is more of a risk factor in overuse injuries than in acute injuries. Foster et al (1989) reported that a lack of quadriceps muscle strength of the non-preferred limb and horizontal flexors of the preferred upper limb were significantly related to 'overuse' back injuries in fast bowlers in cricket. Kowal (1980), in a study of female army recruits, found that those who had reduced leg strength were at greater risk of an overuse injury.

Lysens et al (1989) differentiated muscle strength into dynamic (ballistic) and static (isometric) strength components and found that a lack of static strength is implicated as a risk factor in overuse injuries. Static strength has been identified as a protective factor, probably because of its stabilising effect on a joint (Ekstrand & Gillquist 1983b, Lysens et al 1989). Lysens et al (1989) also found that increased dynamic strength is a risk factor in acute injuries. They postulated that the increased forces generated by individuals with greater dynamic strength were significant in producing these injuries. This research partially validates the model proposed by Richardson (1992). This model states that for appropriate functional and non-stressful movement patterns to be produced, there should be an appropriate balance of synergistic co-activation of muscles that both stabilize and move a joint.

An imbalance of muscle strength between agonists and antagonists has also been implicated in the pathogenesis of injury. Hinton (1988) found in injured baseball pitchers that the pitching arm had relatively weaker external rotators compared to the internal rotators. Further research is required to validate the concept that deficits and imbalances of muscle strength are significant predisposing risk factors to sports injuries.

Lower limb alignment. Poor lower limb alignment has been implicated in the following overuse conditions: sesamoiditis, plantar fasciitis, achilles tendonitis, tarsal tunnel syndrome, shin splints, stress fractures of the leg and foot, patellofemoral pain syndrome and iliotibial band friction syndrome (Bartold 1992, Clement et al 1984, D'Ambrosia & Drez 1982, Greenfield 1990, Hughes 1985, Jackson & Haglund 1991, James et al 1978, Kibler et al 1991, Messier et al 1991, Smart et al 1980, Vitasalo & Kvist 1983, Woodall & Welsh 1990).

Structural foot deformities have been reported to be responsible for compensations that alter the manner in which the lower limb functions (Tiberio 1988). Poor alignment of the lower limb, including structural and functional foot abnormalities, will place the structures that are usually involved in overuse conditions at a mechanical disadvantage during that portion of the stance phase of gait in which maximum vertical ground reaction forces are generated (Bobbert et al 1992, Lafortune 1984 cited by Cavanagh 1990). This is compounded by the increased stress that structures such as the achilles tendon, plantar fascia, talocrural joint, tibia, patellar tendon and patellofemoral joint have been shown to undergo during this phase of the gait cycle (Scott & Winter 1990).

In their prospective longitudinal study, Lysens et al (1989) discovered that pronated feet, leg length discrepancy and an increased Q-angle were significant predisposing factors in overuse injuries. Foster et al (1989) found that cricket bowlers who had a lower longitudinal arch were more likely to develop a stress fracture of the pars interarticularis of a lumbar vertebra than those cricketers who had high arches. Brunet et al (1990), in a study of 1505 long-distance runners, found that leg length asymmetry was significantly associated with the injured runners. Messier and Pittala (1988) found significant associations between pronation velocity, maximum pronation, a lack of dorsiflexion, a limb length discrepancy (> 0.64 cm) and shin splints; and between plantar flexion range of motion and plantar fasciitis. They also found non-significant but strong associations between the amount of total rearfoot movement and a higher arch in plantar fasciitis. This information substantiates the involvement of poor lower limb alignment in the genesis of overuse conditions of the lower quadrant.

Not all studies which have investigated the relationship between poor lower limb alignment and injury have found an association between the two. Reid (1988) described a commonly held clinical belief that insufficient range of external rotation at the hip, in classical ballerinas, will alter lower limb alignment when maximum turnout is attempted, thereby predisposing lower limb structures to injury. Hamilton et al (1992), however, found conflicting evidence. They did find that ballerinas with the highest total number of injuries had less turn out and less bilateral plie, but they also found the opposite to be the case in the male dancers. The males who had the highest number of injuries demonstrated increased amounts of turnout and increased ease of assuming the lotus position. There is a need for further well designed scientific studies into the effect of poor lower limb alignment in the pathogenesis of sports injuries. In the authors' experience, correcting any abnormal lower limb alignment is beneficial in optimizing safe sport participation.

Joint laxity or instability. Instability and hypermobility are different terms that are often used interchangeably. This makes the interpretation of study results difficult at times (Brodie et al 1982). A useful clinical definition of joint instability is an increased range of motion as well as reduced resistance to passive motion testing (physiological, accessory or special orthopaedic test) as a result of disruption of its stabilizing mechanism (usually capsulo-ligamentous structures), whereas hypermobility exists when there is increased range of joint motion in the presence of intact stabilizing mechanisms.

A number of studies have documented that footballers who have specific ligamentous instability have a higher risk of injury (Ekstrand & Gillquist 1983a, Ekstrand & Gillquist 1983b, Nicholas 1970).

Keller et al (1987) stated that 'There is no evidence to suggest that physiologic laxity is associated with any increase in injury rate' (p 236). Grana and Moretz (1978), in a study of secondary school athletes did not find any relationship between ligamentous laxity and injury rates. However Lysens et al (1989) found that ligamentous laxity (in combination with muscle tightness and lower limb mal-alignment) was a significant risk factor in overuse injuries. As seems the case clinically, instability rather than hyper-mobility is a risk factor in sports injury. The reason for this is presented next.

Previous injury

A number of studies have shown that a previous injury significantly predisposes the athlete to another injury. This appears to be true for a large cross-section of the sporting population, including footballers, track and field athletes, runners, gymnasts, ballerinas, and aerobic dancers (Caine et al 1989, Ekstrand & Gillquist 1982, Ekstrand & Gillquist 1983a, Ekstrand & Gillquist 1983b, Garrick et al 1986, Keller et al 1987, Kowal 1980, Lysens et al 1989, Lysens et al 1984, Macera et al 1989b, MacIntosh et al 1972, Marti et al 1988, Martin et al 1987, Steele & White 1986, Walter et al 1989).

The mechanism by which a previous injury increases the risk of further injury is probably mediated via pro-prioceptive deficits and altered central nervous system regulatory mechanisms which result from the initial injury.

Ekstrand and Gillquist (1983b) found in soccer players that a past history of a knee injury that had resulted in instability was frequently noted in recurring knee injuries, usually within two months of the original injury. This is not unexpected because a number of studies have demonstrated that ligament-deficient (resulting from grade III tears) joints display deficits in proprioception and joint position sense (Corrigan 1992, Freeman et al 1965). In the knee, Buchanan et al (1992) have demonstrated that specific patterns of muscle activity are stimulated when a stress is applied to a ligament. They have shown the muscles that contracted were those that were in an anatomical and biomechanical position to oppose the applied force. Therefore it could be postulated that in a joint that has sustained a grade II or III ligament tear, the stimulus for protective muscle contractions is reduced and that further injury to the ligamentous structures and

articular cartilage of the joint is possible (Mow et al 1990, Panush & Brown 1987).

With a reduction of the functional stability the centrode of the instantaneous axes of rotation will deviate from its ideal path and will lead to alterations of the contact areas of the articular surfaces. This will lead to abnormal compressive and shear stresses of the articular cartilage and may eventually predispose the joint to arthritic changes. Thus, the importance of adequate rehabilitation cannot be overstated (Ekstrand & Gillquist 1983b).

At the level of the central nervous system, a study by Bullock-Saxton (1991) found that in patients with chronic ankle sprains there was altered central motor control as reflected by dys-synergistic motor contraction at the hip joint of the affected and unaffected limbs as well as changes in perception of vibration at the hip joint. Whether this alteration in regulation at a central nervous system level and widespread proprioceptive deficit causes an injury of the same or different body region, following an injury, is yet to be determined. Other cortical influences such as psychological and psychosocial factors may also influence the central nervous system because the psychological manifestations of a previous injury, such as mood dis-turbances and lowered self-esteem (Smith et al 1990) may be a precursor to another injury (Grove & Gordon 1992). It is important that rehabilitation should not only focus on the local injured joint but also at related ipsilateral and contralateral body regions.

Physical fitness

Even though it does not have substantial scientific vali-dation, it is a tenet in sports training that athletes who are physically fitter (especially in the cardiovascular system) are less likely to injure themselves (Meeusen & Borms 1992, Stone 1990). Garrick et al (1986) in a study of aerobic dance participants found the dancers who did not par-ticipate in any other form of physical activity were associated with a higher risk of injury. A study of female army recruits who were being inducted into the service found that the recruits who were at risk of injury were those with poorer prior conditioning levels (Kowal 1980). Physiotherapists are well aware of the beneficial adaptations that the musculoskeletal system undergoes when submitted to a sensibly graduated physical fitness program and should continue to advocate for appropriate preparticipation physical fitness levels of all sports participants as a means of preventing musculoskeletal injury.

Demographic and morphological factors

Some of the demographic and morphological factors that are usually considered to predispose the participant to injury are age, gender and somatotype.

Age. The age of a sports participant has been implicated as a significant risk factor in sports injuries. It is generally accepted that adolescents have a greater risk of injury than do pre-adolescents (Backous et al 1988, Backx et al 1989, Gallagher et al 1984, Hoff & Martin 1986, Steele & White 1986, Sugerman 1983) but a smaller risk of injury than do adults, even though the pattern of injuries are similar between adults and adolescents (Keller et al 1987, Schmidt et al 1991).

It would seem that veteran athletes are no more likely than other age groups to injure themselves while undertaking running programs and other general fitness activities (Blair et al 1987, Brunet et al 1990, Macera et al 1989a, Walter et al 1989). However, Marti et al (1988) found that older runners who had greater weekly mileage were more susceptible to achillodynia and calf muscle symptoms. Hamilton et al (1989) found that older elite professional ballet dancers had a higher prevalence of major injuries.

In children, the risk of injury increases as the child becomes older (Keller et al 1987, Schmidt et al 1991, Sugerman 1983). In a series of longitudinal studies of children born at Dunedin's (New Zealand) only obstetric hospital between April 1972 and March 1973, researchers found there was an increase in the proportion of sports-related injuries when the children were aged between 10 and 13 years than when the children were under nine years (Charmers et al 1989, Langley et al 1979, Langley & Silva 1985, Langley & Silva 1987). Further stages of this study are still in progress. Watson (1984) found a slightly different trend in that there was an increase in incidence and severity of injury in boys after the age of 14 and a reduction in girls after the age of 15. They felt this was probably a reflection of extrinsic factors such as higher risk sports and higher level of sport participation for boys rather than girls.

However, in a longitudinal study of a group of 1818 students (age range 8-17), Backx et al (1991) found that age was not a significant predisposing factor to injury and that the majority of the predictor factors were extrinsic in nature.

A criticism of the above studies is that they deal with chronological age. This is a potential problem because chronological age need not be representative of biological age; indeed biological age may be more important in the predisposition to injury than chronological age (Kreipe & Gewanter 1985a, Meeusen & Borms 1992, Stanitski 1989). Stages of specific importance in the growing person are the 'growth spurts' or periods of rapid growth. Caine et al (1989) found that female gymnasts (mean age 12.6 years) who were in a period of rapid growth and were at higher levels of training and competition were more likely to be injured. They recommended that the intensity and amount of training and competition be curtailed during a period of rapid growth.

It has been postulated that during growth spurts there is a lag in the lengthening of the musculotendinous structures compared with the longitudinal lengthening of the bone, which in turn would result in increased tightness of the musculotendinous structures (Micheli 1983).

Tightness in the musculotendinous structures has been linked to an increase in the likelihood of muscle strain or tendonitis (Ekstrand & Gillquist 1983a), to predispose to ankle sprains in the case of tight calf muscles (Lysens et al 1984 cited by Lysens et al 1991) and to increase the likelihood of injury to the growth plate (Caine 1990). Strict control of activity levels of growing children is of paramount importance if potentially serious injuries to the musculo-skeletal system are to be avoided.

Gender. There is an equal risk of injury between male and female athletes when the sporting activities are similar, whereas there is not an equal risk of injury when the sporting activities are dissimilar (Backx et al 1991, Backx et al 1989, Clarke & Buckley 1980, Curtis & Dillon 1985, Durant et al 1992, Hamilton et al 1989, Haycock & Gillette 1976, Johansson 1986, Lanese et al 1990, Macera et al 1989a, Walter et al 1989). The findings from a study by Lanese et al (1990) typifies this. Over a year, they investigated 382 students who participated in sports such as basketball, fencing, gymnastics, swimming, tennis, indoor track, outdoor track, and volleyball. They found in gymnastics, where the sport is different for females and males, the female injury rate was different; but in the sports which are similar for both the female and male participant the injury rates and profiles were similar (Lanese et al 1990). This does not seem to be the case at all age groups because a greater risk of injury was reported in male children and adolescents than in the females of similar ages (Gallagher et al 1984, Watson 1984). However the reason for these findings may not be purely due to a gender difference; it may be due to the possibility that the boys competed at a higher level of competition and in sports that had a greater associated risk of injury.

Strong correlations have been found to exist between amenorrhoea and stress fractures, scoliosis and musculo-skeletal conditions (Brunet et al 1990, Hamilton et al 1989, Warren et al 1986). This is thought to be due to the reduction in bone mineral density (BMD), low bodyweight and hypoeostrogenism that is associated with amenorrhoea.

As well as predisposing the female athlete to injury, amenorrhoea also affects skeletal health after resumption of menses (Drinkwater et al 1990, Drinkwater et al 1986). Drinkwater et al (1986) initially indicated that there was a significant reversal of BMD after resumption of menses. However, in a later study which used a larger sample size of athletes who had experienced longer periods of amenorrhoea, Drinkwater et al (1990) found the BMD had not reversed following the resumption of menses. The cause of amenorrhoea in the female athlete is still largely unknown (Carbon 1992)(See Ch. 34 for further discussion of the female athlete).

Somatotype. Somatotype refers to 'the quantitative description of the morphological structure of an individual' into the ectomorph, mesomorph or endomorph categories

(Oslo 1973, p. 723). The somatotype of an individual is calculated from the measurements of 'height, body mass, four skinfolds, two limb girths and two bone widths' (Ackland & Bloomfield 1992, p. 3). The relationship between somatotype of an athlete and predisposition to injury is equivocal at this stage. Steele and White (1986) found mesomorph to be a risk factor in competitive female gymnasts, a sport in which a high proportion of overuse injuries occur, whereas Lysens et al (1989) found a low score on mesomorph was a predictor in females that experience overuse injuries. Furthermore, Lysens et al (1989) found that endomorphic males were more likely to experience an overuse injury.

Somatotype characteristics of weight and height, when considered separately or when expressed as the body mass index (BMI = weight/height^2 for males and weight/height$^{1.5}$ for females) have been implicated as a contributing factor in sports injuries (Backous et al 1988, Blair et al 1987, Kowal 1980, Macera et al 1989b, Meeusen & Borms 1992, Steele & White 1986, Watson 1984). Lysens et al (1989) and Reilly (1981) have indicated that these factors are not significant predictors in acute injuries and Lysens et al (1989) found they were only implicated as modifiers of other risk factors in overuse injuries.

Disability

The participation of disabled competitors in sport has only recently attracted research interest and therefore not a great deal is known about how or if the disability predisposes a disabled athlete to injury. Ferrara et al (1992) found that athletes with disabilities who competed under the auspices of the National Wheelchair Athletic Association (NWAA), the United States Association for Blind Athletes, and the United States Cerebral Palsy Athletic Association, had approximately the same injury profile and injury incidence as athletes without a disability who competed in similar sporting activities. A study by Curtis and Dillon (1985) found that athletes competing under the auspices of the NWAA were no different in the risk to injury on the basis of their disability.

Psychological/psychosocial factors

When compared with the physical intrinsic factors, the psychological factors have only attracted limited research attention. This may be due to limitations in research methodology (Tenenbaum & Bar-Eli 1992). Nonetheless, several authors have proposed that alterations in psychological or psychosocial aspects of the athlete may predispose them to injury (Bond et al 1988, Grove & Gordon 1992, Lysens et al 1986, Taerk 1977).

In a retrospective study of elite professional ballet dancers, Hamilton et al (1989) found that the dancers who had stress fractures and overuse injuries were more dominant, extroverted and had more practical and scientific lifestyles than non-injured athletes. In addition, the dancers with stress fractures were more enterprising, assertive, adjusted and had interpersonal styles that were more sociable.

Lysens et al (1989) and Watson (1984) have shown that those athletes who demonstrate high risk-taking behaviour by lacking caution are those who are at risk of acute injury. However, no link between emotional and psychosomatic lability have been demonstrated to date (Lysens et al 1991).

Psychosocial factors do not predispose a participant to overuse injuries but they are implicated in the pathogenesis of acute sporting injuries (Lysens et al 1989). Lysens et al (1986) found that a high level of life change would increase the risk of an acute sports injury to an athlete who was not capable of coping with the stress of the change in life. They postulated 'that stress related to life change can lead to a blocking of adaptive responses in potentially dangerous game situations' (p. 83), and thereby predispose the athlete to injury. That the psychological and psychosocial component of the athlete may constitute an injury risk factor should be considered by all practitioners who are concerned with prevention.

Extrinsic factors

The extrinsic factors are those factors that are extrinsic to the participant. They include sport-specific aspects, environmental aspects and the equipment in a sport. The injury profile of a sport consists of the anatomical distribution, the type, and the severity of the injuries characteristically encountered by the participants in that sport. It is usually dependent upon the sport specific skills and requirements of a particular sport (Koplan et al 1982, Van Mechelen et al 1992). Skills that are specific to a sport, either performed correctly or incorrectly, may be a significant factor in the injuries that occur in participants of that sport. Other extrinsic factors that are usually specific to a sport are the rules and aims of the sport, the level of competition, the position of a participant in a sport, the time of the game or season and the training in which the participant engages in preparation for competition. Environmental factors such as temperature, humidity and surface conditions may also affect the participant's health. The equipment that participants use has also been implicated as a causative factor in sports injuries.

Injury profile

There are unique injury profiles in alpine sport (Robinson 1991, Wright et al 1991), badminton (Jorgensen & Winge 1990), ballet (Hardaker 1989), cycling (McLennan et al 1988, Mellion 1991), equestrian events (McLatchie 1979), gymnastics (Garrick & Requa 1980, Pettrone & Ricciardelli 1987), handball (Lindbald et al 1992, Nielsen & Yde 1988), union and rugby league football (Maguire 1990), sailboarding (McCormick & Davis 1988), roller and ice skating (Horner & McCabe 1984, Kvidera & Frankel 1983), sport parachuting (Steinberg 1988), squash (Berson et al 1978), surfing (Draper et al 1987), tennis (Reece et al 1986), weight lifting (Aggrawal et al 1979), wrestling (Marsh 1991), and ultraendurance triathletes (O'Toole et al 1989).

A very popular sport of the past two decades has been distance running. Consequently there has been quite a lot written about injuries in runners. An analysis of running reveals that the essential skill of distance running is alternate leg weightbearing that occurs repetitively for prolonged periods of time at the limits of the runner's physical and mental fatigue level. This type of activity predicts the high incidence of overuse injuries of the lower limb that occur in runners (Clement et al 1984, Jacobs & Berson 1986, Koplan et al 1982, Lysholm & Wiklander 1987, Macera 1992, Marti et al 1988, Maughan & Miller 1983, Walter et al 1989). These overuse injuries are very closely linked to the fatigue and stress created by the successive momentary loading of the lower limb during stance phase by forces that exceed body weight (Eggold 1981). The stress to the lower limb is further compounded if there are faults in the lower limb alignment and biomechanics (see section on intrinsic factors) (James et al 1978, Messier et al 1991, Scott & Winter 1990). In aerobics, which has many characteristics similar to those described for running, Garrick et al (1986) reported a similar anatomical distribution injury profile to running with the majority (82%–88%) of the injuries occurring in the lower limbs. Another sport that is similar to running is orienteering. The major difference from running is that orienteering is held over uneven terrain. Therefore, as well as a high frequency of overuse injuries (57%) in the orienteers surveyed, Johansson (1986) found that 43% of all injuries were traumatic.

Swimming injuries are predominantly overuse in nature because of the distances and the demanding training that competitive and recreational swimmers undergo. A Canadian study of 2496 swimmers found that the area of the body that is most likely to be injured is largely determined by the stroke (Kennedy et al 1978). Most of the shoulder injuries, which accounted for 31% of swimming injuries, resulted predominantly from the freestyle stroke; whereas the knee injuries, which accounted for 28% of all swimming injuries, resulted exclusively from breaststroke. The calf and foot injuries accounted for 32% of injuries and resulted from all strokes. Ten per cent of injuries were from other areas around the body (Kennedy et al 1978).

The anatomical distribution injury profiles of some popular team sports (Australian Rules football, soccer, netball, rugby union and baseball) are presented in Table 7.1. All these sports are land-based and have running and lower limb tasks as fundamental skills, hence the high frequency of lower limb injuries. Soccer requires more emphasis on the lower limbs and therefore has a greater proportion of lower limb injuries. The knee and ankle are the most frequently injured regions of the lower limbs in soccer (Backous et al 1988, Keller et al 1987, Klasen 1984, Schmidt-Olsen et al 1985, Schmidt-Olsen et al 1991). Netball requires sudden explosive accelerative and decelerative manoeuvres superimposed on sudden changes of direction, and consequently has a high incidence of lower limb injuries (Hopper 1986). The upper limbs are less frequently injured, with the exception of baseball where there is a relatively high percentage of upper limb injury compared with the lower limb. This is because the essential skills of baseball involve batting and throwing or pitching the ball. The shoulder accounts for the majority of these upper limb injuries (Polk 1968). The frequency of head and neck injuries are greater in sports such as Australian Rules football and rugby union where tackles are executed with the use of the upper body, shoulder and neck region.

Table 7.1 Anatomical distribution of injuries in some popular sports

Anatomical regions (%)	Head-neck	Upper limb	Trunk	Lower limb	Other
Australian Rules football					
Sali et al (1981)	23	13	10	54	—
Hoy & Kennedy (1984)	23	16	8	53	—
Seward & Patrick (1992)	17	11	14	57	1
Soccer					
Ekstrand & Gilquist (1983b)	—	—	5	88	
Schmidt-Olsen et al (1985)	5	10	4	81	—
Engstrom et al (1991)	—	—	4	88	8
Schmidt-Olsen et al (1991)	4	10	16	69	—
Netball					
Hopper (1986)	—	13	—	74	13
Rugby union					
Sugerman (1983)	25	27	9	39	—
Baseball					
Polk (1968)	9	39	7	45	—

1992b). It is important that participants and organizers of long-distance runs, fun runs and other organised sports should be aware of this (Australian Sports Medicine Federation 1992f). Meir et al (1990) found significant weight loss and body temperature increases in professional rugby league players who played in warm humid conditions. They considered these heat-related changes could reduce performance and predispose the player to heat illness.

Exposure to low temperatures may predispose the athlete to hypothermia and related medical conditions (Australian Sports Medicine Federation 1992a, Pyke 1986). However, the notion that the weather is associated with musculoskeletal injuries has not been substantiated. Studies of elite European soccer players found that the injury rate was not related to the weather (Engstrom et al 1991). Maguire (1990), in a review of injuries in rugby football, reported that the effect of weather on injuries has not been researched.

The playing surface has been shown to be a risk factor in some situations. Hopper (1986), in a study of netball injuries, found that, except for the ankle, surface type had a significant effect on the area that was injured. On grass surfaces the hand was most frequently injured, on bitumen surfaces the knee was most frequently injured, and on synthetic surfaces the other areas of the body with the exception of the ankle, knee and hand were frequently injured. In tennis, Reece et al (1986) found that footwear and the court surface were important predisposing factors to the predominance of lower limb injuries. However, other researchers who investigated the risk factors in sport have found that the injury profile was not related to the playing surface. In aerobics, Garrick et al (1986) found no relationship between surface and injuries, and in an elite female soccer competition Engstrom et al (1991) found that injury was not related to playing surface.

Equipment

In certain circumstances, the equipment that is used in sport can be an injury risk. Protective equipment can be misused and predispose to injury. Helmets can provide a false sense of security because there may be other mechanisms for concussion (head injury) than a direct contact to the skull (Australian Sports Medicine Federation 1992e). They may also be used to detrimental effect, as demonstrated in American football where their introduction protected the head from injury but increased the risk of injury to the neck because they were then used as battering rams in tackling and blocking (Torg et al 1979). However, the failure to wear a protective device has also been shown to increase the risk of injury. In a study of rugby league players Chapman (1988) found a higher incidence of orofacial injury in players that did not wear mouthguards. Ekstrand and Gillquist (1983b) found that soccer players who wore

no shin guards or wore inadequate shin guards were much more likely to suffer traumatic shin injuries.

Some form of footwear is worn in most land-based sports. Cook et al (1990) calculated that between a third and a half of the ability of the running shoe to absorb shock is lost within the first 400 km. They postulated that this was partly due to the runner's perspiration as well as cyclic loading. The runner who uses the same pair of shoes past this distance is at an increased risk of injury.

The study of equipment that is used in sport and its role in the predisposition of the athlete to injury is difficult because of the complex interaction of many variables, only some of which are known. In a study of the effect of the type and tension of tennis racquet string on impact with a ball, Groppel (1987) concluded that there was a complex interaction between string type and racquet size and that the different compounds used in racquet construction, the racquet shape and the stringing method would further compound this interaction. Until further research is conducted into sports equipment, physiotherapists should use their knowledge of the mechanism of injury in conjunction with advice from coaching staff and biomechanists as a guide to appropriate recommendations on this issue.

PREPARTICIPATION EVALUATION

The preparticipation evaluation (PE) is essentially a health screening process that is believed to be beneficial to athletes (Heinzman 1991, Hershman 1984a, Kibler 1990, Maguire 1986, McKeag 1985, Stanitski 1989). The intricate interaction(s) between the intrinsic and extrinsic risk factors need to be considered when performing a PE (Hershman 1984a). Therefore, while the preparticipation evaluation is primarily focused on the athlete (intrinsic factors), it must be conducted in a manner that allows for a recognition of the pertinent sport-specific aspects (extrinsic factors) (Durant et al 1985).

The most important issues of the PE are the goals it seeks to achieve and the significance of its findings. Important logistical issues are the organization and timing of the PE.

Goals

There are several goals that PEs aim to achieve. According to Maguire (1986), the goals of the PE are the identification of impediments, the elucidation of factors predisposing to injury, and the prevention of injury through a prescribed corrective program.

McKeag (1985) states that the objective of the PE is not only to identify any athlete who is at risk of injury but also to optimize performance level, to classify the athlete according to individual qualifications, to fulfil legal and insurance requirements, to evaluate the stage of maturation, to provide opportunities for counselling, and to provide the basis of the practitioner-patient relationship.

Organization

In the authors' experience the most efficient manner in which to conduct a PE is by setting up a number of stations, each staffed by appropriately qualified practitioners. The division of the PE into stations should be primarily guided by the different components of the evaluation that are specifically required for the sport as well as the available expertise of the consulting practitioners. For example, an evaluation of soccer players would focus primarily on the lower limbs. Maguire (1986) believes that the stations should be manned by the appropriate health care professional:

- medical practitioner—examine all body systems
- physiotherapist—musculoskeletal profile
- exercise physiologist—fitness evaluation
- psychologist—psychological testing
- coaches—sport-specific and agility tests
- dentist—dental examination.

Durant et al (1985) compared the results of PEs performed by multiple examiners in a station situation to those performed by single physicians. The two groups being assessed were similar in their previous health status. The result of the comparisons between the two groups showed that the single physician examinations detected significantly fewer abnormalities than did the multiple examiners. This was particularly so in the musculoskeletal system. Because the musculoskeletal system is the system most often injured in sports, Durant et al (1985) felt that it was important to have multiple examiners perform the examination so that all potential risk factors were identified and acted upon.

Timing

The time between the PE and the commencement of competitive participation is critical because there needs to be sufficient time to successfully implement any necessary corrective strategies. The PE should be performed 3-6 weeks before the commencement of the season because most of the focus of the PE is on the musculoskeletal system, and any of the musculoskeletal deficits in strength, endurance, power and flexibility are easily influenced by specific programs within this time (Fisher & Jensen 1990, Heinzman 1991, Hershman 1984b). If required, this time will also allow for further testing and/or counselling about a change of sport or level of competition.

Significance and consequence of findings

There is very little research that proves that the PE is an effective method of ensuring safe participation in sport

(Durant et al 1992, Runyan & Gerken 1989). Kibler et al (1989) believe that combining information from the preparticipation evaluation with injury records is the only way to gain an understanding of the factors involved in the pathogenesis of injury, and therefore the only way to gain an understanding of the factors that are crucial to the prevention of injury. Nonetheless, the PE is essential in order to detect the biological age of the young participant (FIMS 1991) and identify the participant who has a medical condition that could compromise safe participation, such as coronary disease (Kohl et al 1990, McKeag 1985).

In collision sports where physical maturity and size are key factors in participation, it is essential to classify children and adolescents by their biological age and not their chronological age (FIMS 1991, Kreipe & Gewanter 1985a, Watson 1992), because strength and flexibility are better correlated to biological age than they are to chronological age (Pratt 1989). Examples of these types of collision sports are rugby, Australian Rules and American football. The Tanner (1962) staging method is a useful way of assessing physical maturity because it may help to match participants better with respect to their abilities (Kreipe & Gewanter 1985b, Smith & Stanitski 1987). Kreipe and Gewanter (1985b) found that the immature boy (Tanner stage 3) who was likely to be an inappropriate candidate for collision sports had a weaker average grip strength than did the mature boy. The majority of the boys were differentiated by an average grip strength of 24.9 kg.

Caine (1990) suggests that any back pain or pain around a joint in a young athlete may be the symptom of significant growth plate changes. These growth plate changes may be responsible for growth disturbances that may be more prevalent than previously believed. Children experiencing these symptoms should be further investigated.

Guidelines for identifying individuals who should have cardiovascular testing prior to exercise are based on classifying individuals into risk categories based on age, coronary heart disease risk factor status, symptoms, and presence of known disease (American College of Sports Medicine cited in Kohl et al 1990). Individuals over 40 years of age should be routinely assessed for coronary health status (McKeag 1985), as should those who have reached 35 years of age and have not regularly participated in physical activity (Australian Sports Medicine Federation 1992c).

Screening options that may be used, singly or in combination, to identify coronary risk factors are a self-administered questionnaire, a clinical examination, and an exercise electrocardiogram (ECG) (Kohl et al 1990, Shephard 1984). If the self-administered questionnaire or clinical records reveal coronary risk factors, then some sort of patient monitoring is indicated. Breathlessness, sweating and heart rate indicators are some of the indicators that could be used in exercise participation (Shephard 1984).

Exercise ECGs may also be of benefit (Kohl et al 1990), however Shephard (1984) believes that this diagnostic tool is responsible for many misdiagnoses when compared to angiographic criteria.

The participant who has endocrine, metabolic, cardiac, vascular, circulatory, orthopaedic and neurological problems may not be able to participate in some sports, especially collision sports, but may be able to participate in non-collision sports (McKeag 1985). It is important that the participant be referred to a medical practitioner if the participant is a smoker or is overweight; is a regular user of medication; has high blood pressure or cholesterol; has diabetes or any other chronic medical condition that may interfere with safe participation; has a history of chest pain, tightness or discomfort; has a history of indigestion not medically diagnosed; has a history of asthma or other chronic respiratory condition; or has a family history of heart disease or stroke (Australian Sports Medicine Federation 1992c).

Components of the PE

The components of the PE that are appropriate to use in any specific PE depend solely upon the goals of the evaluation, the population within which the evaluation will be conducted and the sporting activities in which the population will participate. The organizational issues and timing constraints will also modify the components used in the PE.

The various components of a PE (Durant et al 1985, Heinzman 1991, Hershman 1984a, Kibler 1990, Kibler et al 1989, Maguire 1986, McKeag 1985) are:

- the history which should include information on: past injury, allergies, illness and medical conditions, head injuries, concussion/knockouts, dizziness or syncope, menstrual details, surgery, medication, drugs, hospitalization, fractures, convulsions, relevant family history;
- nutrition and diet;
- immunization schedule;
- morphological data: weight, height, % body fat, body type, sexual/physical maturity (Tanner staging);
- examination: eyes, hearing, teeth, skin (infections, wounds), ear, nose and throat, lymphatics (including neck and axillary examination);
- cardiac assessment: blood pressure recording, pulse rate, presence of murmurs, arrhythmias, cardiac risk factors, exercise ECG if indicated;
- lung function assessment: this may also include a chest X-ray;
- abdominal assessment: including assessment of genitals (males only) and the presence of hernias;
- laboratory tests as required: urinalysis, full blood and iron status;

- biomechanical assessment, mechanical alignment (posture), flexibility of muscle, neural and joint systems, range of motion, static strength tests of stability muscles (e.g. vastus medialis, gluteus medius, etc.);
- specific orthopaedic tests: ligamentous stability, overuse syndromes (shoulder and ankle impingement etc.);
- neurological assessment: conductivity (reflex, power, sensation), balance, neuromuscular physical assessment, agility, co-ordination, timing, rhythm, steadiness;
- exercise physiology assessment: strength, power, endurance, VO_2 max;
- psychological/psychosocial assessment.

The history of any medical illness or musculoskeletal injury would be detected by a self-administered questionnaire. This questionnaire would be reviewed by the examining practitioners in the presence of the participant. This would allow for the clarification of any issue that arises and would guide the PE on an individual basis. The individual components of the evaluation would then be performed by the suitable health care practitioner. Should any further tests be required the practitioner could refer the participant to the appropriate diagnostic service.

The PE of the musculoskeletal system is important because that system is most frequently involved in sports injuries (Durant et al 1985). The physiotherapists' primary role is in the musculoskeletal evaluation station. The examination findings that should alert the physiotherapist to instigate further management procedures are those that indicate abnormalities of the articular, muscular and neurological systems.

A previous injury to articular structures with the following examination findings would be a strong indication for intervention: grade II or III instability (Andriacchi et al 1987) with specific orthopaedic tests of ligaments, impingement signs with appropriate specific orthopaedic tests (ankle (Crichton et al 1992) and shoulder (Fricker 1992)), reduced proprioception and/or mechanical imbalances. A previous injury of the muscular system, either a contraction or a stretch type tear (Vicenzino 1992), with a residual inability to execute high velocity eccentric-concentric switch-over contractions as is required in sprinting (Stanton & Purdham 1989) or with a residual loss of extensibility of the muscle should also indicate the need for further assessment and rehabilitation. Assessment of muscle function with isokinetic dynamometers is often recommended (Kibler 1990, Kibler et al 1989, McKeag 1985) even though there are unresolved questions about the validity of extrapolating the results of these dynamometer tests to human performance and the ability of the athlete to participate safely (Cabri 1991, Grace 1985, Rothstein et al 1987). Alterations to the normal functioning of the neural system in its primary function as a conductor of impulses or in its important biomechanical properties that allow it to move and elongate to accommodate body movements (Butler 1991) would also indicate a need for further investigation (see chapter 5, on neuromeningeal techniques).

STRATEGIES OF PREVENTION

Physiotherapists have a very important role to play in the prevention of injury. Ekstrand et al (1983) found that close supervision by physiotherapists and doctors of any preventative program markedly increased its effectiveness. Clinical physiotherapists routinely educate their clients (participants, coaches, other health care practitioners, administrators, other associated personnel) on issues relating to the promotion and maintenance of optimum health. The Australian Sports Medicine Federation (1990) has indicated that the role of education is a priority for all personnel involved in sports health care.

Strategies of prevention can be divided into intrinsic and extrinsic categories.

Intrinsic prevention strategies

The most often used strategies that deal with intrinsic factors are remedial programs to rectify any risk factors that have been identified in the PE, specific preparation for a sport, warming up and cooling down. Massage is sometimes advocated as a means of preventing injury and possibly enhancing performance (Meagher & Boughton 1990).

Remedial program

One of the strongest predisposing factor to injury is a previous injury. The rehabilitation of the participant who has a musculoskeletal injury is the traditional role of physiotherapy and utilizes all the management procedures in a therapist's repertoire (see Ch. 10). The emphasis in the remedial program is on an active exercise approach with priority placed on the utilization of therapist-independent techniques. Physiotherapists should give priority to any deficits in functional or structural stability of a joint. Any muscle imbalances consisting of poor proximal stabilizing synergists or tight muscles, if in the presence of joint instability, should be corrected with due care and consideration of the instability.

Proprioceptive retraining is an important part of this rehabilitation, because it is the intrinsic feedback mechanism that participants use to monitor their own ability to maintain stability of a structurally or functionally unstable joint. Ultimately the goal of the participant and the physiotherapist is active safe participation in the chosen sport. Therefore the remedial program must be related to the sports-specific skill requirements. This is important because participants are reassured that the goals of the remedial program focuses on their needs.

Preparation

In essence, the prevention of injury should ultimately be viewed in the context of optimizing performance because a participant who is injured, even if only mildly, is not able to perform fully. In preparation, appropriate components of fitness should be scheduled at the appropriate time of the 'preparation-competition-rest' cycle. Emphasis should be placed on developing the proper sport-specific skill and techniques, primarily to improve performance but also to prevent injury. The combination of input from the training staff, health care professionals and sports scientists should guarantee that the participant has a balanced program that achieves realistic competitive goals while minimizing the risk of injury.

An important planning consideration is the scheduling of activities to reflect the time of the season. This is usually termed periodisation. The season can be divided into three distinct parts: the preparation phase, the competitive phase and the recuperative phase. The preparation phase involves concentrating on the fundamentals to improve the required sports-specific fitness characteristics of the participant. In this phase the focus is on muscle strength, endurance and power. The energy systems that will be used should also be considered so that the preparation can specifically train the aerobic, anaerobic or specific combinations of both these energy systems. The competition phase involves concentration on sport-specific skills. The transition phase between the preparation phase and the competition phase must successfully taper the fitness training and increase the sport-specific skill training. This periodisation not only relates to the entire year but to the different parts of the competitive season and even to each week of the season. For example, in a week the participant should have a period of recuperation, time for higher intensity work to maintain fitness levels and time to concentrate on skill work.

The preparation process should also select those who are not suitable for a sport or particular aspects of that sport. For example, in rugby, Sugerman (1983) believes that the allocation of participants to different team positions should take into consideration the players' somatotype. He states that participants who are mesomorphs are suitable for general team positions whereas those who are endomorphs should be considered for the prop forward positions.

The deleterious effects of overtraining and inadequate recovery periods have been mentioned already. Children are particularly at risk. Bale (1992) cautions that overtraining or too vigorous training may harm children, and that 'Exercise, whether it is short and vigorous or prolonged, may have a minimal effect upon improvement in performance in preadolescents. Strength per unit volume of muscle, stroke volume and cardiac output, and anaerobic and aerobic capacity show only marginal improvements with exercise' (p. 157). Thus there will be no real positive outcome for vigorously training children, but there may detrimental outcomes.

The poor execution of a sports-specific skill or technique has been identified as a significant risk factor. The identification and correction of any potentially harmful idiosyncrasies that appear should be given priority. The role of an astute accredited coach is invaluable, together with the physiotherapist who usually collaborates in this process. In this regard, the biomechanical analysis of movement is very important in developing strategies that identify and alter inappropriate sport specific techniques (Taunton et al 1988).

Warm up

The warm up period involves activities that increase the preparedness of the neuromuscular and articular systems. It usually involves some aerobic activity to the stage of light sweating, some callisthenics and stretching exercises and some sport-specific drills. It is often advocated as a means of preventing injuries.

Preparation for the muscular activity required in sport requires an understanding of the physiological processes involved. Briefly, the repetitive contractions of muscle at a submaximal level produces an initial lag between the creatine phosphate energy system (anaerobic) and the aerobic system which generates an oxygen debt from the anaerobic lactic acid producing energy system. The anaerobic debt is reduced by early delivery of oxygen to the muscle, increased muscle temperature and a reduced local pH. Light aerobic exercise would increase blood flow to the muscle and facilitate these requirements (Fisher & Jensen 1990).

Stretching manoeuvres are usually conducted after the aerobic activity because the increased blood flow to muscles and the increased temperature renders stretching more effective. Proprioceptive neuromuscular facilitation techniques of contract-relax or reciprocal relaxation appear to be more effective in gaining range of motion than static or ballistic techniques are (Wilkerson 1992). However, a lower skill and knowledge level is required for the performance of static stretching techniques and therefore unless supervised by a physiotherapist participants should perform static stretching techniques.

Hopper (1986) demonstrated that netball players who had not warmed up had an increased risk of injury in the first quarter of the game. Seward and Patrick (1992) also found that an important factor in the prevention of hamstring injuries in Australian Rules football players was warming up and stretching. However, Hoff and Martin (1986) in a study of outdoor and indoor soccer injuries in youth found that warmup before the game was not related to injuries that occurred in a game.

Cool down

Cool down consists of a period of activity that 'debriefs' the neuromuscular and psychological system following stressful activity. It should be regarded in the same light as the often vital post-match talks that coaches deliver to the participants. It is highly recommended in participants who are required to participate again within the day or over a number of successive days. The cool down involves some light aerobic activity that will supply blood, oxygen and nutrients to the area that has been used and remove waste products from those areas.

It also involves stretching exercises to restore the muscle (lengths) spindle bias to more appropriate levels of activity as well as provide a stimulus for functional healing following any inflammatory process, should any micro-trauma have occurred.

Massage

In their sport massage textbook, Meagher and Boughton (1990) list many benefits of sports massage, some of which are the prevention of injuries, the enhancement of athletic performance and the extending of both the good health and overall time of an athlete's participation in sport. These are quite substantial claims that have not been conclusively proved (Carfarelli & Flint 1992, Harmer 1991). Despite this, many still believe that massage plays a vital role in the prevention of injury and the enhancement of performance. In a recent review of massage, Carfarelli and Flint (1992) conclude that in the absence of any reports that massage has adverse effects on the participant and in view of the anecdotal evidence in favour of massage, massage should continue to be used.

Massage can be used in many ways in a preparticipation warm up session. The physiological effects of massage that may be beneficial to participation are mechanically, circulatory and neurologically based (Hollis 1987). These effects may be an increase in muscle and connective tissue extensibility, an increase in blood flow to the muscles, and an increased stimulation of the neuromuscular system. This could be achieved by techniques of petrissage, tapoment and/or vibration (Carfarelli et al 1990). The psychological effects of massage that may be beneficial in the preparticipation warm up session relate to the effects on mood states (Weinberg et al 1988). This may be particularly relevant to injury prevention when considering the psychological risk factors that predispose a participant to injury (Lysens et al 1986, Lysens et al 1989). The participant who has had a previous injury may have also experienced lowered self-esteem and mood disturbances (Smith et al 1990) that may respond positively to massage. This may be helpful in preventing a recurrence of the injury.

Post-participation massage may be used to facilitate the recovery from physical exertion and to detect any subclinical injuries of the soft tissues so that prompt appropriate management is instigated. Effleurage techniques may be useful. In terms of the psychological effects of massage post-participation, Weinberg et al (1988) have suggested that the improved mood states observed following massage may be beneficial to the athlete after strenuous and stressful sport. (See Ch. 14 for further discussion of massage.)

Extrinsic prevention strategies

The most often used strategies that involve extrinsic factors are modification of the rules of the sport; better enforcement of the rules of the game; modification of the aims or scoring system of a sport; consideration of the environmental factors such as weather conditions, the surfaces and fixed sport specific equipment; the wearing of well maintained and appropriate sport-specific and protective equipment.

Rules of the sport

In a good example of the value of research in the prevention of injury, Torg et al (1985) identified that spear tackling produced axial loading of the cervical spine and was the major cause of neck injury in American football. Recommendations were made to change the rules so that this tackle was outlawed. This rule change was responsible for a reduction in the incidence of neck injuries (fractures/dislocations) from 34 to 5 from 1976 to 1984 (a reduction of 85%), to 10 in 1985, to 6 in 1986 and 8 in 1987 (Torg et al 1990). A similar tackle in rugby has been banned.

A recent report has suggested that in netball a rule change may be considered by the governing body to allow an extra step to be taken after receiving the ball (Australian Sports Medicine Federation 1990). It is believed that the sudden deceleration and the subsequent generation of high forces on foot contact that is required by the rules of the game after the player has caught the ball has led to the high incidence of knee and ankle injuries. However, Neal and Sydney-Smith (1992) state that the factors surrounding these injuries are not yet fully understood and may be quite complex.

Not only should appropriate rules be instigated but the implementation and enforcement of the rules is also very important. Therefore adequate education and training of referees and umpires are required.

The rules for children's sport should be modified so that the emphasis on competition is realistic. The reduction of playing field sizes, the reduction in the size of the goals and the use of smaller equipment (racquets, hockey sticks, soccer ball sizes) are all changes brought about by rule changes. Likewise, no techniques that are potentially hazardous, proved or anecdotally based, should be allowed; for example, the restriction on the pitching of curve balls by under 14 year olds. The matching of participants on the basis of biological age is important.

Environment

Environmental considerations include weather conditions, sport-specific surfaces and equipment that are part of the environs in which the sport is conducted.

The weather conditions that are of concern are the extremes of heat and cold because they can predispose the participant to heat or cold stress illness. In running, the upper limit of wet bulb globe temperature at which an event should be cancelled is 28°C or higher (ACSM cited by Australian Sports Medicine Federation 1992b). Apart from cancelling an event there are other preventative strategies that can be employed, such as holding the event so that it is concluded by 8 a.m. or commenced after 6 p.m. in the warmer months of the year (Australian Sports Medicine Federation 1992f). The participant's level of hydration must be high at the beginning of the event and maintained with adequate intake of water throughout the event. Therefore, in long-distance running, water stations should be available at the start of the race, at 5 km and thereafter at 2–3 km (Australian Sports Medicine Federation 1992f). The participants should be encouraged to wear loose, light, porous and light-coloured clothing to facilitate evaporation of sweat and to minimize heat absorption (Australian Sports Medicine Federation 1992b).

Heat and humidity are only some of the factors that should be considered. Heat stress is also influenced by a number of factors including age, gender, somatotype, fitness level, state of hydration and level of acclimatisation (Meir 1992).

In colder climates the risk of hypothermia and cold-related illnesses should be considered. Prevention of hypothermia is the key to its management (Australian Sports Medicine Federation 1992a). The guidelines for prevention of hypothermia involve clothing and diet. The clothing should be dry, windproof and well insulated but allow water vapour to escape. It should be sealed about the openings for the hands, feet, and neck. Clothes should be worn in layers and easily adjusted to allow for overheating. It is essential that the participant remains dry and that a suitable wet suit and cap be worn if the participant is competing in a triathlon. Participants should also ensure adequate fluid intake, avoid alcohol, and have available ready sources of energy such as carbohydrate snacks (Australian Sports Medicine Federation 1992a).

The surfaces on which a sport is performed should also be considered. Some of the characteristics of the surface that should be considered are friction and compliance. Ekstrand and Nigg (1989) looked at surface-related injuries in soccer and concluded that there had to be a delicate balance between the amount of friction that the ground and shoe generated. Too high a friction resulted in higher forces at the ankle and knee and too low a friction resulted in slipping and related injuries.

A balanced exposure to surfaces with different compliances is important. For example, medium and long-distance runners should vary their training between concrete, bitumen, grass, cross-country and synthetic surfaces.

Another environmental issue that seems clinically relevant in preventing injury is the gradient of the surface; that is, hilly or flat surfaces and the camber of the surface. Runners should be aware that a balanced exposure to a variety of gradients is recommended.

Sports-specific equipment such as goal posts, walls (squash courts), polevault poles, parallel bars and crowd control barriers may also cause injuries. Softball is a good example of a sport in which the identification of a risk factor and the successful implementation of a preventative strategy has been documented. In a preliminary epidemiological study, Janda et al (1986) found that the majority (71%) of injuries in recreational softball were from sliding-related injuries that resulted from impact with a stationary base. On the basis of those findings, breakaway bases were installed and there was a 98% reduction of serious softball injuries (Janda et al 1992). This resulted in an estimated saving of $2 billion per year in acute medical care costs nationally in the USA (Janda et al 1990).

Equipment

The equipment that is considered in this section is the sport specific equipment that is required for participation in a sport, equipment that is specifically indicated for its protective function and materials such as sports tape that are used for the prevention of sports injuries. The sport specific equipment should be correctly fitted, comfortable, appropriate to the sport and facilitate the maintenance of the participant's health and performance. Probably one of the most basic of all sport-specific equipment is the shoe, particularly in running and running related sports.

Contemporary running shoes are designed with two primary concepts in mind: the prevention of excessive load, and the enhancement of performance (Nigg & Segesser 1992). This is accomplished by the provision of cushioning in the sole of the shoe that at foot strike decreases impact loading, support throughout the mid stance phase and guidance during the push off phase (Nigg & Segesser 1992). The heel counter provides for stability of the calcaneus (Cook et al 1990), which is also improved when shoes are worn (Nigg et al 1984). This reduces the potential for excessive pronation, a movement that has been associated with overuse conditions of the lower limbs in runners. So many different motion control devices are built into the modern shoe that appropriate selection and proper fitting of a shoe must be ensured. An important aspect of fitting a shoe is that the heel pad is appropriately confined by the heel cup. Jorgensen and Ekstrand (1988) have shown that heel pad confinement which is offered by the heel cup increases the shock absorbency of any shoe heel counter.

A view that contrasts with most of the modern day concepts of the sports shoe is presented by Robbins and Gouw (1990). They maintain that the lower limb in barefoot locomotion can maintain itself without footwear and endure the forces involved in running without succumbing to injury. Furthermore, they state that, due to the preoccupation with the minimization of shock, the modern shoe interferes with the body's innate ability to cope with the forces and stresses of running through the interference of the body's sensory feedback mechanisms.

Protective equipment is probably one of the most important when considering the prevention of injury (Fig. 7.1). This equipment has a variety of different properties that may be used in a combined or individual manner. Some of these properties may involve:

- the dispersion of impact energy, as in shin guards for soccer and hockey
- the absorption and reduction in the rate of transfer of energy, as in the high density foam rubber products that are used in shoes and in volley ball knee and football thigh pads
- the deflection of blows, as in helmets
- the transmission of energy to other body parts, as in shin pads or in a baseball catcher's face mask
- the protection of the face and eyes from penetrating equipment, as in fencing face masks and eye protectors in squash

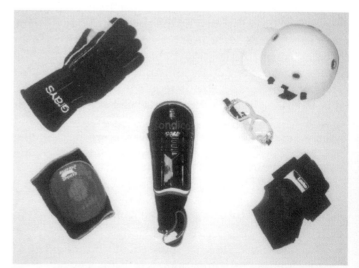

Fig. 7.1 Some examples of protective equipment. (Clockwise) hockey goal keeper's glove, helmet, squash protective glasses, ankle brace, shin guard and knee pad.

- the ability to limit excessive motion by mechanical or proprioceptive mechanisms, as in the use of sports tape, orthotics and braces.

Special attention should be paid to the prevention of severe injuries to participants in high risk sports. Severe injuries, although not frequent, usually involve vitally important body parts such as the eyes, brain and face. The International Federation of Sports Medicine has identified sports in which there is a high risk of eye injury and for which adequate eye protectors are available. They are hockey, racquet sports, lacrosse, handball, baseball, basketball, football, soccer and volleyball (FIMS 1988). The very high risk sports are boxing and karate, for which there are no adequate effective eye protectors available.

Wearing helmets effectively protects the head and brain from injury (Torg et al 1979), and participants of sports in which there is a high risk of head injury should be encouraged to wear them (Australian Sports Medicine Federation 1992e). The helmet should be comfortable, cool, aesthetic and sport-specific. It should distribute the impact forces as widely as possible and have the capacity to absorb some of the energy either on the inside or outside of the shell. It should not compromise hearing, vision or thermal regulation (Australian Sports Medicine Federation 1992e).

Mouthguards should be used in all contact sports because they are important in preventing orofacial injury as well as providing a buffering effect on concussion from impact to the mandible (Australian Sports Medicine Federation 1992d, Chapman 1985a). Their use is especially recommended at higher levels of competition, and for children and adolescents (Chapman 1985b, Chapman 1986). Mouthguards should be custom made and replaced every two years in adults and every year in children and adolescents (Chapman 1985b, Chapman 1986).

The musculoskeletal system features highly when considering the most frequently injured body system in sports participation. The use of materials such as tape and braces to prevent injuries is commonplace in modern sport. The ankle and knee joints tend to be taped or braced most often.

Preventative taping of the ankle has been shown to be very effective in decreasing the severity and frequency of inversion sprains (Bennell & McCrory 1992, Firer 1990, Garrick & Requa 1973). This is accomplished without weakening the ankle or increasing risk of injury to the knee, which was suggested by Ferguson (1973), (Glick et al 1976, Loos and Boelens 1984, and Paris and Sullivan 1992). Tape does loosen during participation after its initial application and to maximize its effect it should be reapplied at the quarter or half time interval of a match. Ankle braces have often been proposed as viable devices to prevent sprains, at a cheaper cost compared with the cost of tape over the lifespan of a brace, and with comparable efficacy. The relative efficacy between tape and braces and between the different braces has been investigated but the results are equivocal (Bennell & McCrory 1992).

Bracing the knee for primary prevention is not recommended because its effectiveness in reducing the severity and incidence of knee injury has not been proved (American Academy of Orthopaedic Surgery 1987, cited in Montgomery and Koziris 1989). However, Veldhuizen et al (1991) have demonstrated that bracing does not reduce the muscle strength about the knee or the performance of the knee. In the absence of any evidence that shows a deleterious effect of bracing its use may be advocated in specific cases.

SUMMARY

Even though the majority of the research dealing with the identification of the risk factors contributing to sports injury and the prevention of injury is still to be conducted, the implementation of strategies to prevent injury should be encouraged. If the strategies used to prevent injuries are not currently validated by research, they should at least be endorsed by sound scientific rationale. These strategies often are based on intuition (Meeuwisse 1991) and a common sense approach. Furthermore, without a comprehensive list of established causative factors of sports injury, the strategies that are employed to prevent sports injuries should be rigorously evaluated at regular intervals to ascertain the outcome of their implementation (Meeuwisse 1991). However, it is important to realise that no matter how methodical and comprehensive the pursuit of identifying risk factors and preventing injury is, there will always be a small risk of injury (Lysens et al 1991).

REFERENCES

Abrams J S 1991 Special shoulder problems in the throwing athlete: pathology, diagnosis, and nonoperative management. Clinics in Sports Medicine 10(4):839—861

Ackland T R, Bloomfield J 1992 Functional anatomy. In: Bloomfield J, Fricker P A, Fitch K D (eds) Textbook of science and medicine in sport. Blackwell Scientific Publications, Melbourne, pp. 2–26

Aggrawal N D, Kaur R, Kumar S, Mathur D N 1979 A study of changes in the spine in weight lifters and other athletes. British Journal of Sports Medicine 13:58–61

Andriacchi T, Sabiston P, Dehaven K, Dahners L, Woo S, Frank C, Oakes B, Brand R, Lewis J 1987 Ligament: injury and repair. In:

Woo S L Y, Buckwalter J A (eds) Injury and repair of the musculoskeletal soft tissues. American Academy of Orthopaedic Surgeons, Illinois, pp. 103—128

Australian Sports Medicine Federation 1990 Sports injuries in Australia: a report to the Better Health Program. Australian Sports Medicine Federation

Australian Sports Medicine Federation 1992a Guidelines for injury due to cold exposure. Australian Sports Medicine Federation

Australian Sports Medicine Federation 1992b Heat stress and exercise. Sport Health 10(4):11–12

Australian Sports Medicine Federation 1992c Medical screening and exercise. Australian Sports Medicine Federation

Australian Sports Medicine Federation 1992d Opinion statement on mouthguards. Australian Sports Medicine Federation

Australian Sports Medicine Federation 1992e Policy statement on head Injuries in sports. Australian Sports Medicine Federation

Australian Sports Medicine Federation 1992f Safety guidelines for fun runs and distance running. Australian Sports Medicine Federation

Backous D D, Friedl K E, Smith N J, Parr T J, Carpine W D 1988 Soccer injuries and their relation to physical maturity. Sports Medicine 142:839–842

Backx F J, Erich W B, Kemper A B, Verbeek L M 1989 Sports injuries in school-aged children. American Journal of Sports Medicine 17(2):234–240

Backx F J, Beifer H J, Bol E, Weitze B M 1991 Injuries in high-risk persons and high-risk sports. American Journal of Sports Medicine 19(2):124–130

Bale P 1992 The functional performance of children in relation to growth, maturation and exercise. Sports Medicine 13(3):151–159

Bartold S 1992 Conservative management of plantar fasciitis. Sport Health 10(3):17–28

Bennell K, McCrory P 1992 The role of ankle support in the prevention of ankle injury. Sport Health 10(3):13–16

Berson B L, Passoff T L, Nagelberg S, Thorton J 1978 Injury patterns in squash players. American Journal of Sports Medicine 6(6):323–325

Blair S N, Kohl H W, Goodyear N N 1987 Rates and risks for running and exercise injuries: studies in three populations. Research Quarterly for Exercise and Sport 58(3):221–228

Bobbert M F, Yeadon M R, Nigg B M 1992 Mechanical analysis of the landing phase in heel-toe running. Journal of Biomechanics 25(3):223–34

Bond J W, Miller B P, Chrisfield P M 1988 Psychological prediction of injury in elite swimmers. International Journal of Sports Medicine 9(5):345–8

Brodie D A, Bird H A, Wright V 1982 Joint laxity in selected athletic populations. Medicine and Science in Sport and Exercise 14(3):190-193

Brunet M E, Cook S D, Brinker M R, Dickinson J A 1990 A survey of running injuries in 1,505 competitive and recreational runners. The Journal of Sports Medicine and Physical Fitness 30:307–315

Buchanan T S, Beckman S, Rymer W Z 1992 Ligament force feedback and the regulation of joint stability. Abstracts of the 15th annual meeting of the American Society of Biomechanics. Journal of Biomechanics 25(6):673

Bullock-Saxton J E 1991 Changes in muscle function at hip and low back following chronic ankle sprain. In: Care in our hands. World Confederation for Physical Therapy, 11th International Congress. London, pp. 1470–1472

Burnett A, Elliott B, Foster D, Hardcastle P 1991 The back breaks before the wicket: the young fast bowler's spine. Sport Health 9(4):11–15

Butler D 1991 Mobilisation of the nervous system. Churchill Livingstone, Melbourne

Cabri J M H 1991 Isokinetic strength aspects of human joints and muscles. Critical Reviews in Biomedical Engineering 19(2–3):231–259

Caine D J 1990 Growth plate injury and bone growth: an update. Pediatric Exercise Science 2:209–229

Caine D, Cochrane B, Caine C, Zemper E 1989 An epidemiologic investigation of injuries affecting young competitive female gymnasts. American Journal of Sports Medicine 17(6):811–820

Calder A 1990 Recovery: restoration and regeneration as essential components within training programmes. Excel 6(3):15–19

Cameron-Tucker H 1983 The neurophysiology of tone: the role of the muscle spindle and the stretch reflex. Australian Journal of Physiotherapy 29(5):155–165

Carbon R J 1992 The female athlete. In: Bloomfield J, Fricker P A, Fitch K D (eds) Textbook of science and medicine in sport. Blackwell Scientific Publications, Melbourne, pp. 467–487

Carfarelli E, Sim J, Carolan B, Liebesman J 1990 Vibratory massage and short-term recovery from muscular fatigue. International Journal of Sports Medicine 11:474–478

Carfarelli E, Flint F 1992 The role of massage in preparation for and recovery from exercise. Sports Medicine 14(1):1–9

Cavanagh P R 1990 Biomechanics: a bridge builder among the sport sciences. Medicine and Science in Sports and Exercise 22(5):546–557

Chapman P J 1985a Concussion in contact sports and importance of mouthguards in protection. Australian Journal of Science and Medicine in Sport 17(1):23–27

Chapman P J 1985b The prevalence of orofacial injuries and use of mouthguards in rugby league. Australian Journal of Science and Medicine in Sport 17(3):15–18

Chapman P J 1986 Prevention of orofacial sporting injuries in children and young adolescents. Australian Journal of Science and Medicine in Sport 18(2):3–6

Chapman P J 1988 The pattern of use of mouthguards in rugby league. British Journal of Sports Medicine 22(3):98–100

Charmers D J, Cecchi J, Langley J D, Silva P A 1989 Injuries in the 12th and 13th years of life. Australian Paediatrics Journal 25:14–20

Clarke K S, Buckley W E 1980 Women's injuries in collegiate sports. American Journal of Sports Medicine 8(3):187–191

Clement D B, Taunton J E, Smart G W, McNicol K L 1984 A survey of overuse running injuries. Sport Health 2(1):25–30

Cook S D, Brinker M R, Poche M 1990 Running shoes. Sports Medicine 10(1):1–8

Corrigan J P 1992 Proprioception in the cruciate deficient knee. Journal of Bone and Joint Surgery 74(2):247–250

Crichton K J, Fricker P A, Purdam C R, Watson A S 1992 Injuries to the pelvis and lower limb. In: Bloomfield J, Fricker P A, Fitch K D (eds) Textbook of science and medicine in sport. Blackwell Scientific Publications, Melbourne, pp. 381–419

Curtis K A, Dillon D A 1985 Survey of wheelchair athletic injuries: common patterns and prevention. Paraplegia 23:170–175

D'Ambrosia R, Drez D 1982 Prevention and treatment of running injuries. Charles B Slack, New Jersey

DeDomenico G 1984 The accuracy of isometric tension production in the flexors of the elbow and terminal joint of the thumb. In: Australian Physiotherapy Association, 2nd International Congress, Asian and Pacific Basin region: Abstracts

Donatelli R 1990 Normal anatomy and biomechanics. In: Donatelli R (ed) The biomechanics of the foot and ankle. F A Davis, Philadelphia, pp. 3–31

Draper J A, Pyne D B, Thompson K M, Fricker P 1987 Injury occurrence in surfboard and surfski paddlers. Australian Journal of Science and Medicine in Sport 19(1):20–22

Drinkwater B L, Nilson K, Ott S, Chestnut C H 1986 Bone mineral density after resumption of menses in amenorrheic athletes. Journal of the American Medical Association 256(3):380–382

Drinkwater B L, Bruemner B, Chestnut C C IIIrd 1990 Menstrual history as a determinant of current bone density in young athletes. Journal of the American Medical Association 263(4):545–548

Durant R H, Seymore C, Lindner C W, Jay S 1985 The preparticipation examination of athletes. Sports Medicine 139:657–661

Durant R H, Pendergrast R A, Seymore C, Gaillard G, Donner J 1992 Findings from the preparticipation athletic examination and athletic injuries. American Journal of Disease in Children 146(1):85–91

Eggold J F 1981 Orthotics in the prevention of runners over-use injuries. The Physician and Sports Medicine 9(3):125–131

Ekstrand J, Gillquist J 1982 The frequency of muscle tightness and injuries in soccer players. American Journal of Sports Medicine 10(2):75–78

Ekstrand J, Gillquist J, Liljedahl S 1983 Prevention of soccer injuries: supervision by doctor and physiotherapist. American Journal of Sports Medicine 11(3):116–120

Ekstrand J, Gillquist J 1983a The avoidability of soccer injuries. International Journal of Sports Medicine 4:124–128

Ekstrand J, Gillquist J 1983b Soccer injuries and their mechanisms: a prospective study. Medicine and Science in Sport and Exercise 15(3):267–270

Ekstrand J, Nigg B M 1989 Surface-related injuries in soccer. Sports Medicine 8:56–62

Engstrom B, Johansson C, Tornkvist H 1991 Soccer injuries among elite female players. American Journal of Sports Medicine 19(4):372–375

Ferguson A 1973 The case against ankle taping. Journal of Sports Medicine 2:46–47

Ferrara M S, Buckley W E, McCann B C, Limbird T J, Powell J W, Robl R 1992 The injury experience of the competitive athlete with a disability: prevention implications. Medicine and Science in Sports and Exercise 24(2):184–8

FIMS 1988 Eye injuries and eye protection in sports: a position statement from the International Federation of Sports Medicine. International Journal of Sports Medicine 9:474–475

FIMS 1991 A position statement from the International Federation of Sports Medicine: excessive physical training in children and adolescents. Sport Health 9(1):23–24

Firer P 1990 Effectiveness of taping for the prevention of ankle ligament sprains. British Journal of Sports Medicine 24(1):47–50

Fisher A G, Jensen C R 1990 Scientific basis of athletic conditioning, 3rd edn. Lea & Febiger, Philadelphia

Fitch S 1984 Influence of muscle strength on fatique. In: Australian Physiotherapy Association, 2nd International Congress, Asian and Pacific Basin region: Abstracts

Foster D, John D, Elliot B, Ackland T, Fitch K 1989 Back injuries to fast bowlers in cricket: a prospective study. British Journal of Sports Medicine 23(3):150–154

Freeman M A R, Dean M R E, Hanham I M F 1965 The etiology of functional instability of the foot. Journal of Bone and Joint Surgery 47B:678–685

Fricker P A 1992 Injuries to the shoulder girdle and upper limb. In: Bloofield J, Fricker P A, Fitch K D (eds) Textbook of science and medicine in sport. Blackwell Scientific Publications, Melbourne, pp. 356–380

Friedlaender G, Joki P, Horowitz M 1990 The autoimmune nature of sports–induced injury: a hypothesis. In: Leadbetter W, Buckwalter J, Gordon S (eds) Sports–induced inflammation. American Academy of Orthopaedic Surgeons, Illinois, pp. 619–627

Fry R W, Morton A R, Keast D 1991 Overtraining in athletes: an update. Sports Medicine 12(1):32–65

Gainor B J, Piotrowski G, Puhl J, Allen W C, Hagen R 1980 The throw: biomechanics and acute injury. American Journal of Sports Medicine 8(2):114–118

Gallagher S S, Finson K, Guyer B, Goodenough S 1984 The incidence of injuries among 87 000 Massachusetts children and adolescents: results of the 1980–81 statewide childhood injury prevention program surveillance system. American Journal of Public Health 74(12):1340–1346

Garrett W E Jr 1990 Muscle strain injuries: clinical and basic concepts. Medicine and Science in Sports and Exercise 22(4):436–443

Garrick J G, Gillien D M, Whiteside P 1986 The epidemiology of aerobic dance injuries. American Journal of Sports Medicine 14(1):67–72

Garrick J G, Requa R K 1973 Role of external support in the prevention of ankle sprains. Medicine and Science in Sports 5(3):200–204

Garrick J G, Requa R K 1980 Epidemiology of women's gymnastics injuries. The American Journal of Sports Medicine 8(4):261–264

Glick J M, Gorden R B, Nishimoto D 1976 The prevention and treatment of ankle injuries. American Journal of Sports Medicine 4(4):136–141

Gossman M R, Sahrmann S A, Rose S J 1982 Review of length associated changes in muscle. Physical Therapy 62(12):1799–1808

Grace T G 1985 Muscle imbalance and extremity injury: a perplexing relationship. Sports Medicine 2:77–82

Grana W A, Moretz J A 1978 Ligamentous laxity in secondary school athletes. Journal of the American Medical Association 240(18):1975–1976

Greenfield B 1990 Evaluation of overuse syndromes. In: Donatelli R (ed) The biomechanics of the foot and ankle. F A Davis, Philadelphia, pp. 153–177

Groppel J L 1987 The effect of string type and tension on impact in mid–sized and over–sized tennis racquets. International Journal of Sport Biomechanics 3(1):40–46

Gross J B 1992 Chronic fatigue syndrome and the sports performer. Sport Health 10(3):25–26

Grove J R, Gordon A M D 1992 The psychological aspects of injury in sport. In: Bloomfield J, Fricker P A, Fitch K D (eds) Textbook of science and medicine in sport. Blackwell Scientific Publications, Melbourne, pp. 176–186

Hamilton L H, Hamilton W G, Meltzer J D, Marshall P, Molnar M 1989 Personality, stress, and injuries in professional ballet dancers. American Journal of Sports Medicine 17(2):263–7

Hamilton W G, Hamilton L H, Marshall P, Molnar M 1992 A profile of the musculoskeletal characteristics of elite professional ballet dancers. American Journal of Sports Medicine 20(3):267–273

Hardaker W P Jr 1989 Foot and ankle injuries in classical ballet dancers. Orthopaedic Clinics of North America 20(4):621–627

Hardcastle P 1991 Lumbar pain in fast bowlers. Australian Family Physician 20(7):943–951

Harmer P 1991 The effect of pre–performance massage on stride frequency in sprinters. Athletic Trainer 26:55–59

Haycock C E, Gillette J V 1976 Susceptibility of women athletes to injury. Journal of the American Medical Association 236(2):163–165

Heinzman S E 1991 Quality physicals that generate funds for the training room. Athletic Training 26(spring):66–69

Herbert R 1988 The passive mechanical properties of muscle and their adaptations to altered patterns of use. Australian Journal of Physiotherapy 34(3):141–149

Hershman E 1984a The profile for prevention of musculoskeletal injury. Clinics in Sports Medicine 3(1):65–84

Hershman E (ed) 1984b The profile for prevention of musculoskeletal injury. W B Saunders, Philadelphia

Hinton R Y 1988 Isokinetic evaluation of shoulder rotational strength in high school baseball pitchers. American Journal of Sports Medicine 16(3):274–279

Hoeberigs J H 1992 Factors related to the incidence of running injuries. Sports Medicine 13(6):408–422

Hoff G L, Martin T A 1986 Outdoor and indoor soccer: injuries among youth players. American Journal of Sports Medicine 14(3):231–233

Hollis M 1987 Massage for therapists. Blackwell Scientific Publications, Oxford

Hopper D 1986 A survey of netball injuries and conditions related to these injuries. Australian Journal of Physiotherapy 32(4):231–239

Horner C, McCabe M J 1984 Ice–skating and roller disco injuries in Dublin. British Journal of Sports Medicine 18(3):207–211

Hoy G A, Kennedy D K 1984 A survey of Victorian Football Association injuries in season 1981. Sport Health 2(2):23–26

Hughes L Y 1985 Biomechanical analysis of the foot and ankle for predisposition to developing stress fractures. Journal of Orthopaedic and Sports Physical Therapy 7(3):96–101

Hunter L Y, Torgan C 1983 Dismounts in gymnastics: should scoring be reevaluated. American Journal of Sports Medicine 11(4):208–210

Jackson D L, Haglund B 1991 Tarsal tunnel syndrome in athletes. American Journal of Sports Medicine 19(1):61–65

Jacobs S J, Berson B L 1986 Injuries to runners: a study of entrants to a 10 000 meter race. American Journal of Sports Medicine 14(2):151

James S L, Bates B T, Osternig C R 1978 Injuries to runners. American Journal of Sports Medicine 6(2):40–50

Janda V 1978 Muscles, central nervous system motor regulation and back problems. In: Korr (ed) Neurobiological mechanisms in manipulative therapy. Plenum Press, New York pp. 27–41

Janda V 1980 Muscles as a pathogenic factor in back pain. In: Proceedings of the 15th International Federation of Orthopaedic Manipulative Therapists. Christchurch, New Zealand, pp. 1–24

Janda D H, Hankin E M, Wojtys F M 1986 Softball injuries, cost, cause, prevention. American Family Physician 33:143–144

Janda D H, Wojtys E M, Hankin F M, Benedict M E, Hensinger R N 1990 A three–phase analysis of the prevention of recreational softball injuries. American Journal of Sports Medicine 18(6):632–635

Janda D H, Wild D E, Hensinger R N 1992 Softball injuries: aetiology and prevention. Sports Medicine 13(4):285–291

Johansson C 1986 Injuries in elite orienteers. American Journal of Sports Medicine 14(5):410–415

Jorgensen U, Ekstrand J 1988 Significance of heel pad confinement for the shock absorption at heel strike. International Journal of Sports Medicine 9:468–473

Jorgensen U, Winge S 1990 Injuries in badminton. Sports Medicine 10(1):59–64

Kamenetz H L (ed) 1985 History of massage. Williams & Wilkins, Baltimore

Van Mechelen W, Hlobil H, Kemper H C 1987 How can sports injuries be prevented? National Institute for Sports Health Care, Oosterbeek, The Netherlands

Van Mechelen W, Hlobil H, Kemper H C G 1992 Incidence, severity, aetiology and prevention of sports injuries. Sports Medicine 14(2):82–99

Veldhuizen J W, Koene F M, Oostvogel H J, Van Thiel T P, Verstappen F T 1991 The effects of a supportive knee brace on leg performance in healthy subjects. International Journal of Sports Medicine 12(6):577–580

Vicenzino B 1992 Sports physiotherapy manual. Department of Physiotherapy, University of Queensland

Vitasalo J T, Kvist M 1983 Some biomechanical aspects of the foot and ankle in athletes with and without shin splints. American Journal of Sports Medicine 11(3):125–130

Walter S D, Hart L E, McIntosh J M, Sutton J R 1989 The Ontario cohort study of running–related injuries. Archives of International Medicine 149:2561–2564

Walter S D, Sutton J R, McIntosh J M, Connolly C 1985 The aetiology of sport injuries. Sports Medicine 2:47–58

Warren B L 1984 Anatomical factors associated with predicting plantar fasciitis in long–distance runners. Medicine and Science in Sports and Exercise 16(1):60–63

Warren B L, Jones C J 1987 Predicting plantar fasciitis in runners. Medicine and Science in Sport and Exercise 19(1):71–73

Warren M P, Brooks–Gunn J, Hamilton L H, Warren L F, Hamilton W G 1986 Scoliosis and fractures in young ballet dancers. New England Journal of Medicine 314(21):1348–1353

Watson A S 1992 Children in sport. In: Bloomfield J, Fricker P A, Fitch K D (eds) Textbook of science and medicine in sport. Blackwell Scientific, Melbourne, pp. 436–466

Watson A W S 1984 Sports injuries during one academic year in 6799 Irish school children. American Journal of Sports Medicine 12(1):65–71

Weinberg R, Jackson A, Kolodny K 1988 The relationship of massage and exercise to mood enhancement. Sport Psychologist 2:202–211

Wilkerson A 1992 Stretching the truth: a review of the literature on muscle stretching. Australian Journal of Physiotherapy 38(4):283–287

Williams P L, Warwick R, Dyson M, Bannister R 1989 Gray's anatomy, 37th edn. Churchill Livingstone, Melbourne

Woodall W, Welsh J 1990 A biomechanical basis for rehabilitation programs involving the patellofemoral joint. Journal of Orthopaedic and Sports Physical Therapy 11(11):535–542

Wright J R, McIntyre L, Rand J L, Hixson E G 1991 Nordic ski jumping injuries. American Journal of Sports Medicine 19(6):615–619

Injury evaluation and management

8. Sporting emergencies

Peter Brukner, Karim Khan

Sporting emergencies are an unfortunate fact of life. They do not occur often, but when they do occur it is imperative that they are immediately recognized and appropriately managed.

In the ideal situation, a doctor would be present to take control of the emergency. If so, the role of the physiotherapist is to render whatever assistance is required under the doctor's instruction. In many cases, however, the physiotherapist is the only health professional present. Therefore, it is essential that all physiotherapists who cover sporting activities are adequately trained in first aid.

The physiotherapist must be able to provide basic first aid on site, including cardiopulmonary resuscitation. The physiotherapist must also be able to recognize life-threatening emergencies and those situations where more expert medical care is required. If there is any suggestion that a serious emergency has occurred, the physiotherapist should not hesitate to arrange immediate transfer to the nearest hospital by any means possible, preferably in a well equipped ambulance. The physiotherapist should always err on the side of caution in these situations and be willing to refer to specialists.

Sporting emergencies may be divided into three categories:

- Trauma to a previously well athlete, e.g. head injury, chest or abdominal injury, spinal injury
- Aggravation of a previously recognized medical problem e.g. heart disease, asthma, diabetes
- Presentation of a previously unrecognized medical problem, e.g. asymptomatic coronary artery disease.

An outline of causes of collapse in the athlete is shown in Table 8.1.

PREPARATION

The secret of success in the treatment of sporting emergencies is adequate preparation. The practitioner responsible for the medical coverage of a sporting event should anticipate sporting emergencies that may occur and be

Table 8.1 The collapsed athlete

Trauma	No trauma
• Head injury	• Cardiac
- severe	- coronary artery disease
- minor	- arrhythmia
• Spinal injury	- congenital abnormality
- cervical	• Hyperthermia
- thoracic	• Hypothermia
- lumbar	• Cerebrovascular accident
• Thoracic injury	• Hypoglycaemia
- multiple rib fracture	• Hyponatraemia
- haemothorax	• Respiratory
- tension pneumothorax	- asthma
- cardiac tamponade	- spontaneous pneumothorax
- cardiac contusion	- pulmonary embolism
• Abdominal injury	• Allergic anaphylaxis
- ruptured viscus,	• Drugs
e.g. liver, spleen, kidney,	- cocaine, morphine etc.
bladder, pancreas, bowel	• Other
• Multiple fractures	- vasovagal (fainting)
• Blood loss	- postural hypotension
	- blood pooling post-exercise
	- hyperventilation
	- hysteria

adequately prepared for any of these. This preparation should include equipment, personnel and training.

Equipment

To treat a sporting emergency, equipment for resuscitation and for safe, rapid transfer of the injured athlete are required. Equipment for cardiopulmonary resuscitation (CPR) should be available at all sporting venues. The Oxy-Viva or Air-Viva contains a mask and a source of oxygen with an adjustable flow rate. An oropharyngeal airway should also be available. A light, strong stretcher should be used to transport unconscious or severely injured athletes. A spine board or Jordan frame is required for the transport of suspected spinal injuries. The Jordan frame may be dismantled and easily stored, and is thus appropriate for any venue. If only one form of transport equipment is to be available, then it should be a Jordan frame as this can also be used to transport athletes with non-spinal injuries.

and mucus removed from the throat immediately. Definitive treatment of laryngeal injuries ranges from monitored observation to surgery in the case of major laryngeal trauma.

Chest injuries

Symptoms associated with chest injuries include pain, shortness of breath and haemoptysis. If there is significant intrathoracic haemorrhage, the patient may show signs of shock, hypotension, tachycardia and poor peripheral perfusion. Rapidly increasing shortness of breath may indicate a tension pneumothorax. Haemoptysis suggests pulmonary haematoma or a ruptured bronchus.

Blunt trauma to the chest wall may result in rib fractures, flail chest, pneumothorax, haemothorax, diaphragm rupture or myocardial contusion. Deceleration injuries, seen in motor sports, may result in injury to the aorta.

Pneumothorax

Pneumothorax (air in the pleural cavity) may occur spontaneously or result from fractured ribs or an open chest wound. Clinical features include shortness of breath, hyperresonance, unilateral diminished breath sounds and tracheal shift to the contralateral side. A pneumothorax should be suspected in all cases of fractured ribs. If the pneumothorax is large enough to cause shortness of breath or takes up the equivalent of one intercostal space on chest X-ray, the athlete should be transported to hospital for insertion of a chest tube. The chest tube allows air to escape from the pleural cavity, enabling the lung to re-expand.

A tension pneumothorax may be indicated by worsening shortness of breath, distended neck veins, cyanosis and diminishing blood pressure. This condition requires urgent transfer to hospital for insertion of a chest tube.

Haemothorax

A haemothorax occurs when blood accumulates in the pleural space, usually as the result of bleeding of thoracic vessels e.g. intercostal, pulmonary or mediastinal vessels. There is often an associated pneumothorax (haemopneumothorax).

Examination of the injured athlete with haemothorax will reveal dullness to percussion, diminished breath sounds and hypotension. The patient requires urgent transfer to hospital, sitting up with oxygen and, preferably, intravenous drip in situ. Definitive treatment consists of chest tube insertion and, occasionally, blood transfusion and even thoracotomy if bleeding continues.

Open chest wounds

Open chest wounds should be sealed with foil, cloth or similar items and taped on three sides only to prevent development of a tension pneumothorax. A chest tube may be inserted later in a hospital.

Flail chest

Multiple rib fractures may result in paradoxical chest wall movement whereby the chest wall moves inwards instead of outwards when the lung expands. This results in decreased air entry and can lead to respiratory failure. The patient should be assisted to sit up and be given oxygen if available.

Cardiac contusion

Crushing and deceleration injuries may result in cardiac contusion. Bruising the cardiac muscle may lead to impaired circulation or cause bleeding into the pericardium, resulting in cardiac tamponade. Clinically this is detectable by the presence of pulsus paradoxus. A fall in blood pressure of greater than 10 mmHg on inspiration suggests cardiac tamponade. Treatment of both conditions requires urgent transfer to hospital.

Abdominal injuries

Any direct blow to the lower rib or abdominal region may cause injury to one of the abdominal organs. When a direct blow is sustained, the athlete should be removed from the field of play and observed closely for signs of damage to abdominal organs and circulatory collapse. The athlete who has sustained damage to one or more abdominal organs may complain of severe pain and develop signs of circulatory collapse almost immediately. Alternatively, if internal bleeding is less severe, the pain may slowly increase over minutes or hours.

The abdomen must be carefully palpated for the presence of tenderness and guarding. If generalized tenderness and guarding is present with abdominal rigidity and absent bowel sounds, peritonitis is present, usually as a result of blood in the peritoneal cavity. The patient should also be assessed for signs of circulatory collapse, by monitoring the pulse and blood pressure.

Increasing abdominal pain, signs of peritonitis or evidence of the development of circulatory collapse are all indications for urgent transportation to hospital. The athlete should not eat or drink prior to hospital evaluation.

Ruptured spleen

Injury to the spleen may occur with trauma to the left lower chest and is often associated with fractures of the overlying ribs. The spleen is particularly prone to damage when it is enlarged (as in infectious mononucleosis).

Clinical features of splenic rupture include left upper quadrant abdominal pain and abdominal distension. Shock may develop rapidly or be delayed by hours or days. Left shoulder pain may occur due to secondary diaphragmatic irritation.

All patients with suspected splenic injury should be admitted to hospital for observation.

performed.
with suspe
perature. (
unreliable
be measur
temperatu
confirm th
indication,
of the seve

If the r
should be
done by a
the major
neck. An
or ice bath
temperatu

In mos
present. T
Evidence
and rapic
rehydratic
be comm
electrolyt

Guid

Most
follow

1. Pe
   m
   cc
2. U
   cc
   ap
3. A
   sl
   e
   o
   cl
   n
4. A
   a
   h
5. V
   t
   l
   v
   t
   (
   l
   l

Kidney injuries

Kidney injuries result from a blow to the flank region. Relatively minor injuries result in a bruise or contusion which manifests as blood in the urine. Clinical features include loin tenderness and swelling, guarding or visible bruising. Urinalysis may reveal gross or microscopic haematuria, or no evidence of blood at all. Extensive retroperitoneal bleeding may result in hypotension and shock.

If renal damage is suspected after a blow to the loin, the athlete should be asked to pass a urine sample. If haematuria is detected, admission to hospital is required.

Pelvic fractures

Athletes who sustain pelvic bone fractures are usually competing in high speed sports, such as motor sports. If the fracture does not destroy the integrity of the pelvic ring and there are no associated injuries, treatment is symptomatic with bed rest for 3 weeks and early limb movement.

If the pelvic ring has been destroyed, there may be associated complications such as ruptured bladder, ruptured urethra, rectal injury or internal haemorrhage. These injuries require urgent hospital admission.

Bladder injuries

Rupture of the bladder is rare in sports unless associated with a pelvic fracture. Clinical features include haematuria, suprapubic pain, pain on voiding or inability to void.

Urethral injury

The most common cause of a urethral injury in sport is a fall-astride injury in cycling, resulting in damage to the membranous urethra. This presents as a drop of blood at the external urethral meatus. If a ruptured urethra is suspected, the patient should be warned not to attempt to pass urine. Urological assessment is required urgently.

Injuries to the external genitalia

Blunt trauma to the scrotum may result in testicular rupture requiring emergency surgery. An associated injury to the pampiniform plexus may cause massive swelling of the scrotum, making diagnosis of the ruptured testicle difficult. Medical examination in the supine position is required and the testicle must be palpated to determine integrity. Cases of ruptured testicle require surgical exploration and repair.

Minor cases of scrotal or testicular contusions may be managed by analgesia, bed rest, scrotal elevation (e.g. rolled towel between legs) and cold packs. Large scrotal haematomas may require surgical drainage.

Rectus abdominis haematoma

The abdominal wall musculature will often bear the brunt of a blow in athletes with conditioned abdominal muscles.

If a direct blow causes haemorrhage into the muscle, rapid swelling may develop. This should be managed with ice and compression. The presence of a stable blood pressure and normal bowel sounds should enable the practitioner to differentiate between a muscle haematoma and an intra-abdominal injury. If the superficial epigastric artery is torn, haemorrhage may be extensive. Operative evacuation of the haematoma and ligation of the bleeding artery may be required.

Injuries to the extremities

Injuries to the limbs may involve damage to the bones, joints, vascular system or nervous system. The initial management of an injured limb includes control of haemorrhage, prevention of further injury and restoration of blood flow to the limb. If the site of the injury is bleeding, this should be controlled by direct pressure. Open wounds should be covered with sterile dressings as soon as possible. Joint dislocations should be reduced if this can be performed relatively easily. Exposed bones, associated with compound fractures, should not be reduced on the field because of the likelihood of contamination.

Closed angulated fractures of the long bones are best straightened prior to splinting. Satisfactory alignment can usually be obtained by applying longitudinal traction to the distal part. If this is not possible at the first attempt, further attempts should be abandoned until the patient is transferred to hospital. The injured area should be splinted, ideally with an air splint but rolled-up blankets, clothing, pillows or adjacent body parts can be used as a splint.

The neurovascular status of a limb should be documented prior to and following any manipulation. This includes palpation of distal pulses such as the dorsalis pedis and posterior tibial pulses of the leg and the radial and ulnar pulses of the arm. Skin pallor, capillary return, temperature and sensation should be noted. Specific motor and sensory testing of the involved limb enables assessment of peripheral nerve function.

Ligamentous injuries to the joints of the upper and lower limbs should be assessed. Often in the case of bony injuries, ligamentous injuries are ignored and consequently cause far more problems than the bony injury. Acute, uncomplicated soft tissue injuries are treated initially with rest, ice, compression and elevation (RICE).

Compound fractures

Open wounds associated with suspected fractures require cleaning and covering with sterile dressings soaked in saline or antiseptic solution. The fracture should be splinted without attempting reduction. It is not advisable to attempt to push the protruding bone back into the wound. The patient must be urgently transported to hospital for management of the fracture, antibiotic therapy and tetanus prophylaxis.

9. Principles of assessment

Murray Hutchison, Jeffrey Oxley

Treatment of even the most straightforward disorder requires a series of very different clinical decisions: decisions about the problem to be addressed; goals and priorities; the timing and intensity of treatment; the methods used; the degree to which athletes will be made responsible for their own treatment; and where and by whom treatment should be administered. To make these decisions prudently, the sports physiotherapist must base them on a thorough and careful assessment of each athlete's needs.

The skill of assessment is one of the most important talents of the sports physiotherapist. An accurate assessment of the neuromusculoskeletal structures will enable a sound pathological diagnosis to be made, the importance of which has been emphasized by Brukner and Khan (1993) and Watson (1993). It is equally important that the physiotherapist have a thorough understanding of the presenting signs and symptoms. Two injured athletes with the same diagnosis may present with very different signs and symptoms depending on the severity and stage of the pathology, and therefore require different management to effectively treat the disorder. However, it must also be remembered that conditions with similar clinical presentations can, by nature of the pathology involved, require quite different management. While focusing on the signs and symptoms has great merit, particularly in treatment selection and reassessment, it should not be done at the expense of a sound pathological diagnosis. This can lead to inefficient treatment and open the physiotherapist to being criticized for treating inappropriately without accurate diagnosis (Watson 1993). Physiotherapists must continually develop their clinical skills to ensure they provide efficacy of treatment and facilitate the earliest possible return of the athlete to the sports arena.

This chapter will cover preseason assessment and the requirements of on-field and detailed clinical assessments.

PRESEASON ASSESSMENT

The organization and preparation of a preseason medical and injury history is an important but often overlooked aspect of sports injury management when working with teams and clubs. Timing of the preseason assessment should consider two points. First, the examination should occur early enough before a particular sport season to allow adequate rehabilitation of injuries, muscle imbalances or other correctable problems including lack of cardiovascular fitness. Second, it should not be so early that time is a factor in the development of any recent problems that may be missed. It is recommended that preseason assessment should be performed approximately six weeks prior to the start of the season (McKeag 1989, Johnson et al 1993).

If possible, a complete medical history should be taken prior to participation in any sport. This assessment should note the athlete's current state of health and condition, and all previous injuries, illnesses and their management, including surgery. Notice should be taken of the response to the previous injuries, such as type and length of rehabilitation. Some athletes have strong opinions on the effectiveness of certain types of treatment or practitioners; consequently, it is important to ascertain such a bias so an appropriate decision can be made if treatment is necessary later.

The examination should identify any conditions that may interfere with the athlete's ability to perform the selected sport or may need special consideration in management.

Regardless of age, sex or sport any screening evaluation should involve an awareness of the stress that exercise places on the musculoskeletal and cardiovascular systems, and psychological factors. Physiotherapists are particularly concerned about the existence, or past history of a musculoskeletal disorder such as subluxing patellae or shoulders, severe scoliosis, the absence of anterior or posterior cruciate ligaments or patellofemoral dysfunction (Reider 1991). There are many tests available to measure criteria such as flexibility measurements, strength, power and endurance testing. Any preseason examination assessing the athlete without an awareness of the demands of the specific sport has major weakness. Clearly, the evaluation of a potential swimmer would be different from that of a

Table 9.1 Suggested areas of sport-specific emphasis (adapted from McKeag, 1989)

Sports	Physical examination emphasis
Football	
Australian Rules	Knee, ankle, lumbar spine
Rugby	Cervical and lumbar spine, head, knee
Soccer	Hip, pelvis, foot
Cricket	Shoulder, lumbar spine
Basketball	Ankle, knee
Squash	Wrist, elbow, eye
Baseball	Shoulder, elbow, arm, cervical spine
Swimming	Ears, throat, shoulder, cervical and thoracic spines, knee (breaststroke)
Gymnastics	Wrist, shoulder, lumbar spine
Running	Lumbar spine, pelvis, hip, knee, ankle, foot
Wrestling	% body fat, shoulder, skin

hockey player. Table 9.1 summarizes the suggested areas of a sports specific examination for various sports. The site of any previous injuries also requires special attention to determine if there are any residual deficits.

Regions and criteria selected for testing may also be determined by selecting a parameter that can be used appropriately for retesting to determine improvement. For example, a screening procedure may be implemented for all members of a team to test for hamstring condition. Flexibility, strength, power and endurance (on a dynamometer), 'slump test' (Maitland 1986) and palpation of areas of scar tissue or defects may be selected for testing. All these criteria must be recorded. Comparisons are made across each limb and with any earlier data that may have been collected. To a lesser extent, comparisons may be made with other participants in the same sport.

The cardiovascular examination should be conducted by a sports physician or team doctor. However, if the physiotherapist becomes aware of a medical condition such as a heart murmur, congenital heart disease, arrhythmia or hypertension it is important to discuss this with the team doctor to be aware of any restrictions placed on the athlete. A history of poorly controlled asthma may be revealed, and may require lung function testing pre- and post-exercise to assess whether the bronchospasm is exercise induced. Seasonal allergy, infections, irritants, weather changes, drugs, and emotional upset also need to be considered (Sonzogni & Gross 1993).

Psychological factors can also be screened prior to the season. Depression should be considered in the diagnosis of an athlete presenting with nonspecific somatic complaints or an inexplicable decrease in level of performance (Sickles & Lombardo 1993). The athlete presenting with prolonged underperformance associated with fatigue following a period of heavy exercise may be developing an overtraining syndrome. This requires early recognition so appropriate rest and stress management can be implemented (Budgett 1990).

The preseason period allows the physiotherapist and other health and fitness professionals prepare assessment records, charts and cards for each athlete that can be readily referenced. These records must be maintained for the whole season to assist with injury statistics, details for insurance claims and ongoing individual injury reference.

ON-FIELD ASSESSMENT

One of the most difficult aspects of assessing sporting injuries is where the physiotherapist must make an assessment on the sporting field. This assessment needs to be swift and accurate, as the game is still proceeding or has been stopped by officials who await a decision. The assessment needs to be comprehensive enough to determine whether the player can remain in the game or must be removed to prevent further injury, to treat or to apply protective bracing or bandaging.

Expertise in this primary assessment skill requires good diagnostic skills, the ability to make decisions in limited time, and often experience of previous practical situations. This process is facilitated if the occurrence of the injury has been witnessed. The physiotherapist must have a good view of the total playing arena and have direct access to the participants. It is extremely important that the physiotherapist view the sport from an injury or potential injury perspective. This requires concentration on the athlete and no distraction by other aspects of the sport. In football, for example, it is necessary to watch the player after the kick and not be tempted to watch the flight of the ball. Many injuries occur as a result of late tackles or falls after contact is made. Once this area of play is cleared for injury, vision must quickly be moved to the next potential injury area, that is, the next player contact with the ball or another player.

If the physiotherapist's vision and concentration are focused, a great deal of information will be known about the injury before entering the playing field. An alert physiotherapist will have noted the mechanism of injury and the region injured, have an idea of the severity of the injury and be starting to formulate a method of coping with the injury even before leaving their seat. Continued concentration on the injured player will provide further valuable assessment information. Mental notes should be made on whether the player has been knocked out initially and, if so, how long he or she takes to rise and the quality of this movement. Actions by the player at this stage will assist in determining the extent of the problem, for example, whether the player immediately begins walking or running. The posture of the player can lead the observant physiotherapist towards an early diagnosis, for example, an acromioclavicular joint injury will usually result in the player holding the affected limb across the body in the least painful position—a posture that is readily recognized from a distance. Consequently, continual visual input will prepare the physiotherapist for the appropriate assessment techniques upon reaching the player.

Of paramount importance is to have an efficient and prioritized plan for the initial assessment and management of the injured athlete while still on the sporting arena (Webb 1990).

One such prioritized plan utilizes the acronym TOTAPS (**T**alk, **O**bserve, **T**ouch, **A**ctive Movement, **P**assive Movements, **S**kill Test). TOTAPS is often taught in first aid programs. It incorporates an ordered and correct procedure to allow the physiotherapist to arrive at a decision in the shortest possible time (Australian Sports Medicine Association 1989).

TOTAPS includes the following:

- **T**: Talk. See if the athlete can talk. If he or she can talk, ask about the mechanism of injury. This will also allow an initial assessment of the state of consciousness. Further questions can be asked at this stage, such as 'What part of the game is it?', or 'What is the score?', to give a more accurate determination of brain function. If possible and necessary, other details should be obtained from the player such as past relevant history, pain (intensity and site) and sensory deficits.
- **O**: Observe. A general observation should be made initially for any life-threatening signs such as airway obstruction, unconsciousness, fitting, cardiac signs or uncontrolled bleeding. These obviously take precedence over any peripheral injuries and require immediate appropriate action. Once these are excluded, observation of the injury site and condition is necessary. A quick comparison with the uninjured side will assist in determining whether there is swelling or deformity.
- **T**: Touch. It may be necessary to palpate the injured part to determine the exact site of injury, the soft tissue feel, including the presence of swelling, change in temperature and tenderness. This may indicate more precisely the exact structure damaged and this knowledge, coupled with experience of the ability of that particular structure to allow appropriate function, will help the decision to allow the athlete to continue or be removed.
- **A**: Active movement. The athlete is asked to actively move the injured limb to ascertain the degree and quality of movement and assess if any limitation exists due to pain or weakness. Comparison can be made between the painfree range and the normal full active range of motion.
- **P**: Passive movement. The injured limb should be taken through its normal range of motion by the physiotherapist to determine joint viability while feeling for laxity and instability. Again, available range of motion should be compared with the other limb for an approximation of loss of normal range. If indicated, special tests for ligament stability are performed at this stage.
- **S**: Skills test. Skills tests should be graduated in difficulty to the full complement required to perform that particular sporting task. These may begin with simply standing unsupported through to walking, running, jumping for the lower limb or swinging a racquet or bat for the upper limb, etc.

The physiotherapist must, based on all the findings, make a decision in a relatively short time on whether the athlete should continue to participate. There may be alternatives to continuing the activity, such as change of position in the sport so as to reduce the activity level for a limited time, or removing the athlete long enough to apply protective bracing or strapping. If the player remains on the playing field, the physiotherapist should watch closely for any signs of limitation due to the injury, that may necessitate removal from the field at a later stage. Irrespective of the injury, where there is any doubt concerning the athlete's ability to continue he or she should be removed from the sports field until further assessment is carried out and the athlete demonstrates fitness.

The indications for reduction of a deformity on the sidelines are extremely narrow. This should only be attempted by a skilled and experienced physiotherapist or physician, and only in certain circumstances such as when the circulatory or neurological status of the limb is in jeopardy (Sonzogni & Gross 1993).

DETAILED CLINICAL ASSESSMENT

A detailed clinical assessment is performed once the athlete has been removed from the sporting field to an area where the athlete can be comfortably positioned and time can be taken for a thorough assessment. This assessment is sometimes referred to as the secondary or subsequent assessment. In many cases the physiotherapist will not have been present on site, at the time of injury, and so this will be the physiotherapist's primary contact with the athlete.

Whether the assessment is performed court side, in a separate room to eliminate distractions, or in the physiotherapy clinic, the physiotherapist should proceed in an ordered manner with a detailed assessment plan. This plan should provide a methodical examination including a thorough subjective and physical investigation. The physiotherapist must remain alert to the particularly relevant factors and the possible relationship between these factors. At this stage it can be determined if there is a necessity for utilizing further assessment tools such as radiographic techniques. The injured player may also require referral to other medical or paramedical personnel for further investigation or treatment.

It is critical that an accurate identification of the presenting problem is made because this will determine the management of the injured athlete and influence the speed of their recovery. Athletes often present with complicated problems and a skilled differential diagnosis will reveal the source of the problem. Where possible an injured joint should be evaluated soon after injury, as information about the severity of the injury is more easily obtained before swelling, reactive muscle spasm and guarding occurs (Maron 1988).

Subjective examination

The athlete is the most valuable source of information and the physiotherapist's ability to extract that information will determine their depth of understanding and, subsequently, their ability to manage the athlete's injury. A thorough subjective assessment is necessary to enable the physiotherapist to formulate a clear picture of the presenting problem, identify the likely source of the symptoms and plan the physical examination.

Establishing good rapport with the athlete and skilful questioning are essential for the physiotherapist to obtain the necessary information while gaining the confidence of a player, who is usually in pain and often unhappy and frustrated about being sidelined by the injury. Through a combination of open-ended and directed questions and active listening, the physiotherapist can guide the subjective examination while letting the athlete give their account of their problems. If the injury is of a chronic nature without a single obvious causative incident, or if there is more than one area of symptoms, the subjective assessment becomes more important in putting together how the problem started and how it has progressed.

It is important during the subjective examination to remember the variations possible with the presentation of a given disorder. This can help the physiotherapist avoid the mistake of assuming the presence or absence of a particular feature, which could lead to missing important information and making incorrect assumptions. Hypotheses formulated throughout the subjective examination, and indeed the physical examination and treatment, are supported or refuted depending how 'the features fit' as the physiotherapist puts all the information together (Maitland 1986). It is when the features do not fit that clarification and further inquiry are necessary. At the end of the subjective examination the physiotherapist should have a good understanding of the problem, and a clear idea about what they expect to find on the physical examination.

History

Current (injury) history. As much information as possible about the present injury should be obtained by encouraging the athlete to describe the injury in detail.

How did the injury occur? It is vital to differentiate initially between a contact and a non-contact injury. This will assist final diagnosis, particularly in differentiating between sprains, strains and haematomae. The mechanism of injury must be determined as accurately as possible and questions continued until adequate answers are obtained. This is more difficult when the examining physiotherapist was not present when the injury occurred.

Information relating to direction of contact, or what body part hit the playing surface, can be invaluable in assisting the diagnosis. If the player remains unsure, it may be possible to obtain relevant information from other players or supporters who were close to the incident, or from viewing a videotape.

When did it occur? The particular injury may not have occurred in one specific incident. It may have slowly developed or indeed been present before the sporting event and aggravated during participation. Timing and length of onset give valuable information on the type of injury sustained.

Was something felt or heard? Most athletes will be able to describe associated sounds, such as pops or cracks, and different types of sensations associated with certain injuries. Not enough notice is taken by physiotherapists of this type of reporting by athletes. It is important to spend some time listening and noting the athlete's feelings and descriptions of the injury.

Where is the injury? Ask the athlete to point to the area of complaint and note how this is done. A single finger point will often indicate a localized injury site, a hand waved over an area may indicate a non-specific and generalized injury. Question carefully the athlete's perception of the depth of the symptoms, that is, whether it is superficial or deep within the limb or joint. It is appropriate at this stage to ask about other areas that could refer to this region. Even if cleared of symptoms this should be noted on the body chart so it can be established later that these areas were considered.

What are the pain characteristics? The type of pain, in the athlete's own words, can give some indicators of the cause of the pain. Pain from deep somatic structures, including muscles, ligaments, other joint structures and neural tissue, is usually described as a deep, dull and diffuse ache. This can often be distinguished from radicular pain which is more characteristically described as shooting, lancinating pain, occurring in a dermatomal distribution. Radicular pain is also associated with other signs of nerve root compression (Bogduk 1984). The athlete may also describe the pain as sharp, throbbing or piercing, usually in the region of the injury. The actual source and cause of somatic pain, whether local or referred, is not revealed by the distribution or description of the pain (Bogduk 1984).

What is the behaviour of the symptoms? The behaviour of the pain should be investigated, and if present greater than twenty-four hours its pattern should be determined. Initially establish whether the pain is constant, intermittent or movement-related. If intermittent, attempt to discern its frequency and duration and question to find out which activities or postures provoke or ease the pain. Information should be obtained on the presence of night pain, latent pain, morning stiffness and pain related to function, posture or activity. Resting or night pain may indicate a significant inflammatory component in the injury or other non-mechanical disorders requiring referral. Morning stiffness is also indicative of an inflammatory component in the injury. Questioning can establish if the stiffness improves as the athlete moves about (suggesting a mechanical disorder), or persists through the morning, which is more characteristic of an underlying inflammatory condition.

What other symptoms are present? Question carefully to ascertain whether other symptoms such as weakness, crepitus, stiffness, feeling of 'giving way' or sensory changes are present. Crepitus is an audible or palpable phenomenon which may indicate joint surface roughening or tenosynovitis. It may be painless but may also be accompanied by pain and represent the main presenting symptom (Cyriax 1982).

What is the level of irritability? Irritability is assessed by determining:

1. the type and amount of activity required to cause an increase in symptoms;
2. the severity of symptoms provoked;
3. the length of time taken for this increase in symptoms to return to its usual level (Maitland 1986).

It is critical the level of irritability be determined accurately so a decision can be made on whether the physical examination should be limited, to prevent any risk of aggravating the condition during the assessment. If irritability is high, it may be necessary to limit the testing to only the more important movements or to spread the examination over more than one visit. The physiotherapist should confirm subjective findings in relation to irritability early in the physical examination.

Information on how the injury has progressed since its onset must also be established. If the disorder has worsened it is important to discover why. This may also indicate the need for being particularly selective with assessment and treatment.

Etiological factors and biomechanical considerations. When the injury has a more insidious onset or is of a chronic or recurrent nature, etiological and biomechanical considerations must be questioned in detail. This is of primary importance if treatment is going to not only alleviate symptoms, but prevent recurrences.

Factors requiring consideration include: training surface, training regime and alterations to it, shoe type, equipment, posture, and requirements of competition.

1. Training surface. Knowledge of the playing surface type and its particular problems may assist with diagnosis and management of the injury. Artificial turf, because of its lack of compliance and increased friction between the foot and playing surface, tends to cause more leg fatigue and shin splints than natural grass (Fried & Lloyd 1992). Hard or uneven running surfaces, rigid gymnasium floors and basketball courts, and inflexible or poorly cushioned floor mats can all produce harmful impact forces resulting in injury (Rzonca & Baylis 1988, Stanitski 1993).

2. Training regimes. An inappropriate training program is the most common significant factor leading to overuse injuries (Zaricznyj et al 1980). Obviously there is a complete spectrum of regimes available, each placing different stresses on the athlete. Many injuries are directly attributable to the style, intensity or duration of training and may arise when there is a significant alteration in the training style. For example a sharp increase in the number of laps being swum in a training session causing fatigue, conversion to an improper stroke technique and consequently injury (Ciullo & Stevens 1989), or the addition of running up and down hills placing greater stresses on muscles and increased impact forces (Andrews 1983). Problems can also arise if there is too much emphasis on one aspect of a training program so that the program is not balanced, such as the inclusion of a great deal of quadriceps exercises with little or no attention to the hamstrings strength. The physiotherapist may need to consult with the coach to obtain detailed knowledge of the training.

3. Footwear. Inadequate footwear, such as ill-fitting, excessively rigid or uncushioned shoes, creates excessive stress in the foot and entire lower extremity (Cook et al. 1990). It is often necessary to examine the shoe type and its condition, and therefore it is important that the athlete always bring sporting footwear to the examination. Understanding that poor shoes can contribute to injuries has led manufacturers to design footwear with added stability and motion control. Assessing foot type and selecting footwear with the appropriate features may be sufficient to alleviate problems (Fick et al. 1992). With more complicated problems the assistance of a podiatrist may be indicated.

4. Equipment. A knowledge of protective equipment, equipment for performing the sport, and orthopaedic braces and supports is often necessary to obtain information about an injury and to prevent an injury or recurrences.

Many sports have specialized equipment, both for protection and improving performance. This necessitates a good appreciation of the sport itself and its physical demands if the physiotherapist is to fully understand a problem. The information can become technical, such as knowledge of tennis racquet styles, material, string tension and grip size. This knowledge can be obtained from an informed tennis coach. Faulty or poorly maintained equipment can contribute to injury.

The physiotherapist must understand the function of equipment, including braces, and be able to recognize when a brace may be contributing to the symptoms. For example, the use of a tennis elbow brace for 'tennis elbow' might be useful, but, if prescribed for other causes of elbow pain such as medial elbow instability it can aggravate the condition (Harding 1992). When the athlete presents, it is important to establish how long the brace has been used, its benefit or otherwise, and who prescribed it.

5. Technique and posture. Poor technique is frequently a major contributing factor in the development of overuse injuries, especially where the athlete performs a repetitive action (Ciullo & Stevens 1989, Elliot and Foster 1984). Proper instruction in the development of good technique should be the goal of every coach. However, the physiotherapist also has a responsibility to emphasize the importance of developing a sound technique. Frequently the athlete places too much emphasis on performance times, for example lap swimming times or speed of cricket ball delivery, and too little emphasis on proper technique. This can lead to injury.

The physiotherapist must understand the various postures that an athlete adopts to perform their sport. These postures are many and varied. For example, cyclists and hockey goalkeepers adopt a forward flexion posture during most of their competition, and this may contribute to spinal derangement. Poor postures at work and during other recreational or leisure activities should also be followed up as these could contribute to the athlete's condition.

6. Requirements of competition. This is a knowledge of the above combined with an understanding of the demands of competition. For example, is the athlete required to perform short fast runs and quick turns as in basketball, which places stress particularly on calf and hamstring musculature and the knee? Or is the athlete involved in body contact sport such as football? This information can be of great value to the assessment.

Past history. Obtaining all relevant past history from the athlete is essential if the physiotherapist is to fully understand the present injury. In situations where the present injury clearly seems part of a long-term problem, inquiring first about the initial injury is useful. However, in most cases taking the current history prior to the past history is advisable as it can help the physiotherapist avoid the irrelevant information.

Details of the previous injury. The cause of the initial injury, its progression, the effect of any treatment and the level of any symptoms remaining should all be ascertained from the athlete. With chronic or recurrent injuries the frequency of recurrences, the ease of provocation and the recovery rate, including the need for and effect of treatment, can assist the physiotherapist to understand the pathology being assessed. The level of symptoms remaining between episodes is a guide to the selection and expectations of treatment and gives an indication of the athlete's tolerance of discomfort.

Relevant past history. Careful questioning is required to elicit any predisposing factors to the current injury. The athlete should always be questioned regarding present or previous spinal symptoms, to help establish whether there could be a spinal component to the current disorder (Maitland 1986). Butler (1991) emphasized that when an athlete presents with an injury without sufficient apparent cause or complaining of a 'run of injuries', it may suggest an adverse neural tension component to the disorder.

Relevant past incidents or activities should be noted and information obtained on illnesses, general state of health, tiredness or familial factors. Symptoms should be plotted over the time period to the present to determine if there is any recognizable pattern which can be related to a diagnosis.

Special questions

These questions constitute a group of questions that must be included in the subjective examination. They are primarily to help the physiotherapist establish any precautions or contraindications to the physical examination and treatment of the athlete and recognize the athlete who presents with a disorder which is not neuromusculoskeletal in origin. It must be borne in mind that serious visceral disease can produce spinal pain which mimics that of relatively innocent vertebral joint problems (Grieve 1988). Henderson (1992) noted that while thoracic or chest pain of musculoskeletal origin occurs regularly with athletes, it can stem from a potentially fatal visceral source. Angina pectoralis, for example, can mimic a muscle strain in the anterior shoulder region. As the physiotherapist may well be the primary contact practitioner it is essential that the special questions are not overlooked or assumed to be negative.

If the athlete complains of pain which appears to be non-mechanical in origin, or where the 'features do not fit', referral to the athlete's local doctor or a sports physician should be organized. Long-standing pain, particularly with a prolonged development and a protracted course, such as chronic groin pain, often has a variable and complex pathogenesis which requires a multidisciplinary approach to management (Ekberg et al. 1988).

General history. Questions relating to weight loss (which may indicate carcinoma), bladder or bowel dysfunction (may indicate cauda equina problems) or bilateral paraesthesia in the feet (possibly indicating canal stenosis or spinal cord compression) are important.

The general health of the athlete should be established. Complaints of ill health associated with prolonged under-performance and fatigue may indicate dietary inadequacies. An overtraining syndrome should be suspected if the symptoms follow a period of heavy exercise (Budgett 1990). Further questioning to eliminate other systemic illnesses, genetic conditions or pregnancy may also be necessary.

Symptoms of vertebrobasilar insufficiency. Recognizing the presence and behaviour of dizziness as a symptom is of great importance when treating an individual with a cervical spine disorder. It is potentially dangerous if dizziness is caused by obstruction of a vertebral artery. While dizziness can be a symptom of numerous disorders, when it is present the physiotherapist must take particular care with cervical assessment and treatment. Dizziness should be further investigated during the physical examination with the vertebral artery screening tests (see Ch. 21). These tests are mandatory before any cervical manipulation is performed and are advisable before using end of range mobilization techniques (Australian Physiotherapy Association 1988, Grant 1988).

Medication. A number of different types of drugs are commonly used in the treatment of sporting injuries. It is important that the physiotherapist is aware of the athlete's use of drugs such as analgesics, non-steroidal anti-inflammatories, and steroidal anti-inflammatories (see Ch. 37). It should be established to what extent the medication has been beneficial. Improvement following the use of non-steroidal anti-inflammatories indicates an inflammatory component in the injury.

With the use of stronger analgesics, such as narcotic analgesics, the physiotherapist must consider that the medication may have the effect of disguising the symptoms. This may indicate a need to exercise particular care during examination to avoid aggravating the condition. The dosage of analgesics required over a twenty-four hour period to give pain relief can provide useful information concerning the athlete's progress.

Rapid relief of symptoms following a corticosteroid injection can result in the overuse of damaged tissues, leading to increased degenerative changes. Therefore, it is important that the athlete rests the affected area for a minimum of two to three days (Brukner & Khan 1993). When repeated injections are administered to the same site there is a risk of rupture of the structure involved. Purdam et al (1992) suggest that when repeated injections have been administered a ten day rest is advisable following an injection. The physiotherapist must take this into consideration during examination and avoid any vigorous assessment procedures involving that part in the initial period following the injection.

X-rays. The athlete should be asked if any X-rays or other radiological investigations have been performed. If so, it is necessary to find out when the investigations were performed and what the results were. This may be useful in determining the diagnosis or providing information relevant to the ongoing management of the athlete's problem.

Planning the physical examination

Having completed the subjective examination, the physiotherapist must analyse the information gained so that the format and priorities of the physical examination can be planned. It is important to recognize that it is generally not possible to perform a comprehensive examination of all structures and consider all etiological factors in the initial assessment. Based on the subjective examination, the physiotherapist must decide what the main priorities are, and ensure that they are included in the initial physical examination. For example, the athlete who has had a traumatic injury involving the knee will require ligamentous stability testing as a priority. On the other hand, examining an athlete presenting with an overuse injury will usually require greater emphasis on muscle imbalances and biomechanical inadequencies.

While planning the physical examination the physiotherapist should consider the format of the examination to ensure it follows a logical and time-efficient sequence. The sequence should also minimize the changing of positions, and consequent discomfort to the athlete. Maitland (1986) emphasized the value of using a planning sheet to assist in planning the physical examination. The following factors must be considered for an appropriate plan to be devised:

1 the structures, both local and those which can refer to the area, which could be responsible for the symptoms
2 the irritability of the symptoms and therefore the strength of the examination. The severity of the injury and/or irritability may be limiting factors to the physical examination
3 the presence of any factors which might contra-indicate any part of the examination, or suggest particular care is required.

The physical examination should proceed in a methodical manner following the assessment plan. If the physical examination is planned, and proceeds accordingly, the physiotherapist is less likely to miss important information or perform an inappropriate or potentially harmful manoeuvre.

Physical examination

The aims of the physical examination are to establish the structures involved in producing the symptoms by:

1 reproducing the athlete's symptoms or finding a comparable sign of restriction in an appropriate joint, muscle or other structure

2 establishing patterns of movement and restriction which match those mentioned during the subjective examination and which are compatible with the structures under consideration
3 finding any associated factors such as biomechanical inadequencies, which may be responsible for the structures becoming symptomatic.

In this way the physiotherapist can investigate the hypotheses formed during the subjective examination, and by confirming, modifying and disproving them can establish an accurate clinical diagnosis on which to base management.

Measurement

Consistency, reproducibility and accuracy in measurement during the physical examination are very important, if the physiotherapist is to make worthwhile comparisons with the contralateral limb, or correctly assess progress at a later date. There are various forms of measurement required during the physical examination.

Joint angle measurement is usually performed visually or with the aid of a measuring device such as a goniometer. The most important point is that it is compared with the contralateral limb to provide 'normal' information for the individual. The use of standardized anatomical landmarks during measurement can help improve consistency. With some movements, such as in the lumbar spine, measurement may be recorded as fractions of normal range.

Linear measurement is often performed to compare one side to the other, for example, comparison between thigh circumferences when measuring an effusion or haematoma. While many linear measurements can be made with a tape measure, some require the physiotherapist to use 'feel', for example estimating the amount of displacement during an anterior drawer test of the ankle. All joints can be tested with linear or accessory movements and, while it is often difficult to record due to the small amount of movement, very valuable information can be gained by comparing to the other side and recording any discrepancies.

Comparative measurements can be very useful to objectively record asymmetries or altered movement patterns. Examples are the comparative measurement of anatomical landmarks such as relative positions of the posterior superior iliac spines to assess leg length discrepancy, or the inferior angle of the scapulae during shoulder abduction to evaluate scapulothoracic movement.

Physiotherapists must be familiar with, and confident of their ability to use, whatever form of measurement they select. Measurements can only be accurate and therefore useful if physiotherapists pay attention to details such as reproducing starting positions and the consistent use of anatomical landmarks and measurement devices.

It is extremely important that the method of recording be easily understood by physiotherapists, and other medical personnel who may be involved in the athlete's management, so it can be valuable at future assessments.

Observation

The physiotherapist should observe for signs that may give some indication of the site, severity and diagnosis of the particular injury. An example of this is the prominence and uneven level of the distal end of the clavicle in an acromioclavicular disruption. Information can be obtained by watching the athlete walking in, looking at arm swing, posture and evenness of weightbearing and when the athlete removes shoes or clothing, seeing if movements are being avoided or protected. The physiotherapist should develop an eye for balance and fluidity of movement. There may be past incidents that have affected normal movement and gait pattern, and consequently are relevant to the etiology or extent of the present injury.

Posture. Does the athlete exhibit a posture that would indicate a particular type or region of injury? This may range from simply holding an arm in the 'collar and cuff' position which may indicate injury to the clavicle, to the typical lumbar lateral shunt that often indicates a lumbar disc injury (McKenzie 1981).

Facial expressions. A large part of communication is non-verbal. In a situation of stress, such as when the injured athlete is in pain, much can be learned from non-verbal communication such as facial expressions and postures. Correct interpretation of facial expressions may indicate the level of pain and consequently the extent of the damage.

Movement quality. Movements which are abnormally slow, jerky or asynchronous may indicate a particular problem, for example, poor quality arm abduction with a rotator cuff tear. During movement assessment, it may become apparent that there is a deviation or tricking to avoid a painful region. To further obtain range, the athlete may utilize trick movements such as trunk lateral flexion while attempting to abduct the shoulder. If the physiotherapist is aware of these movements, additional information can be obtained about the quality and intensity of the injury.

Observation of the part. The physiotherapist must check for any obvious deformity, scars, swelling, wasting or muscle spasm and observe and note any colour changes that may indicate circulatory or inflammatory problems.

Palpation

The experienced physiotherapist can obtain a great deal of knowledge about an injury using a systematic approach to palpation. Beginning with light stroking to discriminate skin temperature, superficial swelling, tone and pain response, the pressure applied can be gradually increased to obtain information about deeper structures. It is often beneficial to begin palpation away from the site of injury and palpate each important structure in turn as the most painful region is approached (Roy & Irvin 1983). This should include joint structures (including bone and ligament), muscles and their tendons, and neural tissue. In this way no area or structure will be overlooked and the limits of the affected area can be determined.

When palpating, the physiotherapist is particularly interested in warmth, swelling, crepitus and pain (Corrigan & Maitland 1983). Warmth indicates increased metabolic activity due to an active inflammatory process or haemarthrosis (Cyriax 1982). Alteration in skin temperature, hot or cold, associated with sweating may indicate sympathetic involvement (Norris 1993).

Swelling can be either intra- or extra-articular, and can vary in consistency from hard to soft. Hard intra-articular swellings are generally the result of osteophytes or osteochondrotic fragments. Soft intra-articular swelling may be due to either fluid from a synovial effusion or synovial thickening. Palpation can confirm whether the swelling is fluid or has the thicker 'doughy' consistency of synovial thickening (Corrigan & Maitland 1983).

Extra-articular swelling can be due to oedema, haematoma, fatty deposits, scar tissue and synovial swelling in tendon sheaths and bursae. Swelling may be localized or diffuse. Diffuse swelling around a joint can implicate an extra-articular structure or may indicate an injury involving the joint capsule, allowing a synovial effusion to escape into the surrounding tissues (Booher & Thibodean 1985).

Crepitus may be heard or felt as a finger is rolled over a structure or a joint is moved. Coarse crepitus in a joint indicates articular cartilage degeneration. Fine crepitus is often indicative of a tenosynovitis (Cyriax 1982).

Although the tenderness produced on palpation can give valuable information, it can provide much misinformation. Tenderness should only be interpreted in conjunction with the other palpatory findings, and comparison should always be made with the other side. Furthermore, tenderness can be a referred phenomenon with the site of the causative lesion being more proximal (Corrigan & Maitland 1983).

Active movement tests

Prior to the initial movement tests, it is important to ascertain whether the patient has any pain in a neutral or rest position. The athlete is then asked to perform the particular movement test while the physiotherapist observes the quality and range of movement and notes whether there are any relevant movement inadequacies or differences from the uninjured side. The athlete is questioned regarding:

1 the nature and location of the symptoms and if there is pain, is it 'their pain'

2 where in the range the symptoms appear, and how the symptoms change during movement

3 if there is any referral of symptoms, and if so, what type and to where.

4 what is limiting the movement, to establish whether the movement is limited by pain, stiffness or muscle weakness.

It may be necessary to perform some of these active tests in more than one position with regard to weightbearing and gravity. By performing the active testing for an ankle problem while standing as well as in a non-weightbearing supine position, the physiotherapist can obtain a more functional measurement of ankle dorsiflexion. Assessment in weight bearing may provide greater information about pain in some intra-articular and periarticular disorders (Maitland 1985a). Another situation where changing the starting position can be valuable is in establishing whether a movement is limited by stiffness or weakness. For example, an athlete may have greater shoulder flexion in lying when compared to their active range in standing or sitting.

Active movements in all directions should be attempted unless the level of irritability suggests otherwise. Further active movement testing is required if there has been insufficient symptoms or movement signs provoked to match those complained of by the athlete. Testing can be more thorough and provocative. The use of combining movements, repeating movements, altering the speed of movement, performing a movement with the addition of a load, or compression or distraction, and sustaining postures at the end of the range can all make the active movement tests more sensitive (Magarey 1986). The selection of additional movement tests will be largely based on the factors previously reported in the subjective examination as being aggravating.

Functional tests

It may be necessary to devise a test or a series of tests that are functionally oriented in order to reproduce the athlete's symptoms. If the athlete can reproduce the symptoms with a particular posture or activity, that posture or activity should be analyzed (Magarey 1988). This may involve replicating some movements contained in the sport such as running, kicking, throwing, or a tennis serve. For example, the tennis serve generally combines thoracic spine extension, rotation and lateral flexion towards the serving arm at the end of the backswing. Therefore if the athlete complained of midthoracic pain at that point in the serve, the physiotherapist can utilize the position to increase individual movements to determine which component provokes the most pain. They may establish, for example, that in neutral extension was painfree, but in the functional position it reproduced the athlete's pain.

On occasions the physiotherapist will require an understanding of the sport's techniques in order to devise a specific test. This may involve performing a backhand stroke with a tennis racquet so that the arc of swing or wrist grip can be altered to reproduce the symptoms. A functional test may have to be repetitive to reproduce the symptoms, for example, swimming laps prior to the examination of a swimmer's shoulder.

Differentiation tests

Often, during the examination of a movement, the source of a symptom provoked is not clear, as it may have originated from one of a number of different structures. Differentiation testing involves examining a painful movement in such a way that one possible structure at fault is stabilized while the position of another implicated structure is altered. Any change in the pain response may help determine the relative contribution of each structure to the symptoms. For example, an athlete may present with limited forearm supination following a fall onto the outstretched hand. Differentiation between the radiocarpal joint and the inferior radioulnar joint can be achieved by provoking the pain then noting any decrease in the pain on releasing the radiocarpal joint component of the movement while maintaining the inferior radioulnar joint on stretch. This can be confirmed by comparing the pain response during the reverse manoeuvre. If a test is designed appropriately, it should be possible to differentiate between the affected structures (Maitland 1991).

Many sporting injuries, particularly overuse injuries, are multifactorial in nature. The physiotherapist can assess the relative contribution to the athlete's symptoms from local joint, muscle and neural tissues using similar principles of differentiation.

Passive movement tests

Passive physiological and/or accessory movements of the joints being examined may be selected when it is necessary to find a particular movement that causes pain, resistance

Table 9.2 Normal endfeels (adapted from Patla 1989, Cyriax 1982)

Structure	Endfeel
Soft tissue approximation	Soft and spongy feel, as with elbow or knee flexion
Muscular	Elastic reflex resistance, for example calf stretch
Ligamentous	Firm arrest of movement with no give, for example, abduction of the extended knee
Cartilaginous	Sudden stop but not hard, for example extreme of extension in a normal elbow
Capsular feel	Firm arrest of movement with a slight creep, for example the extreme of rotation in a normal shoulder or elbow

Table 9.3 Abnormal endfeels (adapted from Patla 1989, Cyriax 1982)

Structure	Endfeel
Bone-to-bone	Sudden hard stop short of range, for example myositis ossificans or a fracture involving a joint
Muscle spasm	'Hard endfeel' accompanies a severe active lesion
	Abnormal elastic resistance, for example, muscle guarding
Capsular	Abnormal creep resistance with a harsh tight limit (chronic inflammation) or painful with muscle spasm (acute inflammation)
Bony grating	Roughing, grating, for example, advanced chondromalacia
Springy block	Slight rebound is seen with an intra-articular displacement such as a torn meniscus in the knee
Loose	Ligamentous laxity, for example, second degree ligament injury
Empty	Boggy, soft, not limited mechanically, for example, synovitis, haemarthrosis

and/or spasm which can then be compared to the athlete's symptoms (Maitland 1991).

During testing, the physiotherapist must continually ask about the presence of pain and record the position when any is reported. The limb can then be taken further into range in an attempt to alter the pain. While taking the limb through range passively, the physiotherapist should note any areas of resistance. An appreciation of the relationship between the pain and the resistance produced during a passive movement is necessary to select an appropriate grade of movement if that passive movement is chosen as a treatment technique (see Ch. 12).

If possible, the joint should be moved to the limit of its available range in order to assess whether the range of movement is full when compared with the other side. The physiotherapist can also establish if there is any joint crepitus during movement and gauge the endfeel of the movement. If pain is not excessive and the level of irritability permits, some over pressure may provide important extra information about the endfeel. This can help determine if there is a normal or abnormal endfeel, and provide some indication of the structures involved in the injury (see Tables 9.2 and 9.3).

Often accessory movements are the earliest detectable changes and therefore the most sensitive indicators of abnormality in joint movement (Magarey 1988). Their inclusion in the examination can be extremely valuable, especially when symptoms are proving difficult to reproduce. It may be necessary to combine an accessory movement with an end of range physiological movement to accurately reproduce the symptoms. If normal passive movement does not elicit pain, the use of combined movements and the application of compression or distraction to joints will help the physiotherapist to further test the integrity of joint structures and ensure that essential information is not missed during the examination.

The testing of passive accessory movement has long been documented for assessing joint stability in many sporting injuries (Reid 1992). Examples are the Lachman's and posterior drawer tests for the knee to determine cruciate ligament viability. There is no substitute for experience. The physiotherapist must continually practise the technique and attempt to grade the movement that is obtained, for example, first, second or third degree depending on the severity of the injury. Further improvement in clinical skills can be achieved by comparing gradings with fellow physiotherapists and doctors on every possible occasion.

Special tests

Special tests are indicated to assist in or confirm the differential diagnosis. They are usually specific in application to a joint or muscle and must be selected accordingly. They are covered in detail in the regional chapters of this book. These tests require practice and skill by the physiotherapist. If the tests are accurately performed immediately after the injury occurs, prior to the onset of spasm or swelling, a great deal of information can be gained, an accurate diagnosis can very often be made, and when indicated referral to an appropriate specialist organized immediately. For example, Lachman's test (Torq et al 1976) for cruciate viability and Thompson's (squeeze) test (Kulund 1982) for achilles rupture are both best performed as early as possible. The sooner an accurate diagnosis is made, the earlier an optimal management program can be instigated.

Muscle examination

Strength testing. It may be necessary to utilize various forms of resistance to assist with a differential diagnosis.

Isometric testing may be indicated when a measure of strength is required at one particular point in the range of motion of the limb. If, for example, pain inhibits part of the range of shoulder movement it may be valuable to obtain a measure of isometric strength at a position outside this painful range.

Isotonic testing is utilized when part or full range of motion is available and a measure of strength is obtained using relatively simple forms of resistance such as manual resistance or free weights.

Isokinetic testing may be indicated when the athlete's symptoms have been difficult to reproduce, or more detailed information is required. Dynamometers are able to provide variable accommodating resistance which enables the physiotherapist to assess and record both concentric and eccentric activity, muscle endurance and muscle balance ratios. This information can be of great assistance when rehabilitating the athlete following a major injury, especially if pre-injury statistics are available for the athlete concerned.

Muscle flexibility and function. The importance of assessing muscle flexibility and function in the pathogenesis of various pain syndromes of the neuromusculo-skeletal system must be emphasized.

Muscle dysfunction is generally recognised in relation to local conditions, however Janda (1988) also stressed the necessity to examine for muscle changes or imbalances which may be remote from the symptomatic region. Muscle imbalances occur when certain muscles become shortened and tight, while others become weak. These muscle imbalances tend to occur in patterns which Jull and Janda (1987) and Janda (1988) have described in detail.

Muscles can be the site of referred pain and may react to pain by inhibition, overactivity or shortness, all of which may in turn contribute to future problems (Jull 1986). Palpation, isometric contractions and muscle stretching can help determine whether a particular muscle is contributing to an athlete's symptoms. Travell and Simons (1983, 1988) provide a detailed description of muscle palpation and trigger points, as well as methods of assessing muscle length. Donatelli and Walker (1989) particularly emphasize the need to assess the flexibility of two-joint muscles as they have a central role in promoting an interdependency of movement and function within the joints of the upper or lower quadrants.

Pathologic change in a muscle is an essential component of dysfunction syndromes of the neuromusculoskeletal system. For example, an athlete with a tight gastrocnemius muscle group may overpronate the foot in order to achieve a greater amount of ankle dorsiflexion during weightbearing activities (Donatelli & Walker 1989). The altered foot posture and biomechanics are likely to cause different and increased stresses in the entire lower limb. Neuromusculo-skeletal problems can also develop secondarily to muscle weakness. For example, it has been proposed that scapulo-thoracic muscle weakness can be a factor contributing to shoulder impingement syndromes (Kamkar et al 1993).

One of the most important aspects in an overall therapeutic program lies in the recognition of factors which perpetuate the dysfunction (Janda 1988). While a muscle imbalance can result in joint dysfunction or poor posture, the reverse can also occur. Once the important factors which perpetuate the dysfunction are recognized an appropriate treatment can be instigated.

Examination of the spine

For the examination of a peripheral musculoskeletal injury to be complete all the structures, both local and remote, from which the pain could arise should be considered. The ability of deep somatic structures to refer pain is often overlooked in the assessment and treatment of peripheral sporting injuries (Niere 1991). The presence of localized clinical signs, such as tenderness on palpation, and painful muscle contraction or stretch, may lead to a premature diagnosis of a local peripheral injury, for example a tennis elbow. This is often reinforced by the temporary benefits of local treatment, whether it involves electrotherapy modalities, manual techniques or injection of a local anaesthetic or corticosteroid (Grieve 1988). However, the examination is incomplete unless the physiotherapist investigates the possibility of a spinal component in the disorder. Even in the absence of complaints of spinal symptoms there may be referred tenderness and increased local muscle activity due to a spinal dysfunction (Grieve 1988). The spinal dysfunction may be solely responsible for the local peripheral signs, may be predisposing the peripheral area to local pathology or may be existing concurrently with, and independent of, the local peripheral disorder (Niere 1991). In this case the relative contributions

from the spinal component and the local peripheral disorder can be determined with careful examination and re-assessment following treatment.

The extent of the examination of a possible spinal component will be determined by the history and nature of the problem. Examination of the lumbar spine in an athlete who presents with a painful swollen ankle following an acute inversion injury would be a far lower priority than in an athlete who presents with recurrent hamstring strains (Niere 1991).

Neurological examination

Following all sporting injuries the integrity of the spinal cord, nerve roots and peripheral nerves must be established. The neurological examination tests for abnormal nerve

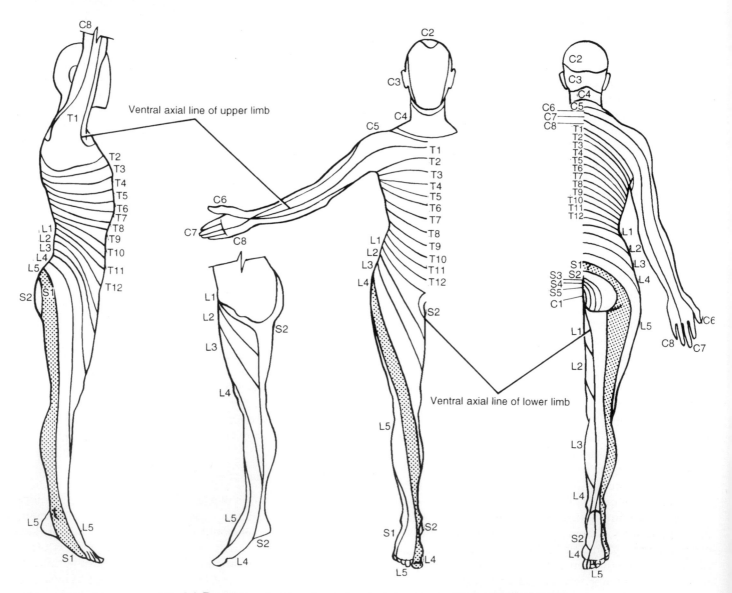

Fig. 9.1 Dermatome chart based on embryological segments. Source: Maitland (1986).

conduction and should be performed on any athlete who complains of referred pain from the spine extending past the shoulder or gluteal crease for the cervical and lumbosacral nerve roots respectively. The injured athlete must be questioned regarding sensory disturbances such as numbness or parathesiae, and responses to the special questions recorded to establish any possible spinal cord or cauda equinae involvement. Following trauma any injured extremities should have immediate and short-term examination of sensory, motor and vascular status. Swelling four to six hours post-injury can cause significant damage to nerves, blood vessels and musculature (Maron 1988), such as in the case of a compartment syndrome.

Positive signs of neurological involvement include diminished or loss of sensation, muscle weakness, muscle wasting, and decreased or absent deep tendon reflex in the distribution of the affected nerve root. In the presence of altered sensation which is bilateral and in a glove/stocking distribution, an upper motor neuron lesion should be suspected. In this case deep tendon reflexes will be hyperflexic, and the athlete will demonstrate ankle clonus and a positive Babinski sign on testing. For a thorough description of the neurological examination the reader is referred to Butler (1991).

A knowledge of dermatomes and myotomes is important with due consideration to the high percentage of anatomical anomalies and individual variations (Figs 9.1 and 9.2). While it is recognized that dermatomes and myotomes are only approximations of nerve root innervation, Jull (1986) suggests that clinical testing can specify the nerve root involved with a reasonable degree of certainty. However, Jull (1986) emphasizes that because of the anatomical position of the nerve roots testing does not necessarily specify the spinal level involved. It is suggested that given the anatomical arrangement of the nerve roots within the thecal sac, as described by Wall et al (1990) (Fig. 9.3), injury at a spinal level may result in compromise of motor and/or sensory bundles of more than one nerve root. This would further complicate the picture.

It is not always clear whether a neurological impairment is spinal in origin or peripheral. Saal et al (1988) reported on forty-five peripheral nerve entrapments which were found to be the cause of leg pain in thirty-six patients who were referred with lumbar radicular syndromes. Many of the patients complained of associated back pain, had spinal range of motion abnormalities and presented with positive neural tension signs. Saal et al concluded that a lower limb peripheral nerve entrapment could mimic a lumbar radicular syndrome. Even in the presence of comparable signs in the spine, a neurological deficit involving a peripheral nerve should not be overlooked. Differentiation between nerve root and a peripheral nerve is generally based on the area of sensory loss and pattern of muscle weakness (Magarey 1986). The majority of athletes presenting to the

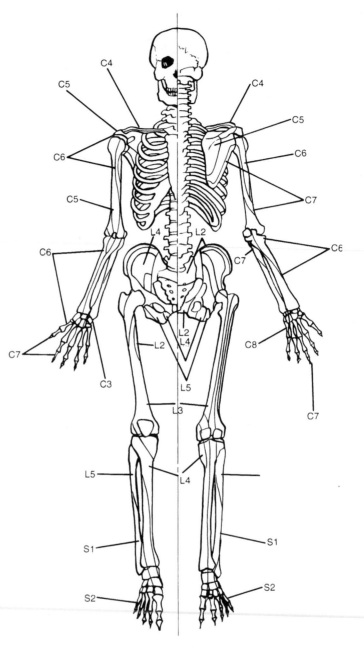

Fig. 9.2 Myotome chart Source:Maitland (1986).

physiotherapist do not require any electrodiagnostic testing such as nerve conduction tests or electromyography (Butler 1991). However, the study of motor and sensory nerve conduction can assist the recognition and accurate localization of peripheral nerve pathology (Brukner & Khan 1993).

Adverse neural tension

Physiotherapists have become increasingly aware of the potential for adverse neural tension to play a role in musculoskeletal disorders. Initially this concentrated on the

a

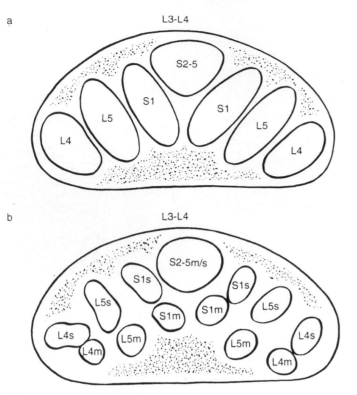

b

Fig. 9.3 (i) Schematic representation of individual nerve roots at L3-4 disc level, (ii) Schematic representation of the placement of motor and sensory bundles within the individual nerve roots. Source: adapted from Wall et al (1990).

movement of pain-sensitive structures in the vertebral canal and intervertebral foramen (Elvey 1979, Cyriax 1982, Maitland 1985b).

A positive tension test is not a definite indicator of a spinal disorder. Rather, it is an indicator of adverse neural tension somewhere in the nervous system. Adverse neural tension is an important component of many sporting injuries, involving the spine and the extremities. This is particularly so in chronic and recurrent injuries and overuse syndromes. In those injuries which resolve slower than expected, occur without sufficient apparent cause, or form part of a 'run of injuries', adverse neural tension should be suspected (Butler 1991).

The mobility of the nervous system of the trunk and limbs can be assessed using the passive neck flexion, straight leg raise, prone knee bend, upper limb tension and slump tests.

Recent refinements to the tests and a greater awareness of our ability to palpate the nervous system have enabled physiotherapists to be far more thorough with their investigation of the nervous system (see Ch. 26 and Butler 1991).

If there is a chronic or recurrent disorder it must also be remembered that there may be a spinal dysfunction or adverse neural tension which is secondary to a peripheral musculoskeletal injury. For example, an athlete presenting with a stiff shoulder due to local shoulder pathology may present with signs of stiffness in the cervical and upper thoracic regions and demonstrate restriction on tension tests. This could be due to the altered shoulder biomechanics resulting in increased stresses on both the spine and neural tissues. It has been suggested that local shoulder stiffness can cause tethering of the upper limb neural structures and act as a site of peripheral entrapment (Watson 1993).

REASSESSMENT

Ongoing assessment of the athlete's problem is essential for the physiotherapist to have a clear understanding of how the problem is progressing. This will enable the physiotherapist to make decisions regarding the likely recovery time and prognosis, which most athletes want to know. It will also enable the physiotherapist to monitor the effects of treatment, thereby establishing which treatment modalities were most beneficial. Knowledge of the response to selected treatment types, such as mobilization or manipulation, can also be useful in assessing irritability. Furthermore, assessment of the effect of treatment may assist in reaching a differential diagnosis.

Assessment of the athlete's progess should be made at various stages including:

- following the initial examination, prior to treatment
- during and/or immediately after the application of a treatment technique or modality
- at the end of a treatment session
- at the commencement of the next session
- at the completion of treatment.

Maitland (1986) emphasizes the value of the retrospective assessment. This should be performed every four or five sessions to ensure that the impression of progress made session to session is correct, and that the overall rate of progress is satisfactory.

The use of asterix signs to highlight the most important subjective and objective examination findings can help make the reassessment process more efficient and ensure it is directed to the most significant factors. The asterix signs should always be interpreted as a comparison with the previous assessment in order to evaluate progress. The physiotherapist must record accurately and in detail, being careful to identify key symptoms or objective measures for reassessment when the athlete next presents.

The emphasis of reassessment will change as the athlete progresses. Assessment may begin in the clinic, but should progress to include functional testing in the gymnasium and eventually on the sports field. Where an injury has been severe, requiring the athlete to be sidelined for a considerable length of time, more fitness aspects require assessment in order for the athlete to maintain their level of fitness while being sidelined. The physiotherapist should determine what modified training the athlete can perform while protecting the integrity of the injured part (Croce & Gregg 1991).

SUMMARY

It is essential that a sports physiotherapist has the ability to assess thoroughly and accurately. There must be an ongoing process of assessment and reassessment in order to select the most appropriate treatment, monitor its effect, and assist with planning future treatment. This process will also enable the physiotherapist to eliminate or identify serious injuries. Furthermore, it will ensure the physiotherapist recognizes limitations in their management of an athlete.

The ability to perform and interpret an accurate assessment is one of the physiotherapist's most important skills. This skill must be practised and refined over the physiotherapist's career. Care must be taken not to become rigid and predictable in the technique of assessment. Physiotherapists need to maintain a fresh and intuitive attitude that is sensitive to the important cues that arise from a comprehensive assessment.

REFERENCES

Andrews J R 1983 Overuse syndromes of the lower extremity. Clinics in Sports Medicine 2(1):137-148

Australian Physiotherapy Association 1988 Protocol for pre-manipulative testing of the cervical spine. Australian Journal of Physiotherapy 34(2):97-100

Australian Sports Medicine Federation 1989 Lecture and practical notes, level 1, 4th edn. Australian Sports Trainers Scheme, Melbourne

Bogduk N 1984 The rationale for patterns of neck and back pain. Patient Management August:13-21

Booher J M, Thibodean G A 1985 Athletic injury assessment. Time Mirror/Mosby College Publishing, St Louis

Brukner P, Khan K 1993 Clinical sports medicine. McGraw-Hill, Sydney

Budgett R 1990 Overtraining syndrome. British Journal of Sports Medicine 24(4):231-236

Butler D S 1991 Mobilization of the nervous system. Churchill Livingstone, Melbourne

Ciullo J V, Stevens G C 1989 The prevention and treatment of injuries to the shoulder in swimming. Sports Medicine 7:182-204

Cook S D, Brinker M R, Poche M 1990 Running shoes: their relationship to running injuries. Sports Medicine 10(1):1-8

Corrigan B, Maitland G D 1983 Practical orthopaedic medicine. Butterworths, London

Croce P, Gregg R 1991 Keeping fit when injured. Clinics in Sports Medicine 10(1):181-195

Cyriax J 1982 Textbook of orthopaedic medicine, vol. 1. Diagnosis of soft tissue lesions. Baillière Tindall, London

Donatelli R, Walker R 1989 Lower quarter evaluation: structural relationships and interdependence. In: Donatelli R, Wooden M J (eds) Orthopaedic physical therapy. Churchill Livingstone, New York, 277-304

Ekberg O, Perrson N H, Abrahamsson P, Westlin N E, Lilja B 1988 Longstanding groin pain in athletes. A multidisciplinary approach. Sports Medicine 6:56-61

Elliot B C, Foster D H 1984 A biomechanical analysis of the front on and side on bowling techniques. Journal of Human Movement Studies 10:83-94

Elvey R L 1979 Brachial plexus tension tests and the pathoanatomical origin of arm pain. Proceedings, Aspects of manipulative therapy, Lincoln Institute of Health Sciences, Melbourne, 105-110

Fick D S, Albright J P, Murray B P 1992 Relieving painful 'shin splints'. Physician and Sports Medicine 20(12):105-113

Fried T, Lloyd G J 1992 An overview of common soccer injuries management and prevention. Sports Medicine 14(4):269-275

Grant R 1988: Dizziness testing and manipulation of the cervical spine. In: Grant R (ed) Physical therapy of the cervical and thoracic spine. Churchill Livingstone, New York, 111-124

Grieve G P 1988 Common vertebral joint problems, 2nd edn. Churchill Livingstone, Edinburgh

Harding W G 1992 Use and misuse of the tennis elbow strap. Physician and Sports Medicine 20(8):65-74

Henderson J M 1992 Ruling out danger. Differential diagnosis of thoracic pain. Physician and Sports Medicine 20(9):124-132

Janda V 1988 Muscles and cervicogenic pain syndromes. In: Grant R (ed) Physical therapy of the cervical and thoracic spine. Churchill Livingstone, New York, 153-166

Johnson M D, Kibler W B, Smith D 1993 Keys to successful pre-participation exams. Physician and Sports Medicine 21(9):109-123

Jull G 1986 Examination of the lumbar spine. In: Grieve G P (ed) Modern manual therapy of the vertebral column. Churchill Livingstone, Edinburgh, 547-560

Jull G, Janda V 1987 Muscles and motor control in low back pain: assessment and management. In: Twomey L T, Taylor J R (eds) Physical therapy of the low back. Churchill Livingstone, New York, 253-278

Kamkar A, Irrgang J J, Whitney S L 1993 Nonoperative management of secondary shoulder impingement syndrome. Journal of Orthopaedic and Sports Physical Therapy 17(5):212-224

Kulund D N 1982 The injured athlete. Lippincott, Philadelphia

Magarey M E 1986 Examination and assessment in spinal joint dysfunction. In: Grieve G P (ed) Modern manual therapy of the vertebral column. Churchill Livingstone, Edinburgh, 481-497

Magarey M E 1988 Examination of the cervical and thoracic spine. In: Grant R (ed) Physical therapy of the cervical and thoracic spine. Churchill Livingstone, New York, 81-109

Maitland G D 1985a Passive movement techniques for intra-articular and periarticular disorders. Australian Journal of Physiotherapy 31(1):3-8

Maitland G D 1985b The slump test: examination and treatment. Australian Journal of Physiotherapy 31(6):215-219

Maitland G D 1986 Vertebral manipulation, 5th edn. Butterworths, London

Maitland G D 1991 Peripheral manipulation, 3rd edn. Butterworth-Heinemann, London

Maron B R 1988 Orthopaedic aspects of sports medicine. In: Appenzeller O (ed) Sports medicine: fitness training injuries. Urban & Schwarzenberg, Baltimore-Munich, 337-394

McKeag D B 1989 Preparticipation screening of the potential athlete. Clinics in Sports Medicine 8(3):373-397

McKenzie R A 1981 The lumbar spine. Mechanical diagnosis and treatment. Spinal Publications, Waikanae, New Zealand

Niere K R 1991 Understanding referred pain. Sports training, medicine and rehabilitation 2:247-256

Norris C M 1993 Sports injuries. Diagnosis and management for physiotherapists. Butterworth Heinemann, Oxford

Patla C E 1989 Extremity dysfunction: principles of management. In: Payton O D, DiFabio R P, Paris S V, Protas E J, VanSant A F (eds) Manual of physical therapy. Churchill Livingstone, New York, 425-439

Purdam C R, Fricker P A, Cooper B 1992 Principles of treatment and rehabilitation. In: Bloomfield J, Fricker P A, Fitch K D Textbook of science and medicine in sport. Blackwell Scientific, Melbourne, 218-234

Roy S, Irvin R 1983 Sports medicine: prevention evaluation management and rehabiliation. Prentice-Hall, New Jersey

Reid D C 1992 Sports injury assessment and rehabilitation. Churchill Livingstone, New York

Reider B 1991 Sports medicine—the school-age athlete. W B Saunders, Philadelphia

Rzonca E C, Baylis W J 1988 Common sports injuries to the foot and leg. Clinics in Podiatric Medicine and Surgery 5(3):591-602

Saal J A, Dillingham M F, Gamburd R S, Fanton G S 1988 The pseudoradicular syndrome. Lower extremity peripheral nerve entrapment masquerading as lumbar radiculopathy. Spine 13(8):926-930

Sickles R T, Lombardo J A 1993 The adolescent basketball player. Clinics in Sports Medicine 12(2):207-219

Sonzogni J J, Gross M L 1993 Assessment and treatment of basketball injuries. Clinics in Sports Medicine 12(2):221-237

Stanitski C L 1993 Combating overuse injuries. A focus on children and adolescents. Physician and Sports Medicine 21(1):87-106

Torq J S, Conrad W, Kalen V 1976 Clinical diagnosis of anterior cruciate ligament instability in the athlete. American Journal of Sports Medicine 4(2):84-91

Travell J G, Simons D G 1983 Myofascial pain and dysfunction. The trigger point manual. Vol. 1 The upper extremity. Williams & Wilkins, Baltimore

Travell J G, Simons D G 1988: Myofascial pain and dysfunction. The trigger point manual. Vol. 2 The lower extremity. Williams & Wilkins, Baltimore

Wall E J, Cohen M S, Massie J B, Rydevik B, Garfin S R 1990 Cauda equina anatomy 1: intrathecal nerve root organization. Spine 15(12):1244-1247

Watson L 1993 Shoulder joint assessment. Proceedings of the Annual Conference of Australian Physiotherapy Association (Queensland Branch), 15-34

Webb D R 1990 Initial assessment and management of acute winter sports injuries. In: Casey M J, Foster C, Hixson E G Winter sports medicine. F A Davis, Philadelphia, 179-190

Zaricznyj B, Shattuck L J, Mast T A, Robertson R V, D'Elia G 1980 Sports related injuries in school aged children. American Journal of Sports Medicine 8(5):318-324

10. Principles of management

Craig Allingham

It is the aim of this chapter to present an overview of the techniques and strategies of managing sporting injuries and conditions in order to optimise recovery. Other chapters contain excellent material illustrating how these principles can be put into practice.

The discussion will not be limited to the technical aspects of physiotherapy or modalities employed, but will encompass the broader questions of a physiotherapist managing an athlete, with all the human strengths and weaknesses incumbent on both parties. Much of the discussion is based on the author's experience and attitudes toward sports physiotherapy. While these may not always agree with those of the reader, exposure to a different viewpoint may stimulate a more critical evaluation of current theory and practice.

This chapter will be divided into three main sections: pathology, physiology and psychology. While each category will be discussed separately, it must be appreciated that all three will operate simultaneously in the physiotherapy/athlete interaction.

PATHOLOGY

The pathological management of an athletic injury falls into three phases: damage control, facilitation of repair, and reconditioning of the recovered lesion. The principles of management for each phase must be considered in light of the type of injury, the structure(s) involved in the lesion, any previous history of similar or associated injury, and whether the recovery process has involved surgical intervention.

Acute management—damage control

In the acute stage of injury the familiar acronym RICE remains applicable. In recent years there have been additions to this acronym, resulting in its extension to PRICER. The words represented are: protection, rest, ice, compression, elevation, referral. This program is recommended as the appropriate acute management of a soft tissue lesion by most first aid and trainers courses (St John Ambulance, 1989).

Protection

Once an injury has occurred, and been identified as involving soft tissue (contusion, sprain, strain), action must be taken to avoid worsening the lesion. Generally this means restricting the athlete's activities to prevent extension of the lesion and placing the injured part in a comfortable and safe position. This may necessitate the use of a sling, crutches or protective padding, strapping or bracing.

Rest

In order to minimise the degree of tissue damage, associated bleeding and pain, the athlete should be instructed to rest the injured part. In the early stage of injury, the athlete may need to rest generally to ensure a lowering of blood pressure and the consequent leaking from damaged blood vessels in the injured tissues (especially if the athlete has just been active in the sport). This also allows time for thorough examination and reassurance of the injured athlete.

Ice

The role of ice is now well accepted in the management of acute soft tissue injury. Its capacity as a pain reliever, reducer of bleeding and swelling, and minimiser of secondary hypoxic injury are recognized in most first aid texts and sports training manuals (Arnheim 1985). The timing of ice application tends to be a matter for personal choice of the therapist, but the recommended maximum duration for continuous ice treatment to an acute soft tissue injury is 20 mins (Arnheim 1985). This maximum is to reduce the intensity of any compensatory reaction by the body to the cooling, in other words to diminish the vasodilatation of the cooled blood vessels as they react to prolonged cooling. Once the ice is removed the injured part is allowed to warm in the ambient conditions. The ice is then replaced for a further 20 mins, after a 20 minute break.

A further reason for limiting the duration of continuous ice application is to reduce the chance of freezing the superficial body fluid and causing an 'ice burn' (frostbite) injury. Particular care in this regard must be taken with commercial ice packs. These should be applied through a moist cloth against the skin to avoid excessive cooling.

Superficial injuries (e.g. collateral ligament sprains of the ankle or knee) are more effectively cooled than those deep to other tissues (e.g. supraspinatus strain or a deep haematoma in the thigh). For such deeper injuries it is imperative that the other techniques of acute soft tissue injury management are not forsaken because ice has been applied.

Compression

The application of an effective compression bandage to an acute soft tissue injury can produce significant results in the control of swelling and minimization of the congestive phase of the inflammatory response to injury. Compression assists in a faster re-establishment of normal circulation and lymphatic drainage in the injured area.

An effective compression bandage is one with elastic threads woven along the length of the fabric. This ensures an even application of pressure without the need to apply the bandage at full tension (as is necessary with a crepe or gauze bandage). The compression can be localized by placing firm padding over the injury site, or the area where swelling may pool, during the application of the bandage. In the ankle, for example, a horseshoe-shaped pad beneath and around the lateral malleolus will give greater pressure over the fossa (Fig. 10.1). Impact injuries to the shin (from ball or boot impact) respond very well to rapid application of a pad and firm compression bandage, which can reduce the periosteal haematoma dramatically.

Once a compression bandage is applied, the athlete should be monitored to ensure adequate circulation is maintained distally to the bandage. If the athlete is leaving

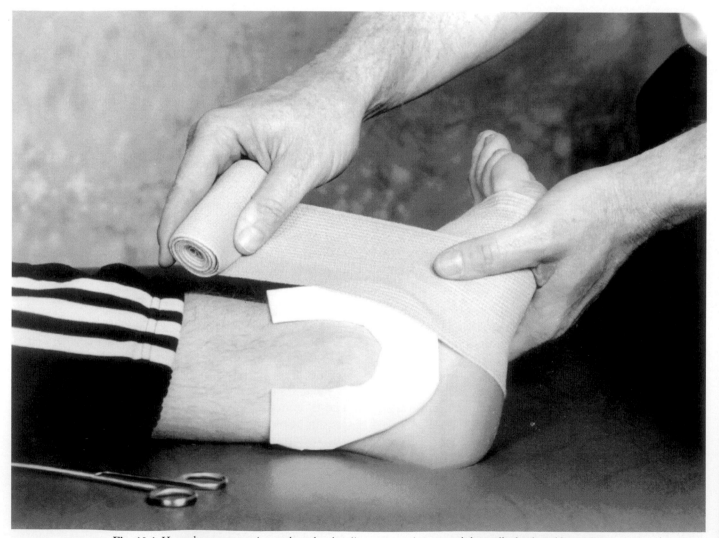

Fig. 10.1 Horseshoe compression pad used to localize compression around the malleolus in ankle sprains

your care, instructions should be given to loosen and reapply the bandage should there be any distal swelling, parasthesia, cyanosis or coldness. Unlike ice, a compression bandage can be used over open wounds (once the wound is suitably dressed) and it can remain on the injury site throughout the acute inflammatory stage. Compression is one of the most valuable modalities of soft tissue injury management.

Elevation

The points of elevating the injured part are to reduce the local intravascular pressure and thus the bleeding from damaged vessels, and to facilitate draining of any accumulating interstitial fluid toward the central circulation. Depending on the site and nature of injury, and the cooperation of the athlete, the value of this technique is variable. In the case of lower limb injury, elevation at least ensures protection and rest for the site. Injuries to the shoulder girdle are unaffected by attempts to elevate them due to their proximity to the heart; more distal upper limb injuries (forearm and hand) can be elevated, relative to the elbow, by a sling.

Head and facial injuries are managed with little regard to elevation due to the necessity of maintaining blood flow to the brain and other organs. Intravascular pressure is regulated closely, and any drop is often accompanied by fainting which undermines any attempt to elevate the part. More important is preventing an increase in blood pressure, by ensuring the athlete is resting.

Referral

The placement of this factor at the end of the mnemonic PRICER reminds all practitioners (trainers, doctors, etc) to be aware of their limitations in managing of acute sports injuries. Referral to a hospital accident and emergency centre, to the athlete's own doctor, to a sports physiotherapist or to a sports physician or specialist should be considered when further investigation, intervention or supervision is required, e.g. when immediate radiological evaluation is necessary, or a player with a head injury needs qualified observation for several hours.

There are several activities which will undermine the effectiveness of the RICE regime, and the athlete should be warned accordingly. They are the application of heat (lamps, rubs, baths or packs); the ingestion of alcohol (a potent vasodilator and suppressor of common sense); vigorous body activity, e.g. running which might cause a rise in blood pressure and increase blood flow to the part; massage to the injured part, which could cause mechanical damage or an increase in blood flow. These four factors were combined into an acronym: the mnemonic becoming—HARM, for heat, alcohol, running, massage.

So remember, RICE is nice, but don't HARM an injury.

Ongoing management—promotion of healing

Following the acute management stage of damage control, attention swings toward facilitating the soft tissue repair processes. This stage constitutes the matrix and cellular proliferation phase of healing and lasts for between 72 hours and 6 weeks (Oakes 1992).

This phase involves continual removal of debris from the injury site by the phagocytic cells (macrophages and monocytes) and the proliferation of fibroblasts. These latter cells are responsible for the synthesis of the collagen/proteoglycan matrix which comprises the healing of the lesion. The migration of these cells to the area may be hampered by the congestion at and around the injury site, and by the reduced blood flow due to vascular damage.

Physiotherapy at this stage is aimed at reducing the congestion (swelling), facilitating oxygenation and nutrition of the injury site and restoring normal movement patterns, while minimizing further deterioration (muscle atrophy, proprioceptive loss) and avoiding re-inflaming the lesion. The early stage of collagen deposition is particularly fragile, in that any decrease in pH of the environment will break down the collagen matrix. The inflammatory reaction is acidic and the enzymes activated are proteolytic, thus dissolving the immature collagen fibrils (Curwin & Stanish 1985). The matrix/proliferative phase of healing must then be re-established.

Physiotherapeutic measures which may be of use in the early stages of this healing phase include massage (gentle stroking and kneading to mobilize the congestion and aid lymphatic drainage), low dose ultrasound (to facilitate transfer of ions or fluids across cell membranes), electrical current (for cell membrane permeability and pain relief), electrical muscle stimulation (to aid drainage by changing pressure in the area and stimulating vascular supply), exercise (for increased blood and lymph flow, and reduction of adhesions and atrophy), and instruction to the patient regarding limitation of activity (to prevent re-inflammation and interruption of the repair process).

Later in the proliferative repair phase, when the collagen cross-linking is more durable and mature, the intensity of exercise, massage and stretching can be safely increased. This provides a more potent stimulus for tissue remodelling and for general body fitness maintenance.

The above suggestions for treatment can be grouped under four headings which make up the basis of most musculoskeletal physiotherapy applications. These are manual therapy (massage, joint mobilization and manipulation, neural mobilization and stretching), exercise therapy, electrotherapy (ultrasound, electrical currents, heat, cryotherapy) and education. More detailed discussions on these and other electrotherapy modalities, manual therapy and exercise therapy can be found elsewhere in this book.

Rehabilitative management— remodelling and conditioning

Once the deposition and primary organization of collagen fibrils has been completed, there remain the tasks of remodelling the repair site to maximize loading tolerance and of conditioning the area around the joint as well as the rest of the body prior to returning the competitive athletic situation. The collagen maturation involves the work of the myofibroblast cells which refine the collagen fibril framework and reorient the fibrils in the direction of loading. This axial loading alignment begins during a well-managed second stage, and continues for some months. In the earlier stage, the fibroblasts lay down type III collagen (small diameter fibrils) which may be converted to type I (large diameter) during this stage of healing (Oakes 1992).

Rehabilitation at this stage becomes more exercise oriented, aimed at progressively loading the new tissue to adapt to the training stimulus. Like any physical training program, rehabilitation exercises rely on the three principles of training theory: the application of stress (imposed demand), specific adaptations for specific stimuli (stresses), and progressive overloading of the stimulus to accommodate the adaptations.

Tendon lesions

Tendon injuries can occur as a result of overuse, in which microtraumatic tears of the tendon establish a chronic inflammatory environment, or as a traumatic event, in which the tendon partially or totally ruptures on one specific effort. The latter case is often preceded by some tendon deterioration over time.

The relatively inelastic nature of tendon structure allows only a 4% elongation before some degree of intermolecular cross-linkage breakdown occurs (Curwin & Stanish 1985, Oakes 1992). Continued application of tensile force then further disrupts the intra- and intermolecular cross-links, leading to gross structural failure of the tendon which may completely rupture.

Healing of tendon lesions progresses according to the general description outlined above, but it should be noted that the quality of the collagen repair is poor compared with the original tendon. That is, the large diameter collagen fibres (type I) of the normal tendon are replaced with small diameter fibres (type III) (Oakes 1992). Physiotherapy techniques useful in the management of tendinitis are discussed below.

Exercise therapy. The role of exercise in managing tendinitis is manifold. First there is the vascular effect whereby exercising the attached muscle produces a demand-induced increase in blood flow, thereby assisting nutrition. Second, the tensile changes in an exercising tendon stimulate a pumping effect whereby blood from the

longitudinal vessels is decreased under tension and forced into the radial vessels, and on relaxation of the muscle the reverse occurs. This occurs even during isometric contractions, and may counter the stasis that develops with the chronic inflammatory process. Third, the application of tensile force provides a stimulus for the newly laid collagen fibres to orient themselves along the longitudinal (loadbearing) axis of the tendon (Oakes 1992). Fourth, exercise can be used to maintain the strength, power, endurance and co-ordination of the muscle as its tendon recovers.

The application of eccentric exercise has been investigated by Curwin and Stanish (1985) and reported by them to be valuable in the management of a tendinitis resulting from a tensile overload. This applies for both overuse and traumatic lesions.

The other type of tendon lesion is from a shearing or compressive load, as with iliotibial band friction syndrome or supraspinatus impingement syndrome. The adaptation sought through exercise of an injured tendon is to improve the intra- and intermolecular cross-linking of the collagen fibres to improve tensile loading capacity. Such cross-link facilitation can occur only through the application of tensile force (specific load for specific adaptation). Eccentric exercise is a vehicle whereby greater tensile stimulus can be applied to a musculotendinous unit by manipulating the speed of the movement, for a given workload: the speed of movement produces different tensile forces depending on whether the movement is performed concentrically or eccentrically (Fig. 10.2).

From their work Curwin and Stanish (1985) developed an eccentric exercise program for the rehabilitation of tendon lesions. It incorporates several important components: the initial stretch of the affected musculotendinous unit, the performance of up to 30 repetitions of a specific eccentric exercise for that tendon, a repeat of the initial stretch, and ice treatment for the tendon upon completion (Table 10.1).

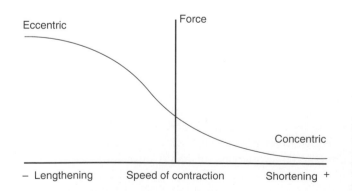

Fig. 10.2 Speed and force of contraction relationship for eccentric and concentric muscle contractions

Table 10.1 Eccentric rehabilitation program for tendon

Stretch	A	Static stretch of injured tendon
	B	Hold for 15-30 seconds
	C	Repeat 3-5 times
Eccentric	A	Three sets of 10 repetitions
	B	Progression:
		days 1-2 slow movement
		3-5 moderate
		6-7 fast movement
	C	Increase external resistance after day 7 and repeat cycle
Stretch		As for prior to exercise
Ice		Crushed ice or ice massage to painful area for 5-10 minutes

Appropriate dose is measured by athlete's pain: there should be some discomfort (slight pain) in the final set of 10. If not, increase the speed. If still no discomfort at fast speed, increase the external resistance and return to slow movement. Source: Curwin & Stanish (1986)

The aim of the exercise is to produce stress along the tendon to stimulate cross-link formation. The only gauge of stress is pain in the tendon, thus the exercise is aimed at producing mild pain to confirm a training stimulus has been applied. The risk is that the stimulus may exacerbate the inflammatory response, the proteolytic effect of which will be counterproductive. So ice is applied at the end of the session to suppress any inflammatory reaction. For this reason, the program must be carefully explained to the athlete in order to avoid overzealousness.

Stretching is another form of exercise that deserves separate mention in relation to tendinitis. Applying tension along the musculotendinous unit and taking that unit to its maximal length is a way of providing the axial stimulation for collagen alignment. An added benefit is that stretching the muscle might decrease the sensitivity of the gamma efferent control of the muscle spindle or the alpha efferent of the golgi tendon organ (Howell et al 1986). Reduction of this hypertonicity reduces the resting tension along the tendon, enabling the unit to perform normally in activities as required. Excessive resting tension of the tendon may reduce the already indifferent blood flow evident in many of the common sites of tendinitis. Stretching can be done passively, actively (muscle energy techniques, Goodridge 1981) or manually by soft tissue manipulation (massage).

Massage. Massage for tendinitis is often useful to stimulate circulation, overcome congestion within a tendon or its synovial sheath, reduce or prevent adhesions within or around the tendon, or manually stretch the musculotendinous unit. Transverse or cross-fibre frictions, when correctly applied and followed by appropriate anti-inflammatory and anti-spasmodic therapy (e.g. ice, stretching, drug therapy, etc), can be most effective in managing chronic tendon problems. Gentle stroking or kneading of the muscle associated with an inflamed tendon can help normalize the resting tone, which may be hypertonic due to muscle guarding or spasm (Howell et al 1986).

Ligament lesions

The structure of ligament tissue is similar to that of tendon, with mainly Type I collagen, a small amount of Type III collagen, and some proteoglycan and elastic fibres in an aqueous gel (Oakes 1992). The progression to failure is likewise similar due to their common crimped collagen structure at the intercellular level. However, the role of the structures is different, with tendons transmitting force to create movement and ligaments stabilizing joints or tendons to prevent undesirable movement.

One decision of ligament repair is whether to mobilize the tissue and, if so, when. Oakes (1992) indicates that ultrastructural repair of ligament tissue occurs best with a period of immobilization followed by early mobilization of the affected joint. A period of 3 weeks immobilization after ligament rupture, followed by controlled progressive mobilization using bracing, is recommended. Presumably, a grade II ligament injury would require less initial restriction, but the principle would remain the same. Advocacy for the role of early mobilization is discussed elsewhere (see Ch. 12).

Muscle lesions

The most dynamic of the soft tissues, muscle, is often subject to impact or tensile injury resulting in a contusion or strain. Occasionally it is injured through vascular compromise (compartmental syndrome or tourniquet trauma), but this is less common.

For *contusions* from blunt trauma, the two components of repair are regeneration of the damaged muscle fibres, and of the intramuscular connective tissue (collagen). This is accompanied by resorption of damaged tissues. Early mobilization of such an injury increases the intensity of the inflammatory reaction which then subsides with extensive scar formation and faster recovery of tensile muscle strength, compared with immobilization of the muscle after injury (Oakes 1992). The greater scar formation (collagen component) results in an undesired stiffness of the muscle, so a mix of immobilizing/mobilizing seems indicated. Oakes (1992) suggests that a significant contusion should be immobilized in the early stage for up to 5 days (depending on severity), and then mobilized (stretched) to assist orientation of the regenerating muscle fibres and the connective tissue along the tensile axis of the muscle. It may also be an advantage to immobilize the muscle in a stretched position to reduce shortening of the connective tissue during repair, thus minimizing stiffness of the healed muscle. However, such a position is not always practical (e.g. for a rectus femoris).

While this might be theoretically the appropriate treatment, there are significant problems in gaining the patient's compliance, and it may not be in the overall best interest of the athlete. For example, immobilization of the muscle in a splint will reduce activity and decrease blood flow, lymphatic return and oxygenation of the resting tissues. Loss of strength, shortening of the antagonist muscle group, slower removal of the cellular debris and an inability to exercise other areas of the body could undermine the apparent benefits of an immobilization program.

A possibility is a semi-active management program for such contusions where, following the initial RICE regime, gradual return to activity is undertaken, guided by pain and an understanding of muscle repair. Forceful stretching through pain is avoided: proprioceptive neuromuscular facilitation techniques are preferred to aid return to full range (Knott & Voss 1968). Electrotherapy modalities and massage are used as indicated.

If, during the course of management of an intramuscular contusion/haematoma, there is a gradual loss of range and a significant hardening of the mass in the muscle, the therapist must alter the aims of treatment. This course of events usually suggests that an inflammatory, fibrotic reaction has occurred in the muscle, which typically becomes irritable. Maintenance stretching only (no attempt to gain movement), medication, ice treatment intermittently through the day, and rest of the affected muscle will assist resolution of this phase of 'unrecovery'. When the range of motion begins to return and pain at the end of range is easing, the active recovery plan can be resumed.

If the muscle injury is a *strain* due to excessive force within the unit, the damage is a tensile failure, often at the transition sites of muscle-bone or muscle-tendon. Tears of the muscle tissue also respond well to initial immobilization combined with stretching to avoid connective tissue shortening and subsequent passive stiffness. Oakes (1992) indicates that only 30 mins per day of passive stretching is necessary to prevent an increase of interstitial collagen in immobilized muscle. He also noted that as little as one maximal muscle stimulation for 10-15 seconds per day was necessary to minimise strength loss and flexibility loss (stiffness). Thus, early isometric or electrical contractions of strained muscles is of clinical value, as is regular (but not frequent) stretching. Purdam et al (1992) note good results treating acute muscle strains using mechanical continuous passive motion combined with ice therapy. Their notes indicate the combination of rest, passive movement through range and anti-inflammatory icing reduces collagen stiffness without compromising muscle fibre regeneration.

PHYSIOLOGY

In addition to managing the physical conditions related to the injury, the sports physiotherapist should take the opportunity to manage the general physiological state of the athlete while he or she is under care. Parameters to be considered include cardiovascular endurance (VO_2 max), anaerobic threshold, muscular strength and power, flexibility, and anthropometric components (body weight, body fat percentage).

Maintenance of fitness

Maintenance of physiological parameters (or fitness) will ensure that the athlete returns to training and competition in the best physical condition, thereby maximizing performance and minimizing risk of further injury. To accomplish this, the sports physiotherapist needs knowledge of training theory and practice, and some experience in applying these principles, either in rehabilitation or in coaching athletes. General information can be found in many texts on exercise physiology (e.g. Astrand & Rohdahl 1986, McArdle et al 1991), and more specific information on sport and fitness is available through coaching and sports science journals and texts (e.g. Rushall & Pyke, 1990). An overview of how to apply these principles is given, to stimulate interest and illustrate utilization.

Baseline parameters

Working with a team or group of athletes on a regular basis presents the opportunity to test the squad during the basic preparatory phase of training (preseason). The testing can comprise physiological measurements or functional assessments relevant to the sport, or a combination of the two. The results for each participant provides a baseline against which to compare tests later in the season. This is particularly useful should the athlete be recovering from injury, in which case the tests can help the decision on when the athlete is fit to return to competition.

For example, working with a basketball team, you might conduct a preseason test that includes anthropometric data (height, weight, body fat percentage), physiological data (predicted maximal oxygen uptake test) and functional tests like distance covered with 10 hops (test each leg), time taken to complete a preset agility run within the stadium, and the number of rapid vertical jump repetitions to the point where fatigue restricts performance to 75% of the difference between standing reach and maximal vertical jump height.

At some stage of the season a player might get injured. (Count yourself lucky if it is only one!) Following treatment of the ankle sprain/groin strain/knee medial ligament repair the player may appear clinically ready to be considered for selection. A repeat of the functional tests will allow a measure of the athlete's ability compared with prior testing. This information may help assess function, and might also be used to direct the later stages of rehabilitation and training. Monitoring body weight and body fat percentage can prevent the incapacitated athlete from undesirable weight gains during the injury layoff. The test for oxygen uptake will give some indication of the player's resistance to fatigue, which is of interest to the coach and to the therapist for performance and safety reasons respectively.

The appropriate tests will vary between sports, and should be developed in conjunction with the coaching staff.

Remember that the functional tests should be suitable to attempt during injury recovery.

Even if a physiotherapist is not working with athletes regularly, when one presents as a patient it provides the opportunity to perform some of these tests. For example, in the case of receiving an athlete who has just had a surgical repair of shoulder, knee or ankle, the first consultation could include a measure of body fat, weight, contralateral strength values across the same joint and a paced cycle (or one leg cycle) heart rate recovery test (Rushall & Pyke 1990). These would provide some baselines to monitor changes throughout the rehabilitation program, and targets to achieve should the athlete 'let himself go' (Fig. 10.3).

Strength training

Many physiotherapy rehabilitation programs utilize strength training for muscle function. It may be useful to note a few principles of strength training to maximize the benefits from the time and effort spent by both the therapist and athlete in the gym. This subject (like conditioning) is extensive, so only a brief overview will be offered. Remember also that these principles can only be applied within the limits of existing pathology.

Critical to the concept of strength gains is the repetition maximum, meaning completing the volume of exercise with maximum effort (see Ch. 13). This parameter is preceded by a number, reading 1RM, 5RM, 10RM, and so on. The interpretation is the number of movements (lifts/squats/leg curls etc.) that are the maximum possible due to fatigue. Thus a 1RM is an athletes maximal strength for one movement, 10RM is 10 repetitions producing fatigue and inability to do an 11th repetition. Obviously the resistance for 10RM will be significantly less than for 1RM, but the end result, fatigue, is common. There are several rules of weight training that involve application of the RM principle (Rushall & Pyke 1990):

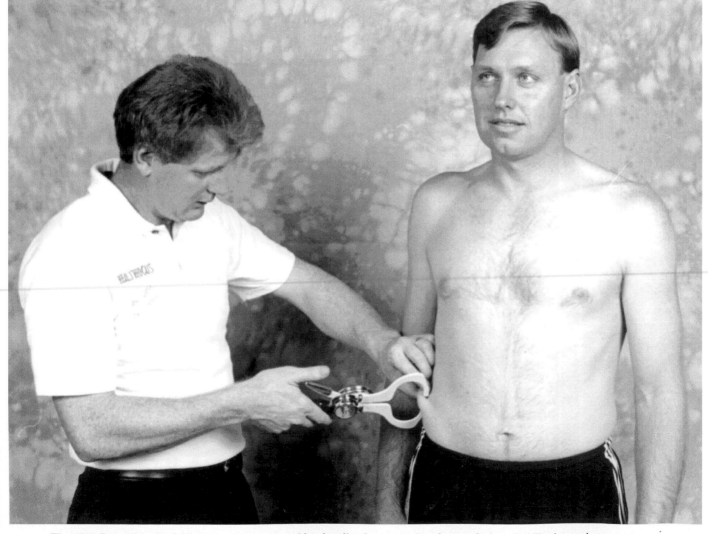

Fig. 10.3 Recording skin fold measurements to provide a baseline for monitoring changes during rehabilitation and return to sport

1 six or fewer RM seems most effective for increasing strength and power;
2 moderate loads of 4-6RM produce larger strength gains than 2RM programs;
3 as the number of RMs progresses beyond six, the strength gains decrease and muscle endurance gains increase;
4 beyond 20RM the strength gains are negligible, but muscle endurance continues to increase.

The above guidelines apply for isotonic strength programs. Physiotherapists often utilize isometric strength training exercises, particularly in relation to stabilization programs with abdominals, vastus medialis, hamstrings, scapular muscles and cervical postural muscles. Some guidelines for these are also summarized by Rushall and Pyke (1990):

1 the level of exertion should exceed 70% of the athlete's maximum;
2 overload increases are made by increasing the number of contractions not their intensity;
3 each contraction should last 6-12 seconds with a total of 90 seconds of muscle work per session;
4 rest intervals should incorporate recovery work, stretching or light aerobic work.
5 to make gains through range, the isometric contraction should be performed at various points through that range (Sale 1986).

Poliquin (1990) makes several points regarding the speed at which strength exercises should be performed in order to maximize gains. Among the points he cites are the following:

1 muscles gain faster in strength if trained at various speeds (periodisation of the stimulus);
2 faster speeds make greater training demands on the neurological component of strength (recruitment of motor units);
3 high-speed strength training should not be attempted until a solid basis of slow-speed strength gains have been made.

While on the subject of neurological aspects of strength training, it is interesting to note that cross-training benefits have been noted, that is, exercising unilaterally produces a gain on the contralateral limb (Sale 1986). This can be particularly useful during the early stages of rehabilitation to minimize disuse atrophy of the affected limb by maximally exercising the opposite limb.

There is much science to strength and power training and the reader is referred to the journals of strength and conditioning associations in Australia and overseas for more detailed information.

Energy systems

When working with an athlete in a program of fitness maintenance or recovery the therapist must not only consider the mechanical and neurological aspects of the sport, but also the energy required to produce that output. Is the sport predominantly aerobic or anaerobic? Are there components of the sport that require specific energy contributions, for example stored ATP for immediate output? Analysis of the energy delivery requirements of the sport and/or occupation of the athlete can help the therapist develop programs that will maintain or retrain those systems.

Full discussion of the immediate (stored phosphate), short-term (glycolytic) and long-term (aerobic) energy pathways is beyond the scope of this chapter (see Ch. 1), however some broad comments based on the author's experience will be made. Further reading is recommended (McArdle et al 1991, Astrand & Rohdahl 1986).

Rehabilitation exercises should be designed with a particular energy pathway in mind. For example, using the stationary bicycle can be done in several ways:

1 slow steady pace for longer periods;
2 intervals of fast pace interspersed with rest periods;
3 intervals of fast pace interspersed with slower paced intervals.

Each of these combinations taxes the energy pathways slightly differently and should be prescribed according to the demands for which the athlete is being prepared. Thus a road cyclist might seem to need the first option (for long races), and a baseball player the second option (as the game comprises bursts of running with frequent recovery times).

On closer examination, however, the road cyclist will be required to vary race speed in order break from a group, chase a leader or tackle varying terrain. Therefore, option three is more suited to the cyclist's needs.

In general, a sound aerobic energy base will assist athletes in several ways:

1 by enabling a longer period of submaximal performance (long, slow distance type exercise);
2 by providing a greater buffer zone in which the oxygen debt incurred during any anaerobic (ATP-CP or glycolytic) burst of energy production can be repaid while maintaining activity at a lower (aerobic) rate;
3 by improving the rate of repayment of oxygen debt during resting recovery.

Accordingly, the baseball player, although involved in a predominantly anaerobic sport, will benefit from faster recovery (oxygen debt repayment) between bursts of activity if he or she has a good aerobic training base as indicated by VO_2 max.

This concept of energy pathway training does not apply only to cycling, running, walking or swimming. It can also be integrated into weight training and circuits of training combining weights, flexibility and endurance activities. The following considerations illustrate this concept.

Heavy resistance training is anaerobic (due to the low repetition rate); light resistance can be used to increase the length and rate of workouts thereby raising the heart rate and placing aerobic demands on the energy pathways; flexibility drills can be used as 'rest' periods in the circuit during which the oxygen debt is repaid prior to another interval of glycolytic or aerobic activity.

The ingenuity of the therapist, combined with advice from the athlete or coach, can produce rehabilitation routines that incorporate training for energy pathways into the activities necessary for musculoskeletal retraining.

Periodization

When undertaking a physiological training program in tandem with the rehabilitation plan, the stage of the training program the athlete is in must be determined, i.e. whether it is a preparatory phase, a pre-competitive phase or a transition phase following peaking (Rushall & Pyke 1990). The balance of volume and intensity of conditioning work varies accordingly (Table 10.2).

Maintenance of skills

During the rehabilitation period, every attempt should be made to maintain the athlete's skills as well as fitness. The therapist should work with the athlete and possibly the coach to ensure that as much as possible is being done within the limits of the pathology.

Motor aspects

Using the principles of motor learning, the athlete can keep in touch with component parts of his or her skill during

rehabilitation. This can be as simple as providing the athlete with the tools of the sport during rehabilitation exercise, for example tossing a netball while doing wobbleboard exercises for an ankle or knee injury, using a golf club for a range of motion exercises to a shoulder, or swinging a tennis racquet to develop endurance of the rotator cuff muscles. As the athlete progresses toward recovery, elements of the sporting activity itself can be integrated into the program, such as jumping for volleyballers, falling for judo players, power kicking for soccer players, or stance phase retraining for kickboxers. Only some discussion with the athlete and imagination from the therapist is required to develop appropriate activities for different sports.

Mental practice

In addition to the physical skill components, there is the opportunity to employ mental practice during injury layoff. The validity of mental practice in the absence of physical practice was reviewed by Richardson (1967) over 25 years ago, so the notion is obviously not a new one.

The idea is to mentally perform the skills, patterns, tactics and strategies of the sport by visualizing their execution. To be maximally effective the mental execution must be perfect, and the athlete should try to simulate all aspects of the skill. For example, the athlete should perceive the stadium/ground, 'hear' the crowd, 'see' opponents and teammates, 'feel' the ball/stick/bat, and so on. The more realistic and perfect the mental practice, the better the retention of optimal skill levels. This requires only 10-15 mins per day of application, but involves strong concentration with minimal distractions. The athlete's coach might be able to help with suggestions of skills or strategies that require extra work in this way.

Fatigue

Fatigue is a very useful tool of rehabilitation. General or local fatigue usually produces a deterioration in the quality and/or quantity of physical activity. Knowing that it becomes more difficult to perform an activity efficiently when fatigued, the therapist can introduce fatigue to stress the athlete and then train the athlete under adverse conditions. For example, in the case of a patellofemoral joint problem which has responded well to a vastus medialis obliquus (VMO) program and is in the later stage of rehabilitation, the athlete can be generally fatigued (e.g. a run, or cycle) or the leg locally fatigued (step-up drill or leg press) and then tested on a biofeedback or manual test for VMO control. Or a netballer with proprioceptive loss following an ankle sprain can be fatigued then given wobbleboard or other balance activities under fatigue conditions. The use of fatigue as an assessment or rehabilitative tool is valuable and applicable for the safe return of the athlete to competitive performance levels.

Table 10.2 Stages of training through the competitive year (from Rushall & Pyke, 1990)

Training phase	Characteristics
Basic preparatory	Pre-season stage High volume Low intensity Non-specific
Specific preparatory	Early season stage Volume decreases Intensity increases Activities become more sport-specific
Pre-competitive	Volume decreases further Intensity becomes very high Sport-specificity paramount May taper before competitive stage events
Competitive	'Peaking' stage Low volume High intensity Totally specific to performance
Transition	Off-season stage Sufficient volume and intensity to prevent 'detraining' Non-specific, may involve other sports or cross-training

PSYCHOLOGY

The material in this chapter has so far concentrated on the physical aspects of recovery and of managing an injured athlete. However, it is also important to consider the mental aspects, for two reasons. First, an understanding of the psychological responses to injury and rehabilitation can be used to maximize the efficacy of physical treatments. Secondly, it helps in recognizing any psychological difficulty the athlete might have in coping with the injury or its implications. In the second case there may be need for referral to a trained psychologist for counselling and support.

Reaction to injury

The reaction of an athlete to injury is similar to the grief response described by Kubler-Ross (1969). This response is characterized by stages of denial, anger, bargaining and acceptance. Injured athletes will display these reaction stages and move through them in different ways. Some may accept the injury and strive to recovery with only a brief anger stage. Others may become preoccupied with anger and resentment, blaming coaches or officials for the injury and have difficulty settling down to purposeful rehabilitation. Still others continue to deny the injury, and keep training and competing despite obvious deterioration, a situation common with overuse injuries.

The efficiency with which an injured athlete moves through these stages is determined by many factors, the interplay of which is difficult to ascertain for any individual case (Grove & Gordon 1992). These include the stress history of the athlete, personality traits and states, coping skills and support available to assist the athlete. The circumstances surrounding the actual injury might also affect the psychological reaction, for example if the injury resulted from a 'professional foul', or was caused by a teammate in training.

An important role for the treating therapist is to try to determine which stage of the grief process the athlete is in, and monitor the progress through the process. If it appears that the athlete is not progressing, some counselling may be required. This may be some active listening by the therapist, or it may involve referral to a psychologist. One strategy found useful in the author's experience is to set appointment times for non-physiotherapy work. On these occasions the therapist sits down with the athlete and listens to the problems and challenges (perceived and real) from the athlete's perspective. Discussion on how to turn these into positive drives for the rehabilitation program, and setting some short- or medium-term goals, follows. The athlete leaves the session with the impression that the therapist cares about his or her ambitions, frustrations and practical difficulties, and a positive feeling regarding the next stage of management. Sometimes such a session does

not achieve this, and the athlete is recommended to seek counselling.

Reaction to rehabilitation

Perhaps one aspect of the psychological side of recovery underestimated by therapists is the anxiety and discomfort many athletes feel when attending for treatment. The highly motivated athlete has been frustrated by an injury that may prevent achievement of performance goals, and must allow a health professional to take control of the next stage toward this goal. This health professional, who may not be well known to nor trusted by the athlete, is encountered in an unfamiliar environment in which the athlete is no longer in control of the activities or outcomes. Not surprisingly, the athlete may be anxious or apprehensive when coming for treatment. This attitude is carried by many athletes when they approach the sports medicine clinic. Obviously this mind-set will be counterproductive to rehabilitation, and must be turned around as quickly as possible. A few minutes in the first consultation for a guided tour of the treatment/gym/pool/waiting areas can help considerably. Clear identification of personnel (reception, aides, other therapists, doctors etc.) will also reduce uncertainty in the environment.

As well as the anxiety created by the perceived threat of an unfamiliar environment, the athlete can feel threatened by other psychological factors. These include fear of pain and disability, worries about self-concept and future plans, and problems with emotional stability and customary social roles and activities (Danish 1986). Identification of the source of the athlete's anxiety is the first step toward resolving it through supply of information, counselling and positive actions to alleviate the problem.

Motivation

A common assumption is to expect a highly motivated athlete to carry his or her performance and training motivation into a clinical rehabilitation setting. This is not always the case, as the new environment may be too far removed from the athlete's motivating goals (medals, financial rewards, applause, media coverage etc.) to provide similar stimulus in rehabilitation. In such situations the therapist can use short- and medium-term goal-setting to show the path through rehabilitation back to the ultimate goal. These intermediate goals are used as a motivating source in themselves, and any competitive athlete enjoys a challenge.

Goal-setting

When the therapist is setting goals, it should be done with the injured athlete rather than for the injured athlete. If the athlete is involved in the discussion and setting of goals it increases the responsibility on that athlete to attain them. It can be easy to ascribe to non-achievement of goals set by someone else, to unrealistic expectations.

As the goals are being set, the intervals at which progress relative to these goals will be reviewed should also be set. This ensures that both the athlete and the therapist are aware of the deadlines and the likely rate of progress. Negotiations with the athlete at the outset should emphasize that the program is flexible not rigid, and may need to be reviewed in the light of unexpected eventualities.

Communication

At all stages of the therapist/athlete relationship communication is critical to maximizing the benefits for the athlete and the professional satisfaction of the therapist. The accuracy, reliability, comprehension and spirit of communication can make the difference between merely treating an injury and comprehensively managing an athlete. One of the most important aspects is to explain the injury and the treatment in terminology understood by the athlete, rather than in technical terms. In the longer term, the athlete will be impressed by treatment outcome, not by vocabulary. The athlete must show comprehension of the diagnosis, management plan, home exercises, gym routine and so on by repeating the information back to the therapist. This process may need to be conducted intermittently as therapists tend to subject the athletes to information overload, and matters can become confused.

Consistency of information given and honesty when answering questions from the athlete will do much to enhance the working relationship. If the physiotherapist does not know an answer, the athlete should be told so. If an answer can be found elsewhere, the physiotherapist should find it or direct the athlete to do so. Reliable information relating to pain, disability, likely rate of progress and possible setbacks can help the athlete in coping with the elations and disappointments common to all rehabilitation courses.

At all stages the therapist should try to perceive the situation from the athlete's viewpoint, understand threats and stressors and communicate this understanding back to the athlete in a non-judgmental, open-ended way. By summarizing and reflecting the therapist is indicating understanding and encouraging a response (Danish 1986). If it becomes necessary to be firm with the athlete, the new tone can be delivered along established lines of communication and rapport.

Compliance

One of the primary aims of goal-setting, communication and support is to increase the compliance of the athlete with the rehabilitation program. Compliance becomes strongest when athletes internalize the behaviour and are motivated toward success because they believe it is in their best interest (Danish 1986). The suggestions made in this section can help achieve this, and see also Ch. 19.

SUMMARY

The overall management of an injured athlete should encompass all aspects affecting health, fitness and performance. This chapter has presented one view, but other strategies may be equally effective. Regular reviews by a therapist of athlete management can often break the cycle of habit that arises in any busy clinic.

REFERENCES

Arnheim D 1985 Modern principles of athletic training, 6th edn. Times Mirror/Mosby, St Louis

Astrand P, Rohdahl K 1986 Textbook of work physiology. McGraw-Hill, New York

Curwin S, Stanish D 1985 Tendinitis: aetiology and management. Collamore, Baltimore

Danish S 1986 Psychological aspects in the care and treatment of athletic injuries. In: Vinger P, Hoerner E (eds) Sports injuries—the unthwarted epidemic 2nd edn. PSG Publishing, Massachusetts

Goodridge J 1981 Muscle energy technique: definition, explanation, methods of procedure. Journal of the American Osteopathic Association 18(4):249-54

Grove J, Gordon A 1992 Psychological aspects of injury in sport. In: Bloomfield J, Fricker P, Fitch K (eds) Textbook of medicine and science in sport. Blackwell Scientific, Melbourne

Howell J, Binder M, Nichols T R, Loeb G 1986 Muscle spindles, golgi tendon organs and the neural control of skeletal muscle. Journal of the American Osteopathic Association 86(9):599-602

Knott M, Voss D 1968 Proprioceptive neuromuscular facilitation, 2nd edn. Harper & Row, New York

Kubler-Ross E 1969 On death and dying. Tavistock, London

McArdle W, Katch F, Katch V 1991 Exercise physiology—energy, nutrition and human performance. 3rd edn. Lea & Febiger, Philadelphia

Oakes B 1992 The classification of injuries and mechanisms of injury, repair and healing. In: Bloomfield J, Fricker P, Fitch K (eds) Textbook of science and medicine in sport. Blackwell Scientific, Melbourne

Poliquin C 1990 Theory and methodology of strength training: at which speeds should repetitions be performed. Sports Coach April-June:35-38

Purdam C, Fricker P, Cooper B 1992 Principles of treatment and rehabilitation. In: Bloomfield J, Fricker P, Fitch K (eds) Textbook of science and medicine in sport. Blackwell Scientific, Melbourne

Richardson B 1967 Mental practice: a review and discussion. Research Quarterly 38:95-107

Rushall B, Pyke F 1990 Training for sports and fitness. Macmillan, Melbourne

St John Ambulance Australia, 1989 Australian first aid. St John Ambulance Australia, Canberra, vol 1

Sale D 1986 Neural adaptation in strength and power training. In: Jones N, McCartney N, McComas A (eds) Human muscle power. Human Kinetics Publishing, Champaign

Evaluation and management techniques

11. Fitness testing

Rod Green, John Lang, Dennis Hatcher

Traditionally, the concepts of fitness and fitness tests are associated with athleticism, however the Oxford definition of fitness is simply 'good condition or good health'. Similarly, the American College of Sports Medicine (1990) describes fitness as 'the ability to perform moderate to vigorous levels of physical activity without undue fatigue'. Thus in sports physiotherapy it should be remembered that, while fitness tests are often described and discussed in terms of their application to the athletic population, many of these tests are relevant to the general population. Generally, a 'fitness test' determines whether individuals are in a state of 'good health' or 'good condition', not only for sporting participation but also to live a healthy life.

The aims of fitness testing could be set out as follows (MacDougall & Wenger 1991):

1. To identify strengths and weaknesses in current performance or state of health
2. To provide feedback regarding the effectiveness of a training/life style modification program
3. To provide the information which will form a basis for the better understanding of the body and its capabilities by the individual concerned.

These aims are appropriate to monitor the progress of individuals, be they athletes or non-athletes. The educational process should be emphasized. The individual must be familiar with the scope of tests (it is inherent in this statement that the test be significant for the individual involved) and the tests need to be conducted on a serial basis to determine the effect of a given change in training or life style.

The fitness tests outlined in this chapter can be divided into the traditional fitness tests, which measure rates of energy production (either aerobic or anaerobic) and a number of other areas including strength, flexibility and medical fitness. Within each of these areas, a number of tests and their relevance for both the athletic and, where appropriate, the non-athletic population will be outlined.

MEASURES OF ENERGY PRODUCTION: THE TRADITIONAL FITNESS TESTS

Although earlier chapters of this book have described energy supply systems in greater detail, it is appropriate to review the salient points of aerobic and anaerobic metabolism as a prelude to describing tests which will measure these abilities.

The contributions of these energy supply systems will vary greatly depending on the intensity and duration of any activity (Table 11.1). This means that for continuous activities of 2 minutes or longer, the aerobic contribution to the activity will become increasingly important (Table 11.2). In devising tests to measure the capabilities of these energy production systems it must be remembered that any activity will utilize a combination of all three systems (Table 11.2), although by manipulation of the intensity and duration of the activity, the characteristics of these systems can be determined with reasonable accuracy.

Aerobic fitness

The maximum oxygen uptake (VO_2 max) is the measure of the maximal rate of aerobic resynthesis of ATP. The measurement of VO_2 max falls into two categories: direct measurement via collection of respiratory gases during maximal exercise, or prediction of VO_2 max by monitoring responses to maximal or submaximal work loads.

Direct measurement of VO_2 max

The most common form of direct measurement of VO_2 during exercise is called 'open-circuit' spirometry. This involves the inspiration of ambient air and the collection of expired gases via a two-way valve system to measure expired ventilation V_E, mixed expired oxygen (F_EO_2) and carbon dioxide (F_ECO_2), concentrations. (This contrasts with the 'closed-circuit' spirometry where the subject inhales from a spirometer bell containing oxygen and expires back to the same bell with the expired CO_2 being removed by a soda-lime canister.) While open-circuit spirometry does not

Table 11.1 Major features of the systems of energy supply[1]

Energy supply system	Max. rate of energy supply (power)[2]	Duration of energy supply (capacity)[2,3]	Substrate utilized	Efficiency of substrate utilization
Aerobic	Limited (135–155 kJ.min⁻¹)	Unlimited (at sub-maximal workloads or 45 000–80 000 kJ)	Carbohydrate, fats, protein	High
Anaerobic: lactic	High (250–500 kJ.min⁻¹)	Limited (30–60 sec at max rate or 200–300 kJ)	Carbohydrate	Low
Anaerobic: alactic or ATP-PC	Very high (400–750 kJ.min⁻¹)	Very limited (10–15 sec at max rate or 55 kJ)	High energy phosphates (ATP + phospho-creatine)	n/a

[1] The external power output and capacity is given for trained athletes and is based on an efficiency of 25%. This has been determined for aerobic metabolism and assumed for anaerobic metabolism, although it is generally thought that the efficiency of some anaerobic activities may be greater than 25% due to a combination of physiological and biomechanical factors.

[2] Compilation from several sources (Howald et al 1978, Bouchard et al 1981, Sale 1991).

[3] Comparison of duration or capacity is difficult for two reasons. First, unlike the aerobic system, a workload of relatively high intensity must be maintained to fully utilize the anaerobic energy systems. Second, the end point of exercise is due to different factors: for example, the end point in the case of the anaerobic lactic system is due to decreasing muscle pH affecting contractile processes, while in the case of the aerobic system the end point may be due to substrate (glycogen) depletion.

allow for the measurement of inspired volume (V_I), the closed-circuit system does not cater for the massive inspired volumes (occasionally in excess of 200 L/min for elite athletes) required during exercise. However, on the basis that the inspired oxygen (F_IO_2) and carbon dioxide (F_ICO_2) concentrations are constant known values, the (V_I) and the VO_2 and other ventilatory parameters, can be determined for a given exercise period using standard gas equations (Thoden 1991).

Equipment requirements. Technological advances have resulted in the use of sophisticated equipment to determine VO_2 in the open-circuit manner. The original technique involved serial collection of expired gas in Douglas bags for a known period of time, subsequent analysis for volume and gas concentrations and manual calculation of VO_2 using gas equations. Recently it has been possible to measure accurately end-tidal gas concentrations and the volume of each breath and with online computerized analysis, determine VO_2 on a breath-by-breath basis in close to real time. For most purposes, however, the 'noise' inherent in the number of data points generated in a breath-by-breath system is an additional complication as is the questionable significance of a peak VO_2 achieved during a single breath. The most readily used online gas analysis systems for determination of VO_2 max therefore use mixed-expired gases and produce data points at intervals of 10–60 seconds.

Table 11.2 Approximate contributions to energy supply during continuous maximal activity

Activity duration	Aerobic energy contribution (%)	Anaerobic energy contribution (%)
5 seconds	5	95
30 seconds	20	80
2 minutes	50	50
10 minutes	90	10
30 minutes	95	5
2 hours	99	1

Equipment requirements to provide this type of analysis are substantial. The major items would include a computerized online gas analysis system, an ECG unit (to measure heart rate as a minimum and, for clinical use, to allow monitoring of the ECG during exercise), and the loading device or ergometer on which the exercise is to be performed. The most common are the treadmill and cycle, however, a range has been used to fulfil specific demands of individual activities, for example the swimming flume or rowing ergometer. The minimum cost for these major items would be $60 000–70 000, but it could be substantially more, depending on the sophistication of the equipment.

Test protocols. The protocols for determining VO_2 max are almost as varied as the number of laboratories conducting these tests. They fall into two major groups: continuous, in which the subject exercises continuously and the work load is incrementally increased; and discontinuous, where a rest period of varying duration is allowed between periods of work at a constant load but which is increased in successive work periods. No significant difference has been found between the VO_2 max when determined using either type of protocol (McArdle et al 1973). The continuous protocol has the advantage of being more time efficient for both subject and tester and the early work loads serve as an effective warm-up for the later maximal loads. The continuous protocol appears to be more commonly used.

The protocol for continuous tests varies considerably in duration and size of work load increments. Test durations can be between 5–15 minutes. Many ergometers are designed so that the work load may be increased either by adjustment of an external resistance (e.g. friction applied to a flywheel) or increase in work rate (e.g. pedalling frequency). However, it is normal for one variable to be kept constant while the other is increased incrementally. This procedure is also adopted on the treadmill, but several standard treadmill protocols (Bruce 1963) involve simultaneous increases in both speed and gradient.

For reasons outlined below the treadmill is the preferred ergometer for determining VO_2 max. A protocol involving speed increments every minute until a respiratory exchange ratio ($R = VCO_2 / VO_2$) of 1.0 is reached (this being indicative of a work load above the anaerobic threshold and therefore limited in duration, see below) followed by increments in gradient until VO_2 max is achieved. This is well tolerated by both athletes and non-athletes, although the size of the increments varies depending on the training state of the individual to result in tests of 8–10 minutes duration for all subjects (Table 11.3). This has the advantage of allowing the response to submaximal speeds to be related to actual walking or running speeds without the complication of the effect of a gradient. This is useful in terms of exercise prescription.

Specificity of VO_2 max. It is generally agreed that the major limitation to VO_2 max is circulatory in nature and, more specifically, due to limitation in the rate of oxygen delivery to working muscle (Saltin 1985). On this basis, a VO_2 max test conducted on a treadmill is usually considered to be maximal, since it requires contribution from the body's major muscle groups and usually results in central (i.e. circulatory) rather than peripheral (i.e. muscle metabolism) fatigue (McArdle et al 1986). The VO_2 max determined on a bicycle ergometer is reported to be 4–7% lower than the treadmill measurement and the VO_2 max for swimming is 15% below the treadmill value for a given individual (Astrand 1984). However athletes specialising in certain events may not follow this trend. Peripheral adaptations in trained muscle result in greater oxygen utilization. Hence, for cyclists, the VO_2 max achieved on a bicycle ergometer will often be equal to or exceed that on a treadmill. Similarly, for swimmers, VO_2 max tested in a swimming flume may approach VO_2 max determined on a treadmill. This concept of specificity of testing is important and means that, where possible, the VO_2 max of an athlete should be determined on an ergometer which simulates as closely as possible the activity in which the athlete participates.

When testing non-athletes the concept of specificity should also be applied. In this instance running or walking, are common activities even for sedentary individuals and so a treadmill test is usually preferred unless there are contraindications (i.e. medical, disability, and so on).

Criteria for VO_2 max. The best criterion for achievement of VO_2 max with an incremental test is regarded generally as no increase or a reduction in VO_2 on successive work loads. This implies a significant anaerobic energy input and partly as a consequence of this significant psychological or motivational input is required. A plateau in VO_2 is deemed to occur when the increase in VO_2 with an increment in work load is less than 150 ml.min^{-1} (Taylor et al 1955) or 2% (Thoden 1991). If the plateau in VO_2 is not observed, other criteria can be applied. These include

reaching: age predicted maximum heart rate (McArdle et al 1986), a ventilatory equivalent (VE/VO_2) in excess of 33 indicating disproportionate respiratory drive associated with maximal exercise, or blood lactate in excess of 10 mmol.l^{-1} (Thoden et al 1982). It has been proposed that a verification of the VO_2 max be conducted (for athletes) after a rest interval by working the subject at a supramaximal load (i.e. above VO_2 max) to exhaustion (Thoden 1991). While this procedure is used with athletes in some laboratories, it is not necessary for the general population.

Advances in technology have led to another issue. As mentioned earlier, a peak VO_2 achieved in a single breath (as measured on a breath-by-breath system) is certainly not considered to be a valid VO_2 max. Peak VO_2 values up to 10 ml.kg^{-1} min higher than surrounding data points with 10 second data points have been noted. However, as the data is progressively smoothed with longer data intervals, the problem rarely occurs. While the units for VO_2 max are expressed per minute, and hence it could be argued that a VO_2 max must be maintained for a full minute, the increased number of data points with 20–30 second data intervals is in fact useful to confirm a plateau in the latter part of the test with little change in the actual VO_2 max score. It is important, therefore, when comparing either intra or intersubject VO_2 max scores that the intervals over which VO_2 data points are calculated is considered.

Prediction of VO_2 max

In some circumstances, tests to predict VO_2 max may be utilized. Without the need for gas analysis equipment, the cost and technical expertise required is substantially reduced and it is possible for testing to be conducted outside the laboratory. Another benefit, particularly for clinical testing, is the submaximal nature of many such tests.

While runs of varying duration and distance carried out in the field have been used to predict VO_2 max (Astrand &

Table 11.3 Sample treadmill protocols for sedentary and athletic subjects

Time (min)	Sedentary Speed (kph)	Gradient (%)	Athletic Speed (kph)	Gradient (%)
1	3	2[1]	6	2[1]
2	4.5	2	9	2
3	6	2	11	2
4	7.5	2	13	2
5	9	2	15	2
6	9[2]	6	17	2
7	9	10	17[2]	6
8	9	14	17	10
9	4.5[3]	0	17	14
10	4.5	0	9[3]	0

[1] To approximate for potential reduced workload relative to flat walking with wind resistance.
[2] R = 1.0
[3] Cool down after achieving VO_2 max

Table 11.4 Maximum oxygen uptake (VO_2) of elite athletes in different sports

Sport	Male			Female		
	n	l.min^{-1}	ml.kg^{-1}.min^{-1}	n	l.min^{-1}	ml.kg^{-1}.min^{-1}
Rowing[1]	10	5.37 ± 0.36	63.3 ± 4.3	6	3.82 ± 0.22	50.6 ± 4.1
Track cycling[1]	7	4.59 ± 0.25	62.8 ± 3.7	9	3.09 ± 0.25	54.3 ± 3.0
Swimming[1]	23	4.70 ± 0.41	61.7 ± 6.0	12	3.30 ± 0.33	50.0 ± 4.3
Road cycling[1]	12	4.81 ± 0.40	66.5 ± 4.5			
8/1500 m running[1]	6	4.52 ± 0.26	64.3 ± 5.0			
Nordic ski[1]	7	4.33 ± 0.57	66.5 ± 3.4			
Weightlifters[2]	11	4.50 ± 0.60	50.7 ± 6.1			
Discus throwers[2]	7	4.90 ± 0.70	47.5 ± 8.0			

[1] Measured using sports specific equipment at the Australian Institute of Sport (Lancaster et al 1986).
[2] Fahey et al 1975.

Rhyming 1954, Fox 1973) these have attracted criticism on the basis that the ability to run at a pace appropriate to the level of individual fitness is difficult for inexperienced runners (McArdle et al 1986). Other tests rely on maximal power output during an incremental test on either bicycle ergometer (Balke 1959) or treadmill (Balke 1959, Bruce et al 1963). In these tests, it is assumed that the VO_2 max and final work load are directly related, however, both motivation which increases the anaerobic input (Thoden et al 1982) and familiarization factors on repeated tests (Froelicher et al 1974) will inflate the predicted result artificially.

The more objective and commonly used tests are based on observing the heart rate response to work performed on a step test (McArdle et al 1972) or, more commonly, a bicycle ergometer (Astrand & Rhyming 1954). These tests rely on two main assumptions:

1. A linear relationship exists between VO_2 and heart rate. This is largely true at the submaximal work loads on which these tests are based.
2. There is a similar maximum heart rate for all individuals of the same age. This is commonly determined as follows:

$$Max HR = 220 - Age$$

Errors will still occur due to intrasubject diurnal variation in heart rate and intersubject variation in mechanical efficiency. The problem of variation in maximum heart rate for subjects of similar age has also been noted in the prediction of VO_2 max (Telford et al 1989). For example, individuals with a higher than predicted maximum heart rate will have their VO_2 max underestimated.

The major advantages of predictive tests are reduced cost; the ability to conduct tests away from the laboratory; and, particularly in some clinical situations, the submaximal nature of some tests. It should be remembered that there are several sources of error in predicting VO_2 max. This becomes relatively minor in grouped data and may not be important in looking at intraindividual changes over time (e.g. to determine the effects of a training program). The margin of error tends to be accentuated in the very low or

very high VO_2 max subjects (Astrand & Rodahl 1986), thus minimizing the benefit of such tests for non-athletes and elite athletes where a true measure of VO_2 max is perceived as being required.

Other measures of aerobic power

Another approach to the measurement of aerobic power involves the determination of a work capacity at a given absolute heart-rate, for example PWC_{170} (Sjostrand 1947, Wahlund 1948) or the Aerobic Power Index (Telford et al 1989). The result is commonly presented as a work load (e.g. Watts or Watts/kg body weight) rather than a VO_2 max score. As mentioned above these tests are probably most suited to intraindividual comparisons over time.

Interpretation of results

The contribution of aerobic energy to endurance events (Table 11.2) is such that the VO_2 max will be a significant indicator of performance in such activities. The VO_2 max is also significant for most team (e.g. basketball, football) or racquet sports where the activity patterns consist of bursts of maximal anaerobic activity separated by relatively longer periods of aerobic recovery. The importance of aerobic power in these sports is the improved ability to replenish anaerobic energy sources during recovery periods.

Table 11.4 shows typical VO_2 max values for elite athletes in a range of sports. This table confirms the importance of VO_2 max in endurance events, but it also raises the issue of units for VO_2 max. The majority of everyday and sporting activities require individuals to overcome the inertia of their own body weight. Thus, as in Table 11.4, the maximum rate of oxygen intake as measured in l.min^{-1} is divided by the body weight of the individual— the unit ml.kg^{-1}.min^{-1}. In sports such as rowing and swimming, the body weight is supported and therefore the VO_2 max expressed in l.min^{-1} is a better indicator of performance.

Table 11.4 shows that the VO_2 max is lower for women. This is partly related to differences in body fat (see below, 'Body composition/fatness') although the VO_2 max for males is still higher when expressed as a function of lean body mass (McArdle et al 1986). Other possible differences include reduced muscle mass, blood volume, haemoglobin levels or stroke volume in females (Fletcher et al 1990) and, particularly for non-athletes, reduced activity levels among females for social or cultural reasons.

In reviewing the importance of aerobic fitness for the general population, it is worth revising the physiological determinants of VO_2 max.

$$VO_2 = CO \times (a\text{-}v)O_2$$

Where CO equals cardiac output and $(a\text{-}v)O_2$ equals the arteriovenous O_2 difference. From this it may be seen that the VO_2 max is proportional to the CO max. Hence aerobic fitness is a very good indicator of cardiovascular fitness and exercise tolerance for everyday activities which are largely aerobic for the general population. Research has indicated the importance of exercise in reducing the risk of cardiovascular disease, through reduction of blood lipids, body fat, blood pressure, improvement in myocardial function, and as an independent risk factor (Fletcher et al 1990, National Heart Foundation 1991). Thus, the concept of fitness being defined as good condition or good health, tells us that, while we do not expect the general population to compete with athletes, an above average VO_2 max score indicates a healthy level of cardiovascular fitness and that an individual is fit to cope with the general demands of living. To determine an appropriate VO_2 max for the general population, we need to consider that the VO_2 max declines with age (Table 11.5) due in part to reduction in maximum heart rate and hence cardiac output. The data collated in Table 11.5 was collected over the period 1987-91 by HBA Health Management. It is limited in that the subjects are almost exclusively white-collar office workers in senior and middle management of Melbourne based companies. It is

well accepted that such a group will probably have healthier activity patterns and therefore a higher VO_2 max than an equivalent population of blue-collar workers (Department of the Arts, Sport, the Environment, Tourism and Territories 1992). Regardless, it is one of the few large samples of the Australian population to have been tested and for that reason worth reporting.

Anaerobic threshold; another measure of aerobic fitness

Until comparatively recently, the major factor determining endurance capacity in exercise was thought to be the VO_2 max. It has since been demonstrated that the anaerobic threshold (AT), that is the maximum oxygen uptake which can be maintained with no detectable onset of lactic acidosis or associated changes in ventilatory parameters, is of far greater importance in this regard (Farrell et al 1979, Tanaka et al 1984). This is consistent with the concept of peripheral factors (i.e. muscle metabolism) limiting prolonged exercise (Gollnick 1982), and the AT being dependent on those same peripheral factors (Hagberg 1984). The VO_2 max is thought to be more dependent on central circulatory factors (Hagberg 1984, Saltin 1985).

Controversy surrounds the point at which such a threshold occurs, the method of determination, and the physiological basis of a 'threshold' work load at which there is a detectable change in the metabolic or ventilatory response to exercise. The use of the term 'anaerobic' has been criticized on the basis that the working muscle is probably not in a state of significant hypoxia (Walsh & Banister 1988). For further detail regarding this controversy several review papers can be consulted (Walsh & Banister 1988, McLellan 1987, Davis 1985, Brookes 1985). There is no doubt that a 'threshold' which occurs at a submaximal

Table 11.5 Maximum oxygen uptake (VO_2 max) of Melbourne-based Australian white-collar workers[1]

Sex	Age group	Age (mean ± sd)	n[4]	VO_2 max (ml.kg⁻¹.min⁻¹)	Poor	Below average	Fitness rating[2,3] Average	Above average	Excellent
Male	<20	18.7 ± 0.4	4	52.8 ± 5.1					
	20-29	26.7 ± 2.2	526	48.3 ± 9.0	<38	38-43	43-53	53-58	>58
	30-39	35.1 ± 2.7	2874	45.0 ± 8.2	<37	37-41	41-49	49-53	>53
	40-49	44.1 ± 2.8	3369	41.6 ± 7.6	<34	34-38	38-46	46-52	>52
	50-59	53.3 ± 2.6	1404	38.1 ± 7.3	<30	30-34	34-42	42-46	>46
	>59	62.5 ± 3.2	156	36.0 ± 8.6	<28	28-32	32-40	40-44	>44
Female	<20	18.5 ± 0.7	11	40.9 ± 9.6					
	20-29	25.9 ± 2.4	241	40.2 ± 8.3	<32	32-36	36-44	44-48	>48
	30-39	34.2 ± 2.8	427	38.3 ± 8.8	<30	30-34	34-42	42-46	>46
	40-49	43.7 ± 2.8	291	34.8 ± 8.6	<27	27-31	31-39	39-43	>43
	50-59	53.6 ± 2.6	81	31.0 ± 7.9	<23	23-27	27-35	35-39	>39
	>59	65.4 ± 4.8	24	37.3 ± 7.0					

[1] Unpublished data collected by HBA Health Management from 1987-1991.
[2] A rating applied by HBA Health Management whereby ratings above average are indicative of a level of cardiovascular fitness consistent with good health.
[3] Categories are determined as follows:
- Average = mean ± 0.5 x sd
- Above average = mean ± 0.5 sd - mean ± 1 sd
[4] Where n<50 fitness ratings have not been determined due to lack of data. The mean and standard deviations have been reported for interest, but it would appear that the data may not be representative of the age group.

or the duration for which a force (either absolute or % MVC) can be maintained. Using isokinetic techniques the fatigue index is measured as the decline in torque produced over a given number of consecutive maximal contractions.

Such tests are essentially a measure of anaerobic capacity and, at least in the case of isometric (Hulten et al 1975) and isokinetic (Thorstensson & Karlsson 1976) techniques, the fatigue index has been related to muscle fibre composition. This is consistent with findings of fibre type selective glycogen depletion (Hatcher et al 1985) and changes in force-velocity properties (Hatcher & Luff 1987) after application of a fatigue regime to isolated muscle preparations.

Interpretation of results

Expression of results. Muscular strength or power is often expressed relative to body weight rather than in absolute terms. Where the force must be applied to an external resistance (e.g. weightlifting), the absolute force is critical in determining performance (although this may be modified in weight restricted categories). Where the force must be applied to moving the body weight, it has been common for the result to be expressed per kilogram of body weight, (Rankin & Thompson 1983, Gregor et al 1979).

Findings of increased development of muscular force with increase in body weight of the individual (assuming similar activity and training patterns) is consistent with the concept that the force developed by a muscle is proportional to the cross-sectional area of the muscle. However, the relationship between force developed and body weight may not be linear. This concept is best understood by comparison of super heavyweight and 'flyweight' weight lifters. The heavyweight is able to lift much heavier weights (produce more absolute force), whereas elite lifters in the lighter classes are now able to lift more than twice their body weight although the absolute weight is less (more force per kilogram of body weight). Therefore, although increases in muscle mass (associated with increase in cross-sectional area) will increase both the total body weight as well as the force developed, there may be some limitations associated with expression of results relative simply to body weight. The possibility that force expressed per kilogram of body weight places heavier individuals at an unfair advantage is discussed in the chapter on Isokinetics.

Determinants of muscular strength and power. The peak torque developed may be related to several factors, all of which are sensitive to training, including muscle fibre size and composition, neuromuscular factors, and neural factors. The effect of fibre type predominance is shown in Figure 11.2 which illustrates a typical graph for peak torque versus velocity for two subjects. The shift to the right of the curve for subject A has been related to a greater percentage of fast twitch fibres (Gregor et al 1979).

If these peak torque values are converted to power, an increase in the power has been found up to velocities of

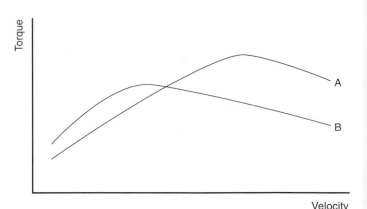

Fig. 11.2 Torque-velocity curves for subjects with a high percentage of fast twitch **A** and slow twitch **B** muscle fibres

400°/sec. for some individuals since the increase in velocity is greater than the reduction in torque developed (Osternig 1986). This effect may be reduced for subjects who have a lower percentage of fast twitch (FT) fibres (Coyle et al 1979). Similarly, the RFD in isometric contractions is also related to the percentage of FT fibres (Viitasalo 1981).

Relevance of strength testing. Not surprisingly muscular strength, power, alactic power and capacity are higher for athletes involved in activities which demand explosive power. This is indicative of the closer relationship between results of muscular strength tests and performance in activities which require significant rapid force development or anaerobic effort. While activities such as field events in athletics, weightlifting and wrestling obviously fit into this category, the ability to perform specific actions in some sports with an otherwise high aerobic component may be indicated by results of tests of muscular force. For example, a soccer player jumping to contest the ball with the head or a 'slam-dunk' by a basketballer also require the development of significant muscular power.

While muscular strength is rarely a limiting factor in everyday life for healthy adults (therefore the relevance of strength testing minimized), there is a loss of muscle mass and associated muscle function with age (Fleg & Lakatta 1988). Substantial benefits have been associated with the restoration of muscular strength through appropriate training in the elderly (Fiatarone et al 1990, Frontera et al 1988) and recommendations made that strength training be prescribed for the maintenance of muscular strength in healthy adults (American College of Sports Medicine 1990). In light of these observations, it is evident that there is a role for strength testing in the general population to prescribe and monitor exercise for the maintenance of minimum muscular strength.

Body composition/fatness

The calculation of a percentage of body fat has been relatively commonplace for both the athletic and the general population. The rationale behind such determinations being that excess body fat is associated clinically with conditions such as hypertension, hyperlipidaemia, diabetes, reduced cardiovascular fitness and other potentially life threatening conditions. For athletes, the primary motivation for minimization of body fat is that, particularly in sports where the body weight must be supported, the fat tissue, unlike muscle, is incapable of producing movement and yet it must be carried—thus reducing the external work produced (hence the unit for VO_2 of $ml.kg^{-1} min^{-1}$) and so having a negative impact on performance.

Measures of body composition

Hydrostatic weighing. This technique involves substantial equipment requirements and detailed techniques which have been described elsewhere (Ross & Marfell-Jones 1991). The subject is weighed both in air and under water and body volume is determined by displacement of water (with correction for residual lung volume). Using appropriate equations, the body density can then be calculated.

Using estimates of fat and fat free weight based on the density determined (Siri 1961, Brozek et al 1963), the percentage of body fat can then be calculated. However, it must be remembered that while the estimation of body fat composition from body density is based on physical principles, it is still an estimate. It appears that for some athletes the density of the 'fat-free' weight is greater than that for the average population (Adams et al 1982) thus invalidating the estimate. Some correction for this has been made by fractionation of 'fat-free' weight into muscle, bone and residual (Drinkwater & Ross 1980), however the inter-individual variations in proportions and density of tissue types still result in inaccuracies when body density is used to calculate a percentage of body fat (Clarys et al 1984, Martin et al 1986).

Anthropometry. Numerous studies have determined body density from the above techniques and related this to various anthropometric measures including soft tissue girths (waist), bony dimensions (styloid process widths) and the thickness of skinfolds at selected sites. Thus the equipment requirements are substantially reduced and include: tape measure, bone calipers and skinfold calipers. Such regression models use the relationship between density and body fat (above) to estimate the percentage of body fat.

A number of different formulae have been determined (Sloan et al 1962, Sloan 1967, Sloan & Weir 1970, Wilmore 1970, Forsyth & Sinning 1973), however most of these formulae have been based on specific population groups in specific countries and their general applicability may be limited. The limitations in using density to calculate a percentage of body fat, outlined above, must also be considered when using these predictions.

For these reasons, many laboratories now prefer to use a sum of skinfolds as an indicator of 'fatness' (Telford et al 1984). These are particularly useful for serial measures on the same individual, but they may not have the same appeal for individuals who are used to the concept of a percentage of body fat (despite its inherent inaccuracies).

Scanning techniques. In an age of technological advance, body fat determinations can be made using methods such as ultrasound, computerized tomography (CT), and nuclear magnetic resonance (NMR) scanning. These techniques require varying degrees of financial cost and are not currently in widespread use.

Interpretation of results. It has been suggested that calculation of body fat from either anthropometric measures or densitometry is inappropriate due to the inaccuracies outlined above (Ross & Marfell-Jones 1991). Both body density, as determined from densitometry, and a sum of skinfolds from a number of specified anatomical sites are useful in themselves as an indicator of body composition and these may be compared to normative data (Telford et al 1984). If measured on a serial basis, these measures are a useful indicator of variation associated with training or life style changes.

Given the widespread use of calculated percentage of body fat, it is likely that this method of determining body fatness will continue to be used for some time. While the calculated percentage should not be taken as an absolute value, changes associated with serial measures (assuming the measurement techniques remain the same) may be just as useful as either body density or sum of skinfolds.

It is well recognized that, for genetic and hormonal reasons, females will have a greater percentage of body fat than males and this fat is distributed to a greater extent in the limbs than the torso. For example, in a Canadian athletic reference population (152 males, 94 females, mean age = 21, Ross & Marfell-Jones 1991), taking into account the fractionation of fat free weight, the body fat of males and females was estimated to be 10.96 and 18.04% respectively. In contrast, a theoretical 'reference' man and woman, based on measurement of 1000 aged between 20–24 were described as having a body fat content of 15 and 27% respectively (Behnke & Wilmore 1974). Calculated body fats below 10% are not unusual for athletes, particularly males, while calculated body fats in excess of 30% are not unusual in sedentary older adults of either sex.

Measures of body weight/shape

Body mass index. The body mass index (BMI) has long been used as an indicator of fatness and may be defined as follows:

$$BMI = weight \ (kg).height^2 \ (m)$$

The National Heart Foundation of Australia concurs with the classification of appropriate weight proposed by Bray (1978) as outlined below (Table 11.9).

Table 11.9 Classification of body weight according to Body Mass Index[1]

Weight classification	Body mass index	
	Male	Female
Normal	20-25	19-24
Overweight	25-30	24-30
Obese	>30	>30

[1] Bray 1978

The BMI is a useful concept for the general population who will have an average muscle mass, however, for athletics in general and particularly in power sports (eg. weight-lifting, shot-put) where a large muscle mass has been developed, a BMI in excess of 30 would be regarded as an advantage rather than unhealthy. As indicated above, the BMI is of little value to athletes since it does not distinguish between fat and muscle, however a combination of BMI and body fat may be useful for the general population. For instance, an individual may have a 'normal' BMI, but an unacceptable level of body fat. The assumption that can be made from this is that the individual probably has a relatively low muscle mass.

Waist-to-hip ratio (WHR). Recent evidence suggests that WHR is a better predictor of risk of cardiovascular and other diseases than other measures of adiposity (Bjorntorp 1988). This association is particularly strong for cardiovascular disease in both men (Larsson et al 1984) and women (Wing et al 1991), although it is also associated with various other diseases (Bjorntrop 1988).

The WHR may be simply calculated as the ratio of the following measurements:

Waist: minimum girth—usually at the level of the umbilicus or above
Hip: maximum girth—usually at the level of the greater trochanter

There has been some variance in these measures in different studies, however the most likely measure to change results significantly is the use of the level of the iliac crest for the hip measurement. It has been suggested that WHR in excess of 0.80 for females and 0.90 for males is associated with an increased risk of disease (Egger 1992).

Somatotype. The Heath-Carter somatotype (Carter 1980) is the most commonly used method to classify physique. By either anthropometric or photographic methods, a rating is determined for each of the three components: endomorphy (fatness), mesomorphy (muscularity) and ectomorphy (linearity). The general population will show a range of physiques (Bailey et al 1982) and, while some sports show very specific somatotype groupings among elite individuals, others are more variable (Ross & Marfell-Jones 1991).

O-Scale. This physique assessment system is based on a series of anthropometric measures (Ross & Ward 1985). The two major variables are size adjusted girths and a proportional weight which are determined by scaling to a common stature and then related to normative values for sex and age group (based on a Canadian reference population). This system has been designed for the health and fitness industry with the emphasis, as with other measures, being on the use of serial measures for comparison.

Flexibility

Flexibility is the joint specific range of movement as opposed to a general characteristic (Harris 1969) that is normally limited by one or more of the following factors:

1. Shape or orientation of the articular surfaces at the joint
2. Tension in ligaments, muscles or other fascia crossing the joint
3. Contact between soft tissues of adjacent joint segments.

While variations in flexibility have not been identified as being a significant factor in determining level of performance (Hubley-Kozey 1991), a 'normal' range of motion at specific joints is required for many sporting and everyday activities. Techniques for the improvement of flexibility and their use in warm-up and cool-down activities are discussed in Chapter 7; however the most significant aspect of flexibility testing in a sports physiotherapy context is the reduced range of motion associated with various articular and soft tissue injuries.

Tests of flexibility

Flexibility can be measured on a dynamic basis during activity using motion analysis systems (VICON) or cinematography. Static tests of flexibility fall into two categories: direct and indirect.

Indirect tests. A number of tests based on a 'sit and reach' approach (Cureton 1941) continue to be used due to their simplicity. Unfortunately, these tests usually measure range of motion at a number of joints (hip, lumbar, thoracic, and cervical spine) and will vary with the anthropometrics of the individual (Hoeger & Hopkins 1992).

Direct tests. Flexibility can be measured at a specific joint and for a specific movement, using either a goniometer or the Leighton flexometer (Leighton 1942). The goniometer has traditionally been subject to error due to difficulty in the location of the axis of movement, particularly for complex movements (Moore 1949). This is exacerbated by the fact that, unlike the goniometer, very few (if any) joints in the body have a fixed axis. It has been suggested that error is reduced by the accurate alignment of the arms of the goniometer with joint segments, with little emphasis being placed on the axis of movement after the initial placement of the goniometer (Miller 1985). Modification of the goniometer to replace the protractor with a potentiometer and hence produce the electrogoniometer (Karpovich

& Karpovich 1959), is useful in terms of analysing dynamic flexibility, but does not eliminate the problems inherent in the goniometer concept as described above.

The Leighton flexometer has proved far more reliable in that it is strapped to the moving limb segment and uses a gravity needle to standardize the starting point for the movement, hence eliminating the two major sources of error inherent in the use of the goniometer. The flexometer has been criticized in that there may be movement of the instrument or difficulty in placement due to soft tissue variations (Miller 1985). However, the flexometer has been proposed as the preferred method for testing because of its greater reliability (Hubley-Kozey 1991).

Interpretation of results

Since the major use of flexibility is as an indication of the rehabilitation of normal motion post injury, in an ideal world the range of motion of all joints susceptible to injury would be assessed prior to participation in activity. As this preventive approach is unlikely in the real world, the remaining options are to compare post-injury range of motion to either:

- 'Normal' values (Miller 1985, Daniels & Worthingham 1986, Hubley-Kozey 1991)
- The same joint in the unaffected limb (where possible).

Comparison to normal results is difficult due to individual variability, however where the injury is not in a limb this may be the only option. Comparison to an unaffected limb of course assumes that the limb is indeed unaffected and has a normal range of motion!

Measurements of flexibility should be taken at regular intervals after injury to monitor the rehabilitation progress. It is also important to remember the significant difference between the active (due to action of muscles) and passive (due to external force applied by the tester) range of movement at a joint; with the latter normally being greater.

Medical fitness

Medical fitness is a particularly important consideration for non-athletes, in part because the life style of most athletes (at an elite level) is consistent with the basic principles of health, that is good nutrition and regular exercise. The medical fitness of athletes or sporting participants at all levels should be neither assumed or ignored.

However, for the non-athlete, a physical examination should be conducted prior to the commencement of an exercise program and at increasingly regular intervals for all individuals as they increase in age. For instance, it has been suggested that for healthy adults under the age of 30 an examination every 2-3 years is adequate, while for those over 50 an annual exam would be appropriate with a range

of intervals in between (Cooper 1982). Others have recommended less frequent intervals for healthy adults (Breslow & Somers 1977). A comprehensive list of appropriate tests to be conducted during such medical examinations can be found elsewhere (Cooper 1982, Couch 1989), however a number of the major tests which will indicate the medical fitness of the individual have been detailed below.

Blood pressure

Elevated resting blood pressure is considered a primary risk factor in the aetiology of cardiovascular disease. Prior to undertaking any test which imposes a significant physiological load, it is prudent to measure blood pressure in any individuals where elevated blood pressure could pose an identifiable risk. Common sense tells us that an athlete who trains intensely 5 days per week is probably subject to no greater risk during testing than is imposed by the daily training regimen. Less fit and less frequent exercisers should be routinely screened for elevated blood pressure. A blood pressure of 140/90 or greater should be followed up with counselling and/or referral. In such individuals, monitoring of blood pressure throughout an exercise test will reveal any inappropriate blood pressure response and may reveal that exercise is contraindicated in some individuals until blood pressure is controlled. An inappropriate response may be defined as either an increase in blood pressure to 260/120 mmHg or greater, or a drop in blood pressure (10 mmHg or greater) with increasing exercise. Either of these responses constitute grounds for the termination of the test (Pollock et al 1978). Heart rate, blood pressure and ECG should be monitored on a regular basis during exercise and at least 5 minutes of recovery. Emergency equipment and qualified personnel should be available.

Heart rate

Resting and maximal heart rates are very useful to determine because they allow the individual to gauge target training zones during future workouts. Although maximum heart rate can be calculated by the formula 220–age, the standard deviation of this prediction is 10 bpm, therefore, one in every three 40-year-olds tested will have maximal heart rates below 170 or above 190.

Spirometry

A basic test of lung function will allow the tester to determine whether inadequacies in ventilatory capacity could limit the exercise performance during a maximal VO_2 test. Forced vital capacity (FVC) and forced expiratory volume in one second (FEV_1) are the most commonly measured variables, however, the mid expiratory flow rate (FEF 25-75) provides a more sensitive indicator of the

probab
predict
analysi
vascula
The ath
determi
speed t
lead EC
on hear
The
modific
are con
Inheren
test is o
exempli
concept
life style
regular a
likely to l
or healt

REFEREN

Adams J, M
    fat con
    Journa
American (
    quantit
    cardior
    and Sci
Astrand P-(
    sports p
Astrand P-(
    capacity
    Applied
Astrand P (
    McGrav
Ayalon A, I
    of explo
    Moreho
    Biomecl
Bailey D A,
    men and
Balke B, Wa
    Force pe
Beaver W L,
    lactate th
    Journal o
Beaver W L,
    detecting
    Physiolog
Behnke A R,
    build and
Berg A, Keul
    exertion
    Internatic
Bjorntrop P 1
    distributi
    723:121–
Bosco C, Kor
    compositi
    Applied P
Bosco C, Kor
    behaviour
    Physiolog

12. Manual therapy: when and why?

Libby Austin, Mary Magarey, Geoffrey D. Maitland

Since the early days of Cyriax, manual therapy has evolved in many different forms, progressing in some schools from an art form to achieving a scientific basis as a result of clinical research. While the broad aim of restoration of normal neuromusculoskeletal function is accepted by all, fundamental differences exist between the various approaches. Such differences are evident in relation to the structures considered at fault and the most appropriate method by which the fault(s) should be remedied. Even when the different schools agree on the structures to be treated, differences exist between the preferred treatments and how to apply them; for example, whether sustained movement is more effective than oscillatory joint mobilization. Further differences emerge in the philosophies behind the choices and progressions of treatment, for example, treatment based on a biomechanical analysis or clinical presentation. This chapter presents one approach in detail. For more information regarding other approaches to manual therapy, a further reading list can be found at the end of the chapter.

THE ROLE OF PASSIVE MOVEMENT IN THE MANAGEMENT OF SPORTING INJURIES

Manual therapy means the 'hands on' treatment used in the management of disorders affecting the musculoskeletal and nervous systems. It includes passive mobilization and manipulation of spinal and peripheral joints, muscle energy techniques, passive stretching of contractile tissues, manual muscle relaxation techniques, 'hands on' muscle rehabilitation techiques, myofascial release, mobilization of the nervous system and massage. In this chapter, the role of passive movement, in the form of mobilization and manipulation, will be discussed as it relates to the successful management of sporting injuries.

Passive mobilization techniques are used predominantly in the treatment of mechanical disorders. These movements include both physiological and accessory movements. Physiological movements are those that the individual can perform actively. Accessory movements are joint movements that cannot be performed actively, but which can be performed on the individual by someone else (Maitland 1986). These techniques, as well as continuous passive motion, can be applied successfully in the treatment of disorders of a number of structures, including spinal and peripheral joints. The application of these techniques may vary from very gentle small amplitude movements, barely perceived by the patient, as a treatment for pain, to large amplitude, through-range movements, or strong, small amplitude, end of range techniques which are aimed at improving range of movement. Firm stretching with passive movement may be used in exceptional circumstances to increase range beyond its normal limits for the purpose of achievement of specific movements or postures. An example is sustained stretching of hip abduction/lateral rotation at the limit of normal range to improve the ability of a gymnast to perform manoeuvres requiring the splits.

Passive movement techniques have other extremely important functions, including a role in the early management of injured structures. Akeson et al (1987), in a review paper, emphasized the growing evidence of clinical and biochemical value of passive motion in a number of experimental and clinical situations. The work of Salter et al (1979, 1980, 1982a, 1982b, 1993) and, more recently, Steptoe and Walton (1989), on continuous passive motion (CPM) has been significant in validating the place of passive motion in repair of hyaline cartilage. Similar work by Woo et al (1981), Woo and Akeson (1987), Salter and Bell (1981), Salter and Minister (1982) and Dahners et al (1989) has shown the value of controlled passive movements in the repair process of ligament and tendons, particularly the rate of healing, fibre alignment and strength of the scar tissue. The benefit of some form of physiologic stress during healing has certainly been reinforced by Jobe (1983). O'Driscoll et al (1983) demonstrated that CPM cleared haemarthrosis at a rate double that in immobilized joints and Skyhar et al (1985) demonstrated similar rapid clearance of synovial fluid with CPM.

Although little research has been completed on the effect of CPM on muscle repair, a retrospective comparative study by Stanton (1988) on the early management of hamstring

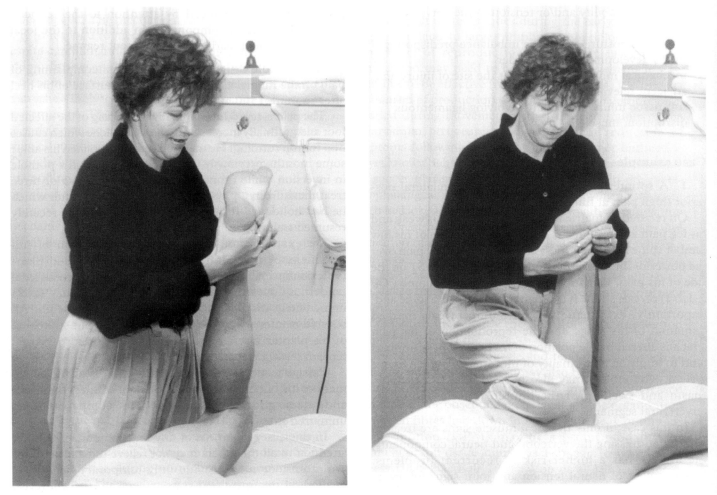

Fig. 12.2 Talocrural distraction combined with medial rotation. A: Grade III-III+, B: Grade IV—using knee on thigh to provide counter resistance

4. A hockey player presents with a vague generalized ache around the ankle mortice exacerbated by playing on artificial turf surfaces.

He has had several ankle sprains in the past and his ankle is thickened and restricted slightly in all directions of movement. He is able to reproduce his pain by running in a figure of eight with his affected foot on the outside of the curve.

Examination reveals that all accessory movements are stiff at his talocrural, subtalar and inferior tibiofibular joints. Treatment aimed at mobilizing these joints with accessory glides is effective in increasing his painfree range of movement but does not alter his symptoms when running. In prone, the ache can be reproduced in dorsiflexion/medial rotation with the addition of compression through his hindfoot. However, treatment with this technique has no effect.

In this instance, the patient appears to have two separate local components. The first problem, periarticular hypo-mobility, has been addressed by the physiotherapist. Consideration must now be given to the second component, that of pain reproduced by joint compression. The potential effect of both the patient's hockey and the joint mobilization

on the articular cartilage should be considered. An athlete with ankle stiffness, playing on an artificial surface, is likely to be placing abnormal compressive stresses through localized areas of the articular cartilage, leading to damage in the form of fissuring as a result of overload. Other areas of the joint surface may receive less compressive force than normal, leading to damage in the form of excessive hydration and an alteration in the synthesis of collagen as a result of underuse (Muir 1988). Consequently, further compression as part of treatment, may have harmful rather than beneficial effects on articular cartilage nutrition and therefore be ineffective as a treatment technique. Treatment with joint distraction, combined with the aggravating physiological movement of dorsiflexion/medial rotation, may have some influence in reversing the degenerative process, although no studies have been undertaken to validate this hypothesis. This technique can be performed strongly, by stabilizing the patient's posterior thigh with the therapist's knee, as Grade IV and III techniques (Figs 12.2a and b), the intention being to alter intra-articular pressure, potentially leading to a reduction of pain on joint compression. Combined with the passive movement approach, shock absorbing footwear, ankle supports and proprioceptive retraining is appropriate for this patient, in an attempt to prevent reinjury on return to hockey.

This patient demonstrates the need to consider more than one component within the intrinsic structures, in this case, both an intra- and periarticular component. Consideration of extrinsic or remote factors is not as significant as recognition of the possibility of multiple structure involvement at the same site.

5. A baseball pitcher presents with intermittent sharp pain and a deep ache in the anterior shoulder region.

The pain is provoked by the late cocking phase of pitching, a position of maximum extension and lateral rotation in approximately 90° of abduction. He has developed the pain during pre-season training including additional training for national championships. He has had similar but less severe and restrictive problems in previous seasons.

On examination, he demonstrates minor anterior instability of the glenohumeral joint and the shoulder quadrant (Maitland 1991) reproduces the deep anterior shoulder ache. Muscle assessment reveals poor control of the scapula during flexion, especially during eccentric movement with resistance, weakness and poor endurance of the middle trapezius and rhomboids on sustained contraction, and of the lower trapezius and serratus anterior on repeated testing. The pectoralis minor and upper trapezius are tight.

In this situation, passive treatment directed at reduction of pain in the quadrant position is appropriate, but not with the intention of increasing range, as the quadrant position stresses the anterior passive restraints, already shown to have diminished integrity. Passive treatment must alter the relationship of pain and joint resistance and restore as normal as possible an endfeel for movement without stretching. In addition, the poor muscular control of the scapula is a significant contributing factor to development of the shoulder problem, as the stress placed on the glenohumeral joint is exacerbated by the lack of a stable base for the joint. Consequently, adequate treatment must include stretching for the tight muscle groups and a functional rehabilitation program for the scapular muscles, working from a position of control to one closer to the functional position required for pitching (Magarey & Jones 1992).

Critical analysis of the contributing factors, in addition to an open attitude allowing the therapist to explore different management options, combined with a thorough reassessment process, will enable determination of the contribution of each factor, whether muscle imbalance, soft tissue, neural, either intra- or perineural, or intra-or periarticular joint and will therefore assist in the accuracy of treatment and speed of resolution.

While passive mobilization and manipulation are often effective forms of treatment, therapists must always remember the necessary precautions and contraindications to strong passive techniques. These are listed in Magarey (1986a) and Maitland (1986) with detailed explanations, and will be presented only briefly here. Although some of the situations in which passive treatment is contraindicated or may proceed only with caution are unlikely to apply to athletes, the complete list of precautionary situations is presented.

CAUTION WITH MOBILIZATION

Caution should be used with mobilization in the following situations.

In the presence of any evidence of vertebrobasilar artery insufficiency (VBI), treatment must be extremely gentle and the symptoms and signs of VBI constantly monitored. Any provocation or exacerbation of symptoms of VBI should lead to an immediate cessation of the treatment technique. Similar care and precautions apply to the less likely situation of symptoms or signs of carotid artery compromise.

Patients with rheumatoid arthritis may have painless weakening of their ligamentous structures, particularly in the upper cervical area. Consequently, treatment should not be directed into joint resistance, as rupture may occur with no warning.

Patients with osteoporosis or elderly patients may have bones which are brittle and readily fractured. Consequently, treatment directed at the ribs, the neck of femur or humerus must be undertaken with care, with particular care needed of local small point pressures or axial rotation forces, which may lead to fractures.

Patients who have taken prolonged courses of corticosteroids for treatment of disorders such as asthma should also be treated with care, as steroid use may lead to a decrease in bone mass. The length of time necessary to produce sufficient alteration in bone structure depends on the pre-treatment status of the subject, the dose of steroids used and the individual's response to corticosteroids, but use of the equivalent of 10 mg of prednisilone for a period of 12 months can lead to sufficient reduction in bone mass that forceful mobilization should be avoided as it can lead to fracture. Following use of corticosteroids for any length of time, a degree of steroid-induced reduction of bone mass remains indefinitely. The degree and significance of such loss varies, depending again on the dose, the length of time taken and the pre-treatment status of the patient. Consequently, any patient with a history of corticosteroid use should be treated with care. Assessment of bone density is cheap and simple and should be undertaken in any patient in whom bone density is a potential management issue. However, as bone density studies may be misinterpreted, physiotherapists should not rely on the patient's report of the results of the tests, but should seek clarification from the relevant medical practitioner. The effect on bone structure of prolonged use of anabolic steroids and other performance enhancing drugs is not known. However, the therapist should be aware of the pharmacological status of the patient before undertaking management.

Patients who have taken aspirin during the previous week, those currently taking aspirin and those on anticoagulant medication should be treated cautiously to avoid excessive strain on any tissue that may respond by bleeding. Aspirin has anticoagulant properties and even in small isolated doses can be responsible for abnormal bleeding following injury or forceful mobilization.

Patients demonstrating structural instability should not have the unstable joint mobilized in such a way that its instability will be increased. Examples include recent dislocation, spondylolisthesis and retrolisthesis. Recent fractures or ligamentous rupture fall into a similar category. Mobilization can be useful to alter the pain response associated with a movement. Even mobilization into joint resistance in the direction of the instability may be necessary to alter the relationship between the pain and joint resistance pattern. However, forceful end of range techniques which will further increase the range of movement in a direction already demonstrating a lack of stability are inappropriate.

Care should be used in treatment of children, particularly in relation to the extremities, as strong mobilization may stress the epiphyseal plates and interfere with normal growth.

Any condition that is worsening should be treated with care. If treatment has already been instigated, strong consideration should be given to reducing the strength of the techniques applied, changing or stopping the technique.

CONTRAINDICATIONS TO MANIPULATION

Any evidence of VBI is a contraindication to manipulation of the cervical spine. A detailed literature review, including signs and symptoms of VBI, may be found in the paper by Grant (1988). The Australian Physiotherapy Association (1988) has produced a protocol for assessment of patients prior to cervical manipulation to determine to the maximum extent possible the presence of symptoms or signs of VBI. This protocol is recommended for use by all physiotherapists undertaking treatment of the cervical spine.

Similarly, during movement of the cervical spine, reproduction or any symptoms or signs that could be attributed to compromise of the carotid artery, although less likely, contraindicate manipulation of the cervical spine.

Any evidence of malignancy of the spine is a contraindication to manipulation.

Manipulation of the upper cervical spine is contraindicated in patients with rheumatoid arthritis as a result of the potential asymptomatic weakening of the supporting ligamentous structures.

Any spinal level demonstrating instability should not be manipulated, as manipulation is likely to further increase the range of movement in an already unstable joint. In the upper cervical spine, where manipulation of an unstable joint may have a catastrophic outcome, manipulation of adjacent levels is also contraindicated. However, in the lumbar spine, manipulation of levels adjacent to an unstable spondylolisthesis or retrolisthesis may be appropriate, provided the manipulation can be sufficiently localized to the correct level. Instability of the upper cervical spine can be tested manually with the tests described by Aspinall (1990), and in other areas of the spine with passive intervertebral movements, particularly those combining a physiological and accessory movement at an individual intervertebral level.

Any suspicion or evidence of a fracture is a contraindication to manipulation in adjacent joints or those in which the manipulation will place stress on the fracture.

Manipulation is contraindicated in the presence of any suspicion or evidence of spinal canal or foraminal encroachment.

Manipulation is contraindicated in the presence of positive neurological signs indicating compromise of spinal cord, cauda equina or spinal nerve roots.

Manipulation is contraindicated following total ligamentous rupture or acute repair of ligaments or tendons. The repair should not be stretched until advised by the surgeon.

PROPOSED MECHANISMS FOR PAIN RELIEF BY PASSIVE MOVEMENT

Athletes present to physiotherapists for many types of problems. They seek advice, education and treatment to facilitate healing and a quick return to their sport. In many cases, pain relief is a priority.

Pain is usually caused by tissue injury or inflammation (Lynn 1984), the damaged or inflamed tissue directly exciting the nerve membranes (Wilson & Ifield 1952, Lance & Bogduk 1982, Wall 1984). This local event precipitates a complex series of reactions in the spinal cord and higher centres of the nervous system which modulate and regulate the experience of pain (Watson 1982). Further discussion regarding the experience of pain is described elsewhere in this book (see Ch. 6). A summary of the main features of the pain modulatory system is shown in Figure 12.3 (Watson 1982).

Experimental research has yet to explain fully the mechanisms for pain relief with passive movement. Such pain relief is less likely to be related to a single mechanism than to the cumulative effects of many processes including neurophysiological and mechanical effects, both at the local cellular level and at sites remote from the symptoms, in conjunction with psychological effects. Several mechanisms have been proposed as hypotheses for the relief of spinal pain with passive movement. This section gives a brief outline of some of these hypotheses. Recent research on

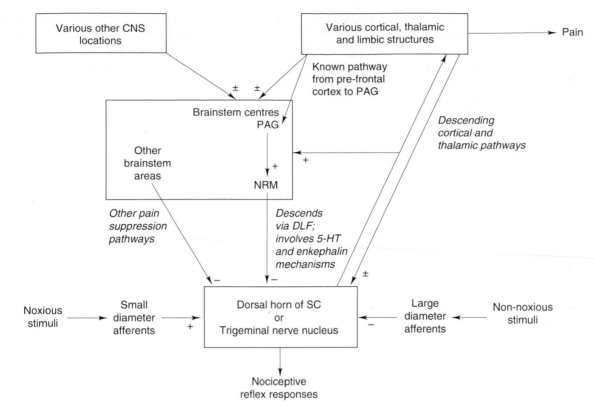

Fig. 12.3 Summary of major features of a pain modulatory system. Source: Watson (1982).
Note: +, facilitatory influence; –, inhibitory influence; CNS, central nervous system; DLF, dorsolateral fasciculus; NRM, nucleus raphe magnus; PAG, periaqueductal grey; SC, spinal cord; 5-HT, 5-hydroxytryptamine (serotonin).

the chemical nature of pain perception and the effect of movement on synaptic chemistry, together with the contribution of the nervous system to the pathophysiology of arthritides (Levine et al 1987), may provide more adequate explanations than are currently available. However, discussion of this complex and relatively unknown area of research is beyond the scope of this chapter.

Neurophysiological mechanisms

Suppression of nociceptive input at the dorsal horn by non-noxious mechanoreceptors

Wyke (1985) proposed a neurophysiological mechanism for the relief of joint pain using passive movement. This mechanism involved stimulation by passive movement of peripheral type I mechanoreceptors which, via their collateral branches, excite inhibitory interneurones which in turn presynaptically inhibit the type IV nociceptors at their afferent terminals.

This theory has since been challenged (Zusman 1986) for the following reasons:

- A weak correlation between the diameter and receptor type in joint nerves found by Andersen et al (1967) does not support the functional specificity of nerve endings suggested by Wyke (1985).

- Based on work by Boyd and Davey (1968) and Langford and Schmidt (1982), the proportion of articular mechanoreceptors in spinal and peripheral joints proposed by Wyke would appear to be inflated.
- Most activity produced in articular nerves with passive movement occurs when the joint is moved at or near the limit of its available range (Grigg 1975, Grigg & Greenspan 1977). Consequently, if Wyke's hypothesis were correct, it would be unable to explain the effectiveness of passive mid-range movements in reduction of pain, a phenomenon frequently observed clinically.
- Passive movement does not selectively stimulate large fibre mechanoreceptors but also a significant number of small myelinated and unmyelinated fibres (Schaible & Schmidt 1983a,1983b).

These observations suggest that any significant neural response which may be evoked by passive movement is likely to involve both large and small diameter joint afferents, rather than only large fibres.

Conduction block effect

A progressive reduction in discharges of large and small diameter normal joint afferents has been found to occur following 1-2 minutes of maintained or repetitive joint movement (Clark 1975, Schaible & Schmidt 1983b). Furthermore, Guilbaud et al (1985) found that approximately 30 seconds of repetitive mechanical stimulation resulted in a rapid and almost complete conduction block of sensitized nociceptors supplying the inflamed ankle joint of a rat. This conduction block lasted for several minutes.

These findings may be used to suggest a mechanism by which passive movement may temporarily decrease pain perception (Zusman 1987). It may also explain how 'after pain' can be minimized with irritable conditions as a result of the blockade temporarily diminishing the release of substance P and other chemical mediators of pain.

Stimulation of endogenous anti-nociceptive system

Rees' (1987) review paper on endogenous opioids emphasized the problems in research related to the action of endogenous opioids in perception of pain, and observed that there are significant species differences in response to opioids, making research in this area difficult, extrapolations from animal experiments dubious and the results inconclusive. Few studies on patients have provided useful information. In one study, patients with inflammatory arthritic conditions demonstrated plasma concentrations of some endogenous opioids lower than those present in control populations (Denko et al 1982), while in a different study, patients with osteoarthritis or ankylosing spondylitis showed no consistent change in levels compared with a control population (Jones et al 1985). Patients in chronic pain have demonstrated increased, decreased or negligible changes in plasma concentrations in different experiments (Millan & Herz 1985).

Despite these difficulties, the hypothesis that passive joint movement relieves pain of spinal origin by arousing a pain control system related to opioid peptides was investigated by Zusman et al (1989) using the opioid—antagonist, naloxone. Subjects with spinal pain were treated with passive movement appropriate for their condition, following which either naloxone or a placebo, physiological saline, was administered and any alteration in the patients' level of pain relief evaluated. The results were not satisfactorily conclusive, with the authors commenting that they may have been influenced by extrinsic factors (Zusman et al 1989). This is certainly likely, as Rees (1987) observed that naloxone is a powerful antagonist to exogenous opioids such as morphine but has little antagonist action against endogenous peptides, thereby leading to the questionable value of naloxone use in such a study. El-Sobky et al (1976) demonstrated that naloxone has no effect on pain threshold/tolerance to electric shock in normal volunteers. A further significant factor in the results of the study of Zusman et al (1989) may be the comparison of reversal of pain relief by naloxone with that of a placebo, given the evidence of the

very real powers of placebos (see Rees 1987, pp. 47-48 for a summary). Even though the significance of opioid peptide concentrations in blood is not clear, Jones et al (1985) demonstrated significant changes in plasma levels during physiotherapeutic exercise and Zusman et al (1989) and other studies have shown that passive movement affords some relief in perceived pain (Hill 1981, Zusman et al 1989), even if its connection to the endogenous opioid system cannot be established.

Inhibition of reflex muscle spasm

The influence of mechanoreceptor input produced by passive movement on the regulation of muscle acting on local as well as distal joints is well documented (Freeman & Wyke 1967, Nade et al 1978). Passive movement may increase the range of movement and reduce perception of pain as a result of inhibition of reflex muscle contraction. Inhibition of reflex contraction about a joint is thought to reduce pain by the dispersion of irritative metabolites accumulated as a result of muscle ischaemia (Wyke 1976). Reduced pain may also be the result of a reduction in muscle tension on periarticular structures and myoaponeurotic peripheral afferent discharge (Grigg 1976).

Jull and Bogduk (1985) demonstrated that abnormal joint resistance or restricted passive range of movement is frequently associated with pain. When muscle spasm is also a factor in the presentation of a painful joint, treatment aimed at improving joint movement is likely to reduce the pain-induced muscle guarding and therefore facilitate normal function (Lewit 1985).

Hysteresis effect on neural discharge

Repeated movement at or to the end of range has been found to increase the natural resting angle of a joint as a result of stretching of periarticular soft tissue. The increase in range is the result of creep deformation occurring in the stretched tissues. In addition, a linear correlation has been observed between the reduction of joint afferent discharge and the relaxation of torque of the capsule when the joint is maintained at a given excitatory angle (Grigg & Greenspan 1977).

Following the onset of creep deformation, the level of discharge at a given position has been found to be substantially reduced or even absent. This phenomenon, known as the 'hysteresis effect', lasts up to 10 minutes and can be produced by sustained or oscillatory passive movements. The cessation of, or reduction in, neural discharge has been noted in large and small diameter joint afferents, including sensitized nociceptors (Schaible & Schmidt 1983b, Iggo et al 1984).

The findings by several authors (Clark 1975, Grigg & Greenspan 1977, Schaible & Schmidt 1983a, 1983b) strongly suggest that deformation by the capsule or other collagenous structures through which the axons pass is a natural stimulus for joint afferents. Zusman (1986) suggested that passive stretching of periarticular tissue with end of range movements may temporarily suppress the natural stimulus, thus reducing the level of joint afferent discharge. This principle can be seen in McKenzie's (1981) advocated management strategy of regular passive or active stretching to assist in the relief of intermittent chronic spinal pain.

Alteration to axoplasmic flow

In 1991, Butler (1991b) presented a plausible mechanism for the production of symptoms and/or a predisposition for the development of disorders at sites remote from that of an initial insult, of both neural and non-neural source, based on an explanation of the significance of axonal transport to the normal functioning of the nerve and its target tissue. While his ideas are still principally hypotheses, they are supported by extrapolation from the results of a number of studies. Axoplasm travels in both an antegrade and retrograde direction along the axon to and from its target tissue and is responsible for nutrition and optimal function of these structures partly as a result of the transmission of nerve growth factor which is responsible for the regulation and production of neuropeptides such as substance P and somatostaten (Otten 1984). Axoplasmic flow is altered by diseases such as diabetes, but also by compression and hypoxia, potentially leading to diminution of synaptic function, impairment of maintenance of the structure of the axon and loss of the chemical contacts between the cell body and the axon and target tissue.

Butler (1991b) suggested that treatment by passive movement may be responsible for alteration of impaired axoplasmic flow in the following ways:

- If the target tissue, e.g. joint or muscle, is treated so that its sensitivity is decreased, the energy demands of the non-neural tissues are decreased, allowing more energy for the axoplasmic flow (Korr 1985).
- Removal or alteration of physical constrictions around the nervous system, such as tightness of overlying muscles (e.g. scalenes) or restriction of joint movement (e.g. wrist stiffness associated with carpal tunnel syndrome), alteration of habitual posture may relieve both the physical constriction on the nervous system and associated hypoxia. Butler (1991b) also suggested that 'treatment of abnormal stresses or distortion of the sympathetic trunk, especially near sites of thoracolumbar outflow may well allow better intraneural circulation.'
- Mobilization of the nervous system, especially its connective tissue components, may alter abnormal elasticity and range of movement of the nervous system, theoretically leading to better nervous system mechanics and blood supply.

Butler (1991b) also discussed other methods of enhancement of axoplasmic flow and these, together with the detail of his presentation, are recommended reading. The concepts of sympathetic maintained pain syndromes and their relationship to adverse neural tension should also be understood by physiotherapists involved with athletes. The paper by Slater (1991) provides a good summary of the current position.

Mechanical mechanisms

Effects on intra-articular pressures

An intra-articular effusion or increased muscular or ligamentous tension on a joint capsule can result in high levels of intra-articular pressure as a result of altered levels of protein content in the synovial fluid, with the small molecules giving evidence of local ischaemia (Simkin 1991). This increased pressure can in turn lead to pain, limitation of joint movement and resultant reflex muscle inhibition and weakness (Levick 1983). Changes in joint position result in intra-articular pressure changes. Maximal pressures are recorded when a joint is fully flexed and further increases are found with an increase of speed of movement into flexion (Nade & Newbold 1983).

Initially, end range passive movements increase intra-articular pressure. However, a joint sustained in flexion or subjected to repeated through range movement will demonstrate diminished pressure levels at other joint angles (Nade & Newbold 1983). Such a reduction may be attributed to loss of fluid as the result of the high intra-articular pressures caused by flexion.

Following studies using CPM equipment, O'Driscoll et al (1983) found that movement increased the rate of clearance of blood from the knee joint. These authors postulated that a pumping effect would occur, facilitating the clearance of fluid (via the lymphatic system) and diffusible particles from the joint space into the interstitial tissues. If these results have been found following CPM, similar results are likely to be found following the application of intermittent passive movement in the form of mobilization. However, no research has yet been undertaken to demonstrate such effects.

In recent human studies, Giovanelli-Blacker et al (1985) demonstrated a reduction in human intra-articular pressure in posterior intervertebral joints following passive oscillatory movement carried to the end of range of joint movement. Grieve (1981) also proposed that a reduction of intra-articular effusion may decrease peripheral afferent discharge and thereby reduce pain perception by decompressing spinal nerves lying close to the joint capsule.

Reduction of joint locking in the vertebral column

Early treatment with high velocity thrusts may be recommended for the correction of an uncommon but intensely painful condition known as acute joint locking, vertebral locking or facet joint fixation (Grieve 1981, Maitland 1986).

A number of mechanisms for acute joint locking have been suggested. The early claims by Lewit (1978) and others that the cause was entrapment of intra-articular meniscoids have not been substantiated by anatomical evidence. Bogduk and Engel (1984) showed that connective tissue rim meniscoids were too short to become trapped between the joint surfaces and that the tension of surrounding soft tissue could protect them from being drawn into the cavity of the lumbar posterior intervertebral joints. Instead, they suggested a mechanism in which the apex of a fibro-adipose meniscoid could be torn from its base to form a loose body which could become trapped between the joint surfaces in the same way as a torn segment of meniscus in the knee. Entrapment of such a loose body would be likely to respond with immediate relief to manipulation. Bogduk and Engel, however, considered that some pathology of the invertebral disc may also be responsible for the acute locked back and that this mechanism should be investigated further.

Bogduk and Engel's work appears to provide the most definitive explanation at this stage. However, other causes of acute joint locking that have been proposed include nipping of synovial folds, as well as heightened intrafusal muscle activity as a result of capsular traction, producing instantaneous muscle spasm and ischaemic pain, as suggested by Droz-Georget (1980). In the latter case, the restriction of movement was attributed to an increase in gamma activity on the affected segments, causing hypertonicity of the segmental muscles which prevent joint movement in one direction but not in another. Korr (1975) suggested that manipulative therapy effects a decrease in gamma activity through its influence on the muscle spindle and the golgi tendon organ.

Whether a joint is locked as a result of entrapment of joint structures or 'blocked' by muscle spasm, a successful manipulative technique may have effect by inhibiting the muscle or freeing the trapped structure.

Reduction in pain following mobilization under joint compression

Reports in the literature related to the mechanisms of production of joint pain do not consider the situation of pain with movement under joint compression that is absent when the same movement is performed without compression. Although the mechanisms of this effect are as yet unknown and in fact do not seem to be considered by commentators in this field (e.g. Harvey 1987), some research into the effects of osteoarthrosis and osteoarthritis on joint structure may provide some indication. An excellent review of the mechanisms of pain production in osteoarthritis can be found in Marks (1992) and, if read with the concept of reproduction of pain under compression and its improvement following passive movement under compression, provides considerable potential support for the phenomenon. In his paper in 1985, Maitland referred to the work of Caterson and Lowther (1978) and Lowther (1979) in relation to the effect of agitation of synovial fluid (surface stirring) on the nutrition of articular cartilage. Lowther (1979) stated that research on movement of synovial fluid indicated that nutrition of articular cartilage was maintained by surface movement of synovial fluid without the necessity for concomitant loading of the joint surfaces. Other work appears to refute that argument, with evidence of articular cartilage damage related to both underloading and overloading (Muir 1988). Palmoski et al (1979) demonstrated that dogs whose foot was amputated and who were allowed to exercise but not bear weight demonstrated a decrease in the quantity and quality of proteoglycans synthesized. This evidence appears to suggest that an optimal amount of loading and unloading is necessary for adequate nutrition of articular cartilage and continued maintenance of its normal structure and function. However, a study by Houlbrooke et al (1990) indicated that movement without weightbearing or weightbearing without movement are both capable of maintaining the normal glycosaminoglycan (GAG) content of articular cartilage in normal sheep radiocarpal joints. Consequently, an improvement in joint mobility resulting from movement under compression could perhaps be explained on the basis of improved joint nutrition related to both the 'surface stirring' effect of Lowther and the sponge-like response of articular cartilage to intermittent compression. However, since articular cartilage is not innervated, this mechanism does not explain the reduction in pain associated with treatment. Indeed, Zusman (1986) highlighted strongly the lack of correlation between joint nutrition and production of or reduction in pain.

Radin and coworkers, in a number of studies, have reported on the relationship between the subchondral bone and articular cartilage in osteoarthrosis, a primary mechanical affliction of the joint, and osteoarthritis, a primary inflammatory affliction of the joint (e.g. Radin & Rose 1986). Primary osteoarthritis will always lead to a secondary osteoarthrosis and primary osteoarthrosis will eventually lead to a secondary arthritis as a result of an inflammatory synovial response to debris in the joint. Therefore, in the advanced state, both will be present and the mechanical and chemical effects may be indistinguishable. However, differentiation in the early stages may be relevant to the clinical picture of athletes with pain provoked on compression. Maitland (1985) referred to the patient with 'minor symptoms with compressive loads', the type of disorder most likely to be seen with a sporting injury. Such patients are unlikely to have developed the pathophysiological changes associated with arthritis, but may be demonstrating the early stages of a mechanical disorder, or arthrosis. Radin and Rose (1986) commented that progression of cartilage lesions probably requires stiffening of subchondral bone, the most likely cause of which is repeated failure of the musculoskeletal peak dynamic force attenuation mechanisms. Such failure may well result from repeated compressive insults or inappropriate muscular support around the joint during athletic activity.

Early osteoarthrosic change has been associated with an increase in intraosseous pressure in the subchondral bone, presumably as a result of venous stasis (e.g. Harrison et al 1953, Arnoldi et al 1966, 1972). In addition, infiltration of the deep layers of the articular cartilage by nutrient blood vessels from the subchondral bone has been demonstrated as an early sign of osteoarthrosis (Bullough & Jaqannath 1983, Radin et al 1991), although this observation is not universally accepted. The nutrient nerves relevant to blood vessels have been shown in other areas of the body to be sensitive to pressure-induced hypoxia (Sunderland 1976). The deep pain characteristic of osteoarthritis has been reproduced experimentally by injection of fluid under pressure into the vessels in the subchondral bone (Gardner 1950, Helal 1965, Phillips et al 1967). As mentioned by Marks (1992), Miller and Kasahara (1963) found small nerve fibres in the epiphyseal region of long bones adjacent to the articular cartilage and Reiman and Christensen (1977) showed that the number of unmyelinated nerve fibres in the subchondral bone marrow of osteoarthritic femoral heads was greater than in a group of control specimens. The nerves were also found in the calcified layer of articular cartilage. Compression of the articular surfaces of a joint with minor disruption of the normal mechanics of the subchondral bone/articular cartilage interface and increased venous pressure in vessels which have infiltrated the calcified layer of the articular cartilage may lead to hypoxia of the nutrient nerves, with the effects registered as pain.

Although strictly hypothetical, this mechanism may provide one possible explanation for production of pain with joint compression. Treatment of such a joint with mid-range movement under a controlled amount of intermittent compression may lead to a stimulation of blood flow in the subchondral vessels, decreasing the subchondral pressure and improving the oxygenation of the associated nerves, thereby leading to a reduction in pain. No studies have been attempted to test this hypothesis.

A second possible explanation for production of pain with mid-range movement under compression and its subsequent relief by treatment using the same mechanism may be related to the synovial membrane, a structure recently confirmed to be innervated (Gronblad et al 1988, Kidd et al 1990, Simkin 1991). Gronblad et al (1988) found neurofilaments immunoreactive for neuropeptides, including substance P, in areas adjacent to the blood vessels

of surgically removed osteoarthritic synovial tissues. Joint movement subjects the synovium to repetitive expansion and contraction (Simkin 1991), which, as a result of its close affiliation with the joint surfaces, is presumably not confined to movement at or near the limit of range. Simkin noted that 'the expansile capabilities of the synovium impose a severe challenge to the lubricating capabilities of synovial fluid'. Improved joint surface nutrition, as a result of passive movement and intermittent compression, may lead to improved nutrition of synovial tissue as well as articular cartilage, thereby reducing the irritative stimulation of the nerve endings within.

Psychological effects

There is no doubt that treatment by passive movement carries inherent psychological benefits through the 'laying on of hands'. This effect does not detract from possible neurophysiological, physiological and mechanical mechanisms of pain relief that may be provided by passive movement but rather is complementary to them.

A thorough examination, followed by an explanation of the reasons for the symptoms and how physiotherapy can help is effective in reducing anxiety and depression and the pain-fear cycle. Most patients, particularly athletes, are concerned, anxious or even fearful of their pain and its consequences in both the short and the long term. Reduction of this anxiety is likely to have a significant effect on the interpretation of symptoms.

Breaking the pain-fear cycle was thought to be a significant factor underlying the immediate and substantial improvement often reported following spinal manipulative therapy (Zusman 1986).

APPLICATION OF PASSIVE MOVEMENT TO TREATMENT

Analysis of movement diagrams

Passive movement techniques can be used as part of the management of most patients with symptoms arising from joints and their associated non-contractile soft tissues. They can also be used successfully to treat symptoms associated with disorders of the nervous system, both in the vertebral and foraminal canals and along the peripheral nervous system (Butler 1991a). As mentioned earlier, treatment of adverse tension in the sympathetic nervous system may also be addressed (Slater 1991). Continuous passive movement has also been shown to be beneficial for gaining range and improving recovery times following muscle tears (Stanton 1988) and for improving the status of articular cartilage following injury (Salter et al 1982b).

One view of selection of passive treatment techniques relates to the concept of treatment of signs and symptoms rather than diagnostic labels or alterations in normal biomechanics. Two patients with a particular diagnosis, for example adhesive capsulitis of the glenohumeral joint, may present with very different symptoms and signs depending on the stage of the pathology. One may present with severe pain but minimal loss of passive range while the other may have marked restriction of movement but minimal pain. If the treating therapist relied only on the diagnosis of adhesive capsulitis when selecting a treatment regime for these patients, clearly that treatment regime would be inappropriate for at least one of the two patients. If, however, the therapist based treatment on the degree of restriction of movement, the amount of pain and the irritability of the disorder, treatment would be different for both patients and therefore more likely to be effective. The symptoms associated with an early acute adhesive capsulitis i.e. severe pain in the joint with any attempt to move the arm but little passive restriction of movement, could also be associated with a different diagnosis e.g. acute subacromial bursitis. The pathological process and therefore the diagnosis is different, but the same set of treatment techniques may be appropriate for the patient with an acute bursitis as for one with early adhesive capsulitis.

Lack of a definite diagnosis does not necessarily restrict the use of passive movement in treatment. While basing the selection for treatment on the presenting signs and symptoms, understanding the underlying pathology and the effect it will have on the signs and symptoms is essential and will assist in prediction of the rate and amount of improvement that can be anticipated from treatment. Consequently, a process of clinical reasoning based on a sound knowledge of recognizable clinical patterns and interpretation of clues from both the subjective and physical examinations forms part of the process of determining the direction treatment should take. Such an approach to examination and management is provided in Jones (1992). With a reasoning approach, the appropriate patient for treatment with passive movement and the appropriate precautions and limitations for such treatment will be determined.

If the two patients' problems are addressed from a biomechanical perspective, similar problems may arise. Treatment directed at altered biomechanics may be appropriate for the stiff, non-painful situation, but not for the patient with severe pain but minimal restriction of movement. Such treatment would be likely to exacerbate this patient's symptoms considerably. However, while the normal biomechanics of the situation may not specifically direct selection of a treatment technique, restoration of normal biomechanics is one of the overall goals of any treatment program for neuromusculoskeletal disorders and should be addressed during management.

Treatment based on the signs and symptoms in this way can be effective even when the precise diagnosis is not known, as the strength of application of a passive technique, the length of time it is applied and the number of times it is repeated are determined by the therapist's assessment of severity and irritability of the pain, the degree of pain provoked during the technique and the response immediately following application of the technique. The concept of 'irritability' relates to the ease of exacerbation of symptoms, the severity of the symptoms provoked and the length of time before they subside. Irritability represents a continuum from the very irritable condition, aggravated by minimal movement, with severe pain taking hours to settle, to the non-irritable condition, where minor discomfort occurs only following extended strenuous activity and disappears immediately the provoking activity is stopped. Understanding the concept of irritability helps the therapist gauge the depth and amount of mobilization that can be used in treatment without provocation of symptoms.

Provided the therapist makes the correct decision about a technique directed into or short of reproduction of pain, the treatment should always be safe, even in the absence of a definitive diagnosis. However, the more that becomes known about the relationship between signs and symptoms and their underlying mechanical and chemical basis and, therefore, the more precise diagnosis can become, the more treatment can be associated directly with particular diagnoses.

If the principle of selection of treatment techniques on the basis of signs and symptoms is accepted, a reliable way to select appropriate techniques must be established in order to protect the patient from inappropriate, particularly forceful, treatment. Maitland (1969) presented a concept of selection of treatment technique, basing it on the relationship between pain and joint resistance. This concept was taken further and applied to analysis of a movement diagram drawn of the most positive passive movement found during examination (Magarey 1985, 1986b, Maitland 1986). This concept will be outlined briefly below, but is presented in more detail in the references cited.

A movement diagram is simply a pictorial representation of a movement on which factors encountered during that movement are recorded and their relationship to each other demonstrated. Pain, resistance to movement and muscle spasm are the most common factors represented, but other factors may also be shown. When a therapist analyses the feel of movement of a structure and its relation to production of symptoms and bases treatment selection on that analysis, the techniques chosen have a greater chance of success than if treatment techniques are selected on the basis of an ad hoc decision (Magarey 1985).

A more recent expansion of the concept of treatment of pain or stiffness was made by Butler (1991a, pp. 185-220), in which he related the selection of pain and stiffness to the underlying mechanisms of production. On this basis, the more the presenting features are dominated by pain, the more inflammation is present and therefore the physiological aspects of the affected structures are involved. Dominance of stiffness, whether of joint or other tissue, indicates a more mechanical involvement of the affected tissue. Consequently, Butler (1991a, p. 188) advocated selection of treatment technique on the basis of dominance of pathophysiological or pathomechanical response. While Butler was referring specifically to the nervous system, the concept applies equally to other structures. This concept in no way alters that of Maitland, but attempts to move Maitland's original concept closer to the current understanding of pathophysiology and pathomechanics.

A basic understanding of the concept of grades of movement is essential prior to any attempt to analyse movement diagrams. While detailed description of the mechanics of drawing a movement diagram is inappropriate in this chapter, it can be found in Magarey (1986a) and Maitland (1986, 1991).

Grades of movement

The original concept of grades of movement is shown in Figure 12.4 (Maitland 1991). This presentation relied on the presence of an endfeel to movement that could be represented on a diagram as a vertical line—i.e. no resistance occurring until the limit is reached. However, even joints with a bony block endfeel (as in elbow extension) display a small amount of extra range where the components of the joint can be moved through a degree of ligamentous resistance. Consequently, in practice, manual therapists frequently referred to grades such as a III- or IV+, which, according to Maitland's definitions, could not exist. Clearly this was not the case, so the original concept was modified to relate it more closely to the true feel of joint movement (Magarey 1985, 1986a, Maitland 1986).

In this modification, grades were related to the presence and degree of resistance to movement, that is, a non-vertical R1-R2 line. For the sake of uniformity of definition, a movement up to the onset of joint resistance was termed a grade IV-- or III--, depending on the amplitude of the movement, while the amount of resistance considered appropriate for a normal joint to withstand was a grade IV++ or III++. Consequently, a grade IV is halfway between a grade IV-- and a grade IV++ (that is, at 50% of the maximum resistance possible in a normal joint). Therefore, grades I and II are unchanged in definition, except with the clarification that a grade II is a large amplitude movement in the resistance-free part of the range. A grade

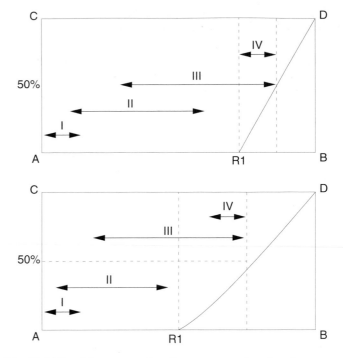

Fig. 12.5 Pictorial representation of new concept of grades of movement. A: Where R1 is close to the end of range. B: Where R1 is a long way from the end of range

I is a small amplitude movement at the beginning of range. Grades III and IV must be redefined to incorporate the concept of movement into joint resistance, with the amount of resistance determined by the addition of + or - signs as appropriate, with a grade III a large amplitude and grade IV, a small amplitude movement, both reaching the same point in range. Consequently, if resistance to movement is felt only near the end of range, the different range at which a grade IV-, a grade IV or a grade IV+ is performed may be very small (Fig. 12.5a). However, if resistance to movement is felt early in range, a grade IV movement may only reach mid-range, and the difference in the point in range at which a grade IV-, a grade IV or a grade IV+ is performed may be much greater (Fig. 12.5b). While the original concept was based on movement predominantly of joint structures, the same principles can equally be applied to movement of the nervous system, with joint resistance replaced by resistance of neural and associated connective tissues.

Selection of treatment based on analysis of movement diagrams

Manual passive movement techniques have an advantage over active movements in many situations, as depth, strength and duration are all directly controlled by the therapist who can also feel the quality of movement and any changes to the quality of movement while performing the technique. The choice of technique is determined in part by symmetry of signs and symptoms, structures

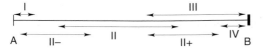

Fig. 12.4 Grades of movement. Source: Maitland (1986)

involved in the disorder and any known pathology (e.g. weakened ligamentous structures, spondylolisthesis).

Two extremes exist, one in which pain is the most significant factor with little or no joint stiffness, therefore with a dominance of pathophysiological response, and the other in which movement is limited by stiffness with no pain, a pathomechanical response. However, the more common presentations include a combination of pain and stiffness in varying degrees.

Treatment of pain

If pain is the dominant feature of a condition, it will be represented on a movement diagram as the limiting factor and movement may be stopped before resistance is encountered. Patients in this category have a disorder which is irritable and causing severe pain, often present at rest. Athletes with acute injuries often fall into this category. In this situation, the affected structure should be placed in its most comfortable position and treatment should be directed at reduction of pain, performed in such a way that it provokes neither pain or discomfort. The initial movement chosen should be performed slowly and smoothly, through as large an amplitude as possible without production of discomfort.

The initial choice of technique is determined partly by factors such as the structures affected, the area of the body, the symmetry of the signs and symptoms, and the pathology, if known (see Magarey 1986b, p. 664). Once those factors have been considered, the final choice is made on the basis of the movement which can be performed through the maximum range of movement without provocation of symptoms. The particular technique can be determined by analysis of the movement diagrams of the most likely movements (Magarey 1985, 1986b, p. 666). For example, if left C2/3 posterior intervertebral joint pain were provoked by both unilateral postero-anterior pressures over the left articular pillar of C2 and cervical rotation to the right, the most appropriate choice of technique would depend on which movement was more restricted by pain. Either technique would be appropriate for treatment of a left C2/3 posterior intervertebral joint problem.

In the spine, the first choice is likely to be an accessory or physiological movement performed in such a way that it does not compress the affected joint or narrow the intervertebral foramen. In the peripheral joints, the first choice is an accessory movement or shaft rotation (about the long axis of the bone forming the distal component of the joint). In relation to the nervous system, treatment of pain may involve movement of a part of the body remote from the site of symptoms, again with the symptomatic part as comfortable as possible, preferably in a tension-relieving position. For example, cervical symptoms of neural origin may be treated with the cervical spine resting in neutral flexion/extension, with the trunk in neutral or slight extension and treatment consisting of through range dorsiflexion/plantarflexion of the ankle, with no provocation of pain or discomfort (Butler 1991a).

As the pain settles, the treatment technique should be progressed according to changes in the movement diagram of the principal passive movement sign. The progression may consist of use of the same accessory movement in a different physiological position, changing the direction of the accessory movement, using a physiological movement and progressing by using the movement in a different part of the range. For example, if the initial treatment for an acute sprain of the C2/3 posterior intervertebral joint were unilateral postero-anterior pressures over the articular pillar of C2, progression may be performance of the same unilateral postero-anterior pressures, but with the cervical spine in a degree of ipsilateral rotation. If the initial technique for a very painful patellofemoral joint was distraction of the patella with the tibiofemoral joint in a neutral position between flexion and extension, progression to a medial glide may be appropriate, with later progression of the same accessory technique, performed with the tibiofemoral joint in a degree of flexion. Progression of the neural example presented above might be continuation of the same technique, but with the leg in a degree of straight leg raise.

When the aim of treatment is still reduction of pain, the choice of the new technique should be based on that which can be performed through the largest range without provoking pain. The rate of progression depends on the severity and irritability of the disorder and the underlying pathology, if known. If the pain is severe and unaltered by the first technique of choice, the next choice may be a different movement performed without resistance rather than progression of the first into pain.

Treatment of stiffness

When choosing a technique to treat stiffness in the absence of pain, a pathomechanical disorder, techniques which stretch the tight structures are necessary. These may include accessory movements and/or physiological movements at the end of range, or a combination of both. All movements of the affected joint are likely to be stiff and so a single treatment may include a number of different techniques all aimed at stretching stiff structures, since pain is not a component of the problem. The movement or combination of movements chosen with the greatest restriction of range should be the first choice of treatment and will again be determined by analysis of movement diagrams drawn for each of the movements. In this situation, use of more than one technique within a single treatment session is often appropriate, the intention of each technique being to increase range. In relation to restriction of movement of the nervous system, techniques are applied at end of range, often in a tension-provoking position such as the slump (Maitland 1978, 1979). When using forceful techniques directed at the nervous system, treatment should always be preceded and followed by examination of neurological status, which should be normal or unchanged from previous assessment.

Care should be taken with the spine, particularly when using techniques which narrow the intervertebral foramina, to avoid compression of the structures within them. No technique should be used that causes symptoms of compression of the spinal cord, cauda equina, vertebrobasilar or carotid arteries or that puts sufficient stress on the intervertebral discs to cause them to rupture or prolapse.

Treatment of pain and stiffness

Most neuromusculoskeletal problems have components of pain and stiffness and therefore the choice of treatment depends predominantly on analysis of the movement diagram of the principal passive movement to determine the dominant feature. In general, if the limiting factor is pain and pain begins much earlier in range than resistance, treatment should initially be directed at decreasing pain as described previously. For example, in the movement diagram represented in Figure 12.6a, pain begins at approximately one quarter of normal range and P2 is the limiting factor, described as severe and irritable. Resistance

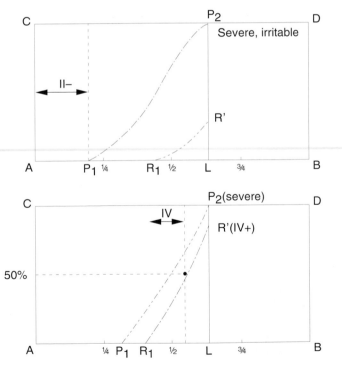

Fig. 12.6 A movement diagram representing a severely painful joint with minimal tissue resistance detectable during the available movement. The appropriate treatment technique, G=grade II-, is indicated

does not start until after half range, at which point the pain is already at 50% of maximum, and only increases to approximately 25% of maximum, or a IV-, at the limit. Clearly, pain is the dominant feature of the movement diagram and treatment should be directed at relief of that pain. The technique of choice is a large amplitude movement short of the onset of pain (P1).

When pain is minimal prior to the onset and initial increase of resistance and then follows a behaviour similar to that of resistance, techniques need to be directed into resistance in order to change the pain. When both pain and resistance change in a similar manner either early or late in range, treatment techniques short of the onset of pain are unlikely to change the pain-stiffness relationship. Therefore, treatment techniques which move into resistance respecting pain should be selected as demonstrated in Figure 12.6b (Magarey 1985, 1986b). The degree of pain the therapist may be prepared to provoke depends partly on the analysis of the movement diagram and partly on the irritability of the disorder. The greater the degree of pain at the limit of range and the more rapidly pain increases through range, the less pain should be provoked during treatment. If the disorder is irritable, provocation of symptoms must be minimal unless long-term benefit can be shown to be worth a short-term exacerbation.

When the limiting factor to further movement is resistance not pain, the dominant feature of the movement diagram is usually stiffness and treatment should be directed towards increasing range. However, since a degree of pain is present, the strength and amount of treatment cannot be the same as in the situation where stiffness is present without pain. The amount of resistance into which the technique is taken is determined by the amount of pain the therapist is prepared to provoke. The factors which will determine the intensity of pain are the same as those outlined above, that is, the greater the pain at the limit and the more rapidly pain increases through range, the less pain should be provoked during treatment. However, treatment must be directed into resistance if it is to be effective in increasing range (Figs 12.7a and 12.7b).

A third situation associated with the relationship between pain and stiffness frequently arises when treating athletes. The athlete presents with a condition which gives severe pain, but only when certain very specific positions or movements are performed. Often, active reproduction of the symptoms in the clinic is difficult as the force or speed involved in provocation cannot easily be replicated. When the involved joint is examined passively, a movement can often be found that is limited by sharp, severe pain only present in the last few degrees of range, so that R' is close to a Grade IV++. This pain is described as a 'bite', a description often used by the patient (Fig. 12.8). The involved movement may consist of a combination of a physiological and an associated accessory movement. The

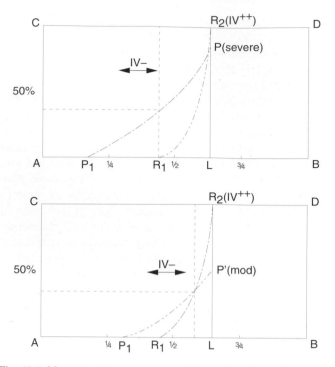

Fig. 12.7 Movement diagrams representing two situations where tissue resistance is the dominant feature of the movement, with a contribution of pain. A: Pain is severe at the limit of range and at the onset of resistance, pain is already at approximately 30% of maximum. Consequently, a technique to the onset of resistance, Grade IV —, is appropriate. B: Pain is moderate at the limit of range and to provoke the equivalent amount of pain, the movement can be taken into more resistance. Consequently, a technique into approximately 30% of resistance, Grade IV-, is appropriate

presentation of a bite of pain on the movement diagram is characteristic and treatment will not be effective unless specifically directed at alteration of the bite.

In this situation, mobilization before the onset of bite or joint resistance will clearly be ineffective, but treatment into resistance immediately causes exacerbation of severe pain. Oscillatory mobilization into pain usually leads to muscle spasm or voluntary holding by the patient who is unable to tolerate movement into such a rapidly provoked and severe pain. Treatment will be more effective if the movement is taken slowly into range to a point just before the final rapid increase of pain to the limit (commonly referred to as 'bite minus'), usually into approximately a grade IV to IV+ resistance, held in that position for a few seconds while the patient becomes accustomed to the pain and is able to relax. It is then taken as close to P2 as the patient can tolerate, as a single movement which is then released slowly back to the point of bite minus. At this point, the patient can recover from the intensity of the pain provoked before a further movement into bite is performed. If the technique is performed in this way, movement can be taken into that part of the range where both the pain and joint resistance can be altered with the co-operation and confidence of the patient who can tell by the handling

that the therapist is able to relate to the intensity of the symptoms provoked. An oscillatory technique, however, is likely to be ineffective as it will not reach end of range because of the protective muscle spasm. An essential component of treatment into pain in this manner is good communication between therapist and patient, so that the patient has confidence in the handling by the therapist and is therefore able to allow the affected joint to be moved into a position which provokes such intense pain.

Treatment of symptoms provoked by joint compression

As discussed earlier, the mechanism responsible for production of pain with mid-range movement during the application of compression perpendicular to the joint surfaces is unclear. However, pain present during mid-range movement with compression of joint surfaces, but absent when the same movement is performed without joint compression, is a phenomenon seen in the physiotherapy clinic.

The patient who tends to demonstrate this phenomenon usually presents with an aching joint, with no specific movement painful or restricted. Symptoms are frequently aggravated by weightbearing and may follow a compression-type injury. In the early stages, pain may be worsened by distraction in addition to compression, but as it settles the only movement able to provoke the symptoms becomes one associated with joint compression.

Treatment should follow the same principles as outlined above, with the only exception related to the direction of progression. If the pain is severe, the first choice of treatment may involve distraction of the joint surfaces, performed with no provocation of discomfort. Progression of this technique may be an increase in grade, then speed and vigour until a sharp grade III+ is tolerated with no exacerbation of symptoms. Further progression would involve the physiological movement most closely associated with the aggravating activity and the strength of technique used for the initial changeover would revert to a slow, smooth, through range movement—i.e. progression in one com-

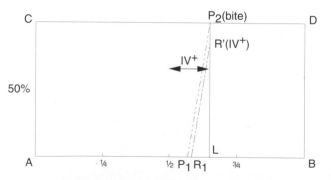

Fig. 12.8 A movement diagram representing a 'bite' of pain with movement and the appropriate treatment technique, Grade IV+

ponent, in this case the movement, should be associated with a temporary regression in another, the vigour. Progression from this point would involve gradual addition of compression through the joint surfaces during movement through range. In lower limb disorders, the final stages of treatment may involve controlled movement in a weight-bearing position, as reproduction by the therapist of the compression force generated by weightbearing is frequently impossible.

Practical application

Acute phase

In the acute phase, the athlete must be informed that he or she has a major role in the success of the treatment by taking the responsibility to report any hint of discomfort with passive movement techniques. No benefit to tissue healing will be gained (in fact the effect may be detrimental) if the athlete allows the therapist to take the movement into pain. In this situation, continued communication between the therapist and patient, Maitland's 'talking to the joint', is essential to monitor the symptoms and adapt rapidly to an increase in discomfort. The movement should be performed very slowly through the maximum painfree range possible, either as a physiological movement in the direction of the injuring movement or an accessory movement associated with the direction of injury. For example, hindfoot plantarflexion/inversion or a postero-anterior glide would be appropriate choices in an acute inversion sprain of the ankle (Fig. 12.9).

Using the example of an inversion sprain of the ankle, the movement would be taken from a position of slight ankle dorsiflexion/eversion and moved smoothly and slowly towards plantarflexion/inversion without provoking any discomfort. This movement is continued for 2-3 minutes during which time, providing there is no increase in the resting ache, the movement is taken slightly further to determine the limit of the painfree range. The technique may be applied while ice and elevation are incorporated, between icing sessions or even with the compression applied, provided it is not restricting the movement or confusing the patient's interpretation of discomfort related to the technique. This movement provides minimal stretching of all the injured structures and should be performed one or two times a day by an educated family member, followed by 2-hourly active movement with the ankle in an ice bath. Gradually the range through which the movement can be taken will increase.

Avoidance of any adverse reaction to mobilization is important. Any latent symptoms of increased resting ache or throbbing indicate that the treatment was performed either for too long or into too great a depth and must therefore be modified, not discarded. If, however, exacer-

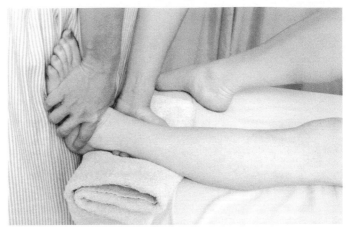

Fig. 12.9 Postero-anterior glide of the talus in the mortise

bation continues, even following modification of the technique to the most gentle, small amplitude painfree technique possible, treatment should be discontinued, as the tissues are indicating a degree of inflammation that is better suited to rest than to movement.

Acute muscle tears may be treated in a similar manner, using continuous passive motion. The commercially available continuous passive motion machines may be used with the athlete positioned so that the muscle being treated may be progressively lengthened as the painfree range increases. If a continuous passive motion machine is not available, a similar effect can be gained by intermittent passive mobilization performed in a way equivalent to that produced by the machine. In this situation, frequent treatment as advocated for the acute sprained ankle by an educated family member is ideal. In addition, active through range movement using the antagonists can also assist relaxation of the injured muscle.

A thorough assessment to determine relative involvement of the gastrocnemius and soleus in a calf tear will enable the therapist to be more specific with the starting position for treatment, thereby making treatment more effective. With biarticular muscles, such as the gastrocnemius and the hamstring group, experience has shown that a more rapid recovery of range is achieved by placing the muscle on stretch over one joint and moving it over the other. For example, with a mid-belly hamstring tear, the patient may be seated, that is, the hip flexed to 90°, and passive movement of the knee through flexion/extension performed. Similarly, for a mid-belly gastrocnemius strain, the knee should be extended and the movement of dorsiflexion/plantarflexion added. However, if the gastrocnemius strain is in the proximal part of the muscle, the patient may regain range more quickly if the foot is positioned in dorsiflexion and then gentle knee extension is applied as a passive movement.

In the initial 48 hours, treatment should also incorporate intermittent application of ice and elevation. Once full and

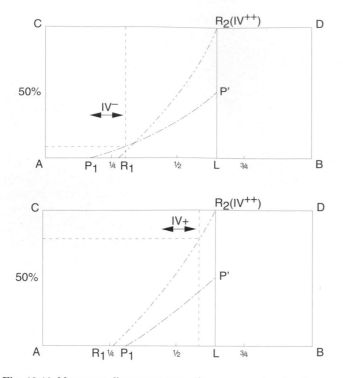

Fig. 12.10 Movement diagrams representing a progressive situation where the relationship between pain and resistance changes and the appropriate treatment technique changes. A: P1 occurs before R1, with approximately 20% of pain provoked by movement into a Grade IV-. B: P1 beyond R1 with considerably more movement into resistance available before significant provocation of pain. Consequently, a technique into considerable resistance is appropriate, as still less than 50% of pain is provoked

painfree range is regained, more active treatment including hydrotherapy and graduated exercise programs may be commenced while healing is enhanced with local massage and electrotherapy modalities to further increase circulation.

An example of an athlete with a severe problem assessed as related predominantly to neural involvement is that of a footballer injured during a tackle, in which his arm was forced into abduction/extension in conjunction with elbow extension, giving severe anterior arm pain. Examination reveals pain in the position of injury, increased with the addition of either contralateral cervical lateral flexion or wrist extension. Treatment with gentle through range wrist extension with the arm in the tension-relieving position of neutral shoulder flexion/extension and abduction/adduction and elbow flexion, should be performed with no exacerbation of anterior arm pain. As with injuries with predominant involvement of non-neural tissues, intermittent application of ice is likely to enhance the treatment.

Subacute phase

Treatment techniques should be progressed according to changes in the movement diagram. How far into range the techniques of progression can be safely taken depends on analysis of the movement diagrams. As long as the diagram is dominated by pain, treatment must have a strong bias towards alteration of that pain. However, if the relationship between pain and resistance alters such that the onset of pain and resistance are close and the two components behave in a similar manner, the assumption can be made that they are related, and treatment into a little resistance in order to alter the pain behaviour may be necessary (Fig. 12.10a and b). The amount of resistance will depend on the pain response; since pain is still dominant, treatment should not lead to significant provocation. However, the disorder is likely to be less irritable and progression can therefore be faster than in the early stages.

Again using the example of an inversion sprain of the ankle, treatment may be progressed by moving further into the range of plantarflexion/inversion as pain settles or it may be augmented by the addition of an accessory movement, e.g. antero-posterior glide of the talus in the ankle mortise, short of pain, with the aim of improving range of dorsiflexion (Fig.12.11).

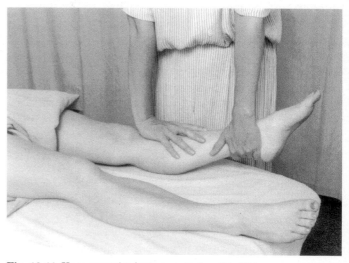

Fig. 12.11 Knee extension/antero-posterior glide IV+

A second example is one of a painful shoulder, where the first choice in the acute stage may have been gentle distraction in the line of the humerus or postero-anterior glides on the head of the humerus with the shoulder positioned in neutral between flexion and extension, abduction and adduction and medial and lateral rotation. As symptoms allow, the therapist may choose to progress this treatment using the same distraction or postero-anterior glides at a larger grade with the arm in slight (e.g. 45°) abduction. An alternative progression would be a physiological movement into flexion or abduction or shaft rotation as a grade II short of any discomfort. In subsequent treatment sessions, these techniques can all be progressed further into range, at a rate determined by analysis of the diagram drawn of the affected movement. At each stage, response to treatment is monitored by assessment of the functional limitations of the athlete and his/her tolerance of the technique, in addition to analysis of the passive movement signs.

Progression of treatment for the footballer with anterior arm pain of neural origin might be performance of the same movement, i.e. wrist extension through range, but with a degree of shoulder girdle depression maintained during the technique. The degree of tension within the system is increased slightly, but the dominant component affected in the injury is still not incorporated.

Treatment of pain and stiffness (increasing dominance of pathomechanics)

As discussed above, the type of approach to treatment depends on the relationship between pain and stiffness as determined by analysis of the diagram of the most positive passive movement. If the dominant feature is stiffness, to be effective, treatment must be directed at its alteration. Therefore, the techniques chosen involve a degree of stretching into resistance in the direction of restriction. How firmly the movement can be stretched and how quickly progressed depends on the amount of pain associated with the movement and its irritability and an understanding of the status of the tissues and their normal biomechanical properties. The more pain is present, the more treatment must be restricted and that pain respected.

An example of the situation where stiffness is dominant but the intensity of pain at the limit is high and P1 occurs before R1 could be that of a knee following a medial collateral ligament strain, with a residual painful restriction of the combined movement of extension/antero-posterior glide (Fig. 12.10a). In this situation, a technique into a grade IV-, that is, into 25% of resistance, provokes approximately 20% of associated pain. Initially, the therapist should not provoke more pain until the response to the movement is known. Treatment of extension/antero-posterior glide at grade IV- should lead to a reduction of pain up to that point in range, and possibly a shift in R1 closer to the limit. As the pain decreases or its onset becomes later in range, movement can be taken into more resistance without provocation of significantly more pain (Fig. 12.10b) until the relationship between resistance and pain changes such that resistance is more dominant and pain is minimal. Treatment can become quite forceful with minimal pain.

If treatment into pain leaves the treated structure with a degree of soreness, this can be reduced by the immediate application of the same treatment technique performed as a large amplitude movement to a point in range just short of that to which the stretching movement was applied. The more pain provoked during the stretching technique, the greater the need for use of an 'easing-off' technique in this manner. For example, if the knee had been stretched into

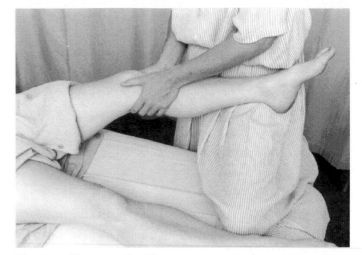

Fig. 12.12 Knee extension III

extension/antero-posterior glide as a grade IV+ (Fig. 12.11), the easing-off technique would be extension, performed as a grade III (Fig. 12.12), initially slowly and rhythmically, gradually increasing the speed and the grade until the movement can be performed quickly through the available range without soreness (Figs 12.13 and 12.14).

At all times, assessment of the functional limitations of the athlete, in addition to assessment of the passive movements, determines progression of treatment. If the analysis of the passive movement signs has been correct, improvement in these signs will be reflected in improvement in the functional activities. However, as a result of the high demands of athletes on their bodies, they may not recognize functional progress until the passive signs have improved to a far greater extent than might be anticipated to be necessary. As the pain settles and range is regained, the athlete must incorporate dynamic rehabilitation progressing

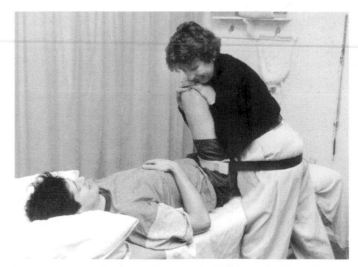

Fig. 12.13 Hip technique making use of a belt. Lateral glide applied at the limit of hip flexion/adduction. Technique can be modified to include longitudinal caudal glide.

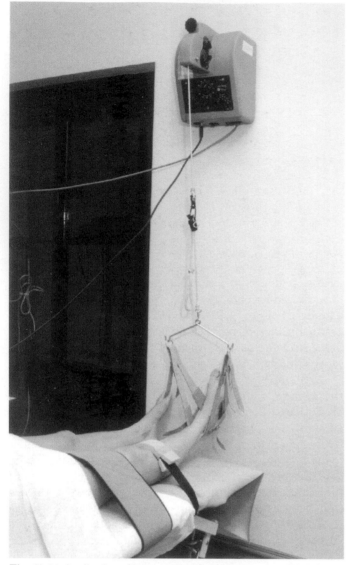

Fig. 12.14 Application of knee extension/antero-posterior glide with a Tru-trac Intermittent Traction Unit

to functional retraining into the treatment program, so that correct neuromuscular patterning, strength and endurance are regained before return to sport.

An example of a situation where treatment into bite is necessary is that of a chronic medial collateral ligament strain of the knee. The athlete presents with a complaint of recurrent episodes of partial giving way without any associated pain. Assessment of functional activities, such as running, cutting and turning does not reproduce the symptoms, but a combination of passive abduction/lateral rotation of the tibiofemoral joint in a position of approximately 30° of flexion provokes a bite of pain and is slightly restricted in range when compared with the unaffected knee. Treatment of the bite as described above would be appropriate. Repeat of this technique three or four times without release from the position of partial stretch at bite minus should be followed by a prolonged session of

easing-off grade III lateral rotation in slight abduction and 30° of flexion to settle any soreness created by the technique. Since immediate functional reassessment is not possible, as the pain could not be provoked actively, reassessment must rely on a reappraisal of the movement diagram of abduction/lateral rotation of the tibiofemoral joint in 30° of flexion. If the treatment has been effective, the range of movement may have increased, the degree of bite at the limit may have decreased or the onset of the bite may be later in range. Clearly, when the abnormality only occurs in the final 2-3° of movement, appreciation of such subtle changes requires critical, fine handling. Assessment of functional improvement can be made between treatment sessions.

If the situation were such that an active movement could be found that reproduced a bite of pain, e.g. end range dorsiflexion in weightbearing, an exercise similar to the mobilizing technique should be taught and implemented at home. Maitland (1991) advocated performance of the same movement, in this example dorsiflexion in weightbearing, as a maximal active-assisted stretch. After sustaining the position until the discomfort starts to subside, the athlete attempts to maintain the position actively. For example, following sustained dorsiflexion in weightbearing, the athlete dorsiflexes the great toe, then the whole foot, and attempts to maintain the range gained by the mobilization as the foot is lifted away from the support. Such an approach to treatment provides good improvement in a functional activity in which a bite occurs or in which pain inhibition leads to functional instability. In conjunction with this approach, strength, endurance, proprioceptive and functional retraining must be given to enable the athlete to use the new range optimally.

Stiffness or loss of range not associated with pain (dominance of pathomechanics)

Treatment of athletes for stiffness without associated pain are few and are usually restricted to the following situations:

- Treatment following immobilization in a plaster or hexalite cast, e.g. following fracture or ligament repair. However, the use of limited motion braces and casts reduces the necessity for this type of treatment.
- Mobilization of stiff but asymptomatic spinal segments to enable better function of adjacent structures. For example, restriction in thoracic extension tends to lead to inadequate rotation of the scapulae with poor positioning of the glenoid, leading to an increased potential for subacromial impingement. Mobilization of the thoracic spine into extension provides better positioning of the scapulae and a potential decrease in stress in the subacromial space. A second example is one of a cricket bowler who requires maximal extension of the trunk to

achieve the desired bowling technique. This movement may be mobilized to provide greater than normal range to facilitate attainment of optimal bowling technique.

- Mobilization of peripheral joints to achieve positions required by the sport which are beyond the normal range of the athlete, e.g. stretching abduction/lateral rotation of the hip in a gymnast to assist in achievement of floor routines; increasing talocrural plantarflexion to improve the 'pointe' position of a dancer; increasing hip flexion in a rower to enable attainment of the optimal position at the catch phase of the stroke without the need for additional lumbosacral flexion; stretching tight muscle and capsular structures in the shoulder if these are preventing a swimmer or thrower achieving optimal technique.
- Mobilization of tight neural structures which prevent the athlete achieving optimal technique, e.g. mobilization of knee extension in the slump position in a hockey player to enhance the ability to trap and run with the ball on artificial surfaces.

Treatment techniques include strong accessory glides at the limit of a physiological movement, for example, antero-posterior glides at the limit of dorsiflexion with variations in the direction of pressure dependent on the most restricted direction of the accessory movement. Treatment of a hip with restricted range of flexion can often be better achieved by the use of belts. The hip is a large strong joint and any change in its range is likely to take a considerable force over a long period of time. A belt tucked into the groin of the patient and around the pelvis of the therapist can provide excellent mechanical advantage to the therapist. The hip is then held at the limit of flexion, while a longitudinal or lateral glide is applied to the joint by pressure of the therapist's body against the belt in the appropriate direction (Fig. 12.13). A similar and extremely effective technique for stiff peripheral joints is intermittent variable traction, used in the same way as the mobilizing technique. For example, a stiff knee following immobilization may be positioned with a strap restraining the lower thigh, a support around the ankle and foot attached to the traction machine and a strap restraining the tibial plateau. The traction force is applied so that the foot is lifted vertically, thus providing an extension/AP mobilization of the knee. With a little ingenuity, similar techniques can be found for other joints. A surprisingly high traction force can be applied to peripheral joints without provocation of any discomfort (Fig. 12.6). Use of a traction device in this manner allows for periods of sustained stretch with intermittent short periods of rest, allowing for a creep effect in the tissues, similar to that described for the lumbar spine (Twomey & Taylor 1982, McGill & Brown 1992) and therefore enhancing the effect of the stretch.

Pain provoked by compression through the joint surfaces

An example of this situation is a netball player with a history of recurrent ankle sprains resulting in minor structural instability of the ankle. Following intensive training on an asphalt court, a particularly hard and unforgiving surface, the netballer develops a deep ache in the ankle. The ache is constant, aggravated by standing, walking and running and partially relieved by gentle shaking of the foot.

Initial treatment consists of distraction of the talocrural joint, short of exacerbation of the ache, following which a dramatic reduction in the constant ache is noted. Treatment progresses rapidly until a grade III+ distraction can be performed on the ankle with no discomfort and the patient only develops the ache following a game or training on the asphalt. Treatment is changed to mid-range plantarflexion/dorsiflexion, initially with no compression, but later with the addition of gradually increasing amounts of compression until the ankle is symptom-free.

Clearly, a stretching technique is inappropriate for this patient as a degree of structural instability is present and end-range movements are only mildly symptomatic, with insufficient changes relative to the degree of symptoms. However, as a result of the structural laxity, a program of proprioceptive rehabilitation, eccentric control and stabilization is instituted once the effect of the passive treatment is determined.

SUMMARY

In this chapter, we have examined the role of passive movement in the management of sporting injuries. Passive movement can be used in all phases of rehabilitation, and if passive techniques are selected in the manner suggested and analysis of movement diagrams used continually to monitor changes, particularly in the relationships between pain and stiffness, the effect of treatment on the structures involved should be optimal.

The appropriate use of passive movement in the ways outlined will be enhanced with continual critical evaluation of the effects of such management. Continuing clinical reasoning throughout management of a patient is essential if treatment is to be progressed appropriately. Experience and a degree of reflection on the responses achieved with each patient seen will assist in enhancing knowledge of appropriate treatment techniques in different situations and where particular approaches varying from the model described are more effective. Modifications to the therapist's knowledge of clinical patterns as they relate to athletes will be made on the basis of such reflective thinking.

The benefit of manual therapy is the ability of the physiotherapist to continually and immediately adapt to the presenting situation by changing the depth, speed or direction of movement while constantly communicating with the injured athlete and monitoring the effect of the treatment. This approach not only helps to develop the confidence of athletes in the therapist, as the therapist is seen to alter the pain with his/her hands, but also includes them actively in the treatment and provides them with a better understanding of the injury and therefore more confidence in the outcome of the management and more willingness to comply with associated dynamic management strategies.

While reference has been made to very specific structures in terms of passive mobilization techniques, the fact that this type of treatment forms only part of the total treatment of the athlete must be remembered. Coincidental to the passive treatment regime should be a strengthening and technique re-education program to enable the athlete to optimally use the increased range of movement. In addition, attention to contributing factors extrinsic to the area of symptoms and a reconditioning program are essential components of the management of the athlete.

REFERENCES

Akeson W H, Amiel D, Woo S L 1987 Physiology and therapeutic value of passive motion. In: Helminen H J, Kiviranta I, Tammi M, Saamananen A-M, Paukkonen K, Jurvelin J (eds) Joint loading: biology and health or articular structures. Wright, Bristol, ch 15, pp 375–411

Andersen H T, Korner L, Landgren S, Silfvenius H 1967 Fibre components and cortical projections of the elbow joint nerve in the cat. Acta Physiologica Scandinavica 69:373–385

Arnoldi C C, Lempberg R K, Linderholm H 1966 Intraosseous hypertension and pain in the knee. Journal of Bone and Joint Surgery 48B:280–288

Arnoldi C C, Linderholm H, Mussbichler H 1972 Venous engorgement and intraosseous hypertension in osteoarthritis of the hip. Journal of Bone and Joint Surgery 54B:409–421

Aspinall W 1990 Clinical testing for the craniovertebral hypermobility syndrome. Journal of Orthopaedic and Sports Physical Therapy 12:2:47–54

Australian Physiotherapy Association 1988 Protocol for pre-manipulative testing of the cervical spine. Australian Journal of Physiotherapy 34:97–100

Bogduk N, Engel R 1984 The menisci of the lumbar zygapophyseal joints. A review of their anatomy and clinical significance. Spine 9:5:454–460

Boyd J A, Davey M R 1968 Composition of peripheral nerves. Churchill Livingstone, Edinburgh

Bullough P G, Jaqannath A 1983 The morphology of the calcification front in articular cartilage. Journal of Bone and Joint Surgery 65B:72–78

Butler D S 1991a Mobilisation of the nervous system. Churchill Livingstone, Melbourne

Butler D S 1991b Axoplasmic flow and manipulative physiotherapy. In: Proceedings of seventh biennial conference of the Manipulative Physiotherapists Association of Australia, Blue Mountains, pp 206–213

Caterson B, Lowther D A 1978 Changes in the metabolism of the proteoglycans from sheep articular cartilage in response to mechanical stress. Biochima et Biophysica Acta 540:412–422

Clark F J 1975 Information signalled by sensory fibres in medial articular nerve. Journal of Neurophysiology 38:1464–1472

Dahners L E, Torke M D, Gilbert J A, Lester G E 1989 The effect of orientation during ligament healing. Orthopaedic Research Society 35:299

Denko C W, Aponte J, Gabriel P, Petricevic M 1982 Serum B-endorphin in rheumatic disorders. Journal of Rheumatology 9:827–833

Droz-Georget J H 1980 High velocity thrust and pathophysiology of segmental dysfunction. In: Glasgow E M, Twomey L T, Scull E R, Kleynhams A M, Idczak R M (eds) Aspects of manipulative therapy. Churchill Livingstone, Melbourne, pp 81–87

El-Sobky A, Dpostrovsky J O, Wall P D 1976 Lack of effect of naloxone on pain perception in humans. Nature 263:783–784

Elvey R L 1979 Painful restriction of shoulder movement: a clinical observational study. In: Proceedings of disorders of the knee, ankle and shoulder. Western Australian Institute of Technology, pp 113–126

Freeman M A R, Wyke B D 1967 Articular reflexes at the ankle joint: an electro-myographic study of normal and abnormal influences of ankle joint mechanoreceptors upon reflex activity in the leg muscles. British Journal of Surgery 54:990

Gardner E 1950 Physiology of moveable joints. Physiological Reviews 30:127–176

Gelberman R H, Amiel D, Gonsalves M, Woo S, Akeson W H 1981 The influence of protected passive mobilization on the healing of flexor tendons: a biochemical and microangiographic study. The Hand 13:120–128

Giovanelli-Blacker B, Elvey R, Thompson E 1985 The clinical significance of measured lumbar zygapophyseal intracapsular pressure variation. Proceedings of the fourth biennial conference, Manipulative Therapists Association of Australia, Brisbane, pp 140–150

Grant R 1988 Dizziness testing and manipulation of the cervical spine. In: Grant R (ed) Physical therapy of the cervical and thoracic spine. Churchill Livingstone, New York, pp 111–125

Grieve G P 1981 Common vertebral joint problems. Churchill Livingstone, Edinburgh

Grigg P 1975 Mechanical factors in influencing the response of joint afferent neurons in the cat knee. Journal of Neurophysiology 38:1473–1484

Grigg P 1976 Response of joint afferent neurones in cat medial articular nerve to active and passive movements of the knee. Brain Research 18:482–485

Grigg P, Greenspan B J 1977 Response of primate joint afferent neurons to mechanical stimulation of the knee joint. Journal of Neurophysiology 40:1–18

Gronblad M, Kontinnen Y T, Korkala O, Liesi P, Hukkanen M, Polak J M 1988 Neuropeptides in synovium of patients with rheumatoid arthritis and osteoarthritis. Journal of Rheumatology 15:1807–1810

Guilbaud G, Iggo A, Tegner R 1985 Sensory receptors in ankle joint capsules of normal and arthritic rats. Experimental Brain Research 58:29–40

Harrison M H M, Schajowicz P, Trueta J 1953 Osteoarthritis of the hip: a study of the nature and evolution of the disease. Journal of Bone and Joint Surgery 35B:598–626

Harvey A R 1987 Neurophysiology of rheumatic pain. In: Bailliere's Clinical Rheumatology. International Practice and Research, vol. 1, no. 1, Pain. Bailliere Tindall, London, ch 1, pp 1–26

Helal B 1965 The pain in primary osteoarthritis of the knee. Its causes and treatment by osteotomy. Postgraduate Medical Journal 41:172–181

Hill R G 1981 The status of naloxone in the identification of pain control mechanisms operated by endogenous opioids. Neuroscience Letters 21:217–222

Houlbrooke K, Vause K, Merrilees M J 1990 Effects of movement and weightbearing on the glycosaminoglycan content of sheep articular cartilage. Australian Journal of Physiotherapy 36:88–91

Iggo A, Guilbaud G, Tegner R 1984 Sensory mechanisms in arthritic rat joints. In: Kruger L, Liebeskind J C (eds) Advances in pain research and therapy, vol. 6. Raven, New York, pp 83–93

Janda V 1983 Muscle function testing. Butterworths, London

Jobe C M 1983 Special properties of living tissue that affect the shoulder in athletes. Clinics in Sports Medicine 2:271–280

Johnson T 1982 Age-related differences in isometric and dynamic strength and endurance. Physical Therapy 62:985–989

Johnstone P A 1985 Normal temperomandibular joint movement— a pilot study. In: Proceedings of fourth biennial conference of Manipulative Therapists Association of Australia, Brisbane, pp 206–220

Jones C A, Rees J M H, Dodds W H, Jayson M I V 1985 Changes in plasma opioid peptide concentrations after physiotherapeutic exercises for arthritic patients. Neuropeptides 5:561–562

Jones M A 1992 Clinical reasoning in manual therapy. American Journal of Physical Therapy 72:875–884

Jull G A, Bogduk N M 1985 Manual examination. An objective test of cervical joint dysfunction. In: Proceedings of fourth biennial conference of Manipulative Therapists Association of Australia, Brisbane, pp 159–170

Kauffman T L 1985 Strength training effect in young and aged women. Archives of Physical Medicine and Rehabilitation 66:223–226

Kidd B L, Mapp P I, Blake D R, Gibson S J, Polak J M 1990 Neurogenic influences in arthritis. Annals of the Rheumatic Diseases 49:649–652

Korr I M 1975 Osteopathic medicine. Stark E H Publishing Sciences Group, pp 28–31, 183–200

Korr I M 1985 Neurochemical and neurotrophic consequences of nerve deformation. In: Glasgow E F, Twomey L T, Scull E R, Kleynhanns A M, Idczak R M (eds) Aspects of manipulative therapy, 2nd edn. Churchill Livingstone, Melbourne, pp 64–71

Lance J W, Bogduk N 1982 Pain and pain syndromes. In: Appel S H (ed) Offprints from neurology, vol 4. Wiley & Sons, New York, ch 8, pp 159–199

Langford L A, Schmidt R F 1982 The medial articular nerve: an electron microscopic examination. Pfleugers Archive European Journal of Physiology 394:R57 (cited by Zusman 1985)

Larsson L, Grimby G, Karlsson J 1979 Muscle strength and speed of movement in relation to age and muscle morphology. Journal of Applied Physiology 46:451–456

Levick J R 1983 Joint pressure-volume studies: their importance, design and interpretation. Editorial article, Journal of Rheumatology 10:3:153–257

Levine J D, Goetz E J, Basbaum A I 1987 Contribution of the nervous system to the pathophysiology of rheumatoid arthritis and other polyarthritides. Rheumatic Disease Clinics of North America 13:369–383

Lewit K 1978 The contribution of clinical observation to neurobiological mechanisms in manipulative therapy. In: Korr I M (ed) The neurobiologic mechanisms in manipulative therapy. Plenum, New York, pp. 3–25

Lewit K 1985 The muscular and articular factor in movement restriction. Manual Medicine 1:83–85

Lowther D A 1979 The effect of compression and tension on the behaviour of connective tissues. In: Grasgow E F, Twomey L T, Scull E R, Kleynhanns A M, Idczak R M (eds) Aspects of manipulative therapy, 1st edn. Churchill Livingstone, Melbourne, pp. 15–21

Lynn B 1984 The detection of injury and tissue damage. In: Wall P D, Melzack R (eds) Textbook of pain, ch I.1, pp 19–33

Magarey M E 1985 Selection of passive treatment techniques. In: Proceedings of fourth biennial conference of Manipulative Therapists Association of Australia, Brisbane, pp 298–320

Magarey M E 1986a Examination of the vertebral column. In: Grieve G P (ed) Modern manual therapy. Churchill Livingstone, London, ch 44, 481–497

Magarey M E 1986b The first treatment session. In: Grieve G P (ed) Modern manual therapy. Churchill Livingstone, London, ch 61, 661–672

Magarey M E, Jones M A 1992 Clinical examination and management of minor instability of the shoulder complex. Australian Journal of Physiotherapy 38:260–280

Maitland G D 1969 Vertebral manipulation, 2nd edn. Butterworths, London

Maitland G D 1978 Movement of pain sensitive structures in the vertebral canal in a group of physiotherapy students. In: Proceedings of first biennial conference, Manipulative Therapists Association of Australia, Sydney, pp. 37–52

Maitland G D 1979 Negative disc exploration: positive canal signs. Australian Journal of Physiotherapy 25:129–134

Maitland G D 1985 Passive movement techniques for intra-articular and periarticular disorders. Australian Journal of Physiotherapy 31:3–8

Maitland G D 1986 Vertebral manipulation, 5th edn. Butterworths, London

Maitland G D 1991 Peripheral manipulation, 3rd edn. Butterworths-Heinemann, London, p. 48

Marks R 1992 Peripheral articular mechanisms in pain production in osteoarthritis. Australian Journal of Physiotherapy 38:289–298

McGill S M, Brown S 1992 Creep response of the lumbar spine to prolonged full flexion. Clinical Biomechanics 7:43–46

McKenzie R A 1981 The lumbar spine, mechanical diagnosis and therapy. Spinal Publications, Waikanae, New Zealand

Milde M R 1982 Accessory movements of the glenohumeral joint— a pilot study of accessory movements in asymptomatic shoulders and the changes related to ageing and hand dominance. Unpublished graduate diploma thesis, School of Physiotherapy, South Australian Institute of Technology

Millan M J, Herz A 1985 The endocrinology of the opioids. International Review of Neurobiology 26:1–83

Miller M R, Kasahara M 1963 Observations on the innervation of human long bones. Anatomical Record 145:13–15

Muir H 1988 Biochemical basis of cartilage degeneration, destruction and loss of function in osteoarthritis. In: Muir H, Hirhota K, Shickikawa K (eds) Mechanisms of articular cartilage damage and repair in osteoarthritis. Hogrefe & Huber, Toronto, pp 31–42

Nade S, Bell E, Wyke B 1978 Articular neurology of the feline lumbar spine. Abstract, Journal of Bone and Joint Surgery 60B:292

Nade S, Newbold P J 1983 Factors determining the level and changes in intra-articular pressure in the knee joint of the dog. Journal of Physiology 338:21–36

O'Driscoll S W, Kumar A, Salter R B 1983 The effect of continuous passive motion on the clearance of a haemarthrosis from a synovial joint. Clinical Orthopaedics and Related Research 176:305–311

Otten U 1984 Nerve growth factor and the peptidergic sensory neurons. Trends in Pharmocology 7:307–310

Palmoski M, Perricone E, Brandt K D 1979 Development and reversal of proteoglyan aggregation defect in normal canine knee cartilage after immobilization. Arthritis and Rheumatism 22:508–517

Phillips R S, Bulmer J H, Hoyle G, Davies W 1967 Venous drainage in osteoarthritis of the hip. A study after osteotomy. Journal of Bone and Joint Surgery 49B:301–309

Radin E L, Burr D B, Caterson D, Fyhrie D, Brown T D, Boyd R D 1991 Mechanical determinants of osteoarthritis. Seminars in Arthritis and Rheumatism 21:12–21

Radin L, Rose R M 1986 Role of subchondral bone in the initiation and progression of cartilage damage. Clinical Orthopaedics and Related Research 213:34–40

Rees J M H 1987 Endogenous opioids. In: Bailliere's clinical rheumatology. International practice and research, vol. 1, no. 1, Pain. Bailliere Tindall, London, ch. 2, pp. 27–56

Reiman I, Christensen S B 1977 A historical demonstration of nerves in the subchondral bone. Acta Orthopaedica Scandinavica 48:345–347

Salter R B, Ogilvie-Harris D J 1979 Healing of intra-articular fractures with continuous passive motion. American Academy of Orthopaedic Surgeons, Lecture Series 28:102–117

Salter R B, Simmonds D F, Malcolm B W, Rumble E J, MacMichael D, Clements N D 1980 The biological effect of continuous passive movement on the healing of full thickness defects in articular cartilage. Journal of Bone and Joint Surgery 62A:1232–1251

Salter R B, Bell S 1981 The effect of continuous passive motion on the healing of partial thickness lacerations of the patellar tendon of the rabbit. Orthopedic Transcripts 5:209

Salter R B, Clements N D, Ogilvie-Harris D, Bogoch E R, Wong D A, Bell R S, Minister R 1982a The healing of articular tissues through continuous passive movement; essence of the first ten years of experimental investigations. Journal of Bone and Joint Surgery 64B:640–641

Salter R B, Minister R R, Clements N, Bogoch E, Bell R S 1982b Continuous passive motion and the repair of full thickness articular cartilage defects—a one year follow-up. Orthopedic Transactions 6:266–267

Salter R B, Minister R R 1982 The effect of continuous passive motion on a semitendinosus tenodesis in the rabbit knee. Orthopedic Transactions 6:292

Salter R B 1993 Continuous passive motion, CPM. Williams & Wilkins, USA

Schaible H G, Schmidt R F 1983a Activation of groups III and IV sensory units in medial articular nerve by local mechanical stimulation of knee joint. Journal of Neurophysiology 49:35–44

Schaible H G, Schmidt R F 1983b Responses of five medial articular nerve afferents to passive movement of knee joint. Journal of Neurophysiology 49:1118–1126

Simkin P A 1991 Physiology of normal and abnormal synovium. Seminars in Arthritis and Rheumatism 21:179–183

Skyhar M J, Danzig L A, Hargens A R, Akeson W H 1985 Nutrition of the anterior cruciate ligament. Effects of continuous passive motion. American Journal of Sports Medicine 13:415–418

Slater H 1991 Adverse neural tension in the sympathetic trunk and sympathetic maintained pain syndromes. In: Proceedings, seventh biennial conference of the Manipulative Physiotherapists Association of Australia, Sydney, pp. 214–219

Stanton P 1988 Continuous passive movement for muscle injuries. In: Torode M (ed) The athlete maximising participation and minimising risk. Cumberland College of Health Sciences, Sydney, pp 95–102

Steptoe D M, Walton M H 1989 The effects of continuous passive motion and immobilization on the repair of displaced intra-articular fractures. Experimental studies on the sheep knee joint. In: Jones H M, Jones M A, Milde M R (eds) Proceedings of sixth biennial conference, Manipulative Therapists Association of Australia, Adelaide, pp 191–196

Sunderland S 1976 The nerve lesion in carpal tunnel syndrome. Journal of Neurology, Neurosurgery and Psychiatry 39:615–626

Thorstensson A, Larsson L, Tesch P, Karlsson J 1977 Muscle strength and fiber composition in athletes and sedentary men. Medicine and Science in Sports 9:26–30

Trott P H 1980 Mobility study of the trapezio-metacarpal joint. In: Proceedings of the second biennial conference of the Manipulative Therapists Association of Australia. Adelaide pp. 9–34

Twomey L, Taylor J 1982 Flexion creep deformation and hysteresis in the lumbar vertebral column. Spine 7:116–122

Walker J M, Bernick S 1987 Natural ageing and exercise effects on joints. In: Helminen H J, Kiviranta I, Tammi M, Saamananen A-M, Paukkonen K, Jurvelin J (eds) Joint loading: biology and health or articular structures. Wright, Bristol, ch. 4, pp. 89–111

Wall P D 1984 Mechanism of acute and chronic pain. Advances in Pain Research and Therapy 76:95–104

Watson J 1982 Pain mechanisms—a review. III. Endogenous pain control mechanisms. Australian Journal of Physiotherapy 28:38–45

Wilson J N, Ifield F W 1952 Manipulation of the herniated intervertebral disc. American Journal of Surgery 83:173–175

Woo S L, Gelberman R H, Cobb N G, Amiel D, Lothringer K, Akeson W H 1981 The importance of controlled passive mobilization on flexor tendons healing: a biomechanical study. Acta Orthopaedica Scandinavica 52:615

Woo S L, Akeson W H 1987 Response of tendons and ligaments to joint loading and movements. In: Helminen H J, Kiviranta I, Tammi M, Saamananen A-M, Paukkonen K, Jurvelin J (eds) Joint loading: biology and health of articular structures. Wright, Bristol, ch. 12, pp. 287–315

Wyke B D 1976 Neurological aspects of low back pain. In: Jayson M (ed) The lumbar spine and back pain. Sector, London, pp 189–256

Wyke B D 1985 Articular neurology and manipulative therapy. In: Grasgow E F, Twomey L T, Scull E R, Kleynhanns A M, Idczak R M (eds) Aspects of manipulative therapy, 2nd edn. Churchill Livingstone, Melbourne, ch. 11, pp 72–80

Zarins B 1982 Soft tissue injury and repair–biomechanical aspects. International Journal of Sports Medicine 3:9–11

Zusman M 1985 Reappraisal of a proposed neurophysical mechanism for the relief of joint pain with passive joint movements. Physiotherapy Practice I:64–70

Zusman M 1986 Spinal manipulative therapy: review of some proposed mechanisms and a new hypothesis. Australian Journal of Physiotherapy 32(2):89–99

Zusman M 1987 A theoretical basis for the short-term relief of some types of spinal pain with manipulative therapy. Manual Medicine 3:54–56

Zusman M, Edwards B C, Donaghy A 1989 Investigation of a proposed mechanism for the relief of spinal pain with passive joint movement. Manual Medicine 4:58–61

FURTHER READING

Brieg A 1960 Biomechanics of the central nervous system. Almquist & Wiksell, Stockholm

Cyriax J, Russell G 1977 Textbook of orthopaedic medicine, vol. 2, 9th edn. Bailliere Tindall, London

Evjenth O, Hamberg J 1988 Muscle stretching in manual therapy: a clinical manual, vols 1 & 2. Alfta, Sweden

Evjenth O, Hamberg J 1989 Auto stretching: the complete manual of specific stretching. Alfta, Sweden

Glasgow E F, Twomey L T, Scull E R (eds) 1984 Aspects of manipulative therapy. Churchill Livingstone, Melbourne

Grieve G P (ed) 1986 Modern manual therapy of the vertebral column. Churchill Livingstone, Edinburgh

Hartman L S 1985 Handbook of osteopathic technique, 2nd edn. Hutchinson, London

Janda V 1978 Muscles, central nervous regulation and back pain. In: Korr I (ed) The neurobiologic mechanisms in manipulative therapy. Plenum Press, London

Janda V 1980 Muscles as a pathogenic factor in back pain. Proceedings of International Federation of Orthopaedic Manipulation Therapy congress, New Zealand

Jayson M I V (ed) 1992 The lumbar spine and back pain, 4th edn. Churchill Livingstone, London

Kaltenborn F M 1976 Manual therapy for the extremity joints. Olaf Norlis Bokhandel, Oslo

Korr I (ed) 1978 The neurobiologic mechanisms in manipulative therapy. Plenum Press, London

McKenzie R A 1990 The cervical and thoracic spine: mechanical diagnosis and therapy. Spinal Publications, Waikanae, New Zealand

Mennell J 1939 The science and art of joint manipulation, vol 1. J & A Churchill Ltd, Edinburgh

Mitchell F L, Moran S, Pruzzo N A 1979 An evaluation and treatment manual of osteopathic muscle energy procedures. ICEOP, Valley Park, Missouri

Payton O D, Difabio R P, Paris S V, Protas E J, VanSant A F (eds) 1989 Manual of physical therapy. Churchill Livingstone, New York

Stoddard A 1977 Manual of osteopathic technique. Hutchinson, London

13. Therapeutic exercise

Henry Wajswelner, Gillian Webb

Exercise is essential in the rehabilitation of sporting injuries to ensure that the sportsperson is able to continue with sport at any level. The ultimate goal of any rehabilitation program using therapeutic exercise is that of symptom free movement and function. The goals of rehabilitating a sportsperson are essentially the same as for a person in the wider community, but the higher functional requirements of the athlete will necessitate a more specific and vigorous program. A balanced exercise program must take into account the needs and desired goals of the athlete, motivation and the extent of the injury.

Therapeutic exercise for injured athletes can be divided broadly into the use of exercise to improve strength (resistance training), range of movement (stretching and mobilizing exercises), balance and co-ordination (proprioceptive training) and finally sporting performance (functional exercises or skill drills). Usually, all of these are used in the comprehensive rehabilitation of an athlete with a serious or long-term injury, and are prescribed and delivered with the individual athlete's goals in mind.

As a general principle, injured athletes should continue with activities which will help maintain fitness for their specific sport, being careful not to hinder recovery. Uninvolved body parts and joints should be exercised daily to maintain cardiorespiratory fitness, muscle strength and endurance, and decrease risk of reinjury. As little as 2 weeks of detraining has been shown to cause significant reductions in cardiorespiratory fitness (Croce & Gregg 1991), while modified training results in only modest reductions in VO_2 max.

In the authors' experience, mantaining or even enhancing aerobic capacity during the rehabilitation period should be encouraged to improve general body fitness and to control weight. This enhances recovery from many athletic injuries, particularly those involving the spine and weightbearing joints. It is also valuable as a psychological tool to enable the athlete to continue with a training schedule despite being injured.

The use of 'good side training', i.e. the transfer of training from the injured to the uninjured limb, may be useful in that it prevents detraining of the unaffected limb and may have carry-over effect to the injured limb.

The sports physiotherapist must have an understanding of how normal and damaged tissues respond to stress and injury, and plan a program accordingly. The muscles need to be returned to full strength and function for protection of joint integrity, including shock absorption. The same principles apply when considering ligaments and tendons, and the time taken for healing and remodelling of the collagen content of injured soft tissue must be taken into account when prescribing exercise (see Ch. 3). Age-related changes, adaptive changes, gender and activity level of the patient must also be considered when designing therapeutic exercise programs.

GOAL SETTING

In the delivery of an exercise program, the long- and short-term goals of the injured athlete should be determined. They will be influenced by the severity of the injury, the stage of healing, the type of treatment (e.g. surgery), pain on movement, swelling, range of movement, strength, any other associated conditions, the demands of the sport and the athlete's own expectations. The short-term goal may be the reduction of pain and disability due to an acute injury, where therapeutic exercise has a limited role. It is in the subacute stage of recovery, or in rehabilitation after surgery or of chronic syndromes, that therapeutic exercise is used to achieve long-term goals, e.g. return to sport.

The final stages of rehabilitation are concerned with re-establishing co-ordination and speed of movement. Before returning fully to sport the athlete should ideally be able to perform at the same level of proficiency and have the same endurance as before the injury. Sometimes this goal may be impossible to attain due to permanent damage, e.g. contact or twisting manoeuvres may always be risky with an anterior cruciate-deficient knee joint, so some sports may be inadvisable and are unrealistic as a goal. The goals that are set co-operatively by the physiotherapist and the athlete should reflect this so that the athlete can achieve a realistic level of participation without risk of further injury.

207

STRENGTHENING PROGRAMS (RESISTANCE TRAINING)

It is generally accepted that athletic injury leads to losses in functional strength, power and endurance, and subsequent decreased performance. Therapeutic strengthening programs aimed at avoiding these results of injury are a major part of rehabilitation of injured athletes. The purpose of progressive resistance exercise in sport and in therapy is to increase muscle strength and size, and to decrease the risk of tissue injury. A number of adaptations occur as a result of strength training. Some of the beneficial changes are increased contractile strength in muscles and increased tensile strength in ligaments, tendons and bones (Fleck & Kraemer 1987).

Strength training enhances muscle contractile strength in two ways:

- It stimulates neural adaptations (Hakkinen & Komi 1983). Strength gains seen during the first 4 weeks of training are primarily due to neural adaptation, not muscle hypertrophy. Proposed mechanisms of this effect include enhancement of the ability to recruit agonist muscles, improved inhibition of antagonist muscles, improved synchronization of the firing pattern of motor units and additional recruitment of motor units.
- It produces more actin and myosin protein filaments, resulting in larger and stronger muscles. This process of hypertrophy takes longer than the neural adaptation (Sale & MacDougall 1981), and is thought to be due to an increase in the size of the existing fibres rather than an increase in the number.

The physiological factors which affect strength are the number, type and frequency of motor units recruited during a contraction and the viscoelastic properties of the contractile and noncontractile tissue. The elastic properties absorb energy and stretch, which can be used to increase the force of contraction.

Too early heavy resistance may lead to an increase in pain and swelling and to a slowing down of the repair process. Isometric type exercises may be more appropriate in the acute stages as long as they do not provoke the symptoms. An example of a functional progression of exercises that can be used as a guide is as follows:

- isometrics
- free active across gravity
- free active against gravity
- resisted active/elastic bands or tubing
- isokinetics/pulleys
- free weights/weight stations/isotonics
- eccentrics
- sport specific drills/plyometrics (i.e. depth jumping).

Principles of strength training

There are a number of basic principles which apply to the development of strength, power and endurance in muscle, which should be taken into account when prescribing therapeutic strengthening exercises. Exercise programs should incorporate these concepts of resisted exercise training, both for performance enhancement or functional gains in rehabilitation. For definitions and relationships between strength, power and endurance see Wilson (1992).

Overload

To effect gains in strength, the muscle must be progressively overloaded. This is done when a demand is put on the muscle which is greater than that normally required or used, such as a maximum voluntary contraction. The physiological changes in the muscle which results in an increase in strength are detailed in Fleck and Kraemer (1987). Overload in strength training can be achieved by manipulation of the following variables: the number of repetitions; the number of sets; the loads used and type of muscle action; the speed of movement; the rest interval between sets (Wilson 1992).

The way these variables are used forms the basis of many of the 'systems' for producing specific gains in resistance training, such as muscle hypertrophy, definition, power or endurance (Fleck & Kraemer 1987).

When deciding on protocols for strengthening muscle the physiotherapist must devise a safe and effective program that progressively overloads the muscles and allows adequate time for adaptation to each level of stimulation. The muscle or group of muscles should be exercised to the point of fatigue, not pain, in order to obtain adaptive changes. The type of program used will vary according to the needs of the athlete.

Specificity

Specific adaptation to imposed demands (SAID) is the body's response to exercise, in that the more specific the demands made the more specific are the adaptations that occur. Research has shown that isometric, isotonic and isokinetic strength gains are specific to the type of contraction used during training (Atha 1981). It has also been demonstrated that using a combination of isometric, concentric and eccentric contractions in an exercise routine results in larger strength gains than any one alone (Atha 1981).

According to Wilson (1992), weight training regimes used by many athletes are often very non-specific to their competitive requirements. Specificity must be observed to ensure the carryover of strength gains in rehabilitation to functional activities on the playing field. The type of training emphasis followed will also determine whether there are increases in muscle strength, power or endurance.

A repetition maximum (RM) is the maximum number of repetitions that can be performed maintaining good form, i.e. without tricking. The weight or load for a given RM (usually 10) is the load that can be lifted 10 times maintaining correct form. RMs of 6 or less predominantly cause gains in strength/power, and require the use of heavier loads than training with RM of 20, which produces gains mainly in muscle endurance (Fleck 1989). Power athletes (e.g. throwers) need to be strong but must generate this strength quickly. Their therapeutic exercise should emphasize speed of movement within limits imposed by the stage of rehabilitation. Endurance athletes need prolonged exercise at low resistances when returning from injury.

Many athletes overtrain one muscle group and undertrain its counterpart, which leads to muscle imbalance and injury (Janda 1978). Resistance training exercises should be prescribed to specifically strengthen the weak muscle groups. This often means going back to basics in terms of simple dumbbell or leg raise movements initially, before using gym equipment, which may be less specific to the muscle groups in question.

Speed specificity of muscle strength training is another concept that has some scientific basis from the use of isokinetics (Moffroid & Whipple 1970, Coyle & Feiring 1980). Theoretically, exercises should be performed at the same velocity as that required for performance. In practical terms, however, this is often impossible to achieve so these functional speeds can only be approximated. For sport movements performed at high velocity, supplementary training at lower speeds may be useful (Sale & MacDougall 1981). For more general strength gains, an intermediate training velocity should be used (Fleck & Kraemer 1987).

In summary, strength training exercises should simulate the requirements of the sport as closely as possible, in terms of movement pattern, velocity, type of contraction, contraction force, muscle groups, joint angles, repetitions and energy systems used (Sale & MacDougall 1981).

Variation

The training stimulus to the muscle or body part should be varied, e.g. by alternating high repetitions at low loads with sessions using heavier loads and fewer repetitions. This is to avoid the decreased efficiency and diminished training gains that come with an athlete becoming 'stale' (Wilson 1992). This approach has lead to the concept of cycling or periodization, originally developed by Eastern European weightlifters, to combat staleness in training.

Periodization involves changing loads and number of repetitions periodically in an attempt to optimize strength and power gains. This is based on the phases of the body's adaptation to a stress stimulus, known as Selye's general adaptation syndrome (Fleck & Kraemer 1987). The first phase is shock and soreness, the second is adaptation to the stimulus and increase in performance, the third phase is staleness. The body or muscle has already adapted to the new stimulus, further adaptation will not take place and performance will actually decrease unless the stimulus is changed.

Other methods of introducing variation in stimulus in strength training include variations in starting positions, range worked through or positions of the body parts. Hakkinen and Komi (1981) showed that combinations of concentric and eccentric contractions produced better strength gains than did concentric contractions alone. These ideas can easily be incorporated in a therapeutic strength training program.

Recovery

It is important to allow adequate recovery between exercise sessions so that muscles can adapt to training without breaking down. Generally there should be 48–72 hours between sessions of exercising the same muscle group (Wilson 1992). Delayed muscle soreness is an indication of inadequate recovery and overtraining of a particular muscle group, which is why split routines are popular in strength training, e.g. upper body one day followed by lower body the next (Fig. 13.1).

Rest between sets

The rest periods between sets of strengthening exercises should be determined by the goals of the exercises. For maximal strength gains, long rest periods between maximal contractions are used. For aerobic endurance, brief rest periods between sets of high repetitions at low resistances are used (Fleck & Kraemer 1987).

Strength training methods

The following is a brief discussion on each type of strength training exercise used in therapy. The order in which they are described can be used as a guide to progression of exercises, i.e. as healing progresses a greater variety can be introduced. For example, when isometrics become too easy the patient can progress to the next stage, such as isotonics or pulleys.

Isometric exercise

Isometric or static strength training involves a muscular contraction performed without movement or change in length of the muscle. This is probably not totally realistic, since all muscle action is accompanied by some joint movement, though this may not be visible to the naked

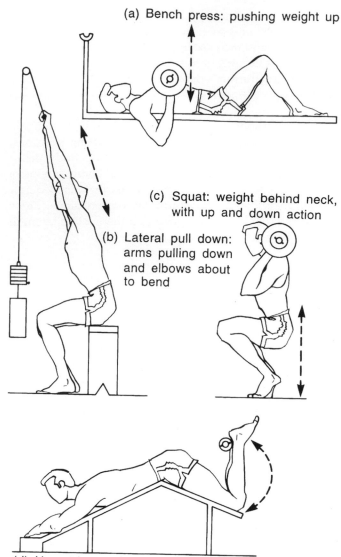

(a) Bench press: pushing weight up

(b) Lateral pull down: arms pulling down and elbows about to bend

(c) Squat: weight behind neck, with up and down action

(d) Hamstring curl: knee bending action

Fig. 13.1 Examples of common resistance training exercises for upper body (a,b) and lower body (c,d)

eye. However, isometrics are commonly prescribed in the early or acute stages of injury because the basic characteristic of this form of exercise is the limitation of joint movement, which makes the exercise less likely to cause aggravation in the early stages of recovery.

The length of time the contraction is held and the amount of force used will depend on the state of the muscle and the amount of tissue damage. Strength gains have been demonstrated with isometric training, related to the number of contractions performed and their duration, intensity of contractions, frequency of training and joint angle. A number of recommendations regarding the use of isometric training are justified in the light of research findings (Fleck & Kraemer 1987).

Maximal voluntary contractions have been found to be superior to submaximal isometric holds for strength gains.

In the case of the injured athlete, the strongest maximal contraction possible within appropriate limits of pain should be encouraged. The majority of research has utilized isometric contractions of 3–10 seconds duration. A small number of long duration contractions or a higher number of short contractions per day will give optimal strength gains. Thus if contractions are painful or irritable, it is better to do a little often than a lot once. One contraction per day has been shown to be ineffective (McDonagh & Davies 1984). Atha (1981) demonstrated the superiority of daily isometric training for maximum strength gains. Isometric exercise can bring about increases in muscle hypertrophy and neural adaptations, leading to strength gains (Fleck & Kraemer 1987). These gains are joint angle specific, with a carry-over of about 20°. A greater number of contractions leads to a greater carry-over, so that if isometric training is intended to increase strength throughout range, training must take place at several joint angles with a large number of contractions (Fleck & Kraemer 1987).

Isometric exercises are easily performed without elaborate equipment, so are very suitable for a home exercise regime. However, they are not very functional for most of the demands of sport. In fact, they have been shown to reduce the maximum speed of a limb's movement and do not increase motor performance ability. For these gains, more dynamic exercise is required.

Pulleys, slings, springs, elastic tubing and bands

Sling or suspension therapy is often used in the early stages of rehabilitation because the weakened limb can be supported while it is exercised across gravity (Hollis 1989). By manipulating the position of the axis of joint motion, a movement can be either assisted or resisted by gravity, i.e. axial versus displaced suspension. It is most often used for weak proximal limb muscle groups, e.g. hip or shoulder. As strength returns but guidance of movement is still required for safety and to avoid trick movements, pulleys are often prescribed for controlled resisted exercise. If more resistance is desirable, springs can be used, but for a home exercise program, elastic bands or tubing of varying thicknesses are the most convenient and are safer and easier to handle than free weights (Fig. 13.2A–E).

Isotonic exercise (dynamic constant resistance)

Isotonic exercise is technically defined as exercise with constant tension. Thus, free weights are not purely isotonic, because muscle tension will vary according to joint mechanics and gravity through range. A better definition would be that the weight or resistance does not vary, and Fleck and Kraemer (1987) used the term 'dynamic constant resistance' (DCR). DCR improves motor performance to a greater extent than does isometric training (Fleck & Kraemer 1987).

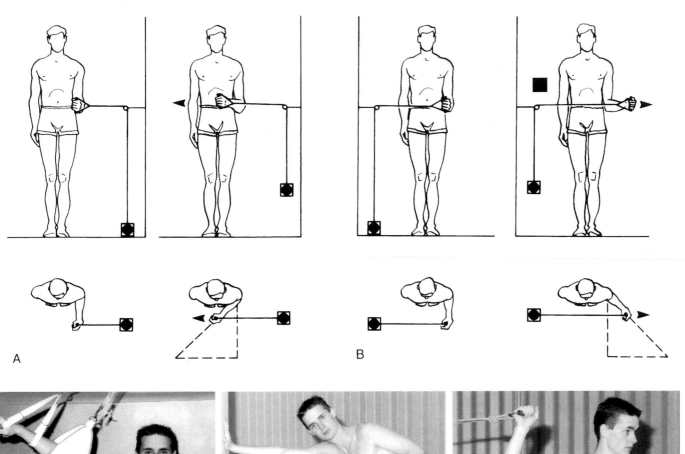

Fig. 13.2 The use of pulleys for therapeutic exercise of the upper limb. Source: adapted from Hayes et al (1990) (a) Pulley set up to exercise internal rotation of the shoulder (b) External rotation of the shoulder (c) Suspension therapy for shoulder mobilization exercises (d) Spring used for resisted shoulder extension (e) Elastic tubing used to resist the throwing action.

The use of free weights, pulley weights and weight loaded machines or stations have been used widely in rehabilitation. Delorme first used a weighted boot to provide the overload needed to gain increases in strength and called the program 'progressive resistance exercises'. The amount of resistance was varied for the individual and a program developed which took into account the weight to be lifted, determined from the 10 repetition maximum (10 RM), plus the number of repetitions and the frequency of exercise needed per week.

Delorme's strengthening program or progressive resistance exercise (PRE) followed the protocol in Table 13.1.

Many modifications to this system have occurred over the years, including the daily adjusted progressive resistance exercise (DAPRE), in which daily adjustments are made to the progressive resistance depending on the number of repetitions done and the weight lifted. The major problem associated with this type of exercise is that by using a fixed weight throughout the movement no account is taken of the effective resistance that the muscle is able to provide throughout the range of movement. The other major problem is specificity, and whether strength gains with a weight or a machine can be transferred to the sporting activity. However, as a progression in rehabilitation, weight boots, sandbag cuffs and hand-held dumbbells are often used to add resistance when free active exercises become too easy.

Fleck and Kraemer (1987) reviewed the literature and have made the following recommendations regarding dynamic constant resistance training:

Table 13.1

Determine the 10 RM		
Set	**Weight**	**Repetitions**
1	one half of 10 RM	10
2	three quarters of 10RM	10
3	full 10RM	10

The 10RM is increased weekly as strength increases

- The optimum number of repetitions for strength improvement is 2-10 RM and the optimum number of sets 2-5. Maximal voluntary contractions are needed for maximal strength gains.
- Three training sessions per muscle group per week is the minimum which causes maximal strength gains. DCR increases motor performance and to optimally improve motor performance, direct practice of the skill and resistance training should be combined, e.g. using a weight or pulleys to resist the throwing action or tennis stroke.

Eccentric exercise

Muscles can develop more tension when they contract eccentrically than either isometrically or concentrically (Hakkinen & Komi 1981). They also require less energy to develop the equivalent force and are more efficient metabolically when contracting eccentrically.

Unaccustomed intense eccentric contractions cause myofibrillar damage and delayed onset muscle soreness (DOMS) (Friden et al 1983a). This post-exercise soreness tends to peak at 48 hours after training, and is greater than that experienced following other types of resistance training. However, Friden et al (1983b) showed that DOMS due to eccentric exercise can be reduced or prevented by specific eccentric training, and because eccentric contractions play a significant role in the dynamics of muscle actions in sports, eccentrics should be considered as an important part of therapeutic exercise. Eccentric contractions are common in athletic activity. Many ballistic movements are preceded by a short countermovement in the opposite direction to utilize stretch reflex; these are usually eccentric (Bosco et al 1981).

A muscle-tendon unit has a contractile element and a series elastic component (SEC), located mainly in the tendon area but also within the muscle belly. The SEC is made up of connective tissue consisting mainly of collagen and elastin (see Chs 2 and 3). In eccentric contractions, the SEC is stretched and contributes to force produced. In many sports downward motion precedes the upward, and as a result the muscle is stretched before it contracts, allowing the SEC to contribute.

Curwin and Stanish (1984) introduced the concept of a graduated eccentric exercise for tendinitis, specifically targeting the SEC. Such a program is designed to strengthen tendons, whereas rest or immobilization leads to tendon atrophy. Muscle becomes stronger if exercised, but because of the continuity of the muscle-tendon unit (MTU), tendon is also affected. Previously tendon was thought to be inert tissue, but now it is known that it responds positively to exercise. The role of exercise is firmly supported by experimental studies and forms the basis of the Curwin and Stanish (1984) therapeutic program using eccentric contractions for the management of tendinitis.

The program is based on four major components:

- The MTU is thoroughly warmed up and stretched, as increasing its resting length helps decrease the strain by spreading tension over a greater length
- The load is progressively increased within pain limits
- The speed of contraction is also progressively increased
- There are set rest periods to allow the stressed tissues to recover, adapt and become stronger.

Eccentric exercise programs are therefore used to strengthen the MTU using three variables:

- Length of the MTU
- Load: 'progressive overloading' forms basis of progression of the program.
- Speed of contraction.

The safe application of eccentric training requires a controlled lowering of the load or body weight.

THE ECCENTRIC EXERCISE PROGRAM

1. Warm up 5 minutes. (Use exercise that does not aggravate the injury).
2. Stretch. Static stretch, hold 15-30 seconds, × 3 each side.
3. Eccentric exercise. Do 3 sets of 10 repetitions, days 1 and 2 slowly. Days 3 to 5 moderate speed. Days 6 and 7 faster. Increase resistance after day 7 and repeat.
4. Stretch again as before.
5. Apply ice.

Discomfort should only be experienced in the last set of 10 repetitions. This indicates slight overloading which is necessary to increase tendon strength. Pain or discomfort through all 30 repetitions is undesirable as too much overloading is occurring, and load or speed should be reduced. The discomfort experienced is the yardstick for progression of the program. Incorrect evaluation of this discomfort is a major cause of program failure (Curwin & Stanish 1984). The program is continued for 6 weeks, but there may be no appreciable change in symptoms for the first 2-3 weeks. Patient compliance is the single largest factor determining the success or failure of an eccentric program. As strength increases the discomfort will decrease, and force can be increased till discomfort recurs, usually by increasing the speed. Ice is used after every session to decrease inflammation.

The eccentric program is suitable for achilles tendinitis, jumper's knee (patellar tendinitis), tennis elbow, hamstring tendonitis and triceps tendinitis.

Patellar tendinitis

The program is designed to increase the tensile strength of the patellar tendon. Warm-up and flexibility are important, as many patients have tight quadriceps which may need stretching and massage to improve resting length first. To stress the tendon, the patient drops to a semisquatting position (Curwin & Stanish 1984). Progress is made by adding weight or increasing speed.

The patient's discomfort is used as a monitor of progress. In the final stages of rehabilitation the patient should be able to drop rapidly and freely and stop the movement with an eccentric quadriceps contraction. The sudden reversal of the downward motion is the important feature of the program. No resistance is added until the patient can drop and stop with little or no discomfort. The load can be increased further with dropping from a height, initially onto a mat, then onto sport-specific surfaces, as in volleyball and basketball.

Hamstring tendinitis

All the above principles apply. For lower hamstring tendon lesions (biceps femoris, semitendonosis) the eccentric exercise is done by rapidly extending the knee and 'catching' just short of full extension (Stanton et al 1989). Progress with speed and load can be done in standing, prone lying, or inclined prone lying. Usually 6 sets of 10 are used. For upper hamstring lesions pulleys can be used to apply eccentric load and progression is made via speed and weight. Because the tendon is much thicker than those previously described, many more repetitions are used, e.g. up to 100. In the author's experience, the exercise can be done with the knee held in slight flexion to better localize the force to the upper hamstring. Another position that can be utilized for the upper hamstring is in prone with the leg over the side of a plinth. The main movement used is hip flexion/extension rather than knee flexion/extension. The affected leg is allowed to drop down with gravity into hip flexion and 'caught' with eccentric control utilizing the upper hamstrings and gluteals.

Isokinetic exercise

This is exercise that uses equipment that produces an accommodating variable resistance in which the speed of motion is set and the resistance accommodates to match the force applied. Isokinetic machines can be used as an evaluative tool and as a means of exercising using a progressive program individualized to suit each person. However, they suffer from the same problems as other machines in that they cannot replicate sporting patterns of movement accurately, and are costly compared to more simple resistance training systems (see Chapter 17, Isokinetic dynamometry).

Variable resistance

This type of training requires specialized equipment that uses a system of pulleys, cams or levers to vary resistance through the range in an attempt to correct for the effects of gravity and human mechanics, e.g. the force generated by a muscle varies through a range of motion due to its length/tension relationship (Wilson 1992). Although this concept is logical, it is not possible for currently available equipment to match the body mechanics of all individuals. Also, in the author's opinion, this type of equipment is not particularly suited to therapeutic exercise or rehabilitation, because the variations in resistance through range are designed around a supposedly normal body, while in an injured limb, weakness may be present at points in a range of motion different from those described as normal.

In comparing types of strength training programs, Fleck and Kraemer (1987), Hakkinen and Komi (1981) and Atha (1981) all concluded that several types of contractions were desirable to bring about maximal gains in strength. It is recommended that the physiotherapist consider the wide range of options available in the progression of therapeutic strength training, using the common principles as outlined above, to achieve maximal benefit to the injured athlete.

SPECIAL PROGRAMS

Proprioceptive neuromuscular facilitation techniques

PNF patterns improve motor skill through positive motor transfer (Voss et al 1984) and use four major neurophysiological principles:

- Facilitation and inhibition
- Irradiation or reinforcement which refers to a strong voluntary muscle action against resistance, that will bring about a response in other muscle groups.
- Sherrington's law of successive induction that indicates that flexion augments extension and extension augments flexion (Voss et al 1984).
- Sherrington's law of reciprocal innervation, which states that each voluntary or reflex contraction of a muscle is associated with a simultaneous relaxation of its antagonist muscle because of an inhibitory response in the muscle spindle.

The major muscle and joint reflexes used are the muscle spindle, which is activated by stretch, the Golgi tendon organ which is activated by pressure and concerned with muscle tonus, deep pressure receptors in joints and the righting reflex. PNF techniques in rehabilitation commonly used for the purposes of facilitating strength are repeated contractions, slow reversals, rhythmic stabilizations and patterns of movement. The diagonal patterns of movement used in PNF programs often mirror the functional movement patterns of athletes and the physiotherapist should consider the use of PNF patterns as the athlete progresses to the functional exercise or 'skill drill' stage. Because the resistance is provided manually by the physiotherapist, this is also an excellent method of assessing for arcs of pain or weakness through range, and appreciating which components of combined movements remain problematic. This allows ongoing therapy to be more specifically targetted.

Kinetic chain exercises

Kinetic chain concepts in rehabilitation have evolved from studies in the rehabilitation of knee reconstructions. Henning et al (1985) studied the strain on the anterior cruciate ligament (ACL) *in vivo* in two subjects during various lower limb exercises. They found that isometric knee extension at 0 and 22° produced 5–17 times more strain on the ACL than weightbearing exercise such as the half squat or stationary cycling. This decrease in ACL strain has been explained by the fact that the hamstrings are active in weightbearing and that this hamstring/quadriceps cocontraction prevents anterior translation of the tibia (Palmitier et al 1991). This small but important study showed that the quadriceps could be exercised safely without jeopardizing the reconstructed ACL, using what has come to be known as 'closed kinetic chain' exercises.

In mechanical engineering, a closed kinematic system is where both ends of a linked chain are fixed, so that movement of one of the rigid linked segments causes predictable movement of other segments. By this definition, only isometrics are true closed chain exercises, but the definition has broadened to include dynamic exercises wherever the hand or foot meets resistance, such as in squats, leg press, stepups, pushups or chinups. An open kinetic chain exists when the peripheral joint of an extremity can still move freely and resistance is applied more proximally, as in leg extension or leg curls. In practical terms, closed chain exercises usually involve movement while weightbearing through the limb, while in open chain work the limb is moving against resistance but is not weight bearing.

The many exercises used for rehabilitating the knee joint can thus be divided into open or closed chain categories. With the accelerated ACL rehabilitation protocols described by Shelbourne and Nitz (1992), closed kinetic chain exercises are emphasized and open chain quadriceps exercises are avoided. One of the advantages of closed chain quadriceps exercises is that patellofemoral joint forces are less than those experienced with open chain exercises between 30° and 90° of knee flexion (Arms et al 1984). Closed kinetic chain exercises place functional stresses on a limb that are similar to weightbearing activities, give joint compression that provides stability, produce less postoperative anterior knee pain and more patient confidence in ambulation (Shelbourne & Nitz 1992). These exercises are commenced as soon as full unsupported weightbearing is allowed (Fig 13.3).

Palmitier et al (1991) also described a 'concurrent shift'. This is the 'pseudoisometric contraction' around the knee joint caused by the simultaneous lengthening of the rectus femoris across the hip as it shortens at the knee, while the hamstrings lengthen at the knee but shorten over the hip in rising from the squat position. This synchronous combination of concentric and eccentric contractions within the same muscle is often used in functional activities and cannot be reproduced with open kinetic chain exercises (Fu et al 1992).

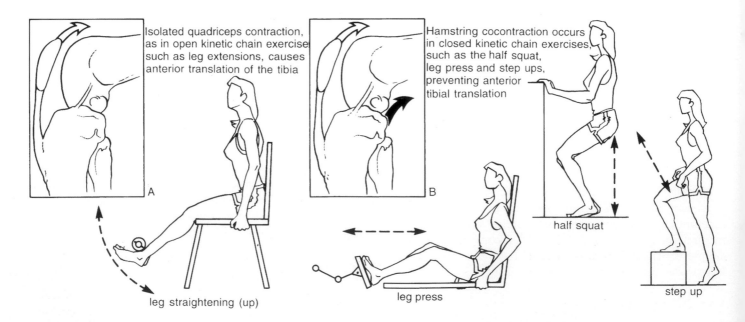

Isolated quadriceps contraction, as in open kinetic chain exercise such as leg extensions, causes anterior translation of the tibia

Hamstring cocontraction occurs in closed kinetic chain exercises, such as the half squat, leg press and step ups, preventing anterior tibial translation

A

leg straightening (up)

B

leg press

half squat

step up

Fig. 13.3 The kinetic chain concept at the knee joint. Source: adapted from Palmitier (1991)

The concept of closed kinetic chain exercises in the knee joint can also be applied to other regions in the body, as in the upper limb across the shoulder joint (Fig. 13.4).

Where the stability of the shoulder is compromised, weightbearing exercise involving joint compression, such as the pressup, can induce cocontraction around the glenohumeral joint and of the scapular muscles. This approach may aid functional stability in a more effective way than isolated open chain type exercises.

Flexibility and stretching exercises

Stretching techniques and exercises for the musculotendonous unit and other soft tissues have been used extensively in rehabilitation programs. Stretching is also used by athletes in a warm up routine, which enhances skilled movements both physiologically by increasing body and muscle temperature, and biomechanically by enabling forces to be applied over greater distances and time. Stretching exercises are an important part of athletic training and are critical for skilled performance. Increase in flexibility and decrease in muscle imbalance with a stretching program will help improve the athlete's exercise tolerance and decrease the likelihood of injury. Athletes often have muscle imbalances due to the nature of their sport and the types of training regimes they follow. Faulty loading and overexertion of the locomotor system due to this imbalance leads to injuries. Correction of muscle imbalance involves reducing the emphasis in training of strengthening muscle groups that are already hypertrophied (Janda 1978). Tight muscles must be stretched, while their weakened and elongated antagonists must be specifically strengthened in isolation.

Flexibility at a joint is specific to that joint or series of joints and is dependent on factors such as muscle bulk, structure of bony articulations, the functional requirements of the joint, and the person's age and body type. It has two components:

- static flexibility or the ability to move through a range of motion with no emphasis on speed or time
- dynamic flexibility or the ability to move through a range of movement with emphasis on speed of motion.

It is important when devising a flexibility program to analyse the movements and range required by the athlete. If there is limitation of movement a detailed assessment must be made of the tissues involved to differentiate which factors may be causing the decrease in movement. These include adaptive changes in the soft tissues surrounding a joint, limitation due to adverse mechanical tension of the neuromeningeal system, ageing effects on the connective tissues, the effects of immobilization or an increased efferent

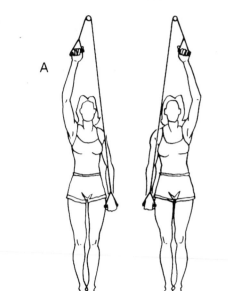

A

Moving arms up and down with overhead pulley

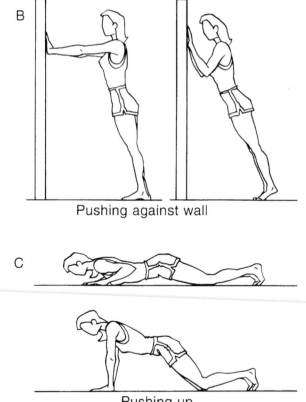

B

Pushing against wall

C

Pushing up

Fig. 13.4 Examples of closed kinetic chain exercises for the upper limb. Source: adapted from Hayes et al (1990)

output to the muscles causing spasm with subsequent increased stiffness. Tight muscles and adaptive changes in connective tissues can alter an athlete's style, reducing biomechanical efficiency and predisposing the athlete to injury. Tightness may vary the length tension of the muscle and alter the limb's shock-absorbing properties.

The question of whether stretching should be performed before or after exercise or both has been investigated by Cornelius (1988), who found no flexibility regime to be superior in improvement. In the authors' experience, more permanent gains in flexibility are achieved when stretching is performed after exercise, when the tissues in question are well warmed up.

In order to consider the most appropriate way to increase the range of movement it is necessary to understand the properties of all tissues being treated (see Chs 2 and 3).

There is agreement in the literature that static or slow stretching is preferable to ballistic stretching as it is less likely to cause trauma. Ballistic stretching activates the stretch reflex which may prevent the required lengthening of muscle fibres and cause muscle strain (Wilkinson 1993). Permanent lengthening of tissues is enhanced by the application of a low force over a long period of time to a tissue that has been warmed up. Stretching is not as effective when done rapidly. The type of static stretching used should be selected according to the individual. It is most important that the athlete understands exactly how a stretch is to be done and that stretching should be used both in the prevention of injury as well as in the treatment of damaged tissues. Connective tissue being stretched passively should have the stretch maintained for a prolonged period and should be warmed and allowed to cool in a lengthened position for better long-term effects.

According to Wilkinson (1993), the 'best' form of stretching is to use the benefit of reciprocal inhibition (or relaxation), where the agonist produces the stretching force on its antagonist, with or without the assistance of a passive force. This is sometimes referred to as active stretching, PNF stretching or the 'buddy system' where a partner is used. The two most commonly used methods are contract-relax and reciprocal inhibition. Reciprocal inhibition is based on Sherrington's law of reciprocal innervation, that states that as a muscle actively contracts, its antagonist will be inhibited so that movement can occur. The contraction of the agonist causes a reflex inhibition of the antagonist to allow increased range of motion. This stretching technique may also be preceded by a voluntary contraction against resistance (contract/relax). The force applied should be held statically for approximately 15 seconds and should not be painful. This should be repeated two to four times per session and be done three times per week (Wilkinson 1993). Kisner and Colby (1985) showed no significant difference in muscle elongation with PNF stretching compared to passive stretching.

Passive stretching

In passive stretching an external force is applied to the limb or muscle. Passive stretching is used to lengthen soft tissue such as muscle, tendon or ligament beyond its resting length. It is applied to tissues that are shortened due to immobilization, spasm, surgical procedures and scarring, or contracted due to pain-induced hypomobility or muscle hypertrophy. It is one of the techniques used most often in the treatment of injuries to athletes. It is usually applied to soft tissues in a relaxed state, so that an appreciation of the end feel or resistance to stretch is possible. Passive stretch is applied by the physiotherapist, by the patient or by mechanical means, e.g. pulleys, or weights. The direction, speed, intensity and duration of the passive stretch are controlled, either by the physiotherapist or the patient, so that stretch is applied to the point of discomfort, not pain. The stretch should be held for 15 seconds (Wilkinson 1993). This type of stretching is often used to good effect in the team setting with the help of a partner. In this case, the passive stretches should be explained and demonstrated carefully first to the group so that the person applying the stretch and the recipient are aware of the safety factors and the stretches are performed in an effective and controlled manner.

Neuromeningeal stretching

Adverse mechanical tension of the neuromeningeal chain anatomically associated with a site of injury may prolong disability by preventing the return of full flexibility. There may be a plateau in improvement of range with the use of traditional active and passive stretching techniques aimed at the muscle-tendon unit alone. In the comprehensive management of muscle injuries in athletes, attempts should be made at maintaining the range of motion of the neuromeningeal structures by mobilization of the nerves local to the site of injury, and proximal and distal to that site (Wajswelner 1993).

Application of stretching

The effectiveness of the stretching exercise will depend on the physiological and biomechanical properties of the tissues being stretched. Injury within soft tissues heals by replacement with scar tissue initially and the effective application of stretching requires a knowledge of the biomechanical properties of collagen. Scar tissue is formed mainly from collagen and elastin and to gain permanent increase in range of movement there must be conditions conducive to plastic deformation. This requires increased tissue temperature which allows the tissue to elongate or 'creep'. Low forces over a period of time should then be applied and the tissues allowed to cool on the stretch to obtain a more permanent elongation (Safran et al 1988).

Therefore 'warm up, stretch slowly, cool' is the formula that can be applied for the most effective stretching.

A number of other principles can be applied.

- Safety should always come first. The starting position, method and dosage should be specific for the athlete and must be understood completely by the athlete.

Prevention of further injury due to unsafe or overly vigorous stretching is of primary importance. To prevent overstretching the intensity and duration of stretch, the frequency of movements performed in a given period and the velocity or nature of the stretch should be carefully explained.

- Stretching exercises should be done after the athlete is warm as an increase in tissue temperature increases the flexibility of the tissues. They should also be done when the athlete is cooling down to allow the fatigued muscles to return to their normal resting length.
- Passive stretching should be done slowly as its effectiveness depends on the development of tension and time of stretch. Less tension over more time appears to be most appropriate.
- Each muscle should be taken to the end of its range, then taken a little further within pain limits.
- The dosage of progressive stretching and mobilizing techniques used depends on the degree of primary tissue damage and the resulting time needed for repair. After injury, muscles must not be stretched if there is a likelihood of increasing tissue damage. The formation of dense connective scar tissue post trauma is lessened if early mobilization occurs within the limits of pain.

Contraindications to stretching

Stretching is contraindicated where there is a bony block to movement, recent or unstabilized fracture, acute inflammatory or infectious process, sharp acute pain, recent haematoma or other indications of tissue trauma, e.g. myositis ossificans. When contractures or shortened soft tissues are giving stability to a joint in the absence of structural stability or muscle strength, care must be taken not to decrease the functional capabilities of a joint by overstretching. This is particularly important in chronically hypermobile joints where repeated trauma has led to capsular scarring and thickening. These joints stiffen with time and injudicious stretching or mobilizing may cause symptoms to recur.

Exercises done too vigorously or functional activities started too early may damage new tissues and delay recovery. Signs of excessive stretching include resting pain, loss of range, tenderness and spasm. However, if movement is not progressed, new tissues may adhere to surrounding structures and become the source of pain and limitation of movement. The dosage of active exercise depends on the patient's response; if inflammatory signs increase, e.g. morning stiffness, the dosage or intensity must be modified.

Return to full activity should coincide with a full painfree range of motion, adequate strength, good endurance and normal movement patterns.

Mobilizing exercises

When there is a limitation in joint range of motion, it can be treated with passive mobilization applied by the physiotherapist or with equipment. It can also be worked on by the patient using active or passive movement to apply a mobilizing force to the joint. An example of this is to do a weightbearing lunge exercise for the talocrural joint that is limited in dorsiflexion. The patient is doing an active exercise but using a passive force to mobilize the joint. The patient can be instructed to perform the mobilizing exercise with an appropriate grade of force, as with passive mobilizing. It is, of course, possible to use an active or assisted active movement to mobilize a joint, as with a shoulder wheel or a pulley arrangement.

Proprioception exercises

Proprioception is the sense of position and movement of the body, in particular the limbs, assisting with maintenance of balance and co-ordination. It is hence vital in the rehabilitation of athletic injury. Proprioceptive sensations are mediated by mechanical displacements within peripheral joint and muscle receptors, which can be damaged with injury. Whether injury is acute or chronic, the proprioceptors will most likely have been affected.

Limb proprioception is mediated primarily by muscle afferent receptors, the muscle spindles, which are slowly adapting mechanoreceptors wound around a specialized muscle fibre. These muscle spindles are sensitive to minute changes in muscle length, thereby deriving information on joint angle and movement (kinaesthesia). Joint mechanoreceptors within the connective tissue of the joint capsule are sensitive to extremes of range. People with total joint replacements can still detect static position, but their kinaesthetic awareness is reduced (Kandel et al 1991).

Occluded circulation in a limb reduces the perception of movement, and patients with impaired sensation in the limbs show deficits in both feed-forward and feedback control of movement (Kandel et al 1991). Proprioception is profoundly affected by damage to large diameter sensory fibres, as in a peripheral nerve injury, and is dramatically illustrated in the condition of large-fibre sensory neuropathy. Unless they can see their limbs, these patients cannot detect position or motion, and tactile sensation and tendon reflexes are impaired. Pain and temperature sensation, carried by small diameter fibers, are not affected, but rapid movements to points in space are profoundly inaccurate due to loss of feed-forward control (Kandel et al 1991). Athletes often complain of reduced performance and inaccuracy of movements following injury, even when the original pathology has healed, and the possibility of prolonged disability due to peripheral receptor damage needs to be borne in mind by the physiotherapist and addressed clinically.

Exercises to increase the athlete's proprioceptive awareness should be incorporated into rehabilitation early and continued throughout the program. These may include the use of rocker or wobble boards, balance activities, balls thrown and caught while balancing, jumping and landing from and onto gradually more unstable surfaces, and proprioceptive neuromuscular facilitation patterns (see Ch. 32). More advanced proprioceptive work such as mimicking limb position with vision occluded and eye-hand co-ordination tasks bring the rehabilitation of athletes toward more functional activities and skill drills.

Functional activities

The final stages of a rehabilitation program should ensure that co-ordination and speed of motion has been re-established, along with strength, flexibility, balance and proprioception. The athlete must also have confidence in his or her ability to perform at the level required. There is often a gap in a rehabilitation program between the activities performed in the physiotherapist's rooms and the return to a sports training situation. At this stage, the athlete has recovered sufficiently to return to sport in a gradual progression but is often unsure of how far to go in training. At this point detailed discussions with the coach should take place so that a 'back to basics' approach can be taken to relearn the basic motor skills required for the sport. The coach and athlete should be counselled on the warning signs of doing 'too much too soon'. Measures such as ice after training should be routine. Both the athlete and coach must be aware of their limitations, as there is a high risk of reinjury or aggravation at this crucial stage. It is insufficient to allow a return to light training without this detailed instruction.

Exercise prescription

When prescribing exercises, objective measurements should be made and baseline data collected that is retestable, such as the maximum number of repetitions of a particular exercise before fatigue, maximum voluntary isokinetic strength testing, goniometry etc. Assessment is an ongoing process: as the athlete improves the exercise program must reflect this improvement and be progressed accordingly. This also assists in the motivation of the injured athlete, who may become discouraged if there is no tangible sign of improvement with therapeutic exercise.

Commencement of exercise

Exercise should be started as soon as possible in the rehabilitation program within the limits of the demands for healing, irritability of the injured part, surgeon's instructions and general physical condition of the injured athlete. It is important to accurately assess the injured area for signs of heat, redness, swelling, ecchymosis, exudate or pain that may indicate inflammation, bleeding or infection. If exercise is deemed appropriate, it is important to expose the part being rehabilitated, stabilize the body around the part being used and to prevent trick or compensatory movements so that the athlete can demonstrate that he or she can perform the exercise correctly. The appropriate dosage and an explanation of what the athlete should be feeling during and after exercise should be provided. Only then can the athlete commence a regime which may include some unsupervised exercise.

Appropriate mode of exercise

When choosing an exercise it should be safe, appropriate to the stage of recovery and well understood by the athlete. As a general rule, the sequence of progression of types of therapeutic exercise can follow that described above: resistance, speed, range and degree of difficulty are gradually progressed. In special cases, certain types of exercise are introduced sooner. For example, eccentric exercise is used early in the rehabilitation of tendon injuries, and closed chain weightbearing exercises are used early in the rehabilitation of the lower limb. This will depend on the forces that can be safely generated at affected joints and demands a knowledge of the applied anatomy of the ligamentous and other soft tissue structures. The level of difficulty and resistance must also be tailored to the particular requirement of the injured part at the time, e.g. cycling is not possible until the knee joint has acquired an adequate range of motion.

Equipment

It is important to consider the type of strengthening equipment that is to be used. Consideration should be given to safety, availability, cost and what can be achieved with the apparatus. For example, free weights strengthen not only the prime mover muscles but also the synergists and stabilizers. They can also be used in a variety of planes. They can be used to simulate functional activities and therefore carry over into the sporting activity. It must be remembered that not all athletes have access to the latest gym equipment and need to have programs designed to their situation. Elasticized rubber is a relatively cheap and effective resistance that can be used for many exercises and is easy for the athlete to use at home or work.

Speed selection/appropriate velocity of exercise

It is important to strengthen through the whole spectrum of velocities but also to concentrate on the specific requirements of the athlete's sport in terms of training speed. Slow movement is characterized by greater force output, but this may be inappropriate in a power event such as throwing or jumping. Usually there will be a combination of high and low speed repetitions with varying resistances according to the needs and goals of the athlete.

Facilitation

It may be possible to facilitate greater motor unit recruitment by a prior contraction of the antagonist or by stretching (Bosco et al 1981). Warm-up sessions including an aerobic component and stretching prior to a strengthening program are recommended to optimize body temperature so that muscles can work more efficiently.

Training effects

These are the product of frequency, duration and intensity. The recommended frequencies for therapeutic exercises will depend on the stage of rehabilitation and the type of exercise being prescribed. As a general rule, 2-3 evenly spaced sessions per week initially, increasing to 3-4 per week can be used as a guide. Duration refers to the length of hold on contraction and the optimum periods have been described above. Progression to encourage training effects depends on the relationship between the weight load and the number of repetitions, but in general 8-12 repetitions per set are safe and effective with 75% of their maximum resistance (see Ch. 9).

Recovery

It is important to allow time for rest between sets to allow the muscle to recover prior to exercising again. Time must be allowed in the program for tissue repair and protein synthesis to occur. Muscle recovery is an important part of muscle growth and strength building. Most people need 48 hours to recover from a hard muscular workout.

Progression

Therapeutic exercise should be progressively directed to provide painfree movement, full strength, power, and full extensibility of muscles. The affected ligamentous tissue should become painfree, have full tensile strength and full range of motion. Some guidelines for progression include:

- In the acute stage of injury, swelling needs to be controlled before exercise can be progressed.
- Pain is a safe guideline for progression. If there is no pain after exercising or it is of very short duration (less than 30 min), and there is no swelling or stiffness the next morning, it is safe to move on to the next stage. It is also advisable to restore and maintain strength in surrounding muscles to restore optimal function to the entire affected limb or region.
- Intermediate exercise phase. Painfree muscle contraction has been achieved with up to 50% ROM and strength and near normal co-ordination.
- Advanced exercise phase. At least 90% of ROM and strength has been restored. The primary goal now is to fully restore power, flexibility, endurance, speed and agility of the affected part as well as to encourage total body conditioning.

- Return to sport should be gradual and carefully monitored by the physiotherapist and coach (see Ch. 10). Ongoing exercise plans such as gym programs must also fit in with what is required for full recovery from an injury.

Full range of movement, strength, proprioception, co-ordination, speed and cardiovascular fitness in a gym program are important considerations, and the professional assistance of a coach or personal fitness trainer within the gym setting is advisable. The athlete must have gained full confidence to perform to his or her best on return to sport, and the advice of a sports psychologist may be of assistance.

Criteria for recovery and return to full training

1. Range of motion the same as the unaffected side and painfree.
2. Strength is equal to or greater than the other side.
3. Proprioception restored.
4. Full function restored using sport-specific drills.
5. Confident attitude.

OTHER CONSIDERATIONS

Chronic recurring pain

A premature return to sport before full healing of injured tissues may lead to chronic recurring pain. This may also be due to scar tissue improperly aligned to the lines of stress while healing. Contractures or poor mobility occurs in structures that become stressed with premature repeated or vigorous activity, resulting in a painful and enlarged but weak scar. Sometimes a focus of degenerative or necrotic tissue forms which acts as a source of irritation that will not respond to conservative treatment, despite a carefully planned and well executed rehabilitation. Cortisone injection or surgical excision and repair may be required. Specific passive stretching or mobilizing exercises will then be required. This is common in chronic achilles and patellar tendonitis, where an eccentric program may have failed initially due to presence of necrotic tissue, but is beneficial postoperatively in rehabilitation.

Less recognized reason for chronic recurring pain and dysfunction is adverse mechanical tension of the neuro-meningeal structures associated with the site of injury (Wajswelner 1993). Specific assessment and treatment procedures are described elsewhere in this book (see Chs 26 and 33).

Women and strengthening programs

Programs for women, like those for men, should be tailored for the individual. Strength training programs have been under-used for females and need to be incorporated into their programs if female athletes are to achieve full potential in their sport and protect themselves against injury. Recent research appears to suggest that strength differences between men and women are related to differences in normal body proportions and daily activities and that when adjusted to body weight the strength differences are not so great (Wilson 1992).

Older athletes and strengthening programs

Maximum strength is gained during the 20s, after which there is a gradual diminution of strength each year. However, research shows that most of the diminutions of strength shown in the older population are due to disuse rather than physiological changes of muscle (Chapman 1985). The older athlete may need lighter loads and more repetitions, but the program can be tailored to the individual's needs and aimed towards general conditioning. Research has shown conclusively that strength gains with exercise are possible in the elderly population.

Young athletes and strengthening programs

Very intensive exercise or 'too much too soon' may damage epiphyseal growth plates, but strengthening programs are essential for the adolescent in rehabilitation. Adolescents need to be taught good training techniques, should be well supervised if using a weight training program and should be encouraged to use lighter weights with more repetitions so that exercises can be performed in a controlled manner without trick movements. The use of circuit training with the incorporation of the use of body weight as the resisting force can be used successfully and safely with adolescents. Young athletes should be encouraged to take note of their bodies' reaction to exercise, and to recognize the warning signs of overuse, modifying their training accordingly.

SUMMARY

Therapeutic exercise is one of the main contributions a physiotherapist makes to the success of recovery from athletic injury. In the modern approach to management of sports injuries, therapeutic exercise can be commenced virtually immediately in modified forms such as continuous passive motion or isometrics to avoid the secondary insult that goes with immobility and lack of normal use of an injured part. These early simple exercises are gradually progressed and resistance training, passive and active stretching and mobilizing can be introduced with the athlete's specific goals in mind. The sports physiotherapist should have a thorough appreciation of the principles of resistance training to be able to take advantage of the gains to be made by using strengthening exercises in the rehabilitation of the injured athlete.

REFERENCES

Arms S W, Pope M H, Johnson R J 1984 The biomechanics of anterior cruciate ligament rehabilitation and reconstruction. American Journal of Sports Medicine 12(8):8-18

Atha J 1981 Strengthening muscle. Exercise and Sports Science Reviews 9:1-73

Bosco C, Komi P V, Ho A, 1981 Prestretch potentiation of human skeletal muscle during ballistic movement. Acta Physiologica Scandinavica 111:135-140

Chapman A E 1985 The mechanical properties of human muscle. Exercise and Sports Science Review 13:443-501

Cornelius W L 1988 A study on placement of stretching within a workout. Journal of Sports Medicine and Physical Fitness 28:234-236

Coyle E F, Feiring D 1980 Muscular power improvements: specificity of training velocity. Medicine and Science in Sports and Exercise 12(2):134

Croce P, Gregg J R 1991 Keeping fit when injured. Clinics in Sports Medicine 10(1):181-195

Curwin D, Stanish M 1984 Tendinitis: its etiology and treatment. Collamore Press, Massachusetts

De Carlo M S, Shelbourne D, McCarroll R, Rettig A C 1992 Traditional versus accelerated rehabilitation following ACL reconstruction: a one year follow-up. Journal of Orthopaedic and Sports Physical Therapy 15(6):309-316

Fleck S J 1989 Designing a resistance training session. State of the Art Review, National Sports Research Centre. Australian Sports Commission, Canberra

Fleck S, Kraemer W 1987 Designing resistance training programs. Human Kinetics, Illinois

Friden J, Sjostrom M, Ekblom B, 1983a Myofibrillar damage following intense eccentric exercise in man. International Journal of Sports Medicine 4(3):170-176

Friden J, Seger J, Sjostrom M, Ekblom B 1983b Adaptive response in human skeletal muscle subjected to prolonged eccentric training. International Journal of Sports Medicine 4(3):177-183

Fu F H, Woo S L-Y, Irrgang J J 1992 Current concepts for rehabilitation following anterior cruciate ligament reconstruction. Journal of Orthopaedic and Sports Physical Therapy 15(6):270-278

Gould J, Davies G (eds) 1985 Orthopedic and sports physical therapy. C V Mosby, St Louis, vol 2

Hakkinen K, Komi P V 1981 Effect of different combined concentric and eccentric muscle work regimens on maximal strength development. Journal of Human Movement Studies 7:33-44

Hakkinen K, Komi P V 1983 Electromyographic changes during strength training and detraining. Medicine and Science in Sports and Exercise 15:455-460

Hayes M, Dalton S, Wajswelner H 1990 Common shoulder problems in sport. Australian Sports Medicine Federation, Canberra

Henning C E, Lynch A, Glick K R 1985 An in vivo strain gauge study of elongation of the anterior cruciate ligament. American Journal of Sports Medicine 13:22-26

Hollis M 1989 Practical exercise therapy, 3rd edn. Blackwell Scientific, Oxford

Janda V 1978 Muscles, central nervous regulation and back problems. In: Kerr I M The neurobiologic mechanisms in manipulative therapy. Plenum Press, New York

Kandel E R, Shwartz J H, Jessell T M 1991 Principles of neural science, 3rd edn. Prentice Hall, London

Kisner C, Colby L, 1985 Therapeutic exercise: foundations and techniques. F A Davis, Philadelphia

Mangine R E 1988 Physical therapy of the knee, vol 19. Clinics in Physical Therapy. Churchill Livingstone, New York

McDonagh M J N, Davies C T M 1984 Adaptive responses of mammalian skeletal muscle to exercise with high loads. European Journal of Applied Physiology 52:140

Moffroid M T, Whipple R H 1970 Specificity of speed of exercise. Physical Therapy 50:1693-1699

Palmitier R A, An K N, Scott S G, Chao E Y S 1991 Kinetic chain exercise in knee rehabilitation. Sports Medicine 11:402-413

Safran M R, Garrett W E, Seaber A V, Glisson R R, Ribbeck B M 1988 The role of warm up in the muscle injury prevention. American Journal of Sports Medicine 16:123–128

Sale D, MacDougall D, 1981 Specificity of strength training: a review for the coach and the athlete. Canadian Journal of Applied Sport Science 16(2):87–91

Shelbourne K D, Nitz P 1992 Accelerated rehabilitation after anterior cruciate ligament reconstruction. Journal of Orthopaedic and Sports Physical Therapy 15(6):256–264

Stanish W, Curwin D 1986 Eccentric exercise in chronic tendonitis. Clinical Orthopaedics and Related Research 208(July):65–68

Stanton P, Purdam C, LaFortune M 1989 Hamstring injuries in sprinting—the role of eccentric exercise. Journal of Orthopaedic Sports Physical Therapy 10:347

Voss D E, Ionta M K, Myers B J 1984 Proprioceptive neuromuscular facilitation patterns and techniques, 3rd edn. Harper & Row, Philadelphia

Wajswelner H 1993 Neural tissue stretching in the rehabilitation of sports injuries. Proceedings of the long and short of stretching symposium. Manual Therapy Special Group and Sports Physiotherapy Group of NSW, pp 31–35

Wilkinson A C 1993 Stretching and muscle stiffness. Proceedings of the long and short of stretching symposium. Manual Therapy Special Group and Sports Physiotherapy Group of NSW

Wilson G 1992 Strength training for sport. State of the Art Review. National Sports Research Centre, Australian Sports Commission, Canberra

14. Massage

Colleen B. Liston

Definitions of massage refer to a repair movement (Rawlins 1930), a healing art (Krieger 1973), and the mechanical stimulation of the tissue by rhythmically applied pressure and stretching (Wood & Becker 1981).

The use of massage in conjunction with sporting pursuits is reported by Graham (1902) as being referred to by Homer in the *Odyssey* c. 8th century BC, Herodotus in the 5th century BC and Hippocrates c. 460–375 BC. Massage was given to prepare those indulging in severe activities to test strength. It was purported to make the tissues more supple and prevent ruptures and strains. After strength tests and games the gladiators used massage to relieve pain and bruising, to stroke away swelling and to refresh them. In gymnasia massage was given by 'anointers'—usually medical practitioners or slaves—to wrestlers before and after they performed their exercises.

Sports massage, sometimes called 'apotherapy' was revived from its Greek origins with gladiators in the 20th century. Two French books by Coste (1906) and Ruffier (1907) specifically addressed 'massage sportif' (Kamenetz 1985). Muller and Schutze am Esch (1966) reported that the value of sports massage in hastening recovery for muscle fatigue had been confirmed by numerous investigators, (Kamenetz 1985).

With the increasing involvement in sporting pursuits by the majority, sports massage is gaining recognition as an important preventive and treatment modality. Investigations into its efficacy and uses continue, and at the Australian Institute of Sport a leading masseur, Clews (1990), has written a book about self-massage techniques for sporting activities.

EFFICACY AND INDICATIONS FOR MASSAGE IN SPORT

In this section, the variety of techniques relevant for use by those undertaking sports massage will be presented. For each the physiological basis, effects and indications will be given support by scientific evidence.

In general sports massage can:
- decrease the detrimental effects of training, for example strain and discomfort
- improve training consistency
- prevent muscle and tendon injuries
- assist acute injury healing—complete and proper healing prevents acute problems becoming chronic.
- assist chronic injury healing by breaking down adhesions therefore, restoring mobility. The cycle of tight → tear → tighter → more tearing can be avoided.
- reduce muscle spasm leading to restoration of normal muscle function
- engender a relaxed mental attitude, enhance confidence and increase the possible length of a person's sports career.

Through rhythmically applying pressure and stretching to the soft tissues of the body, there is stimulation of exteroceptors, both deep and superficial; proprioceptors in tendons and muscles; and, interoceptors in the deeper tissues and the organs.

The effects that ensue are based on physical, psychological and physiological events, through reflex and mechanical mechanisms.

Graham (1913) suggests that studying the effects of massage is indeed the study of physiology. The facilitation of capillary circulation and lymph flow points increases nutritive supply and removal of waste products. Swelling and induration are reduced, adhesions are broken down, contracted tendons and ligaments are stretched and the skin is warmed and mobilized on the underlying tissues (Maggiora 1891, Starling 1894, Graham 1913, Kleen 1921, Krogh 1929, Drinker 1939, Drinker & Yoffey 1941, Pemberton 1945, Wakim et al 1949, Ladd et al 1952).

Reflex effects (MacKenzie 1923, Mennell 1945, Ebner 1956, Jacobs 1960, Bugaj 1975, Mattson Porth 1986) such as capillary vasodilation or constriction, relaxation or stimulation of voluntary muscle contraction, and pain reduction or exacerbation with sensory input variations also occur. In massage the hands stimulate sensory receptors in the skin, the resultant stimuli passing along afferent fibres to the spinal cord through the automatic and central nervous systems. The aforementioned effects occur in the segmentally related body zones. Barrow, in Graham (1913), also suggests an explanation for the visceral effects which may accompany the reflex effects of massage.

The touching of another person communicates an intention, in the case of therapeutic massage, to heal, recruit inherent energy or share energy, or promote relaxation. An increase in haemoglobin has been reported (Pemberton 1945, Krieger 1973, Krieger 1976) as has release of acetylcholine and histamine (as well as histamine-like substances) (Skull 1945). Furthermore, Siegel (1986) believes that is it possible to activate the body's immune system through a loving healing touch and self healing.

Hyperstimulation analgesia can be achieved through acupuncture, acupressure, trigger point stimulation, myofascial techniques, cupping and the use of TENS (Anderson et al 1974, Fox & Melzack 1976, Lewit 1979, Melzack 1981, Travell & Simons 1983, Melzack 1985).

Table 14.1 provides a list of massage techniques and a brief statement of major effects and indications. It may be used as a guideline for selection of the most appropriate technique to fulfil an aim.

SAFETY

For all types and applications of massage in sport there are few age or gender specific considerations. Baby massage is well recognized as an ideal way to introduce touch as well as being shown to have a beneficial influence on development, alertness and emotional status (Leboyer 1976, Prudence 1984, Rice 1975, Schneider 1982). Massage is also of use for relaxation and pain relief in the elderly and dying when the constantly changing needs of the client should be taken into account (Levine 1982). The person's tolerance and skin condition—such as dryness, tightness or frailty—must be taken into account whenever massage is performed, so it applies for sports massage.

Massage does not take the place of stretching and warm-up but is used as an adjunct to these important requirements prior to undertaking any sporting pursuit.

For acute injuries, the regime of ice, compression and elevation must be used at once. Massage should not be used for complete tears, newly strained muscles in the first 48 hours and where there is a high level of pain. Masseurs should be alert to signs of inflammation where there is a pocket of fluid in muscle tissue with a 'dent' in it indicating intramuscular bleeding (such as a 'corked' thigh). Rest is essential in this situation.

When administering acupressure, an adverse autonomic or psychophysiological response may occur in children under seven whose autonomic nervous system is immature, and those with severe cardiac conditions (Armstrong 1972, Tappan 1988). Acupressure should not be given over contusions, scar tissue or where there is irregularity of the skin (such as moles, warts or acne).

The use of lubricants, creams and gels cannot be supported by the literature. Peripheral vasodilation and an increase in peripheral blood flow during massage has been noted by Skull (1954). Acetylcholine is released and histamine and histamine-like substances produce the vasodilation. There is local counter-irritation produced as any agents that penetrate are absorbed by the blood in the cutaneous capillary system. The subject may feel a pleasant warmth and glow as a result, but the only effect on deeper tissues is a lessening of the blood flow there as blood rushes

Table 14.1 Massage techniques, effects and indications

Choice of technique	Likely effects	Indications for use
Swedish remedial effleurage	• Lymphatic drainage • Relaxation or stimulation	• Oedema • Psychological stress • Immobility and lethargy
Petrissage • Kneading • Wringing • Picking up • Ironing • Skinrolling	• Increase in stimulation of blood flows thereby improving removal of wastes and provision of nutrients • Mechanical—deep movement of soft tissues	• Retention of waste products • Poor circulation • Immobility • Adhesions • Contractures
Frictions • Circular	• Break down adhesions	• Adhesions • Contractures
Tapôtment • Hacking • Pounding • Beating • Clapping • Vibrations and shaking	• Stimulation of peripheral nerve endings and circulation • Respiratory effects— removal of sputum	• Poor circulation • Interactive stretch reflex • Sputum retention
Cyriax frictions • Transverse	• Prevention and breakdown of adhesions and movement • Trauma hyperemia pain relief	• Sub-acute muscle and ligamentous lesions • Chronic adhesions • Tenosynovitis • Tendonitis • Vaginitis
Connective tissue massage • Basic section • Long and short strokes • Balancing strokes	• Stimulation of somatic and autonomic nervous system • Reflex effects therefore vascular changes	• Peripheral vascular disease • Adhesions • Circulatory insufficiency
Acupressure/Shiatsu • Finger pressure to acupuncture points	• Homeostasis — balance of Chi (Ki) (energy) • Pain	• Pain with functional disorders
Trigger point Icing • Stretching • Pressure	• Muscle reflex responses and muscle relaxation • Referred pain	• Local pain • Muscle tension • Referred pain
Myofascial release • Stretching	• Constriction • Pain	• Pain • Fascial and muscular restriction

to the skin. However, the penetrating substances are quickly removed from the local area and so do not have a lasting or systemic effect (Tappan 1988).

Oily substances may reduce friction too much so that for deeper techniques there is an inability to grasp the tissues as the hands slide on the skin, rendering the treatment ineffective.

Contraindications

General contraindications to massage of all types are obvious because of the physiological effects of the techniques utilised. No massage technique should be given in the presence of:

1. General illness: pyrexia as massage will further increase the overall body temperature
2. Acute inflammation with pus: to avoid spread of the inflammatory process with the increase in circulation
3. Haemophilia: to ensure that bleeding does not occur
4. Early stages of lymphangitis: to decrease the risk of facilitating the production of excessive lymph
5. Acute neuritis: so that further sensory irritation does not occur
6. Skin disease, or
7. Acute or active rheumatoid arthritis, infective or gouty arthritis: so that the inflammatory process is not aggravated.

Local contraindications include:

1. Thrombosis, aneurysm, phlebitis, marked varicosity in the limb being massaged
2. Open wounds in the area of the massage
3. Recent fracture sites: to ensure movement does not take place. Massage may be applied elsewhere
4. Calcifications in the soft tissues: massage may spread to the deposits to other areas and lead to myositis ossificans
5. Local cancer: to avoid movement of abnormal cells to other areas
6. Panniculitis—fatty lobules: to reduce the risk of fat embolus
7. Poisonous foci—snake bites, stings: so that poison is not released into the circulation
8. Foreign bodies: to avoid their movement in the circulatory system.

Specifically, where autonomic responses may be elicited such as connective tissue massage, acupressure and trigger point technique, contraindications include pregnancy (because of the autonomic response), cardiorespiratory conditions and psychological disorders such as panic attacks.

ASSESSMENT AND EVALUATION

Sports massage is the skilful selection and application of the wide range of reflex and mechanical stimuli available in the form of massage.

An understanding of structure and function, together with an ability to assess, identify dysfunction and changes in posture and tissues, then plan safe effective treatment, is important in choosing massage techniques.

Aims to be achieved with sports massage are:

1. Prevention of injury by maintaining optimal resting length of muscles
2. Lasting treatment for acute and chronic injuries (Hannaford et al 1988)
3. Pain free training.

The methods suggested to ensure these aims are achieved include massage during training; use of deep techniques e.g. connective tissue massage, frictions (especially deep transverse) and myofascial stretching; and conditioning e.g. pre-event/warm-up massage.

Assessment

Knowledge of the massage techniques themselves, their likely effects and thus their indication for use can be applied after assessment. Attention to the age and attitude of the client as well as the precautions and contraindications should also be part of the rationale used in selection of techniques. Observation and palpation of soft tissue to indicate areas of oedema, induration and changes in temperature should be followed by assessment of muscle length and strength, joint mobility and range. Functional assessment and pain charting will provide information relevant to the massage chosen.

Application

Table 14.1 gives information relevant to the application. Specific massage techniques may be chosen where there is found to be oedema, poor circulation, adhesions, contractures and so on. The massage may be used as part of the whole treatment program. For example, it may follow or precede application of a hot or cold pack and may facilitate joint mobilization or manipulation. Exercise regimes to maintain the effects achieved in massage should be complementary.

Evaluation

Evaluation of swelling (e.g. circumference or fluid displacement techniques), joint range and muscle tension (by goniometry and similar measurement methods), skin temperature and other relevant assessments will provide evidence of the effects of the massage applied and guidance for continuance or the employment of alternative modalities to achieve the planned outcomes.

TECHNIQUES

Pre-event massage

In order to promote speed, power, endurance and to prevent injury it is reasonable to use massage to break down

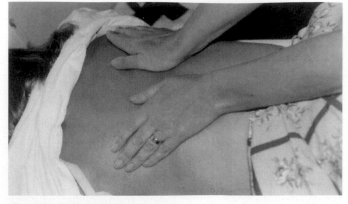

Fig. 14.1 Petrissage

adhesions, increase cellular nutrition, increase circulation and reduce muscle spasm.

Massage should be given 20–30 minutes before the warm-up and stretching of body parts that will undergo the greatest stress in the event (Calder 1990). It should be preceded by a brief 'needle' shower to stimulate peripheral nerve endings. Warm (45°C) ending in cool (25°C) water temperature leaves the sensory receptors stimulated and the core temperature at a normal level (Tappan 1988). It is important that the massage does not of itself increase the overall body temperature, yet warms the part to maximize the effects of the ensuing warm-up and stretching. Preceding marathon type events, special attention to climate and core temperature should be given, i.e. less warm-up on warmer days and rectal thermometer testing of core temperature.

Begin with the client lying prone in a comfortable resting position. Give effleurage to the back, starting lightly and progressing more deeply for relaxation. Relevant petrissage techniques follow (Fig. 14.1). These may include kneading for trapezius, erector spinae, latissimus dorsi, levator scapulae and rhomboids, picking up and wringing for upper fibres of trapezius, ironing, skin rolling and frictions on either side of the spinous processes (Beard & Wood 1964). Areas of tension and/or pain can be identified during the effleurage and dwelt on during the petrissage.

Deeper techniques for the specific muscles to be used will include frictions to tendons and ligaments and other petrissage techniques such as kneading to muscle bellies. Frictions should include musculotendinous junctions. Clients may be taught to give themselves pre-event massage for some of the muscles specific to their sport. This is relatively easy for the lower limb, more difficult for the upper limb where only one hand is available and requires imagination for the back and buttocks (Prentice 1986, Tappan 1988, Clews 1990).

Conclude with brisk tapôtment, e.g. hacking, to provide stimulation and a sense of well being. That is, administer:

- relaxation
- conditioning
- stimulation.

This will ensure the athlete is ready to go and enhance the preparation of the body and mind for warm-up and stretching prior to optimum performance.

Acute injuries

It is important to encourage the development of an orderly fibrillary network early, in order to produce strong pliable connective tissue. Deep transverse frictions can be used to 'spin' the fibres (like separating individual strands in a piece of string rolled under the finger) that are present 48 hours after injury (Stearns 1940). Fibroplasia can be prevented by inhibiting an inflammatory reaction (Ketchum 1977). However, since this is rarely completely effective, another mechanism to reduce the formation of tight scar tissue resulting from fibroplasia is required (Noyes et al 1974, Akeson et al 1977). Immobility has been shown to lead to scar tissue in structures, and pain when movement recommences (Mason & Allen 1941, Tipton et al 1970, Woo et al 1975, Noyes 1977, Cooper 1986).

Stearns (1940), Akeson et al (1977) and Vailas et al (1981) have found that movement seems to prevent scar formation by stimulating proteoglycan synthesis, providing mechanical stress which assists orderly laying down of new collagen fibres and preventing intermolecular cross-linking which results in tight, short collagen fibres. Thus, the connective tissue is lubricated and fibres are kept separate to ensure efficient remodelling.

Cyriax developed a specific regime for the application of transverse frictions (Chamberlain 1982). Based on a thorough examination, the treatment is applied to acute ligamentous and muscle injuries, inflammatory conditions and chronic adhesions. Cyriax (1980) insists that the massage must be given to the right spot and in the most effective way. That is, the small area treated must be that from which pain in a muscle, ligament, tendon, joint capsule or the fascia originates. Areas of referred pain are ignored. Partial muscle ruptures, ligamentous sprains, tenosynovitis and tendonitis respond well to deep frictions. The technique employed is dependent upon the correct identification of pathology. For muscle or musculotendinous junction the affected muscle should be in a relaxed position. To prevent scar tissue from matting muscle fibres together during healing, deep transverse frictions are applied across the fibres for up to 20 minutes about three times a week (Cyriax 1977). Active movement of the muscle is permitted but passive stretching and resisted movement will strain the healing breach.

Ligaments recently sprained (minor rupture or tear of the ligamentous fibres) respond well to less vigorous frictions applied immediately to passively maintain mobility in the ligament. While the fibroblasts are newly formed and not strongly attached, light transverse frictions are given (Fig. 14.2). For chronic sprains, vigorous deep frictions are

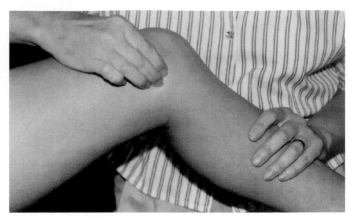

Fig. 14.2 Cyriax frictions

employed to induce the numbing effect of hyperemia acheived when, through enhancing the blood supply, Lewis' P-substance is destroyed more rapidly so pain is reduced during the treatment (15–20 min) and beyond (up to 30 min) Tappan (1988). Adhesions binding ligaments to underlying bone may then be broken down and a normal acute healing process can proceed. As rationalized earlier, the importance of movement during healing prevents the formation of scar tissue thus maintaining the length of the structure involved.

In tenosynovitis it is necessary to place the tendon on stretch to provide a base on which to move the sheath. The friction must be given across the components comprising the structure, with sufficient sweep and depth. The two gliding surfaces are then 'smoothed off' by the breaking down of inflammatory exudates on the inner surface of the sheath and outer surface of the tendon resulting in full and pain free mobility (Chamberlain, 1982). Tendonitis may result from scar tissue forming after tearing any number of the small tendon bundles or collagen fibres which are bound by loose connective tissue to make larger bundles and thus the tendon itself (Chamberlain 1982). Deep transverse frictions are applied to the tendon on stretch. The pain associated with scar tissue in tendons may be treated with steroidal infiltration but deep frictions enhance breaking down of the scarring and promote correct healing (Cyriax 1977).

Other conditions responding well to deep frictions are painful and immobile traumatic scar tissue, tenovaginitis and indurated subcutaneous areas.

For the specific Cyriax regimes readers are referred to Cyriax (1980).

Chronic injuries

Maxwell et al (1988) attribute muscle soreness after high levels of exertion to local muscle spasm. Although stretching reduces pain where there is spasm, stretching torn muscle produces increased pain levels and further tearing. Physiologically, in the presence of muscle spasm there is capillary restriction which reduces blood flow. The circulatory restriction results in limitation of the flow of nutrients and

oxygen to the area and retention of waste products. More spasm leads to more pain and less flexible tissues. This vicious cycle can be broken by massage. Where joint range is affected the muscles and tendons above and below the joint should be treated (Wiktorsson-Möller et al 1983), including agonistic and antagonistic groups.

Delayed muscle soreness has been described as a dull aching type of pain in conjunction with tender, stiff muscles (Ebbeling & Clarkson 1989). It is not related to fatigue and occurs when performing unaccustomed exercises. Studies into this phenomenon cite muscle trauma associated with eccentric muscle work, tonic muscle spasm and connective tissue damage as occurring (Abraham 1977, Armstrong 1984, Armstrong 1990, Ebbeling & Clarkson 1989, Ferstat & Davidson 1990, Hasson et al 1989, Maxwell et al 1988).

Massage has been shown to provide faster, more graded recovery from delayed muscle soreness when compared with an untreated control group (Ferstat & Davidson 1990, Hill & Richardson 1989, Wiktorsson-Möller et al 1983).

Compression of the tissues with relaxed palms will spread the fibres, intensify the hyperemia and increase blood flow to and from the area (Fig. 14.3). Broad thumb strokes may be applied generally to muscle fibres to assess for adhesions. The thumb is used as it is more sensitive than other areas such as the heel of the hand. Normal muscle will spread but where there are adhesions the whole muscle moves away and snaps back after the stroke.

Deep thumb stroking may be used to stimulate flow of lymph and hyperemia in deeper tissues. Thumbs may work side by side or one behind the other. Some therapists use an elbow, multiple fingers, or the heel of the hand for the strokes which move in line with the muscle fibres, as do the full hand strokes applied in Swedish techniques. The depth reached depends on the bulk of the tissues and acceptance by the athlete. Deep transverse frictions, as previously described, are applied to specific chronic injuries.

Other massage and associated techniques which may be used in the treatment of sports injuries include connective

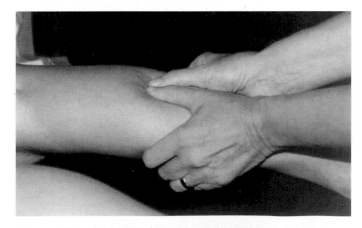

Fig. 14.3 Thumb strokes for delayed muscle soreness

tissue massage, acupressure (Shiatsu), trigger point stimulation and myofascial techniques (Tappan 1988).

The particular application of connective tissue massage to chronic sports injuries may be its ability to produce pain relief and increase the microcirculation in vascular beds. Kaada and Torsteinbo (1989) measured the concentration of plasma ß-endorphins before and 5, 30 and 90 minutes after 30 minutes of connective tissue massage. There was a 16% increase in the ß-endorphin levels from 20.0 to 23.2 pg/0.1 ml (p = 0.025) with a maximum at 5 minutes after the end of the massage. The effect lasted for about one hour. Developed by Elizabeth Dicke of Germany in 1929, bindegewebsmassage or connective tissue massage is the application of short and long deep strokes aimed at the connective tissue between the skin and the muscle. Findings support claims that a large number of disabilities respond to a system of stroking over reflex areas (head zones), especially on the trunk (Baker & Taylor 1954, Ebner 1956, Kisner & Taslitz 1968, Langen 1959, Mahoney 1957). Ebner (1962) points to the segmental development of the body as the underlying scientific basis. The orderly basic section of strokes to the low back prepares the body for other stroking, depending upon the condition of the connective tissue. Where there are areas bound down in muscle, the flat long pulls and shorter hooking strokes may be used locally (Counsilman & McAllister 1986, Hannaford et al 1988, Scher 1988).

Studies of the effects of connective tissue massage demonstrate that the four measures of autonomic activity—heart rate, blood pressure, galvanic skin resistance and peripheral skin temperature—reflect increased sympathetic activity (Burch & De Pasquale 1965, Kisner & Taslitz 1968, Lazarus et al 1963, Wang 1958). Using psychophysiological parameters, McKechnie et al (1983) report that symptoms of tension are alleviated when connective tissue massage is applied. In their study the heart rate slowed, skin resistance increased and levels of muscle tension decreased (p = <0.001) and the subjects were more relaxed and willing to talk about their physical problems.

It is of interest to note the overlap in the reflex zones stroked in connective tissue massage and the sites of acupuncture points which, when stimulated, claim relief of symptoms for the same pathologies and disabilities. In comparing Japanese Shiatsu, Chinese acupuncture/pressure and connective tissue massage there is an obvious relationship between the systems applied (Fig. 14.4).

More than 4500 years ago the first text on acupuncture, the Nei Ching, was written by Huang Ti (Tappan 1988). Pieces of stone and bone were used to press points on the skin. The response from stimulation to some points corresponds to that associated with the head zones mentioned previously (Armstrong 1972).

Finger pressure to acupuncture points is administered with one finger—the middle finger or thumb for preference

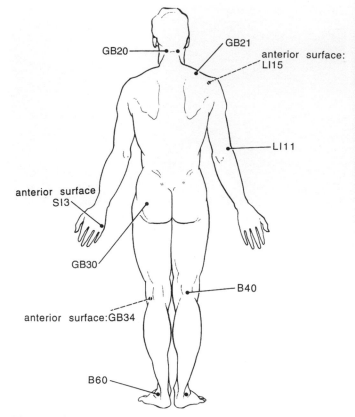

Fig. 14.4 Common acupuncture points

(Prentice 1986). Limited circular frictions progressing more deeply to static pressure over the point are given for 1–5 minutes. Prescriptive texts are available, which give information about point location and indications in applying acupressure for orthopaedic conditions (Chaitow 1979, Tappan 1988) . Table 14.2 adapted from these two authors and the Academy of Traditional Chinese Medicine (1975) provides examples of useful points for sports injuries and related problems.

Some acupuncture points correspond with the head zones and some with motor points: 50% of acupuncture points are directly over nerve trunks, 50% are within 0.5 cm and 71% coincide with trigger points (Manheim & Lavett 1989).

Trigger points—called 'myofascial triggers' by Travell and 'myodysneuric points' by Gutstein—are sensitive points or areas producing pain some distance away (Travell & Simons 1983). Active trigger points produce referred pain when palpated. There may be localized sharp pain which may radiate to the referred or target area some distance away (Fig. 14.5). The point is sensitive and may be associated with any or all of the following:

- movement restriction
- muscle weakness
- protective muscle spasm
- lowered skin resistance
- fibrositic nodules

Table 14.2 Points of sports injuries

Point	Location	Indications
B40 (bladder 40 Wei-Chung)	• Centre of popliteal fossa	• Leg cramp • Low back pain • Sciatica • Knee joint pain • Heat stroke
B60 (bladder 60 Kun lun)	• Midpoint between posterior margin of lateral malleolus and achilles tendon	• Low back pain • Sciatica • Ankle joint disorders—soft tissue sprains
GB20 (gall bladder 20 Feng-chih)	• Midpoint of line from tip of mastoid to posterior mid-line groove between trapezius and sternocleidomastoid	• Tension headache • Migraine • Stiff neck • Vertigo
GB21 (gall bladder 21 Chieng-ching)	• Midpoint between the C7 and the acromion process	• Shoulder pain • Neck pain with rigidity • Upper extremity motor problems
GB30 (gall bladder 30 Huan-tiao)	• Point at outer one-third of a line from greater trochanter to base of coccyx	• Hip joint pain • Soft tissue disorders of the hip • Low back pain
GB34 (gall bladder 34 Yangling Chuan)	• Anterior to the neck of the fibula	• Knee and lower extremity pain
LI11 (large intestine 11 Chu-chih) of the elbow	• At radial end of flexed elbow fold	• Shoulder pain • Elbow pain • Soft tissue disorders
LI15 (large intestine 15 Chien-yu)	• Acromial depression in mid deltoid with arm abducted to 90°	• Pain and motor problems of arm and elbow • Shoulder joint and soft tissue disorders
SI3 (small intestine 3 Hou-chi)	• Apex of the distal palmar crease on ulnar side of a clenched fist	• Low back pain • Neck pain and rigidity • Upper extremity weakness

- the 'jump' sign on palpation
- secondary trigger points in agonistic and antagonistic muscles overloaded through 'splinting' the injured muscle in compensation
- autonomic responses.

By releasing the active primary point the referred pain, motor, sensory and autonomic responses are also ameliorated, so the treatment of trigger points can be a useful adjunct to treatment of chronic sports injuries. Careful palpation and awareness of acupuncture points assists in the assessment of related soft tissue (Fischer 1988, Goldenberg 1989).

1. Localize the trigger point. It will be found in tight/taut fascial or muscular bands. It could be in the skin (scar tissue), a ligament, a tendon or even deeper at the joint capsule or periosteal level.

2. Treat more recent injuries and the generated trigger first, then work on older injuries. There will be more secondary triggers associated with chronic injuries.

3. Fast ice with the edge of an ice block or give parallel sweeps of vapocoolant spray, give at 4 cm/s 50 cm away from the skin (Simons 1985, Mance et al 1986, Wolfe 1988). Simons (1985) claims that Flouri-Methane sprays are safe.

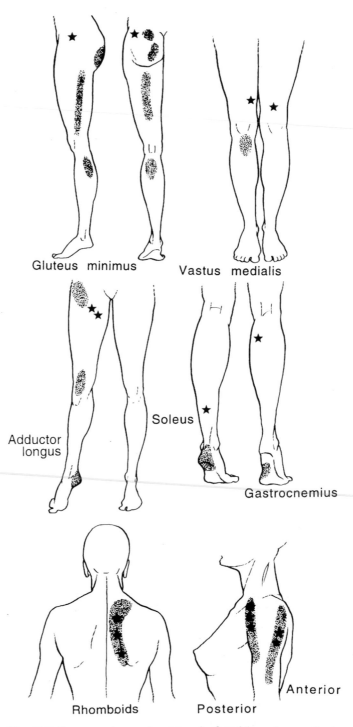

Fig. 14.5 Common trigger points (x) and referred (target) areas of pain

4. Gentle sustained stretch—with relaxation the muscle lengthens.
5. Apply 1 minute of sustained pressure (as for acupressure) over the trigger point. Increase the depth gradually or give intermittently.
6. Ice or spray again.

Sustained pressure may be given with one finger, two or more fingers, a knuckle, an elbow, or by 'strumming'—as in applying connective tissue massage—with the fingers extended (Manheim & Lavett 1989, Peppard 1983, Travell & Simons 1983).

A home program incorporating post-isometric relaxation can be used to maintain gains after trigger point treatment. This should involve stretching gently to resistance, contracting against gentle pressure for 10 seconds, maintaining this range and relaxing, then gently passively taking up the 'slack' to gain new range. The cycle should be repeated three to five times and may be used with self-administration of trigger point stimulation (Chaitow 1981).

The type of gain in range referred to is achieved by myofascial release. Fascia is a type of connective tissue with three layers—superficial, potential space and deep. It assists in maintaining muscle force. Whereas a fasciotomy to release tight fascia results in a 15% loss of muscle strength (Manheim & Lavett 1989), myofascial release techniques reduce constriction and pain without compromise to muscle strength (Manheim & Lavett 1989). Myofascial release in conjunction with trigger point stimulation is vital because the fascia tightens with inflammation (as the potential space swells), heals slowly (because of a poor blood supply), and is a pain focus (because of its overabundant nerve supply).

In chronic sports injuries the importance of proper assessment of postural alignment, and awareness of the proprioceptive feedback between the therapist and the athlete during myofascial release, is essential. The technique involves the hands of the relaxed therapist being placed at each extreme of muscle attachments. The subject should be encouraged to relax. Firm pressure is applied to provide stretch to the muscle for about 10 seconds then eased off. The slack should be taken up and a further stretch applied. After three to five repetitions the stretch should be slowly released and the subject reassessed. This process may be repeated up to five times dependent upon progress as gauged by the reassessment. Manheim and Lavett (1989) provide postural assessment methods and a detailed description of techniques used in myofascial release.

The role of myoglobin in myofascial pain and its dispersion with associated pain relief by massage techniques has been studied by Brendstrup et al (1957), Krusen et al (1965) and Danneskiold-Samsøe et al (1986). Melzack (1985) has reported on the similarity of the neural mechanisms involved in the relief of pain produced by acupuncture, acupressure, ice massage and trigger point stimulation. This hyperstimulation analgesia is one of the oldest recorded remedies and should become a useful technique in pain relief for the management of those with sports injuries, especially where chronic conditions have affected posture, gait and other functional activities.

Training/post-event massage

Massage techniques that slowly stroke the tissues and knead the muscles are widely used, particularly by the Russians, in training sessions (10–30 min for relaxation) or events for their ability to improve potential performance and recovery. It is reported by Calder (1990) that researchers publishing results in the *Soviet Sports Review* found increased performance for massaged athletes in sports ranging from track and field to wrestling. The area showing most gain was that of strength. Furthermore, massage techniques (light after heavy activities, deeper for light workloads and lasting 30–60 min) have been shown to be two to three times more likely to promote recovery than resting (Crampton & Fox 1987). During recovery physiological and psychological states return to pre-event levels (Blake et al 1989, Danneskiold-Samsøe et al 1982). This results in restoration of plasma myoglobin, hormone, enzyme and metabolic levels, i.e. a return to homeostasis (Arkko et al 1983, Barr & Taslitz 1970). Studies into the physiological effects of massage have been extensive and are continuing as improved sensitivity for measuring those parameters used as indices become available.

Psychologically and emotionally, massage can be used to enhance a feeling of well-being and relaxation. It should be given up to eight hours after the event when lighter techniques are used and one or two days later for heavier techniques (Calder 1990).

SUMMARY

Various types of massage can be undertaken by those involved with all fields of sports activities.

Massage is best combined with other techniques and modalities such as stretching, passive and active movements, proprioceptive neuromuscular facilitation, free and resisted exercise, ice, heat, electrical stimulation and hydrotherapy. The importance of touch as a means of communication, and to impart a sense of well being and confidence should not be ignored. There are approximately 18 000 square cm of skin, the principal seat of touch (as indicated by the large sensory homunculus). Massage is a delightful sensation (in most cases!), can have a soothing or stimulatory effect, promote increased flexibility and elasticity in the skin and underlying tissues and improve interaction between the client and the therapist (Montague 1978, Pratt & Mason 1981). Hippocrates (c. 460–375 BC) wrote of mobilizing the body's natural recuperative powers.

With increased mechanization and improving pharmacology there has been a move to dehumanization. The lack of contact and aloofness perceived by clients has led to the search for health practitioners who will provide closer contact, touch and massage. Physiotherapists have a licence to touch and must ensure that massage has a place in their practise of physiotherapy. Those working with athletes from all sports are ideally placed to use massage pre-event for prevention, for acute and chronic injuries, for restoration and to improve their clients' quality of performance.

REFERENCES

Abraham N M 1977 Factors in delayed muscle soreness. Medicine and Science in Sports 9(1):11-20

Academy of Traditional Chinese Medicine 1975 An outline of Chinese acupuncture. Foreign Language Press, Peking

Akeson W H, Amiel D, Mechanic G L, Woo S L, Harwood M L 1977 Collagen-cross-linking alterations in joint contractures: changes in the reducible cross-links in periarticular connective tissue collagen after nine weeks of immobilization. Connective Tissue Research 5:15-19

Anderson, D G, Jamieson J L, Man S C 1974 Analgesic effects of acupuncture on the pain of ice water: a double-blind study. Canadian Journal of Psychology 28:239-244

Arkko P J, Pakarinen A J, Kari-koskinen O 1983 Effects of whole body massage on serum protein, electrolyte and hormone concentrations, enzyme activities and haematological parameters. International Journal of Sports Medicine 4:265-267

Armstrong M E 1972 Acupuncture. American Journal of Nursing:1582

Armstrong R B 1984 Mechanisms of exercise-induced delayed onset muscular soreness: a brief review. Medicine and Science in Sports and Exercise 16(6):529-535

Armstrong R B 1990 Initial events in exercise-induced muscular injuries. Medicine and Science in Sports and Exercise 22(4):429-435

Baker L M, Taylor W M 1954 The relationship under stress between changes in skin temperature, electrical resistance and pulse rate. Journal of Experimental Psychology 48:361-366

Barr J S, Taslitz N 1970 The influence of back massage on autonomic functions. Physical Therapy 50:1670-1691

Basmajian J V (ed) 1985 Manipulation, traction and massage, 3rd edn. Williams & Wilkins, Baltimore

Beard G, Wood E C 1964 Massage principles and techniques. W B Saunders, Philadelphia

Blake B, Anthony J, Wyatt F 1989 The effects of massage treatment on exercise fatigue. Clinical Sports Medicine 1:189-196

Brendstrup P, Jespersen K, Asboe-Hansen G 1957 Morphological and chemical connective tissue changes in fibrositic muscles. Annals of Rheumatoid Diseases 16:438-440

Bugaj R 1975 The cooling, analgesic, rewarming effects of ice massage on localised skin. Physical Therapy 55:11

Burch G E, De Pasquale 1965 Methods for studying the influence of higher central nervous centers on the peripheral circulation of intact man. American Heart Journal 70:411-422

Calder A 1990 Sports massage. In: Third Report on National Sports Research Program July 1988-June 1990. Australian Sports Commission CPN, Canberra

Chaitow L 1979 The acupuncture treatment of pain. Thorsons, Northamptonshire

Chaitow L 1981 Instant pain control. Thorsons, Northamptonshire

Chamberlain G J 1982 Cyriax's friction massage: a review. Journal of Orthopaedic and Sports Physical Therapy 4(1):16-22

Clews W 1990 Sports massage and stretching. Bantam, Sydney

Cooper B 1986 Massage of the forearms for male gymnasts. Sports Science and Medicine Quarterly 2(3):4-6

Counsilman J, McAllister B 1986 Breaking up shoulder problems. Swimming Technique Feb/Apr:14-18

Crampton J, Fox J 1987 Regeneration vs burnout: prevention is better than cure. Sports Coach 10(4):7-10

Cyriax J 1977 Deep massage. Physiotherapy 63(2):60-61

Cyriax J 1980 Textbook of orthopaedic medicine, 10th edn, vol 2. Baillière Tindall, London

Danneskiold-Samsøe B, Christiansen E, Lund B, Anderson R B 1982 Regional muscle tension and pain ('fibrositis'). Scandinavian Journal of Rehabilitation Medicine 15:17-20

Danneskiold-Samsøe B, Christiansen E, Anderson R B 1986 Myofascial pain and the role of myoglobin. Scandinavian Journal of Rheumatology 15:175-178

Drinker C K 1939 The formation and movements of lymph. American Heart Journal 18:389

Drinker C K, Yoffey J M 1941 Lymphatics, lymph and lymphoid tissue: the physiological and clinical significance. Cambridge University Press, Cambridge

Ebbeling C B, Clarkson P M 1989 Exercise-induced muscle damage and adaptation. Sports Medicine 7:207-234

Ebner M 1956 Peripheral circulatory disturbances; treatment by massage of connective tissue in reflex zones. British Journal of Physical Medicine 19:176-180

Ebner M 1962 Connective tissue massage. Theory and therapeutic application. Livingstone, Edinburgh

Ferstat A, Davidson C 1990 The effectiveness of massage on delayed muscle soreness induced by consecutive days of eccentric and concentric muscle activity. Unpublished undergraduate research paper, Curtin University

Fischer A A 1988 Documentation of myofascial trigger points. Archives of Physical Medicine and Rehabilitation 69:286-291

Fox E J, Melzack R 1976 Transcutaneous electrical stimulation and acupuncture: comparison of treatment for low back pain. Pain 2:141-148

Goldenberg D L 1989 Treatment of fibromyalgia syndrome. Rheumatic Disease Clinics of North America 15(1):61-71

Graham D 1902 Treatise on massage. Its history, mode of application and effects. Lippincott, Philadelphia

Graham D 1913 Massage, manual treatment, remedial movements: history, mode of application and effects, indications and contraindications. Lippincott, Philadelphia

Hannaford P, Clews W S, Fardy E, Wajswelner H 1988 Effects of therapeutic massage versus physiotherapy modalities on interstitial compartment pressure. In: Proceedings of the 25th National Annual Scientific Conference. Australian Sports Medicine Federation, Sydney

Hasson S, Barnes W, Hunter M, Williams J 1989 Therapeutic effect of high speed voluntary muscle contraction on muscle soreness and muscle performance. Journal of Orthopaedic and Sports Physical Therapy June:499-507

He L 1987 Involvement of endogenous opioid peptides in acupuncture analgesia. Pain 31(1):91-121

Hill D W, Richardson J D 1989 Effectiveness of 10% trolamine salicylate cream on muscular soreness induced by a reproducible program of weight training. Journal of Orthopaedic and Sports Physical Therapy July:19-23

Jacobs M 1960 Massage for the relief of anatomical and physiological considerations. Physical Therapy Review 40:96

Kaada B, Torsteinbo O 1989 Increase of plasma ß-endorphins in connective tissue massage. General Pharmacology 20(4):487-489

Kamenetz HL 1985 History of massage. In: Basmajian J V (ed) Manipulation, traction and massage, 3rd edn. Williams & Wilkins, Baltimore

Kerr F W L, Wilson P R, Nijensohn D E 1978 Acupuncture reduces the trigeminal evoked response in decerebrate cats. Experimental Neurology 61:84-95

Ketchum L D 1977 Primary tendon healing: a review. Journal of Hand Surgery 2:428-435

Kisner C D, Taslibz N 1968 Connective tissue massage: the influence of the introductory treatment on autonomic functions. Physical Therapy 48(2):107-119

Kleen E A G 1921 Massage and medical gymnastics, 2nd edn. Trans Mina L Dobbie. Wood, New York

Krieger D 1973 The relationship of touch with intent to help or heal, studies in-vivo haemoglobin values. In: Proceedings of the American Nurses Association 9th Nursing Research Conference. Kansas City

Krieger D 1976 Nursing research for a new age. Nursing Times 72:1-7

Krogh A 1929 The anatomy and physiology of capillaries. New Haven Press, New Haven

Krusen F H, Kottke F J, Ellwood P M 1965 Handbook of physical medicine and rehabilitation. Saunders, Philadelphia

Ladd M P, Kottke F J, Blanchard R S 1952 Studies on the effect of massage on the flow of lymph from the the foreleg of a dog. Archives of Physical Medicine 33:604-612

Langen D 1959 Study on the mechanism of action of massage of reflex zones in connective tissue. Psychotherapy and Medical Psychology 9:194-201

Lazarus R S, Speisman J C, Mordkoff A M 1963 The relationship between autonomic indicators of psychological stress: heart rate and skin conductance. Psychosomatic Medicine 25:19-29

Leboyer F 1976 Birth without violence. Knopf, New York

Levine S 1982 Who dies? Anchor Press/Doubleday, Garden City, New York

Lewitt 1979 The needle effect in the relief of myofascial pain. Pain 6:83-90

MacKenzie J 1923 Angina pectoris. Hodder & Stoughton, London

Maggiora A 1891 De l'action physiologique du massage sur les muscles de l'homme. Archives of Italian Biology 16:225-246

Mahoney L 1957 Massage of reflex zones. Physiotherapy 43:74-76

Major R H 1954 A history of medicine. Blackwell, Springfield, Oxford

Mance D, McConnell B, Ryan P A, Silverman M, Master G 1986 Myofascial pain syndrome. Journal of the American Podiatric Medicine Association 76(6):328-331

Manheim C J, Lavett D K 1989 The myofascial release manual. Slack, New Jersey

Mason M L, Allen H S 1941 The rate of healing tendons. Annals of Surgery 113:424-456

Mattson Porth C 1986 Pathophysiology: concepts of altered health states, 2nd edn. Lippincott, Philadelphia

Maxwell S, Kohn S, Watson A, Balnave R J 1988 Is stretching effective in the prevention of or amelioration of delayed-onset muscle soreness? In: Proceedings of the 25th National Annual Scientific Conference of the Australian Sports Medicine Federation, Sydney

McKechnie A A, Wilson F, Watson N, Scott D 1983 Anxiety states: a preliminary report on the value of connective tissue massage. Journal of Psychosomatic Research 27(2):125-129

Melzack R 1981 Myofascial trigger points: relation to acupuncture and mechanisms of pain. Archives of Physical Medicine and Rehabilitation 62:114-117

Melzack R 1985 Hyperstimulation analgesia. Clinics in Anaesthesiology 3(1):81-92

Mennell J B 1945 Physical treatment by movement manipulation and massage, 5th edn. Blakiston, Philadelphia

Montague A 1978 Touching. Harper & Row, Toronto

Noyes F R, Torvik P J, Hyde W B et al 1974 Biomechanics of ligament failure. Journal of Bone and Joint Surgery 56-A:1406-1418

Noyes F R, 1977 Functional properties of knee ligaments and alterations induced by immobilization. Clinical Orthopaedics 123:210-242

Pemberton R 1945 Physiology of massage. In: AMA Handbook of Physical Medicine. American Medical Association, Chicago

Peppard A 1983 Trigger-point massage therapy. Physician and Sports Medicine 11(5):159-162

Pratt J W, Mason A 1981 The caring touch. Heyden, London

Prentice W E 1986 Therapeutic modalities in sports medicine. C V Mosby, Missouri

Prudence B 1984 Pain erasure. Evans, New York

Rawlins M S 1930 Textbook of massage: for nurses and beginners. C V Mosby, St Louis

Rice R D 1975 Premature infants respond to sensory stimulation. American Psychological Association Monitor 6(II):8

Scher 1988 Scarred stiff. Using massage to reduce muscular scar tissue. Triathlete 18-19:63

Schneider V 1982 Infant massage. Bantam, New York

Siegel B S 1986 Love, medicine & miracles. Harper & Row, New York

Simons D G 1985 Myofascial pain syndromes due to trigger points: 2 Treatment and single-muscle syndromes. Manual Medicine 1:72-77

Skull C W 1945 Massage—physiologic basis. Archives of Physical Medicine 261:159-167

Starling E H 1894 The influence of mechanical factors on lymph production. Journal of Physiology 16:224

Stearns M L 1940 Studies of the development of connective tissue in transparent chambers in the rabbit ear II. American Journal of Anatomy 67:55-97

Tappan F M 1988 Healing massage techniques. Appleton & Lange, Connecticut

Tipton C M, James S L, Merger W, Tcheng T K 1970 Influence of exercise on strength of medial collateral knee ligament of dogs. American Journal of Physiology 218:894-902

Travell J G, Simons D G 1983 Myofascial pain and dysfunction: the trigger point manual. Williams & Wilkins, Baltimore

Vailas A C, Tipton C M, Matthes R D, Gart M 1981 Physical activity and its influence on the repair process of medial collateral ligaments. Connective Tissue Research 9:25-31

Wakim K G, Martin G M, Terrier J C, Elkins E C, Krusen F H 1949 The effects of massage on the circulation in normal and paralyzed extremities. Archives of Physical Medicine 30:135

Wang G H 1958 The galvanic skin reflex: a review of old and recent works from a physiologic point of view. American Journal of Physical Medicine 37:37-57

Wiktorsson-Möller M, Öberg B, Ekstrand J, Gillquist J 1983 Effects of warming up, massage and stretching on range of motion and muscle strength in the lower extremity. American Journal of Sports Medicine 11(4):249-252

Wolfe F 1988 Fibrositis, fibromyalgia and musculoskeletal disease: the current status of fibrositis syndrome. Archives of Physical Medicine and Rehabilitation 69:527-531

Woo S L, Matthew J V, Akeson W H, Amiel D, Convery F R 1975 Connective tissue response to immobility. Arthritis and Rheumatism 18:257-264

Wood E, Becker P 1981 Beard's massage, 3rd edn. Saunders, Philadelphia

15. Electrotherapy

Joan McMeeken

In this discussion, electrotherapy encompasses thermal, electrical, mechanical, photobiological, magnetic and biofeedback devices used in sports physiotherapy practice. Electrotherapy modalities may constitute about 60% of patient treatment time (Dennis 1987) and are likely to be perceived by athletes as playing a significant role in the management of the presenting problem. Ultrasound and electrical stimulation devices are used more frequently than other equipment such as shortwave, microwave or laser (Lindsay et al 1990, Robinson & Snyder-Mackler 1988). Electrotherapy must be integrated to assist in the total management program of the athlete's problem. Its role should be put into perspective for the athlete; electrotherapy normally plays a minor role in the rehabilitation of sporting injuries or injuries sustained by sports persons in other environments. Electrotherapy may contribute to tissue healing by minimizing continuing damage and facilitating repair, may reduce pain and act as an adjunct to what is usually the key therapeutic modality—exercise. Chronic problems are unlikely to resolve with electrotherapy unless the precipitating factor is removed, although an athlete may continue to participate while active treatment keeps symptoms partially controlled. Both athlete and therapist should consider the long term implications to the athlete of this form of management.

SAFETY ISSUES

Sports injury may be due to trauma or over-use. Surgery may be required following a sports injury. However the tissue trauma occurs, electrotherapy can affect the response to pain, the inflammatory response to injury and contribute to minimizing tissue damage, facilitating repair, mobilization and strengthening and maintaining tissue health during enforced inactivity. To ensure that this is achieved, electrotherapy modalities need to be applied at the appropriate dosage and frequency. Nonetheless, devices which have the capacity to affect pathophysiological processes in a favourable direction may also cause tissue damage, as is evidenced by the production of tissue burns

by many modalities. Particular attention must be paid at all times to ensure the safety of athletes being treated with electrotherapy. Expediency cannot excuse a lack of elementary safety requirements such as checking for contraindications to the use of specific modalities, and ensuring that athletes are not subjected to the risk of thermal or chemical burns. Contraindications are summarized in Table 15.1.

The athlete will burn as easily as any other patient, and therapists must be aware of the population of athletes who think that the strongest stimulus will be the most effective. Risks are increased when problems of communication are a real or potential issue such as with children and intellectually disabled athletes. Concurrent disabilities require consideration, such as in the case of a spinal cord injured athlete who may be unable to perceive stimulation from thermal and electrical devices. In these situations any device used must be continuously monitored by the therapist. Provided risks and contraindications are addressed prior to treatment, there are no special electrotherapy difficulties in dealing with older athletes. During pregnancy, forms of electrotherapy that have the potential to reach or traverse the developing fetus should be avoided: these include all deep heating modalities, ultrasound and non-co-planar electrical stimulation.

Safety should be of the highest priority at all times. There is the potential for compromise in the club room environment or when travelling with teams. The electrical wiring of areas used for electrotherapy should be checked for safety. Where this is not possible, such as when travelling, the use of a portable earth leakage detector between the mains outlet and the equipment will decrease the potential for electrical accidents (De Domenico et al 1990). The environment should be checked to minimize risks: electrotherapy equipment should be used away from other electrical or earthed objects, and where the floor is dry. Whenever possible the therapist should use familiar equipment for which the service record is known. Portable devices are available for nearly all types of modalities: hot and cold packs (chemically generated if desired), electro-

Table 15.1 Contraindications related to specific modalities (each patient must be assessed individually)

	Cold	Wax	IR	MW	SW	US		ES		UV	LA
						Athermal	Thermal	Sensory	Motor		
Circulatory insufficiency	A	A	A	A	A	R	A	R	R	U	R
Inability to detect heat	-	U	U	A	A	U	A	R	R	R	R
Treatment over areas containing metal	R	R	R	A	A	R	R	R	R	R	R
Treatment of open wounds	R	A	R	R	R	R	R	U	U	R	R
Treatment of eyes	-	-	A	A	-	A	A	-	-	A	A
Inflammatory conditions —acute	R	A	U	A	A	R	A	R	U	U	R
Infective disorders—acute	R	A	U	A	A	A	A	U	U	U	R
Areas of increased fluid tension	R	U	U	U	U	R	U	R	R	R	R
Haemorrhagic conditions	R	U	U	A	A	U	A	R	U	A	R
Patients with severe cardiac or renal disease	U	R	A^{1}R^2	U	U	R	R	R	R	A^{1}R^2	R
Patient with cardiac pacemaker	R	R	R	A	A	R	R	A	A	R	R
Benign/malignant tumours, TB, osteomyelitis	R	R	R	A	A	A	A	R	U	A	U
Skin disorders, e.g. eczema, dermatitis	U	A	U	A	A	U	U	U	U	U	R
In the area of the pregnant uterus	R	-	R	A	A	A	A	U	U	R	U
Hearing aids (remove if A)	R	R	R	A	A	R	R	R	R	R	R
Inability to communicate	U	U	U	A	A	U	U	U	U	U	U

NOTE: Contraindication: A = always; U = usually; R = rarely; IR = infrared treatments; MW = mainly continuous microwave treatment; SW = continuous shortwave; UV = general applications of ultravoilet radiation; LA = laser; US = Ultrasound; ES = electrical stimulation.

myographic, electrical stimulation, lasers and ultrasound equipment. Battery powered equipment can be particularly useful when carrying capacity and weight are important considerations. The use of electrotherapy apparatus by untrained personnel should not be counselled by the physiotherapist.

Acute injuries require careful assessment and frequent review. The usual management is local rest, with compression and elevation of the injured area in conjunction with cold to minimize continuing tissue damage and reduce the acute inflammatory response. Athermal ultrasound, athermal pulsed shortwave, laser or magnetic fields may contribute to tissue healing. When the risk of bleeding is minimal, heat aids the healing process in conjunction with continuous passive movement and/or gentle active movement.

Pain management requires careful consideration. Pain may be derived from the initial injury itself, such as an abrasion which damages many nerve endings, or from later surgery. Pain may be as a consequence of the healing process, an example is the swelling associated with an inflammatory response, or it may occur during some treatment techniques.

The type of pain experienced by the athlete helps to indicate the nature of the injury and the structures that may be damaged, such as when fluid under tension causes a throbbing sensation. Pain may also be used as an indicator of the suitability of treatment techniques, so total masking of pain may make it difficult to determine the most appropriate time to advance treatment. It is essential that a thorough, careful assessment is made of the injury before using analgesic or anaesthetic techniques. More than mild pain during an activity indicates that the activity is too strenuous or complex; residual pain the next day indicates that the previous day's activity was excessive. Pain which makes it difficult for the athlete to obtain adequate rest and/or sleep should be reduced or eliminated (McMeeken & Stillman 1987). Various electrotherapy techniques can assist, particularly those which lead to:

1. Segmental 'gating' of pain sensation such as vibration, comfortable transcutaneous electrical nerve stimulation and warmth
2. Analgesia or anaesthesia, with the use of cold or iontophoresed or phonophoresed analgesics
3. Reduced inflammation with athermal ultrasound, or anti-inflammatory drugs iontophoresed or phonophoresed into the affected tissue
4. Counter-irritant techniques, such as uncomfortable transcutaneous electrical nerve stimulation and acupuncture, which probably release endogenous opiates.

Particular care must be taken to prevent burns. Ice burns and fatty necrosis are a hazard of vapour-coolant sprays and commercial ice packs cooled to below freezing in deep freeze units. (McMeeken 1982). The physiotherapist is responsible for informing the athlete of the risks of excessive heat with any heating modality. The physiotherapist should be particularly diligent in the application of high frequency apparatus, ensuring that there is no risk of burns from leads resting on the athlete, from compressing and devascularizing tissue, from metal within the treatment area, or from excessive fat in the area being treated. When applying ultrasound, it is essential that an efficient coupling medium be used, and that the sound head be moved continuously to avoid a concentration of energy within the tissue increasing the risk of tissue damage.

The principal risk of electrical stimulation is a burn which may occur with excessive current intensity or excessive current density due to uneven contact or stimulation with impulses of an unnecessarily long duration. Burns have been common with quadripolar electrodes delivering electrical stimulation from interferential machines. Small electrodes covered with a thin layer of cloth soaked in tap water increase the risk of burns threefold: small electrodes relative to large electrodes increase current density, a thin layer of cloth relative to several layers of sponge or cloth over the metal electrode provides for little retention of conducting medium, and tap water compared to a more concentrated saline solution or electroconductive gel, provides few ions for conduction of current requiring a higher current intensity. Athletes having electrical stimulation may be burned when close to operating high frequency apparatus such as shortwave or microwave.

The most common problem of electrical stimulation is skin irritation, due to allergy to the tape or electrode gel, or traction by the tape on the skin during application. Change of tape or gel, variation of electrode sites, and care not to exert traction on the skin will usually alleviate these problems. Athletes should be questioned about known allergies to any tapes or gels so that these can be avoided. The skin under electrode sites needs to be monitored. Chemical burns may occur due to passage of direct current and adverse reactions to drugs introduced by iontophoresis.

Ultraviolet irradiation either from electrotherapy apparatus or natural sunlight carries short term risks of sunburn and long term risks of skin cancer. These risks should be outweighed by the potential benefits of treatment. There are risks to the eyes with ultraviolet, as there is with lasers. The eyes of both the operator and the athlete should be protected by goggles when using ultraviolet or laser irradiation.

Electromyography (EMG) presents few dangers, but skin irritation may occur as a reaction to the electroconductive gel or the tape affixing the electrodes. More importantly, proximity to operating shortwave or microwave machines may cause burns to the athlete on the EMG.

Some techniques used in electrotherapy, such as the use of heat or cold packs, can be satisfactorily performed by the athlete or another responsible person. It is the physiotherapist's responsibility to teach the techniques safely and efficiently. Written instructions are recommended to support any technique which has been taught to the athlete. The physiotherapist should give careful consideration of the potential medico-legal implications of teaching or advising unqualified personnel in the use of electrotherapy or other physiotherapy techniques.

PATHOPHYSIOLOGY

Research related to the physiological and biophysical effects of electrotherapy modalities and their interaction with pathological processes is continuing, and physiotherapists need to be alert to new developments in the area. Despite these activities, it is not unusual for new devices to be promoted on the market with little fundamental or applied research to support the manufacturer's claims. In some instances where studies have been undertaken, experimental equipment is dissimilar to that used clinically, such as water cooled ultrasound heads or air cooled microwave. Valuable research contains sufficient information to be replicable and physiotherapists must ensure that clinical studies yielding statistically significant results also yield clinically significant results. Double blind, placebo controlled trials are not always possible to undertake with electrotherapy equipment, and more studies with clinically relevant controls are required.

THERMOTHERAPY

Local temperature change from normal body temperature up to about 45°C and down to less than 10°C, can usefully affect metabolic processes, blood flow, flexibility and elasticity of collagen containing structures and fluid viscosity. Temperature change in either direction facilitates a reduction in pain and protective muscle spasm.

Cold

Local application of cold decreases metabolism, circulation, pain, muscle spasm and inflammation but increases stiffness (see Knight 1985 for an extensive review of the literature). Following injury, ice is initially applied to reduce the metabolic demands of the tissue during the period of hypoxia, to decrease bleeding and minimize oedema. In the opinion of the author, simultaneous application of compression is essential to minimize the oedema likely as a result of all but very brief ice application (Michlovitch 1990). Although ice application is initially painful, within the space of a few minutes pain decreases and the part becomes relatively anaesthetized. Athletes habituate to the initial pain sensation and those who regularly use cryotherapy rarely complain of continued discomfort. In the first aid management of acute injuries, compression and rest take priority over ice if there is a risk of bleeding or effusion. Compression and rest should be maintained continuously while risk of bleeding or effusion continue.

Ice, if available can be applied over the first compressive bandage, initially for 30 minutes and then intermittently for 20-30 minutes every 2 hours for the first 12-24 hours post injury. Reflex vasodilation may be observed after the application of ice. This may produce a marked increase in blood flow measurable in the fingers after exposure to cold (Lewis 1930) and in the forearm after immersion in an ice bath (Clarke et al 1958).

Ice can be further applied at any stage in a sports injury for pain relief and to aid in rehabilitation. Ice massage, packs or immersion are optional methods of application depending on the part and the degree of cooling required. Both massage and ice immersion have the potential to cool the tissues to a greater degree than ice packs. Ice massage has been used successfully in the treatment of local sensitive areas of soft tissue such as for myofascial trigger points or tendinitis. Commercial ice packs are usually the least effective method of reducing tissue temperature due to rapid warming. The application of cold prior to exercise permits pain-free or pain reduced activity. Cold is applied until numbness or decreased sensation is reported by the athlete who then commences active exercise or controlled stretching. Recooling may be required after several minutes and the activity is undertaken again. This cycle may be repeated several times in an exercise session, if required. Ice application is frequently used to reduce pain with overuse injuries such as tenosynovitis, and after training. It has not been established whether this reduces inflammation or masks further pain, but it will usually permit the athlete to continue training or competing. Risks of increasing the pathology must be balanced against the need or desire to continue with the athlete's activity.

Contrast baths are a popular method of treatment following soft tissue and joint injury. The alternation of warmth and cold stimulates blood flow and may assist in the reduction of swelling. It is recommended that contrast baths alternate hot (up to 45°C) and iced water in a ratio of approximately 3:1 minutes. The routine should be commenced and finished with iced water, and it is advisable to exercise the part while in the baths in order to minimize swelling.

Heat

Local temperature increase from normal body temperature up to about 45°C may be achieved with therapeutic heating devices. Heating above 45°C will burn tissue. As most people can tolerate temperatures sufficient to destroy tissue, it is critical to emphasize that heat must be no more than comfortable and not hot. The location of maximal tissue heating will depend on the specific modality used, the technique of application, and the thermal properties of the tissues. Heat has the capacity to accelerate metabolic processes, thus stimulating an increase in blood flow. Flexibility and elasticity of collagen containing structures

is increased and fluid viscosity reduced. The primary effects of heat lead to reduced joint stiffness, enhanced relaxation, enhanced resolution of inflammatory processes, reduction of pain, and increased tissue healing (Lehmann & De Lateur 1990, Wadsworth & Chanmugam 1988).

Mobilization and stretching is most effectively achieved while the tissues are warmed (Lehmann et al 1970). Heating collagen containing tissue such as ligament, joint capsule or tendon up to 45°C will decrease the amount of force required to stretch to a given length, and allow the tissue to stretch further before tearing. It should be noted that heat also increases the likelihood of damage if force is applied very quickly. Slow sustained stretch during warming is optimal (Lehmann et al 1970). Intramuscular temperature is also raised with active exercise, and temperatures about 39°C are obtainable. Preparatory activity or 'warm-up' before competition has potential for tissue stretching. Golgi tendon organs increase sensitivity with increased temperature (Fukami & Wilkinson 1977). The most effective stretching is likely to be after a prolonged period of exercise.

The author recommends that to obtain maximum benefits from heating using electrotherapy devices, tissue structures should be in a stretched position during heating. Alternatively, the physiotherapist can perform small amplitude movements (active or passive) at the end of range while heating.

Superficial tissue heating may be achieved with simple techniques such as infrared lamps, hot packs or whirlpool baths. The main precaution is to ensure that the applied modality is perceived by the athlete as no more than comfortably warm so that tissue temperature is not greater than 45°C.

Shortwave or microwave employ high frequency alternating currents to heat superficial and deeply located soft tissues, particularly where there is only a thin layer of subcutaneous fat (Lehmann & De Lateur 1990). Both modalities increase muscle blood flow (De Lateur et al 1970, McNiven & Wyper 1976, Sekins et al 1980, Sekins et al 1984) and blood flow remains elevated for up to 20 minutes following exposure (McMeeken & Bell 1990). Microwave applicators can be quickly applied for efficient tissue heating and are particularly useful for tissues of high water content such as muscle, where there is little subcutaneous fat (Ward 1986). A relatively thick layer of subcutaneous fat limits the effective penetration of high frequency energy (Emery & Sekins 1990), and energy may be concentrated in the blood and lymph vessels within the fatty tissues (Ward 1986).

Pulsed shortwave may or may not cause measurable temperature rise in tissue, depending on the current parameters set. Pulsed shortwave has been shown to facilitate regeneration in mammalian nerve tissue (Raji 1984, Raji & Bowden 1983, Wilson & Jagadeesh 1974, Wilson & Jagadeesh 1976) and may help in reduction of swelling and tissue healing (Barclay et al 1983, Goldin et al 1981, Nadasdi 1960). Evidence to suggest pulsed shortwave is valuable in reducing pain has been given (Barclay et al 1983), although other investigators do not support these findings (Barker et al 1985, Pasila et al 1978). The available evidence indicates that further investigation of the effects of pulsed shortwave is warranted particularly in the acute phase of soft tissue injury.

Ultrasound is a valuable local heating modality with maximum effective penetration depth of 40 mm in muscle and 220 mm in fat and preferential absorption in protein (Ward 1986).

MECHANICAL ENERGY

Vibration

Simple, inexpensive massage vibrators can be used for facilitation of muscle activity or for pain relief. Mechanical vibration of muscle tendon using a frequency >50 Hz produces a normal reflex asynchronous muscle contraction with relaxation of its antagonists. This is suitable for facilitation of muscle strengthening and endurance and joint mobilization (Hagbarth 1969). The reflex may be evoked with the athlete relaxed or during voluntary contraction or attempted contraction. When superimposed on an already contracted muscle, the initial and superimposed reflex contractions are summated such that the combination may cause a much greater muscle tension than that achieved by voluntary or artificial means separately. The associated inhibition of antagonists can be used to relax muscle spasm. Vibration should be transmitted to the muscle belly by firm application over the tendon of the stretched muscle. The effects of the tonic vibration reflex persist for at least 5-10 minutes after vibration ceases, and it is therefore possible to vibrate specific muscles or muscle groups prior to exercise (Hagbarth 1969, Johnston 1970, Stillman 1970).

Vibration has additional benefits in relation to pain relief. It may be effectively used as a form of transcutaneous nerve stimulation for pain relief and should be applied at any point within the dermatome/s corresponding to the innervation of a painful area (Lundberg 1984). Vibration should not be used over fracture sites.

Mechanical compression

Soft tissue oedema of the limbs may be reduced by rhythmical mechanical compression using a pressure pump with inflatable sleeves. Sequential compression commencing with the proximal limb segment then moving more distally to compress the next segment has the potential to be more effective when swelling is extensive. Simultaneous limb elevation and electrical stimulation of the appropriate muscle, or voluntary exercise may be incorporated inside the inflatable sleeves. Continuous compression bandaging is essential at other times for any problem for which mechanical compression or other electrotherapy is considered appropriate as a means of reducing swelling.

Ultrasound

The primary uses of therapeutic ultrasound in sports medicine are for pain reduction, facilitation of healing, and to increase tissue extensibility. It can be used for athermal effects and as a deeply penetrating heating modality within a fairly selected area (Kitchen & Partridge 1990). Preferential absorption in proteinaceous tissue such as intermuscular interfaces, tendon sheaths, fibrotic muscles and periosteum occurs (Cartensen et al 1953). There is little influence on blood flow (Paaske et al 1973, Wyper & McNiven 1976). Absorption in fatty tissue is minimal, permitting penetration below the subcutaneous fat layer (Ward 1986).

Non-thermal effects of ultrasound are due to cavitation, acoustic streaming and standing wave formation. Stable cavitation induces micron sized bubbles which vibrate in response to the ultrasound energy, producing a streaming effect which influences membrane permeability and facilitates diffusion of ions and metabolites (Dyson 1985). High levels of ultrasound cause the bubbles to implode, producing tissue destruction and the release of reactive free radicals. Standing waves are produced when reflected waves summate with incident waves increasing the local energy to potentially destructive levels. Moving the ultrasound head during all forms of treatment prevents the production of standing waves.

At therapeutic levels ultrasound has been shown to reduce inflammation, increase rates of protein synthesis, and promote healing in normal and slowly healing tissues. Dosage should be kept to the minimum necessary to achieve the desired results as excess energy can increase tissue damage. Recent work by Young and Dyson (reviewed in Kitchen & Partridge 1990) suggests that athermal ultrasound accelerates the inflammatory stage of the healing process.

During the acute inflammatory stage mast cells may release chemotactic agents which attract monocytes to the injured area (Fyfe & Chahl 1984). These develop into macrophages which phagocytise the injured tissue and also stimulate the formation of new connective tissue (Dyson 1989). Bruising and swelling can be minimized with early ultrasound. During the proliferative phase of healing, the rate of wound contraction is increased with ultrasound. This may be due to stimulation of myofibroblasts (ter Haar et al 1978). Angiogenesis is also facilitated (Martin et al 1981). Dyson (1989) suggests that ultrasound can assist in the development of stronger, more elastic scar tissue.

Chronic problems are unlikely to resolve with ultrasound unless the cause is removed, although treatment may keep symptoms, such as that of chronic tendinitis, partially controlled.

There has been uncertainty about the use of ultrasound over epiphyseal growth plates. Lehmann and de Lateur (1990) imply that this is safe at therapeutic levels, but may be detrimental at higher dosages. Lowden (1986) has indicated that a pain response to ultrasound may be of value in supporting the diagnosis of stress fracture, and Dyson and Brookes (1983) claim that bony union can be accelerated if low dose pulsed ultrasound (duty cycle 20%) is applied for the first 2 weeks after fracture.

Local phonophoresis of analgesic and anti-inflammatory salicylates is an appropriate alternative to systemic administration of these drugs. Corticosteroids and compounds containing heparin and hyaluronidase may also be administered phonophoretically. Heparin and hyaluronidase containing compounds aid in the resolution of haematoma. Injected analgesics and anti-inflammatory agents may be dispersed within the local tissue area with ultrasound (Griffin 1981). Phonophoretically applied drugs should be used at the same dosage as is advised for topical application. The advised quantity of drug can be mixed with an ultrasound gel if the drug base is too viscous or fluid for ultrasound application.

Diagnostic ultrasound may be available in radiological practices for imaging of soft tissues. This normally employs frequencies in the range of 2-10 MHz. Diagnostic ultrasound relies on the computerized processing of reflected pulses of ultrasound from tissue interfaces which are used to produce a grey scale image of the cross-section of tissues traversed by the ultrasound beam. Ultrasound images are increasingly used for accurate measurement of muscle cross-sectional area.

ELECTRICAL STIMULATION

Action potential generation is the therapeutically significant physiological response to electrical stimulation which occurs as a result of the modification of cellular activity by changing membrane excitability. Sensory, motor and autonomic responses can have beneficial therapeutic effects. Muscle contraction can produce secondary effects on muscle strength, contraction speed, reaction time, and fatigability. The muscle action stimulates blood and lymph flow. Kinaesthetic awareness is increased by motor and sensory stimulation. Analgesic responses are associated with sensory stimulation due to the release of endogenous polypeptides and neurotransmitters. It has been claimed that electrical stimulation can modulate autonomic nervous system activity.

Effects on non-excitable cells and tissues are not well established, but there are indications that mitachondrial activity and protein synthesis may be influenced and stimulation of fibroblast and osteoblast formation is beneficial to collagen and bony tissue regeneration and remodelling (Weiss et al 1990).

Generally, electrical excitation of peripheral nerves across the skin is perceived as sensory, followed by motor, and then painful stimulation. These responses can be most easily discriminated with pulse durations <200 µs. The shape of the pulse used is not critical provided there is adequate pulse charge (product of intensity of output and pulse duration) for the desired stimulation. Pulse frequency < 20 Hz will produce twitch contractions whereas frequencies >25Hz cause a tetanic muscle contraction. Pulse frequency may also influence the type of endogenous analgesic mechanism.

When using electrical stimulation, the electrode sizes and number should be chosen to facilitate the desired response. Point electrodes will generate localized responses, whereas larger electrodes reduce the concentration of current, but also reduce the specificity of stimulation. Current requirements will be minimized if an electroconductive gel or saline solution is used with all forms of electrical stimulation. All current requires some ions for conduction, and ultrasound gel or water are unsuitable (Ward 1986).

Advertising literature provided by proponents of microelectrical stimulation at subthreshold intensities state, that by altering the body's internal electrical signals with an external signal it may be possible to regulate growth, development and repair of injured tissues and reduce pain. It is claimed that, by adding a current similar to the currents endogenous to the body's electric currents, homeostatic or healing mechanism may be facilitated. No clinical research supporting these claims has been sighted.

Whilst it is well established that any form of electrical stimulation which induces muscle contraction will increase blood flow, it has been specifically suggested that sensory stimulation with interferential therapy may influence blood flow by inhibition of the sympathetic nervous system (De Domenico 1987, Nikolova 1987, Wadsworth & Chanmugam 1988). Nussbaum et al (1990) have recently shown that interferential currents applied to the cervical sympathetic chain, the stellate ganglion, the dorsolumbar sympathetic outflow, and peripheral sympathetic nerves do not produce any vasodilation as measured by surface thermography.

Electrical current may be used in sports physiotherapy for:
1. Pain relief
2. Muscle contraction for muscle strengthening and endurance, prevention of muscle wasting, re-education of muscle action, reduction of oedema or effusion, reduction of muscle spasm, stimulation of the circulation and increasing range of movement
3. Tissue healing including stimulation of bony union in slowly or non-uniting fractures
4. Iontophoresis
5. The management of nerve lesions, from assisting in diagnosis, providing lively orthoses, to augmenting muscle strength and retraining.

Many types of electrical stimulator have been used for pain relief, from continuous direct, faradic and sinusoidal current to the more recent diadynamic, interferential and high voltage currents. The most critical feature of an electrical stimulator is the available current paramenters. Now, short pulse duration, low frequency currents providing comfortable sensory stimulation are most commonly used for pain relief, although painful intensities may be necessary in some circumstances. Electrodes chosen should be as large as reasonably possible and situated around the painful site, within the dermatome, or along the peripheral nerve supplying the source of pain. Electrical stimulation should be the minimum intensity required for pain relief, and can be used continuously (McMeeken & Stillman 1987).

Although electrical stimulation can strengthen muscle without voluntary effort (Currier 1987, De Domenico & Strauss 1986) the torques developed will usually be less than those obtained from active exercise and will make no contribution to skill development. In order to strengthen muscle, it should be positioned on slight stretch against moderate resistance, and the athlete encouraged to perform voluntary contractions with the electrically induced contractions. The dosage is comparable to active exercise with machine parameters set with a phase duration at 200 μs, frequency at 30-60 Hz, with an on-time of 5-15 seconds and a duty cycle of 20%. A minimum of 10 to 20 contractions are performed daily at 60% of the athlete's maximum voluntary tetanic contraction. Overdosage will be indicated by excessive muscle soreness approximately 24 hours after stimulation. Muscle atrophy after surgery or immobilization may be prevented by the use of electrical stimulation (Williams & Street 1976), for example quadriceps stimulation post surgically enhances the efficiency in recruiting motor units (Moritani & Devries 1979). Electrical stimulation appears to maintain or increase the levels of oxidative enzymes (Eriksson & Haggmark 1979). Compared to voluntary activation, electrical activation of muscle tends to reverse the recruitment order from largest to smallest motor units and all units reaching threshold are activated synchronously. Once threshold for muscle contraction is reached, small increments in power have the capacity to substantially increase the number of motor units recruited and physiotherapists should advance the power control slowly.

Clinical reports are not available on the effects of electrical stimulation on endurance and muscle fatigability in athletes. However, it has been found that long term stimulation of muscle at frequencies naturally occurring in the nerves of supply converts predominantly anaerobic fast glycolytic fibres to aerobic slow oxidative fibres (Pette 1975, Hudlicka et al 1982). Short term high intensity electrical stimulation fatigues muscle, whereas long term chronic stimulation induces metabolic changes and increased capillarization within the muscle. There is minimal fatigue with electrical stimulation $\leq$ 20 Hz in experimental situations permitting the use of stimulators for several hours daily if desired. Capillarization increases to the level in slow oxidative muscle fibres with 10-14 days of stimulation. The potential for use in injured athletes or to enhance endurance performance warrants further investigation.

Oedema reduction using electrical stimulation requires muscle contraction to effectively pump fluid by alternating compression and relaxation on the veins and lymphatics. This can be augmented with a pressure pump, and the affected part elevated above the athlete's heart level.

Muscle spasm may be treated by continuous contraction in order to fatigue the muscle. A biphasic wave form, phase duration of 20-200 μs, at 50-150 Hz with electrodes placed over the affected muscles for 30-60 minutes has been recommended (Alon 1987).

Range of joint movement may be increased by electrical stimulation. One method is to stimulate the muscle antagonist to the tight structure in order to produce reciprocal relaxation in the agonist. Alternatively, strong electrical stimulation of a tight muscle group may be followed by active or passive stretching (Baker et al 1979).

A key factor in tissue healing is an adequate oxygen supply which requires an efficient blood flow (Niinikoski 1980). Transient increases in peripheral blood flow have been described with electrical stimulation (summarized in Snyder-Mackler 1989) and Kaada and Eielsen (1983a, 1983b) demonstrated a reflex vascular vasodilatory response which lasted 4-8 hours. It required local electrically induced muscle contraction. Note that rhythmic exercise increases muscle blood flow up to 40 times during exercise (Wesche 1986), and a vigorous post exercise hyperaemia occurs after sustained isometric contractions (Barcroft & Millen 1939). Increased perfusion and tissue temperature may be reproduced by electrical stimulation provided muscle contraction occurs, and may be more efficient at increasing muscle blood flow than heating (McMeeken & Bell 1988). Similar muscle blood flow responses can be achieved with a variety of stimulators including high voltage stimulators (Mohr et al 1987, McMeeken & Bell 1988). Electrical stimulation for chronic wound healing has been undertaken but evidence is awaited to support its use for routine soft tissue healing in athletes. The techniques used to stimulate bony union in slowly or non-uniting fractures include implanted and external application of a variety of electrical stimulators and the use of pulsed electromagnetic fields from high or low frequency sources (Ganne 1988, Snyder-Mackler 1989).

Iontophoresis introduces charged substances through the skin with direct current. There appears to be a resurgence of interest in this modality (Glick & Snyder-Mackler 1989). Antihistamines have been used locally as anti-inflammatory agents, and analgesics may be applied in this way as an alternative to injection. Iontophoresis with the positively charged hyaluronidase has been recommended for oedema reduction (Magistro 1964). Glas et al (1980) showed penetration of radio labelled dexamethasone through primate skin. The application of corticosteroids has been recommended in musculoskeletal inflammatory conditions, particularly tendinitis (Bertolucci 1982, Harris 1982). To ensure introduction of electrically charged substances through the skin, the active agent must be in solution positioned under the electrode of opposite polarity. The active agents of dexamethasone sodium phosphate and lidocaine hydrochloride are positively charged, sodium salicylate is negatively charged. Any medication used must be water and lipid soluble. A small active electrode with a large dispersive is suitable for treating localized lesions.

Strength duration testing can be undertaken if a nerve lesion is suspected following sports injury. A lack of response to the maximum pulse width of about 200 µs on a small battery operated stimulator is cause for suspicion. Electrical stimulation can be used to provide dynamic splinting for retraining and to augment muscle strength (Delitto & Robinson 1989).

Many items of equipment can be used for electrical stimulation: battery operated devices, and high voltage galvanic, interferential, impulse, diadynamic and multi-purpose apparatus. Provided the desired stimulus parameters for a particular purpose are available, all these machines are essentially interchangeable (McMeeken & Stillman 1987, Alon 1987). Manufacturers have traded on the gullibility of physiotherapists to produce a wide variety of variously named devices. Unless the physiotherapist specifically desires a variety of machines, it is advisable to determine the electrical parameters required for pain reduction, muscle re-education and tissue healing, and to purchase a machine which encompasses all these requirements.

Applying the principles of strength duration testing prior to treatment allows selection of the optimal pulse durations and frequencies to determine sensory and motor requirements for electrical stimulation. It is recommended that the narrowest pulse duration and the minimal intensity be used for the desired clinical result. Recent work indicates that square biphasic symmetrical pulses achieve the most comfortable muscle contractions with minimal energy input (Baker 1988). Unipolar techniques are recommended for point stimulation, otherwise the use of bipolar application with electrodes of equal surface area applied over the area to be treated, for maintenance of muscle strength, correction of muscle weakness, to maintain or increase range of movement, facilitation of motor control, muscle spasm or reduced circulation (Alon 1987). Consistency in application is strongly recommended to enable comparison of results of treatment.

Electrical stimulation may be used in athletes with previous spinal injuries in prevention of muscle wasting and restoration of muscle bulk. For example, restoration of gluteal muscle bulk may increase sitting tolerance for extended wheelchair events. Standing protocols using electrical stimulation have been used for people with paraplegia to benefit kidneys and bladder function, and stimulate osteogenesis in the weight bearing skeleton. Morale may be improved by using walking, assisted by electrical stimulation, as an exercise. To reduce abdominal spasm, gluteal and lower back stimulation may be effective, and electrical stimulation combined with passive movement may relieve contractures (Baker 1988).

Electrical stimulation may be combined with heat or ultrasound to improve blood flow or enhance pain relief, although there is little research evidence to support a synergistic effect by combining two modalities (Robinson & Snyder-Mackler 1988).

Electromagnetic fields

Magnetic field therapy employs an alternating magnetic field to generate an electric current inside the tissues. This current, however, is too small to generate either neuromuscular action potentials or heat. Fracture repair is stimulated by electromagnetic fields (Brighton & McCluskey 1983) and appears to stimulate osteogenesis for bony regrowth in non-union and osteonecrosis.

Little work has been undertaken on connective tissue and cartilage, although Binder et al (1984) showed improved pain relief, range of movement and pain on resisted movement by treating patients who had persistent rotator cuff tendinitis with pulsed electromagnetic fields. By contrast there has been considerable non-clinical investigation suggesting enhanced neural repair (Sissken 1988) although no clinical trials have been reported.

Manufacturers claim that some benefits of magnetic fields are secondary to changes in blood flow, with low frequencies (< 6 Hz) having a vasoconstrictor effect and higher frequencies (> 25 Hz) a vasodilator effect. Anaesthetized dogs did not show a significant change in blood flow with several combinations of frequency and intensity (McMeeken & Bell 1987). In normal human subjects, high frequency (99 Hz) and high intensity (10 mT) magnetic field exposure of the forearm did not change blood flow measured by venous occlusion plethysmography, although a small increase in skin temperature under the applicator may be achieved using this maximum output (McMeeken 1992). Despite some promising in vitro and experimental results, there is little clinical evidence to support the use of pulsed electromagnetic fields in soft tissue injuries at this stage (Brighton & McCluskey 1983, Sissken 1988).

Phototherapy

Ultraviolet irradiation is suitable for the treatment of superficial infections and dermatological conditions as it has the capacity to induce mutations in nuclear genetic material and is a potent agent for clearing superficial infection and stimulating healing of superficial wounds (Stillwell 1983). Exposure of sports induced skin lesions such as blister bases to ultraviolet irradiation should be undertaken at times when they are not required to be covered.

Laser (light amplification by stimulated emission of radiation)

Low powered therapeutic lasers are being used in physiotherapy for the relief of pain, reduction of swelling and inflammation, and the promotion of healing. These are areas where scientific research indicates they may be useful, although there does not yet appear to be any generally agreed or scientifically validated dose for laser treatment in humans (De Domenico et al 1990, Kitchen & Partridge 1991a, Kitchen & Partridge 1991b).

The penetration and absorption characteristics of most therapeutic lasers have not been fully characterized, but penetration depth increases as the wavelength increases. In 1967, Carney et al indicated that of the incident light 40% absorption occurs in the skin, 20% is reflected and 40% passes through the skin to subcutaneous tissue. Anderson and Parrish (1981) indicate that penetration depth for optical radiation in fair skin ranges from 6μm at a wavelength of 300 nm to 2200 μm at a wavelength of 1200 nm, but that penetration depth at any one site will always be influenced by factors such as skin pigmentation, scattering from fibrous tissue, and tissue characteristics. A penetration depth of 1–4 mm has been suggested (King 1989, Kolari 1985). Haker and Lundeberg (1990) state the penetration depth as 0.62 mm for HeNe and 1.4 mm for GaAs lasers. Recent work has shown that HeNe laser (0-5MW, 0-1800s) cannot penetrate sufficiently into the rabbit cornea to influence evoked responses of A∂ or C fibres and that penetration was inadequate to alter sensory changes or transmission in these nociceptors (Jarvis et al 1990).

Laser devices typically emit one wavelength, although some units have diode and HeNe lasers in a single unit where the visible HeNe laser is often used to aim the invisible infrared diode laser. Photons of energy are absorbed by tissue electrons and the excited electrons may cause chemical changes stimulating cellular processes (Karu 1988). Irradiation may influence intercellular communication and hormone systems (Ohshiro & Calderhead 1988).

Physiological effects that have been determined from experimental data have used dosages which are highly variable, and there is a lack of rigour in some reports making it difficult to verify the physiological effects claimed and to determine useful clinical protocols. A number of studies indicate therapeutic lasers influence cell cultures. Cell division has increased in mouse fibroblasts (Hardy et al 1967). The amount of radio labelled proline incorporation into cultured skin from guinea pigs is increased under the influence of laser light (Carney et al 1967). Collagen gene expression has been stimulated in human skin fibroblasts (Lam et al 1986). Dyson has shown that macrophages can be stimulated to release chemicals that either stimulate or inhibit collagen production in fibroblasts by using different wavelengths of laser or non-coherent light (Dyson quoted by Perera 1988). Lasers may increase the vascular supply to healing tissue. In 1985, the Mesters showed that both total skin defects and burns in mice healed more quickly than controls. Dyson and Young (1986) indicated this is due to stimulation of cellular activity and development of a new blood supply in the damaged tissues. Conversely, Surinchack et al (1983) did not show an increased rate of healing of skin defects and incisions in rabbits.

There are mixed results from laser application for problems relevant to sports medicine: wound and bone healing may be stimulated and pain reduced (Walker 1983, 1988), but recent studies showed no superiority of real laser compared to sham laser treatment for tennis elbow (Lundeberg et al 1987, Haker & Lundeberg 1990), tendinopathies (Seibert et al 1987), low back pain (Klein & Eek 1990) or orofacial pain (Hansen & Thoroe 1990). Vasseljen (1992) showed the overall superiority of ultrasound and deep friction massage over laser in the treatment of tennis elbow. Devor (1990) argues that any proposed treatment for pain must be evaluated in controlled, blind trials and that it is irresponsible to use lasers for pain relief in the light of the present scientific research.

Greguss (1984) concluded that low level continuous laser irradiation may replace the needle in acupuncture therapy. Anecdotal reports indicate it is valued as a form of treatment for pain relief. Lundeberg et al (1987) investigated claims that laser is useful in pain management, by experiments in rats. They compared the effects of HeNe (continuous wav 632.8 nm), and GaAs (pulse wave 904 nm at 73 Hz) laser treatment with electrical stimulation, via needle acupuncture, and morphine, on the response to a noxious stimulus. Both electrical stimulation and morphine showed significant changes in response to a noxious stimulus, but the laser was no different from control responses. The authors suggest that pain relief in humans may be due to placebo.

Physiotherapists using lasers are advised to use the manufacturers' dosage guidelines and to ensure a full record for each treatment with lasers: diagnosis, type of laser, manufacturer/supplier, machine parameters, wavelength, beam spot size, frequency, average power, techniques used, dose per unit area, dosage details, time, pulse rate, area treated, frequency, number of treatments, distance from skin, summary of other treatment techniques used and outcome (De Domenico et al 1990). Research based on such information has the potential to provide a relevant guide to the clinical effectiveness of lasers.

BIOFEEDBACK

Biofeedback is 'the use of appropriate instrumentation to bring covert physiological processes to the conscious awareness of one or more individuals' (Wolf 1978). This generally means the transduction of a physiological event into auditory and visual signals which are proportional to the event. Biofeedback may be used to control a variety of functions, but is most valuable in the athlete to control muscle activity and joint movement. Electromyography (EMG) provides immediate, quantified visual and/or auditory information representing the overall muscle activity. The source of the EMG is the movement of ions between the muscle cell and the extracellular fluid during depolarization and repolarization of muscle fibres (Basmajian 1983).

Physiotherapists normally use disposable pre-gelled electrodes (once only) or silver-silver chloride electrodes with electroconductive gel to record EMGs. Skin should be prepared by brisk rubbing with soap and water or alcohol, and electrodes chosen with consideration of muscle size. Electrodes are placed over the midpoint of the target muscle belly. A third earthing electrode is used to avoid recording extraneous electrical signals. To reduce movement artefact the electrode leads should be taped to the skin surface. A very small contraction requires high sensitivity settings, whereas a large contraction will require low sensitivity with the meter level set to read about the middle of the scale. The signal may be presented as a raw or integrated signal.

Machines may be single, dual or multichannel allowing for simultaneous recording from one, two or several muscles or muscle groups. Most devices used in physiotherapy have a rectified, integrated signal. A threshold or level detector, if present, can be incorporated into the training program. To increase activity, the threshold is set progressively higher as the athlete reaches the pre-set goal. To achieve a progressive increase in muscle strength in a muscle such as quadriceps following knee surgery, initially an attainable threshold is set with electrodes spaced widely on the muscle mass and sensitivity setting high. As more muscle activity is recruited sensitivity is lowered, electrodes are more closely spaced, and the athlete must generate more activity to trigger the threshold level for feedback.

Training in muscle relaxation using biofeedback, as may be desired following low back injury, requires widely spaced electrodes to sample many muscles. The time constant of the integrated signal may be altered in some devices so that relatively long integration times (0.1-0.5 s) can be used for relaxation (Turner & Chapman 1982, Wolf et al 1982) or postural control. Shorter integration times facilitate dynamic activity.

EMG is particularly useful for assessment of the ability to contract or relax particular muscles. When comparing the response from different muscles, or of the same muscles on different occasions, special care must be taken in making interpretive decisions. For repeat testing of the same muscles it is essential that the electrodes are precisely relocated in the previous position.

The immediate feedback of effectiveness of muscle contraction and relaxation may be used in general and localized relaxation training, facilitation and strengthening exercises, and in exercises and functional activities where the key element is co-ordination. Biofeedback has the potential to be a valuable tool in developing greater control and more efficient movement patterns. The athlete should be encouraged to work independently with portable equipment once the tasks are understood. Telemetric apparatus may be used for monitoring of athletes during sporting activities and EMG may be coupled with video recording for more sophisticated movement analysis.

Pressure sensing devices may be incorporated into shoes or seats to indicate weight bearing characteristics or to retrain appropriate distribution of pressure. There are many other options that may be explored for feedback such as the use of auditory stimuli in timing of movements. In the author's opinion the use of the video camera and recorder to capture information on movement performance in the training and retraining of athletes following injury or surgery has the potential to be used as a powerful form of biofeedback.

Summary

The use of electrotherapy in the management of the injured athlete requires consideration of safety at all times. The choice of modality and dosage should be based on the pathophysiology of the problem, its anatomical location and the potential for the modality to be the most effective and efficient in restoring the athlete to the sporting arena.

REFERENCES

Alon G 1987 Principles of electrical stimulation ch 3. In: Nelson R M, Currier D P (eds) Clinical electrotherapy. Appleton & Lange, Norwalk

Anderson R, Parrish J 1981 The optics of human skin. Journal of Investigative Dermatology 77:13–19

Baker L 1988 Personal communication

Baker L L, Yeh C, Wikson D, Waters R L 1979 Electrical stimulation of wrist and fingers of hemiplegic patients. Physical Therapy 59:1495–1499

Barclay V, Collier R J, Jones A 1983 Treatment of various hand injuries by pulsed electromagnetic energy. Diapulse Physiotherapy 696:186-188

Barcroft H, Millen J L E 1939 The blood flow through muscle during sustained contractions. Journal of Physiology 97:17-31

Barker A T, Barlow P S, Porter J, Smith M E, Clifton S, Andrews L, O'Dowd W J 1985 A double-blind clinical trial of low power pulsed shortwave therapy in the treatment of a soft tissue injury. Physiotherapy 7112:500-504

Basmajian J V 1983 Biofeedback principles and practice for clinicians, 2nd edn. Williams & Wilkins, Baltimore

Bertolucci L E 1982 Introduction of antiinflammatory drugs by iontophoresis: double blind study. Journal of Orthopaedic and Sports Physical Therapy 4:103

Binder A, Parr G, Hazelman B, Fitton Jackson S 1984 Pulsed electromagnetic field therapy of persistent rotator cuff tendinitis. The Lancet 31:695–698

Brighton C T, McCluskey W P 1983 The early response of bone cells in culture to a capacitively coupled electrical field. Transactions of the Bioelkectrica Repair and Growth Society 310

Carney S A, Lawrence J C, Ricketts C R 1967 The effect of light from a ruby laser on the metabolism of skin tissue culture. Biochemica Biophysica Acta 148:525–530

Cartensen E L, Li K, Schwan H P 1953 Determination of the acoustic properties of blood and its components. Journal of Acoustic Society of America 25:286-289

Clarke R S J, Hellon R F, Lind A R 1958 Vascular reactions of the human forearm to cold. Clinical Science 17:165

Currier D P 1987 Electrical stimulation for improving muscle strength and blood flow ch 7. In: Nelson R M, Currier D P (eds) Clinical electrotherapy. Appleton & Lange, Norwalk

De Domenico G 1987 New dimensions in interferential therapy: a theoretical and clinical guide. Reid Medical Books, Lindfield

De Domenico G, Strauss G R 1986 Maximum torque production in the quadriceps femoris muscle group using a variety of electrical stimulators. Australian Journal of Physiotherapy 32 51-56

De Domenico G, Ford I, McMeeken J M, Richardson C 1990 Electrotherapy standards. Australian Journal of Physiotherapy 36:39–52

De Lateur B J, Lehmann J F, Stonebridge J B, Warren B J, Guy A W 1970 Muscle heating in human subjects with 915 MHz microwave contact applicator. Archives Physical Medicine and Rehabilitation 51:147–151

Delitto A, Robinson A J 1989 Electrical stimulation of muscle: techniques and applications. Snyder-Mackler L, Robinson A J (ed) Williams & Wilkins, ch 4

Dennis J K 1987 What physiotherapists in private practice do: the effects of sex and training on clinical behaviour. Australian Journal of Physiotherapy 33:181–191

Devor M 1990: What's in a laser beam for pain therapy? Pain 43:139

Dyson M, Brookes M 1983 Stimulation of bone repair by ultrasound In: Lerske R A, Morley P (eds) Proceedings of the third meeting of the World Federation in Ultrasound in Medicine and Biology. Pergamon, Oxford pp 61-66

Dyson M, Young S 1986 Effect of laser therapy on wound contraction and cellularity in mice. Lasers in Medical Science 1:125-130

Dyson M 1985 Therapeutic applications of ultrasound. In: Grisogono V (ed) Sports injuries. International Perspectives in Physical Therapy 4. Churchill Livingstone, Edinburgh ch 10, p 213

Dyson M 1989 The use of ultrasound in sports physiotherapy. In: Nyborg W L, Ziskin M C (eds) Biological effects of ultrasound. Clinics in Diagnostic Ultrasound. Churchill Livingstone, New York ch 11, p 121

Emery A F, Sekins K M 1990 Computer modelling of thermotherapy ch 3. In: Lehmann J F Therapeutic heat and cold, 4th edn. Rehabilitation Medicine Library series. Williams and Wilkins, Baltimore pp 113-149

Eriksson E, Haggmark T 1979 Comparison of isometric muscle training and electrical stimulation supplementing isometric muscle training in the recovery after major knee ligament surgery. American Journal of Sports Medicine 7:169

Fukami Y, Wilkinson R S 1977 Responses on isolated golgi tendon organs of the cat. Journal of Physiology 265:673-689

Fyfe M, Chahl L A 1984 Mast cell degranulation and increased vascular permeability induced by 'therapeutic' ultrasound in the rat ankle joint. British Journal of Experimental Pathology 65:671–676

Ganne J-M 1988 Stimulation of bone healing with interferential therapy. Australian Journal of Physiotherapy 34:9-20

Glas J M, Stephen R L, Jacobsen S C 1980 The quantity and distribution of radiolabelled dexamethosone delivered to tissue by iontophoresis International Journal of Dermatology 19:(9):519-525

Glick E, Snyder-Mackler L 1989 Iontophoresis, ch 8. In: clinical electrophysiology electrotherapy and electrophysiologic testing.

Snyder-Mackler L, Robinson A J (eds) Williams & Wilkins, Baltimore

Goldin J H, Broadbent N R G, Nancarrow J D, Marshall T 1981 The effects of diapulse on the healing of wounds: a double-blind randomised controlled trial in man. British Journal of Plastic Surgery 34:267-270

Greguss P 1984 Low-level laser therapy—reality or myth? Optics and Lasers Technology 81–85

Griffin J E 1981 Phonophoresis—a review In: Proceedings of an international symposium on therapeutic ultrasound. Canadian Physiotherapy Association, Winnipeg

Hagbarth K-E G 1969 The muscle vibrator: a useful tool in neurological therapeutic work. Scandinavian Journal of Rehabilitation Medicine 1:26

Haker E, Lundeberg T 1990 Laser treatment applied to acupuncture points in lateral humeral epicondylalgia: a double blind study. Pain 43:243-247.

Hansen H J, Thoroe U 1990 Low power laser biostimulation of chronic oro-facial pain: a double-blind placebo controlled cross-over study in 40 patients. Pain 43:169-179

Hardy L B, Hardy F S, Fine S, Sokal J 1967 Effect of ruby laser irradiation on mouse fibroblast culture. Federal Proceedings 26:668

Harris P 1982 Iontophoresis: clinical research in musculoskeletal inflammatory conditions. Journal of Orthopaedic and Sports Physical Therapy 4:109-112

Hudlicka O, Dodd L, Renkin E M, Gray S D 1982 Early changes in fibre profile and capillary density in long term stimulated muscles. American Journal of Physiology 243:H528

Jarvis D, MacIver M B, Tanelian D L 1990 Electrophysiological recording and thermodynamic modeling demonstrate that helium-neon laser irradiation does not affect peripheral A∂- or C-fiber nociceptors. Pain 43:235-242

Johnston R M et al 1970 Mechanical vibration of skeletal muscles. Physical Therapy 50:499

Kaada B, Eielsen O 1983a In search of mediators of skin vasodilation induced by transcutaneous nerve stimulation: II Serotonin implicated. General Pharmacology 14:635–641

Kaada B and Eielsen O 1983b In search of mediators of skin vasodilation induced by transcutaneous nerve stimulation: I Failure to block the response by antagonists of endogenous vasodilators. General Pharmacology 14:623–633

Karu T I 1988 Molecular mechanisms of the therapeutic effects of low intensity laser radiation. Lasers in Life Science 2:53-74

King P R 1989 Low level laser therapy–a review. Lasers in Medical Science 4:141-150

Kitchen S S, Partridge C J 1990 A review of therapeutic ultrasound. Physiotherapy 761:593-600

Kitchen S S, Partridge C J 1991a A review of low level laser therapy. Physiotherapy 773:161-163

Kitchen S S, Partridge C J 1991b The efficacy of level laser therapy. Physiotherapy 773:163-168

Klein R, Eek B 1990 Low energy laser treatment and exercise for chronic low back pain: double blind controlled trial. Archives of Physical Medicine and Rehabilitation 71:34-37

Knight K L 1985 Cryotherapy: theory. Technique and Physiology. Chattanooga Corporation, Tennessee

Kolari P J 1985 Penetration of unfocused laser light into the skin. Archives of Dermatological Research 277:342-344

Lam T S, Abergel R P, Meeker C A, Castel J C, Dwyer R M, Uitto J 1986 Laser stimulation of collagen synthesis in human skin fibroblast cultures. Lasers in the Life Sciences 1:61–77

Lehmann J F, De Lateur B J 1990 Therapeutic heat in therapeutic heat and cold, 4th edn. Rehabilitation Medicine Library series. Williams & Wilkins, Baltimore pp 417-581

Lehmann J F, Masock A J, Warren C G et al 1970 Effect of therapeutic temperatures on tendon extensibility. Archives of Physical Medicine and Rehabilitation 51:481-487

Lewis T 1930 Observation upon the reactions of the vessels of the human skin to cold. Heart 15:177-208

Lindsay D, Dearness J, Richardson C, Chapman A, Cuskelly G 1990 A survey of electromodality usage in private physiotherapy practices. Australian Journal of Physiotherapy 36:249–256

Lowden A 1986 Application of ultrasound to assess stress fractures. Physiotherapy 72:160-161

Lundeberg T 1984 Pain alleviation by vibratory stimulation. Pain 20:25–44

Lundeberg T, Haker E, Thomas M 1987 Effects of laser versus placebo in tennis elbow. Scandinavian Journal of Rehabilitation Medicine 19:135-138

Magistro C M 1964 Hyaluronidase by inotophoresis. Physical Therapy 44:169

Martin B M, Grimbone M A Jr, Unanue E R, Cotran R S 1981 Stimulation of nonlymphoid mesenchymal cell proliferation by a macrophage-derived growth factor. Journal of Immunology 126:1510-1515

McMeeken J M 1982 Practical aspects of electrical safety. Australian Journal of Physiotherapy 28:21–22

McMeeken J M 1992 Magnetic fields: effects on blood flow in human subjects. Physiotherapy Theory and Practice 8:3-9

McMeekin J M, Bell C 1987 Effects of therapeutic doses of magnetic fields on blood flow in the dog hind leg. Proceedings of World Confederation of Physical Therapy. Book 1 WCPT Sydney 347-350

McMeeken J M, Bell C 1988 The effects of electromotor stimulation and other modalities on blood flow in dog hind limb. Proceedings of the Post-Congress Symposium of the World Confederation of Physical Therapy on Exercise Rehabilitation CARESR, pp 70–78

McMeeken J M, Bell C 1990 Microwave irradiation of the human forearm and hand. Physiotherapy Theory and Practice 6:171-177

McMeeken J M, Stillman B C 1987 Transcutaneous nerve stimulation.. In: Burrows G D, Elton D, Stanley G V (eds) Handbook of chronic pain management Elsevier. Amsterdam.

McNiven D R, Wyper D J 1976 Microwave therapy and muscle blood flow in man. Journal of Microwave Power 11:168–170

Mester E, Mester A F, Mester A 1985 The biomedical effects of laser application. Lasers in Surgery and Medicine 5:31–39

Michlovitch S L M 1990 Thermal agents in rehabilitation, 2nd edn. F A Davis Company, Philadelphia

Mohr T, Akers T M, Landry R G 1987 Effect of high voltage stimulation on edema reduction in the rat hind limb. Physical Therapy 67:1703-1707

Moritani T, Devries H A 1979 Neural factors versus hypertrophy in the time course of muscle strength gain. American Journal of Physical Medicine 58:115

Nadasdi M 1960 inhibition of experimental arthritis by athermic pulsating short-waves in rats. American Journal of Orthopaedics 2:105-107

Niinikoski J 1980 The effect of blood and oxygen supply on the biochemistry of repair. In: Hunt T K (ed) Wound healing and wound infection: theory and surgical practice. Appleton-Century-Crofts, New York pp 56–69

Nikolova L T 1987 Treatment with interferential currents. Churchill Livingstone, Edinburgh

Nussbaum N E, Rush R P, Disenhaus D L 1990 The effects of interferential therapy on peripheral blood flow. Physiotherapy 76:803-807

Ohshiro T, Calderhead R G 1988 Low-level laser therapy: a practical introduction. Wiley, Chichester

Pasila M, Visuri T, Sundholm A 1978 Pulsating short-wave diathermy: value in treatment of recent ankle and foot sprains. Archives of Physical Medicine and Rehabilitation 59:383–386

Perera J 1988 Lasers offer ray of hope for healing burns. New Scientist 19 May

Pette D et al 1975 Influence of intermittent long term stimulation on contractile histochemical and metabolic properties of fibre population as in fast and slow rabbit muscles. Pfluegers Archives 3611

Raji A R M 1984 An experimental study of the effects of pulsed electromagnetic field diapulse on nerve repair. Journal of Hand Surgery 9B:105-112

Raji A R M, Bowden R E M 1983 Effects of high peak pulsed electromagnetic field on the degeneration and regeneration of the common peroneal nerve in rats. Journal of Bone and Joint Surgery 65B:478-492

Robinson A J, Snyder-Mackler L 1988 Clinical application of electrotherapeutic modalities. Physical Therapy 68:1235-1238

Seibert W, Seichert N, Seibert B, Wirth C 1987 What is the efficacy of 'soft' and 'mid' lasers in therapy of tendinopathies? Archives of Orthopaedic and Traumatic Surgery 106:358-363

Sekins K M, Dundore D, Emery A F, Lehmann J F, McGrath P W, Nelp W B 1980 Muscle blood flow changes in response to 915 MHz diathermy with surface cooling as measured by Xe^{133} clearance. Archives of Physical Medicine and Rehabilitation 61:105–113

Sekins K M, Lehmann J F, Esselman P, Dundore D, Emery A F, de Lateur B J, Nelp W B 1984 Local muscle blood flow and temperature responses to 915 MHz diathermy as simultaneously measured and numerically predicted. Archives of Physical Medicine and Rehabilitation 65:1–7

Sissken B F 1988 Effects of electromagnetic fields on nerve regeneration. In: Mariino A A (ed) Modern bioelectricity. Marcel Dekker, New York

Snyder-Mackler 1989 Electrical stimulation for tissue repair. Snyder-Mackler L, Robinson A J (eds). Williams & Wilkins, Baltimore

Stillman B C 1970 Vibratory motor stimulation: a preliminary report. Australian Journal of Physiotherapy 16:118–123

Stillwell G K 1983 Therapeutic Electricity and Ultraviolet radiation, 3rd edn. Williams & Wilkins, Baltimore

Surinchack J S, Alago M L, Bellamy R F, Stuck B E, Belkin M 1983 Effects of low level energy laser therapy on the healing of full thickness skin defects. Lasers in Surgery and Medicine 2:267–274

ter Haar G R, Dyson M, Talbert D 1978 Ultrasonically induced contraction of mouse uterine smooth muscle in vivo. Ultrasonics 16:275-276

Turner J A, Chapman C R 1982 Psychological interventions for chronic pain: a critical review. 1 Relaxation training and biofeedback. Pain 121

Vasseljen O 1992 Low-level laser versus traditional physiotherapy in the treatment of tennis elbow. Physiotherapy 78:329–334

Wadsworth H, Chanmugam A P P 1988 Electrophysical agents in physiotherapy, 2nd edn. Science Press, Marrickville

Walker J 1983 Relief from chronic pain by low power laser irradiation. Neuroscience Letters 43:339-344

Walker J 1988 Photobioactivation. In: Ohshiro T, Calderhead R D (eds) Low-level laser therapy: a practical introduction. Wiley, Chichester

Ward A R 1986 Electricity fields and waves in therapy, 3rd edn. Science Press, Marrickville

Weiss D S, Kirsner R, Eaglestein W H 1990 Electrical stimulation and wound healing. Archives of Dermatology 126:222-225

Wesche J 1986 The time course and magnitude of blood flow changes in the human quadriceps muscle following isometric contractions. Journal Physiology 377:445–462

Williams J G P, Street M 1976 Sequential faradism in quadriceps rehabilitation. Physiology 62:252

Wilson D H, Jagadeesh P 1974 The effects of pulsed electromagnetic energy on peripheral nerve regeneration. Annals of the New York Academy of Science 238:575-585

Wilson D H, Jagadeesh P 1976 Experimental regeneration in peripheral nerves and the spinal cord in laboratory animals exposed to pulsed electromagnetic fields. Paraplegia 14:12-20

Wolf S L, Nacht M, Kelly J L 1982 EMG feedback training during dynamic movement for low back pain patients. Behavioural Therapy 13:395

Wyper D J, McNiven D R 1976 Effects of some physiotherapeutic agents on skeletal muscle blood flow. Physiotherapy 62:83–85

Young S R, Dyson M 1990 Macrophage responsiveness to therapeutic ultrasound. Ultrasound in Medicine and Biology 16:809-8164

16. Hydrotherapy

Margaret Reid Campion, Peter W. Hamer

PART 1
OVERVIEW
Margaret Reid Campion

The use of water in sports medicine has a history dating back to early Grecian and Roman times. Through the ages whirlpool baths, hot springs and the sea have been advocated for the treatment of sports injuries. Today, with a greater number of pools available and the increasing interest and awareness of the possibilities for activity in water, hydrotherapy has taken on new dimensions.

Hydrotherapy is defined as a physiotherapy treatment carried out in water by a physiotherapist and involves the use of the medium in the treatment of disease using the hydrodynamic principles to the maximum.

The treatment of sports injuries in water is more than a non-specific swim or a session in water because it is a 'nice thing to do'. The value of exercise in water for the injured athlete is appreciated as a means of maintaining fitness as well as for the treatment of the specific injuries.

It is essential that when treating patients in water the physiotherapist understands the properties pertaining to water, utilizes them to the full and recognizes that to take land-based exercise into water is to deny the uniqueness of the medium.

The physiotherapist should be in the water with the patient; especially when treating a specific body part. This permits appropriate observation of the exercises, and guidance can be provided to facilitate accuracy of the movement pattern. However, when running or swimming activities form the fitness components of the rehabilitation program careful supervision from the poolside can enhance the benefits of the session.

In an age when health and fitness are considered of such importance sport is undertaken by people of all age groups. It is not only the elite athlete who sustains injury and needs rehabilitation, but also the large numbers of amateurs and recreational athletes. Hydrotherapy has a unique and important role to offer for all injured athletes (Reid Campion 1990).

Rehabilitation programs in water can be commenced in the early stages of the injury, otherwise rest or non-weightbearing would be advised. In addition, the injured athlete can use the pool to train and maintain fitness related to a particular sport (Hopper 1990).

Indications and contra-indications and safety

The indications and contra-indications for hydrotherapy have undergone change in recent years (Davis & Harrison 1988). Most disorders of the locomotor system can be treated in the hydrotherapy pool. A few co-existing disorders or complications such as infections and contagious skin conditions and large open wounds which cannot be covered form contra-indications to pool treatment.

The physiotherapist must ensure that all safety measures are taken. The confidence and ability of the athlete in water can be ascertained during the assessment. Where anxiety is a factor, mental adjustment to water and instruction in balance restoration can do much to ameliorate concern (Reid Campion 1990). The presence of the physiotherapist in the water can act as further reassurance.

Assessment

Land assessment is essential and the details must be noted by the physiotherapist conducting the hydrotherapy treatment. Assessment based on the same criteria is required for water, but additional issues which have particular relevance to activity in water must be considered, such as the athlete's attitude to water, including perceived ability in water and details of previous water activity. Any contra-indications to hydrotherapy should be observed and recorded (Reid Campion 1990).

PHYSIOLOGY OF IMMERSION

Immersion in water affects the major systems of the body—the cardiovascular, respiratory, metabolic and nervous systems—along with the effects on the skin and kidneys (Rowell 1974, Swannell et al 1976, Kirby et al 1984, Koga 1985, Hall et al 1990).

It is recognized that exercise in warm water brings about the physiological effects of exercise in combination with those effects brought about by water and its warmth (Skinner & Thomson 1983). However, Hall et al (1990) suggest that further research is necessary to support the theory that treatment in warm water is therapeutic due to physiological changes brought about by combining exercise and immersion in water.

The uniqueness of water lies mainly in its buoyancy which relieves stress on weightbearing joints and allows movement to take place with reduced gravitational forces. The magnitude of the reduction in weightbearing is dependent on the depth of immersion. Harrison and Bulstrode's (1987) study showed that with immersion to the C7 level only 8% of body weight was experienced. This is increased to approximately 30% at the xiphisternum and to 50% at the anterior superior iliac spines.

Turbulence, which may be used to assist or resist movement and can be produced in several ways, comes about through irregular movement of the molecules of water. Its use is not only effective in treatment techniques but may also affect pain by acting like a soft tissue massage when the turbulence is strong and rapid. Gentler turbulence brings about relaxation and may ease muscle tension or spasm (Skinner & Thomson 1988).

The fact that skin friction on movement through the water is 790 times greater in water than in air was established by Froude (Massey 1979) and Zahm. This results in more energy being required for moving in water than through air, and ensures that exercise in water demands considerably more effort with resultant effects on the body systems (Evans et al 1978, Kirby et al 1984, Johnson et al 1977).

The warmth of the water plays a part in the physiological effects of immersion. The temperature of hydrotherapy pools should be maintained at 35°C . However, a range between 32°C and 34°C caters for the many different conditions treated in the pool and is suitable during rehabilitation of sports injuries. Lower temperatures are advisable for water-running and swimming, however, it is impractical to continual changing the water temperature.

HYDROTHERAPY: ITS USE IN SPORTS INJURIES

According to Hopper (1990), the use of hydrotherapy in the treatment of sports injuries is not sufficiently valued nor appropriately implemented. The hydrotherapy pool has been used for the maintenance of fitness in athletes who have sustained an injury (Buss 1976, Gatti 1978, Gibson 1981, McWaters 1988).

Hydrotherapy is indicated in the subacute and chronic phases of rehabilitation of sports injuries. Early treatment can take place where weightbearing is undesirable and appropriate levels of fitness can be maintained simultaneously.

Techniques

Apart from the 'conventional' method of buoyancy assisted neutral and resisted exercise, Bad Ragaz patterns, buoyancy and gravity dominant exercise, turbulence assisted and resisted techniques, hold-relax, repeated contractions, rhythmic stabilizations, and the recently devised hydrodynamic exercise can be utilized.

'Conventional' method

Exercises from the 'conventional' method require that the person's position allows the achievement of the required action, assisted, supported or resisted by buoyancy. These exercises can be progressed by altering the lever arm, by the addition of floats and by the usual means of an increase in speed and the number of repetitions. Manual resistance may also be applied (Bolton & Goodwin 1974, Skinner & Thomson 1983).

Bad Ragaz patterns

The Bad Ragaz patterns which have been described in detail by Skinner and Thomson (1983) and Davis and Harrison (1988) utilize the properties of water and encourage normal anatomical and physiological function of joints and muscles. Buoyancy is used for flotation only with further flotation provided by the application of a neck, pelvis and ankle floats where appropriate. Resistance to movement is provided by the 'bow wave' and turbulent effects created as the body or body parts move through the water.

The physiotherapist, who must be in the water with the person receiving treatment, provides fixation in three ways. Firstly, the physiotherapist acts as the fixation and the person moves through the water towards, away from or around the physiotherapist. Secondly, while again acting as a stabilizing point, the person is pushed by the physiotherapist in the direction of movement producing turbulence and thereby increasing the impedance to the movement. Thirdly, a position is chosen which the person holds as the physiotherapist pushes the body through the water (Bolton & Goodwin 1974).

Bad Ragaz patterns are designed to provide isotonic and isometric muscle work for the upper and lower limbs and the trunk. They are carried out mainly in supine lying although there are trunk patterns performed in side lying (Egger & Zinn 1990).

Increasing range of movement and the strengthening of muscle power are the two main aims of the Bad Ragaz patterns. Appropriate holds are most important and vary from proximal to distal depending on the action required. Irradiation or overflow from stronger to weaker muscle groups can be implemented as well as specific techniques of stabilization, repeated contractions, slow reversals and quick stretch (Skinner & Thomson 1983, Davis & Harrison 1988).

Buoyancy and gravity

The use of buoyancy and gravity dominated depths depends upon the purpose for which an exercise or technique is employed and the condition of the person being treated.

Hydrodynamic exercises

These exercises are specifically related to changes of shape and are based on the hydrodynamic principles of buoyancy, turbulence and metacentre (balance in water) (McMillan 1976, Reid Campion 1990). They provide a useful means of rehabilitation of sports injuries.

Shape and density of a body or body part influence hydrotherapy techniques. When changes of shape are made an alteration in the balance of the body in water occurs due to the metacentric principle.

When an object, human or otherwise, is immersed in water it is subjected to opposing forces—gravity acting downwards and buoyancy acting upwards. When gravity or buoyancy are equal and opposite each other the body is balanced and in equilibrium. However, any action which makes the forces unequal means that the body is no longer balanced. Movement takes place and it is always a rotational movement, the body rotating until the two forces are once more equal and opposite to each other.

Movement of any kind in water produces turbulence which is a disturbing force. Buoyancy is the other disturbing factor.

The process whereby hydrodynamic exercise is achieved requires assuming a stable shape, changing that shape, which creates turbulence, balancing against the turbulent effects, and finally balancing in the new shape. These techniques produce muscle work and demand balance and co-ordination.

The four main starting positions of standing, sitting, kneeling and lying are used with these being modified to change muscle work and control of balance. The depths at which these exercises in standing, sitting and kneeling are undertaken varies with the condition of the person being treated and the aim of the techniques used for the condition. In standing generally a depth of two-thirds the person's height would be used, but deeper or shallower water may be chosen depending on the degree of balance and co-ordination or increased weightbearing needed. The sitting position may vary from minimal flexion at the hips and knees to a right angle at all lower limb joints, moving from

deeper to shallower water as the condition improves but the water should always cover the shoulders. The same situation as sitting applies to the kneeling position.

While hydrodynamic exercise can be brought about by taking one arm or both arms above the water, changes of shape below the water produce greater reactions. Not only is it possible to work symmetrically and asymmetrically but muscle work can be finely graded by controlling the degree to which the body part or parts are taken above the water, and by the changes of shape undertaken below the surface. Static and dynamic activity as well as balance can be developed (Reid Campion 1990).

GENERAL INDICATIONS FOR HYDROTHERAPY IN SPORTS INJURIES

Sporting injuries are frequently treated by traditional land-based treatment. Water has the advantage of buoyancy which reduces the stress of weightbearing, particularly through the lower limb musculoskeletal system (Skinner & Thomson 1988).

Where pain and muscle spasm are present, the part affected should be immersed in warm water so that the heating effects and the support of the water will bring about relaxation (Skinner & Thomson 1983). It is suggested that the warmth of the water may aid the circulation and assist the dispersal of haematoma and oedema. Swelling may be further reduced by the pressure of water on the limb. Hydrostatic pressure increases with depth, suggesting that a swollen part where practicable should be exercised in as great a depth as possible (Skinner & Thomson 1983).

Musculoskeletal conditions with limitation of movement, muscle weakness, decreased balance, unco-ordination and alterations in the gait pattern exist may all benefit from activity in the pool.

SPECIFIC INDICATIONS

Stress fractures

When high impact loading such as running is curtailed, activity in water is the means by which the athlete can maintain specific aerobic and anaerobic fitness levels. Swimming and water-running (supported by a flotation device) are useful to reduce an interruption to the athlete's participation in sport. As healing occurs at the fracture site, increased impact loading can be gradually introduced by reducing the depth of immersion in relation to the guidelines of Harrison and Bulstrode (1987) or decreasing the impedance to movement.

Specific treatment would include the use of the 'conventional' method and Bad Ragaz patterns (Skinner & Thomson 1983) for the joints above and below the fracture. Even from very early stages of repair the introduction of

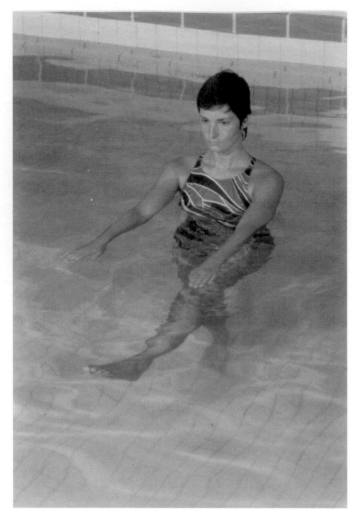

Fig. 16.1 Hydrodynamic gait training

hydrodynamic exercise and turbulence deliberately created by the physiotherapist and suitably placed around the athlete will strengthen and stimulate balance mechanisms.

Hydrotherapy is indicated in the subacute and chronic phases whether the injury of bony or muscular origin. Exercises in water should commence with buoyancy neutral since buoyancy-assisted exercise may produced undue stretching. The progression would be to buoyancy assisted and then to buoyancy resisted activities. Bad Ragaz isometric abduction and adduction patterns may be initiated, dorsiflexion/plantarflexion and knee flexion and extension isotonic patterns carefully applied to appropriate body parts. As healing occurs the conventional exercises and Bad Ragaz patterns may be progressed.

Gait re-education should be commenced with water at C7 level, progressing gradually to shallower water. Hydrodynamic techniques of gait training are conducted with straight legs and the patterns involve balance and co-ordination as well as increased range of movement (Fig. 16.1). 'Cossack dancing' is a means of developing knee extension with dorsi-flexion, and may be introduced towards the end

of the program; this can lead into an effective backstroke kick for swimming (Fig. 16.2). These techniques are described by Reid Campion (1990).

Injuries to the hip region

Sub-acute and chronic injuries to the hip and groin areas can be effectively strengthened using hydrotherapy, which provides variety to the athlete's program.

Supine and standing are commonly used starting positions (Fig. 16.3). Strengthening can be progressed by the addition of flotation to the limb. For example, with an adductor strain, in standing starting leg abducted and adducting to the mid line. Controlled eccentric action is required on the return to the starting position.

Injuries to the knee

Hydrotherapy is indicated in the subacute phase. Gentle exercises for the knee within the limitations of pain would be used while more active and vigorous activity would be employed for the trunk and unaffected limbs. It should be remembered that the warmth and support of the water allows an increased range of movement to take place and the physiotherapist needs to instruct the athlete carefully, especially where pain is present. Bad Ragaz patterns should be applied to the affected limb extremely carefully so that the freedom of movement which occurs in water does not aggravate the condition. Control can be obtained by the use of proximal holds and modification of the patterns. Initially, patterns that have a marked rotatory component should be avoided.

In the chronic phase all exercises and patterns can be progressed. Hydrodynamic exercises may be introduced as the range of knee flexion and extension increases and the strength of the quadriceps and hamstring muscle groups

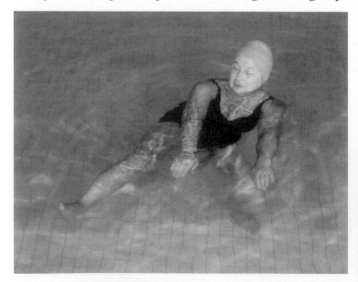

Fig. 16.2 Cossack dancing

out at decreasing depths to allow more weightbearing to occur. A hydrodynamic exercise for the ankle would be that of 'sitting' with the hips, knees and ankles at right angles and the arms forward, stretching the fingers forwards so that the body falls forwards and the heels rise, then returning to the starting position. Dropping the hips down to the heels, causes the body to fall backwards and the toes to rise from the floor of the pool. In controlling the forwards and backwards falling action the plantarflexors and dorsiflexors work strongly. Where only one direction is required the body is only caused to fall in the desired direction and to return to the starting position repeatedly.

Hydrotherapy is ideal for the athlete suffering from achilles tendonitis, as it allows aerobic fitness to be maintained by water-running and swimming (Hopper 1990). Specific techniques would include conventional exercises, Bad Ragaz patterns and later hydrodynamic exercise, always aiming to correct muscle imbalance such as tightness of gastrocnemius and soleus muscles.

Spinal injuries

Hydrotherapy is a valuable modality to achieve mobility, stability, dynamic control and relaxation of all regions of the spine.

Relaxation may be obtained in water in various ways. Conscious relaxation can be encouraged if the person is placed in supine lying fully supported by neck, pelvic and ankle floats and awareness of the support of the floats and water is developed (Skinner & Thomson 1988). Alternatively, the physiotherapist can support the person in this position. The head is on the physiotherapist's shoulder with the physiotherapist's upturned hands being placed as low down under the body as possible to support the trunk and give balance to the lower limbs. Gentle passive swaying from side to side by the physiotherapist of the person's body and lower limbs or passive or gentle active movements of the limbs often assists in relaxation.

On occasion pain and muscle spasm may prevent the assumption of the lying position even when supported by floats. Altering the position of the pelvic float may overcome this, but there are some people who cannot achieve comfortable float support lying wherever the floats are placed. In such cases where the thoracic and/or lumbar areas are affected but not the cervical region, it is possible for the athlete to 'hang' from the poolside (Fig. 16.4). This must take place in deep water so that the feet are clear of the floor of the pool. (If there is insufficient depth of water the athlete would bend the knees.) The forearms and flexed elbows are placed on the poolside and the body is lowered into the water facing the wall of the pool. The warmth of the water reduces pain and brings about relaxation. This position can be maintained for as long as is required to bring about relief. 'Hanging' with ring floats under the

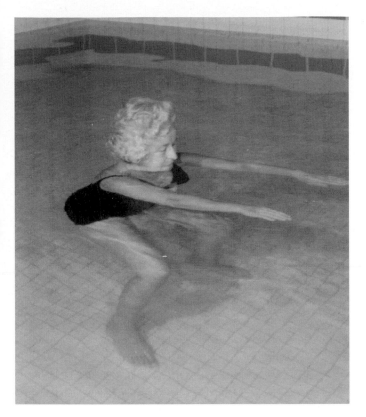

Fig. 16.3 'Sitting'—a starting position for hydrodynamic exercise

improves. As an example of hydrodynamic exercise, Cossack dancing may be used.

Swimming can also form part of the program, strokes being modified where necessary, particular attention being given to the breaststroke kick to ensure the movement is a 'narrow' one avoiding excessive abduction and knee pain during the extension phase of the kick which may be due to tension in the medial collateral ligament from external rotatory and valgus forces (Rovere & Nichols 1985, Hopper 1990).

Ankle problems

Soft tissue injuries to the ankle are very common, inversion sprains forming 80% of all ankle injuries (Roy & Irvin 1983).

Treating an ankle injury in the pool has a number of advantages. Hydrostatic pressure may reduce swelling and a buoyancy dominated water depth allows exercise in standing on the affected leg to take place. Turbulence around the athlete requires balance control and having the athlete standing on one leg can make this more critical. The technique simulates the wobble board on land and improves proprioception in addition to balance and co-ordination.

Bad Ragaz patterns such as dorsiflexion and plantar-flexion and other leg patterns which include ankle movements could be used. As weightbearing is allowed so ankle exercises such as heel and toe raising could be added, such land-based exercises being valuable because they are carried

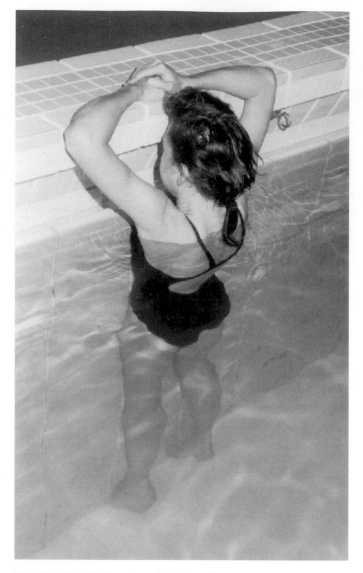

Fig. 16.4 'Hanging' on the wall of the pool

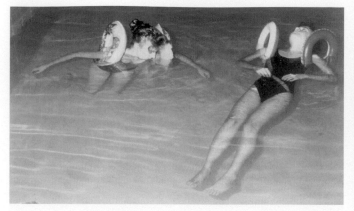

Fig. 16.5 Hanging in floats. The head controls the position of the body and lower limbs

axillae can provide an alternative to wall hanging or supine floating (Fig. 16.5).

Conventional exercises and Bad Ragaz arm and leg patterns are used initially, with trunk patterns being introduced gradually, commencing with static work and moving to more active patterns as the condition improves. It should be remembered that conventional exercises for the trunk cannot always be buoyancy assisted, supported or resisted.

Hydrodynamic exercises which require considerable static trunk work with fine muscular adjustment are valuable. An example is when supported by the physiotherapist in supine the position is maintained and rotation controlled when one arm is lifted upwards above the water.

These techniques require the physiotherapist to be in the water to support the athlete and indicate where the corrections should be made.

The cervical spine

The cervical region is not easily treated in water. However, specific techniques can be used to produce all movements of the cervical spine with immersion of the part as full as possible. Walking sideways in the water can initiate some side flexion if carried out at C7 water level and becomes more effective as direction is changed. Full immersion of the cervical spine can be obtained in supine, either supported by neck and ankle floats or by the physiotherapist supporting the athlete as described for relaxation and rolling the body to one side requesting the athlete to turn the head away from the side being rolled under to bring the body back to a flat position. This rotation of the head can be increased if following the body back to a flat position again is resisted by the physiotherapist (Reid Campion 1990).

Flexion and extension can be induced if the athlete is held in the curled up position—knees to chest and hands around the knees. The physiotherapist holds the athlete with one arm around the athlete's back at waist level and the other hand over the athlete's hands (Fig. 16.6). In this position the physiotherapist passively rocks the athlete backwards and forwards, inducing cervical flexion and extension. The body is held away from the physiotherapist's body to allow it to swing freely. As the condition improves the athlete can initiate the rocking action by the use of the head. Side flexion can also be produced in this position by tilting the body sideways.

To develop rotation in the cervical spine the physiotherapist supports the athlete as described for relaxation and rolls the body to one side, requesting the athlete to turn the head away from the side being rolled under to bring the body back to a flat position. This rotation of the head can be increased if rolling the body back to a flat position again is resisted by the physiotherapist (Reid Campion 1990).

Where pain and muscle spasm is marked, this may be reduced effectively by passive rotation of the body on the head. Two methods can be employed. The athlete may be supported by the physiotherapist in supine lying as described above, the physiotherapist fixing the athlete's head with the shoulder and own head, or the athlete's head may be supported by a neck collar with the physiotherapist standing to one side of the athlete's hips. In both instances the athlete's body is passively rotated by the physiotherapist, the athlete's head being maintained in mid-position.

Thoracic and lumbar spine

These areas of the spine are treated as indicated in the introductory remarks to treatment of the spine. Specifically for these regions hanging either on the poolside or suspended at the axilla by two inflated rings is useful. As pain decreases, small slow movements of the head in any direction may be made, with time being given for the body to react as the altered head position will be 'noted' by the water and the body's position altered. Flexion, extension, side flexion and rotation of the trunk can be developed in this way. Later, movements of the lower limbs can be introduced along with the head movements. Balance and co-ordination can also be improved by the use of turbulence judiciously created around the athlete by the physiotherapist, the athlete holding different shapes, for example, sitting, kneeling and standing.

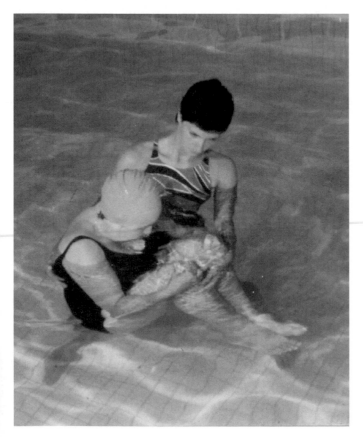

Fig. 16.6 The 'curled' position for flexion, extension and side flexion of the cervical spine

Swimming for athletes with spinal trauma needs to be considered carefully and strokes modified. Initially a bilateral arm movement in the backstroke may be possible, gradually moving into a unilateral arm pattern. Breast stroke is often difficult for spinal injuries because of the amount of cervical and trunk extension (Blades 1990).

Shoulder injuries

Hydrotherapy would be introduced in the subacute phase. If the athlete is reluctant to move the arm away from the body this can be achieved in water by inducing relaxation in specific ways. By supporting the athlete in float lying the physiotherapist, standing behind the athlete's head and holding the athlete under the back at waist level, walks slowly backwards gently swaying the athlete's body from side to side. When the arm is relaxed it will tend to move away from the side of the body due to turbulence which facilitates movement. Buoyancy assisted arm movement is then introduced which is later progressed to buoyancy neutral. As healing occurs exercise can be progressed and Bad Ragaz isometric patterns introduced, followed by isotonic patterns initially using proximal holds.

In the chronic phase, strength and muscle control become important and all the techniques given above are extended. The holds for the Bad Ragaz patterns could become distal, particularly if pain has decreased. Slow reversal, stabilizations, successive inductions and repeated contractions may be employed (Skinner & Thomson 1983).

The above treatment would certainly apply to the rotator cuff impingement syndrome with emphasis in the treatment regime on the correction of training and technical errors (Hopper 1990). Strengthening exercises can also be progressed with the addition of a paddle or enlarged glove to the hand, to increase the surface area of the limb, and/or increase in speed or movement of the exercise.

To treat sports injuries effectively in the pool, the physiotherapist must understand and utilize the medium to its fullest extent, handling and guiding the athlete to optimal recovery and speeding the return to sport.

PART 2
WATER RUNNING
Peter Hamer

An important component in the rehabilitation of injured athletes is the maintenance of the athlete's cardiovascular fitness. In the past, swimming and cycling have been prescribed for those athletes forced to avoid full weightbearing activities due to injury of their locomotor system. More recently, water-running has been prescribed to replace the athlete's normal land-based running activities. Water-running is a generic term that can cover a wide range of running-type activities in the water. Most commonly, water-running refers to running in water while maintaining a normal running style and posture. It can be performed in shallow water (0.8-1 m deep) or, when supported by a flotation device, in deep water (>1.8 m deep) (Hamer & Morton 1990).

The indications for the use of water-running are wide and varied. Most commonly it has been used during the rehabilitation of stress injuries of the lower limbs. These have included stress fractures, medial tibial stress syndrome and the various lower limb compartment syndromes. The applications suitable for water-running have been extended to include its use as a recovery activity after hard workouts, e.g. an aerobic water-running workout following intensive basketball training. Water-running is also used as a substitute training so that it becomes a regular workout during the training week, e.g. as a replacement for the 8 km run the day after a 20 km hard effort.

Water-running, which may progress from walking in water through to running and sprinting in the water, may also be progressed from a non-weightbearing activity (using flotation) to a partial weightbearing activity at the shallow end of a pool. This has important implications not only for injuries requiring graduated weightbearing activities, e.g. fractures, stress fractures and ligament sprains, but also for other populations. The elderly, the obese and the arthritic are all likely to benefit from the increase in activity level without the stress of impact on the lower limbs.

WATER-RUNNING TECHNIQUE

The premise of water-running is an attempt to replicate the metabolic and neuromuscular specificity of running on land. This premise requires that the action of water-running should involve the same muscle groups and should simulate the movement patterns required during the over-ground running action.

DEEP WATER-RUNNING

When running in deep water a flotation device is required so that there is no impact of the lower limbs on the pool floor. A variety of flotation devices have been utilized, including waterski belts, kayak/canoe vests and polystyrene floats, with the commercial products, e.g. Wet Vest (Bioenergetics Inc., Birmingham AL), Hydro-tone belts (Hydro-tone International, Inc.) being the ultimate flotation for water-running. It is important that the flotation device, which is imperative to ensure optimal running action, does not interfere with the proper running action. Without flotation the running action deteriorates so that there is an increased forward trunk lean associated with a cycling action of the legs and an improper reciprocal arm action. The correct action encourages an upright body posture (10-15° forward trunk lean) with a reciprocal arm action concentrating on replicating the normal excursion of the arms. The hands should be lightly clenched to prevent a 'dog paddle' type action. The lower limb action should be emphasized using the cues 'lift the thigh, straighten the knee in front and then drive the leg back through the water'. This action results in the foot becoming plantarflexed during the recovery phase of the running action with this plantarflexion being maintained through the drive phase of lower limb extension which correlates with the stance phase of the running gait. Allowing dorsiflexion to occur will result in a cycling action rather than a running style. This cycling action may of course be that required for an injured cyclist wishing to avoid any impact on the lower limbs. It is equally important to stress the lifting of the thigh and leg extension component to prevent a running on the spot technique (Fig. 16.7 a,b,c,d).

The water-running technique has been studied using high speed cinematography at 100 frames per second and compared with treadmill running (Hamer et al 1984). The lower limb kinematics of a trained uninjured runner, who

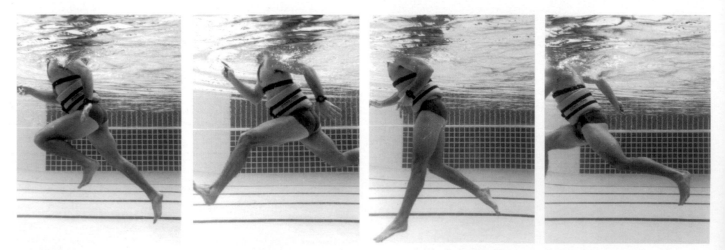

Fig. 16.7 Deep water-running technique, emphasizing: (a) the slight forward body lean with hip flexion during the late stage of recovery; (b) knee extension during the stride forward; (c) the plantarflexed foot with knee extension during the drive phase; (d) the hip extension and knee flexion just prior to leg recovery

was familiar with both treadmill running and the deep water-running action, was compared running on the treadmill and running in the water using a flotation vest for support. The intensity of exercise was determined as a target heart rate of 160 bpm (using Karvonen's formula), resulting in a rating of perceived exertion (RPE) (Borg 1982) of Hard (15-16) while running in water and Somewhat Hard (13-14) while running on the treadmill. Biomechanical analysis indicated that the angular velocities for the thigh and leg did reach similar magnitudes in both running actions, with the angular accelerations being of a lower magnitude and less variable during water running. The joint angles at which the peak angular velocities occurred were also similar (Hamer et al 1984). These factors would serve to provide some evidence of the specificity of the deep water-running action to the treadmill running action.

Dissimilarities between treadmill running and deep water-running do exist, mainly relating to the action about the knee. During the 'drive' phase of deep water-running the knee joint may achieve a hyperextended position so that not until thigh recovery is initiated is there any marked degree of flexion of the knee joint (Hamer et al 1984). During the stance phase of treadmill and overground running the resultant knee flexion is a function of shock absorption and the action of the hamstring muscle group (Dillman 1975, Elliott & Blanksby 1979). During deep water-running the hyperextension that does occur will largely be a function of there being no supporting surface, while the hamstring group will be functioning synergistically as hip extensors against the accommodating resistance of the water. The degree of hyperextension seen at the knee joint, while uncomfortable on dry land, is not noticed by the athlete during the deep water-running action (Hamer et al 1984), and may only pose a problem if excessive genu recurvatum or cruciate laxity is present.

During the leg recovery phase, the action is similar to that of overground and treadmill running, with the deep water-running technique tending to exhibit the characteristics of the faster overground running action of greater knee flexion accompanying higher knee lift during the thigh recovery phase of running.

SHALLOW WATER-RUNNING

Shallow water-running is most commonly used in athletes as a transition from deep water-running to the land. This transition is most pertinent to athletes using the pool for rehabilitation and training during injuries that have required reduction of impact shock, e.g. stress fractures, medial tibial stress syndrome, patella tendonitis. Flotation is not required, but it is worthwhile to wear some form of footwear to prevent damage to the feet. Suitable footwear may be old running shoes, diving neoprene bootees, or windsurfing bootees. Dunlop Volley tennis shoes with their soft rubber ripple sole provide excellent protection and grip. The running action should be as similar as possible to over-ground running with the leg action emphasized to ensure a striding action rather than a running on the spot technique. Care must also be taken to ensure a reciprocal arm action.

THE POOL ENVIRONMENT

The pool environment should be conducive to performance of moderate to intense physical activity. Indoor or outdoor swimming pools and diving pools, maintained at a temperature of 22°-27°C, are ideal. Hydrotherapy pools at a temperature at 36°C compromise the body's thermo-regulation during moderate to intense exercise (Craig & Dvorak 1966), resulting in cardiovascular drift as evidenced by gradually increasing heart rate at any given submaximal workrate (Gleim & Nicholas 1989).

In pools where it is not possible or acceptable to transverse lengths or widths, tethered water-running may be employed. This entails either a direct rope or strong elastic cord attachment from the runner to the side of the pool, or a more elaborate pulley and weight system so that different workloads can be administered (Hamer & Morton 1990, Welsh & Rhodes 1988). The disadvantage of tethered water-running is a loss of the true water-running action and a reduction in the resistive forces of drag and viscosity friction. A further alternative for shallow water-running is the water-running treadmill (Carlson et al 1985, Gleim & Nicholas 1989, Welsh & Rhodes 1988), which although offering the benefit of a controlled workrate may be influenced by both the greater flight time of the water-running action and differences in the dispersion of turbulence. The turbulence created while running on a treadmill immersed in water would create a reduced pressure area in front of the runner resulting in less resistance to movement. A person running freely through the water experiences greater drag forces and therefore greater resistance to forward movements.

EXERCISE PRESCRIPTION

Water-running offers a unique environment for running training, however, direct transfer of training routines from land to water-running is not completely possible. The form of training most appropriate to water-running is interval training. This allows a training program to be developed to specifically stress each of the energy systems as required (Fox 1979, Hamer & Morton 1990). A program may entail prescription of sets of 10 sec, 30 sec and 60 sec sprints allowing almost complete recovery between each sprint. This would develop anaerobic power and capacities, whereas the prescription of longer intervals of 3-6 minutes at a work to recovery ratio of 1:0.5 or 1:1 would be used for aerobic power development. Continuous running can be utilized, e.g. 45 minutes (Bishop et al 1989); however boredom and lack of variety can become a problem affecting the compliance of athletes to the program.

The setting of the intensity, duration, and frequency of the workouts should initially follow accepted training principles dependent on the energy system being maintained or developed (Fox 1979). The basic principles of exercise prescription do, however, need some modification due to the physiological effects of immersion. In principle the effects of increased hydrostatic pressure on the immersed body (Pascal's Law) will increase venous return thereby increasing stroke volume (SV) resulting in a lower heart rate for any given submaximal oxygen consumption (Hamer & Morton 1990). It is generally accepted that for shallow water-running the target heart rate should be set between 6-10 bpm lower than that used for overground running (Hamer & Morton 1990). For deep water-running the target heart rate should be set 12-17 bpm lower than that for land training (Hamer & Slocombe 1991, McWaters 1988). While the heart rate is depressed during submaximal deep water-running, the HR/RPE relationship maintains a linear relationship and is parallel with the HR/RPE relationship derived from treadmill running (Hamer & Slocombe 1991).

A further important factor to consider is the effect of the temperature of the water on the heart rate response to exercise. Exercise in thermoneutral water (32-34°C) results in cardiovascular adjustments very similar to those experienced on dry land (McArdle et al 1976). At higher temperatures (> 35°C) a thermal stimulus is responsible for increasing the heart rate at comparable metabolic workrates—cardiovascular drift (Craig & Dvorak 1966, Gleim & Nicholas 1989). At lower water temperatures (< 25°C) a significant reduction in the heart rate (15 bpm) is induced when compared with equivalent workrates in thermoneutral water. This is compensated for by a proportionate increase in the stroke volume of the heart (Weston et al 1987). This bradycardia response has also been found to be dependent on body composition parameters as well as acclimatization to the cool water environment (McMurray 1983).

The heart rate-oxygen consumption relationship (HR/VO_2) may also be affected by the type of water-running, i.e. between tethered water-running versus water-running treadmill versus free water-running. Much of the research has been collected using either underwater cycle ergometers, tethered water-running or underwater-treadmill ergometer tests (Avellini et al 1982, Gleim & Nicholas 1989, Hamer & Morton 1990, McMurray et al, 1983, Welsh & Rhodes 1988). It is from these studies that many of the recommendations have been derived. Where free water-running has been investigated, and compared with treadmill running (Gleim & Nicholas 1989, Moore 1990), the HR/VO_2 relationships, although remaining linear, are contrary to the generally accepted guidelines. These studies have demonstrated that at exercise intensities greater than 60% of VO_2 max the heart rates at similar oxygen consumption levels were approximately 6-7 bpm higher during water-running through deep water compared to the heart rate response observed during water-running through shallow water, which were in turn greater than that the heart rates observed during dry treadmill running. This antithesis to that generally accepted may be due to the fact that during free water-running the limbs are exposed to undisturbed water with each limb excursion. This means that the forces of viscosity friction and turbulence will be greater than when the limb recovers forward in the turbulent hole in the water left by the limb during the stance phase of running either on a treadmill in water or during tethered water-running. This appears to affect the cardiac output side of the oxygen consumption equation ($VO_2 = HR \times SV \times a\text{-}\bar{v}O_2\Delta$), where $HR \times SV$ equals cardiac output. A further explanation may be due to the method of setting a controlled rate of exercise, as in a speed of a treadmill or a cadence for free-water-running. This may result in entrainment of the heartrate to an inefficient gait cycle, culminating in an elevated heart rate response to the activity (Paterson et al 1986).

RECOVERY HEART RATES

The rate of recovery is also affected by the water environment. Due to the effects of immersion on the cardiovascular system the heart rate recovers to resting levels at a greater rate than after land running (Hamer & Morton 1990). This has been proposed to be due to the increase in intrathoracic blood volume increasing stroke volume, resulting in a decreased heart rate for any given submaximal VO_2 (McArdle et al 1976). It is generally accepted and utilized that the greater rate of return to resting heart rate will allow a reduction in the duration of the rest interval within an interval training program. This may reduce the work (W) to rest (R) ratio from a 1:3 W:R ratio on land to a 1:2 W:R ratio for sprinting activities in the water. Further research to investigate the rate of metabolic recovery as externally expressed and measured by VO_2 and lactate (HLa) is necessary to ensure that athletes are being given adequate recovery. The external manifestation of the rate of recovery as evidenced by the heart rate may not be concomitant with recovery at the muscle cell level. Some level of exercise recovery may be needed to prevent excessive central shunting of blood volume during rest periods. This central shunting of blood volume may prevent muscle level glycogen repletion and lactate resynthesis. A further important consideration is the water's thermal effect on heart rate. The rate and magnitude of the drop in heart rate may well be in response to the temperature of the water.

Monitoring of the intensity of water-running training heart rate

To monitor the training heart rate during water-running the traditional method of palpation of the carotid pulse may be used. Most heart rate monitors utilizing the electrical activity of the heart do not work very well in water, as the conductivity of the water interferes with differentiation of the electrical activity of the heart through the skin. This is compounded by many of the monitors not being waterproof. The Sportstester PE4000, is available for use in water environments, but precautionary measures to reduce the total immersion of the unit should be undertaken. This may entail wearing a headband to which the monitor is attached and the use of the approved accessory (or plastic food wrap) to minimize the saturation of the transmitter. Other types of heart rate monitoring as used by swimmers (Chivers 1988) may be used.

Ratings of perceived exertion

It has been documented that when land exercises are performed in water the result is a higher metabolic cost and a greater rating of perceived exertion (Johnson et al 1977, Kirby et al 1984, Moore 1990). The use of ratings of perceived exertion as a prescriptor of exercise intensity is influenced by the greater metabolic cost of the activity in the water; the lower heart rate at equivalent metabolic workrates; possible thermal effects of the water; and the greater resistive forces to limb movement—viscosity friction, drag and turbulence.

McWaters (1988) has utilized the ratio scale of perceived exertion of Borg (1982) in prescribing intensities for water-running. McWaters (1988) outlines that 'competitive runners can perform long sustained runs (45 min) at an RPE of 7 while interval training consisting of hard running for 2-5 minutes can be sustained at an RPE of 8-9. All-out efforts (RPE = 10) can usually be sustained for no longer than 30 seconds at a time'. These RPE values compare with RPE values of 13, 15-17 and 19, respectively, when using the original RPE scale (Borg 1982).

BENEFITS OF WATER-RUNNING

Psychological benefits

One of the important benefits gained from placing injured athletes into a correctly constructed and administered water-running program is the effect on the psychological reaction to being injured. A water-running program satisfies not only the requirements of the clinician i.e. decreased impact loading and accommodative resistance with low accelerative components, but also satisfies the running athlete. Athletes are still actively involved in training using running as the mode of activity. This results in compliance with the rehabilitation program and will engender a positive attitude to rehabilitation, maintaining a closer affinity to the visualization of the athlete's successful return to competition (Williams 1986). The use of water-running within this framework provides an ideal protected environment for the setting of short-term and long-term goals for rehabilitation and training.

When water-running is used as a recovery activity or as supplementary training, the psychological benefits of hydrotherapy and relaxation (Reid Campion 1990) can be built into the program to aid in the prevention of over-training.

Physiological benefits

The increasing popularity of water-running as a training mode for running activities has largely been prompted by the anecdotal evidence from athletes and coaches. The use of the water by high profile athletes, e.g. Steve Scott, Mary Decker-Slaney and John Walker, encourage other athletes to use the water when injured and as a recovery or supplementary training session. Research into the physiological aspects of water-running has centred on improvements or maintenance of training status or aerobic power as measured by VO_2 max (Buss 1976, Gatti 1978). Many of the studies have suffered from a low number of subjects, short periods of training stimulus, and a low number of parameters describing cardiovascular fitness. Controlled studies of shallow and deep water-running that have utilized 8-12 week training programs (Chivers 1988, Hamer & Morton 1990) have demonstrated aerobic improvements of 10-13% increase in VO_2 max, 13% increase in maximal oxygen pulse (HR/VO_2), a decrease in the submaximal heart rate at any given submaximal workrate and a decrease in maximal heart rate, with the change in the parameters being attributable to the training program. An important finding from these training studies has been that water-running elicits short-term and long-term cardiovascular responses similar to land-based running. The short-term responses include similar VO_2 max values being achieved during graded exercise testing on both a dry-land treadmill and during tethered water-running (Hamer & Morton 1990). The long-term responses are similar in magnitude to the change expected from comparable training frequencies, intensities and duration of a land-based training program (Chivers 1988, Hamer & Morton 1990). This has lead to the inference that water-running satisfies the metabolic requirements of specificity of training (Hamer & Morton 1990)

It is also interesting to note that although the training stimuli of the water-running programs were designed to improve the aerobic capabilities of the subjects within the guidelines of the American College of Sports Medicine (ACSM 1990), there were concomitant improvements, in the region of 14-16%, in anaerobic capacities and power output that were attributable to the water-running training program (Hamer & Morton 1990).

Biomechanical benefits

There is a paucity of published research directed to the biomechanical action and benefits of water-running.

Cinematographical studies have demonstrated some variation in the angular kinematics and joint angles of water-running when compared with those of treadmill running (Glass 1987, Hamer et al 1984). As has already been detailed, the running style in the water must be as close as possible to the running action on land. When this is achieved there is some anecdotal evidence that demonstrates the biomechanical and kinaesthetic value of water-running.

It has been observed by the author on several occasions that athletes that display a poor running technique on land, e.g. arms crossing the body when sprinting, lower limb external rotation at impact and stance phase followed by internal rotation and abduction of the lower limb during recovery phase, can benefit from water-running. The external forces offered by the water environment can be useful firstly in alerting the athlete to the faulty technique, and secondly to increase the kinaesthetic input to the neuromuscular system. These two factors enable the athlete to work at slower angular velocities for the same, if not greater, perceived effort which, particularly if captured on video, can be used to give feedback to the athlete. The pseudo-slow-motion action of the limb excursions in the water allow cognition of the components of limb movement and identification of technical errors. The increased kinaesthetic feedback will allow athletes to appreciate their established movement patterns and, using this increased feedback, establish optimal motor patterns to help correct faulty technique. The water thus provides an ideal environment to facilitate the stages of motor control as outlined by Fitts and Posner (1967). The cognitive and associative stages require controlled environments with initially high levels of sensory input in establishing sub-routines for new or modified motor patterns prior to the automatization of these patterns that are then transferred to overground running.

The importance of using the water to firstly analyze technique and secondly to optimize running techniques is particularly relevant to the injured runner. The faulty technique, identified and corrected in the water, may well have been a contributing factor to improper impact loading and/or overuse type injuries.

The principles of hydrodynamic exercise ensure the greater use of proximal and distal dynamic joint stabilizers. Activation of these joint and limb dynamic stabilizers are important in the smooth execution of limb movement to ensure controlled mobility and static dynamic capabilities. This improved control allows an improved functional control of movement e.g. the control of femoral internal/external rotation during the hip flexion of the recovery phase of running. The water's unique environment encourages the activation of this part of the neuromuscular system and may be useful in the prevention of injury during land-based running. Anecdotal evidence also supports the use of these principles across many different sporting populations e.g. ballet dancers or gymnasts working at improving their control and execution of a leap, or footballers needing to improve proximal control about the hip, pelvis and groin during kicking actions.

RISKS AND UNKNOWNS

The uniqueness of the water environment has many advantages, however, water-running is not completely free of risks or unknowns. Aside from the obvious risks associated with the water that need to be addressed for the safety of athletes (e.g. drowning, hygiene and supervision) there appears to one group of musculoskeletal injuries that may not respond well to water-running. Lower limb compartmental pressure syndromes tend to be unpredictable in their reaction to water-running. In particular, the anterior compartmental pressure syndrome may be exacerbated, most commonly with shallow water-running. This may be due to ankle dorsiflexion prior to impact being subjected to increased viscosity friction and drag. This resistance may be enough to exacerbate a pre-existing compartmental pressure syndrome. Deep water-running, however, does not appear to aggravate this condition as the ankle is maintained predominantly in plantarflexion throughout the running action (Hamer et al 1984).

While there is still some controversy over the heart rate response to water-running, caution must be respected when prescribing this mode of exercise for any of the 'at-risk' populations, specifically cardiac patients.

As has been demonstrated, water-running does have many benefits for the injured athlete, however, further research is required to investigate anaerobic benefits; biomechanical and physiological correlates with respect to technique; and document beneficial skill changes occurring due to the unique kinaesthetic and resistive features of the water environment.

REFERENCES

American College of Sports Medicine 1990 The recommended quantity and quality of exercise for developing and maintaining cardiorespiratory and muscular fitness in healthy adults. Medicine and Science in Sports and Exercise 22(2):265-274

Avellini B A, Shapiro Y, Fortney S M, Wenger C B, Pandolf K B 1982 Effects of heat tolerance of physical training in water and on land. Journal of Applied Physiology 53 (5):1291-1298

Bishop P A, Frazier S, Smith J, Jacobs D 1989 Physiological responses to treadmill and water-running. The Physician and Sportsmedicine 17(2):87-95

Blades K 1990 Hydrotherapy in orthopaedics. In: Reid Campion M (ed) Adult hydrotherapy: a practical approach. Heinemann Medical, Oxford

Bolton E, Goodwin D 1974 An introduction to pool exercises, 4th edn. Churchill Livingstone, Edinburgh

Bonnette A R 1978 Use the swimming pool to rehabilitate injuries. Athletic Journal 59(3):62-63

Borg G 1982 Psychophysical bases of perceived exertion. Medicine and Science in Sports and Exercise 14(5):377-381

Buss R 1976 Keeping the injured athlete fit. Track Technique 63:2001

Carlson J S, Snow R J, Jones C J, Payne W R 1985 Examination of cardiovascular and metabolic adjustments to exercise on a treadmill immersed in water (abstract). Medicine and Science in Sports 17(2):252

Chivers L 1988 Deep water running: changes in selected body composition, cardiorespiratory and biochemical variables following a twelve week training programme. Unpublished Masters thesis, University of Western Australia, Perth

Craig A B Jr, Dvorak M 1966 Thermal regulation during water immersion. Journal of Applied Physiology 21(5):1577-1585

Davis B C, Harrison R A 1988 Hydrotherapy in practice. Churchill Livingstone, Edinburgh

Dillman C J 1975 Kinematic analyses of running. In: Wilmore J H, Keogh J F (eds) Exercise science and sports reviews, vol 3. Academic Press, New York

Egger B, Zinn W M 1990 Aktive physiotherapie in wasser. Gustav Fischer Verlag, Stuttgart

Elliott B C, Blanksby B A 1976 A cinematographical analysis of overground and treadmill running by males and females. Medicine and Science in Sports 8(2):84-87

Evans B W, Cureton K J, Purvis J W 1978 Metabolic and circulatory responses to walking and jogging in water. Res Q 48(4):442-448

Fitts P M, Posner M I 1967. Human performance. Wadsworth, California

Fox E L 1979 Sports physiology. Saunders, Philadelphia

Franchimont P, Juchmes J, Lecomte J H 1983 Hydrotherapy mechanisms and indications. Pharmacology and Therapeutics 20:79-83

Gatti C J 1978 Maintaining endurance in injured runners. Track Technique, 72:2289

Gibson K 1981 Shallow water conditioning/rehabilitation for track. Scholastic Coach 50(9):58, 52

Glass R A 1987 Comparative biomechanical and physiological responses of suspended deep water running to hard surface running. Unpublished thesis, Auburn University, USA

Gleim G W, Nicholas J A 1989 Metabolic costs and heart rate responses to treadmill walking in water at different depths and temperatures. American Journal of Sports Medicine 17(2):248-252

Hall J, Bisson D, O'Hare P 1990 The physiology of immersion. Physiotherapy 76(9):517-521

Hamer P W, Morton A R 1990 Water-running: training effects and specificity of aerobic, anaerobic and muscular parameters following an eight-week interval training programme. Australian Journal of Science and Medicine in Sport 22(1):13-22

Hamer P W, Slocombe B 1991 The perceived exertion-heart rate relationship for deep water-running. 1991 Annual Scientific Conference in Sports Medicine, Canberra, October

Hamer P W, Whittington D, Spittles M, Yakovina M 1984 Cinematographical comparison of water running to treadmill running. Unpublished paper

Harrison R, Bulstrode S 1987 Percentage weightbearing during partial immersion in the hydrotherapy pool. Physiotherapy Practice 3(2):60-63

Hopper D 1990 Hydrotherapy for sports injuries. In: Reid Campion M (ed) Adult hydrotherapy. Heinemann Medical, Oxford

Johnson B L, Strømme S B, Adamczyk J W, Tennøe K O 1977 Comparison of oxygen uptake and heart rate during exercises on land and in water. Physical Therapy 57(3):273-278

Kirby R L, Sacamano J T, Balch D E, Krielaars D J 1984 Oxygen consumption during exercise in a heated pool. Archives of Physical Medicine and Rehabilitation 65:21-23

Koga S 1985 The regional difference of thermal response to immersion during rest and exercise. Annals of Physiological Anthropology 4(2):191-192

McArdle W D, Magel J R, Lesmes G R, Pechar G S 1976 Metabolic and cardiovascular adjustment to work in air and water at 18°, 25° and 33°C. Journal of Applied Physiology 40(1):85-90

McMillan J 1976 The role of water in rehabilitation. Fysioterapeuten 45(5):237

McMurray R G, Hovarth S M, Miles D S 1983. Hemodynamic responses of runners and water polo players during exertion in water. European Journal of Applied Physiology 51:163-173

McWaters J G 1988 Deep water exercise for health and fitness. Publitec, Laguna Beach, California

Massey B S 1976 Mechanics of fluids, 4th edn. Van Nostraud Rheinhold, New York

Moore J-A 1990 The relationship between oxygen consumption, heart rate and perceived exertion during water-running at different depths of immersion. Unpublished Honours thesis, School of Physiotherapy, Curtin University of Technology, Western Australia

Paterson D J, Wood G A, Morton A R, Henstridge J D 1986 The entrainment of ventilation frequency to exercise rhythm. European Journal of Applied Physiology 55(5):530-537

Reid Campion M 1990 Adult hydrotherapy: a practical approach. Heinemann Medical, Oxford

Reid Campion M 1991 Hydrotherapy in paediatrics, 2nd edn. Heinemann Medical, Oxford

Rovere G D, Nichols A W 1985 Frequency, associated factors and treatment of breaststroker's knee in competitive swimmers. American Journal of Sports Medicine 13(2):99-104

Rowell L E 1974 Human cardiovascular adjustments to exercise and thermal stress. Physiological Review 54(1):75-159

Roy S, Irvin R 1983 Sports medicine: prevention, evaluation, management and rehabilitation. Prentice-Hall, Inglewood Cliffs

Skinner A T, Thomson A M (eds) 1983 Duffield's exercise in water, 3rd edn. Baillere Tindall, London

Skinner A T, Thomson A M 1988 Hydrotherapy in pain: management and control in physiotherapy. Wells P, Frampton V, Bowsher D (eds). Heinemann Medical, London

Swannell A J, Fenkem P H, Hughes A O, Trussell E C 1976 Changes in arterial blood pressure in patients undergoing routine pool therapy. Physiotherapy 62(3):86-88

Welsh D G, Rhodes E C 1988 Comparison of cardiorespiratory parameters during treadmill and simulated immersion running. Canadian Journal of Sports Sciences 13(3):94P-95P

Weston D F M, O'Hare J P, Evans J M, Corrall R J M 1987 Haemodynamic changes in man during immersion in water at different temperatures. Clinical Science 73:613-616

Williams J 1986 Applied sport psychology: personal growth to peak performance. Mayfield, Palo Alto, California

17. Isokinetic dynamometry

Tim Wrigley, Margaret Grant

Isokinetic testing and exercise equipment has been available for almost twenty years, and it has been in wide use for over a decade. A task analysis survey of the sports physical therapy section of the American Physical Therapy Association in 1980 concluded that such equipment was 'essential to very essential' in the practice of sports physiotherapy (Skovly 1980). As of 1994, the literature on isokinetic dynamometry amounts to over 2000 articles and research abstracts. Clearly, therefore, isokinetic testing and exercise has established a major place in the assessment and rehabilitation of sports injuries.

The use of isokinetic dynamometers and the practice of sports medicine have evolved together; the link is more than simply coincidental. In sports medicine, objective assessment of muscle-joint performance became imperative, with the need to refine clinical decisions and expedite the injured athlete's rehabilitation and return to competition.

Despite the established position of isokinetic testing and exercise, some of the 'tenets' of isokinetic clinical practice are unproven, poorly understood by users, or patently false. Furthermore, a substantial portion of the published literature is scientifically unsound. However, a growing realization of this state of affairs hopefully heralds a new, more critical phase for the practice of isokinetic dynamometry. This development is vital if users are to keep up with the expanding capabilities of the isokinetic dynamometers, and the additional data now available for interpretation as a result of computerization. Failing this, it is likely that isokinetic dynamometry will fail to achieve its full potential or, worse still, fall into disrepute.

The material presented in this chapter reflects this more critical perspective. First, general principles are outlined and problem areas are identified, then the principles for clinical application of isokinetic testing and exercise are described, with particular reference to the knee and shoulder joints and the back. Because of the suspect validity of some existing aspects of isokinetic practice, 'question everything' is a useful maxim in relation to isokinetic dynamometry. Where research evidence for practice is lacking, this is clearly indicated. However, in such instances, clinical experience is occasionally cited as the basis for the recommendations made. Sound isokinetic practice can only be learnt by experience in applying valid principles to various pathologies. In many areas, the most efficient ways of using isokinetic testing and exercise remain to be determined. These will be elucidated by innovative clinicians in the future, based on sound scientific and clinical principles as outlined in this chapter.

GENERAL PRINCIPLES OF ISOKINETIC DYNAMOMETRY

PHYSIOLOGY AND BIOMECHANICS OF MUSCLE AND JOINT FUNCTION

The ability of a muscle to generate torque (rotational force) about a joint is a function of a number of physiological and biomechanical factors: muscle length, velocity and cross-sectional area, muscle moment arm, motor unit recruitment and firing frequency. Each muscle-joint complex has a characteristic relationship of torque versus joint angle, also known as its 'strength' curve (Kulig et al 1984). The shape of this curve reflects the maximal joint torque generating capability throughout the range of motion, which is primarily determined by the muscle length-tension relationship, and the muscle moment arm (distance from the muscle's line of action to the axis of joint rotation). It is important to realize that the angle at which maximum torque is generated does not necessarily represent the point of maximum muscle tension; rather, the maximum torque is achieved at the point where the optimum combination of muscle length-tension and moment arm length occurs.

Factors that may decrease the torque-generating capability include fatigue, pain, lack of motivation, joint effusion, and mechanical derangements or neurological disorders that affect the normal function of muscle and joint.

The variation in muscle tension with contraction velocity is characterized by the well-known force-velocity relationship. The torque-velocity relationship has a similar shape: concentrically, joint torque declines exponentially as velocity increases; eccentrically, peak torque has been shown to remain relatively constant (at a level similar to isometric torque) regardless of velocity (e.g. Dudley et al 1990, Westing 1990), at least for lower limb muscles. This is in contrast to isolated animal muscle, where the eccentric tension-generating ability continues to increase with increasing velocity, plateauing only at up to twice the isometric tension (Katz 1939) (Fig. 17.1).

Metabolic energy supply

In the context of sports physiotherapy, it is important to understand the physiological basis of an injured athlete's sporting activity. Most protocols employed in isokinetic testing and exercise are based on the exertion of maximal strength, with energy supplied mainly by anaerobic processes. The relative emphasis in a rehabilitation program on this form of intense, maximal exercise in comparison to submaximal, aerobic forms of exercise (using other exercise equipment, as well as submaximal isokinetic exercise) should be predicated upon the relative importance of strength and anaerobic/aerobic metabolism in the athlete's sport. (See Ch.1 for more information on metabolic energy supply systems, and Ch. 2 for the physiological changes that accompany injury.)

DEFINITIONS OF BASIC TERMINOLOGY

One condition for the establishment of the legitimacy and maturity of any form of technology in biomedicine is a rigorously defined and unambiguous terminology. Unfortunately, the practice of isokinetic dynamometry is characterized by nebulously defined or incorrect ter-

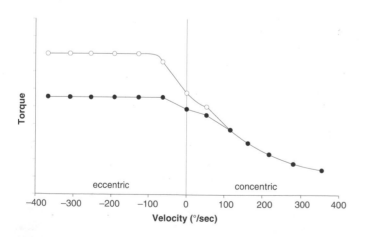

Fig. 17.1 Apparent difference between the 'intrinsic' torque-velocity relationship [open circles] (consistent with in vitro studies of isolated animal muscle) and the in vitro human torque-velocity relationship [closed circles]. Note especially the discrepancy for eccentric contractions. The divergence in the low velocity-high torque concentric region is somewhat contentious (e.g. Yates & Kamon 1983).

minology in a number of areas. This section introduces and defines several basic terms. Isokinetic measurement parameters—with which most of the terminological problems exist—are covered in the Measurements section.

In utilizing isokinetic dynamometry, the clinician is usually attempting to get an indication of a patient's 'strength'; there is, however, no universally-agreed definition of 'strength'. Although the ability to develop force is a generic capability of muscle, this ability varies with muscle length, contraction velocity, and direction (shortening or lengthening). Therefore, the conditions under which strength is measured should be operationally defined in terms of these mediating factors. Most authors who have put forward definitions of strength have contended that the entity that comes closest to being a generic measure of the force-generating capability of muscle is isometric strength, since the number of potential confounding variables (e.g. changes in muscle length and velocity) is minimized. An example of such a definition is that of Atha (1981), who suggested that strength be defined as 'the ability to develop force against an unyielding resistance in a single contraction of unrestricted duration' (p. 7), that is, an isometric contraction.

However, in practice, isometric strength is less commonly measured by instrumented means than other forms of strength. This reflects the assumption that a static measure of strength is less likely to be indicative of 'functional' strength than a dynamic measure. Thus, a typical operational definition of 'strength' (that might be stated in an isokinetic research study) would be: 'concentric knee extension strength was measured as the peak torque achieved at 60°/second on an isokinetic dynamometer'.

To put isokinetic dynamometry within its broad context of muscle joint performance testing and exercise, it is necessary to contrast it with other forms, namely, isometric and isotonic. The three terms (isometric, isotonic, isokinetic) have literal translations from the Greek, which are included below with operational definitions. Some of these terms, in particular 'isotonic' and 'isokinetic', are often imprecisely defined and/or understood, so considerable detail is included. It is also worth noting that the term 'isokinetic' dynamometer is now perhaps too narrow, in that all current dynamometer models in fact support isometric, isotonic and isokinetic modes.

Isometric: 'constant (muscle) length'

This term was initially used to describe muscle physiology experiments on isolated animal muscle, in which muscle length was held constant while the muscle was electrically stimulated and force measured (Carlson & Wilkie 1974). When applied to human muscle function, an appropriate operational definition is 'muscle contraction without movement at the joint'.

Isotonic: 'constant (muscle) tension'

This term was also initially used in the context of isolated muscle physiology experiments; in this case, the stimulated animal muscle shortened against a constant weight load (attached to its tendon)—hence constant muscle tension—while the change in length was measured.

This discussion is particularly relevant now that some isokinetic dynamometers have an isotonic mode, although the term has traditionally been applied to loading methods that involve a constant external weight load. However, the use of the term to describe such an external weight resistance implies a constancy of loading that does not in fact occur. Thus, the use of the term 'isotonic' in the human context is not entirely appropriate. The only consistent feature of most exercises that have been termed 'isotonic' is not constant loading, but variable velocity. With variable velocity comes acceleration, and thus unquantified inertial forces. The magnitude of forces involved in these types of exercises are thus the least readily controlled (and quantified) of all testing/exercise modes. For example, in a typical 'isotonic' bench press exercise, the resistance experienced by the subject may vary from the actual weight of the barbell by about 20%, due to inertial forces induced by acceleration/deceleration (Wilson et al 1989).

Isotonic devices (including the isotonic mode of isokinetic dynamometers) can generally be considered, at best, to achieve maximal test/exercise loading only at the weakest point in the range of motion, since if the load cannot be moved through the weakest point the movement cannot be completed. The seated, weighted boot knee extension exercise is possibly a 'worst case' example, because the point at which the maximum loading is experienced (full extension) corresponds to a relatively weak point in the range of motion for the knee extensors. Therefore, throughout the rest of the range, this muscle group is relatively underloaded (Fig. 17.2).

The term 'isoinertial' has been suggested as a more appropriate term to describe many of the methods that are currently termed isotonic (Kroemer 1983), as the only properties of the load that remain constant with such methods are the inertial properties. However, this description does not convey any information about the pattern and magnitude of the loading experienced. The determination of the actual joint torques imposed by such variable loading requires biomechanical test methods that are not amenable to routine clinical use. There is, as yet, no general agreement on the term 'isoinertial' as an alternative to 'isotonic'. Some physiotherapists may be familiar with another class of dynamometers, specifically for back testing, that have gone by the name 'isoinertial' (or 'isodynamic'(*sic*)). Since the total loads actually experienced by the subject cannot be readily quantified or controlled (McIntyre 1987), caution should be exercised in the interpretation of data from such devices.

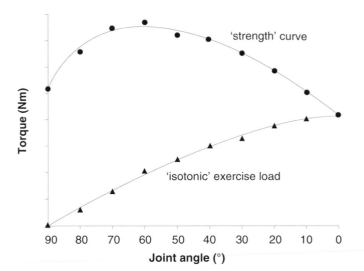

Fig. 17.2 The 'isotonic' exercise load resisting seated knee extension with a weighted boot, contrasted with the maximum 'strength' curve for the knee extensors

Isokinetic: 'constant movement (velocity)'

The youngest of the three terms, the term 'isokinetic' has come to be applied to muscle contraction in which constant joint angular velocity is maintained by an 'accommodating' resistance (see explanation below). Muscle velocity is not constant in such an isokinetic movement, but varies with muscle length, moment arm, etc. (Hinson et al 1979). By maintaining constant angular velocity, an isokinetic dynamometer achieves a condition of dynamic equilibrium, where the torque applied to the limb by the dynamometer is equal in magnitude and opposite in direction to that developed by the patient. This is an example of Newton's first law of motion. Thus there is no acceleration, and the resistance torque applied by the dynamometer 'accommodates' to changes in torque-generating capacity throughout the range of motion, due to physiological (muscle length-tension) and biomechanical (moment arm) changes, pain, fatigue and motivation. The range of velocities offered by isokinetic dynamometers are in the low to medium physiological range. The relevance of velocity in relation to several issues is discussed further in later sections. Some published definitions of 'isokinetic' confuse the characteristics that are always present in an isokinetic movement with those that may be present: the only obligatory characteristic of an isokinetic movement is constant velocity (since this is the literal derivation of the term). Maximal resistance is not an obligatory characteristic of the loading imposed by an isokinetic dynamometer; maximal resistance may be an indirect consequence of the constant velocity imposed, but such resistance is only applied by the dynamometer if the patient exerts a maximal effort.

Isotonic and isokinetic methods can be considered as requiring 'dynamic' muscle contractions, in contrast to the 'static' isometric contraction. Such dynamic muscle contractions can be further characterized as either 'concentric' (shortening) or 'eccentric' (lengthening). Muscle physiology research over the last century has concentrated on concentric contractions. Likewise, the history of isokinetic dynamometry has been dominated by concentric testing; eccentric capabilities have only recently become available on all except one of the current models of isokinetic dynamometers. Much is now written in the isokinetic clinical literature about eccentric contractions, given the important role that such contractions play in normal functional activities and in the aetiology of some injuries (particularly those of muscle and tendon). However, the basic explanations of eccentric contraction in such clinical literature have often been physiologically non-sensical. Authors have suggested, for example, that the greater tension seen in eccentric contraction is due to non-contractile tissue being 'pulled apart' (this is quoted in one of the dynamometer manufacturer's manuals), or that the extra tension comes from the series elastic components, not the contractile component. A full explanation of why these notions are not sound is beyond the scope of this chapter. However, the most tenable explanation for the greater tension of eccentric contraction is that a cross-bridge can sustain greater force before releasing when stretched in an eccentric contraction than it can develop in an isometric or concentric contraction (Cavagna et al 1985).

As well as the greater tension of eccentric contraction, other characteristics that appear to distinguish such contractions from isometric and concentric contractions include non-uniform sarcomere lengthening (Morgan 1990), low ATP usage (Curtin & Davies 1975), possible selective recruitment of fast motor units (Nardone et al 1989), and possible neurally-mediated inhibition (Dudley et al 1990, Westing 1990). Much, however, remains to be learnt about eccentric contractions (Huxley 1980, Noble 1992, Stauber 1989).

It has been suggested that the word 'contraction' should no longer be used, as it is contradictory in the case of an eccentric (i.e. lengthening) contraction (implies shortening) (Cavanagh 1988). The alternative proposed by Cavanagh was 'muscle action', but it is not certain whether this alternative is likely to gain universal acceptance. There is another school of thought that sees little reason to discard 'contraction' (Raven 1991).

ADVANTAGES AND DISADVANTAGES OF ISOKINETIC TESTING AND EXERCISE

In the 1960s, the concept of the isokinetic dynamometer was put forward in a US patent by James Perrine, an American bioengineer. The commercial introduction and subsequent popularity of isokinetic dynamometers were a result of the fact that the existing means of muscle testing (generally manual) were insufficiently sensitive, and the existing exercise modalities (isometric and isotonic) were incapable of dynamically exercising muscles to their maximum tension-generating capacity. The measurement sensitivity and maximal accommodating resistance of isokinetic dynamometers remain the primary advantages of this form of testing and exercise for muscle-joint systems. The relative advantages and disadvantages of isometric and isotonic exercise are covered elsewhere (e.g. Sapega 1991).

High velocity exercise

Ironically, the maximum velocities that can be achieved by isokinetic dynamometers have been portrayed both as advantages and disadvantages of isokinetic dynamometry. On the one hand, it has been argued that specificity to high velocity functional activities is conferred by high velocity isokinetic exercise. In apparent contradiction, it has been suggested that isokinetic dynamometers are deficient in not allowing sufficiently fast maximum velocities to approach the very high joint angular velocities seen in many sporting activities. It is likely that both positions reflect exaggerations and/or misunderstandings by their proponents. The relevant considerations are discussed in this section.

The ability to exercise effectively at moderately high velocities (in relation to functional velocities) with isokinetic devices does confer an advantage over other forms of exercise in some situations. With an 'isotonic' resistance, when an athlete attempts to exercise at high velocity the exercise becomes ballistic. Significant muscle activation is involved primarily only at the beginning (agonist) and end (antagonist) of the range of motion; the momentum imparted to the load at the start of the range of motion by concentric agonist contraction carries it through the range, until an eccentric antagonist contraction decelerates the load as the end of range is approached. While this type of high-velocity, ballistic, isotonic exercise has a place in the training of healthy athletes in explosive sporting activities, its use in a rehabilitation program is both relatively ineffective and potentially damaging to joint and muscle. It may, however, have application late in such a rehabilitation program, when return to full function for the athlete is imminent. In contrast to the phasic nature of muscle activation in high-velocity, ballistic, isotonic exercise, the maximal resistance of an isokinetic dynamometer implies maximal muscle activation (for a given velocity) throughout the range of motion. Thus, even at high velocities, there is consistent agonist muscle activation throughout the range of motion (Osternig et al 1986).

The availability of useful higher velocity concentric exercise (several hundred degrees per second or greater) with isokinetic devices has particular advantages in some pathologies. Unlike isotonic exercise, isokinetic resistance continues to accommodate to muscle tension-generating capability as dynamometer velocity settings are increased, so that acceleration does not predominate and the exercise does not become ballistic. Because of the exponential decline in concentric muscle tension development capability with increasing velocity (the characteristic force-velocity relationship of muscle), the resultant joint forces will also generally be lower at higher isokinetic velocities (Nisell 1985). Therefore, in patients with patellofemoral pain syndrome, for example, the patellofemoral compressive force during concentric isokinetic knee extension should be lower at higher velocities (Nisell & Ericson 1992, Kaufman et al 1991). Of course, the patient's pain should always guide the use of such high velocity isokinetic exercise. Since the eccentric torque-velocity relationship does not decrease with increasing velocity settings (Westing 1990), high velocity eccentric exercise does not possess this advantage. However, as with concentric contractions, the fact that high velocity movements are completed more quickly will mean that the muscle-joint system is under load for a shorter length of time, which may be desirable in patellofemoral problems.

Discussions of the advantages of isokinetic dynamometers have often stressed a perceived specificity of high isokinetic velocities to functional activities. This contention is, at best, probably overemphasized. The usual examples given in an attempt to support the specificity contention reflect a misunderstanding of human muscle function in functional activities. For example, Wyatt and Edwards' (1981) report of knee extension angular velocities in normal gait—reaching 233°/second in late swing phase (in their example)—has often been cited to justify the need for high velocity concentric isokinetic exercise of the quadriceps. This assertion fails to recognize the fact that peak knee extension velocities are seen during gait when the knee is extending largely under its own momentum rather than as a result of actual concurrent quadriceps muscle activity that is, the movement is substantially ballistic. During late swing phase, at the point when this velocity was measured, the lower leg is actually beginning to slow down, decelerated by the eccentric action of the quadriceps' antagonists, the hamstrings (Winter 1991). There is some quadriceps activity recommencing at this time, but such activity is in preparation for eccentric absorption of the forces following footstrike, rather than generating further knee extension. The motion of the leg in swing phase is largely the result of hip flexor and knee extensor activity early in the forward range of motion of the leg, when joint angular velocities are relatively slow.

Ironically, if the exaggerated suggestion of velocity specificity were extended to its seemingly logical conclusion for high velocity sporting activities—many of which occur with joint angular velocities approaching (or even exceeding) 1000°/second—we would be led to conclude that isokinetic exercise (or any other form of resistance exercise) would not be particularly useful for such sports, since no dynamometers are capable of reaching these velocities ! Clearly this is not so. Such false logic again ignores the ballistic nature of these high velocity activities—such angular velocities are not solely due to concurrent agonist muscle activity across one joint. Extreme functional angular velocities are usually seen at distal joints, and are the result of summation of velocities from proximal to distal joints (Chapman & Sanderson 1990). Two research results further highlight the fallacy of these assertions. First, Houston et al (1988) found that the maximum velocity that could be achieved in maximum free knee extension was only approximately 700°/second. Secondly, Davies (1992) tested isokinetic knee extension-flexion of normal subjects from 300-600°/second on a modified Cybex II+ dynamometer, noting that a substantial number of subjects failed to record any torque at all at 600°/second. Both findings thus suggest that the common achievement of knee extension velocities exceeding 1000°/second at the knee during sprinting (unpublished observations), for example, is not inconsistent with much lower isolated-joint maximum velocities (i.e. when only the knee is extending). Thus, it is unreasonable to extrapolate uncritically from observed functional joint angular velocities when prescribing appropriate isokinetic testing and exercise velocities.

Safety

The relative safety of isokinetic testing and exercise over isotonic exercise is often cited. This is due to the accommodating nature of the resistance provided by an isokinetic device. For example, a sudden episode of pain in the middle of a range of motion will not leave the patient with a heavy load on the limb that must be returned to the starting position, as could occur with an isotonic device. Rather, when the patient experiences any pain, their natural reduction in muscle-generated torque will cause the dynamometer resistance torque to be proportionally reduced. This is not to say that patients cannot experience significant pain during testing and exercise on an isokinetic dynamometer (Lysholm 1987), given that maximum torques are more readily generated than with other methods. Therefore, it is important that the perceived safety advantage of isokinetic dynamometry is not exaggerated; the indications for isokinetic testing and exercise need to be carefully assessed in light of the potential for pain resulting from overstressing particular structures.

The special case of eccentric isokinetic testing and exercise warrants particular mention in relation to safety. Eccentric isokinetic dynamometry is probably the most precise and controlled means of assessing maximal eccentric muscle performance. However, because the maximum eccentric tension that an intact human muscle can develop is generally the greatest tension that it can develop under any circumstances, there is an inherently greater risk of injury with eccentric testing than with concentric testing. Therefore, the decision to test or exercise a patient eccentrically must be made carefully. Maximum eccentric testing and/or exercise is not appropriate for an acutely weakened muscle-joint complex.

Other advantages?

Some clinicians assume certain perceived advantages of isokinetic exercise that are in fact false. For example, it may be falsely assumed that slow-velocity isokinetic exercise preferentially recruits slow-twitch fibres, and that fast-velocity isokinetic exercise preferentially recruits fast twitch muscle fibres. The vast majority of the physiological evidence indicates that this is not the case; rather, the recruitment of muscle fibres is based on the relative force requirements of a given isometric or concentric contraction, regardless of velocity (Burke 1981, Sale 1987). The slow twitch fibres are recruited first, at low forces, followed by the fast twitch fibres as the force requirement increases. In a submaximal concentric contraction, the force requirement will therefore be met predominantly by the slow twitch fibres, regardless of velocity. In a true maximal concentric isokinetic contraction, we could reasonably assume that all muscle fibre types will be recruited, again regardless of velocity. There is, however, some evidence that healthy individuals do vary in their ability to recruit their entire motoneuron pool for a given muscle (Bigland-Ritchie et al 1986).

The intrinsic maximum shortening velocities of slow twitch fibres are less than those of fast twitch fibres (Close 1972). Therefore, the decline in concentric force development as velocity is increased is most likely due to the fact that cross-bridge cycling time becomes limiting in an increasing proportion of the available muscle fibres. Initially, at relatively slow velocities, this may occur for some slow twitch fibres, while at very fast velocities it will have occurred for almost all muscle fibres. That is, even though all fibres may be recruited, their cross-bridges may not be capable of cycling fast enough to contribute appreciable tension to the contraction.

Motor unit recruitment during eccentric contractions is not as well understood as that during concentric contractions. However, there is some evidence that eccentric contractions in humans may be inhibited to some extent (Dudley et al 1990, Westing 1990), and that preferential fast twitch recruitment may occur (Nardone et al 1989).

Disadvantages

One of the most obvious disadvantages of isokinetic devices is their high cost. As far as rehabilitative exercise is concerned, there are certainly less expensive means of exercise that may be similarly effective in improving muscle performance. The choice of the most appropriate exercise modality should most often be based on which equipment allows the performance of the desired movement pattern in the most appropriate fashion (e.g. contraction mode), rather than the specific type of resistance provided. However, for muscle-joint performance testing, only isokinetic dynamometers provide a theoretically optimal means of controlling potentially confounding variables (i.e. velocity), for a range of dynamic isolated movement patterns, with objective quantitative data feedback.

Motivation

In the definition of an isokinetic accommodating resistance, it was mentioned that resistance would vary with motivation. This is a potential disadvantage of isokinetic testing and exercise, as maximal patient motivation may be difficult to ensure. Furthermore, where motivation is not maximal, this may sometimes be difficult to detect. This potential limitation of isokinetic dynamometry can be minimized to some extent by emphasizing appropriate instructions and strong verbal encouragement, plus visual feedback (e.g. computer graphic displays). Where the dynamometer allows, a judicious choice should be made of torque thresholds that the patient must initially exceed and then maintain in order for the lever arm to begin and continue movement.

Other disadvantages?

An argument has come from some quarters (often with commercial motives) that isokinetic testing and exercise is inappropriate, because constant velocity movements are rarely seen in any functional activities. This is debatable. The ability to contract is a generic capability of muscle. In the context of exercise or testing of maximal muscle function, the actual conditions under which a muscle is called upon to contract are not especially important (see e.g. Westing et al 1991) as long as those conditions allow maximal activation of muscle and sufficient control over potentially confounding variables so that measurement reliability and validity are reasonable expectations. The conditions that most readily meet these criteria are isokinetic. The operating modes of non-isokinetic devices do not meet these criteria; problems with such devices include the fact that unquantified inertial torques (due to acceleration) confound valid measurements, and/or that both torque and velocity may be allowed to vary.

Perhaps the strongest argument for the functional relevance of isokinetic testing is the large number of studies that have shown associations between such test results and a wide range of functional athletic performances (Genuario & Dolgener 1980, Podolsky et al 1990, Pedegana et al 1982, Miyashita & Kanehisa 1979, Anderson et al 1991, Sjodin

1982, Bosco et al 1983, Wiklander & Lysholm 1987, Mascaro et al 1992, Cisar et al 1987, Bartlett et al 1989, Ciccone & Lyons 1987, Narici et al 1988, Cabri et al 1988, Morrow et al 1979, Pawlowski & Perrin 1989, Fleck et al 1992, Alexander 1990, Galbreath et al 1989, Lephart et al 1987, Picconatto et al 1989, Russum & Cisar 1989, Delitto et al 1988, Guskiewicz et al 1993, Oddsson & Westing 1991, Perrine & Edgerton 1975, Poulmedis et al 1988). Given a number of factors that might be expected to militate against such associations, such as the obvious multifactorial nature of athletic performance and the methodological problems of some of these studies, the weight of evidence of the studies cited is compelling. It would seem that the rarity of constant velocity movements in functional activities is probably largely irrelevant to the functional significance of isokinetic testing and exercise.

ISOKINETIC DEVICES

Testing devices

It is important that potential isokinetic users are able to judge the relative merits of the various dynamometers on the basis of the relative importance of a given machine's 'strengths' to their clinical needs. An isokinetic dynamometer may represent the single most expensive piece of equipment that a clinician contemplates acquiring. On the other hand, a clinician without such equipment, who is considering the referral of a patient for an isokinetic test, needs to be sure that the device chosen is capable of providing the most relevant clinical information. Unfortunately, the different isokinetic dynamometers that are currently (1994) commercially available do not possess consistent features. Neither do the collection of features possessed by any given dynamometer give it clear superiority over its competitors.

As of 1994, there are five isokinetic dynamometers available commercially and widely used (either in their current or earlier models). In alphabetical order, these are the Biodex, Cybex (currently 6000 series), Kin-Com, Lido, and Merac; all are of American origin. There are several more obscure devices available in Europe and Japan. Initially, the Cybex I, and then the Cybex II, were the only dynamometers available from the early 1970s until the early 1980s. The Cybex II device is still the most commonly used, although it has now been superseded and is no longer commercially available. The vast majority of the published research literature concerns studies that were performed with the Cybex II.

All but one of the latest models of isokinetic dynamometers mentioned above are capable of testing both concentrically and eccentrically, although some companies also produce simpler versions of their more sophisticated models that provide only concentric testing. All isokinetic dynamometers now come with computer systems (all IBM compatible) that collect, display and store the isokinetic test data. In some cases, these computers also control the movements of the dynamometer. The various dynamometers differ greatly in their support for direct calibration of the transducer systems with which torque, velocity and joint angle measurements are made.

The features of isokinetic dynamometers have changed considerably since the original models. Rather than list the current features of each device, the major categories of features common to machines will be described. In some instances, feature comparisons between isokinetic dynamometers have tended to focus on factors that are not particularly important, such as the maximum velocity achievable. Conversely, the considerable variation in the quality of the dynamometers' computer software has generally been ignored, although this aspect is extremely important. The way in which the software operates tends to determine the type of environment a particular dynamometer is best suited to, and what it is not suited to. For example, some systems are particularly suited to testing patients quickly; thus they are ideal for a busy clinic environment. However, one consequence of this type of operation is that the software may not allow the clinician sufficient time to closely monitor the patient's performance, and thus ensure quality control. Conversely, another system, although allowing close attention to quality control and precise prescription of patient testing and exercise protocols, is rather time-consuming to use in a busy clinic. Some software systems almost overwhelm the clinician with data, while others do not provide enough data while the test is in progress, or afterwards. There is happy medium, with both of these extremes incorporated for different user requirements, but at the time of writing no vendor has achieved it.

Angular velocity (speed)

Isokinetic devices, by definition, are capable of operating at a range of constant angular velocities. At the low end of the velocity scale, all devices are capable of operation at $0°$/second, that is, isometrically. Some devices are capable of relatively modest maximum velocities (just over $200°$/s), while others have maximum velocities more than double those of their counterparts (over $500°$/s). The clinical usefulness of such high velocity capabilities is questionable.

In devices that are capable of both concentric and eccentric operation, the maximum velocity may not be the same for both modes. In such cases, the maximum eccentric velocity is often less than the maximum concentric velocity. However, this is not of great concern, as the maximum useful eccentric test velocity will probably invariably be lower than the maximum useful concentric test velocity. There are several reasons for this. First, when we try to exert a maximal eccentric contraction at a fast velocity on an isokinetic dynamometer, we immediately realize that it is a rather unusual sensation and one that may not be particularly similar to the type of fast eccentric contractions that occur functionally. Consequently, fast eccentric isokinetic movements can be very difficult to master. Secondly, the human eccentric torque-velocity relationship appears to be relatively 'flat', that is, torque varies little from slow to fast velocities (see Fig. 17.1). Therefore, muscle and joint will be exposed to similarly high forces, regardless of the eccentric isokinetic velocity used. Thus, the utility of high velocity isokinetic eccentric contractions is questionable.

Contraction modes

As mentioned earlier, all but one of the latest models (1994) of isokinetic dynamometers are capable of testing both concentrically and eccentrically. However, the dynamometer that has historically been the most commonly used, the Cybex II (now superseded), is a concentric-only device. This means that the vast majority of isokinetic testing and exercise performed over the last two decades has been concentric. The ability to test eccentrically has been available for less than a decade. Consequently, the relative role and relevance of eccentric testing in clinical practice is still evolving, however its use is increasing all the time. This trend reflects what is a relatively common eccentric aetiology for many injuries, particularly those of muscle and tendon. The second consequence of the longer history of concentric testing is that the vast bulk of the published literature concerns concentric-only testing and exercise.

Some dynamometers, although capable of testing both concentrically and eccentrically, place particular restrictions on the combinations of modes that can be accommodated. Other dynamometers, although allowing all possible combinations and ordering of modes for reciprocal movements (concentric/concentric, eccentric/eccentric, concentric/eccentric, eccentric/concentric), place greater restrictions on maximum torque or velocity when certain combinations are employed.

Torque limits

Some dynamometers allow the clinician to precisely control the maximum and minimum torque limits within which the patient is allowed to exercise. Ideally, the clinician should be able to set these limits independently for each movement direction.

Several dynamometers have maximum allowable torque limits that may preclude testing large muscle groups of strong athletes, especially eccentrically. Not only is eccentric strength usually greater than concentric, but it does not usually decrease as velocity increases like concentric strength does (Westing 1990), so we cannot simply test at a faster eccentric velocity to come under the machine's maximum torque limit.

Exercise training devices

All the isokinetic dynamometers discussed above can also be used for rehabilitative exercise. The extent to which they are used in this role varies from clinic to clinic, and between dynamometers.

As with testing capabilities, dynamometers vary greatly in their usefulness as exercise devices. The more sophisticated facilities allow the exercise parameters to be precisely set and controlled. Obviously there is no substitute for direct patient supervision, but this is not always possible. Therefore, the ability to set maximum and minimum torque limits, goals to be achieved (in terms of torque, work or exercise time) and range of motion limits is a significant advantage. With such capabilities, there may also be graphic performance feedback to the patient while they are actually exercising, and recording of patient performance for subsequent assessment by the clinician.

In addition to the adjunct exercise capabilities of the test dynamometers, there is a range of isokinetic devices designed solely for exercise; that is, they have no testing capability. In this category are devices that mimic the exercise movement patterns supported by their more sophisticated testing counterparts, as well as devices that allow exercise patterns that are not possible with any of the test devices. Among the former are multi-movement-pattern devices and dedicated knee extension-flexion devices, for example. Amongst the latter group are isokinetic 'ergometers' for the upper body and, for the lower body, in the form of bicycle ergometers. Also in this second group are unique devices such as the Cybex Kinetron (Porche 1988, Delitto & Lehman 1989), that have no counterparts in other areas of exercise technology.

ISOKINETIC TESTING

Protocols

Isokinetic testing protocols have been proposed and adopted on a largely arbitrary basis. Currently, the protocols possible on a given dynamometer are substantially dictated by the software, and not all systems have equivalent protocols. While angular velocities can be set with reasonable flexibility, this is not true of other aspects. This is unfortunate, as it is unlikely that these software-enforced protocols are ideal in all circumstances. This section outlines general considerations with respect to protocols. Specific details for particular joints and movements are discussed later.

The most common test protocol involves three to five continuous reciprocal concentric contractions, first at a slow velocity, and then at a moderately fast velocity. For example, for knee extension-flexion testing, these velocities are most commonly 60°/second and 240°/second. This protocol originated with the Cybex II dynamometer. It has always been normal practice to test the slow velocity first; recent evidence has shown that this may indeed be the most reliable sequence (Wilhite et al 1992). Tests at slow and fast isokinetic velocities were once erroneously termed 'strength' and 'power' tests respectively. Joints with smaller ranges of motion require slower velocities. This is because, at faster velocities, a greater portion of the range is necessary for the limb to reach the (higher) isokinetic velocity at the start of the movement, and to slow the limb at the end of range. If the total range of motion is small, too great a proportion will be taken up in this way and little time will be spent at the isokinetic velocity. Athletes—particularly those in sprint or explosive-type sports—may be tested at faster velocities than non-athletes. Some patients may have trouble 'catching the machine' at faster velocities; this ability should return as rehabilitation progresses.

There are no standards for eccentric test protocols. A single, slow eccentric test velocity (e.g. 60°/s) is probably adequate, for the following reasons. Firstly, experience indicates that eccentric contractions, particularly fast contractions, are more difficult for patients to master. Secondly, the eccentric torque-velocity relationship is essentially flat across all velocities (Westing 1990), so there is little reason to believe that different eccentric test velocities test different properties of the muscle-joint complex. Finally, there is the increased risk of delayed onset muscle soreness if the number of sets of eccentric contractions is excessive.

The test is typically preceded by a warm-up, usually performed on an appropriate ergometer, combined with stretching of relevant muscle groups. The uninjured limb is tested first. Once the patient is on the dynamometer, it is important to provide a period of familiarization with the requirements of the test, as isokinetic resistance is a somewhat novel experience. This familiarization phase typically involves a gradual increase in effort on the part of the patient with each practice repetition, proceeding to at least one maximal or near-maximal effort after several submaximal efforts. Patients with little experience of maximal muscle contractions may take longer to grasp the intense level of contraction required for a valid test. Familiarization is repeated at each test velocity. Eccentric contractions are more difficult for patients to master than concentric contractions. This probably reflects the novelty and anxiety of attempting to resist an isokinetic machine that is moving of its own accord. Also, the greater torque involved in an eccentric contraction means that pain is more likely to be evoked. For these reasons, eccentric testing may require greater familiarization than concentric testing.

As mentioned above, the software that is supplied with isokinetic dynamometers currently restricts the flexibility of the protocols that can be utilized. In one case, the standard protocol requires that movements be performed in each direction one at a time. When a given movement (e.g. knee extension) is completed, the clinician inspects the torque graph and chooses to save or reject the data for that movement. Then the patient performs the reciprocal movement (e.g. knee flexion), and the inspection process is repeated. Physiologically, this discontinuous protocol will result in less fatigue than continuous protocols. The sequence continues until the clinician is satisfied with the number of repetitions collected. Other dynamometer software assumes that movements will be performed in a continuous reciprocal fashion, with no pauses. Computer software support for test protocol flexibility is clearly an area of isokinetic technology that needs improvement, so that protocols may be chosen on clinical or physiological grounds rather than be dictated by inflexible software.

The above discussion mainly concerns the protocols used for assessment of strength-related parameters, over a small number of repetitions. Isokinetic dynamometers are also sometimes used to assess muscle endurance. Such tests typically involve twenty to forty contractions at a relatively fast velocity. It is often difficult to ensure maximum effort throughout such a test; patients often pace themselves to some extent, thus confounding a valid assessment. This will be evident when inspecting the sequence of torque curves, which often do not show a consistent decline in peak torque; instead, short sections of increased or decreased effort may be apparent. Physiologically, this type of intense effort is a test of the ability of muscle to perform anaerobically for the duration of the test. The relevance of this type of maximal anaerobic endurance effort to athletes not involved in pure sprint or sprint endurance type activities that include efforts of this intensity and duration is questionable. However, in certain instances such tests may still have some clinical utility. For example, recent evidence has suggested an association between swimmers' shoulder problems and decreased external rotator endurance (Falkel & Murphy 1988, Beach et al 1992). Experience with this type of shoulder test suggests that it may also function as a pain provocation test, and thus be clinically useful in identifying the source of symptoms.

Reliability

A number of studies have shown that the isokinetic dynamometers themselves are capable of measuring applied torques with high reliability (e.g. Farrell & Richards 1986, Taylor et al 1991). Unfortunately, human reliability—of both patient and clinician—is somewhat less than that of the dynamometers (e.g. Byl et al 1991, Greenfield et al 1991).

While there are many studies of the reliability of isokinetic testing of normal subjects (see Nitschke 1992 for a review), there are few that have investigated reliability of patient groups. It is simplistic to assume that patients should be as reliable as uninjured individuals (Henke 1987). It is also unlikely that a single test protocol—such as have been examined in reliability studies—will be optimal for all types of pathology. Physiological differences between patients may dictate modifications to standard protocols. For example, deconditioned individuals, or athletes with high anaerobic glycolytic power who generate large amounts of lactic acid (e.g. sprint-type athletes), will require longer rest intervals for recovery between test bouts.

If reliability studies are to be clinically useful, their results must include a standard error of measurement (SEM) which is in the units of the actual measurement (e.g. Harding et al 1988). This allows the clinician to decide whether a change in isokinetic test score between two tests reflects a 'true' change or whether it is within the bounds of error (that is, human or dynamometer variability). For example, Delitto (1990) reported the results of retesting subjects for isokinetic trunk strength where the SEM for peak torque was found to be 27 Nm (20 ft lbs). This means that a given peak torque score recorded by a subject in this group was probably somewhere in the range between the subject's 'true' score and plus or minus 27 Nm (the SEM)—this is in fact the 68% 'confidence interval'. If a patient were retested on multiple occasions over a short period of time, the test results would be expected to fall within this range for about two-thirds (68%) of the test sessions (central limit theorem). A more conservative range for the 'true score' is given by the 95% confidence interval, which is equal to about twice the SEM. The implication of this example for clinical practice is that, if the clinician wished to be about 95% sure that the patient had really improved in strength over a period of time, then the patient's score would have to have improved by over 50 Nm (40 ft lbs). An improvement of less than this would not allow the clinician to rule out the possibility that the change had been due to other, sources of variation, including the normal variability of human performance. There is little information currently available on which to base the estimation of such confidence intervals for clinical patients; therefore, it is unclear whether the above example might be typical. In any case, if the significance of a patient's test result is uncertain, the test should be repeated at a subsequent visit.

Maximizing reliability

Given the inadequacies of the literature in relation to actual patient reliability, it is suggested that clinicians choose a standard protocol and vary it only with good reason. For example, a patient may need additional practice repetitions to grasp the test requirements, or additional rest to recover between bouts. General principles likely to maximize the chances of high test reliability are described below.

The clinician must ensure that the patient is adequately stabilized so that movement occurs only about the joint being tested. Accurate alignment of the joint rotational axis with the dynamometer's rotational axis should be checked,

although this often shifts unavoidably when resisted motion commences (especially for reciprocal test movements with the same contraction mode).

One of the advantages of using torque rather than force as the primary measurement criterion is that it is theoretically independent of dynamometer lever arm length. By simple physics, the torque generated against a long machine lever arm should be unchanged with a shorter lever arm, because the shorter lever length is associated with a greater force at the point of contact. Although such length independence may generally be assumed to be the case, in certain instances this may not hold (e.g. Otis & Gould 1986, Kramer et al 1989). Therefore, as a general rule, it is a good idea to standardize the length of the lever arm for both limbs tested and for all subsequent tests of the same patient, to minimize the potential for artefactual variation in torque measurement. Where force measurements are the only measures taken, these will certainly vary if lever length is not constant between limbs and tests.

To maximize patient reliability, it is particularly important that every effort is made to ensure that extraneous influences that might produce a less-than-maximal patient performance are minimized. Pre-test procedures should be consistent with the nature of the intense physical exertion required in the test. Thus, patients should be tested in a rested state and should not have eaten immediately prior to the test. A specific warm-up of the involved area (including stretching and light exercise) has already been mentioned, as has the importance of adequate familiarization of the patient with the test requirements. It is particularly important that the clinician exhort the patient to maximal effort with strong verbal encouragement. Clinicians find that some patients need more motivation than others. Observing the patient's facial expression usually gives an indication of the patient's intensity of effort; it also allows the clinician to ensure that the patient is breathing normally during the test, rather than holding their breath. Results should be inspected immediately following each phase of a test; repetitions should be repeated if the clinician doubts the validity of the results for any reason. Patients should be questioned regarding the occurrence of pain at any point in the range of motion during the test. This should be accurately noted, particularly for reports to referring physicians.

MEASUREMENTS

The ability of today's computerized muscle-dynamometry systems to generate quantitative data has far surpassed the average clinician's ability to interpret that data properly (Sapega 1991, p. 1562).

The primary parameters from which all other isokinetic measurement parameters are derived are torque, joint angle, angular velocity (at which the test is performed) and time.

In most dynamometers, torque is measured directly. In others, it is derived from the product of independent measurements of force (perpendicular to the lever arm) and distance (from the point of force application to the rotational axis of the dynamometer); the latter must be measured by the user.

The different types of measurements that can be made from an isokinetic test at a given velocity can be usefully divided into three categories:

1 'peak' measures, e.g. peak torque, angle-specific torque and peak power
2 'average' or 'whole curve' parameters, e.g. average torque, average power and work
3 'time-based' or 'rate' parameters, e.g. time to peak torque, rate of torque development, 'torque acceleration energy'(*sic*) and acceleration time.

Figure 17.3 and Table 17.1 show the most common isokinetic measurement parameters for a hypothetical torque vs angle curve generated at 60°/second, over a range of motion of 90°. Peak torque is the highest torque achieved in the movement. With the older non-computerized systems (i.e. Cybex II), this was the only parameter that was readily measured (from the chart recording). The following measurements are generally only made with a computer system for data acquisition and calculation. Some dynamometer software provides all these parameters, while in other systems only one parameter is readily available.

In addition to peak torque, 'angle-specific torque' may also be measured at a specified angle in the range of motion. The choice of angle may reflect the particular clinical significance of a given angle and/or an attempt to make all torque measurements at a relatively constant muscle length (e.g. Yates & Kamon 1983). Average torque is the mean level of torque for the whole torque curve. This is the simplest of the 'whole curve' measures (category 2 above). However, the majority of the dynamometer software systems, most of which calculate a large range of isokinetic measurement parameters, paradoxically omit average torque.

The derivation of work has been a major source of misunderstanding (Wrigley 1989). Work done in a rotational movement is analogous to its linear form, force multiplied by displacement: work in an isokinetic contraction is derived from average torque multiplied by the range of motion ('angular displacement', in radians rather than degrees). This is equivalent to the area under the torque vs angle curve, not the area under a torque vs time curve, as has often been stated. Because the calculation of work includes angular displacement, comparison of work values between limbs or tests should not be made unless the measured ranges of motion are numerically and anatomically equal.

Interestingly, no mechanical work is done in an isometric contraction, as there is no displacement. This may seem

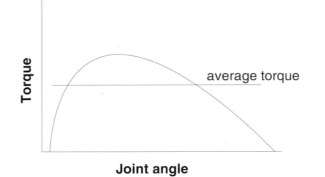

Angular velocity 60°/sec (1.05 radians/sec) **Angular displacement** 90° (1.57 radians)

Fig. 17.3 The most common isokinetic measurement parameters, for a hypothetical torque vs angle curve generated at 60°/sec, over a range of motion of 90°. Example calculations are shown in both imperial and metric/SI units

Table 17.1 Most common isokinetic measurement parameters*

Parameter	Value	
	Imperial	Metric/SI
Peak torque	180 ft lbs	244 Nm
Average torque	111 ft lbs	151 Nm
Work	= force × displacement	
	= torque × angular displacement (radians)	
	= area under torque vs angular displacement curve	
	111 × 1.57	151 × 1.57
	= 174 ft lbs	= 237 Nm
		= 237 joules
Average power ('rate at which work is done')	= work/time	
To determine time (i.e. duration of contraction), use the fact that:		
• angular velocity	= angular displacement/time	
therefore		
• time	= angular displacement/angular velocity	
	= 90/60	= 1.5 sec
Average power	174/1.50	237/1.5
	= 116 ft lbs/sec	= 158 Nm/sec
		= 158 Joules/sec
		= 158 watts

*for a hypothetical torque vs. angle curve generated at 60°/s, over a range of motion of 90 degrees. Example calculations are shown in both Imperial and the preferred Metric/SI units.

illogical, as clearly there is physiological effort expended in an isometric contraction. However, this highlights the fact that when we are measuring muscle performance, we are dealing with measures that have their basis in physics, not physiology. Furthermore, the relationship between physics and physiology is not always intuitive!

Average power is the rate at which work is done. Therefore it is derived by dividing work by the time (duration) of the contraction. Mathematically inclined readers will realize that this is equivalent to multiplying average torque by the velocity (in radians/second). Thus average power is essentially independent of range of motion, so it and average torque are the preferred whole curve measures of isokinetic performance (category 2 above), in preference to work. Since there is no mechanical work done in an isometric contraction, there is also no power developed in such a contraction.

Unfortunately, the use of 'average power' is complicated by the fact that some dynamometer software calculates it as the highest average power in a single torque curve, while other software calculates it as the average power over all curves. Usually, a clinician will wish to know the maximum average power from a single curve. However, in an endurance test, a clinician may actually prefer the average power from all curves.

As the quote from Sapega indicated, the plethora of data now available from computerized isokinetic dynamometers raises concerns regarding accurate interpretation. It is possible that some of the above-mentioned parameters are redundant. That is, the information that they convey may be contained in other parameters. A number of studies have examined this question (e.g. Kannus 1992, Kannus & Jarvinen 1989), generally by calculating the correlation between parameters that were hypothesized to contain similar information. However, if we consider the association between peak torque and work, for example, there is a proportion of patients who demonstrate torque curve shapes that differ from the 'norm', for whom peak torque and work will not follow the usual association. Because this group represents a minority, it is effectively lost in the generally high correlations between torque and work reported by the above-mentioned studies. However, such patients are likely to be of particular clinical significance. Therefore, it is probable that such studies have prematurely concluded that high correlations between parameters such as peak torque and work indicate redundancy of information, and therefore no need to measure more than one of the parameters.

Until the importance of these exceptions to the generally high correlations between some parameters can be determined, it is suggested that at least one measure be taken from each of the first two categories outlined at the start of this section, from which an assessment of the test is made. The 'time' or 'rate' measures in the third category tend to be the least reliable requiring an 'explosive' effort to be stressed. These measures are the least often used of the three measurement classes, and they are not described in further detail here.

For all measurement parameters, an important question is whether to take the maximum value or the average value from a set of torque curves at a particular test velocity. This has been a perennial question among statisticians and scientists in human performance measurement. It is best resolved by asking the purpose of the test. In essence, if the test is being performed to determine an individual's best current performance, then the maximum score is the most appropriate measure (Johnson & Meeter 1977); alternatively, if an indication of an individual's average performance is desired, then the average score is the most appropriate. Almost invariably, the former is the case.

Note that the measurements in Figure 17.3 are expressed in both imperial and the preferred metric/SI units. However, isokinetic test results are still most commonly expressed in imperial units as these remain common in the United States, where most dynamometers originate, most isokinetic tests are performed and most of the literature published.

Further information on isokinetic measurement parameters and related issues may be found in Knuttgen (1978), Laird and Rozier (1979), Sale (1991) and Sapega and Drillings (1983).

Problems with isokinetic measurement terminology

There are particular areas of isokinetic terminology where the laws of physics have regularly been transgressed. However, isokinetic users are not the only culprits; one dynamometer manufacturer currently has an isometric test mode in which values for work and power are displayed. That mistakes of this magnitude have occurred is nothing short of astounding (see definitions of work and power above). The confusion regarding the derivation of work was mentioned above. One of several other such areas of confusion is discussed below.

Incorrect use of 'strength' and 'power'

The Cybex company's early misdefinition of slow velocity tests as 'strength' tests and fast velocity tests as 'power' tests is not acceptable terminology. The erroneous association of power with fast movements reflects a false assumption that high velocity and high power are synonymous; this misperception is common among coaches and athletes. The concentric power-velocity relationship shows that high power and high velocity are not in fact synonymous; maximum power is reached at an intermediate velocity then declines as velocity continues to increase (e.g. Hall & Roofner 1991, Tihanyi et al 1982) (Fig.17.4).

Fortunately, this incorrect usage of 'strength' and 'power' has almost disappeared from the isokinetic literature. In addition to the erroneous association of power and high velocity, Cybex's terminology also ignored the fact that the parameter measured in both the so-called 'strength' and 'power' tests was peak torque. The main problem with this was in the use of the term 'power' when peak torque was actually measured. The association of 'strength' and peak torque in the slow velocity test is not so specious; there is no universally accepted definition for 'strength' and it must be operationally defined for the context in which it is being used. As such, strength might be justifiably defined

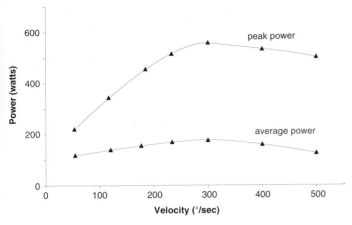

Fig. 17.4 Concentric power-velocity relationship

as peak torque at a slow velocity. 'Power', however, is a standard mechanical parameter and is strictly defined in physics as 'the rate at which work is done' (see above); thus, power cannot be peak torque. Note that the two derivations of average power that were outlined above (work/time and average torque x velocity) are mathematically equivalent. They are not arbitrarily chosen alternative ways of expressing a measure of 'power'. Some authors appear to erroneously believe that several nebulous mathematical concoctions can be termed 'power' (e.g. Moffroid & Kusiak 1975).

Gravitational torque

An article entitled 'Errors in the use of isokinetic dynamometers' (Winter et al 1981), drew attention to the fact that isokinetic torque measurements may require compensation if the clinician wishes to account for gravitational torque. Torque measurements for muscle contractions exerted in the direction of gravity (i.e. downwards) are artefactually inflated by the assistance of gravity acting on the mass of the limb segment (distal to the dynamometer axis) and dynamometer arm. Conversely, measurements from upwardly directed contractions omit some of the torque actually generated by the subject, as the torque necessary to move the limb and lever arm at the constant velocity against gravity is not registered.

The magnitude of this gravitational torque depends on the mass of the limb segment and the distance of its centre of mass from the dynamometer axis of rotation. On most dynamometers, the mass of the machine lever arm is also part of this gravitational torque. The significance of gravitational torque is dependent on its relative magnitude compared to the muscle-generated torque. As such, this phenomenon has a relatively small effect on the individual absolute values actually measured for most joint movements by healthy individuals (e.g. Richards 1981), with some exceptions (e.g. trunk flexion-extension). However, it has

a relatively large effect on reciprocal muscle group ratios for large limb segments that are tested in the vertical plane (e.g. knee extension-flexion). Failure to recognize this led, for example, to false conclusions being made regarding the changes in relative strength of the quadriceps and hamstrings as velocity increases.

Thus, there is a good theoretical basis to gravitational torque compensation, and it can probably be concluded that this procedure is usually desirable. However, there are practical considerations that must be borne in mind.

1 Not all dynamometers, particularly older systems, can easily measure and compensate for gravitational torque. Among those that have this capability, most do not provide the choice of displaying data for a given test with or without the gravitational compensation. This makes comparison of data recorded on systems with gravitational compensation with older uncompensated data, difficult.
2. Most of the published literature concerns testing that has been performed without gravitational torque compensation. However, most new studies being published generally include such compensation.
3. The validity of the methods used to determine the gravitational weight of a limb segment prior to isokinetic testing has not been subjected to scrutiny. Where a gravitational torque measurement is made at a single joint angle, an assumption is made that the only source of measured torque is gravitational torque (so that the compensation necessary at other angles can be calculated by simple trigonometry). That is, it is assumed that the patient has relaxed their muscles completely, and that there is no other passive torque from tissues spanning the tested joint within the range of motion.

DATA INTERPRETATION

Normative data

Before covering the various ways in which isokinetic data may be assessed, it is worth introducing the issue of 'normative' data. Isokinetic technology has a relatively long history, so it would perhaps be reasonable to expect that valid normative data should be available for all forms of isokinetic data. Unfortunately, this is not the case, as will be explained.

The discussion of 'normative' isokinetic data first requires consideration of how to define 'normal'. 'Normal' may have a purely statistical definition, for example 'within two standard deviations of the mean' for a given population sample. Alternatively, 'normal' may have a clinical definition that implies a relationship between a patient's isokinetic data and the probability of satisfactory performance of particular functional activities, with minimal risk of reinjury.

This definition suggests an inferential or predictive ability for isokinetic data, in relation to functional activities. The bulk of existing published isokinetic normative data studies have not attempted to address the possible inferential validity of isokinetic data—they have merely presented descriptive statistics of the data collected (i.e. mean, standard deviation. At best, such data may satisfy only the first notion of normality. However, it is apparent that some clinicians over-interpret their patients' test results in relation to such normative data, as if that data somehow also has implicit inferential validity with respect to predicting likely functional status and the potential for reinjury.

A number of common ways of expressing a patient's results are discussed below: absolute values, relative values (body weight ratios), reciprocal and bilateral muscle group ratios. Purportedly normative data have been published for each of these forms of expression, for most major joints and movements. However, even if only the statistical definition of normality is adhered to, there are other issues that raise serious questions regarding the utility of some of these expressions. As such issues have generally been ignored in the publication of normative data, much of this data is of questionable value. For this reason, no normative data is included here.

Absolute vs relative values

Isokinetic strength data can be considered in two ways: absolute strength and relative strength. The range of absolute strength levels in the population is obviously large. This large range is due to such factors as body size, age, sex, and activity/injury history. Variation due to all of these factors could be accounted for by collecting reference isokinetic data on discrete population samples that differ on these factors. However, the large number of subjects required for this purpose means that it is not a straightforward exercise, and it is not surprising that it has only rarely been attempted (e.g. Molnar & Alexander 1974).

Without such categorization of the population, we are left with the large population range of absolute isokinetic strength values, which are of little or no use as normative data against which to judge patients' results. The only exception to this is the assessment of athletes or workers who are required to apply force to external objects (see Delitto 1990), where absolute strength is the performance criterion of interest. However, in clinical settings, isokinetic test data is not commonly interpreted in relation to external force requirements. Rather, the clinician generally wishes to judge isokinetic test results in light of less clearly defined functional requirements for a given patient. It is logical to assume that these requirements are in some way related to the patient's body size and the type of athletic activity in which they are engaged, thus, data may be expressed in relation to a patient's body weight, for example. Un-

fortunately, judging the exact nature of this relationship is probably less clear than has generally been assumed. Note the use of the adjective 'exact': if the way in which clinicians wish to employ normative data is considered, namely judgements regarding rehabilitation success, readiness for return to competition etc., it is clear that a reasonably high degree of specificity and sensitivity is required of normative data. Note also that these sorts of inferences are currently unsupported by any research evidence. However, some clinicians do use normative isokinetic data in this way. Because of this, and so that future studies can more adequately explore the inferential potential of isokinetic data, it is important that the potential inadequacies of the current forms of such relative data expressions are understood.

A common school of thought contends that differences in torque-generating capability due to differences in body size can be accounted for simply by dividing isokinetic results by the patient's body weight (or, more correctly, body mass); this is therefore an expression of relative strength. The most common relative strength expression derived in this way is the peak-torque-to-body-mass ratio. Most isokinetic parameters can in fact be expressed in the form of such body mass ratios; the following discussion is relevant to all such expressions. This section will conclude that the use of such relative strength measures as normative data against which to judge patient performance is at best questionable. In order to reach this conclusion, the two rationales that underlie attempts to justify the use of peak-torque-to-body-mass ratios by their proponents will be reviewed.

The first rationale generally suggested or implied for the use of relative strength measures, such as the peak-torque-to-body-mass ratio, is that body mass is related to muscle mass, and therefore strength (peak torque). An expanded reasoning for the assumed relationship between torque production and body mass, along the lines of that suggested by Delitto et al (1989), would be that: (1) a certain proportion of total body mass is muscle mass; (2) muscle mass is related to muscle cross-sectional area; (3) cross-sectional area is directly related to muscle force production; and (4) force production is related to torque production. While these relationships are at least approximately true, some are possibly sufficiently tenuous to confound a direct linear relationship between body mass and torque production. For example, by 'dimensional analysis' (assuming 'geometric similarity' of human body shapes) an area and a mass, such as muscle cross-sectional area and muscle mass, are not directly proportional to each other (Astrand & Rodahl 1977). A complete analysis of these relationships is beyond the scope of this chapter, but it is suggested that this rationale be viewed with caution.

The second suggested rationale for the use of isokinetic values expressed relative to body mass is the contention that a level of strength proportional to body mass is necessary to adequately support and move that mass in normal daily and sporting activities (Davies 1987). Implicit in this argument is the expectation that differences in body mass between individuals should be associated with proportional differences in torque generation capability. Thus, this argument assumes that there is a linear relationship between torque and body mass. If this linear relationship does not exist, then individuals in certain body mass classes simply have less torque-generating capability to move their body mass than those in other body mass classes. If so, then expecting the same torque-to-body-mass ratios for all body mass classes is not realistic.

What does the research literature show regarding the relationship between body mass and torque ? Most studies that have published data for torque-to-body-mass ratios have ignored this issue, or have not even realized that it was an issue. Others have argued that without a demonstrated strong linear relationship between torque and body mass, the use of body mass ratios is not valid (Delitto 1990, Delitto et al 1989, Brown et al 1991). While a strong linear relationship has been found for some populations (e.g. young children—see Gilliam et al 1979), in many instances the association between torque and body mass has not been found to be close (e.g. Delitto et al 1989). The lack of a strong correlation between torque and body mass in a given population reflects the presence of additional sources of variance that explain differences in torque production, other than just body mass. The lower the correlation between torque and body mass in a population sample, the greater the range of torque-to-body-mass ratio values in that group. With such a wide range, it is unlikely that the simple torque-to-body-mass ratio will possess the sensitivity and specificity for detecting muscle-joint weakness. In light of these considerations, it is suggested that comparison of a patient's relative strength measures—derived from simple torque-to-body-mass ratios—to so-called normative values be made with extreme caution. In their current form, these relative measures are unlikely to allow clinicians to validly make the sort of clinical judgements that they would like to.

Reciprocal and bilateral ratio comparisons

Once the absolute values for the measurement parameters have been derived for each direction of movement and each limb, it is routine practice to derive certain ratio (percentage) comparisons between muscle groups and between limbs. In fact, the overall interpretation of a patient's test results is often based largely on these ratio comparisons (i.e. intra-individual comparisons).

Reciprocal (agonist/antagonist) muscle group ratios are derived by expressing the values for the expected weaker group (e.g. knee flexors) as a percentage of the expected stronger muscle group values (e.g. knee extensors).

Although there is little evidence that such ratios have any inferential predictive capability in relation to function or injury, some clinicians adhere to notions of 'expected' values for major muscle group ratios calculated in this way. For example, the concentric knee flexor/extensor peak torque ratio (hamstring/quadriceps) at 60°/second usually falls in the range of 60%-80% (e.g. Wyatt & Edwards 1981). In the standard seated test position, concentric knee extension is resisted by gravity (in addition to the isokinetic resistance) and knee flexion is assisted by gravity; compensation for this gravitational torque effect lowers the flexor/extensor ratio (Fillyaw et al 1986).

In a screening context, there is little evidence to suggest that reciprocal ratio values outside the presumed 'normal' range are any more likely to suffer injury—such as hamstring or anterior cruciate ligament injury—than those that fall within this range (Grace et al 1984, Grace 1985, Knapik et al 1991). This is partly due to the fact that very few studies have examined the issue of such an inferential capability for reciprocal isokinetic ratios. However, it can also be argued that many of the existing isokinetic test protocols, and/or the measures of agonist and antagonist muscle function used in such ratios, may not sufficiently reflect the way in which muscles and joints function in the activities where injuries occur. In this regard, Rothstein et al (1987) have questioned the widespread use of reciprocal contractions, where a maximal concentric contraction of an agonist muscle group is immediately followed by a maximal concentric contraction of the antagonist muscle group. This protocol has essentially been imposed by the way in which most of the dynamometers operate. Dvir and colleagues (Dvir et al 1989, Dvir 1991) have suggested a more 'function-specific' approach to the derivation of reciprocal ratios for the anterior cruciate ligament-deficient knee. These authors suggested that the ratio of eccentric hamstrings to concentric quadriceps average torque may reflect the ability of the hamstrings to eccentrically restrain anterior tibial displacement induced by concentric quadriceps contraction (as the hamstrings may potentially do during functional activities). This notion, and other possible more 'function-specific' ratios, await further study.

It is important to consider the possibility that athletic success may to some extent be the result of reciprocal muscle function that is different from the norm. Such a departure from expected values may be the result of specific adaptation to the functional demands of an athlete's sport, or the particular type of training employed, or may reflect the genetic endowment that has made the athlete successful. In this light, clinicians should be particularly wary of attempting to modify an athlete's agonist-antagonist muscle balance, simply because it does not fit the notion of a supposed 'norm'. In this regard, there is a growing tendency in some quarters to regard an apparent relative enhancement of shoulder internal rotator strength in relation to external rotator strength in upper limb athletes (e.g. throwers, swimmers, tennis players) as causative with respect to various shoulder pathologies. While 'low' external-to-internal rotation torque ratios are found with some pathologies (e.g. Warner et al 1990), they are also found among apparently asymptomatic athletes (e.g. Chandler et al 1992, Fowler & Webster 1985, McMaster et al 1991). Since no prospective studies have been done, it is too early to conclude whether low external-to-internal rotator torque ratios are the cause or the effect of pathological conditions, and may also exist without pathogenic consequences. Therefore, in the absence of symptoms, prophylactic attempts to alter a low external-to-internal ratio in an upper limb athlete would seem unjustified.

'Bilateral' (injured/uninjured limb) ratios are computed that express each measure from the injured limb as a percentage of its counterpart from the uninjured limb. There are a number of limitations on the use of such ratios. Attaching a high level of significance to this procedure is obviously inappropriate in the case of bilateral injury histories. The procedure is impossible in the case of trunk extension-flexion testing. Limb dominance is generally less of a confounding factor than might be assumed, at least for the lower limbs (Wyatt & Edwards 1981, Hageman et al 1988); strongly unilateral sporting activities are likely to be exceptions. The literature on the effect of dominance on upper limb isokinetic strength (mainly shoulder strength) is somewhat equivocal, even for healthy athletes in unilateral shoulder sports (Brown et al 1988, Calahan et al 1991, Chandler et al 1992, Cook et al 1987, Connelly-Maddux et al 1989, Wilk et al 1993, Alderink & Kuck 1986, Hinton 1988, Ivey et al 1985, Perrin et al 1987, Otis et al 1990, Reid et al 1987).

It is common to regard a 10% inter-limb difference as the threshold for clinical significance, but there is little evidence to support this assumption (Grace et al 1984, Grace 1985). Given some evidence that inter-limb differences of 10% may be relatively common in 'normals' (e.g. Daniel et al 1982), it is suggested that a more conservative inter-limb difference, such as 15%, should perhaps be adopted as the threshold for potential clinical significance. Such differences are usually most evident at slow velocities, but their significance is further confirmed if they are also present at faster velocities (although often not to quite the same extent).

Subjective assessment of torque curve shape

Considerable differences in torque curve shapes occur among patients. Therefore, in addition to the quantitative analysis of numerical test data, it is likely that further information is present in these shape variants. Experienced clinicians become used to the typical torque curve shapes expected of healthy muscle-joint complexes. For example,

normal concentric knee extension-flexion curves generated at a slow velocity (e.g. 60°/s) have a typical skewed appearance, with convex downslopes after peak torque is reached early in the curve. The significance of departures from such apparently normal curve shapes are currently unknown. Some patients with some pathologies exhibit specific curve shapes, which initially led to the suggestion of pathology-specific torque curves, particularly for the knee (e.g. Davies 1987). However, the general suggestion that these are common in many pathologies, are of consistent clinical utility, or have any diagnostic or prognostic significance, is not supported by any evidence (see e.g. Stratford et al 1987).

CLINICAL APPLICATION

PREPARTICIPATION SCREENING

Isokinetic testing of appropriate areas can provide information regarding neuromuscular dysfunction that can predispose the athlete to injury (Wallace 1978, Kibler 1990). This dysfunction, usually due to previous injury, may be identified as a deficit in peak torque values compared to the contralateral limb, or as a change in the pattern of development and maintenance of torque through the range of movement. Clinicians should be conservative in considering differences in peak torque between limbs as deficits if an athlete participates in a predominantly unilateral sport, because such differences may be an adaptation to activity (Ng & Kramer 1991, Wyatt & Edwards 1981). Further research is required to determine the magnitude of difference between limbs which may predispose to injury.

Post injury/surgery

Isokinetic testing may be included in assessment of muscle-joint performance to identify neuromuscular deficits following injury or surgery. If results of preparticipation isokinetic testing are not available, torque values and curves may be compared to the those obtained from tests of the uninjured limb. Contralateral differences may be an adaptation to unilateral sports rather than deficits due to injury. Often, performance of specific functional tasks, such as the distance an athlete can jump or throw, or a football player can kick a ball, compared to pre-injury levels may provide alternative indications of residual muscle-joint performance deficits.

Progress testing during rehabilitation

Results of progress isokinetic tests at regular intervals during rehabilitation provide objective feedback regarding improvement and recovery status of muscle-joint performance.

This information can be used as an objective basis for appropriate modification of rehabilitation programs.

PRECAUTIONS AND CONTRAINDICATIONS TO ISOKINETIC TESTING

Little information has been published regarding precautions and contraindications specific to isokinetic testing. Care should be taken when testing muscle-joint performance of a recently injured area and the test should be terminated if the patient experiences pain as continuation of the test may cause further injury. Pain and swelling of a joint can reflexly inhibit the muscles around the joint, resulting in decreased torque values not indicative of the force generating capacity of the uninhibited muscle (Spencer et al 1984, Arvidsson et al 1986). Care must be taken when testing patients whose condition may be exacerbated by the test position or test movements. Testing in a restricted range of joint motion may avoid excessive stress on healing soft tissues, for example, external rotation of the shoulder following anterior dislocation, and knee extension following medial collateral or anterior cruciate ligament injury/surgery. An ice pack should be applied following maximal isokinetic testing of a recently injured area to minimize possible inflammatory responses to maximal exercise. Contraindications to maximal isokinetic testing include conditions where maximal resistance to movement is contraindicated, such as unconsolidated fractures, bone tumours, acute joint or soft tissue inflammation, muscle spasm and joint effusion.

Cardiovascular responses to maximal isokinetic testing are similar to those observed during maximal exercise treadmill testing (Solomon 1992). Several authors have documented increases in systolic pressure during maximal isokinetic testing (Greer et al 1984, McMasters et al 1987, Solomon 1992). Isometric contractions cause a marked increase in systolic and, to a lesser extent, diastolic blood pressure (Greer et al 1984). Changes in blood pressure during maximal isokinetic exercise may be expected to be greatest at velocities less than 60°/second as maximal isokinetic contractions at slow velocities are likely to place similar stresses upon the cardiovascular system as isometric contractions, particularly when the upper limb is being exercised (Solomon 1992). Heart rate responses appear to depend on the number of repetitions (duration of the test) and resting heart rate of the patient (Solomon 1992). In light of these responses, Solomon (1992) recommends screening of each patient prior to maximal isokinetic testing. Perrin (1993) suggests examination of the area prior to testing and recommends medical screening of the obese and/or severely deconditioned patient, sedentary men over forty years of age and sedentary women over fifty years of age. Richter (1992) suggests that patients receiving anticoagulant therapy may be at risk of haemorrhagic complications during isokinetic exercise.

PRINCIPLES OF CLINICAL TESTING

Factors which can influence the accurate and reliable performance of maximal isokinetic tests have been discussed earlier in this chapter. It is important to apply this information to clinical isokinetic testing.

Familiarization and warm up

Familiarization with isokinetic exercise is required to obtain reliable and valid test results. Familiarization may involve a practice session prior to the test session (Helgeson & Gajdosik 1993) or warm-up repetitions prior to assessment (Perrin 1993). Warm-up repetitions should progress from submaximal to maximal at each test velocity, to ensure the patient is capable of performing a maximal contraction.

A general body warm-up of 5 minutes easy stationary cycling followed by a 5 minute rest interval should be included before isokinetic testing of the knee (Perrin 1993). A short warm-up activity for the upper limbs may precede testing of shoulder internal rotation (IR) and external rotation (ER).

Positioning and stabilisation

Extraneous body movements may contribute to torque generation and confuse results during isokinetic testing and exercise. Positioning and stabilization should isolate movement to the joint to be tested (Perrin 1993). Details of position and stabilization should be recorded for accurate reproduction of test conditions during subsequent test sessions and valid comparison of results between tests.

Stabilization, usually achieved by restraining extraneous movement of the trunk and limbs with straps, has been identified as a key factor affecting reproducibility of isokinetic testing of knee extension/flexion (Hart et al 1984, Mayhew & Rothstein 1985). Testing knee extensors and flexors with the athlete seated with stabilizing straps for the thigh, pelvis and chest usually provides adequate stabilization (Harding et al 1988, Stratford 1991). Although there is less extraneous body segment movement if the arms are folded in front of the body (Perrin 1993), the hands can be placed in the lap or can grasp the sides of the test table or pelvic strap without significantly affecting torque production (Kramer 1990).

Good reliability of isokinetic testing of the shoulder can be obtained with healthy subjects, careful attention to stabilization and strictly enforced protocols (Walmsley & Pentland 1993). During testing of the shoulder rotators, it is important to prevent trunk rotation and extraneous movements of the elbow and glenohumeral joints. Specific methods of stabilization may include an upper chest strap, a strap placed around the forearm and a strap across the front of the elbow (Perrin 1993). The elbow is usually flexed to 90°, with the forearm placed on a support or strapped to the lever arm to ensure adequate stabilization. A handpiece at the distal end of the lever arm is grasped during testing.

An inherent consideration in selecting an appropriate position for each isokinetic test is the length-tension relationship of the muscle groups involved, because length-tension relationships influence the shape of the strength curve (Garrett & Duncan 1988). To have the potential to produce a maximal torque during testing or exercise of biarthrodial muscle groups, the muscle group to be tested should be in a relatively lengthened position at some point of the contraction cycle.

Studies which have compared hamstring peak torque values obtained from the seated, supine and prone positions have reported higher peak torque values with lower motor unit activity in the sitting than in either supine or prone positions (Currier 1977, Figoni et al 1988, Lunnen et al 1981, Worrell et al 1989). Controversy remains regarding whether to test knee flexor isokinetic performance of athletes involved in running and sprinting activities from a position facilitating maximal torque production (sitting), or from a position simulating a functional position (prone or supine). Isokinetic testing of knee flexion in the seated position is preferred because it is difficult to stabilize the hip joint during maximal contractions in prone and supine (Worrell et al 1990, Perrin 1993). Worrell et al (1989) suggest it may be appropriate to test the hamstring muscle group in 10° of hip flexion to simulate the action of knee flexors in athletic activities such as running and sprinting. It is difficult to comprehend why this angle is suggested when, in a later paper, Worrell et al (1990) state that at ground contact during sprinting the hip is in 30-45° of flexion. Further research is required to investigate reproduction of a functional length-tension relationship for hamstring and quadriceps muscles during isokinetic testing and whether this relationship will affect test results.

Traditionally, the shoulder rotators are tested in supine with the shoulder joint in a starting position of either 90° flexion or 90° abduction (Hageman et al 1989). These joint positions have been associated with rapid fatigue of shoulder musculature resulting in pain on movement (Hagberg 1981) and with increased intramuscular pressure causing muscle ischaemia and pain (Jarvholm et al 1988). Rotator cuff injuries and shoulder subluxations may be caused by maximal exercise in these positions (Hageman et al 1989). Alternative positions include prone (Falkel et al 1987), sitting with the glenohumeral joint in a midposition of 45° flexion and abduction (Soderberg & Blaschak 1987), sitting with the glenohumeral joint in 45° abduction (Greenfield et al 1990), standing with the glenohumeral joint in neutral, and standing with the glenohumeral joint in 90 degrees abduction (Miniaci & Fowler 1993).

Isokinetic testing of the shoulder in different positions may yield significantly different peak torque and work values (Ng & Kramer 1991, Walmsley & Szybbo 1987).

Movement in the plane of the scapula will enhance activity of the shoulder abductors and rotators by improving the length-tension relationship of the muscles responsible for these movements (Perrin 1993). Greenfield et al (1990) reported greater strength values for the external rotators in the plane of the scapula compared to the frontal plane, but Hellwig and Perrin (1991) found no difference in torque values between these positions for IR or ER of the shoulder.

When formulating testing protocols for shoulder muscle-joint performance, the clinician should consider the muscular 'force couples' (Maddux et al 1989), the particular movements involved in each athlete's sporting activity (Kramer et al 1991) and the position of the arm during symptomatic activity. For example, isokinetic testing of shoulder IR and ER in a baseball pitcher is likely to be performed in 90° of abduction, whereas similar testing of a tennis player may involve less abduction if pain is experienced during the forehand or backhand strokes. Although selection of a test position for shoulder rotators may vary, position must remain constant whenever test results are to be compared within or between individuals.

Axis placement

Although the instantaneous centre of rotation of many joints changes during movement, the axis of rotation of the dynamometer must approximate as closely as possible the axis of rotation of the joint being tested (Perrin 1993). To minimize relative changes in axis position throughout range, alignment of the joint and machine axes should be observed and adjusted during passive movement of the joint prior to testing.

Axis alignment is difficult for movements such as lumbar spine extension/flexion and relatively straightforward for other joints such as the knee. During isokinetic tests of knee flexion and/or extension, the axis of the testing device is commonly aligned with either the lateral epicondyle of the knee (Durand et al 1991) or with a point at the centre of the lateral knee joint line (Bishop et al 1991). Clinicians should select either the joint line or the lateral epicondyle and use it consistently when conducting isokinetic tests of the knee. For shoulder IR and ER testing, the long axis of the upper arm is usually aligned with the rotational axis of the dynamometer (Perrin 1993). Consistent axis placement appears important in the performance of reliable isokinetic test protocols (Stokes et al 1990), but further research is required to establish the effects of altering axis position on isokinetic test results.

Other considerations

Consistent methods of instruction, verbal encouragement and performance feedback during isokinetic assessment will increase the reliability of test procedures. The importance of these factors has been explained earlier in this chapter and strategies to encourage maximal patient effort have been suggested. Other considerations include whether the test repetitions are reciprocal, continuous or single, whether the contraction is eccentric or concentric, the angular velocity of the test, the range of movement tested, duration of rest periods between test repetitions and sets and the preload settings employed (Nitschke 1992).

Types of contraction

The sequence when muscle contracts eccentrically then immediately contracts concentrically has been termed the stretch-shortening cycle (SSC) (Komi 1986). The SSC concentric contraction exhibits greater torque than a concentric contraction not preceded by an eccentric contraction. Maximal loading of the muscle-tendon complex during the SSC usually occurs at the end of range as the muscle exerts a momentary isometric contraction as it changes from an eccentric to a concentric mode of contraction, for example as the hamstring muscle group resists end range knee extension (eccentric), then flexes the knee (concentric). If an SSC occurs during functional activity of a muscle group, testing eccentric/concentric cycles may provide a better indication of functional deficits than conventional isokinetic testing (Helgeson & Gajdosik 1993).

Many studies have recommended the inclusion of eccentric testing following injury to the hamstring muscle group in athletes (Knapik et al 1983, Worrell et al 1991). Few studies have considered the need to test the SSC of the knee extensors in athletes, yet this muscle group utilizes an SSC during countermovement jumping, such as the basketball rebound. Helgeson and Gajdosik (1993) reported the effect of the SSC on knee extension torque at 60°/second in healthy subjects. Results showed a significant increase in concentric peak torque during five maximal contractions of eccentric/concentric knee extension compared to five repetitions of concentric knee extension without preload. Helgeson and Gajdosik (1993) suggest further study of the SSC is required at different angular velocities. Further research is required to establish reliable protocols to test the SSC of knee extensors and flexors.

Most available studies of shoulder IR/ER focus on concentric contractions, but eccentric contractions are extremely important in control of glenohumeral rotation during throwing and racquet sports, and may be incorporated into some shoulder IR/ER test protocols (Ng & Kramer 1991). Ellenbecker et al (1988) reported greater eccentric than concentric peak torques of shoulder rotators. Further research is required to quantify the relationship between functional SSC and isokinetic eccentric/concentric cycles, particularly for knee and shoulder musculature.

Test velocities

Generally, testing velocity will depend on the specific sport requirements of the individual (Perrin 1993). For example, a baseball pitcher may be tested at higher velocities than a swimmer, and a sprinter may be tested at higher velocities than a recreational jogger. Reliability of testing knee flexion/extension at velocities above 180°/second appears to be low in subjects who are unfamiliar with isokinetic exercise (Nitschke 1992, Wilhite et al 1992) and Perrin (1993) suggests initial testing at slow velocities (up to 180°/s) to familiarize the patient with isokinetic resistance. Tests of knee extension/flexion are usually performed at 60° and either 180° or 240°/second. If the athlete is unable to generate maximum force with minimal discomfort at 60°/second, a faster testing velocity may be utilized. Experience indicates that some conditions (e.g. patellofemoral dysfunction) may reveal greater deficits at low angular velocities and others (e.g. some hamstring conditions) may cause greater deficits at higher angular velocities.

Miniaci and Fowler (1993) recommend initial testing of shoulder IR and ER at 60°/second and 240°/second. Clinical experience suggests that 60°/second may be too slow for many patients to perform a maximal painfree movement. In many cases, testing shoulder IR and ER at 120°/second is less likely to cause pain and may therefore achieve more valid results. Testing shoulder IR/ER to fatigue at 240°/second may be useful in overuse conditions to correlate the onset of pain with a change in relative peak torque of the IR and ER.

Further research comparing angular velocities, concentric and eccentric contractions and different muscle groups is required to quantify the magnitude of measurement errors at different velocities and to determine optimal angular velocities for assessment of specific musculoskeletal conditions. The suggestion that testing at high velocities may provide more information about functional performance than testing at low velocities has been discussed earlier in this chapter.

Specific considerations

Anterior cruciate ligament injury/surgery

Usually, the distal aspect of the resistance pad is placed 2 cm proximal to the tibiotalar joint line when testing knee extension/flexion. Controversy exists regarding the placement of this pad for patients following ACL injury or surgery. Some authors (Nisell et al 1989, Wilk & Andrews 1993) suggest that a more proximal placement of the resistance pad on the leg for patients following ACL injury or surgery will decrease anterior tibial displacement during maximal knee extension efforts. Howell (1990) reported that anterior tibial displacement during maximum knee extension efforts was less than the displacement produced during ligament laxity testing, and questioned whether the anterior tibial displacement reported by earlier studies was detrimental to a recently reconstructed ACL. More recently, Maitland et al (1993) have reported that a single maximal isokinetic test of knee extension performed at least six months after surgery did not affect anterior tibial displacement.

It remains unclear whether isolated knee extension exercises with a distal tibial resistance pad have the potential to cause excessive anterior shear forces and deformation of the healing graft in the last 40° of extension. The tensile strength of the healing graft in vivo has not been adequately studied and quantification of excessive stress on the reconstructed ACL has not been determined. It is suggested that care be taken when performing isokinetic testing of the knee following ACL reconstruction. Clinicians may choose to use a more proximal pad placement or anti-shear device (Li et al 1993, Wilk & Andrews 1993), higher angular velocities (Li et al 1993, Nisell et al 1989, Wilk & Andrews 1993) or limited range of extension at 30° of flexion (Frndak & Berasi 1991, Halling et al 1993, Kaufman et al 1991, Nisell et al 1989, Wilk & Andrews 1993) during isokinetic testing following ACL injury/surgery. Each of these strategies will decrease anterior tibiofemoral shear forces by decreasing the knee joint extensor moment. Further research is required in this area to assist clinicians in formulating appropriate and safe isokinetic testing protocols following ACL reconstruction.

Shoulder impingement syndrome

Evaluation of muscle-joint performance is an important component of the prevention and management of shoulder pain and dysfunction (Jobe & Jobe 1983). Thein (1989) recommends the inclusion of isokinetic testing and exercise in the conservative management of shoulder impingement syndrome. In particular, valuable assessment information may be gained from testing of shoulder IR and ER in athletes presenting with signs and symptoms of rotator cuff impingement (Warner et al 1990).

In addition to measuring torque values of each movement, isokinetic test results can be used to calculate the ratio of shoulder IR to ER strength. Because significant differences in IR/ER ratios represent imbalances in the muscles that act as a force couple to maintain correct position of the humeral head in the glenoid cavity (Warner et al 1990), IR and ER results may provide a basis for including appropriate strengthening exercises in shoulder rehabilitation programs (Miniaci & Fowler 1993, Warner et al 1990).

Isokinetic testing of the trunk

Activity of the trunk muscles contributes to balance, stability and control of the upper body relative to the lower limb, so strength of the abdominal muscles and erector spinae can play a significant role in athletic performance. Isokinetic testing of trunk musculature was first performed in the late 1970s using custom-modified Cybex II dynamometers. Since the mid 1980s, trunk testing attachments designed for use with isokinetic dynamometers have been commercially available (Flory et al 1993). There is limited literature related to isokinetic testing of trunk movements and, probably because few dynamometers allow testing of trunk rotation or lateral flexion, most studies have reported results for trunk flexion and extension only.

Specific contraindications to isokinetic testing of the trunk musculature are neurological symptoms, acute or unstable fractures and acute intervertebral disc injury (Flory et al 1993). Pathology of posterior structures, including spondylolytic conditions and posterior element stress fractures occurring in joggers and dancers, may be aggravated by excessive or forceful extension. Athletes who participate in racquet sports are more likely to have intervertebral disc pathology which may be irritated by excessive or forceful flexion (Haher et al 1993). Testing should be terminated if the athlete experiences pain and range of movement may need to be restricted in some conditions, such as disc pathology and following posterior element stress injuries.

Several papers report high variability in peak torque measurements of trunk extension and flexion (Bygott et al 1993, Delitto et al 1991, Friedlander et al 1991, Stokes et al 1990) and variation is consistently greater for trunk extension than trunk flexion (Bygott et al 1993, Delitto et al 1991, Friedlander et al 1991, Grabiner et al 1990). Grabiner et al (1990) noted a concomitant increase in variability with increased angular velocity for trunk flexion and extension at 60°, 120° and 180°/second. The magnitude of variability reported in several papers means increases of up to 30% in peak torque values between tests must be achieved for results to indicate that improvement in performance was real and not a result of the measurement error associated with trunk testing (Bygott et al 1993, Friedlander et al 1991, Grabiner et al 1990). Further research is required to identify influences upon variability in isokinetic performance of trunk flexion and extension to enable clinicians to minimize the effects of these factors and to obtain clinically useful test results. Factors suggested as contributing to poor reproducibility include axis alignment, fatigue, stabilization and inability to isolate movement to the lumbar spine (Bygott et al 1993, Flory et al 1993, Grabiner et al 1990).

Positioning and stabilization of the patient during isokinetic testing of trunk flexion and extension must ensure maximum stabilization of the pelvic girdle, and minimize contributions from hip flexors and extensors which may augment the torque values of trunk flexion and extension respectively (Perrin 1993, Thortensson & Nilsson 1982). Langrana et al (1984) suggest sitting will best fulfil these requirements. Further research is required to establish the effect of position on the reliability of results obtained during testing of trunk flexion and extension.

The instantaneous centre of rotation of the vertebral column is not fixed during trunk flexion and extension (Grabiner et al 1990, Haher et al 1993, Perrin 1993), and identification of the trunk axis for dynamometer alignment is largely subjective as the actual vertebral axes for flexion and extension are nonpalpable and movement occurs at many joints (Grabiner et al 1990). Most reported studies use a reference point such as the anterior superior iliac spine (ASIS), the posterior superior iliac spine (PSIS), the greater trochanter of the femur, or a variety of levels associated with these points, and suggest the reference point approximates a vertebral level, for example a point 2.5 cm distal to the ASIS is nominally the L5/S1 intervertebral space (Calé-Benzoor 1992, Grabiner et al 1990, Stokes et al 1990). Changes in axis alignment may effectively alter relative moment arms and thus the contribution of muscle groups to the net flexion and extension torque. Thortensson and Nilsson (1982) reported consistently higher values for trunk flexion and extension torques when the dynamometer axis was aligned with the greater trochanter than the ASIS, but Grabiner et al (1990) reported more reliable measurements of trunk flexion and extension when the dynamometer axis of rotation was aligned with the ASIS. Stokes et al (1990) reported significant changes in torque values for trunk flexion and extension when the axis placement was varied in a horizontal (+/- 0.5 cm) or vertical (+/- 1.0 cm) direction about a point located 2.5 cm distal to the ASIS.

It is recommended that clinicians use consistent axis placement during testing of trunk flexion and extension (Stokes et al 1990), and that the anatomical reference point used be palpable and easily identified to increase the reproducibility of the axis alignment (Flory et al 1993).

Effects of angular velocity on trunk flexion and extension torque values are not clear. Testing at 30°/second may be too slow to predict any functional performance, and may cause pain as the athlete is required to generate excessive force (Flory et al 1993, Thortensson & Nilsson 1982). No significant difference between trunk peak torques recorded at velocities of 30°, 60° and 90°/second have been reported (Wessel et al 1989, Hoens et al 1990), but Grabiner et al (1990) found a concommitant decrease in torque as angular velocities rose from 60°/second to 120° and 180°/second.

It has been suggested that faster velocities can cause whiplash-type stresses on the cervical spine during isokinetic flexion/extension cycles (Hoens et al 1990), and that acceleration of the mass of the trunk against gravity is difficult at higher velocities (Perrin 1993). In light of these suggestions and the trend to increased variability of results at higher velocities, suitable angular velocities for isokinetic testing of trunk flexion and extension may be between 60 and 120°/second.

Further research is needed to investigate many aspects of isokinetic testing of trunk movements including the effects of axis alignment, stabilization, pelvis and chair position, motor learning and gravity correction method on reliability of results (Bygott et al 1993), as well as the functional significance and interpretation of results (Grabiner et al 1990), the effects of changes in angular velocity, and the role of eccentric contractions. Until this information is available, the clinical value of isokinetic testing of trunk flexion and extension remains limited.

Summary

Many factors influence the selection of specific test protocols, including the muscle group to be tested, the nature of the injury or pathology and the athlete's level and type of sports activity. While quantitative measurement of muscle strength may assist in the identification of specific deficits and enhance the implementation of appropriate exercise programs for athletes, test procedures must be sensitive, precise, reliable and predictive of functional performance to be of real value. Consistency in selection and application of isokinetic test protocols and further research is needed in many areas to provide clinicians with sound bases for design and implementation of isokinetic test protocols.

PRINCIPLES OF ISOKINETIC EXERCISE

Isokinetic exercise is often effective in improving the strength and endurance aspects of muscle-joint performance and is valuable in the rehabilitation program if the patient has sufficient range of motion and healing will not be compromised by resistance exercise. Many strengthening protocols begin with isometric maximal contractions against resistance for 5 seconds. As strength increases, healing progresses and treatment pain decreases, the patient is graduated to isotonic the isokinetic exercises (Miniaci & Fowler 1993). Early training of any type may be expected to produce gains in both strength and endurance and it is not uncommon in the clinical setting for patients to demonstrate significant improvement in the initial stages of an isokinetic rehabilitation program and a subsequent plateau in strength gain after several weeks (Jackson & Dickinson 1988). Each program must be directed to the individual's deficits, pathology and intended outcome (Garrett & Duncan 1988). They may be modified by varying angular velocity, range of movement, number of sets and repetitions, and body position as well as introduction of eccentric exercises and progression from submaximal to maximal effort (Perrin 1993).

Selection of training velocities

Although reports of velocity-specific effects of concentric training conflict, it appears that isokinetic training may improve performance across a limited range of velocities around the training velocity. Strength gains have been found at and below the training velocity (Moffroid & Whipple 1970), only at the training velocity (Moffroid & Whipple 1970), at angular velocities higher than the training velocity (Rutala & Kogon 1982, Timm 1987) and at angular velocities above and below the training velocity (Sherman et al 1981). Davies et al (1986) suggest that speed-specific adaptations may differ between muscle groups. Most studies have used healthy subjects and it may expected that the response of athletes with musculoskeletal disorders may differ from these due to pain, swelling and scar tissue, as well as the effects of immobilisation and disuse following trauma. In selecting a training velocity, factors such as increased joint loading at low angular velocities must be considered. Where a joint is irritable, particularly the patellofemoral joint, initial training should be at higher angular velocities to lessen possible aggravation of the condition (Perrin 1993).

In clinical practice, training usually commences with intermediate and slow angular velocities until the patient is familiar with the performance of an isokinetic contraction. Usually a minimum of three angular velocities are chosen for a training program, e.g. 90°, 120° and 180°/second for knee extension/flexion or 120°, 150° and 210°/second for shoulder IR/ER (Davies 1987). 'Spectrum' training (Davies 1987) is performed in an ascending, then descending, manner from slow to fast angular velocites and from fastest to slowest. Garrett and Duncan (1988) suggest ten reciprocal repetitions of at intervals of 60°/second, whereas other protocols are based upon ten repetitions at 30 degree/second increments (Davies 1987).

Concentric and eccentric exercise

Isokinetic exercise protocols usually commence with concentric contractions and, depending on the functional requirements of the athlete, may be progressed to include eccentric exercise. Individual isokinetic exercise protocols should address deficits identified during each isokinetic test and the physiological demands of the athlete's sport (Perrin 1993). As rehabilitation progresses and return to competition approaches, exercises must address the specific needs of each athlete. Inappropriate training effects may hinder return to maximum performance (Nelson et al 1990).

The principal specificity of exercise suggests that concentric training increases concentric strength and eccentric training increases eccentric strength, but the documented effects of concentric and eccentric exercise on strength gains are controversial (Perrin 1993). Consistent findings are that eccentric exercise is mechanically more efficient than concentric, that eccentric peak torque is greater than concentric peak torque, that eccentric peak torque does not change significantly with increasing velocity, that concentric peak torque decreases with increasing velocity, that at a constant velocity an eccentric contraction produces more force, and that at the same force value eccentric EMG is less than that of a concentric action.

Clinically, muscular pain and tenderness typically occurs twenty-four to seventy-two hours after initial unaccustomed eccentric exercise; this response usually disappears after several training sessions (Armstrong 1984, Cleak & Easton 1992). Although the mechanism of delayed onset muscle soreness (DOMS) is not well understood, suggested causes include muscle and connective tissue damage, muscle spasm and osmotic changes with resultant fluid retention and sensory nerve stimulation (Armstrong et al 1983, Bobbert et al 1986, Friden et al 1986). Clinicians should inform patients about DOMS following performance of initial eccentric exercise protocols. Maximum voluntary force production is reduced after exercise which causes soreness, so eccentric strength gains may be greater if training sessions are not on consecutive days (Clarkson & Tremblay 1988).

Further research is needed to quantify the effects of various factors—angular velocity of training, muscle fibre type, differences in functional activity of muscle groups, and changes in the length-tension relationship of the muscle—on strength acquisition during concentric and eccentric exercise protocols for healthy and injured athletic populations (Duncan et al 1989, Friden et al 1983, Ryan et al 1991). It is suggested that isokinetic exercise should focus upon the functions of the muscle group during the specific activities. If a muscle group functions predominantly in an eccentric contraction during sports activity (e.g. shoulder rotators in a throwing athlete), eccentric exercise should be emphasized, whereas muscles which mainly function concentrically (e.g. quadriceps in kicking sports), should be exercised concentrically. Eccentric contractions may be limited to the part of range in which the muscle acts eccentrically during function, for example the last 20-30° degrees of external rotation with the shoulder abducted to 90° for a pitching athlete (Perrin 1993).

Sets and repetitions

For adaptive changes to occur in dynamic muscular performance, the demands of the exercise must exceed the athlete's regular motor unit activation (Perrin 1993). Conditions which will affect performance include patient position (relative length-tension relationship of the muscle), selection of appropriate speeds for exercise in the early rehabilitation program, and use of reciprocal exercise and eccentric/concentric cycles to potentiate a more forceful concentric contraction (Perrin 1993). Either endurance training with fatigue overload during many repetitions of submaximal exercise (e.g. 3 sets of 15 repetitions of concentric knee extension/flexion at 180°/s), or strength training with high loads/resistance and less repetitions (e.g. 3 sets of 5 repetitions of concentric knee extension/flexion at 60°/s) (Jackson & Dickinson 1988).

Positioning and stabilization

Positioning and stabilisation for isokinetic exercise protocols are based on similar principles to those outlined for isokinetic testing and should aim to maximize isolated activity of the muscle groups to be exercised. Position of the athlete during isokinetic exercise is an important consideration in the first ten to fourteen days following muscle injury. Position of the limb and associated joints may alter the length-tension relationship of muscles around the moving joint and affect stresses on the healing tissue (Garrett 1990). If a muscle passes over two joints, the limb position should allow exercise in a painfree range of movement by ensuring sufficient extensibility is afforded by the position of the immobile joint, for example, biceps femoris passive tension may be decreased during knee extension/flexion by decreasing the angle of hip flexion (Garrett & Duncan 1988). It is recommended that clinicians warn patients of the adverse effects of pain during isokinetic exercise, particularly in the early healing phase following musculoskeletal trauma, and modify positions, angular velocities, range of movement and patient effort to maximize performance during painfree exercise.

Other considerations

Rehabilitation protocols must consider the mechanism(s) of injury and respect soft tissue healing in relation to the relative tensile strength of damaged muscle and the stresses placed upon injured tissues, particularly by eccentric exercise (Garrett & Duncan 1988). In cases such as grade I muscle strains, isokinetic exercise may commence in painfree range as early as forty-eight to seventy-two hours following injury. Isokinetic training may be a useful means of improving or maintaining muscle-joint performance in the early stages following ligament injury when functional activities are restricted by decreased weightbearing ability. Initiation of isokinetic training must be carefully gauged, and is usually based upon assessment findings such as pain on stretch or resisted contraction of the affected muscle, or joint pain during or at end-range of movement (Garrett 1990). To minimize the risk of aggravating the injury during early rehabilitation, exercise may need to be performed submaximally at intermediate angular velocities, in a limited range of movement (Perrin 1993).

Much of the research on the effect of isokinetic exercise protocols has been performed on healthy subjects and whether findings can be generalized to pathological states is largely unknown. While clinicians may attempt to apply the principles of musculoskeletal training, much more research is needed to investigate the effects of strength and endurance isokinetic exercise protocols following musculo-skeletal trauma. It should be remembered that exercises involving functional movement patterns and activities related to sport are important and must be included in specific rehabilitation protocols for each athlete (Perrin 1993).

CONCLUSIONS

Isokinetic technology and its use continue to evolve. Many areas of existing isokinetic practice require further investigation and validation. Taking the 'devil's advocate' position, Rothstein et al (1987) challenged many current practices and assumptions. The American Physical Therapy Association defined the requirements that must be met by both manufacturers and clinical users of all clinical tests, including isokinetic dynamometry (Task Force on Standards for Measurement in Physical Therapy 1991); many of the requirements specified are not currently met by either group. The following comments concern some of the major isokinetic issues that are likely to be addressed in the coming years.

Clinical reliability

As noted earlier, there are many studies of the reliability of isokinetic performance by normal, uninjured individuals. However, the literature lacks studies of the isokinetic reliability of patients with various pathologies. Therefore, although 'normals' appear to be relatively reliable isokinetic performers, it is unlikely that patients are equally consistent, given the additional factors that are present in a clinical context. It is hoped that clinicians will focus on this subject as an important area for future research studies.

Normative data

A relatively pessimistic perspective on the use of 'normative' data in clinical practice has been presented in this chapter. Unfortunately, there is a relative lack of critical thought on this issue in the literature and in the clinical community.

In relation to the statistical definition of 'normative', future studies that purport to provide such data must improve in a number of areas if this data is to be clinically useful and valid. Such studies must characterize as comprehensively as possible the population sample used; the sample must be particularly homogenous with respect to sex, age, activity level and injury history. Sample size should be as large as possible. Test reliability for the population sample should be assessed and reported. A statistic describing the distribution of the data must be quoted (e.g. standard deviation), ideally with a test of Gaussianality. If the latter is not satisfied, either the distribution should be transformed or distribution-free statistics (such as percentiles) should be used when reporting the data. If the data is also reported relative to body mass, the correlation with body mass should be reported.

Inference

The ability of isokinetic test data to tell us anything about a patient's ability to perform functional activities, or the likely risk of injury, has generally been assumed rather than demonstrated. It is suggested that future investigations of the inferential ability of isokinetic testing in relation to functional activities should be considered as a three-phase process. Firstly, the physiology and biomechanics—both normal and pathological—of the activities about which inferences are desired must be understood. Secondly, on the basis of this understanding, the muscle actions that are deemed most relevant should be tested isokinetically in the population in question. Thirdly, univariate or multivariate associations between the isokinetic data and performance criteria for the functional activity of interest should be examined. In the case of desired inferential capability regarding injury predisposition in a healthy test population, or post-injury prognosis in a clinical group, the test population must be followed for a reasonable period of time to record injury occurrence or natural injury history, respectively.

Eccentric testing and training

The relative importance of eccentric isokinetic testing and training is yet to be fully determined. Although some pathologies appear to have eccentric-related aetiologies, it does not necessarily follow that rehabilitation should emphasize eccentric exercise, although this may often be the case. Clinical studies must compare different re-habilitation programs for various pathologies to resolve this issue. In any case, the incorporation of eccentric exercise in rehabilitation must be subject to greater precautions than concentric exercise, because of the higher levels of joint torque generally involved and the possibility of delayed-onset muscle soreness.

It is important that clinical principles are not drawn too readily from single studies in relation to the role of eccentric exercise, and indeed all areas of isokinetic practice. In other areas of scientific research, a particular research finding must be replicated several times before a given principle can be assumed to hold widely. Contradictory findings of subsequent studies are common in science, and often highlight methodological inadequacies of earlier work. For example, Bennett and Stauber (1986) contended that an eccentric knee extensor deficit was pathognomic in their group of patients with anterior knee pain; however,

Trudelle-Jackson et al (1989) presented evidence that suggested that such deficits were relatively common among healthy subjects. It is thus likely that the conclusions of clinical relevance by Bennett and Stauber were premature. In fact, both studies may have been flawed. Therefore, the importance of such deficits remains uncertain.

Isokinetic software

The lack of consistent capabilities and quality among isokinetic software systems has been mentioned throughout this chapter. Currently there are no standards on the capabilities expected of such software; some suggestions have been made in this chapter. Users must realize that software is a critical aspect of the performance of an isokinetic dynamometer.

User education

Training in the use of isokinetic dynamometers has tended to focus only on procedural aspects of their operation. Appropriate use of isokinetic dynamometers involves much more than simply being able to set up a given dynamometer and operate the associated computer system or chart recorder. Unfortunately, users cannot simply be directed to the existing published literature for the source of improved education, as many dubious practices are perpetuated in much of the clinical literature.

Back testing

Isokinetic testing and exercise has until recently been largely concerned with peripheral joint testing. Now, all of the major manufacturers of isokinetic dynamometers also market equipment for isokinetic back dynamometry, either as stand-alone systems or attachments to their existing peripheral joint dynamometers. For several reasons, the use of these back testing devices is likely to be more contentious than peripheral joint testing.

Firstly, while much of a peripheral limb joint assessment is based on bilateral comparison with the uninjured limb, this is obviously not possible with back testing. This places increased importance on absolute data values, values expressed relative to body mass, and reciprocal muscle group ratios. As indicated in the Measurement section, these types of data are among the more contentious forms of data expression on which to base a test interpretation. A further complicating factor is the much greater contribution of the gravitational weight of the upper body segment (in extension-flexion testing) than is seen for limb segments in peripheral joint testing. Especially if a patient is overweight, the upper body is more likely to change mass significantly during a rehabilitation program than would be the case for a peripheral limb segment. If such a change is not accounted for in the test data by gravitational torque compensation, it will be impossible to separate improvements in muscle strength from changes in segment mass. Improved extensor function (concentric) may thus be exaggerated, while improved flexor function may be underestimated. Currently, not all back dynamometers allow compensation for gravitational torque. The most suitable procedure for determination of this gravitational torque is also problematical.

The final reason why back testing is likely to prove especially contentious is that the context in which such testing is contemplated is often a medico-legal one. Rightly or wrongly, clinicians and insurance or legal interests will turn to back dynamometry as a means of determining the legitimacy of an individual's back injury claim. There is currently no evidence to support such a practice.

Comparison of results between dynamometers

Despite the ostensibly similar basic operating principles of the different makes of dynamometer, the small number of studies that have examined the agreement between dynamometers when testing the same individuals have found some differences (although some studies have had methodological problems and others have not been reported in full). Such differences have sometimes been large enough to preclude the automatic interchangeability of test results from different dynamometers. The generality of results between dynamometers may vary among the different measurement parameters; for example, one study found generality for peak torque between two dynamometers, while others parameters were more variable (Thompson et al 1989). Whether some dynamometers produce data that is particularly specific to that dynamometer, while another group of dynamometers produce relatively homogeneous results, is not currently known; particular dynamometer comparisons have, however, found especially poor agreement between results (see e.g. Timm 1989). The explanations for these differences are undetermined, except of course where manufacturers have deliberately chosen to calculate a particular parameter in a fashion that is not consistent with other dynamometers (e.g. average power). Until the issue of generality versus specificity of isokinetic test results among all dynamometers is fully resolved, isokinetic dynamometry cannot be considered as a generic assessment modality.

NOTE

This chapter is an abridged version of a longer original document. The authors have omitted or condensed certain topics.

REFERENCES

Alderink G J, Kuck D J 1986 Isokinetic shoulder strength of high school and college-aged pitchers. Journal of Orthopaedic and Sports Physical Therapy 7:163-172

Alexander M J L 1990 The relationship between muscle strength and sprint kinematics in elite sprinters. Canadian Journal of Applied Sport Science 14:148-157

Anderson M A, Gieck J H, Perrin D, Weltman A, Rutt R, Denegar C 1991 The relationships among isometric, isotonic, and isokinetic concentric and eccentric quadriceps and hamstring force and three components of athletic performance. Journal of Orthopaedic and Sports Physical Therapy 14:114-120

Armstrong R B 1984 Mechanisms of exercise-induced delayed onset muscle soreness: a brief review. Medicine and Science in Sports and Exercise 16:529-538

Armstrong R B, Ogilivie R W, Schwane J A 1983 Eccentric exercise-induced injury to rat skeletal muscle. Journal of Applied Physiology 54:80-93

Arvidsson I, Eriksson E, Knutsson E, Arner S 1986 Reduction of pain inhibition on voluntary muscle activation by epidural analgesia. Orthopaedics 9:1415-1419

Astrand P-O, Rodahl K 1977 Body dimensions in muscular work. In: Textbook of work physiology. McGraw-Hill, New York, ch 11, pp. 369-388

Atha A 1981 Strengthening muscle. In: Miller D I (ed) Exercise and sport sciences reviews, vol 9. Franklin Institute, Philadelphia, pp. 1-73

Bartlett L R, Storey M D, Simons B D 1989 Measurement of upper extremity torque production and its relationship to throwing speed in the competitive athlete. American Journal of Sports Medicine 17:89-91

Beach M L, Whitney S L, Dickoff-Hoffman S A 1992 Relationship of shoulder flexibility, strength, and endurance to shoulder pain in competitive swimmers. Journal of Orthopaedic and Sports Physical Therapy 16:262-268

Bennett J G, Stauber W T 1986 Evaluation and treatment of anterior knee pain. Medicine and Science in Sports and Exercise 18:526-530

Bigland-Ritchie B, Bellemare F, Woods J J 1986 Excitation frequencies and sites of fatigue. In: Jones N L, McCartney N, McComas A J (eds) Human muscle power. Human Kinetics, Champaign, Illinois, pp. 197-213

Bishop K N, Durrant E, Allsen P E, Merrill G 1991 The effect of eccentric strength training at various speeds on concentric strength of quadriceps and hamstring muscles. Journal of Orthopaedic and Sports Physical Therapy 13:5-8

Bobbert M F, Hollander A P, Huijing P A 1986 Factors in delayed onset muscle soreness in man. Medicine and Science in Sports and Exercise 18:75-81

Bosco C, Mognoni P, Luhtanen P 1983 Relationship between isokinetic performance and ballistic movement. European Journal of Applied Physiology 51:357-364

Brown L P, Niehues S L, Harrah A, Yavorksy P, Hirshman H P 1988 Upper extremity range of motion and isokinetic strength of the internal and external shoulder rotators in major league baseball pitchers. American Journal of Sports Medicine 16:577-585

Brown M, Kohrt W M, Delitto A 1991 Peak torque to body weight ratios in older adults: a re-examination. Physiotherapy Canada 43:7-11

Burke R E 1981 Motor units: anatomy, physiology, and functional organization. In: Brooks V B (ed) Handbook of physiology. Section 1: The nervous system. Vol. II: Motor control, Part 1. American Physiological Society, Bethesda, Maryland, pp. 345-422

Bygott I-L, McMeeken J, Carroll S, Baker P 1993 Reliability of dynamometric trunk strength measurement. Presented at the

Australian Sports Medicine Federation Annual Scientific Conference in Sports Medicine, Melbourne

Byl N N, Wells L, Grady D, Friedlander A, Sadowsky S 1991 Consistency of repeated isokinetic testing: effect of different examiners, sites, and protocols. Isokinetics and Exercise Science 1:122-130

Cabri J, DeProft E, Dufour W, Clarys J P 1988 The relation between muscular strength and kick performance. In: Reilly T, Lees A, Davids K, Murphy W J (eds) Science and football. E & F N Spon, London, pp. 186-193

Calahan T D, Johnson M E, Chao E Y S 1991 Shoulder strength analysis using the Cybex II isokinetic dynamometer. Clinical Orthopaedics and Related Research 271:249-257

Calè-Benzoor M, Albert M, Grodin A, Woodruff L D 1992 Isokinetic trunk muscle performance characteristics of classical ballet dancers. Journal of Orthopaedic and Sports Physical Therapy 15:99-105

Carlson F D, Wilkie D R 1974 Muscle physiology. Prentice-Hall, Englewood Cliffs, New Jersey

Cavagna G A, Mazzanti M, Heglund N C, Citterio G 1985 Storage and release of mechanical energy by active muscle: a non-elastic mechanism? Journal of Experimental Biology 115:79-87

Cavanagh P R 1988 On 'muscle action' vs 'muscle contraction'. Journal of Biomechanics 21:69

Chandler T J, Kibler W B, Stracener E C, Ziegler A K, Pace B 1992 Shoulder strength, power, and endurance in college tennis players. American Journal of Sports Medicine 20:455-458

Chapman A E, Sanderson D J 1990 Muscular coordination in sporting skills. In: Winters J M, Woo S L-Y (eds) Multiple muscle systems: biomechanics and movement organization. Springer-Verlag, New York, pp. 608-620

Ciccone C D, Lyons C M 1987 Relationships of upper extremity strength and swimming stroke technique on competitive freestyle swimming performance. Journal of Human Movement Studies 13:143-150

Cisar C J, Johnson G O, Fry A C, Housh T J, Hughes R A, Ryan A J, Thorland W G 1987 Preseason body composition, build, and strength as predictors of high school wrestling success. Journal of Applied Sport Science Research 1:66-70

Clarkson P M, Tremblay 1988 Exercise-induced muscle damage, repair, and adapation in humans. Journal of Applied Physiology 65:1-6

Cleak M J, Easton R G 1992 Muscle soreness, swelling, stiffness and strength loss after intense eccentric exercise. British Journal of Sports Medicine 26:267-272

Close R I 1972 Dynamic properties of mammalian skeletal muscles. Physiological Reviews 52:129-197

Connolly-Maddux R E, Kibler W B, Uhi T 1989 Isokinetic peak torque and work values for the shoulder. Journal of Orthopaedic and sports Physical Therapy 10:264-269

Cook E E, Gray V L, Savinor-Nogue E, Medeiros J 1987 Shoulder antagonistic strength ratios: a comparison between college-level baseball pitchers. Journal of Orthopaedic and Sports Physical Therapy 8:451-461

Currier D 1977 Positioning for knee strengthening exercising. Physical Therapy 57:148-151

Curtin N A, Davies R E 1975 Very high tension with very little ATP breakdown by active skeletal muscle. Journal of Mechanochemistry and Cell Motility 3:147-154

Daniel D, Malcom L, Stone M L, Perth H, Morgan J, Riehl B 1982 Quantification of knee stability and function. Contemporary Orthopaedics 5:83-91

Davies G J 1987 A compendium of isokinetics in clinical usage, 3rd edn. S & S, Onalaska

Davies G J 1992 A descriptive study of isokinetic knee flexion extension testing from 300-600°/s. Presented at the 67th Annual Conference of the American Physical Therapy Association, Denver

Davies G J, Bendle S R, Wood K L, Rowinski M J, Price S, Halbach J 1986 The optimal number of repetitions to be used with isokinetic training to increase average power (abstract). Physical Therapy 66:794

Delitto A 1990 Trunk strength testing. In: Amundsen L R (ed) Muscle strength testing. Instrumented and non-instrumented systems. Churchill Livingstone, New York, pp. 151-162

Delitto A, Rose S J, Crandell C E, Staube M J 1991 Reliability of isokinetic measurements of trunk muscle performance. Spine 16:800-803

Delitto A, Crandell C E, Rose S J 1989 Peak torque-to-body weight ratios in the trunk: a critical analysis. Physical Therapy 69:138-143

Delitto A, Lehman R C 1989 Rehabilitation of the athlete with a knee injury. Clinics in Sports Medicine 8:805-840

Delitto R S, Rose S J, Delitto A, Welkener J, Kurfman K, Kaufman C 1988 Isokinetic measures as predictors for maximal lift capacity (abstract). Physical Therapy 68:801

Dudley G A, Harris R T, Duvoisin M R, Hather B M, Buchanan P 1990 Effect of voluntary vs. artificial activation on the relationship of muscle torque to speed. Journal of Applied Physiology 69:2215-2221

Duncan P W, Chandler J M, Cavanaugh D K, Johnson K R, Buehler A G 1989 Mode and speed specificity of eccentric and concentric exercise training. Journal of Orthopaedic and Sports Physical Therapy 11:70-75

Durand A, Malouin F, Richards C L, Bravo G 1991 Intertrial reliability of work measurements recorded during concentric isokinetic knee extension and flexion in subjects with and without meniscal tears. Physical Therapy 71:804-812

Dvir Z 1991 Clinical applicability of isokinetics: a review. Clinical Biomechanics 6:133-144

Dvir Z, Eger G, Halperin N, Shklar A 1989 Thigh muscle activity and anterior cruciate ligament insufficiency. Clinical Biomechanics 4:87-91

Ellenbecker T S, Davies G J, Rowinski M J 1988 Concentric versus eccentric isokinetic strengthening of the rotator cuff: objective data versus functional testing. American Journal of Sports Medicine 16:64-69

Falkel J E, Murphy T C, Murray T F 1987 Suggestion from the clinic: prone positioning for testing shoulder internal and external rotation on the Cybex II isokinetic dynamometer. Journal of Orthopaedic and Sports Physiotherapy 8:368-370

Falkel J E, Murphy T C 1988 Case principles: swimmer's shoulder. In: Shoulder injuries. Sports injury management, vol 1, no 2. Williams & Wilkins, Baltimore pp. 109-125

Farrell M, Richards J G 1986 Analysis of the reliability and validity of the Kinetic Communicator exercise device. Medicine and Science in Sports and Exercise 18:44-49

Figoni S, Christ C, Massey B 1988 Effect of speed, hip and knee angle, and gravity on hamstring to quadriceps torque ratios. Journal of Orthopaedic and Sports Physical Therapy 9:287-291

Fillyaw M, Bevins T, Fernandez L 1986 Importance of correcting isokinetic peak torque for the effects of gravity when calculating knee flexor to extensor muscle ratios. Physical Therapy 66:23-30

Fleck S J, Smith S L, Craib M W, Denahan T, Snow R E, Mitchell M L 1992 Upper extremity isokinetic torque and throwing velocity in team handball. Journal of Applied Sport Science Research 6:120-124

Flory P D, Rivenburgh D W, Stinson J T 1993 Isokinetic back testing in the athlete. Clinics in Sports Medicine 12:529-546

Fowler P J, Webster M S 1985 Rotation strength about the shoulder. Establishment of internal to external strength ratios. Presented at the American Orthopaedic Society for Sports Medicine Annual Meeting, Nashville, July. Cited in: Fowler P J 1988 Shoulder injuries in the mature athlete. In: Grana W A, Lombardo J A, Sharkey B J, Stone J A (eds) Advances in sports medicine and fitness, vol. 1. Year Book Medical, Chicago, pp. 225-238

Friden J, Sejer J, Sjostrom M, Ekblom B 1983 Adaptive responses in human skeletal muscle subjected to prolonged eccentric exercise. International Journal of Sports Medicine 4:177-183

Friden J, Sfakianos P N, Hargens A R 1986 Muscle soreness and intramuscular fluid pressure: comparison between eccentric and concentric load. Journal of Applied Physiology 61:2175-2179

Friedlander A L, Block J E, Byl N N, Stubb H A, Sadowsky H S, Genant H K 1991 Isokinetic limb and trunk muscle performance testing: short term reliability. Journal of Orthopaedic and Sports Physical Therapy 14:220-224

Frndak P A, Berasi C C 1991 Rehabilitation concerns following anterior cruciate ligament reconstruction. Sports Medicine 12:338-346

Galbreath R W, Goss F L, Robertson R J, Metz K F, Burdett R 1989 The relationship between selected isokinetic variables and sprint times (abstract). Medicine and Science in Sports and Exercise 21(2, suppl):S51

Garrett W E 1990 Muscle strain injury: clinical and basic aspects. Medicine and Science in Sports and Exercise 22:436-443

Garrett W E, Duncan P W 1988 Muscle rehabilitation. In: Muscle injury and rehabilitation. Sports injury management, vol. 1, no. 3. Williams & Wilkins, Baltimore pp. 43-71

Genuario S E, Dolgener F A 1980 The relationship of isokinetic torque at two speeds to the vertical jump. Research Quarterly for Exercise and Sport 51(4):593-598

Gettman L R, Pollock M L 1981 Circuit weight training: a critical review of its physiological benefits. Physician and Sports Medicine 9:44-60

Gilliam T B, Villanacci J F, Freedson P S, Sady S P 1979 Isokinetic torque in boys and girls ages 7 to 13: Effect of age, height, and weight. Research Quarterly 50:599-609

Grabiner M D, Jeziorowski J J, Divekar A D 1990 Isokinetic measurements of trunk extension and flexion performance collected with the Biodex Clinical Data Station. Journal of Orthopaedic and Sports Physical Therapy 11:590-598

Grace T G 1985 Muscle imbalance and extremity injury. A perplexing relationship. Sports Medicine 2:77-82

Grace T G, Sweetser E R, Nelson M A, Ydens L R, Skipper B J 1984 Isokinetic muscle imbalance and knee-joint injuries. A prospective blind study. Journal of Bone and Joint Surgery 66A:734-740

Greenfield B H, Donatelli R, Wooden M J, Wilkes J 1990 Isokinetic evaluation of shoulder rotational strength between the plane of the scapula and the frontal plane. American Journal of Sports Medicine 18:124-128

Greenfield B H, Catlin P A, George T W, Hastings B J, Mees K A 1991 Intra- and interrater reliability of reciprocal, isokinetic contractions of the quadriceps and hamstrings as measured by the MERAC. Isokinetics and Exercise Science 1:207-215

Greer M, Dimick S, Burns S 1984 Heart rate and blood pressure responses to several methods of strength training. Physical Therapy 64:179-183

Guskiewicz K, Lephart S, Burkholder R 1991 The relationship between sprint speed and hip flexion/extension strength in collegiate athletes. Isokinetics and Exercise Science 3:111-116

Hagberg M 1981 Electromyographic signs of shoulder muscular fatigue in two elevated arm positions. American Journal of Physical Medicine 60:111-121

Hageman P A, Gillaspie D M, Hill L D 1988 Effects of speed and limb dominance on eccentric and concentric isokinetic testing of the knee. Journal of Orthopaedic and Sports Physical Therapy 10:59-65

Hageman P A, Mason D K, Rydlund, K W, Humpal, S A 1989 Effects of position and speed on eccentric and concentric isokinetic testing of the shoulder rotators. Journal of Orthopaedic and Sports Physical Therapy 11:64-69

Haher T R, O'Brien M, Kauffman C, Liao K C 1993 Biomechanics of the spine in sports. Clinics in Sports Medicine 12:449-464

Hall P S, Roofner M A 1991 Velocity spectrum study of knee flexion and extension in normal adults: 60 to 500 deg/second. Isokinetics and Exercise Science 1:131-137

Halling A H, Howard M E, Cawley P W 1993 Rehabilitation of anterior cruciate ligament injuries. Clinics in Sports Medicine 12: 329-348

Harding B, Black T, Bruulsema A, Maxwell B, Stratford P 1988 Reliability of a reciprocal test protocol performed on the Kinetic Communicator: an isokinetic test of knee extensor and flexor strength. Journal of Orthopaedic and Sports Physical Therapy 10:218-223

Hart D L, Strobe T J, Till C W, Plummer R W 1984 Effect of trunk stabilisation on quadriceps femoris muscle torque. Physical Therapy 64:1375-1380

Helgeson K, Gajdosik R L 1993 The stretch shortening cycle of the quadriceps femoris muscle group measured by isokinetic dynamometry. Journal of Orthopaedic and Sports Physical Therapy 17:17-23

Hellwig E V, Perrin D H 1991 A comparison of two positions for assessing shoulder rotator peak torque: the traditional frontal plane versus the plane of the scapula. Isokinetics and Exercise Science 1:1-5

Henke P 1987 Muscle strength testing—physiology or psychology. In: Russo P, Balnave R (eds) Muscle and nerve. Factors affecting motor performance. Proceedings of 6th Biennial Conference. Cumberland College of Health Sciences, Sydney, pp. 34-44

Hinson M N, Smith W C, Funk S 1979 Isokinetics: a clarification. Research Quarterly 50:30-35

Hinton R Y 1988 Isokinetic evaluation of shoulder rotational strength in high school baseball pitchers. American Journal of Sports Medicine 16:274-279

Hoens A, Telfer M, Strauss G 1990 An isokinetic evaluation of trunk strength in elite female hockey players. Australian Journal of Physiotherapy 36:163-171

Houston M E, Norman R W, Froese E A 1988 Mechanical measures during maximal velocity knee extension exercise and their relation to fibre composition of the human vastus lateralis muscle. European Journal of Applied Physiology 58:1-7

Howell S M 1990 Anterior tibial translation during a maximum quadriceps contraction: is it clinically significant? American Journal of Sports Medicine 18:573-578

Huxley A 1980 Reflections on muscle. Liverpool University Press, Liverpool, p. 85

Ivey F M, Calhoun J H, Rusche K, Bierschenk J 1985 Isokinetic testing of shoulder strength: normal values. Archives of Physical Medicine and Rehabilitation 66:384-386

Jackson C G R, Dickinson A L 1988 Adaptations of skeletal muscle to strength or endurance training. Advances in Sports Medicine and Fitness 1:45-60

Jarvholm U, Palmerud G, Styf J, Herberts P, Kadefors R 1988 Intramuscular pressure in the supraspinatus muscle. Journal of Orthopaedic Research 6:230-238

Jobe F W, Jobe C M 1983 Painful athletic injuries of the shoulder. Clinical Orthopaedics and Related Research 173:117-124

Johnson R, Meeter D 1977 Estimation of maximum physical performance. Research Quarterly 48:74-84

Kannus P 1992 Normality, variability and predictability of work, power and torque acceleration energy with respect to peak torque in isokinetic muscle testing. International Journal of Sports Medicine 13:249-256

Kannus P, Jarvinen M 1989 Prediction of torque acceleration energy and power of thigh muscles from peak torque. Medicine and Science in Sports and Exercise 21:304-307

Katz B 1939 The relationship between force and speed in muscular contraction. Journal of Physiology 96:45-64

Kaufman K R, An K-N, Litchy W J, Morrey B F, Chao E Y S 1991 Dynamic joint forces during knee isokinetic exercise. American Journal of Sports Medicine 19:305-316

Kibler W B 1990 Clinical aspects of muscle injury. Medicine and Science in Sports and Exercise 22:450-452

Knapik J J, Mawdsley R H, Ramos M U 1983 Angular specificity and test mode specificity of isometric and isokinetic strength training. Journal of Orthopaedic and Sports Physical Therapy 5:58-65

Knapik J J, Bauman C L, Jones B H, Harris J M, Vaughan L 1991 Preseason strength and flexibility imbalances associated with athletic injuries in female collegiate athletes. American Journal of Sports Medicine 19:76-81

Knuttgen H G 1978 Force, work, power, and exercise. Medicine and Science in Sports 10:227-228

Komi P V, Buskirk E R 1972 Effects of eccentric and concentric muscle conditioning on tension and electrical activity of human muscle. Ergonomics 15:417-434

Kramer J F 1990 Effect of hand position on knee extension and knee flexion torques of intercollegiate rowers. Journal of Orthopaedic and Sports Physical Therapy 11:367-371

Kramer J F, Hill K, Jones I C, Sandrin M, Vyse M 1989 Effect of dynamometer application arm length on concentric and eccentric torques during isokinetic knee extension. Physiotherapy Canada 41:100-106

Kramer J F, Leger A, Morrow A 1991 Oarside and nonoarside knee extensor strength measures and their relationship to rowing ergometer performance. Journal of Orthopaedic and Sports Physical Therapy 14:213-219

18. Acupuncture

Peter Selvaratnam, Kay Knight

Needle acupuncture to specific acupoints can be beneficial in treatment and management of some sports injuries. Acupuncture may be used to alter pain threshold and/or pain perception (Gaw et al 1975, Katz et al 1974, Leung et al 1974, Matsumoto et al 1974, Strauss 1987), either in the acute or chronic stage of an injury. When indicated, acupuncture can be used either on its own or in combination with manual therapy or electrotherapy (see Chs 12 and 15).

The neurophysiological mechanisms of acupuncture have been evaluated and accepted by the National Health and Medical Research Council of Australia (1989) in the treatment of musculoskeletal conditions. However, therapists should be aware that acupuncture is also used in management of other disorders (Baldry 1989, Jayasuriya 1981).

Indications for treatment

Acupuncture may be indicated as the primary treatment if the athlete's injury is determined (on subjective and objective examination) to be 'irritable' (Maitland 1986) and cannot be treated with manual therapy or exercises. Since acupuncture promotes analgesia at regions remote from the site of stimulation, it can be applied without aggravating the injured region. For instance, if an athlete experiences acute neck and right shoulder pain, acupuncture could be administered to acupoints in the hand such as LI4, SI3 and SI6 (Fig. 18.1). This type of analgesia might be explained by the physiological phenomenon referred to as 'diffuse noxious inhibitory controls' where transmission of nociceptive information can be blocked by the application of a second new noxious stimulus at acupoints remote from the region of injury (Le Bars et al 1979). The second noxious stimulation may then activate brain stem centres and descending modulatory pathways (Le Bars et al 1983).

Therapists could also use acupuncture for soft tissue injuries when there is considerable muscle spasm associated with pain in the injured region. Acupuncture is considered

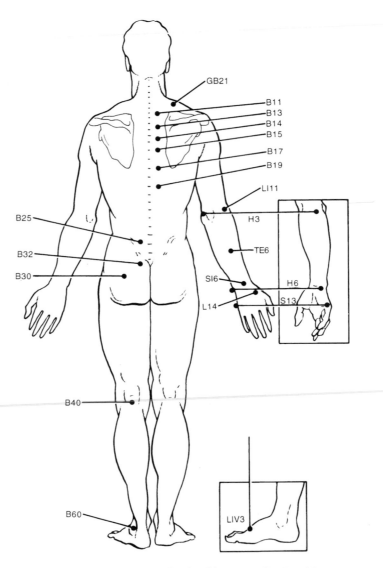

Fig. 18.1 Acupoints that were stimulated in case studies 1 and 2

to have a local segmental effect since it depolarizes large diameter afferents in lamina V of the dorsal horn and thereby inhibits nociceptive information (Le Bars et al 1979, Han and Terenius 1982, Bogduk 1989). This

289

segmental effect might account for local analgesia and reduction of muscle spasm in the affected region (Han & Terenius 1982).

Acupuncture could be indicated in the chronic stage of an injury, especially when other therapeutic modalities have been less effective. The effect of acupuncture in the chronic stage (as well as in the acute stage) could be due to its neurophysiological effects, mentioned previously. Other neurophysiological effects include release of opiate peptides such as beta-endorphins, enkephalins and dynorphins (Akil et al 1984, Fields & Basbaum 1984, Terenius 1985, He 1987). These neurotransmitters block the transmission of nociceptive information between primary afferent fibres and spinal cord neurons, and thereby prevent the central experience of pain from being activated (Besson & Chaouch 1987, Fields & Basbaum 1984, Le Bars 1983). Beta-endorphins may also activate the descending modulatory systems (Le Bars 1983). Opiate antagonists such as naloxone reduce the effectiveness of acupuncture analgesia, indicating that acupuncture increases endorphin levels (He & Dong 1983, He 1987).

Athletes suffering from headaches (Katz et al 1974), migraine (Loh et al 1984), neck pain (Katz et al 1974, Matsumoto et al 1974), back pain (Coan et al 1980), sciatica (Leung et al 1974), brachialgia (Leung et al 1974), frozen shoulder (Gaw et al 1975, Moore & Berk 1976) or lateral epicondylitis (Katz et al 1974) could benefit from acupuncture since clinical studies have demonstrated its efficacy in altering pain perception. Other clinicians (Baldry 1989, Jayasuriya 1981) have reported that acupuncture may be used for the return of function in conditions such as Bell's palsy, trigeminal neuralgia, neuropraxias (for example, the lateral popliteal nerve), disorders of the autonomic nervous system, temperomandibular joint dysfunction, acute cervical torticollis, de Quervain's tenosynovitis, plantar fascitis and metatarsalgia.

The indication for pain relief with acupuncture was supported by Pomeranz and Stux (1988) following an extensive review of the literature. They reported that 55%–85% of patients treated with acupuncture gained some pain relief, while the effects of placebo control benefited only 30%–35% of cases. These findings compare favourably with potent drugs such as morphine which afford pain relief in 70% of cases (Pomeranz & Stux 1988, Pomeranz 1989). Other clinicians have reported that acupuncture may be used to produce sedation (Brattberg 1986, Wei 1986), a tranquillizing effect (Jayasuriya 1981, Wei 1986) and modulation of the sympathetic and parasympathetic nervous system (Jayasuriya 1981).

Wei (1986) inferred from experimental work on nerve axons that sedation was due to stimulation of nerve membranes, while Jayasuriya (1981) reported that it was due to the influence on the mid-brain reticular formation. However, there have been no controlled clinical studies on these effects, only the report of clinicians.

Precautions

Athletes need to be assessed prior to acupuncture therapy. Therapists need to take great care with athletes who carry blood-borne infections, due to the risk of contagion.

Needling acupoints in the thoracic region must be performed carefully since there is a potential for the lung to be punctured, causing a pneumothorax. Similarly, great care is required while needling acupoints near vital organs and blood vessels.

Contraindications

Certain conditions do not respond to or are adversely affected by acupuncture (Jayasuriya 1981). See list of potential contraindications to acupuncture below. For such conditions it is advisable to avoid acupuncture and recommend the athlete to seek other medical treatment. Some of the rare side effects of acupuncture are listed below.

ASSESSMENT AND EVALUATION

Traditional Chinese practitioners assess a patient's condition by examining the patient's appearance, tongue and radial pulse, and by questioning the state of the patient's daily functions (e.g, sleep, thirst, bowel action and emotions). These findings are integrated into the principles of yin and yang, the five element theory, and are reassessed at each treatment (The Academy of Traditional Chinese Medicine 1980, 1987).

Some therapists assess the presence of 'trigger points' (Baldry 1989) in athletes. These points are small hypersensitive regions on the muscle origin, insertion, muscle belly, ligaments, skin or periosteum (Baldry 1989, Travell & Simons 1983). Melzack et al (1977) demonstrated that 71% of acupoints are trigger points, which are referred to as painful 'Ah Shih' points.

Therapists should also actively and passively move and assess the injured region, and if required, perform a neurological examination, in order to identify the nature of the injury and potential structures involved. For instance, if an athlete presents with arm pain, the neck, thoracic region and upper limbs should be examined as described elsewhere in this book. Trigger points in the affected region should be palpated following treatment to evaluate if they have been deactivated (Baldry 1989). Active and passive movements of injured regions must be reassessed.

TECHNIQUES

The needle is the primary instrument used in acupuncture and it can be inserted at acupoints in various ways (The Academy of Traditional Chinese Medicine 1987). The technique for a particular acupoint will depend on its anatomical location and the length of the needle. Needles may be inserted perpendicularly, obliquely or horizontally. Generally, a combination of acupoints for each sporting injury is selected from points that are local or adjacent to the injury and from appropriate distal points.

Potential contraindications to acupuncture

1. Conditions that clearly call for medical management e.g. a fractured neck of humerus, a dislocated joint, severed tendons, ruptured ligaments or bleeding wounds.
2. Cancer and other malignant disorders, since acupuncture has no curative effect. However, secondary effects such as pain and lack of sleep may be safely managed by acupuncture.
3. Nipples or the umbilicus, which should not have needles inserted.
4. Athletes with fulminating infections. Antibiotics are preferable in such conditions, although acupuncture is sometimes combined with drug therapy to relieve symptoms.
5. Athletes with haemorrhagic diseases.
6. Athletes receiving drug treatment
   a anticoagulants.
   b drug treatment for hypertension. A patient may experience a sudden fall in blood pressure when needled at Liver 3 (Fig 18.1). In such patients this point should be avoided.
   c anti-diabetic medication. Athletes may become hypoglycaemic following acupuncture.
7. Athletes who are intoxicated or emotional may have an adverse sedatory effect following acupuncture.
8. Retention of needles in children.
9. The first trimester of pregnancy and the last trimester in female athletes since needling may cause abortion or premature delivery. The second trimester is considered to be relatively stable for acupuncture. However, the authors avoid administering acupuncture during pregnancy due to the possibility of potential complications.

Source: Jayasuriya (1981)

Side-effect of acupuncture

1. Vasovagal attacks
2. Convulsions
3. Damage to viscera
4. Haemorrhage
5. Post-treatment drowsiness

Source: Baldry (1989)

The athlete should be treated while lying down although the sitting position could be adopted. In rare instances, a vasovagal response has been observed in athletes treated in the sitting position. Therefore, athletes treated while sitting should be constantly observed.

Needle or electroacupuncture

Needles are inserted into acupoints and left in situ or stimulated in certain acute and chronic conditions. Stimulation is conducted manually by using a 'lifting', 'thrusting' or 'rotatory technique' (Baldry 1989).

Electrical stimulation can be applied by connecting two different needles to alligator callipers attached to a stimulator with a variable frequency. More than one circuit can be used along pertinent meridians. However, acupoints that are stimulated on the same output should always be ipsilateral since crossing the midline could lead to cardiac arrhythmias, especially when stimulation is performed across acupoints in the chest and upper abdomen (Jayasuriya 1981). Chan (1982) also recommended that electrodes from the same output should never be placed across the spine above the third lumbar vertebra. Although the rationale for such precaution was not discussed, therapists should take heed and avoid stimulation across the spine.

Athletes with chronic pain would benefit from low frequency electroacupuncture stimulation (0–4 Hz) (Strauss 1987). The intensity of the current should produce a strong but comfortable tingling sensation. In acute or irritable conditions frequencies above 200 Hz are recommended. The intensity of the current in such conditions should produce a mild comfortable tingling sensation. Strauss (1987) reported that below 4 Hz the periaqueductal grey zone in the mid-brain is stimulated to release enkephalins. Above 200 Hz, the inhibitory mechanisms of the mid-brain are stimulated directly, thereby bypassing the endorphin system but also inhibiting pain perception.

Trigger point acupuncture

Some Western physicians apply needles to deactivate 'trigger points' (Baldry 1989, Travell & Simon 1983). The needle is left in situ for 1–3 minutes, and then rotated between the thumb and middle finger until the sensation of 'te-chi' is developed (Bauldry 1989). Once te-chi is produced the needle is withdrawn; if not, the needle is left in place till the sensation is produced but for no longer then 10 minutes. Baldry (1989) deactivates all trigger points related to an injured region while Travell and Simons (1983) deactivate specific trigger points, then stretch the affected muscle. For instance, the trapezius muscle is stretched following deactivation of GB21 (see Fig. 18.1). However, in the authors' experience trigger point therapy may exacerbate the athlete's pain and therefore must be carefully administered.

Dosage guidelines

Generally, athletes with acute injuries need frequent treatment. They may require treatment daily or on alternate days (The Academy of Traditional Chinese Medicine 1980). Needles are left in situ for approximately 15–20 minutes. Athletes with chronic pain require longer retention of needles for 30–45 minutes, and may require treatment less often, ie. once or twice per week. These are general guidelines for needle acupuncture and electropuncture but may not be always practicable.

A course of treatment generally consists of 6–10 sessions. Chronic conditions may require more than 10 sessions. After the first course of acupuncture, the athlete should be reassessed after two weeks to ascertain if further treatment is required (Chan 1982).

TREATMENT MODIFICATIONS

The athlete's response to acupuncture should be evaluated prior to combining it with other therapeutic modalities. For instance, the effect of acupuncture should be first ascertained in athletes whose injuries are too 'irritable' for treatment with manual therapy. Manual therapy could be considered once the irritability of the athlete's condition is significantly reduced with acupuncture.

Acupuncture therapy may need to be modified if the athlete's pain is significantly increased during or after treatment. In such instances, needles could be inserted on the non-affected limb or at sites distal to the affected region. The duration of treatment may need to be reduced if athletes feel drowsy after therapy.

Athletes who are sensitive to needle acupuncture may benefit from acupressure, laser or transcutaneous electrical stimulation (TENS). Acupressure may be applied briskly at acupoints in a rotatory direction for up to 1 minute (Blate 1976). Similarly, low power laser may be applied to acupoints or trigger points. Laser is thought to have a therapeutic effect at cell level (Kert & Rose 1989). It has been demonstrated in rats subjected to a crush injury of the sciatic nerve that low power laser irradiation increases the number of astrocytes and oligodendrocytes in the spinal cord (Rochkind et al 1990). This investigation suggests that laser therapy produces higher metabolism and the ability to produce myelin (Rochkind et al 1990). However, laser technology to date is unable to reach the penetration depth required in some acupoints, and it may not have the neurophysiological effects that acupuncture offers.

TENS may also be used on acupoints. It has been the authors' experience that TENS combined with acupuncture has greater therapeutic effects in some athletes with lateral epicondylitis and low back pain than TENS or acupuncture used on its own.

CASE STUDY 1

A 23-year-old Australian Rules footballer was referred by his team therapist with a 1 week history of pain in the left hamstring muscle belly. The injury occurred while bending to pick up the ball. The athlete previously had massage, laser and passive stretches to the low back and hamstring muscle. This treatment reduced the pain intensity by 50% but the athlete was experiencing pain while jogging and sprinting.

Examination showed myofascial trigger points in the hamstring muscle belly, the left buttock and the lower lumbar region. Straight leg raise (SLR) was 80° bilaterally; the pain in the hamstring was reproduced on addition of 10° of left ankle dorsiflexion (DF). There was restriction in movement at the left L1–L2 and L4–L5 zygapophyseal joints. X-rays and CT-scans of the lumbar spine were unremarkable. Magnetic resonance imaging demonstrated hypertrophy of the left hamstring muscle.

Clinical decision making

The athlete had a hamstring component with a possible involvement of the lumbar region and the left sciatic nerve. It was decided to treat the athlete with acupuncture due to the presence of myofascial trigger points.

Management

Day 1
Acupuncture needles were inserted at left B25, B30, B32, B40, B60 (Fig. 18.1) and two myofascial trigger points in the left hamstring muscle belly. Electroacupuncture (200 Hz) was administered to myofascial trigger points in the hamstring for 30 minutes. Following stimulation, left ankle DF improved to 20° in the SLR position (80°). On palpatory examination the tenderness in the trigger points was unchanged as were the lumbar signs.

Day 2 (5 days later)
The athlete reported that he was able to jog for 30 minutes. Acupuncture was administered as per Day 1; left ankle DF at 20° was pain free on overpressure. The tenderness at trigger points had reduced. Lumbar spine signs were unchanged.

General grade 4 lumbar rotation (in right side-lying) with left SLR was performed for 60 seconds and repeated twice. Postero-anterior movement at L4–L5 improved following treatment.

Day 3 (5 days later)
The athlete reported that he was able to run and sprint. Since he had decided to play in another two days he was advised on a warm-up and cool-down program for the spinal and lower limb musculature. The treatment of Day 2 was repeated.

Day 4 (2 weeks later)
The athlete reported that he had participated in two football games and had minimal discomfort while sprinting. He was advised on stabilizing exercises to the gluteus medius muscle and had one further session of acupuncture. He was recommended to continue

manual therapy by his team therapist until he could play without experiencing pain.

CASE STUDY 2

A 38-year-old tennis player had developed pain in the right lateral epicondyle while playing tennis two years previously. He was pain free following injection to the tendon of the right common extensor origin. He returned to play after a month but had an exacerbation of the injury 14 months later. A second cortisone injection was uneventful. He stopped playing tennis due to the pain intensity.

On examination he was tender in the region of the right lateral epicondyle and had myofascial trigger points in the right forearm extensor muscle belly, the right trapezius and infraspinatus. Shoulder, elbow and wrist active and passive movements were full and pain free. The right grip strength was tested manually and was 50% compared to the left. Anterior palpation in the region of the right C6 transverse process reproduced the elbow pain, as did manoeuvres of the upper limb tension test (ULTT).

Clinical decision making

The condition appeared to involve components from the common extensor tendon origin and from the cervical region.

Management

Day 1

The athlete requested an exercise program and was given an active flexibility and strengthening program to the forearm flexors and extensors, the biceps and triceps, trapezeii and levator scapulae.

Day 2 (1 week later)

The athlete reported that the condition was unchanged with the exercise program. Objective signs were also unchanged. It was decided to administer acupuncture due to the presence of myofascial trigger points.

Acupuncture needles were inserted on the right arm at LI4, TE6, LI11, H3, H6, GB21 (Fig. 18.1) and to two myofascial trigger points in the right forearm extensor muscle belly. Electro-acupuncture (200 Hz) was applied to these two trigger points for 30 minutes. Following acupuncture the grip test produced minimal elbow pain. The ULTT and the referred pain on palpation of the C6 transverse process were unaltered.

Day 3 (1 week later)

The athlete reported that he had no pain with functional activities but experienced tenderness on palpation of the right lateral epicondyle. The grip test was pain free but the ULTT and cervical palpatory sign were unaltered.

The treatment of Day 2 was repeated. There was no change in the objective signs.

Day 4 (2 weeks later)

The athlete reported that he had noted no significant change since the previous treatment. The ULTT and cervical palpatory signs were unchanged.

Treatment was changed to include points in the thoracic region B11, B13, B14, B15, B17, B19 (Fig. 18.1) and the trigger point in the infraspinatus muscle in addition to the treatment given on Day 2. Following acupuncture for 30 minutes the ULTT was pain free. The palpatory cervical sign was unaltered.

Day 5 (2 weeks later)

The athlete reported that he was pain free and had played a game of tennis the previous week. The ULTT was pain free but the palpatory cervical sign was unaltered. The acupuncture treatment of Day 4 was repeated. Since the cervical palpatory sign was unaltered following treatment, antero-posterio mobilization (grade II-) was performed at the right C6/C7 level. Following treatment, firm palpation of the right C6 transverse process did not reproduce the right elbow pain. The athlete was also advised on technique modifications while playing tennis and recommended to perform active flexibility movements as a warm-up and cool-down program.

This case study illustrates the use of acupuncture when exercises failed to alter the athlete's condition, and the role of manual therapy in clearing cervical signs.

SUMMARY

In summary, needle acupuncture is useful in treating sports injuries which cause pain and dysfunction. Acupuncture may be indicated at any stage of the injury although in the opinion of the authors it should be used in the acute stage of an injury and, if indicated, combined with other therapeutic modalities.

REFERENCES

Akil H, Watson S J, Young E 1984 Endogenous opioids: biology and function. Annual Review of Neuroscience 7:223-255

Allen M 1983 Activity generated endorphins; a review of their role in sports science. Canadian Journal of Applied Sports Science 8(3):115-133

Baldry P E 1989 Acupuncture, trigger points and musculoskeletal pain. Churchill Livingstone, Edinburgh

Besson J M, Chaouch A 1987 Peripheral and spinal mechanisms of nociception. Physiological Reviews 67(1):67-186

Blate M 1976 The natural healer's acupressure handbook. Kegan Paul, Routledge

Bogduk N 1989 Understanding pain pathways. Current Therapeutics 30(1):25-40

Brattberg G 1986 Acupuncture treatment: a traffic hazard? American Journal of Acupuncture 14(3): 265-267

Chan P 1982 Electroacupuncture its clinical applications in therapy. J F Chow (ed) Chan's Corporation. Monterey Park, California

Coan R M, Wong G, Ku S L 1980 The acupuncture treatment of low back pain: a randomized controlled study. American Journal of Chinese Medicine 8:181-192

Fields H L, Basbaum A I 1984 Endogenous pain control mechanisms. In: Wall P D, Melzack R (eds) Textbook of pain. Churchill Livingstone, Edinburgh, 142-152

Gaw A C, Chang L W, Shaw L C 1975 Efficacy of acupuncture on osteoarthritic pain. New England Journal of Medicine 293:375-378

Han J S, Terenius L 1982 Neurochemical basis of acupuncture analgesia. Annual Review of Pharmacology and Toxicology 22:193-220

He L 1987 Involvement of endogenous opioid peptides in acupuncture analgesia. Pain 31(1):99-121

He L F, Dong W Q 1983 Activity of opioid peptidergic system in acupuncture analgesia. Acupuncture Electrotherapy Research 8(3-4):257-266

Jayasuriya A 1981 Clinical acupuncture. The Acupuncture Foundation of Sri Lanka, Colombo

Katz R L, Kao CY, Spiegel H, Katz G J 1974 Pain, acupuncture, hypnosis. Advances in Neurology 4:819-825

Kert J, Rose L 1989 Clinical laser therapy—low level laser therapy. Scandinavian Medical Laser Technology, Copenhagen

Le Bars D, Dickenson A H, Besson J M 1979 Diffuse noxious inhibitory controls (DNIC) II. Lack of effect on non-convergent neurones, supraspinal involvement and theoretical implications. Pain 6(3):305-327

Le Bars D, Dickenson A H, Besson J M 1983 Opiate analgesia and descending control systems. In: Bonica J J, Lindblom V, Iggo A (eds) Advances in pain research and therapy. Raven Press, New York, vol 5, 341-372

Leung S J, Fan C-F, Sechzer P H 1974 Acupuncture therapeutics. Anesthesia and Analgesia 53:942-950

Loh L, Nathan P W, Schott G D, Zilkha K J 1984 Acupuncture versus medical treatment for migraine & muscle tension headaches. Journal of Neurology Neurosurgery & Psychiatry 47:333-337

Maitland G D M 1986 Vertebral manipulation, 5th edn. Butterworths, London

Matsumoto T, Levy B, Ambruso V 1974 Clinical evaluation of acupuncture. American Surgeon 40:400-405

Melzack R, Stillwell D M, Fox E J 1977 Trigger points and acupuncture points for pain: correlations and implications. Pain 3:3-23

Moore M E, Berk S N 1976 Acupuncture for chronic shoulder pain: an experimental study with attention to the role of placebo and hypnotic suggestibility. Annals of Internal Medicine 84:381-384

National Health and Medical Research Council 1989 Acupuncture. Australian Government Printing Service, Canberra

Pomeranz B 1989 Acupuncture research related to pain, drug addition and nerve regeneration. In: B Pomeranz (ed) Scientific bases of acupuncture. Springer-Verlag, Berlin, 35-53

Pomeranz B, Stux G 1988 Basics of acupuncture. Springer-Verlag, Berlin

Rockhind S, Vogler I, Barr-Nea L 1990 Spinal cord response to laser treatment of injured peripheral nerve. Spine 15(1):6-10

Sechzer P H, Leung S J 1975 Acupuncture: surgical aspects. Bulletin of the New York Academy of Medicine 51:922-929

Sjolund B, Eriksson M 1980 Relief of pain by TENS. John Wiley, Chichester

Strauss S 1987 The scientific basis of acupuncture. Australian Family Physician 16(2):166-169

The Academy of Traditional Chinese Medicine 1980 Essentials of Chinese acupuncture. Foreign Languages Press, Beijing

The Academy of Traditional Chinese Medicine 1987 Chinese acupuncture and moxibustion. Foreign Languages Press, Beijing

Terenius L 1985 Families of opioid peptides and classes of opioid receptors. In: Fields H L, Dubner R, Cervero F (eds) Advances in pain research and therapy. Raven Press, New York, vol 9, 463-477

Travell J G, Simons D G 1983 Myofascial pain and dysfunction. The trigger point manual. Williams & Wilkins, Baltimore

Wei Ly 1986 Physical mechanism of tonification and sedation by acupuncture. American Journal of Acupuncture 14(4):317-324

Psychology of injury rehabilitation

19. Understanding and managing the injured athlete

Christopher Horsley

Physiotherapists can provide a positive contribution to the mental management state of injured athletes. To do so in an effective manner requires an understanding of the psychology of injured athletes and mechanisms for management. Not only does the athletes' mental state contribute to successful rehabilitation, it also determines the confidence with which they return to competition.

The objectives of this chapter are to provide an overview of factors that influence athletes' behaviour when injured and guidelines for the psychological management of injured athletes. The author does not intend to provide an encompassing psychological manual for physiotherapists. There will be times when referral to a psychologist will be appropriate. Of importance for physiotherapists is an awareness of the psychology of the injured athlete and basic management skills. If rehabilitation can be directed towards the achievement of physiological as well as psychological goals then it is to be hoped that controllable disruptions will be avoided.

Three theoretical models of athletes' responses to injury are outlined. The first is adapted from a model proposed by Kubler-Ross. It details five stages of 'grieving' that injured athletes may be expected to follow. Physiotherapists should be able to associate behaviours and responses with each stage. The second model conceptualizes injury as a loss, and proposes that the psychological reaction of injured athletes is a function of perceived loss. In the final model, injury is conceptualized as a function of stress. This model proposes that athletes' thoughts determine athlete behaviour. Each model provides a framework for understanding the psychological reaction of athletes to injury.

Common psychological responses experienced by injured athletes are outlined next. Reactions such as loss of motivation to attend appointments or complete exercises, negative and destructive emotions, loss of confidence, and irrational behaviours can be detrimental to rehabilitation.

It is proposed that the most effective way of preventing undesired psychological responses to injury is by exerting control over factors that influence the thinking and behaviour of athletes.

Thirdly, a range of factors that mediate athletes' reactions to injury are detailed. Athletes' psychological reactions to injury and the rehabilitation process often depends on the nature of the injury, the characteristics of the individual, the available social support and the context within which the athlete operates.

Lastly, a management program for physiotherapists is proposed. The dual objectives of this program are to reduce possible problems during rehabilitation and to assist the athlete's mental preparation for return to competition.

There is much a physiotherapist can do to assist athletes' mental well being during rehabilitation. An understanding of the mechanisms of psychological rehabilitation is important. Creating a system that controls the influencing factors is even more appropriate. Assisting the physiotherapist to gain an understanding of the mechanisms and guidelines to operating an effective system is the goal of this chapter.

THEORIES OF ATHLETE RESPONSE TO INJURY

Three models are presented to explain the way athletes typically respond when injured: the Kubler-Ross grief model, Peretz's model of loss, and a stress model proposed by Weiss and Troxel (1986). The models will provide the physiotherapist with an understanding of athletes' psychological response to injury and principles that can be used in the management of an injured athlete. It is important to recognize that while the models outline generalized responses, they do not suggest that each athlete will respond in exactly the same way. Athletes vary in their response to injury.

Two principles are important when considering general models of behaviour. Firstly, within each athlete exists a person with a life away from sport. The psychological management of the injured athlete must take into account more than just the athlete's sporting existence. Secondly, each person will respond differently to the stress of injury and needs to be managed accordingly. The application of both principles is important for the mental well-being of the injured athlete and the effectiveness of a mental management program.

Kubler-Ross grief model

Kubler-Ross (1969) proposed that when an individual suffers a significant loss such as death of a family member, the individual will typically proceed through five stages of grieving. The stages are denial, anger, bargaining, depression and acceptance. Writers in sport psychology have adapted this model to sport where parallels of loss and trauma exist. Researchers have collected data supporting the view that injured athletes will typically experience five similar stages of grieving (Gordon et al 1991). Each stage can be characterized by specific moods and behaviours. During most of the grieving process athletes will experience moods, thoughts and behaviours that are dysfunctional and exacerbate the difficulties of rehabilitation (Table 19.1). Initially athletes may deny an injury, or the ramifications of an injury. Only after they progress to the stage of acceptance can the injured athletes behave and think in a way that can be considered productive and constructive.

Stage1: Denial

An athlete's first response to injury is denial. Athletes will typically deny the injury exists, accept the diagnosis but reject the extent of the prognosis and/or refuse to accept the limitations it will place upon training and competition. During this denial phase an athlete may react against the injury to prove nothing is wrong, or argue unrealistically that a future competition is not beyond reach. Some injuries are easier to deny than others. An Australian javelin champion had no choice but to accept her injury because 'I was wrapped in a cast from calf to toe'. A world junior

Table 19.1 Typical thoughts and behaviours at each stage of the Kubler-Ross model

Stage of reaction	Thoughts and behaviours
1. Denial	'I can tough it out. It'll be OK'. Continue training and/or competing.
2. Anger	'Why didn't the physio warn me!' 'Bloody typical of me to get injured just before the trials.' Storm away; kick and scream.
3. Bargaining	'If I do what they (doctor and physio) say, I should be OK by the trials. What would they know.' Fail to follow advice of medical staff; aggravate injury.
4. Depression	'This is hopeless. Why do I bother with treatment.' Lethargy; lack of motivation; depression.
5. Acceptance	'OK, they were right after all. I must follow advice and be professional.' Positive, controlled emotions; committed; accepting situation.

champion hurdler trained through the pain of an inflamed achilles tendon in preparation for the 1989 European season, only to miss the entire season due to chronic tendinitis.

The culturally conditioned attitude to deny pain and train on regardless sanctions, if not encourages, athletes to deny the injury. The more astute and experienced athletes tend to differentiate the danger signals of injury pain from the less-threatening pain of muscular and physiological stress. Less mature and inexperienced athletes find it more difficult to make the differentiation and/or have the conviction to hold back.

Stage 2: Anger

An athlete's emotional reaction can be extreme and abrupt when faced with the implications of the injury. It is a response characterized by anger, rage and resentment. The anger will often be directed towards someone or something considered responsible for the injury. Responsibility may be attributed to an opposition player, a coach, teammate or physiotherapist who previously treated the recurring injury. At times athletes may direct the anger internally. The anger is often accompanied by irrational beliefs such as 'It is the coach's fault. It is his job to know when I am fatigued and should have pulled me off the court'.

Stage 3: Bargaining

A phase of rationalisation is entered, replacing blind emotion with negotiation. Athletes will attempt to bargain a position in order to postpone loss. The bargaining may be with a significant other, such as doctor or physiotherapist, or be a series of arguments conducted within an athlete's own head.

The significant features of this stage are attempts to place the injury into perspective and a diminution of anger. Athletes may become inflexible as they strive to salvage the best position possible. Their thinking can be irrational and rigid. They rarely achieve a lasting position or peace of mind.

Stage 4: Depression

The full realization of the extent of the injury dawns upon the athlete. This is the stage of depression. It is characterized by feelings of lethargy, apathy, disappointment, and lack of satisfaction. Depressed athletes tend to take a negative view of themselves, the world and their future. Instead of focusing on overcoming the injury their focus is turned inwards with accompanying attacks upon self-concept (image of self), self-esteem (feelings of self-worth) and self-confidence (belief in self) (Gordon 1986).

Irrational beliefs and thoughts, that undermine functional moods and behaviours are common among depressed

Table 19.2 Therapist's perceptions of behavioural symptoms of psychological responses to injury

Negative psychological responses		Positive psychological responses	
Behaviour*	Rank**	Behaviour*	Rank**
Failure to take responsibility for own rehabilitation	1	Ask questions of therapist to understand injury	1
Non-acceptance of injury	2	Listens well to advice	2
Non-compliance and lack of co-operation with treatment	3	Co-operation and compliance with therapist	3
Denial of seriousness or injury	4	Receptive of physical restrictions	4
Displays of depression	5	Initiates progression rehabilitation at home	5
Bargaining with therapists over treatment and time out of competition	6	Early acceptance of injury	6

N = 66
* Behaviour more than 'moderately indicative' of a negative or positive response
** Ranked in order of high to lower indication of positive/negative psychological response to injury. I = most highly indicative; 6 = least indicative

athletes. Examples include 'My body owes me', or 'If I am not a successful athlete I am a nobody'.

The depth of an athlete's depression will depend upon the length and severity of the previous stages of denial, anger and bargaining. An athlete who trains regardless of advice and pain may experience depression more severely than an athlete who moves more quickly through the previous stages. Athletes recovering from acute injuries, such as knee reconstruction, may experience numerous bouts of depression during the prolonged rehabilitation process.

Rehabilitation is disrupted when an athlete is depressed too often or for a prolonged period of time. Chronically depressed athletes look for an outlet from the bad feelings. They may lose motivation for treatment, train inappropriately in an attempt to gain some positive feelings or become involved in unwarranted activities to 'release the pressure'.

Stage 5: Acceptance

This stage is rarely characterized by happy acceptance, but rather a realistic acceptance of the extent of the injury and the implications it will have upon training and performance. The athlete's focus is directed towards the work that needs to be done before returning to full training and competition. The injured athlete's view of him/herself, the world and the future is more positive, realistic and flexible. Gordon (1990b) questioned physiotherapists on their perceptions of the behavioural symptoms of a poor psychological response to injury. Their reports exhibit a strong similarity to the five stages proposed by Kubler-Ross (Table 19.2).

It is important to recognize that the Kubler-Ross model is an ideal representation of how the majority of athletes typically respond to injury. Rarely is the transition from denial to acceptance sequential or progressive. Athletes may return to a previous stage or may fluctuate between two stages. Also, athletes differ in the way they negotiate each stage. For example, Rottella (1982) noted that although one athlete may perceive an injury as disastrous, another may perceive it as undesirable, but also as an opportunity to work on existing weaknesses and to display self-discipline and courage to fight back. Consequently the athletes will move through the stages at different rates and with different impact. Situational factors such as the type of injury, closeness to major competition, age of the athlete, and the extent of the athlete's social support system will influence how the athlete moves through each stage.

Peretz model of loss

Peretz (1970) views the psychological response of grief as a 'function of loss'. To many athletes an injury represents a loss: loss of mobility, opportunities, finances and possibly self-confidence. Peretz (1970) defines loss as 'a state of being deprived of or being without something one has had'. For an athlete this sense of loss can precipitate the grieving process.

Peretz (1970) outlines four different types of loss, three of which athletes can experience when injured.

The most common loss for the injured athlete is a loss of some aspect of self. Peretz (1970) describes the self as 'the over-all mental representation or image each of us has of his body and of his person. This self-representation includes ideas and feelings about the self, its worth, attractiveness...and capacities'. Loss to an injured athlete can be physical, such as the loss of strength or mobility. Loss can be in the form of self-representation such as self-image and self-worth. An athlete's self-image and self-worth is inextricably tied to his or her athletic pursuit and successes. When denied the opportunity to train, compete and achieve success, athletes experience loss. Loss through injury can be more dramatic for the professional athlete than for the casual athlete as illustrated by Peretz (1970): 'loss of...social roles such as occupation, profession, position in the family, and the status associated with each...frequently has dramatic impact upon the person's life'.

Tied to self-image is the strong attachment athletes have to their body. 'To an athlete who is accustomed to moving his or her body in a controlled, smooth fashion, the loss of this control can be terribly upsetting' (Astle 1986, p. 280).

The second form of loss experienced by injured athletes is described by Peretz (1970, p. 5) as 'developmental loss, or that loss which occurs in the process of human growth and development'. Injured athletes are often denied the opportunity of training benefits. They can lose speed, strength, cardiovascular fitness, and flexibility. Athletes also experience a 'loss by comparison': while injured athletes stagnate, competitors have the opportunity to develop.

Examples of the third category of loss, of external objects, include the loss of financial rewards, scholarships, sponsorship and endorsements. While the loss of external objects may not be as emotionally disruptive as loss of some aspect of self, it can add to the stress experienced by injured athletes.

It can be expected that at some stage injured athletes will proceed through Kubler-Ross' five stages and/or experience loss outlined by Peretz. Both models provide the physiotherapist with an overview upon which to understand the fluctuating moods and behaviours often experienced by injured athletes. Understanding and empathy are crucial ingredients when helping athletes deal with the trauma of injury. However, neither model specifies the processes underlying athletes' responses. A more functional model is proposed by Weiss and Troxel (1986). Their stress model is based upon the premise that athletes' thoughts determine their moods and behaviours.

Cognitive stress model

The role of beliefs and thoughts in determining moods, physiological responses and behaviours has been a popular, empirically supported relationship over the past 20 years. Athletes who think 'this is going to hurt' are likely to perceive treatment as more painful than athletes who think 'I'm good at dealing with pain'. Understanding the relationship between thoughts (cognitions) and behaviour is of great benefit when working with athletes who are attempting to deal with the difficulties of injury.

The stress model, as proposed by Weiss and Troxel (1986) is based upon the cognitive concept that people's experience of stress is a function of their thoughts about stressful situations (Fig. 19.1). A certain amount of stress

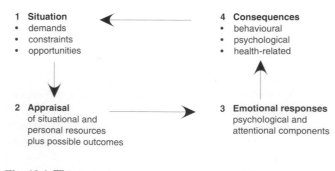

1 **Situation**
• demands
• constraints
• opportunities

4 **Consequences**
• behavioural
• psychological
• health-related

2 **Appraisal**
of situational and
personal resources
plus possible outcomes

3 **Emotional responses**
psychological and
attentional components

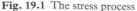

Fig. 19.1 The stress process

is necessary for daily functioning. As the number of stressors increase and become more intense, individuals are required to deal with them in the most productive manner. Stress can therefore be productive and beneficial. It can also be unproductive and harmful to the well being of an individual if excessive or mismanaged.

A **stressor** (point 1) is any situation or influence that places a demand upon the organism. Illness and injury are common sources of stress for athletes, with injury placing obvious physiological demands. Once injured there are many sources of stress which an athletes must control.

Dealings with professional staff, the treatment process, relations with coach and teammates, an uncertain future, financial difficulties, and pain can be sources of stress for injured athletes. The impact each source has upon athletes depends upon how the athlete perceives the stressor.

Cognitive appraisal (point 2) refers to the thinking athletes will engage in when faced with a stressor. Athletes weigh the demands of the situation against some assessment of personal capabilities to deal with the situation. The cognitive appraisal is a conscious, active thinking process.

An athlete's response will be dependent upon the outcome of the cognitive appraisal. Two issues influence this outcome. The first is the athlete's perception of the stressor. For example, a strained hamstring can have different implications for different athletes. To a young, inexperienced athlete a strained hamstring may mean nothing more than a minor inconvenience. For an athlete in final preparations for the Olympic Games a strained hamstring can cause great anxiety. The meaning an athlete attaches to an event will influence his or her appraisal.

A second influencing factor is the result an athlete comes to after weighing up the demands of the situation with perceived resources to deal with the situation. When demands overwhelm resources athletes feel incapable of effectively dealing with the situation, and are likely to experience anxiety and lack of confidence. However, if athletes perceive that they have the resources to deal effectively with the situation they will respond to the injury with composure and confidence.

The third phase of the stress model is the **emotional response** (point 3) that follows cognitive appraisal. The athletes' appraisal of a situation will determine their emotional, physiological and psychological response to injury. For example, an athlete can respond emotionally, with anger or frustration; physiologically, with increased muscle tension and elevated heart rate; or attentionally such as narrowing of attention resulting from the pain or fear.

Two questions should be considered by the physiotherapist. Are the athlete's responses negative and dysfunctional? Is there a significant change from what can be considered 'normal' behaviour by that athlete? The vigilant physiotherapist should become aware of prolonged or extreme states of anger, worry, uncertainty, fear, anxiety or depression. They are the signs of an inappropriate and negative cognitive appraisal. Conversely, an appropriate and positive cognitive appraisal will produce states of determination, optimism, effective attention and composure.

The link between emotions and physiological states is not linear nor unidirectional, but a circular feedback system. Anxiety and anger will produce an increase in heart rate and blood pressure, which will affect the emotional response. In such a way a negative cycle is created.

The final stage of the stress process is the **behavioural consequence** (point 4). An athlete's emotions and physiological state will affect the choice of behaviour. A depressed and demotivated injured athlete is more likely to miss a physiotherapy appointment than is an athlete who is striving to achieve specific goals and to derive something positive from each day.

Common stress responses include chronic tension in the affected area, loss of appetite or sleep, lack of motivation, and adverse effects on the healing process (Weiss & Troxel 1986).

Although the model outlines a sequential process from stage 1 to stage 4, in reality the process is neither sequential nor progressive. Emotions may feedback to thoughts before a decision for action is taken. However, the model does provide an intuitive and pragmatic understanding of the stress process, in which situational demands interact with the individual's cognitive appraisal. It also highlights the important role cognitions play in determining the emotions and behaviour of injured athletes. This point is significant for the physiotherapist involved in the psychological management of injured athletes.

Each of the three models provides the physiotherapist with a framework within which to understand the generalized psychological response of athletes to the stresses of injury. In particular, the stress model details the processes underlying an athlete's moods and behavior. It sensitizes the physiotherapist to points within the process where intervention would be most effective.

Early recognition of unproductive and undesired reactions to injury is important if a negative pool of moods and behaviours is to be prevented. Physiotherapists need to acquaint themselves with the work of researchers who have identified common reacions of athletes when injured.

ATHLETES' REACTIONS WHEN INJURED

Athletes exhibit a range of psychological reactions when injured. Some reactions are productive, giving the athlete the best possible chance of a speedy recovery. Other reactions are unproductive, causing problems with physical rehabilitation and ultimately return to competition. It is proposed that the focus of prevention and management should be on positive productive reactions, however, an understanding of the unproductive and undesired reactions to injury is helpful.

Table 19.3 Psychologically related reactions to physical injury

Emotional signs
- Distractibility
- Hyperexcitation
- Depression
- Boredom
- Restlessness
- Difficulty relaxing
- Feeling people don't appreciate you; feeling used
- Inability to laugh at yourself
- Increased feeling of expression of anger or being cynical
- Inability to concentrate
- Feeling life is not much fun
- Denial that anything is wrong
- Reduced body image
- Reduced self-esteem
- Feeling vulnerable (physical impairment or loss of position on team)
- Distrust
- Feeling afraid (loss of position on team, permanent injury, reduction of physical activity)
- Free floating anxiety (being afraid of something but don't know exactly what it is)
- Feeling under pressure to always succeed
- Automatic expression of negative feelings
- Obsession
- Fault finding

Behavioural signs
- Continuing to train even though medically, vocationally and socially contraindicated
- Tendency to overtrain
- Isolation
- Increased use of alcohol
- Increased use of various medications, such as tranquillizers or amphetamines
- Less time for intimacy with people around you
- Overworked, but can't say no to more work without feeling guilty
- Inability to take a physically relaxed attitude, sitting quietly in a chair or lying on a sofa
- Feeling sexually inadequate
- Speaking up less at gatherings, and then only speaking negatively
- Difficulty setting goals
- Forgetting deadlines, appointments etc.
- Making foolish mistakes
- Decay in interpersonal relationships

Physical signs
- Pain
- Hypersensitivity to pain
- Insomnia; an inability to fall asleep or stay asleep; early awakenings
- Frequent or lingering colds
- Grinding the teeth
- Increase or decrease in appetite
- Indigestion, queasiness
- Vomiting
- Missed menstrual cycle
- Headache
- Increased pitch in voice
- Nervous laughter
- Muscle tension
- Soreness

Most research attention has focused upon the unproductive emotional behaviours. Summarized from May and Sieb (1987), Table 19.3 is an extensive list of psychologically related reactions to physical injury. The list is categorized into three sections: emotional, behavioural and physical. Not listed but also relevant are the cognitive reactions.

Table 19.4 Behavioural responses indicative of attitude towards treatment and rehabilitation

Negative psychological responses		Positive psychological responses	
Behaviours	Degree of negative attitude[a] (average)	Behaviours	Degree of positive attitude[b] (average)
1. Does not follow rehabilitation program at home.	5.95	1. Athlete works hard in rehabilitation	6.21
2. Does not turn up for appointments	5.42	2. Assumes personal responsibility for rehabilitation	6.15
3. Does not listen attentively	5.21	3. Provides feedback to therapist about injury and the rehabilitation program	6.06
4. Denies the extent of the injury	5.06	4. Questions in a cheerful manner on how to assist in rehabilitation	5.76
5. Does not accommodate the injury by making changes in life style	5.04	5. Compliance and co-operation with therapist	5.62
6. Goofs around during rehabilitation	5.03		
7. Seeks multiple opinions about the injury	4.34		
8. Believes that if pain is absent there is no further need for treatment	4.26		
9. Questions therapist's ability and diagnosis	4.20		
10. Overdoes rehabilitation	3.68		

N = 66
[a] 1 not at all indicative of a negative attitude
   4 indicative of a moderately negative attitude
   7 indicative of a very negative attitude
[b] 1 not at all indicative of a positive attitude
   4 indicative of a moderately positive attitude
   7 indicative of a very positive attitude

Gordon et al (1991) found that physiotherapists' perception of athletes' behavioural responses to treatment and rehabilitation were both positive and negative (Table 19.4).

Cognitive reactions to injury

Despite the generally accepted view that cognitive appraisal is the crucial factor in determining an athlete's response to a situation, little research has been conducted into how athletes think when injured. There is little direct evidence to indicate that injured athletes think differently from uninjured athletes, or that athletes who rehabilitate successfully think differently from athletes who encounter problems when rehabilitating. Any understanding that does exist derives from general psychology, case studies and anecdotal evidence. It suggests that athletes who experience difficulties during rehabilitation can be characterized by their thought content and thinking processes.

Three characteristics highlight the thinking processes of problem rehabilitators: irrational and unrealistic beliefs, negative thinking, and excessive worry about problems beyond their control.

Irrational and unrealistic beliefs

The role of irrational and unrealistic beliefs upon thinking and behaviour has been popularized by the work of the psychologist Beck (1976). Beck, like Weiss and Troxel (1986), proposed that thoughts determine emotions and behaviour, but went one step further by proposing that underlying beliefs determine thoughts (Fig. 19.2). Instead of there being a direct link between thoughts and response, beliefs intercede. A hypothetical example is provided in Table 19.5 to illustrate how the relationship affects the response of an injured athlete.

It is important to recognize that the source of the problem is not only negative thoughts, but also the irrational beliefs that underlies the thoughts. When athletes think irrationally and unrealistically they may exaggerate the meaning of the injury, disregard particularly important aspects of the injury, over simplify the injury as good or bad or right or wrong, overgeneralise from this single event, or draw unwarranted conclusions when evidence is lacking or contradictory (Beck, 1976). Irrational negative beliefs correlate with dysfunctional emotions and attacks upon an

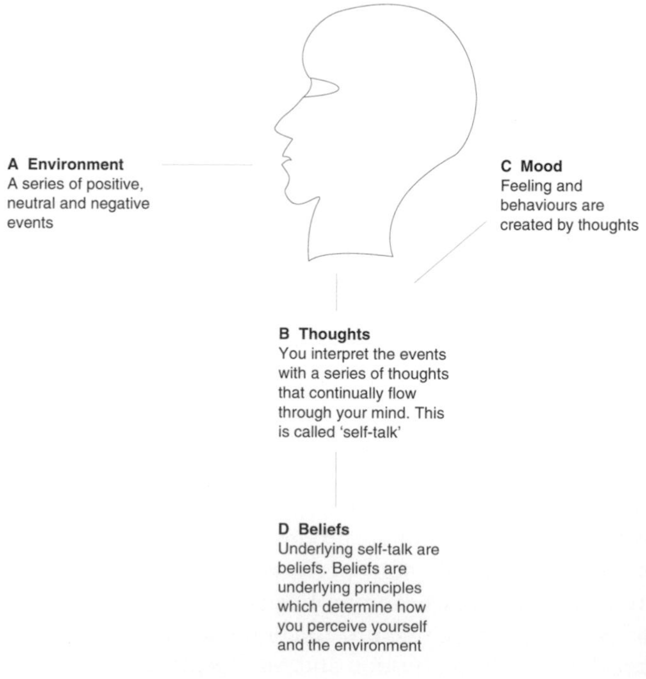

A Environment
A series of positive, neutral and negative events

C Mood
Feeling and behaviours are created by thoughts

B Thoughts
You interpret the events with a series of thoughts that continually flow through your mind. This is called 'self-talk'

D Beliefs
Underlying self-talk are beliefs. Beliefs are underlying principles which determine how you perceive yourself and the environment

Fig. 19.2 Relationship between beliefs, thoughts and mood
Source: adapted from Kidman (1988)

Table 19.5 Hypothetical example of the impact an athlete's belief has upon thoughts, mood and behaviour

Situation	Belief	Thoughts	Mood	Behaviour
Athlete is told to stay off his/her leg for another 3 weeks. A setback in recovery of 3 weeks	The world should be a perfect place and allow me to achieve what I want without setbacks and when it doesn't I can't stand it	The doctors and physios don't understand how how important it is to me	• Resentment • Anger • Frustration	• Overtrains • Doesn't do all exercises prescribed

athlete's self-esteem and self-confidence. An injured professional footballer whose self-identity is tied to athletic achievement can experience great difficulties if operating on the irrational belief that 'I am a nobody if I am not performing well each week'. Such a belief indicates a narrow self-concept and an over-reliance upon sporting performance for self-confidence.

Tendency to engage in negative thinking

The second cognitive characteristic of problem rehabilitators is the tendency to engage in negative thinking. When athletes think: 'This is going to hurt', 'All this rehab work is getting me nowhere fast', 'I might as well be depressed. There is nothing to look forward to' there is a good chance they will fulfil the prophecy.

The power of positive thinking is a popularist notion at present. A number of paperback books on the subject can be found at any newsagent. Positive thinking does work. Conversely, negative thinking also works. Athletes who think negatively about themselves or their situation will respond with destructive emotions and behaviour accordingly. We cannot expect an injured athlete to be a model of consistency or positiveness. However, injured athletes can strive to reinforce their positive attributes and to derive something positive from each situation.

Worry about the uncontrollables

The third characteristic of problem rehabilitators is their tendency to worry about things beyond their control. Rather than focus on things over which they can exert some control, they expend time and energy worrying about things over which they have little control. The result is often a feeling of uncertainty, doubt and lack of control. In fact, control and certainty are achievable if athletes can learn to ignore the uncontrollables and deal only with the controllables. However, they need to accept that a small degree of uncertainty is inherent in the future.

Emotional responses to injury

Athletes experience many positive emotional benefits from participation in sport. It has been found to relieve tension, to reduce anxiety and depression (Dishman 1985), to be a source of fun, competence and positive self-concept, to provide excitement and positive sources of stress and to be

a platform for the development of self-esteem and the enhancement of self-confidence (Deutsch 1985). For many athletes, especially the elite, athletic success shapes their self-identity. Sport provides a degree of control and certainty in the lives of athletes. When injured, many of these positive benefits are lost. It is therefore understandable that injured athletes are susceptible to emotional fluctuations.

Most studies into the psychology of injured athletes have focused on the emotional response of athletes to injury. Rottella (1982) claimed that perhaps the single most important coping skill athletes can have at their disposal is emotional self-control. Eldridge (1983) identified three athlete characteristics that tend to exacerbate an athlete's emotional reaction to injury:

1. Individuals with a narrow self-concept. This often results from an early socialization into the athletic role or when the athlete's experience in life is limited primarily to the athletic environment. They view themselves as athletes and that is about all.
2. People who perceive themselves as failures in other areas of life and rely excessively upon athletic success.
3. Personality types oriented toward work, ambition, competitiveness and social achievement.

Role of self-identity

A powerful factor highlighted by Eldridge (1983) is the important influence of self-identity confirming roles in determining emotions and behaviours. Self-identity is a person's definition of him or her self. Athletes will engage in activities and perform roles that confirm/support their self-identity. In effect, they attempt to maintain congruence between the roles they perform daily and their own perception of themselves. Athlete's self-identities (and this is particularly true at the professional levels), are strongly linked to their athletic pursuits, expectations and successes. Injury can temporarily or permanently eliminate identity-confirming roles. 'This often results in emotional frustration, internal conflict, depression and fear concerning unratified ideal self-image' (Eldridge 1983, p. 272).

Another group of athletes who experience non-adaptive emotional responses to injury are those who are negatively addicted to exercise—the fitness junkies. They have developed a compulsive need for exercise. It serves a dependent function in their emotional well-being. When people who are negatively addicted are unable to train they may experience one or more of the following symptoms: depression, increased irritability, decay of personal relationships, anxiety, restlessness, insomnia, generalised fatigue, muscle tension and decline of appetite (May & Sieb 1987).

Common emotional responses to injury

There appears to be broad common ground of dysfunctional responses of athletes to injury. Depression, anger and frustration are common emotional responses (Chan & Crossman 1988, Smith et al 1990a, Smith et al 1988, Weiss & Troxel 1986, Wiese & Weiss 1987). Tied to the notion of lost self-identity are reported feelings of lowered confidence and self-esteem, inadequacy and loss of control. Chan and Crossman (1988) found injured runners exhibited significantly more depression, anxiety, confusion and lower self-esteem than a group of uninjured runners. Morgan (1977) also found injured runners scored higher on negative mood scales of depression, tension and confusion than uninjured runners.

Subjects who were part of a study by Weiss and Troxel (1986) indicated an inability to cope with injury because they felt externally controlled by the injury. The feeling of being externally controlled is anathema to what is known of the characteristics of successful athletes. Anshel (1990) proposed that successful athletes tend to be internally controlled. They know what they want to achieve and believe they have the capabilities and opportunity to significantly influence outcome. Injury can undermine perceived control. If the prognosis is not definite and specific, the future uncertain, or the athlete is denied important information, perceived control is passed from the athlete to others. From a managerial perspective it is important to recognise that athletes differ in their need for control. This topic is covered in further depth later in the chapter.

The athlete's perception of recovery and the seriousness of an injury also appears to influence the emotional response. Smith et al (1990b) found commonality within a group of seriously injured athletes. They reported simultaneous elevations in depression, anger, tension and frustration. Crossman and Jamison (1985) found that the overestimation of the seriousness or disruptive impact of the injury, by the athlete and/or medical staff, was significantly correlated with reports of more pain, a higher state of anxiety and greater feelings of anger, apathy, loneliness and inadequacy. The response was more common for athletes competing at the non-elite low standards. From a managerial perspective it is important to clearly and specifically inform athletes of the extent of the injury and ensure that their understanding of the diagnosis and prognosis equals reality.

Influence of the caregiver's emotions

Also important is the transference of emotion from the caregiver to the injured athlete. Dugan (1987) found that the emotional state of the caregiver (physiotherapist) influences the caregiver's perception of the emotional state of the athlete. The nature of the emotional communication between caregiver and patient was also affected. The study highlighted the importance of objectivity and emotional control when working with injured athletes. The conflicting issue of proactive direction versus empathy faces each health professional, and needs careful balancing.

Research indicates that adverse emotional responses are common among injured athletes. In many cases (and this is only inferred) extreme and/or prolonged emotional reactions interfere with successful rehabilitation. However, not all athletes respond negatively to injury. Post-injury mood disturbance cannot be assumed.

This marked individual variation in response underscores the importance of neither assuming mood disturbance nor overlooking a serious emotional response to the injured athlete. Awareness of the emotional responses of athletes to injuries and employment of appropriate coping strategies should facilitate optimal rehabilitation and return to sport. (Smith et al 1990b, p. 353).

Athletes' reactions when injured do not occur in isolation. They are a function of a number of interacting variables both within and outside the individual. For the physiotherapist to play an effective role as psychological manager, it is important to be aware of significant intervening variables.

INTERVENING VARIABLES

Weiss and Troxel's (1986) stress model is based upon the premise that an athlete's reaction to injury and the recovery process will be determined by perceptions of internal and external stressors. It would appear that an injured athlete's ability to deal effectively with stress is crucial for the success of rehabilitation.

The stress response

Andersen and Williams (1988) argue for the link between stress, cognitive appraisal and athlete reaction (Fig. 19.3). As with Weiss and Troxel (1986), cognitive appraisal is the central function. Athletes balance the perceived demands of the situation against their perceived capabilities to deal with the situation. The result of the appraisal will determine emotions and behaviours. Athletes who decide that knee reconstruction is the most terrible catastrophe anyone could endure and that it signals the end of their career is more likely to become depressed and angry than athletes who believe they have the capabilities to deal with the difficulties and get back to competition. Athletes' reactions to stressors will be determined by their perceived ability to cope.

Andersen and Williams (1988) contend that stress is experienced not just emotionally but physiologically and

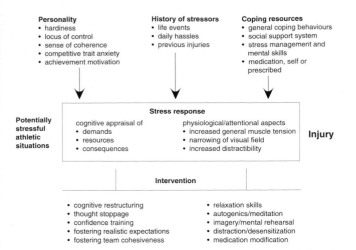

Fig. 19.3 A model of stress and athletic injury. Source: Andersen & Williams (1988)

attentionally as well. Physiological stress is manifested in heightened generalized muscle tension and muscle soreness, disturbed muscle co-ordination, reduced flexibility and stomach upsets. Similar physical signs were found by May and Sieb (1987) in their study of psychologically related reactions to physical injury (Table 19.3).

Stress has also been found to affect the attentional effectiveness of athletes. Nideffer (1980) concluded that heightened stress produces a narrowing of athletes' attentional fields. Peripheral vision is reduced and awareness of important auditory and tactile stimuli is reduced. This is particularly significant for athletes during competition. Athletes can fail to attend to peripheral information they would process when functioning in a more relaxed state.

When injured, athletes can become so consumed with their own physical and emotional state that they tend to lose touch with the purpose of rehabilitation. Stressed athletes can become preoccupied with feelings of pain and discomfort rather than maintaining a broad awareness of environmental cues. Coupled with the tendency to narrow, injured athletes often find it difficult to maintain attentional focus. Concentration becomes scattered, jumping from one cue to another. Stressed injured athletes can become distracted by irrelevant cues and influences. Even during the recovery process athletes need to control their focus and avoid distractions.

Influencing variables

It is all very well for psychologists and physiotherapists to understand how, and possibly why, athletes will react when injured. However, to be of practical benefit to athletes, it is important to know what, out of a myriad of possible factors, can be controlled, managed and/or changed. From the discussion so far it should be obvious that an individuals' beliefs, thoughts and moods can be changed and managed,

although not easily. Andersen and Williams (1988) recognized that there existed many factors that affected athletes' cognitive appraisal. They are factors, outlined in Figure 19.3, that influence an athlete's appraisal of stressful situations. The intervening factors are classified into three groups: personality factors, history of stressors, and coping resources.

Personality

Personality variables, commonly referred to as traits, are relatively enduring and stable characteristics that predispose an athlete to behave in a certain way under most, but not all, conditions. Psychologists, using personality inventories to classify and map an individual's personality, have attempted to link personality traits with athletic performance. The results have been far from conclusive. Investigations into the personality-injury relationship have proved to be just as equivocal. Crossman (1986) claims 'caution should be exercised in drawing conclusions from...studies linking personality traits to athletic injury' (p. 55). Many of the studies reviewed by Crossman investigated the relationship between personality and the occurrence of injury. While this relationship may be inconclusive, it would appear that personality factors play a role in an athlete's reaction when recovering from injury.

One relevant personality factor that has been demonstrated as useful in stress-illness related research is locus of control. A comparison of the characteristics of athletes with differing loci of control is outlined in Table 19.6. Locus of control explains the extent to which a person feels responsible for the outcome of his or her behaviour (or performance), and is reinforced by behaviour outcomes (or performance outcomes) (Anshel 1990). The main issue is the extent to which individuals perceive the results of their behaviour (performance) to be under their control. 'Internals' perceive that their experiences in life are attributable to their own actions. 'Externals', on the other hand, claim little responsibility for the results of their actions. Externals are more likely to consider themselves pawns at the mercy of powerful others or subject to chance (Levenson et al 1983). In terms of injury research, Dalhauser and Thomas (1979) found athletes with an internal locus of control had fewer injuries than those athletes with an external locus of control. Once an athlete is injured, the perceived locus of control will affect the responsibility an athlete will take for recovery, and the attribution leads to success or failure.

Andersen and Williams (1988) highlighted the trait of hardiness as a influencing variable in the stress-injury relationship. Psychological hardiness is a combination of characteristics such as curiosity, willingness to commit, seeing change as a challenge and stimulus to development, and having a sense of control over one's life (Kobasa 1979). Athletes with a strong hardiness factor are more likely to

Table 19.6 Characteristics that distinguish internal from external loci of control

Internals	Externals
Perceive positive and negative events as a consequence of their own actions	Do not connect the events in their lives with their own actions
Feel they can regulate and be held responsible for most events in their lives	Feel that events are beyond their control
Are markedly affected by environmental factors such as external feedback or performance outcomes	Are not affected physically or emotionally by external feedback or outcomes (which they explain as being caused by luck or chance)
Prefer situations in which they can employ skill, rather than chance situations	Prefer luck or chance situations
Set relatively high performance goals	Set relatively less challenging goals
Have higher self-confidence and self-esteem	Are lower in self-confidence and self-esteem
Reinforcement and recognition for performance are very important in increasing the chance of recurring success	Reinforcement and recognition for performance are not as important because they do not tend to take responsibility for success or failure
Persist longer at tasks	Have relatively short persistence
React more adversely to continued failure	Are somewhat less upset by failure

Source: adapted from Anshel 1990

deal effectively with the difficulties of injury than those who perceive change as a threat, find it difficult to stay committed to a course of action or a single goal, and perceive they have little control over their lives. Tough-mindedness, a trait similar to hardiness, was found by Jackson et al (1978) to differentiate footballers who were likely to get injured. They found that tough-minded football players were less likely to be injured than tender-minded players.

Studies investigating athlete susceptibility to injury have found differences based upon self-concept. Lamb (1986) found that athletes with a low self-concept tended to have more injuries than athletes with a high self-concept. 'Self-concept influences one's behaviour. It encompasses the individual's response to the predictions of others, events in the environment, and internal factors such as emotions and values' (Lamb 1986, p. 220). Young and Cohen (1979) on the other hand, using the Tennessee self-concept scale, found no significant difference in self-concept between injured and uninjured female college basketball players. The Tennessee self-concept scale assesses identity (i.e. how an individual describes their basic identity), self-satisfaction (how satisfied the individual is with their perceived image) and behaviour.

It is unfortunate that most of the studies conducted to date have investigated personality factors that differentiate injured from uninjured athletes. Although injury prevention is a primary objective, many problems that prolong recovery and are preventable, occur during rehabilitation. Further research needs to be conducted to determine the relationship between personality traits and reactions when injured. It is sufficient to say at this stage that the traits of locus of control, self-concept and hardiness appear relevant to the reaction of the injured athlete.

History of stressors

Three factors within the category of history of stressors are significant: stressful life events, daily hassles and previous injuries. Each has been shown to influence an athlete's predisposition to injury and an athlete's reaction to injury.

Stressful life events

Stress is not necessarily negative and destructive. Without stress there is no motive to achieve, interact or derive satisfaction. However, there is a level of stress, when demands exceed resources, beyond which negative consequences result. An individual can only endure a finite amount of stress before the human system begins to break down. Excessive stress, resulting in negative, undesired consequences, is rarely the result of one specific event or stimulus. Rather, it is the result of accumulated stress over a period of time involving a number of stimuli.

The concept of life event stressors was developed by Holmes and Rahe (1967), formalized in a questionnaire 'The Social Readjustment Rating Scale' (SRRS) and used to investigate the relationship between cumulative life stressors and proneness to illness. Rahe (1968) found a significant and positive relationship between life stressors and illness. He found that people were more likely to fall ill after a period of heightened accumulated stress. Bramwell et al (1975) extrapolated that same relationship to sport, and developed a sport specific version of the SRRS, the 'Social and Athletic Readjustment Rating Scale' (SARRS—Table 19.7) and found that athletes experiencing stressful life events are more likely to become injured than those with less stressful life events. Bramwell et al concluded 'that heightened stress may impact upon muscle tension, attentional effectiveness and block responses and coping mechanism that assist athletes deal with frustrations and anger' (1975, p. 12). Crosswell (1986) also found that accumulated life event stresses increased the likelihood of injury. Deutsch (1985) provides anecdotal evidence of a racquetball player who reported that he sprained his ankle because he was 'pressing too hard on the courts, probably because I'm having troubles at home'.

Injury is both a physical and a mental stressor for athletes. The pain and shock of injury is stressful. For an elite tennis player the uncertainty and constant physical

Table 19.7 Social and athletic readjustment rating scale

Rank	Life Event
1	Death of spouse
2	Death of close family member
3	Marriage
4	Death of close friend
5	Divorce
6	Marital separation
7	Being fired
8	Marital reconciliation
9	Change in health of family member
10	Begin or cease formal schooling
11	Change in financial state
12	Jail term
13	Outstanding personal achievement
14	Changing to different kind of work
.	
16	Sexual difficulties
.	
.	
.	
.	
25	Change in living conditions

Ranking by USA college football players. Injury not included
Source: Bramwell et al (1975)

pain during recovery, appointments with doctors and physiotherapists to discuss the prognosis, and missing an important competition such as Wimbledon are stressful injury-specific events. Associated with the injury are a range of contextual stressors with which the athlete must contend. Issues such as a change in financial position, change in living conditions, difficulties with transportation, change in routine and changed relationship with coach and teammates can be stressful events for injured athletes. Injured athletes need to deal with the stress of the injury, the associated uncertainty of recovery and normal life stressors that can become exacerbated due to the difficulties associated with injury.

The impact stressful events have upon rehabilitating athletes is relevant to physiotherapists. The SARRS scale indicates that injury itself is stressful to an athlete. With prolonged rehabilitation such as follows a knee reconstruction, athletes must negotiate further stressful life events. Athletes often need assistance to manage their stress levels. They need to be aware of real and potential sources of stress, and have strategies to deal with the stress effectively.

Daily hassles

Specific major stressors such as divorce or family death are identifiable, quantifiable and capable of being related to illness or injury. Less poignant are the many hassles that comprise daily existence. A list of daily hassles was compiled from athletes at the Australian Institute of Sport (AIS) (Albinson 1989) (Table 19.8). Although not representative of the general population, given the eliteness of the athlete group and the conditions of institutional living at the AIS, the list is comprehensive and is indicative of the small—

and insignificant when taken in isolation—hassles athletes have to deal with on a daily basis. An accumulation of daily hassles can elevate athletes' stress levels to that comparable to daily life events.

As with life events physiotherapists need to be aware of the many minor hassles an athlete has to contend with on a daily basis. The objective for the physiotherapist is to assist the athlete to identify and address minor hassles. Sometimes direct action is required to resolve the hassle. For example, if a basketball player is concerned about the expectations of his coach when he returns to training, some direct intervention by the physiotherapist may be of benefit. The player may need encouragement to discuss the issue with the coach, and strategies to use. Direct communication to clarify the issue may resolve the stress and worry. In another situation, and for some individuals, denial is appropriate.

Table 19.8 Examples of the types of daily hassles experienced by AIS athletes

Accommodation
- noise and rules of place of residence
- going home to live
- paying household bills
- lifestyle of the people lived with

Financial
- having to get money from parents
- not having money to buy things peers buy
- being owed money/owing money
- being behind peers in establishing a career

Competition and training
- conflicts with coach
- training with people athlete has to compete against
- lack of short term success opportunities
- getting to training
- not being able to talk to coach

Education/work
- too tired to do well at school
- transportation to/from school/work
- getting time off school/work
- prejudice of people at school/work because of being an athlete

Injury
- getting injured/being injured
- playing/training with a minor injury
- paying for physio and/or massage
- playing/training with pain
- setting appropriate athlete/physio care

Social support
- being away from home
- losing contact with friends
- not having someone to talk to about personal matters
- difficulties in establishing a relationship
- non-athlete friends who do not understand
- commitment needed to be élite

Time
- not having time to do things athlete wants to do
- managing time
- not enough time to socialise with school/work mates

Other
- others' perception of the training for sport
- expectations placed upon self
- dealing with the media
- dealing with other athletes' problems

That is, to ignore the hassle and focus on productive aspects of life. Issues beyond the control of the athlete can, as a general rule, be ignored. The training and competition performances of other athletes are common issues of concern that are best ignored. Alternatively, resolution can be achieved by the reordering of priorities and eliminating the less important. The job of sorting out what is important and what action needs to be taken is a task athletes, especially when confused, depressed or demotivated, find difficult. In such situations athletes need support, direction and guidance.

Previous injury

It has been reported anecdotally that athletes often experience a lag between physical rehabilitation and psychological rehabilitation. One rugby union player, a national squad member, described how he experienced a lack of confidence when returning to competition after knee reconstruction. Although advised by the doctor that his knee was strong and fully repaired he lacked confidence in both his knees, to withstand the rigours of top-class competition, and his football skills. He stated, in hindsight, that he should have asked questions of both the doctor and physiotherapist when uncertain about the strength of his knee.

Previous injury can produce doubt and uncertainty in the minds of athletes. Hesitancy, anxiety, doubt and a lack of rhythm and timing are the hallmarks of athletes who lack confidence. Athletes are then susceptible to further injury or reinjury. Injured athletes can be assisted to mentally prepare for a return to competition. Although assistance from a sport psychologist would be most appropriate, physiotherapists can be helpful to athletes. Knowledge about the development of self-confidence and the processes of performance are important.

Coping resources

General coping mechanisms

'Coping resources comprise a wide variety of behaviours and social networks that help the individual deal with the problems, joys, disappointments, and stresses of life' (Andersen & Williams 1988, (p. 303).

Everyone has coping resources and stratagems. They are learnt from the hard lessons of experience, acquired vicariously and based upon suggestions from others. Age, life experiences and support from others contribute to an array of coping resources.

Coping strategies can be functional or dysfunctional. Sleep is a functional response to fatigue; excessive use of alcohol is a dysfunctional response. To deal effectively with the stresses of life we need an array of coping resources plus awareness of timing. Coping strategies need to be used at the appropriate time. For example, an Australian track athlete used social isolation as a coping mechanism when injured. She isolated herself when the emotional disappointment associated with a stress fracture of the tibia became too much. However, she found that if she did not start to interact with others within 24 hours her feelings of depression and self-pity strengthened. She had to make the effort to interact with others in a positive manner. She used social isolation as an effective coping strategy, while at the same time recognizing its limitations.

Table 19.9 Coping strategies used by athletes

Coping Strategies	Method of coping		Focus of coping		
	Active Cognitive	Active Behavioural	Avoidance	Problem focused	Emotion focused
Tried to see a positive side	X				X
Tried to step back from situation and be more objective	X				X
Took things one step at a time				X	
Considered several alternatives for handling the problem	X			X	
Drew on past experiences; has been in a similar situation before	X			X	
Tried to find out more about the situation		X		X	
Took some positive action		X		X	
Talked with a friend about the situation		X			
Prepared for the worst			X		
Sometimes took it out on other people when felt angry or depressed			X		
Kept feelings to self			X		
Tried to reduce tension by eating more			X		X

Source: Billings & Moos (1981)

The important role that coping resources play in the stress-illness relationship has been well established. However, only limited research has been conducted into the role that coping resources play in relation to athlete well being during recovery from injury. Andersen and Williams (1988) proposed coping resources as a mediating influence upon the stress response based upon extensive and supportive stress-illness literature. Billings and Moos (1981) reviewed the interactions of coping resources and life stress and proposed an extensive range of effective coping mechanisms commonly used by athletes (Table 19.9).

Implications for physiotherapists

Injured athletes need a range of coping strategies to stay positive and focused during the stresses of rehabilitation. Their coping resources moderate the impact of stressors. Personality traits also affect athletes' uses of coping resources. For example, an athlete with a high external locus of control may be reluctant to take responsibility for any outcome, and to avoid a stressful issue rather than deal with it directly.

Young athletes in particular find it emotionally difficult to cope with injury. It may be a new experience, thereby presenting a new set of problems which are difficult, at first, to handle. Young athletes are often hamstrung by a lack of coping stratagems and, simply because of age and inexperience, lack sophistication in the use of their limited resources. They often need assistance to broaden their range of coping strategies and guidance to use them effectively. A strong social support mechanism and role models are important for athletes in need of assistance.

Social support systems

Athletes' social support systems comprise the family, teammates, coach, school and work friends, and sports medical staff. The social support system buffers athletes' attempts to cope with the problems, disappointments and difficulties of athletic injury. The relative importance of each group is dependent upon the situation. For elite athletes, the coach and family provide significant support. For an injured athlete, the role of the medical staff becomes important, not only for medical services but also for the provision of psychological support. 'It is not so much friends' help that helps us as the confident knowledge that they will help us' (Epicurus, 13th century BC).

Sarason et al (1990) proposed that an athlete's ability to cope was enhanced by simply knowing that social support was available. Their research focused on two factors related to perceived support. 'Sense of support' was a belief that supportive others will provide support, regardless of sacrifice and demands. 'Sense of acceptance' is the comfort of knowing that supportive others are accepting, including best

Table 19.10   Types of social support

Listening
  Characterized by active listening, i.e. listening without giving advice or making judgements

Emotional challenge
  Characterized by challenges and questions to the recipient concerning whether she/he is doing her/his best to fulfil goals and overcome obstacles

Technical appreciation
  Characterized by acknowledgment of task effort

Emotional support
  Characterized by the willingness to be on the recipient's side in a difficult situation, even if the supporter is not in total agreement with her/him

Shared social reality
  Characterized by the sharing of similar experiences, priorities, values and views (the supporter serves as a social reality 'touchstone' with whom perceptions of the social context are checked)

Technical challenge
  Characterized by questions and challenges that keep the recipient from becoming stale or superficial by stretching, encouraging and leadinghim/her to greater involvement,excitement and creativity

Source: Hardy et al (1989)

and worst points. A sense of acceptance is related not only to the athletes' view of others but the view they have of themselves. Sense of acceptance is 'related to the individual's belief concerning personal control in significant areas of life. People feel in control when they have opinions and wherewithal' (Sarason et al 1990, p. 119). Even if contact or direct intervention by coach or medical staff did not occur, athletes were buoyed by knowing that support was available if needed.

However, the role of the social support team is to provide a service. Members of the social support system listen without judgement, have a technical appreciation of the sport, share the social reality of the athlete, provide emotional encouragement and challenges, and challenge the athlete technically. Types of social support are outlined in Table 19.10. Rarely can one person provide each and every type of social support. Richman et al (1989) found coaches were more likely to provide technical challenges, have a technical appreciation of the sport and provide emotional challenges. They were less likely to provide emotional support, to listen and to have a shared social reality. Physiotherapists are in a position to provide listening support, emotional and technical challenges and emotional support.

Alberecht and Adelman (1984) concluded from a review of the social support literature, that the network 'serves to meet a recipient's needs for venting feelings, reassurance, and improved communication skills. It also serves to reduce uncertainty during times of stress, provides resources and companionship, and aids in mental and physical recovery' (p. 8).

Sarason et al (1990), following extensive studies into the relationship between social support and health, concluded that social support increased the coping efforts of the individual. In effect, social support was perceived as a stress buffer. They found that a sense of acceptance buoyed the person with a willingness to explore and take reasonable risks, with a sense of self-efficacy leading to effective management of stressors, low levels of anxiety, positive self-image, expectations of desirable outcomes from social interactions and a benign view of people (Sarason et al 1987). Sarason et al (1990) explained the sense of support as 'the belief that there are supportive others who are willing and able to provide support, regardless of what may be required or the sacrifice that may have to be made to provide it' (p. 121).

Hardy et al (1987) found a direct influence of social support on injuries. They found that athletes with a high level of social support had a lower incidence of injury. However, the notion that social support buffers the effect of life stress by serving as a mediating variable in the life stress injury relationship has yet to be conclusively supported (Andersen & Williams 1988).

Implications for physiotherapists

Physiotherapists form part of an injured athlete's social support system and perform a social support function. What is relevant is the effectiveness with which the physiotherapist is able to listen, provide a technical challenge, and so on. The function of social support is a skill acquired with training and experience. It is the responsibility of the physiotherapist to develop the skill to a level whereby it becomes effective in the psychological management of injured athletes.

While each of the intervening factors—personality, history of stressors and coping resources—are significant in their own right, the interaction between the three is also important. Personality factors affect an athlete's range and use of coping resources. Coping resources in turn affect an athlete's ability to deal with stressful life events. The athlete's personality determines, in part, what is perceived as stressful. The interaction of personality factors, the athlete's history of stressors and coping resources should be kept in mind when considering the role of each variable group. However it is important to understand the role of each variable in the stress response.

PSYCHOLOGICAL MANAGEMENT

The primary purpose of this section is to propose that physiotherapists can and should play a vital role in the psychological well being of injured athletes. It has been explained why athletes react the way they do; what generalized reponses athletes exhibit when injured; and what factors influence the reaction of athletes. This comprises guidelines for information gathering, engineering the environment and management of athletes.

Firstly, a clarification is needed. Terms such as 'management of athletes' and 'engineering of the environment' are not intended to imply an Orwellian domination of the athlete population by the tribe of physiotherapists. The long term objective of athletic development is mature, independent and emotionally secure athletes. However, a snapshot of reality reveals a large percentage of athletes who, because of age, personality factors and situational variants, need guidance, direction and encouragement. Gordon et al (1991) found the most prominant factors that appeared to heighten athlete reactions to injury were related to timing of the injury, intensity/importance of sport involvement, personality of the athlete and the athletes level of competition (Table 19.11).

In such situations physiotherapists can play a productive managerial role. The role will vary depending upon circumstances and may change over time. In some cases a supportive role may be required. Other times, physiotherapists may have to be directive and authoritative. The management skill of physiotherapists is in fulfilling the role the situation demands, and being adaptable. Managing does not mean controlling. In this context, it refers to the function of influencing interpersonal and situational factors to ensure the mental well being of injured athletes.

Referral

There will be times when physiotherapists will consider the mental state of athletes is such that referral is necessary. A referral point is not easy to define. Short term and minor disruptions to psychological well being are common for injured athletes. Referral becomes an issue when the disruptions are prolonged or are extreme enough to significantly interfere with athletes' daily functioning. Example of referral signs include prolonged or severe

Table 19.11 Factors affecting the degree of psychological response to injury

	Average degree of effect on response
Injury occurs just prior to major competition/finals	6.45
Intensity/importance of sport involvement	6.27
Personality of athlete	6.11
Level of competition	6.10
Athlete's faith in therapist	6.09
Confidence in therapist's diagnosis	5.91
Severity of injury	5.82
Previous injury of similar type	5.56
Athlete is close to the end of career	4.88
Injury caused by athlete's lack of preparation	4.38
Injury to a young inexperienced athlete	4.37
Injury occurs in mid-season	4.36
Injury occurs in pre-season	4.18

N = 66
1   no effect on degree of response
4   moderate effect on degree of response
7   significant effect on degree of response

depression, extreme mood swings, a breakdown in what can be considered normal communication, severe weight loss or gain, insomnia or heightened anxiety.

Objectives

The objectives of the psychological management program are:

1. A positive, constructive mental set that contributes to the physical rehabilitation program
2. A confident optimistic athlete
3. Assistance to the athlete to deal with the stresses associated with rehabilitation
4. Reduction of extreme behaviours, emotions and attitudes that interfere with successful recovery.

Successful rehabilitation: the ideal

Even the most successful rehabilitation has peaks and troughs. Athletes do become emotional, demotivated and uncertain about the future. In cases of successful rehabilitation the setbacks are short-lived and have minimal impact upon the rehabilitation process. Successful cases maintain realistic expectations and rational thinking under difficult circumstances. They exhibit a positive, optimistic approach to rehabilitation, life in general and setbacks. Injured athletes use their time productively. They may become involved in alternative activities outside their sport, take on administrative or coaching responsibilities, or work on aspects of their performance that have been neglected in the past, such as physical strength or mental skills. They use the time to their benefit, returning after injury with confidence and enthusiasm.

Athletes who successfully rehabilitate have clear and specific goals for both rehabilitation and their return to competition. They use professional support staff as a source of information and as a referral for short term goal-setting. They establish a self-management system that incorporates rehabilitation objectives and guidelines for feedback. Their goal-setting system helps them to quickly recognise improvements. Their expectations are realistic and their thoughts are focused upon imporovements they wish to make rather than problems that may occur.

Injured athletes need to be mentally flexible. They need to be willing to adapt to changing circumstances and setbacks. The more effective athletes deal with setbacks positively and with composure, adapting to changed circumstances, maintaining control and being free of anxiety and worry. They exhibit a high degree of control—control of thoughts, emotions and behaviours. Coupled with a high level of control is a faith in the advice and instructions of the medical staff. They ask for, and often demand, information about their condition and the rehabilitation

process. They are able to maintain positive and constructive communication with medical professionals, coaches and teammates.

Athletes who successfully rehabilitate maintain a high level of self-confidence and positive self-esteem. They are able to handle setbacks because of a high belief in their capabilities to be successful, to achieve a task and to fulfil a goal. In doing so they exhibit patience, rarely becoming flustered or negative when their recovery plateaus.

The ideal is the objective of the athlete, medical staff and sport psychologist. Achieving the ideal requires discipline from the athlete, assistance from support staff and method.

Psychological management program

Guidelines

Establish positive relationship for information gathering. An assessment of the athlete's psychological well being should be conducted simultaneously with the physical assessment. It is helpful to understand the athlete's current emotional state, immediate implications of the injury and expectations of recovery. Listening, empathy and reassurance are important factors at this stage. The physiotherapist should establish a postive relationship with the athlete, and an understanding that there will be a continuity of care.

Physiotherapists need to discuss and understand the role of sport for athletes. Specifically, these include the role sport plays in the athlete's self-identity and self-esteem, the significance of sport in the athlete's social network, and the importance of non-sporting activities in the athlete's life. In other words, the physiotherapist must discover the meaning and connotations of the injury.

During the process of information gathering the physiotherapist should be sensitive to signs of irrational beliefs and unrealistic interpretations of reality. These can be determined by listening to the athlete's interpretations and thoughts on specific situations. Being non-judgemental is important. At this stage of the relationship the objective is to gather information and gain understanding of the athlete, not challenge or change.

Identifying sources of stress in the athlete's life will assist management later. Information should be gathered on the nature of the family system and relationships within the family; the impact of the injury on relationships; interruptions to relationships connected with the athletic activity; financial difficulties or changes. Table 19.11 provides a list of stressors an injured athlete may encounter.

What is the extent of the athlete's social support network? Who is involved and what role do they play? Can the athlete rely upon these people to provide the required emotional, technical and material support? If the social support network needs to be expanded, who would the athlete choose?

An athlete's range of personal strengths and competencies, fears and concerns, and existing coping strategies all form the fodder for future management. How has the athlete dealt with personal difficulties in the past? What are the immediate fears and worries? What concerns does the athlete have for the future? Has the athlete had a previous injury? How severe? How did the athlete deal with it emotionally? What did the athlete learn from the experience? What does the athlete intend to do differently this time? If the physiotherapist is willing to listen, and the athlete trusts the physiotherapist not to reveal confidential information, this type of information will be available.

Nideffer (1983) highlighted the importance of understanding certain personality characteristics of the athlete to assist the therapeutic relationship and management process:

1. Athletes vary in their need to seek information. Athletes with a high need for information will want to know what is happening and may become stressed when denied information. Conversely, athletes with a low need for information will become quickly overloaded when presented with too much information too quickly.

2. Differing levels of self-esteem will affect the trust athletes have in the physiotherapist, and compliance with instructions. Athletes with confidence in themselves will frequently have difficulty trusting and listening to the opinion of others. They have a tendency to do things on their own, which may be exacerbated when injured. The input from the physiotherapist may be disregarded or devalued.

3. Varying speeds of decision-making will affect how athletes assimilate information and the speed with which they put the information into action. Slow decision makers will become pressured when asked to make quick decisions. Instinctive, reactive athletes will become frustrated with others who are slow when giving decisions or ponder decisions.

4. Quiet, more socially withdrawn athletes tend to become even more withdrawn when injured. The physiotherapist may have to probe to gather information, especially if the athletes also lack confidence. Nideffer (1983) warns that the introverted athletes' tendency to withdraw enhances their susceptibility to the development of depression. 'The athlete will need to be brought out of her/himself' (p. 374). Conversely, extroverts may become socially involved and employ denial to avoid the possible realities of injury. While denial can be helpful it can be destructive if it 'interferes with the individual's ability or willingness to make a decision about treatment...or to accept reality' (p. 375).

5. Athletes vary in willingness to express themselves. Those with strong intellectual expressiveness will provide the physiotherapist with information about the injury and themselves as it relates to the injury. They are at ease expressing ideas and opinions logically and rationally. They become stressed when denied the opportunity. Individuals with little expressiveness will withhold information. The physiotherapist will have to work hard to elicit information.

Nideffer's (1983) categories will help the inquisitive physiotherapist to identify personality characteristics that will affect management and treatment.

Maintain non-judgemental stance. Non-judgemental listening is important during the initial stage of the consultative process. Information is the basis upon which future decisions are made. In extreme cases, such as unrealistic denial, a more direct and forceful approach may be necessary to avert futher physical damage. Effective confrontation, where the desired outcome is achieved, is an important skill. Dealing with confrontation can be stressful. It can be less stressful, and more successful, if the physiotherapist is skilled in the area.

Reduce uncertainty. An injury creates uncertainty in the mind of athlete: How long? What impact? What will the coach think? The further uncertainty is reduced the less chance there is of behavioural or emotional problems. Physiotherapists can reduce uncertainty for athletes by providing the appropriate amount of information at the right pace and helping the athletes to plan for the future. Athletes need information about the nature of the injury, and the impact it will have upon training and competition: Can I do weights? Can I run at half pace? Will I be ready for the trials? Is a tear worse than a rupture? Why was David training again within a week and I am out for a month?

The amount of information athletes want, and the amount they can absorb, varies. The physiotherapist must be sensitive to the signs of overload and the desire for more information. Information can be provided by verbal explanations, written materials and role models. Information will be required at the time of injury and during the recovery process as athletes learn to understand what can, and what cannot, be achieved.

Information alone is only part of the confidence building process. Injured athletes need a plan for the future. Some athletes need a detailed, highly structured plan. Others are able to complete the picture from a generalized outline. Athletes need a plan for recovery and goals to achieve.

Goals are important. They provide athletes with a purpose. When injured, athletes are denied the opportunity to work towards or achieve their athletic goals. To maintain purpose and direction in their life their athletic goals must be replaced with goals that are achievable and rewarding.

Applicable goals include rehabilitation goals, training goals, professionalism goals, mental goals and social/personal goals. Physiotherapists have to assist athletes to set specific, achievable and relevant goals. The goals should be written in a training diary and reviewed weekly.

Address fears and concerns. It is important to deal immediately with the fears and concerns of athletes. They should not be magnified or dramatized. Fears and concerns are simply challenges to overcome. In many cases a strategy is needed to bring the fear under the control of the athlete. A physiotherapist can assist athletes to identify and isolate the concern, devise a strategy and monitor progress. Often the concern is simply a function of the athlete's perception of the situation. A physiotherapist can serve an important function by listening to the athlete, understanding how the athlete perceives the situation, and providing an alternative view that may be more realistic, rational or positive. This is a process known as reframing—changing or 'turning around' a certain point of view already in existence to one that is more constructive and positive. Assisting athletes to reframe requires listening skills, patience and the willingness to not provide the answer but to ask the right questions so as to guide athletes to the solution.

Establish a system to build self-confidence. The primary concern for the sport psychologist and coach is the loss of confidence in injured athletes. Although they may be recovering physically, their confidence lowers. Consequently, when athletes return to competition their mental readiness lags behind their physical preparedness. A few specific guidelines are worth following.

1. Clearly specify the stages of recovery and ensure athletes recognize when these are achieved. Create a system that provides feedback to athletes that progress has been achieved.
2. Ensure the athletes are achieving in areas of their life other than injury rehabilitation. Athletes should also be setting goals in a social and interpersonal context.
3. Have athletes incorporate expanded physical capabilities into a training program. For example, only a few injuries restrict athletes from any sort of training. Often athletes can undertake restricted work in the pool and gym, on the cycle and treadmill. Specific programs and goals should be set, progress monitored and evaluated, and the program and physical loads increased as recovery progresses. The objective is for athletes to derive confidence from the fact that they have maintained, and hopefully progressed, in specific physical areas.
4. To stay in touch with the feel and intensity of their activity injured athletes need to watch videos of themselves, or their role models, performing. They need to attend training sessions to be aware of tactics and absorb from others. They need to regularly visualize themselves training and performing at competition level. After injury, the middle distance runner loses touch with the rhythm of running and the awareness of race tactics; hockey players lose touch with the feel of ball on stick when moving at full pace. They do not lose total awareness or feel for their craft, but it diminishes. The image is less vivid. Their sensitivity to the kinesthetic, tactile, auditory and visual cues is reduced.
5. Confidence is determined largely by the beliefs and thoughts in the mind of injured athletes. Beliefs of injured athletes need to be realistic, rational and optimistic. Thoughts need to be positive, constructive and task-related. Physiotherapists can assist athletes by regularly asking how they think and feel about specific situations.

Assist in monitoring of stress levels. Excessive stress will affect athletes' self-confidence, emotional control, ability to cope with adversity, tolerance, muscle tension and interpersonal relations. Athletes, with the assistance of the physiotherapist, need to monitor stress levels. If the signs of stress appear all sources of stress should be identified and action taken to eliminate and/or alleviate the number and intensity of each source of stress.

Assist in developing range of coping strategies. Athletes' ranges and uses of coping strategies will determine the effectiveness with which they deal with stress and difficulties during the recovery process. Physiotherapists can assist athletes to develop their range of strategies and the effectiveness with which they use the strategies.

Assist with anticipation of setbacks. The best managed athletes anticipate setbacks, plateaus and distractions and determine how they will successfully deal with each. This is not a negative or pessimistic approach. They do not dwell on the problem. They identify the situation, determine a strategy and get on with recovery. If the setback does occur they are prepared to deal with it. If it does not occur, little is lost.

Distractions need to be anticipated and dismissed. Injured athletes with spare time, little structure and few sources of satisfaction tend to be distracted by unproductive and dysfunctional influences. The distractions may be concrete, such as going to the beach rather than having treatment. The distraction may be abstract, such as a comment by a coach upon which athletes dwell and worry.

SUMMARY

Assisting injured athletes to deal with distractions, stresses and threats to their self-confidence is a role that can, and should, be performed by a physiotherapist. Ideally, the physiotherapist should work in partnership with a psychologist. However, in a less than ideal world, the physiotherapist becomes the mental manager.

The first attribute of a mental manager is common sense. The second attribute is an understanding of human behaviour in relation to injury—the models of athlete response when injured. The third is a knowledge of research findings of athletes' reactions when injured and variables that influence the athletes reaction.

Once armed with common sense, understanding and knowledge, it is up to the physiotherapist to assist athletes to deal with the emotional ups and downs of injury rehabilitation.

Accepting the role of mental manager requires the physiotherapist to accept partial responsibility for the psychological well being of injured athletes. The responsibility must ultimately be held by the athlete but the physiotherapist can accept the challenge to positively influence the rehabilition of athletes.

REFERENCES

Alberecht T L, Adelman M B 1984 Social support and life stress: new directions for communication research. Human Communication Research 11:3-22

Albinson J 1989 The daily hassles of elite athletes. Unpublished study, Australian Institute of Sport

Andersen M B, Williams J M 1988 A model of stress and athletic injury. Prediction and Prevention 294-306

Anshel M H 1990 Sport psychology: from theory to practice. Gorsuch Scarisbrick, Arizona

Astle S J 1986 The experience of loss in athletes. Journal of Sports Medicine 26:179-284

Beck A T 1976 Cognitive therapy and the emotional disorders. Penguin Books, London

Billings A G, Moos R H 1981 The role of coping resources and social resources in attenuating the stress of life events. Journal of Behavioral Medicine

Bramwell S T, Masuda M, Wagner N N, Holmes T H 1975 Psychosocial factors in athletic injuries: development and application of the social and athletic readjustment rating scale (SARRS). Journal of Human Stress 6-20

Chan C S, Crossman H Y 1988 Psychological effects of running loss on consistent runners. Perceptual and Motor Skills 66:875-883

Crossman J E, Jamison J 1985 Differences in perceptions of seriousness and disrupting effects of athletic injury as viewed by athletes and trainers. Perceptual and Motor Skills 71:848-850

Crossman J E 1986 Psychological and sociological factors supporting athletic injury. Coaching Review May/June:54-58

Dalhauser M, Thomas M D 1979 Visual disembedding and locus of control as variables associated with high school football injuries. Perceptual and Motor Skills 49:254

Deutsch R E 1985 The psychological implications of sports related injuries. International Journal of Sport Psychology 16:232-237

Dishman R K 1985 Medical psychology in exercise and sport. Medical Clinics in North America 69(1):123-142

Dugan D O 1987 Death and dying: emotional, spiritual and athical support for patients and families. Journal of Psychosocial Nursing 25(7):21-29

Eldridge P 1983 The importance of psychotherapy for athletic-related orthopedic injuries among adults. Comprehensive Psychiatry 24(3):271-277

Gordon S 1986 Sport psychology and the injured athlete: a cognitive-behavioral approach to injury response and injury rehabilitation. Sports:Science Periodical on research and technology in Sport March

Gordon S, Milios D M, Grove J R 1991 Psychological aspects of the recovery process from sport injury: the perspective of sport psychotherapists. The Australian Journal of Science and Medicine in Sport 23(2):53-60

Hardy C J, Prentice W E, Kirsanoff M T, Ricjman J M, Rosenfeld L B 1987 Life stress, social support, and athletic injury: in search of relationships. In: Williams J M (chair) Psychological factors in injury occurrence. Symposium conducted at the meeting of the NASPSPA, Vancouver

Holmes T H, Rahe R H 1967 The social adjustment rating scale. Journal of Psychosomatic Research 11:213-218

Jackson D W, Jarret H, Bailey D, Kausek J, Swanson J, Powell J 1978 Injury prediction in the young athlete: a preliminary report. American Journal of Sports Medicine 6(1):6-14

Kidman A 1988 From thought to action: A self help manual. Biochemical and General Consulting Service, Sydney

Kobasa S C 1979 Stressful life events, personality and health: an inquiry into hardiness. Journal of Personality and Social Psychology 37:1-11

Kubler-Ross E 1969 On death and dying. Macmillan, New York

Lamb M 1976 Self-concept and injury frequency among female college field hockey players. Athletic Training Fall:220-224

Levenson H, Hirschfeld L, Hirschfeld A, Dzubay B 1983 Recent life events and accidents: the role of sex differences. Journal of Human Stress 10:4-11

May J R, Sieb G E 1987 Athletic injuries: psychosocial factors in the onset, sequelea, rehabilitation, and prevention. In: May J R, Asken M J (eds) Sport psychology. PMA Publishing 157-185

Morgan W P 1977 Psychologic characteristics of the elite long distance runner. Annals of the NY Academy of Sciences 301:382-403

Nideffer R M 1980 The ethics and practice of applied sport psychology. Mouvement, New York

Nideffer R M 1983 The injured athlete: psychological factors in treatment. Orthopedic Clinics of North America 14(2)

Peretz D 1970 In: Schoenberg B, Carr A C, Peretz D, Kutscher A H (eds) Loss and grief: psychological management in medical practice. Columbia University Press, New York

Rahe R H 1968 Life change as a predictor of illness. Proceedings of the Royal Society of Medicine 61:1124-1126

Rottella R J 1982 Psychological care of the injured athlete. In: Kulund D N (ed) The injured athlete. Lippincott, Toronto

Rotter J B 1966 Generalized expectancies for internal versus external control of reinforcement. Psychological Monographs 80(1)No 609

Sarason B R, Shearin E N, Pierce G R, Sarason I G 1987 Interrelations of social support measures: theoretical and practical implications. Journal of Personality and Social Psychology 52:813-832

Sarason I G, Levine H M, Basham R B, Sarason B R 1983 Assessing social support: the social support questionnaire. Journal of Personality and Social Psychology 44:127-139

Sarason I G, Sarason B R, Pierce G R 1990 Social support, personality, and performance. Journal of Applied Sport Psychology 2:117-127

Smith A M, Scott S G, Young M L 1988 The emotional responses of athletes to injury. Canadian Association of Sport Sciences Proceedings September:83-85

Smith A M, Scott S G, O'Fallon W, Young M L 1990a The emotional responses of athletes to injury. Mayo Clinical Proceedings 65:38-50

Smith A M, Scott S G, Wiese D M 1990b The psychological effects of sports injuries. Sports Medicine 9(6):352-369

Weiss M R, Troxel R K 1986 Psychology of the injured athletic training. Summer:104-110

Wiese D M, Weiss M R 1987 Psychological rehabilitation and physical injury: implications for the sportsmedicine team. The Sport Psychologist 1:318-330

Regional assessment and management

20. The temporomandibular region

Guy Zito

The structures of the temporomandibular (TM) region are seldom considered as sources of symptoms in sports injuries in the absence of definite evidence of trauma. Furthermore, recognition of injury to this area is difficult because, as with other parts of the body, when the affected tissues are put under stress, they give rise to either local or referred symptoms similar to those originating from other structures such as the cervical spine, the ears and the teeth, and X-rays are often normal.

ANATOMY

The mobility required by the TM joint for normal function is provided at the expense of stability by the articular components which create a hinge joint with a movable socket (Du Brul 1980). It is a synovial joint formed by an oval-shaped glenoid fossa and a knuckle-shaped mandibular condyle, and its articular surfaces are covered by fibro-cartilage.

Articular disc

A fibrous, sparsely innervated and vascularized disc divides the joint cavity into upper and lower compartments (Fig. 20.1). It is often likened to a schoolboy's peaked cap and is attached to the condyle like a handle to a bucket by collateral discal ligaments (Du Brul 1980).

Anteriorly the disc fuses with the articular capsule and has some indirect connection with fibres of the superior head of lateral pterygoid muscle (Wilkinson 1989), while posteriorly it fuses with the densely innervated retrodiscal ligament which is highly elastic and allows the disc to move anteriorly.

Capsule and ligaments

The capsule, with the synovial membrane, surrounds the joint and is reinforced laterally by the temporomandibular ligament, though is deficient anteriorly (Rees 1954). It is loose as it encircles the upper part of the joint and taut around the lower part, holding the disc firmly on the condyle (Oberg & Carisson 1979). The stylomandibular and sphenomandibular ligaments are accessory ligaments and have little influence on joint function.

The disc's attachments combined with the different laxities of the capsule allow the condyle to rotate on the disc in the lower compartment and the disc/condyle complex to translate in the fossa in the upper compartment (Williams et al 1989) (Fig. 20.1).

The disc commonly displaces anteriorly relative to the condyle and interferes with function. In this abnormal position the disc may still permit movement while moving on and off the condyle during movement (disc derangement with reduction), or may block movement significantly (disc derangement without reduction).

Muscles

The muscles of mastication consist of medial and lateral pterygoid, temporalis and masseter. They contribute to the stability of the joint, and with the assistance of the suprahyoid muscles, the digastric, mylohyoid and genio-hyoid control jaw movements. The masseter and medial pterygoid act with the temporalis to prevent the jaw from

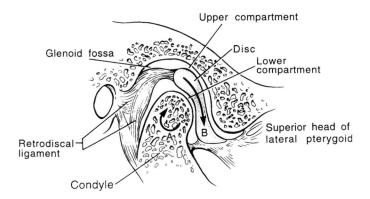

Fig. 20.1 The temporomandibular joint (sagittal section)
  a Direction of condylar rotation in the lower compartment
  b Direction of translation of the disc/condyle complex in the upper complex

317

dislocating when the mouth is fully open (Basmajian & De Luca 1985, MacDougall & Andrew 1953), whereas the superior head of lateral pterygoid, assisted by the other masticatory muscles, seats the condyle upward and forward against the posterior slope of the eminence in the final part of closure (Wilkinson 1989, Du Brul 1980).

Movements

The movements of the mandible are influenced by the shape and position of the teeth and result from the co-ordinated and simultaneous movement of both TM joints. They consist of depression (opening), elevation (closing), protrusion and retrusion, and lateral deviation.

- *Depression* (range 45–55 mm) is a combination of rotation and translation, produced with the help of the lateral pterygoid, digastric, mylohyoid and geniohyoid. The movements occur simultaneously after an initial relaxation of the masticatory muscles which allows the condyle to rotate relative to the disc in the lower compartment, opening the jaw approximately 1 cm.
- *Elevation*, which is limited by the contacting tooth surfaces, is the reverse of depression. It is produced by contraction of the temporalis, masseter and medial pterygoid, with the assistance of the superior head of lateral pterygoid to control the position of the condyle and disc during the closing phase.
- *Protrusion* (5 mm) is a downward and forward slide of the disc/condyle complex and is produced by the medial pterygoid along with the inferior head of lateral pterygoid and masseter, whereas *retrusion* (3–4 mm) the opposite movement, is produced by digastric and posterior temporalis.
- *Lateral deviation* (10–12 mm) involves downward, forward and medial movement of the disc/condyle complex on the contralateral side while the disc/condyle complex on the ipsilateral side rotates laterally about a vertical axis. It is performed by ipsilateral temporalis and masseter and contralateral medial and lateral pterygoid.

MECHANISM OF INJURY

The TM region may be injured directly or indirectly and consequently the cause of the symptoms is not always obvious. A detailed account of the mechanism of injury may provide a better understanding of the nature and extent of the injury. Common causes of TM disorders in sport include the following:

- Trauma to the jaw. A posteriorly directed force on the chin such as a blow from a squash racquet or hitting the ground with the point of the chin, may drive the condyle superiorly and posteriorly into the fossa. This may result in soft tissues injury, damage to the joint surfaces if the force is great enough to impact the condyle into the glenoid fossa, internal derangement of the disc, or fracture of the neck of the mandible. A blow on the side of the jaw may cause a compression injury to the contralateral joint.
- Trauma to the head. Injuries to the TM region as a consequence of trauma to the head may cause the masticatory muscles to spasm. The resultant parafunctional activity of the mandible to avoid a broken maxillary tooth or to favour one side while chewing for instance, predisposes the joint to internal derangement and degenerative change.
- Injuries to the cervical spine. Hyperextension of the cervical spine as may result from a vigorous rugby tackle may cause the mandible to open forcibly, leading to subluxation or dislocation of the jaw, disruption of the disc/condyle complex, stretching the retrodiscal ligament and straining the periarticular tissues.
- Non-use of mouth guards. Trauma to the mandible without the buffering effect of a mouthguard could result in damage to the teeth and TM joint as a result of the compressive and shearing forces to which they are subjected.

Predisposing factors

In the absence of obvious reasons for the TM region becoming symptomatic, factors which may predispose it to injury need to be taken into account:

- Emotional tension. Stress may cause increased tone in the muscles of the head and neck which in turn alters the resting position of the mandible and increases the intra-articular pressure. Chronic bruxism (grinding) may also overload the joint, giving rise to symptoms.
- Poor craniocervical posture. The forward head posture alters the position of the atlanto-occipital joints and increases the tension in the hyoid musculature. The resultant increase in muscle tone affects the resting position of the mandible and the occlusal contact pattern (Rocabado & Iglarsh 1991, Bell 1990, Kraus 1988).
- Occlusal disharmony. The increase in load on the TM joint due to a malocclusion may lead to dysfunction.
- Previous trauma. Studies have noted the prevalence of TM disc derangement following whiplash type injury of the neck due to the forces that are placed on mandible (Weiberg & LaPointe 1987) and intra-articular damage to both TM joints following mandibular fractures (Goss & Bosanquet 1990).
- History of dislocation or subluxation. Damage from recurrent or traumatic dislocations or subluxations

may result in loss of congruence of the articular surfaces (Bell 1990).

- Tooth loss. Loss of teeth, especially the molars, alters the chewing pattern. The resultant increase in load on the TM joint during mastication predisposes it to degenerative joint disease (Werner et al 1991, Hansson et al 1979, Weinberg 1976).
- Inflammatory arthritis. Rheumatoid arthritis and its variants frequently affect the TM joint and interfere with normal mandibular mechanics (Bell 1990).

SIGNS AND SYMPTOMS

The signs and symptoms may be obtained from a thorough examination and will vary depending on which structures are affected and whether they are intra- or extracapsular. Throughout the examination, all structures likely to be at fault should be assessed and consideration should also be given to their functional interdependence.

Subjective examination

In the subjective examination the clinician should aim to get a detailed description of the symptoms and their behaviour. The symptoms may include:

- Pain—frequently felt over the TM joint itself, though may radiate anteriorly, superiorly, inferiorly and posteriorly.
- Headaches—these tend to be located over the temples though it is not uncommon for patients to complain of occipital, frontal or retro-orbital symptoms.
- Neck pain—neck and shoulder pains are commonly associated with TM disorders, and may occasionally extend as far as the low back.
- Ear symptoms—ear pain, tinnitus, impaired hearing, blocked ears, vertigo and dizziness.
- Toothache—pain is commonly felt in the region of the molar or wisdom teeth.
- Throat symptoms—these include sore throat or difficulty swallowing (dysphagia).
- Functional limitations—difficulty yawning, biting and/ or chewing due to muscle guarding or mechanical dysfunction resulting from an internal derangement.
- Clicking—reciprocal clicking (both on opening and closing the mandible) is often associated with internal derangement of the disc, though a duller sound, louder on closing, may indicate subluxation of the joint.
- Crepitus—this is characteristic of degenerative joint disease (Widmalm et al 1992).
- Locking—the two types of locking occurring in the TM joint include a 'closed locked' joint (usually due to disc derangement without reduction) and an 'open locked' joint (dislocation) where the mouth cannot be closed once opened wide, as in yawning.

PHYSICAL EXAMINATION

With the exception of the craniocervical assessment, all tests should be performed with the patient in a semi-recumbent position, with the head and neck well supported. It is recommended that sterile gloves be worn by the clinician for all intra-oral procedures.

Signs to confirm the involvement of the TM area may be found when performing the following routine tests.

- Observation. Poor craniocervical posture characteristically includes forward head posture with a poking chin, elevated and protracted shoulder girdles.
- Muscle testing. Tenderness and increased tone in the masticatory and suprahyoid muscles may be elicited by isometric contraction, passive stretching and/or palpation.
- Joint line palpation. Joint tenderness may be provoked on palpation around joint line or through the external auditory meatus which provides good access to the posterior aspect of the joint.
- Oral examination. The resting position of the mandible should be assessed with the orofacial muscles relaxed. An inspection of dentition, occlusal pattern, tooth enamel for signs of wear and tongue position at rest may provide useful information. Malalignment of the incisors at rest may confirm a laterally deviated mandible.
- TM joint test movements. Opening, closing, left and right lateral deviation, protrusion and retrusion need to be assessed. Observation of movement relative to the incisors is an easy guide to the quality and quantity of movement. Palpation of the condyles as the mandible moves may detect abnormalities of movement. Abnormal movement patterns such as lateral deflections are most evident in the opening phase and may be seen in the frontal plane, while hypertranslation may be picked up in the sagittal plane. The most common pattern of restriction of movement is opening and contralateral lateral deviation.
- Accessory movements. These movements should be assessed for stiffness and reproduction of symptoms. They consist of distraction, performed with the therapist's thumb over the ipsilateral molars (Fig. 20.2), and lateral glide, with the thumb against the medial aspect of the ramus of the mandible.
  Medial glide and postero-anterior glide may be performed extra-orally with pads of thumbs as close to the joint as practically possible.
- Auscultation. Joint sounds include clicking and crepitus which may be loud enough to be heard in a quiet environment, may be heard with a stethoscope or may be felt with the fingers over the joint.
- Craniocervical palpation. Examination of the upper cervical spine is essential with all TM disorders as the

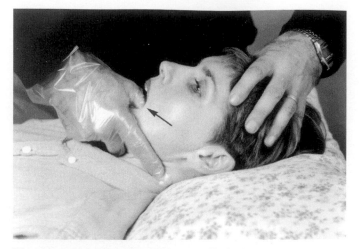

Fig. 20.2 Distraction of the temporomandibular joint

two regions are closely linked anatomically and biomechanically. Palpatory findings include pain and restricted movement in the upper cervical joints and suboccipital muscles.

Radiological examination may be indicated when considering osteoarthritis, rheumatoid arthritis, fractures and tumours as possible causes of the symptoms. It should be noted, however, that imaging of this region is difficult and various techniques may be required to obtain useful information. Standard radiographs are frequently useless in this region.

DIFFERENTIAL DIAGNOSIS

The following points should be taken into consideration when trying to differentiate between symptoms arising from TM structures and from other structures.

- Upper cervical spine. This may involve ear symptoms. The atlanto-occipital joint may refer pain to the ear which usually presents as post-auricular pain, while ear pain from the TM joint tends to be pre-auricular. There may be headaches. The areas affected by the upper cervical spine include occipital, frontal or retro-orbital (Jull 1986), whereas the temporal area is characteristically TM. Palpation of the upper cervical spine, posterior TM joint through the external auditory meatus and muscles of mastication may confirm the origin of the symptoms.
- Vertebral artery. Tinnitus, dizziness and dysphagia may be associated with vertebral artery insufficiency. A thorough examination of the cervical spine and vertebral artery testing may assist with differential diagnosis.
- Dentition. Caries, abscesses, gum disease, pulpitis and impacted wisdom teeth are common causes of toothache. Odontogenic pain may be aggravated by hot or cold beverages, or by percussion of the suspected tooth. A thorough assessment, including evaluation of the occlusion, should be undertaken by a dental surgeon to help confirm the origin of the symptoms.
- Sinuses. Frontal headaches and maxillary tooth pain originating from the sinuses may be diagnosed if the symptoms are altered with changes in head positions, and by radiological examination of the sinuses.
- Auditory apparatus. The proximity of the TM joint to the inner ear makes it difficult to distinguish the origin of such symptoms as ear pain, dizziness, tinnitus, blocked ears or impaired hearing. Clearance from an ear, nose and throat specialist may be necessary to eliminate involvement of the auditory apparatus.
- Intracranial lesions. Following trauma to the head, e.g. as in boxing, symptoms of persisting or worsening headaches, nausea, vomiting, loss of strength and affected cognitive powers should be referred promptly for further medical investigations.

PHYSIOTHERAPY MANAGEMENT

Treatment should be directed at the cause of the symptoms and will vary according to the stage and state of the pathology.

Acute stage

Having eliminated any medical or dental causes, physiotherapy management in the acute phase will usually include the following.

- Rest. The jaw should be used as little as possible, and chewy foods should be avoided. In severe cases, a liquid diet and a resting splint supplied and fitted by a dentist may be necessary. To suppress painful yawning, the patient should be taught to place the index finger horizontally between the lips and maintain the contact throughout the yawn.
- Cryotherapy. In the early stages cold applications using ice packs or towels soaked in cold water for up to 15 minutes several times per day are useful to decrease pain, swelling and spasm.
- Ultrasound. In the acute phase the dosage range is 0.05 to 1.5 W/cm^2 for 5 minutes. No heat should be felt throughout the treatment.
- Laser therapy. The therapeutic use of lasers is rapidly gaining popularity and may be used to assist tissue healing and for pain control. Dosage usually ranges from 1–8 joules/cm^2 for 5 minutes though care must be taken not to apply the beam directly into the eye.
- Exercise. If appropriate, gentle exercise should be encouraged to promote good healing. To avoid stressing the damaged soft tissues movement in the

early stages should be pain free and should be limited to rotary or hinge opening, performed with the tongue on the roof of the mouth.

Associated soft tissue injuries, particularly to the cervical spine, need to be assessed and treated concurrently, following the guidelines for management of any soft tissue injury.

Considerations for specific pathologies in the acute phase

- Dislocated joint (open locked). If self-reduction is unsuccessful, the technique of choice is a longitudinal caudad movement of the mandible in combination with a backward movement of the disc/condyle complex. Forceful reduction of the joint must not be attempted due to the possibility of the presence of a fracture of the mandibular neck or of further damaging the joint, and should be referred to an oral surgeon. No exercises should be prescribed for the open locked joint in the acute situation due to the instability.
- Disc derangement without reduction (closed locked). While some authors describe techniques for recapturing an anteriorly displaced disc (Friedman & Weisberg 1985, Kraus 1988), it is not advisable to attempt such a manoeuvre as not only is there doubt about the efficacy of the procedure, but also, if it is reduced easily, the disc may displace again just as easily unless an adequate occlusal splint to hold the condyle down and forward is available immediately. A difficult reduction may cause more damage to the disc and the articular surfaces. Management of the closed locked joint in the early stages is as for other acute injuries in this region.

Later stage

Treatment progression depends on the residual signs and symptoms.

Pain and swelling

Ultrasound (up to 3.0 W/cm^2 for 15 minutes), laser (up to 8 joules/cm^2 for 10 minutes), transcutaneous nerve stimulation [TNS], and interferential therapy may be used. Shortwave diathermy is also beneficial in the later stages, though dryness of the eyes may be a side effect, especially for wearers of contact lenses.

Muscle spasm

Ice and/or heat and gentle passive stretching will aid in the reduction of muscle spasm. A simple, effective hold-relax technique for reduction of muscle spasm involves asking the patient to bite down on spatulas which are placed between the teeth to keep the mandible opened maximally (Fig. 20.3). As the patient relaxes the jaw muscles and tries to open the mouth further, more spatulas are carefully inserted (Kraus 1988, Trott 1986).

With chronic spasm, the patient must be made aware of the resultant parafunctional activity and must identify the precipitating factors, such as emotional stress, mental or physical concentration if he or she is to control it. More persistent presentations may necessitate other strategies such as relaxation techniques, biofeedback and nocturnal splinting or even stress management.

Hypomobility

Mobilization. Tight periarticular structures require mobilization and exercise (Maitland 1991, Rocabado & Iglarsh 1991, Kraus 1988, Trott 1986). Initially mobilization should consist of accessory movements as described previously, in the direction of greatest restriction, and should be performed gently with the TM joint in the rest position (relaxed, with teeth slightly apart). Depending on the symptoms, the state of the pathology and the response to treatment, mobilization should be progressed to where firmer techniques are performed with the TM joint in different parts of the range.

Exercises. These should complement the mobilization techniques to help maintain the newly gained range. To improve opening, patients are instructed to stretch the mouth open with the tips of their index finger and thumb on the lower and upper incisors respectively (Fig. 20.4).

This exercise may be done passively or following contraction/relaxation of the depressors or contraction/relaxation of the elevators.

Lateral deviation and protrusion are best exercised with spatulas placed across the incisors to hold the

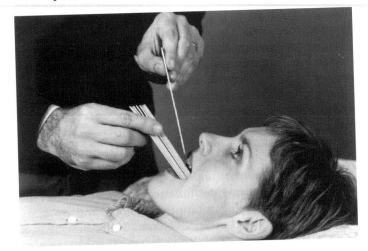

Fig. 20.3 Hold/relax technique

usually involving positioning of the neck, shoulders and arms. The limitations of the thoracic outlet tests are that they are often positive in asymptomatic individuals and are not particularly sensitive. That is, they stress many other pain sensitive structures in the cervicothoracic region which are possible sources of 'thoracic outlet' symptoms. These may include the intervertebral discs and zygapophyseal joints and their surrounding ligaments, the joints of the first or second ribs or the musculature of the area. It is vital when confronted with an athlete presenting with 'thoracic outlet syndrome' to bear these other structures in mind and include them in the physical examination as appropriate. Treatment will then be based upon examination findings rather than a nebulous diagnostic label, in this case 'thoracic outlet syndrome'. As Phillips and Grieve (1986) point out, such labels create difficulties by initiating a 'wild goose chase' for a single site of impingement when none may exist.

Age changes in the cervical spine

With increasing numbers of 'veteran competitions' and larger numbers of older people enjoying competitive and recreational sport, the physiotherapist should be aware of the effects of ageing on the cervical spine.

Clinical observation suggests that with increasing age there is a tendency for increased cervicothoracic kyphosis and reduced cervical lordosis. Loebl (1967, cited in Dalton & Jull 1989) showed an increasing upper thoracic incline in women from about 40 years of age. Dalton & Jull (1989), in a normal female population, showed an increased craniovertebral angle and decreased mobility of antero-posterior gliding of the neck with age. This may be due to poor postural habits over many years leading to adaptive soft tissue shortening. Age changes in the intervertebral discs and degenerative changes affecting the cervical vertebrae could also contribute to these abnormalities. The incidence of cervical degenerative changes shown on X-ray increases with the ageing process and would appear, clinically at least, to be associated with a reduction in the range of cervical movement.

The ageing process of the cervical intervertebral disc is of particular interest. In the second decade of life, the nucleus pulposis is replaced by firm fibrocartilage (Oda et al 1988) and horizontal fissuring of the adult disc is universal, beginning towards the end of the first decade (Twomey & Taylor 1989). In the mid to lower cervical spine horizontal fissures extend medially from the unco-vertebral joints. These fissures by the fifth or sixth decade may extend throughout the disc, establishing a gliding joint between the disc's upper and lower parts. This allows translation of several millimetres anteriorly and posteriorly in full flexion and extension respectively (Twomey & Taylor 1989).

SUBJECTIVE EXAMINATION/HISTORY

Butler (1991) reported that the subjective examination should contain information which can be categorized as follows:

- the source of the symptoms
- contributing factors
- precautions and contraindications
- management
- prognosis

The kind of disorder

The different kinds of disorder may include pain, stiffness, weakness, instability, giving way or loss of function (Maitland 1986). Athletes are very performance oriented and often present with symptoms other than pain as their main problem. Therefore, it is important to establish the kind of disorder early in the examination in order to make questioning more specific for each athlete (Magarey 1988).

The site of the symptoms

The sports physiotherapist should attempt to accurately record the location (area and depth) and nature of the symptoms on a body chart. Structures supplied by the upper three cervical nerves may refer pain to the face or head via connections in the trigemino-cervical nucleus (Kerr & Olafson 1961, Bogduk 1986). Although the upper cervical joints are commonly found to be symptomatic in headache sufferers (Jull 1986), the dura mater and cervical muscles including the upper trapezius, levator scapulae and sternocleido-mastoid are partially innervated by the upper cervical nerves and may therefore be a source of headaches (Kimmel 1961, Travell & Simons 1983).

The cervical spine may also refer pain to the upper limb either as somatic referred pain from the stimulation of the deep somatic structures (fascia, muscles, ligaments, zygaphophyseal joints, intervertebral discs) or as radicular pain from the irritation of a cervical nerve root (Bogduk 1988). Anaesthesia or paraesthesia may be present with either somatic or radicular pain (or even in the absence of any pain) due to disturbances of neural conduction. The location of these symptoms must be carefully mapped.

In addition, Cloward's investigations (1959) demonstrated that the cervical intervertebral discs can refer pain to the interscapular region and upper thoracic area. Therefore, it is important for the therapist to check these regions for symptoms which may originate in the cervical spine (Fig. 21.4).

The behaviour of the problem

This section of the subjective examination will give the therapist an indication of how the injury responds to

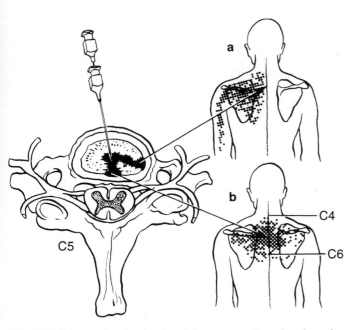

Fig. 21.4 Discogenic pain: **A** referred from postero-lateral surface of cervical discs. **B** referred from central disc ruptures

different kinds of mechanical stress and if there are other factors, such as an inflammatory process, which are contributing to symptom production.

It will help the therapist to determine how much examination will be appropriate for the athlete and whether or not mechanical treatment is indicated.

Aggravating and easing factors

'Symptoms which respond to mechanical stimuli in a predictable manner tend to have a mechanical cause' (Magarey 1988, p 85). Information regarding activities or postures which aggravate or ease the athlete's symptoms will help to determine the type and extent of the physical examination. Mechanical problems may be aggravated by movement or sustained postures. For instance, the swimmers who experiences ipsilateral neck pain while turning their head to breathe but can continue swimming are likely to have a non-irritable, mechanical disorder involving cervical rotation. Physical examination would certainly include a detailed assessment of cervical rotation, possibly in some degree of extension.

Following the collapse of a scrum, a rugby player with constant cervical, interscapular and arm pain which is aggravated by the slightest movement in any direction and takes considerable time to settle, could be regarded as having an irritable condition. Physical examination and treatment would be limited and should proceed with great caution.

24-hour behaviour

A non-mechanical, inflammatory condition may be present if the athlete reports that the symptoms are unrelieved when resting, causing him or her to wake at night and get out of bed. Further support for an inflammatory condition would be present if the athlete complains of prolonged morning stiffness and pain.

A mechanical problem may wake the athlete at night if the pillow provides inadequate support, or if turning causes pain. With mechanical problems morning stiffness is usually eased fairly quickly and will show a consistent response to mechanical stimuli throughout the day.

History

Where the injury is due to recent trauma or of relatively acute onset it is usually easier to establish the history early in the subjective examination. When the problem is long-standing or of gradual onset, the history is best left until last in order to tailor questions to information which becomes apparent with other questioning (Maitland 1986, Magarey 1988).

Traumatic causes of injury (extrinsic)

Mechanism of injury. If the injury is of traumatic origin it is important to ascertain the exact mechanism because that knowledge will help the therapist to predict the possible structures at fault, the severity of the injury and the likelihood of serious damage.

Traumatic injuries to the neck are usually associated with tackling sports such as rugby, Australian Rules football and American football, but also may be experienced in other contact sports such as wrestling, boxing, ice hockey or lacrosse (Scher 1991). Sports such as gymnastics or trampolining may lead to traumatic cervical injuries following falls from or onto the relevant equipment or apparatus (Bailes & Maroon 1989).

The physiotherapist should be able to determine from an accurate history the magnitude and direction of the applied force. The mechanism of injury may assist in identifying the possible cervical structures contributing to pain and dysfunction and the extent of the soft tissue damage. For example, a hyperflexion injury could produce compression of the anterior spinal elements and stretching or possible tearing of the posterior cervical muscles, ligaments, posterior annulus and zygapophyseal joint structures.

The collapse of a scrum in rugby may lead to hyperflexion or hyperextension injuries where the athlete's head is driven into the ground by the weight of the players behind (Myers 1980, Scher 1987, Silver & Gill 1988). Compressive forces or forced cervical rotation may also cause trauma to cervical structures. Direct blows to the head can transmit forces to the cervical spine. Blows to the neck itself may be responsible for soft tissue haematomas or ligamentous sprains and could even contribute to vertebral fractures (Marks et al 1990).

Fractures of the lower cervical spinous processes, known as 'clay shoveller's fractures' may occur from strong contraction of the musculature attaching to the spinous processes or from direct blows (Marks et al 1990, Pavlov & Torg 1987, Sparks 1985). These fractures are considered to be stable and may occur in tackling sports such as American football (Nuber & Schafer 1987) or even in power lifting (Herrick 1991).

The literature on cervical injuries (Bailes & Maroon 1989, Marks et al 1990) cites the more disastrous cervical sporting injuries as death or quadriplegia following cervical fractures or dislocations. The identification and on-field management of these incidents is beyond the scope of this chapter and has been dealt with elsewhere in this volume (see Chapter 8). Although the actual incidence of these serious injuries varies, two sports in which they occur most are rugby and American football. This is the result of the frequency and style of tackling and the heavy body contact common to both (Silver & Gill 1988, Torg et al 1985).

Despite the possibility of cervical fractures and dislocations, it appears that the most common athletic injuries to the cervical spine can be classified as sprains or strains of the cervical soft tissues (Jackson & Lohr 1986). This is still the case in contact sports such as rugby (Addley & Farren 1988, Silver & Gill 1988, Sugerman 1983) and wrestling (Wroble & Albright 1986).

Severe trauma to the cervical muscles, joints and ligaments during sporting events may resemble the hyper-flexion/hyperextension injuries caused by motor vehicle accidents. The work by Twomey and Taylor (1989, 1991) on cervical spine pathology following motor vehicle accidents may be of assistance when managing traumatic sporting injuries to the neck. Those authors found injury to be focused on the intervertebral discs, particularly at the end plate/vertebral body region with extension into the annulus and/or the vertebral body. Appreciation of pathology of this type and the length of time needed to recover from these injuries should help the physiotherapist to plan appropriate rehabilitation in an extended time-frame for athletes who suffer injuries of similar magnitude. Repeated micro-trauma to the neck as a result of sporting endeavours may also require a prolonged recovery time.

Another type of cervical injury is trauma to the brachial plexus or its roots resulting in neurological signs and symptoms. These injuries are often referred to as 'stingers' or 'burners'. There appears to be some debate as to the exact pathology. Speer and Bassett (1990) studied 19 American footballers who complained of deadness, numbness, heaviness and/or tingling and burning in the involved upper limb. They found that the symptoms abated within 5 minutes in 13 of the players and were associated with a normal neurological examination. The remaining six players reported that their symptoms abated after 15–45 minutes. The neurological findings in these athletes varied on physical examination. Mechanisms of injury were given as direct blows to the supraclavicular area or stretching of the brachial plexus with a combination of cervical contralateral flexion and shoulder depression (Speer & Bassett 1990). Poindexter and Johnson (1984) examined 12 patients with this syndrome and found that all but one had C6 radiculopathy of the nerve root rather than a more distal stretch of the brachial plexus. The most frequent mechanism of injury was hyperextension or hyperflexion of the neck. From the point of view of the sports physiotherapist, the direction of trauma may indicate whether the injury is likely to involve the nerve root or the brachial plexus itself. Hyperextension or hyperflexion injuries are more likely to damage cervical discs, zygapophyseal joints and ligaments with a secondary effect on the spinal nerve (Poindexter & Johnson 1984). Direct blows to the neck, the supraclavicular area or forces resulting in cervical lateral flexion or traction through the upper limb may cause direct injury to the brachial plexus, with or without damage to other cervical structures (Speer & Bassett 1990).

It is envisaged that radiculopathy secondary to cervical hyperflexion/hyperextension strains would be more amenable to physical therapy directed at the cervical spine than neuropraxia or axonotmesis of the brachial plexus.

Non-traumatic causes of injury

Sporting injuries to the cervical region are not always due to a single traumatic incident. The sustained postures required for archery, pistol shooting or rifle shooting may lead to neck pain and stiffness. In sailing, neck positioning for checking and adjusting the sail trim could have similar consequences. Cervical pain or dysfunction which can develop as a result of occupational or postural stresses may be triggered or aggravated by the athlete's sport.

Incorrect technique or a poorly designed weightlifting program could lead to muscle imbalance and then to cervical dysfunction. Sports involving throwing (e.g. baseball, cricket, field events) or racquet sports involve the transmission of forces through the upper limb to the neck and can lead to cervical problems through overuse or poor technique.

An example of cervical injury due to poor technique was reported by Paley and Gillespie (1986) where cervical instability was seen in a 17-year-old female high-jumper as a result of repetitive flexion loading of her cervical spine due to incorrect landing technique.

Other factors which need consideration in the history include the results and type of previous treatment, the duration of the disorder and whether it is getting worse, better or remaining the same. These factors will influence the physiotherapist's expectations of treatment outcome. For an athlete whose disorder is getting worse, a stabilization in the condition after treatment may be seen as a positive result, whereas a stabilization would be unacceptable for an athlete whose conditon was already improving. In the latter case the treatment would need to be modified or changed (see Chapter 12).

Past history

It is useful to determine the past history of previous neck problems, their duration and any treatment received. A recurring problem will obviously need more than simply treating the acute episode. In these cases, patient education, identification of predisposing or precipitating factors and technique modification become more important.

Screening questions

The athlete's history should include specific questions regarding general health, medication taken, recent weight loss and X-ray findings to indicate the presence of any factors which may contraindicate or require special caution in the provision of physical treatment.

General health

The possibility of systemic disease such as rheumatoid arthritis should be discounted. In cases where the athlete does have a history of rheumatoid arthritis and presents with neck pain, the physiotherapist must be aware of the possibility of upper cervical instability and proceed with extreme caution in examination and treatment. Care should also be taken with patients who appear generally unwell due to undetected co-existing systemic disease. A history of malignancy, particularly breast cancer when dealing with upper quarter problems, requires caution.

Medication

Long-term cortico-steroid therapy for a variety of diseases can lead to osteoporosis, thereby warranting care with stronger techniques. It is useful to know whether the patient is taking analgesics or anti-inflammatory medication because a sudden aggravation in the condition could be due to the athlete stopping the medication rather than to the physical treatment. Conversely, these drugs may mask the full extent of the injury.

A good response to anti-inflammatory medication may indicate a significant inflammatory component in the condition, possibly limiting the role of manual therapy. Non-response to these drugs may indicate that the condition could be a mechanical problem and may respond well to manual therapy.

Forceful manual techniques may be contraindicated for patients on anti-coagulant medication.

Unexplained weight loss

This may be associated with systemic disease or malignancy. While primary neoplasms of the cervical spine are rare, Golding (1969) reported three cases of meningioma that presented with cervical and occipital pain and restricted cervical flexion. Pancoast tumours of the apex of the lung may cause neck and arm symptoms through irritation or compression of somatic structures or the cervicothoracic nerve roots.

X-rays

It is better to actually view the X-rays if they have been taken to establish the quality of the films and the various views taken. For instance, open-mouth views are important to visualize the upper cervical spine. Oblique foraminal views should be included where nerve-root compromise is suspected and functional views should be performed where instability or hypermobility is suspected. Webb et al (1976) and Herkowitz and Rothman (1984) have detailed cases where cervical instability following flexion injury was detected on X-ray when initial examination was considered normal. These cases highlight the need for flexibility and open-mindedness in examination, particularly where previous testing has proven negative.

It is the view of the authors that cervical X-rays are mandatory after sporting injuries to the cervical spine when:

1. the force of the injury is significant, e.g. a forceful, direct blow or a fall onto the neck or head or after a strong tackle
2. the condition is irritable
3. there are consistent neurological signs or symptoms
4. the condition is not improving
5. movement is restricted by muscle spasm which is out of proportion to the presenting symptoms.

These precautions will speed the identification and recognition of serious pathology or instability and minimize the likelihood of medico-legal repercussions.

Spinal cord

Unsteadiness of gait, anaesthesia or paraesthesia in both hands or both feet and positive Babinki reflex can indicate cervical spinal cord involvement. If the sports physiotherapist suspects trespass of the spinal cord an urgent medical referral is advised.

Vertebral artery

As discussed previously the vertebral artery may be damaged by sports injuries or decreased blood flow may exist concurrently with neck pain and dysfunction. Death or stroke following inappropriate manipulative treatment are the most serious consequences of spinal manipulative therapy. Sports physiotherapists treating the cervical region must be able to identify the athlete at risk and have appropriate skills to minimize the likelihood of complications from mobilization or manipulation.

Dizziness is the most common symptom of vertebrobasilar insufficiency but may also arise from a number of other sources, including disorders of the upper cervical spine (Bogduk 1986). Other symptoms such as drop attacks, dysphagia (difficulty in swallowing), diplopia (double vision) and dysarthria (difficulty with speech) may help the physiotherapist differentiate between vertebrobasilar insufficiency and dizziness of cervical origin. However, Grant (1988) reported that such differentiation may be difficult when dizziness is the only presenting symptom. If there is a possibility that vertebrobasilar insufficiency exists the therapist must take great care with examination and treatment procedures that could further compromise blood flow, particularly cervical rotation and extension, or a combination of these two manoeuvres. Cervical manipulation and any other technique which reproduces the dizziness is contraindicated in these patients.

PHYSICAL EXAMINATION

From the information gained in the subjective examination the therapist can determine the extent, type and direction of the physical examination. If the condition is irritable, as in many acute sports injuries, only one or two cervical movements may be examined to the onset of pain. For a more chronic, non-irritable condition combined movements and overpressure at the limit of range may be more appropriate (Edwards 1988).

At this stage it is worth remembering that the cervical spine should be considered as a possible source of symptoms in all upper limb syndromes. The emphasis and timing of the cervical examination will obviously vary from patient to patient.

As stated previously, it is the authors' opinion that the cervicothoracic region should be examined in all sporting problems of the upper quarter. The cervical spine should not be discarded as a source of symptoms until a thorough examination of passive intervertebral movement has been performed. Such examination must be performed even if there is no history of neck pain or stiffness and active movements are full range and pain free with overpressure.

Chadwick (1987) claims that when there is a central component to a peripheral problem, treatment of the spinal component enhances the effect of ensuing peripheral treatment. Grieve (1988) agrees noting that mobilization and manipulation of the spine can eradicate peripheral changes. Accurate reassessment will help to determine the efficacy of each technique.

Indicators which suggest a significant cervical component to an upper limb problem may include a chronic or recurring condition despite appropriate local treatment. Examples commonly seen are tennis elbow and shoulder tendonitis. A cervical component may also be suspected if the athlete presents with an atypical level of local pain or more tenderness than could be expected from the degree of the injury. The athlete may present with more than one symptom. For instance, an athlete with 'tennis elbow' may complain of intermittent lateral elbow pain which may be associated with a constant ache in the arm or forearm. The constant ache is frequently cervical in origin and abates with treatment directed to the neck. Treatment may then be focused on the peripheral lesion.

In the treatment of 'swimmer's shoulder' Popov (1989) considered that normalizing cervicothoracic movement and improving scapular control are of equal importance as symptomatic treatment of the shoulder. He indicated that the continued treatment of the central component, both in a given treatment session and in the long term, seems to yield the best results.

Schneider (1989) indicated that when shoulder stiffness is present in a non-proportional pattern (i.e. some movements far more limited than others), there may be a causal relationship with cervical somatic structures.

Throughout the physical examination the physiotherapist must evaluate the effect of each procedure on the athlete's condition. Questioning should be precise and unambiguous. The tests performed should be precise and reproducible. The physiotherapist needs to be aware of any overall change in the athlete's condition as the examination proceeds.

Observation

The total posture of the athlete in sitting and standing is observed since thoracic and lumbar posture can affect cervical positioning. Special attention should be paid to the head-on-neck and neck-on-thorax postures. An athlete with an acute wry neck or locked zygapophyseal joint may present with the head tilted away from the side of the pain. A poking chin may be associated with tightness of the upper cervical extensors and weakness of the deep neck flexors in an athlete complaining of upper cervical pain and headaches. An increased cervicothoracic kyphosis associated with a forward head posture may indicate thickened soft tissues or articular stiffness in the lower cervical region while a straightening of the neck/shoulder curve when viewed from the front may indicate tightness of the upper trapezius and levator scapulae muscles (Janda 1988).

An athlete's poor sitting posture may be a factor in pain reproduction during prolonged sitting or may even delay recovery after trauma. In some cases assessment of specific postures required in the course of the athlete's sport is necessary to gain an appreciation of the demands of the activity on the neck or to assist in reproducing the symptoms during the physical examination.

Active movement tests

The standard movement tests for the cervical spine are flexion/extension, rotation and lateral flexion. The following features should be noted with these cervical movements and with subsequent movement tests:

- range
- quality
- onset/change of pain or other symptoms (e.g. paraesthesia)
- behaviour of symptoms through range
- limiting factor (e.g. pain, spasm, resistance)
- quality of the end feel (if appropriate).

The standard movement tests can be altered by combining different cervical movements as described by Edwards (1980, 1988), altering the speed of the movement, sustaining or repeating the movement or adding cervical compression. The movements may also be localized to different areas by specific handling and overpressures (Maitland 1986). In cases where only one or two movements or positions aggravate the athlete's symptoms it may be informative to ask the athlete to demonstrate the specific activity which aggravates the symptoms. For example, the head position during a golf swing or archery stance, the combination of cervical movements during a tennis serve or a badminton smash can help the therapist modify the examination to suit the athlete's injury. The provoking activity or position is a useful sign to reassess after treatment. Repeated cervical movements and cervical protraction/retraction may help the therapist using the approach advocated by McKenzie to achieve a mechanical diagnosis of the cervical injury (Stevens & McKenzie 1988).

Palpation

Palpation of the vertebrae and soft tissues of the cervical region is an integral part of the physical examination and may be performed with the athlete in prone and/or supine.

The bony prominences of the cervical vertebrae must be palpated and any malalignments or asymmetries should be noted. Anomalies of the bifid spinous processes of the cervical vertebrae and differences in their spacing are not uncommon and may not be clinically significant. The clay shoveller's fracture of the spinous process will show marked tenderness on palpation although the diagnosis of this fracture needs to be confirmed radiologically.

Palpation of the soft tissues of the neck should include the vascular and neural tissues at the root of the neck, the trachea and the oesophagus if these areas are related to the injury or the symptoms. The deep and superficial cervical muscles are palpated for increased tension or spasm (discrete or generalized) and the presence of trigger points as described by Travell and Simons (1983).

The sports physiotherapist should beware when an athlete presents with excessive cervical muscle spasm or rigidity following trauma as these may be protective of underlying pathology such as fracture, dislocation or instability.

Passive intervertebral movement tests

Passive physiological intervertebral movements (PPIVMs)

These movements can be tested with the athlete in the sitting position but the supine position usually enables better relaxation necessary for accurate feel of the movement by the therapist. Magarey (1988) pointed out that PPIVMs can be used to confirm any restriction of motion seen on active movement tests, to detect restriction of movement not discovered by the active movement tests and to detect hypermobility. A loss of the normal end feel may be associated with instability. For a detailed account of the positioning and handling required for PPIVMs the reader is referred to Maitland (1986).

Passive accessory intervertebral movements (PAIVMs)

Examination of PAIVMs usually involves postero-anterior (p-a) pressures on the spinous processes centrally and laterally on each articular pillar or facet joint-line. The direction of pressure may be directed cephalad, caudad, medially, laterally or in any combination of these. PAIVMs can also be tested with the neck positioned in different combinations of physiological movements of the neck. PAIVMs may also be tested from the anterior aspect of the vertebra in an antero-posterior direction. The presence of abnormality of movement, pain or other symptoms (local or referred), end feel and relationship of pain and resistance through range are all noted. Maitland (1982, 1986) offers a comprehensive account of the techniques and findings of cervical palpation.

Muscle tests

As mentioned previously the cervical musculature may be a source of neck pain or dysfunction or the muscles may contribute to symptoms from other structures such as the cervical zygapophyseal joints.

Testing muscles as a source of pain may include palpation of the muscle and its attachments, isometric contraction and stretching the muscle. Janda (1988) described a situation in the cervical region where certain muscles become short and tight while others become weak, thereby creating muscle imbalance. In the upper quarter this imbalance is known as the 'proximal crossed syndrome'. It involves tightness of the upper trapezius, levator scapulae and pectoral muscles with weakness of the lower scapular stabilizers and the deep neck flexors. This imbalance can lead to cervical problems by accentuating the cervicothoracic kyphosis with a compensatory increase in the mid-cervical lordosis and upper cervical extension. Janda (1988) discussed the implication of this syndrome on scapular and glenohumeral function. Watson and Trott (1991) found that cervical headache sufferers were more likely to exhibit a forward head posture and have loss of strength and endurance in the upper cervical flexors than a non-headache population.

Athletes are often prone to developing muscular imbalance, such as the proximal crossed syndrome due to the participation in weight-training regimes which over-emphasize pectoral and upper trapezius strength at the expense of the lower scapular stabilizers and deep neck flexors. Muscular imbalance should be suspected in athletes participating in weight training regimes and should be routinely assessed in athletes with chronic or recurring neck or shoulder problems, particularly when treatment directed at the cervical joints is not improving the condition or giving long term relief.

Evaluation of muscle imbalance is commenced by observing the overall posture of the athlete, noting hypertrophy, wasting and tightness of the soft tissues . The physiotherapist should also examine for fibrous bands, tightness within the muscles, myofascial trigger points and other anomalies. Details of testing for tight muscles and evaluation of inhibition and weakness is beyond the scope of this section and may be found in Janda (1983, 1988) and Travell and Simons (1983).

Neurological examination

It is necessary to perform a neurological examination when there is a possibility of neural compromise. When considering injuries to the cervical spine possible levels of involvement are:

- spinal cord
- spinal nerve-root
- peripheral nerve.

Spinal cord

Sporting injuries resulting in spinal cord trespass must be diagnosed at the time of injury and receive the appropriate care. Fractures, dislocations, instabilities and, less commonly, massive posterior cervical disc herniation may lead to cord signs as many subacute instabilities, particularly if occurring with a congenitally narrow spinal canal. As mentioned previously, patients with suspected spinal cord involvement should be referred immediately for medical opinion.

Spinal nerve roots

Injury to the spinal nerve roots is possibly the most common neurological problem associated with sporting injuries to the neck. A segmental neurological examination includes testing of sensation, deep tendon reflexes and muscle power.

Because of the variability of dermatomes and the common co-existence of somatic referred pain (which is deep and poorly localized) and radicular pain, it is difficult to predict a level of nerve root involvement solely on the distribution of symptoms (pain, anaesthesia or paraesthesia) (Grieve 1988).

Dalton and Jull (1989) examined 42 subjects with neck and arm pain and reported their inability to predict the likelihood of neurological findings based on the distribution and characteristics of the pain. For this reason a segmental neurological examination is recommended in patients complaining of numbness, tingling, weakness or pain extending into the upper limb. A neurological examinaton is also recommended in athletes with cervical pain only when the condition is worsening. Details of the neurological examination for the upper quarter may be found elsewhere (Butler 1991, Grieve 1988, Maitland 1986).

Neurological findings should be closely monitored with regard to the treatment given. Any deterioration in neurological function should be noted and appropriate medical opinion sought.

Peripheral nerves

In chronic or recurring arm symptoms examination of the whole extent of the peripheral nerve is warranted. This would include muscle strength and sensory testing, palpation along the course of the nerve and tests of neural mobility via the relevant upper limb tension tests (Butler 1991, Selvaratnam et al 1989, Selvaratnam 1991) (see Chapter 26).

Vertebral artery testing

Vertebral artery testing must be performed to assess the relationship between neck movements and symptoms which may be vertebrobasilar in origin. Such examination should be performed when the subjective examination suggests that blood flow may be affected (complaints of dizziness, diplopia, drop attacks, dysarthria and dysphagia) or prior to a manipulative technique which may compromise the blood flow to the brain (Australian Physiotherapy Association 1988, Grant 1988).

Physical tests of the vertebrobasilar system most commonly include components of rotation and/or extension as these movements have been found to be most likely to affect blood flow (Tatlow & Bammer 1957, Toole & Tucker 1960).

Tests advocated by the Australian Physiotherapy Association protocol (1988) include the following manoeuvres:

- Sustained rotation to the left and right
- Sustained extension
- Sustained rotation and extension to the left and right
- Any position described by the patient that causes dizziness.

These tests are sustained for at least ten seconds and are discontinued if symptoms are reproduced. If negative in the sitting position, testing can be performed in supine where the non-weightbearing position affords a greater range of cervical mobility.

Grant (1988) recommended that two further tests should be carried out before cervical manipulation is attempted. First, to increase rotatory stress at the C1–C2 level, unilateral postero-anterior pressure is applied to the C1–C2 zygaphophyseal joint with the patient prone and the neck in ipsilateral rotation. Second, the patient's neck is held in the position of manipulation and the response noted.

It should be noted that a positive response to these tests does not necessarily indicate vertebrobasilar dysfunction. Other cervical structures including the muscles, joints and ligaments of the upper cervical spine may cause dizziness on these tests (Bogduk 1986). Hutchison (1989) investigated 50 patients with cervical pain and found that those with upper cervical dysfunction were significantly more likely to have a positive vertebral artery test than those with lower cervical dysfunction. This finding indicates either that vertebrobasilar insufficiency exists more commonly in patients with upper cervical dysfunction (which has not yet been proven) or that the positive test (i.e. reproduction of dizziness) is due to the upper cervical dysfunction in at least some of these patients. More investigation needs to be conducted on these tests to determine their sensitivity. It should also be borne in mind that the tests do not reproduce the high velocity thrust component of cervical manipulation reported to be a significant factor in vascular complications after manipulation (Bogduk 1986).

In summary, cervical manipulation is contraindicated in athletes in whom the subjective examination or physical tests indicate the possibility of vertebrobasilar insufficiency. To minimize the risk of complications, sports physiotherapists should avoid large amplitude and forceful manipulation, particularly involving cervical rotation. Specific manipulation using minimal force is recommended.

Spinal canal and foraminal tension tests

Restriction of motion of the pain sensitive structures in the spinal canal and the intervertebral foraminae can contribute to neck pain and referred cervical pain patterns. These structures include the dura mater, the nerve roots and their dural sheaths and blood vessels within the canal and intervertebral foramen (Maitland 1979). These structures are more likely to be implicated when the cervical injury is chronic in nature, when it is associated with thoracic or lumbar symptoms or when it is not responding as anticipated to manual treatment aimed at the cervical joints or muscles. The tests which are most likely to be positive in these cases include the slump test, the upper limb tension tests or the passive neck flexion test. These tests are described in detail in Chapters 26 and 33.

Performing the active and passive movement tests outlined earlier in a position which produces increased tension on the dura or brachial plexus may give substantially different results when compared to the same tests performed in the neutral position, e.g. cervical movements may be tested in the slumped position with and without the addition of knee extension. Similarly, the assessment of a unilateral postero-anterior PAIVM may be performed with the upper limb in a position of increased tension of the brachial plexus (Fig. 21.5). This type of testing may not be appropriate for every athlete with a cervical injury, but may give valuable information regarding the relationship between neural mobility and dysfunction of other cervical structures.

MANAGEMENT

The management of sports injuries of the cervical spine will depend on the nature of the injury, the aims and expectations of the athlete and the physiotherapist and the examination findings. The therapist should always be aware of external pressures exerted on the athlete by coaches, family, peers and others. To avoid a premature return to

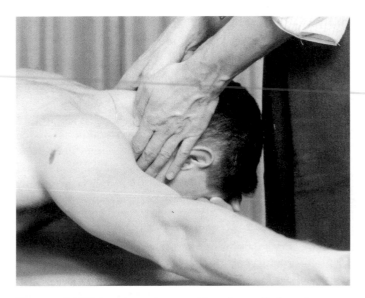

Fig. 21.5 PAIVMs performed in a position of upper limb tension may give different results from the same test performed with the arm in neutral

activity or competitive sport the athlete should be fully informed of the nature of the disorder and, where appropriate, liaison between the therapist, athlete and coach encouraged.

The main aim of the initial treatment session should be to address the immediate cause of the symptoms and, if necessary, the main predisposing or precipitating factors. Once pathology necessitating medical intervention has been ruled out the following modalities are available to the physiotherapist:

- Rest
- Support
- Ice
- Electrotherapy
- Manual therapy
- Education
- Exercises.

These will be discussed in relation to acute, chronic and recurrent sports injuries of the neck.

Acute injuries

In many sporting injuries, particularly those traumatic in nature, the most effective treatments in the early stages are those which restrict the inflammatory response and relieve pain. Electrotherapy modalities such as electrical stimulation, interferential, magnetic field therapy or lasers are often used in the treatment of acute cervical injuries. Their indications and use are detailed in Chapter 15. The application of ice packs is also a useful adjunct to treatment at this stage. They can be applied by the athlete at a frequency and duration specified by the physiotherapist. Non-steroidal anti-inflammatories, analgesics and muscle relaxants, when not contraindicated, can be of great benefit in the relief of inflammation, pain and swelling (see Ch. 37).

In more severe injuries to the cervical intervertebral discs and joints, where there is no bony damage, Twomey and Taylor (1991) recommend an initial period of immobilization for a few days. This facilitates the resolution of effusion and ensures that bleeding into the damaged area has ceased. They advocate that gentle, small amplitude active movements in the pain free range should be started after this time and active movement should then be steadily progressed over a number of weeks, depending on the patient's response.

The use of a cervical collar may be indicated in the acute stage of cervical injuries, particularly if the condition is irritable or range of movement is drastically reduced by pain. Collars may be firm or soft depending on the degree of support required. They are made from a variety of materials, ranging from sponge rubber to firm plastic reinforced with metal struts.

Collars can be beneficial when the athlete comments that supporting the head gives relief or that the neck feels like it needs support. Neck injuries in contact sports such as Australian Rules or American football, rugby or sports resulting in falls onto the head and neck such as gymnastics, trampolining, wrestling, surfing or sailboarding, may be severe enough to warrant the temporary use of a cervical collar. The athlete should be warned not to drive a motor vehicle while wearing the collar as restriction of neck mobility will reduce vision. If the collar is not beneficial or it makes the condition worse it should be discarded. The collar should be viewed as temporary assistance only and the athlete gradually weaned off it. As Grieve (1988) notes, a cervical support should never be provided without a plan to eliminate it.

Manual therapy used judiciously will often lead to decreased pain and increased range of movement. The type and direction of the manual technique will depend largely on the examination findings. A localized unilateral problem may be best treated with a PAIVM to the affected level. In comparison, an injury affecting a number of cervical levels may respond to a more generalized physiological technique (see Ch. 12). If the athlete experiences severe pain or has an irritable condition the technique should be performed short of reproducing the symptoms. Careful positioning of the neck by the physiotherapist may be necessary to achieve a pain-free starting positon and the subsequent technique should be performed without producing pain.

Where severe nerve root pain is present the technique should be aimed at opening the intervertebral foramen on the affected side. This may be achieved with a longitudinal technique (traction), contralateral rotation or possibly a combination of movements which lead to decreased impingement of the nerve root.

Manual techniques aimed at the cervical muscles may also be useful, particularly gentle massage or muscle energy techniques which involve' minimal contraction and subsequent relaxation, followed by gentle stretching (Lee 1986) (see Chs 12 and 14).

The use of heat can be useful in the acute phase of neck injuries although it is contraindicated in the initial stages due to the presence of inflammation. Muscle relaxation and pain relief can be achieved with electromedical equipment such as ultrasound, shortwave and microwave. Clinically, hot packs can be equally effective and are easily mimicked by the athlete at home with the common hot water bottle (see Ch. 15).

Advice to an athlete and education regarding the injury is very important, especially in the acute stage. With severe injuries, avoidance of the sport or activity is essential while less significant injuries may not restrict the athlete at all.

Most athletes are very keen to know the nature and extent of the injury and how it will limit their participation in their sport. With some neck injuries it is impossible to give an accurate answer to these questions, particularly in the early stages. The physiotherapist should take into account the following factors when planning a return to sport for an athlete with an acute neck injury.

The nature and severity of the injury

The more severe the initial injury the longer the athlete is likely to take to recover. A rugby player with widespread musculoligamentous damage following a hyperflexion injury is likely to take a number of weeks to recover. However, a gymnast with a localized joint strain after twisting her neck at training will most likely be 100% fit in a matter of days.

The demands of the sport

The physiotherapist should consider how the particular sport affects the athlete's cervical region. Certain sports may place particular stress on the cervical region while others may not require involvement of the neck at all. Rotation flexibility is required for freestyle swimming while the ability to cope with sustained postures is required for rifle shooting or sailing. In rugby and wrestling, strength and flexibility are required for the demands of the sport.

Predisposing factors

Poor postural habits, muscle imbalance, lack of mobility, strength and endurance and poor technique are factors which may have predisposed the neck to injury. These will need to be addressed in the treatment program and possibly eliminated before a successful return to sport by the athlete.

The risk of reinjury

The physiotherapist must weigh up the above factors to decide the likelihood of reinjury upon the athlete's return to sport. Ideally, there should be no risk or minimal risk but this is not always the case. Some athletes will return to sport prematurely despite advice to the contrary. The risks of early return to sport must be clearly spelt out to the athlete by the physiotherapist.

Chronic and recurring injuries

The physical management of chronic or recurring sporting injuries to the neck requires a different approach to the treatment of acute injuries. Control of the inflammatory response is usually not a high priority and the injuries are less likely to be irritable. The athlete may still be participating in the sport, albeit with reduced effectiveness. The physiotherapist should look beyond the immediate source of the symptoms and identify and treat any underlying factors. An abnormality in any or all of these factors could contribute to symptoms arising from the neck. Thus, for long term relief, an effective treatment regime for chronic or recurrent neck injuries will need to incorporate assessment and management of following aspects:

- Upper quarter posture
- Upper quarter muscle length/strength/endurance
- Upper quarter joint mobility
- Postural requirements of the sport
- Specific technique of the athlete.

Upper quarter posture

Poor postural habits may predispose the cervical spine to dysfunction and pain or perpetuate pre-existing pathology. The most common abnormality is the forward head posture (Stevens & McKenzie 1988). It is important that athletes are taught to recognize the times when their posture is poor. These are likely to include periods of prolonged sitting at work, when driving a car or even when relaxing in front of the television at night.

The posture adopted after sport may also be a factor in symptom production. McKenzie (1981) reported that pain after activity is often caused by the subsequent faulty posture rather than the activity itself. The athlete should be encouraged to correct faulty cervical posture at regular intervals throughout the day. The technique of over-correcting into retraction or posterior gliding as described by McKenzie (1983) is recommended. Correction of sitting posture may be limited by cervicothoracic joint stiffness or muscular tightness. Techniques to improve joint mobility or muscle length may be necessary before postural correction can be attained.

Postural correction may also extend to the sleeping position, particularly if the athlete wakes with pain at night or has morning pain and stiffness of mechanical (as opposed to inflammatory) origin. Alteration of the sleeping position may be necessary, particularly if the athlete sleeps in prone position with the neck in rotation or extension. The physiotherapist should evaluate whether the athlete's pillow provides adequate support for the cervical region in all sleeping positions. Feather pillows of sufficient density for support are recommended, although the choice of pillow will often depend on the individual requirements and preferences of the athlete.

Upper quarter muscle length/strength/endurance

As Janda (1988) contends, dysfunction in the muscular system in the upper body may be closely related to the joint dysfunction which is often seen in athletes presenting with chronic or recurring cervical problems. This appears to be more common in athletes who undertake weight training programs or whose sports involve repetitive or sustained muscular contraction e.g. swimmers, sailboarders and archers.

Treatment of the muscular component of the disorder may involve the stretching of tight muscles, which in cervical problems are most commonly the upper trapezius, the pectorals and levator scapulae (Janda 1988). Strengthening or retraining of weakened muscles (deep neck flexors and lower scapular stabilizers) may also be required to regain muscular balance and co-ordinated movement. A home program of specific exercises will be necessary to achieve optimum results (Janda & Schmid 1980).

Other techniques affecting muscles and surrounding soft tissues may be used in the treatment of neck injuries. These include the various forms of soft tissue massage and associated rhythmic techniques (Hartman 1983) and the deep transverse frictions as described by Cyriax (1974) (see Ch. 14).

Upper quarter joint mobility including neck, thorax, shoulder complex and shoulder girdle

Clinically, cervical zygapophyseal joint stiffness is common in many athletes with chronic or recurring neck injuries. Spinal manipulative therapy involving passive mobilization and manipulation may form part of the treatment of these patients. The selection of technique will rely on the nature and direction of movement restriction and the degree of any associated pain. For more detail in the selection of passive movement techniques the reader is referred to Magarey (1985), Maitland (1986) and Grieve (1988) (see Ch. 12). A program of exercises may be necessary to maintain any increase in range following treatment and to improve muscular control of the newly gained range.

Hypermobility

In acute or recurring neck problems hypermobility or minor instability can often be overlooked, particularly if adjacent levels are stiff or the patient appears to improve with therapy aimed at increasing joint range. As mentioned previously under 'examination', careful subjective questioning, close observation of active movements and precise passive testing of intersegmental mobility can alert the physiotherapist to the presence of hypermobility or instability.

Hypermobility has been defined by Maitland (1986, p viii) as 'an excessive range of movement for which there is complete muscular control'. Similarly, instability is defined as 'an excessive range of abnormal movement for which there is no protective muscular control' (Maitland 1986, p viii).

Certain features in the examination may alert the physiotherapist to the possibility of hypermobility or instability as a source of the symptoms. The patient may use the terms 'unstable' or 'weak'.

Previous treatment aimed at joint mobilizing may have had little or no lasting effect and investigations such as plain X-rays, CT scans and MR imaging are usually normal. Functional views are often useful in detecting segmental hypermobility and minor instability in these athletes.

The athlete needs to understand the nature of the problem in these cases because rehabilitation tends to be prolonged. Aggravating activities should be initially avoided. Later they are gradually reintroduced as tissue healing takes place and the athlete builds up muscular strength and endurance to support and protect the injured segment. This is illustrated by the following case study.

A 19-year-old boxer presented with bilateral mid-lower cervical pain of 6 months' standing, following a blow on the head by a falling piece of timber. The patient had been treated with passive mobilization and manipulation in conjunction with generalized range of motion exercises. This therapy had given relief until the boxer had restarted sparring, when punches to the head would re-aggravate the pain.

Cervical active movements were full range and pain-free although increased range of flexion/extension at C5–C6 was noted. Passive physiological movements confirmed the suspected increased movement at C5–C6. Assessment of accessory movements revealed hypomobility in the C6–T2 region and excessive movement at the C5–C6 level.

It was hypothesized from the clinical findings that the athlete's symptoms were related to the hypermobility at the C5–C6 level, while the stiffness in the lower levels (C6–T2) contributed to increased mechanical stress at C5–C6. It was further hypothesized that the boxer did not have the muscular control necessary to absorb the shock of the punches taken to the head, leading to further stress on the C5–C6 level.

Treatment consisted of passive mobilization and manipulation directed specifically at the hypomobile C6–T2 region. An exercise program was devised to strengthen and re-educate the cervical musculature, particularly the cervical flexors and rotatators. It was felt that control of these movements was necessary to withstand the forces applied from anteriorly or antero-laterally due to the punches.

The exercises were performed in the upright position and resistance was applied by the patient with his fist under his chin for the flexion exercises and with his hand on the side of his face for those involving rotation. Initially, the exercises were performed as an isometric contraction, holding for 5 seconds for 10 repetitions and performed at least three times per day. As the isometric strength improved, the flexors and rotators were worked concentrically and eccentrically. Initially, the contractions were slow and controlled, but the speed of the movement was increased as the control and strength increased over a number of weeks. The athlete returned to boxing after

12 weeks and had no recurrences after a further 6 months of normal training and fighting.

Specific postural requirements of the sport

Sports such as archery, shooting and sailing all require static positioning of the head and neck which may lead to cervical pain and dysfunction. If poor cervical posture is a contributing factor to the cause of the injury or is hampering recovery, the physiotherapist and the athlete should analyse the specific positioning required and discuss how to modify or regularly interrupt these postures.

Specific technique of the athlete

Technique modification may also help to reduce the strain on cervical structures. Faulty technique may be a contributing factor to cervical injuries in swimming, racquet sports or throwing sports.

Bower (1989) described anterior neck pain in backstrokers, often precipitated by an increase in the distance swum while holding the neck in a flexed position. On examination tenderness was evoked on palpation of the scalene and sternomastoid muscles. Treatment involved stretching of the tight muscles, electrotherapy and, more importantly, technique correction to improve mid to lower cervical extension (see Ch. 23).

Bower (1989) also recommended that in freestyle swimmers, unilateral breathing may be valuable in the short term if performed away from the side of the neck problem or shoulder impingement. A possible explanation for this is that patients with unilateral neck or shoulder problems commonly present with painful ipsilateral neck rotation due to compression or closing down of the cervical structures on that side. Unilateral breathing away from the painful side would ease the strain on these structures and allow the swimmer to continue training or competing without aggravating the condition. Part of the physiotherapy treatment should be directed at normalizing the ipsilateral rotation as well as appropriate local measures to the shoulder itself.

Instruction in correct tackling techniques may reduce the incidence of cervical injury in sports such as rugby, Australian Rules football and gridiron. Bailes and Maroon (1989), Sugerman (1983), and Wroble and Albright (1986) reported that instruction regarding correct holds and falls in wrestling may decrease the likelihood of injury.

PREVENTION

The prevention of sporting injuries to the cervical region and recurrence of such injuries are high priorities for physiotherapists working with sporting teams or with individual athletes. Ideally, before returning to sport, an athlete should have full painless range of active and passive cervical movement and normal muscle strength and control. Wroble and Albright (1986) reported that wrestlers returning to a new season with persisting symptoms had a higher risk of reinjury than those who had made a full recovery. If athletes insist on returning to competition with less than full function the physiotherapist must make them aware of the increased risk of reinjury or aggravation of the condition.

Many authors (Jackson & Lohr 1986, Wroble & Albright 1986, Bailes & Maroon 1989) advocate the use of muscle strengthening exercises to prevent cervical spine injuries. Programs for cervical muscle strengthening should be specific for that athlete's condition and for the particular sport. A non-specific strengthening program may lead to or aggravate muscle imbalance in the cervical region and cause rather than prevent cervical injury.

The importance of correct technique has already been discussed in relation to the prevention of sporting injuries to the cervical region. The therapist may have to work closely with the athlete's coach or trainer to make changes in this area. Videotaping performance may also help to pick up technique deficiencies which require correction. This allows athletes to watch their own performance and helps to reinforce the need to alter technique.

Other factors not directly under the control of the therapist may also help prevent cervical sporting injuries. Alteration of the rules of the game and the strict policing of these rules by referees may help prevent injuries. For example, the eradication of spearing in gridiron and rugby, where the opponent is 'speared' headfirst into the ground, appears to have reduced the incidence of severe neck injuries in these sports (Silver & Gill 1988, Bailes & Maroon 1989, Fine et al 1991). Similarly, the prevention of high tackles in contact sports will help decrease the incidence of trauma to the neck (Scher 1987). The prevention of illegal holds in wrestling which may cause the wrestler to be thrown to the mat without any control can help prevent injuries to the neck (Wroble & Albright 1986).

SUMMARY

Although sporting injuries to the cervical region are not as common as to other areas of the body the consequences of injury to this area are often great. Severe injury, resulting in fracture or dislocation and subsequent neurological complications, must be diagnosed immediately and appropriate action taken. Less severe injuries to the cervical joints, muscles or nerves can be incapacitating and require careful management for optimal recovery.

In sporting injuries of the upper quarter, the cervical spine should always be considered as a possible source of the symptoms and not discarded until active and passive movements have been proven to be full range and pain-free.

Specific questioning regarding the mechanism of injury and behaviour of the symptoms is important, as is a knowledge of the requirements of the athlete's sport. A thorough and detailed assessment of both the source of the symptoms and any predisposing factors is essential. This assessment allows the athlete and the physiotherapist to plan a program of management with short and long term goals.

Precise physical examination of the structures which may be affected will lead to the most appropriate treatment. The effectiveness of passive movement in the treatment of sporting injuries to the cervical region should not be underestimated although other techniques and modalities may be necessary to achieve an optimal result.

REFERENCES

Addley K, Farren J 198–7 Irish rugby injury survey: Dungannon football club. British Journal of Sports Medicine 22(1):22–24

Australian Physiotherapy Association 1988 Protocol for pre-manipulative testing of the cervical spine. Australian Journal of Physiotherapy 34(2):97–100

Bailes J E, Maroon J C 1989 Management of cervical spine injuries in athletes. Clinics in Sports Medicine 8(1):43–58

Bakay L, Leslie E V 1965 Surgical treatment of vertebral artery insufficiency caused by cervical spondylosis. Journal of Neurosurgery 23:596–602

Bogduk N 1986 Cervical causes of headache and dizziness. In: Grieve G P (ed) Modern manual therapy of the vertebral column. Churchill Livingstone, Edinburgh, pp 289–302

Bogduk N 1988 Innervation and pain patterns of the cervical spine. In: Grant R (ed) Physical therapy of the cervical and thoracic spine. Churchill Livingstone, New York, pp 1–13

Bower K 1989 Swimming injuries of the cervical spine. Newsletter of the National Sports Physiotherapy Group 89(4):9–10

Butler D S 1991 Mobilization of the nervous system. Churchill Livingstone, Melbourne

Chadwick P 1987 The significance of spinal joint signs in the management of groin strain and patellofemoral pain by manual techniques. Physiotherapy 73(10):507

Cloward R B 1959 Cervical discography. A contribution to the aetiology and mechanism of neck, shoulder and arm pain. Annals of Surgery 150:1052–1064

Cyriax J 1974 Textbook of orthopaedic medicine, 8th edn. Baillière Tindall, London, vol. II

Dalton M B 1989 The effect of age on cervical posture in a normal female population. In: Jones H M, Jones M A, Milde M R (eds) MPAA sixth biennial conference proceedings, Adelaide: 34–44

Dove C I 1982 The occipito-atlanto-axial complex. Manuelle Medizin 20:11–15

Dalton P A, Jull G A 1989 The distribution and characteristics of neck-arm pain in patients with and without a neurological deficit. Australian Journal of Physiotherapy 35(1):3–8

Edwards B 1980 Combined movements in the cervical spine: their value in examination and treatment choice. Australian Journal of Physiotherapy 26:165-171

Edwards B C 1988 Combined movements of the cervical spine in examination and treatment. In: Grant R (ed) Physical therapy for the cervical and thoracic spine. Churchill Livingstone, New York, pp 125–151

Fast A, Zinicola D F, Marin E L 1987 Vertebral artery damage complicating cervical manipulation. Spine 12(9):840–842

Fielding J W, Fietti V G, Mardam-Bey T H 1978 Athletic injuries to the atlanto-axial articulation. The American Journal of Sports Medicine 6(5):226–231

Fine K M, Vegso J J, Sonnett B, Torg J J 1991 Prevention of cervical spine injuries in football. Physician and Sports Medicine 19(10):54–64

Golding D N 1969 Cervical and occipital pain as presenting symptoms of intracranial tumour. Annals of Physical Medicine 10:1

Grant R 1988 Dizziness testing and manipulation of the cervical spine. In: Grant R (ed) Physical therapy of the cervical and thoracic spine. Churchill Livingstone, New York, pp 111–124

Grieve G P 1988 Common vertebral joint problems, 2nd edn. Churchill Livingstone, Edinburgh

Hanus S H, Homer T D, Harter D H 1977 Vertebral artery occlusion complicating yoga exercises. Archives of Neurology 34:574–575

Hartman L S 1983 Handbook of osteopathic technique. NMK, Hadley Wood

Herkowitz H N, Rothman R H 1984 Subacute instability of the cervical spine. Spine 9(4):348–357

Herrick R T 1981 Clay shoveller's fracture in power lifting: a case report. American Journal of Sports Medicine 9:29–30

Hutchison M S 1989 An investigation of pre-manipulative dizziness testing. In: Jones H M, Jones M A, Milde M R (eds) MPAA sixth biennial conference proceedings, Adelaide, pp 104–112

Jackson D W, Lohr F T 1986 Cervical spine injuries. Clinics in Sports Medicine 5(2):373–386

Janda V 1983 Muscle function testing. Butterworths, London

Janda V 1988 Muscles and cervicogenic pain syndromes. In: Grant R (ed) Physical therapy of the cervical and thoracic spine. Churchill Livingstone, New York, pp 153–166

Janda V, Schmid H J A 1980 Muscles as a pathogenic factor in back pain. In: The treatment of patients, proceedings of fourth IFOMT conference, Christchurch, New Zealand

Jull G 1986 Clinical observations of upper cervical mobility. In: Grieve G P (ed) Modern manual therapy. Churchill Livingstone, Edinburgh

Kerr F W L, Olafson R A 1961 Trigeminal and cervical volleys. Archives of Neurology 5:171–178

Kimmel D L 1961 Innervation of the spinal dura mater and dura mater of the posterior cranial fossa. Neurology 11:800

Kovacs A 1955 Subluxation and deformation of the cervical apophyseal joints. Acta Radiologica Stockholm 43:1–16

Lee D 1986: Principles and practice of muscle energy and functional techniques. In: Grieve G (ed) Modern manual therapy. Churchill Livingstone, Edinburgh, pp 640–655

Lindgren K A, Leino E, Lepantalo M, Paukku P 1991 Recurrent thoracic outlet syndrome after first rib resection. Archives of Physical Medicine and Rehabilitation 72:208–214

Lyness S S, Simeone F A 1978 Vascular complications of upper cervical spine injuries. Orthopaedic Clinics of North America 9(4):1029–1039

Magarey M E 1985 Selection of passive treatment techniques. In: Proceedings of MTAA fourth biennial conference, Brisbane, pp 298–320

Magarey M E 1988 Examination of the cervical and thoracic spine. In: Grant R (ed) Physical therapy of the cervical and thoracic spine. Churchill Livingstone, New York, pp 81–109

Maitland G D 1979 Negative disc exploration: positive canal signs. Australian Journal of Physiotherapy 25(3):129–133

Maitland G D 1982 Palpation examination of the posterior cervical spine: ideal average and normal. Australian Journal of Physiotherapy 28(3):3

Maitland G D 1986: Vertebral manipulation, 5th edn. Butterworths, London

Marks M R, Bell G R, Boumphrey F R 1990 Cervical spine fractures in athletes. Clinics in Sports Medicine 9(1):13–29

McKenzie R A 1981 The lumbar spine. Mechanical diagnosis and treatment. Spinal Publications, Waikanae, New Zealand

McKenzie R A 1983 Treat your own neck. Spinal Publications, Waikanae, New Zealand

Mimura M, Moriya M, Watanabe T, Takahashi K, Yamagata M, Tamaki T 1989 Three dimensional motion analysis of the cervical spine with special reference to the axial rotation. Spine 14(11):1135-1139

Myers P T 1980 Injuries presenting from rugby union football. The Medical Journal of Australia 2:7–20

Nichols H M 1986 Anatomic structures of the thoracic outlet. Clinical and Related Research 207:13–20

Nuber G W, Schafer M F 1987 Clay shovellers' injuries. A report of two injuries sustained from football. American Journal of Sports Medicine 15(2):182–183

Oda J, Tanaka H, Tsuzuki N 1988 Intervertebral disc changes with ageing of the human cervical vertebrae. From the neonate to the eighties. Spine 13(11):1205–1211

Paley D, Gillespie R 1986 Chronic repetitive unrecognized flexion injury of the cervical spine (high jumper's neck). American Journal of Sports Medicine 14(1):92–95

Pavlov H, Torg J S 1987 Roentgen examination of cervical spine injuries in the athlete. Clinics in Sports Medicine 6(4):751–766

Phillips H, Grieve G P 1986 The thoracic outlet syndrome. In: Grieve G P (ed) Modern manual therapy of the vertebral column. Churchill Livingstone, Edinburgh, pp 359–369

Poindexter D P, Johnson M D 1984 Football shoulder and neck injury: a study of the 'stinger'. Archives of Physical Medicine and Rehabilitation 65:601–602

Popov V 1989: Shoulder injuries in swimmers. Newsletter of the National Sports Physiotherapy Group 90(4):12–13

Pratt N E 1986 Neurovascular entrapment in the regions of the shoulder and posterior triangle of the neck. Physical Therapy 66(12):1894–1900

Rogers A W 1992 Textbook of Anatomy. Churchill Livingstone, Edinburgh

Scher A T 1987 Rugby injuries of the spine and spinal cord. Clinics in Sports Medicine 6(1):87–99

Scher A T 1991 Catastrophic rugby injuries of the spinal cord; changing patterns of injury. British Journal of Sports Medicine: 25(1):57–60

Schneider G 1989 Restricted shoulder movement: capsular contracture or cervical referral? A clinical study. Australian Journal of Physiotherapy 35(2):97

Schneider G, Pardoe M 1985 Translation of the facets during coupled motion in the cervical spine: a pilot study. Australian Journal of Physiotherapy 31:39–44

Selvaratnam P J 1991 The brachial plexus tension test in patients and cadavers. Unpublished PhD thesis

Selvaratnam P J, Glasgow E F, Matyas T A 1989 Differential strain produced by the brachial plexus tension test on C5–T1 nerve roots. In: Jones H M, Jones M A (eds) MPAA sixth biennial conference proceedings, Adelaide, pp 167–172

Silver J R, Gill S 1988 Injuries of the spine sustained during rugby. Sports Medicine 5:328–344

Sparks J P 1985 Rugby football injuries, 1980-1983. British Journal of Sports Medicine 20:71–74

Speer K P, Bassett F H 1990 The prolonged burner syndrome. American Journal of Sports Medicine 18(6):591–594

Stevens B J, McKenzie R A 1988 Mechanical diagnosis and self treatment of the cervical spine. In: Grant R (ed) Physical therapy for the cervical and thoracic vertebral column. Churchill Livingstone, New York, pp 271–289

Sugerman S 1983 Injuries in an Australian schools rugby union season. Australian Journal of Sports Medicine and Exercise Science 15(1):5–14

Tatlow W F T, Bammer H G 1957 Syndrome of vertebral artery compression. Neurology 7:331–340

Toole J F, Tucker S H 1960 Influence of head position on cerebral circulation. Archives of Neurology 2:616–623

Torg J S, Vegso J J, Sennett B, Das M 1985 The national football head and neck injury registry. 14 year report on cervical quadriplegia 1971 through 1984. Journal of the American Medical Association 254:3439–3443

Travell J G, Simons D G 1983 Myofascial pain and dysfunction. The trigger point manual. Vol. 1, The upper extremity. Williams & Wilkins, Baltimore

Trott P H, Ruston S A, Pearcy M J, Fulton I 1991 Coupling of movements on the cervical spine-an in vivo study. MPAA seventh biennial conference proceedings, Blue Mountains New South Wales, pp 33–39

Twomey L T, Taylor J R 1989 Joints of the middle and lower cervical spine: age changes and pathology. In: Jones H M, Jones M A, Milde M R (eds) MPAA sixth biennial conference proceedings, Adelaide, pp 215–220

Twomey L T, Taylor J R 1991 Damage to the cervical discs and facet joints following severe trauma. In: MPAA seventh biennial conference proceedings, Blue Mountains, New South Wales, pp 25–32

Valencia F 1988 Biomechanics of the thoracic spine. In: Grant R (ed) Physical therapy of the cervical and thoracic spine. Churchill Livingstone, New York, pp 39–50

Watson D H, Trott P H 1993 Cervical headache: an investigation of natural head posture and upper cervical flexor muscle performance. Cephalagia 13:272-284

Webb J K, Broughton R B, McSweeney K T, Park W M 1976 Hidden flexion injury of the cervical spine. Journal of Bone and Joint Surgery 58B(3):322–327

White A A, Panjabi M M 1978 The clinical biomechanics of the occipito atlantal complex. Orthopaedic Clinics of North America 9(4):867–878

Williams P L, Warwick R, Dyson M, Bannister L H (eds) 1989 Gray's anatomy, 37th edn. Churchill Livingstone, Edinburgh

Worth D R 1985 Kinematics of the cranio-vertebral joints. In: Glasgow E F, Twomey L T (eds) Aspects of manipulative therapy, 2nd edn. Churchill Livingstone, Melbourne, pp 39–44

Worth D R, Selvick G 1986 Movements of the craniovertebral joints. In: Grieve G (ed) Modern manual therapy of the vertebral column. Churchill Livingstone, Edinburgh, pp 53–63

Wroble R R, Albright J P 1986 Neck and low back injuries in wrestling. Clinics in Sports Medicine 5(2):295–325

22. The thoracic and abdominal region

Peter Howley

Sporting injuries in the thorax and abdomen, while not as common as in other areas of the body, can be extremely serious and may be life threatening.

The thoracic spine is the region of the spine least likely to be injured in sport when compared to the cervical and lumbar regions (Cruess & Rennie 1984). Haycock (1986) surprisingly reports that abdominal injuries make up 10% of sports injuries, and can result in the internal organs, particularly spleen, kidneys and liver, being involved. The thorax may sustain superficial musculoskeletal injuries, particularly in contact sports, but may also suffer internal injury such as pneumothorax.

It is therefore of paramount importance that the examining physiotherapist be able to differentiate a local lesion, referred pain from another source (particularly the thoracic spine) and a visceral injury or disease.

ANATOMY AND BIOMECHANICS

When discussing the thorax and abdomen a few anatomical features are worthy of note. The obvious feature which distinguishes the thoracic spine from the cervical spine is its attachment to the ribs. The 12 thoracic vertebrae, articulating with the ribs, and the sternum anteriorly combine to form the thorax.

It must be remembered that the upper seven ribs, when articulating anteriorly with the sternum, do so through their costocartilages. The costochondral junction forms a fibrocartilaginous joint in which the ribs and cartilage are slotted together (Corrigan & Maitland 1983). Injuries peculiar to these joints occur in sport, usually from direct contact. The 8th, 9th and 10th ribs are unlike the previous seven ribs; they do not attach to the sternum, but attach to the costocartilage of the ribs above. The 11th and 12th ribs have no anterior attachments to either cartilage or bone. These anatomical considerations are of functional importance when palpating the thorax during examination.

The first rib can be palpated in the anterior aspect of the neck, just superior to the clavicle as well as posteriorly under the suprascapular musculature just below the transverse process of C7. The author suggests this area should be considered as a potential source of arm pain. The T1 sclerotome extends into the upper limb and it is believed that the upper few ribs can also cause symptoms in that area (Grieve 1986).

The intercostales run between the ribs to occupy the intercostal space. The intercostales externi are the superficial and the intercostales interni are the innermost layer (Warrick & William 1973). These muscles may be injured in isolation or in conjunction with rib fractures.

The intercostal nerve, running through the intercostal space and supplying the muscles and skin, may be a source of pain when irritated or compressed at its origin in the thoracic spine.

The structure of the thorax is such that it tends to limit motion of the spine, particularly extension due largely to the dorsal convexity. The spine itself also has firmly-bound vertebrae due to the various ligaments in various planes, and this adds to the stability.

Functionally there are differences in normal mobility of the thoracic spine. Age and sex differences exist. Grieve (1986) stated that male mobility is greater than female mobility when performing sagittal movements, while female mobility is greater than males when side bending. He also points out that in right-handed individuals there is a slight right convex curve and a left convex curve in left-handed individuals. These factors are important when assessing 'normal' appearance and movement patterns.

Movements of the upper limb produce movement of the thorax via its muscle attachments and the shoulder girdle. These muscle attachments also provide stability for the upper limbs and cervical spine. Upper limb movement specifically stresses the costovertebral joints, which is functionally significant when considering the causes of strain and prevention of further strain in these joints.

The thoracic spine is the site of the sympathetic plexus which gives segmental sympathetic supply of the head and neck (from T1–5) and of the upper limbs (T2–7). This is important when considering the T4 syndrome, which will be discussed later. The anatomical connection between the blood supply to the head and upper limb and the thoracic segments of the spinal cord via the sympathetic nervous system is well documented. A sympathectomy, or removal of various parts of the sympathetic system surgically, is performed for the relief of pain and in the treatment of a number of clinical conditions. For example, the arteries of limbs may be denervated surgically in conditions of vascular spasm (Raynaud's disease) by cutting the sympathetic trunk below the third thoracic ganglion, severing the rami communicartes connected with the second and third thoracic spinal nerve. The white ramus to the cervico-thoracic ganglion is not cut, mainly because it contains most of the preganglion fibres that pass up to the superior cervical ganglion. Destruction of this nerve would result in Horner's syndrome, ie the pupil in the affected eye does not dilate to shade and there is a reduction of sweating on the same side of the face (Houston et al 1978).

Thus it is logical to summarise that local pathology in the region of the upper thoracic sympathetic ganglion may cause aberration of the vascular pattern in the head, neck and upper limbs (Newland 1989).

The following muscles cover the thorax: pectoralis major and minor, rectus abdominis, external oblique, internal oblique, serratus anterior, latissimus dorsi, trapezius, rhomboideus major and minor, levator scapulae, serratus posterior and erector spinae. These muscles produce trunk and, in most cases, upper limb stability and movement, and may be injured by a direct contusion or strained during sporting activity.

The specific muscles forming the anterior abdominal wall are the anterolateral group consisting of external oblique, internal oblique, transversus abdominis and rectus abdominis. The muscles act to retain the abdominal viscera in position as well as flexing, rotating and laterally flexing the trunk (internal oblique rotates the trunk to the side where the muscle is contracting and external oblique rotates to the opposite side–this is important to remember when differentiating in examination).

Studies have shown that the abdominal muscles also have a role in increasing intraabdominal pressure and thereby helping with trunk stabilization (Zettenburg et al 1987).

EXAMINATION

Subjective examination of the thorax and abdomen

Athletes presenting with symptoms in the thoracic and abdominal areas provide physiotherapists with the challenge of differentiating between musculoskeletal and non-musculoskeletal causes. For this reason a thorough examination is crucial.

When commencing the subjective examination the first aim is to establish the area and the nature of the symptoms. It is best to ask the athlete to physically indicate the most localized area of discomfort, however, assistance from the physiotherapist may be needed in mapping the extent of symptoms, especially in the upper thoracic region. Once established, the site of the symptoms will help in identifying the possible anatomical structure involved. In the author's opinion, the area the pain radiates or refers to is very important. Radiating directly out from the spine, or following the line of the ribs or shooting centrally through to the front of the chest, may indicate an intervertebral joint, costovertebral joint or disc lesion respectively.

Knowing the behaviour of the athlete's pain helps in assessing whether the pain is of a mechanical or in-flammatory nature. If the pain is aggravated only by certain movements, such as a golf swing, a musculoskeletal origin for the pain should be expected. If the symptoms occur at rest and are not aggravated by activity or certain postures, the physiotherapist should suspect inflammatory or visceral causes. Exploring aggravating factors such as pain on deep breathing, coughing, twisting, movement from a reclined position and arm movements (especially in the case of lower rib symptoms) should help the physiotherapist with the diagnosis. If the symptoms are associated with certain postures, these should be demonstrated to help provide clues of possible structural causes.

As in all cases, the irritability of the condition should be established before proceeding with the objective examination.

A precise history, taking into account the nature of the athlete's sport and the specific movements and postures involved, will help establish not only the possible structures at fault but what objective tests need to be explored. Where a specific trauma has occurred, the mechanism of the injury and the progress of the condition leading up to the athlete's presentation need to be clarified.

Finally, and of utmost importance in managing conditions of this area, the physiotherapist needs to ascertain a profile of the athlete's general health, to screen for cord and cauda equina lesions, previous relevant conditions or surgery, past and present use of medication and investigative procedures already performed.

Radiological findings

Radiological examination of the thorax is important to help in the management of injuries in this area, particularly when trauma is involved. Plain chest X-rays will help detect a pneumothorax, rib or sternum fracture and any bony change in the thoracic spine.

Compression-type fractures must be checked for in traumatic episodes involving the thoracic spine, for example landing on the head in gymnastics, football and high jumping.

Osteoporotic changes in the thoracic spine may lead to spontaneous compression fractures and their presence must be investigated in middle-aged or older females or in those taking long term oral corticosteroids.

Objective examination of the thorax

The objective examination of the thoracic spine is best performed in the sitting position. This should follow a quick appraisal of the appearance of the spine in standing. The contours of the thoracic spine can vary greatly among individuals and common findings are increased kyphosis and scoliosis. When assessing the latter, the athlete should be asked to flex forward to ascertain whether there is a rib hump on the side of the convexity. Its presence signifies vertebral rotation and therefore a structural scoliosis. Kulund (1988) believes that young athletes with curvatures greater than 20° may experience spinal problems when participating in contact sports. Large curves will need referral to an orthopaedic specialist.

Thoracolumbar movements should also be assessed in standing (see Ch. 27) before moving on to the tests of sitting (for further detail the reader is referred to Maitland 1986).

Flexion

This movement is often asymptomatic, but when used as part of the slump test the author finds it to be a more helpful procedure (see Ch. 33). In the author's experience flexion, combined with protraction of the scapulae as in reaching forwards, is a more sensitive test. This position stimulates the position adopted in rowing and may reproduce pain experienced by these athletes.

The author has also found that pure thoracic spine flexion usually produces sharp pain in the presence of a disc lesion.

Extension

While a most helpful movement to examine in the lumbar spine, extension in the thoracic spine is occasionally limited and/or painful in the thoracic spine. In the author's experience, extension is painful and restricted in the presence of a disc lesion.

Lateral flexion

Injuries in the thorax in general will usually be painful when a lateral flexion movement is performed. The author has found that rib fractures, intercostal muscle injuries and thoracic spine joint injuries will be painful during this test.

Rotation

This is the most valuable movement from an assessment point of view, as almost all of thoracic spine lesions cause either pain or restriction of movement upon rotation. Sports such as cricket, tennis, discus and javelin throwing will be difficult if thoracic rotation is painful. In many cases rotation will help the physiotherapist discriminate between symptoms of thoracic origin and those arising from the neck or lumbar regions. It is also a useful movement in reassessment procedures, when gauging response to treatment.

Rotation of the thorax stresses the ribs, costochondral junction and sternum. Kapanji (1974) states that the ribs are elastic and distort during rotation, as do the costochondral junction and sternum. Therefore any injury to these areas will be painful upon rotation.

Flexion/rotation

Flexion/rotation is a combined movement performed in sitting. Overpressure is important to elicit the true findings when testing flexion/rotation. This test will often cause pain and restrict movement in conditions that are more difficult to assess, and helps in differentiating between a musculoskeletal and visceral cause of thorax pain.

The combined movement simulates the actual movements involved in several sports such as golf, cricket and football, and is a good way of assessing an athlete's readiness to resume sport following injury.

Having completed the active movements of the thoracic spine, examining the patient's chest expansion is a quick way to ascertain if there is any limitation in the range of motion of the thorax. Chest expansion is usually painful with intercostal muscle injury, rib fracture or thoracic disc lesion. It may also point to an internal injury, if the breathing expansion is extremely difficult to produce and pain is severe. This is also important, to exclude rheumatoid variant diseases such as ankylosing spondylitis (see Ch. 27).

Neurological testing

Neurological deficit in the thoracic spine is rare, in the author's experience, but when seen may be an indication of severe spinal cord pathology. The physiotherapist must be aware of any cord signs such as disturbances in gait, weakness, pain and a sensory deficit in the lower limbs. A neoplastic disease or canal stenosis may be the cause of such symptoms (Chusid 1970).

Neurological testing in the case of spinal cord involvement will reveal ankle clonus, exaggerated lower limb reflexes and dorsiflexion (Babinski's sign) together with lower limb sensory loss and muscle weakness. Occasionally local sensory loss along an intercostal space may occur in the presence of a nerve root compression from a thoracic disc lesion. If the therapist has any suspicion of neurological involvement the athlete should be referred for medical opinion.

Palpation of the thorax

With the patient lying face-down on the examination couch, the physiotherapist should observe the appearance of the thoracic spine. Notice should be taken of any apparent deviation from the normal, such as scoliosis, increased kyphosis and any prominent, depressed or absent spinous process. A general observation of the musculature should be performed for any spasm or increased development unilaterally. Palpatory examination is then commenced. Postero-anterior pressures, central, unilateral and transverse pressures as described by Maitland (1986) are performed to detect symptomatic intervertebral joint lesion (to be discussed later).

Postero-anterior pressures are then applied along the posterior aspect of the ribs and along the intercostal spaces at regular intervals in an attempt to ascertain bony and/or intercostal muscle tenderness.

With the patient lying on his/her back, palpation is continued around the ribs and intercostal spaces as before, particularly over the costochondral junctions and the articulations with the sternum. 'Springing' the thorax by compression directed laterally on the rib cage will usually cause pain if there is a rib fracture. Compression centrally over the sternum will cause pain with sternum fractures, costochondral junction injuries and injuries to the articulation with the sternum.

Pain may also be felt in the thoracic spine in the absence of any injury or disease. Minucci (1987) found pain on passive accessory intervertebral movement tests in 37% of subjects, and pain was found to be significantly more frequent at T3, T4 and T5 in a study on normal (non-symptomatic) subjects. Similarly, hypomobility was detected in these normal (non-symptomatic) subjects, particularly at T3/4.

It is therefore important to take into account all the findings from both the subjective and objective examination when making a diagnosis.

Passive physiological intervertebral movement tests (PPIVMs) may also be used, but the author finds them of dubious significance due to the subjective nature of the interpretation. Minucci (1987) again found a high incidence of abnormal findings with PPIVMs in normal subjects, particularly when examining the extension movement.

Examination of the abdomen

An objective examination should be performed to determine if the abdominal muscles have been injured and to check for internal injury that may require medical intervention.

The rectus abdominis is tested for injury by resisting the patient's attempts to sit up from the supine position. Resistance is applied to the anterior thorax (over the sternum) by the therapist. The sit-up is performed with the hip and knee joints in the extended position, then with the hips and knee joints flexed and the feet flat on the couch. This may help differentiate between a hip flexion injury (hip/knee extension) and a true abdominal muscle injury (hip/knee flexion).

The internal oblique and external oblique are tested with the patient seated over the edge of the couch. The patient's legs are stabilized by the therapist and resistance applied by placing both hands on the patient's anterior shoulder area. If pain is felt when rotating towards the painful side the internal oblique is involved, if pain is felt on the opposite side the external oblique is involved.

Palpation of the abdomen

With the patient lying supine the abdominal muscles are palpated for tenderness and any disruption to the usual muscular contour, as with a muscle rupture or swelling from a local haematoma. Particular attention should be directed to palpation over the attachment to the ribs and distally to the iliac crest, where tenderness and swelling is evident in the 'hip pointer' injury (see Ch. 28).

Rectus abdominis diastasis is a condition occasionally present in the female athlete during pregnancy and in the early months after childbirth. This condition will be detected during the above mentioned testing procedures where a distinctive 'gap' in the linear alba can be seen and readily palpated. In the fit prima gravida, who continues to exercise more than four times a week during her pregnancy, the condition should be screened for after 20 weeks gestation. In the multigravida, a past history of the problem predisposes the athlete to recurrences. In these cases it may appear as early as at 17 weeks gestation (Cooper 1992). In the presence of diastisis rectus, advice must be given to the athlete to ensure excessive overloading of the muscle does not occur. Abdominal muscle exercises must be modified and after 20 weeks gestation should not be performed in the supine position (see Ch. 34).

Palpation of the lower abdominal area should be performed to detect the presence of an inguinal hernia. The examiner palpates over a precise area (the inguinal ring) along the inner half of a line between the pubic tubercle and the anterior superior iliac crest, for swelling and tenderness. The athlete should also cough while the examiner is palpating over the inguinal ring. If there is a hernia, a bulge will be produced.

Should any signs and symptoms of a visceral injury be present specific palpation should be performed over the organs most likely involved. The spleen is palpated on the left side under the diaphragm and is often associated with fractures of the 9th and 10th ribs; the liver is palpated on the right and in the upper aspect of the abdomen; and the kidneys to the right or left of the spine above the pelvic girdle.

Differentiation between conditions of the anterior abdominal wall and the underlying viscera may also be aided by a simple test during palpation in supine. Once the tender area is located, the athlete should be asked to lift the head, which will contract and firm the abdominal wall. If the tenderness disappears the painful structure may be visceral, if it increases the muscles may be more at fault.

Radiological investigations such as plain films, ultrasound, CT scanning and an IVP should be performed for a more precise diagnosis (Haycock 1986). Although plain films may be ordered by the physiotherapist, these and more detailed investigations should be performed under the direction of a medical practitioner. Close liaison with other medical workers is essential, particularly when diagnosis is unclear.

CONDITIONS AND MANAGEMENT OF THE THORAX AND ABDOMEN

Good management of the thoracic and abdominal region depends on making a diagnosis based on accurate and thorough assessment of the athlete. As stated earlier, these areas present the greatest challenge to the physiotherapist when differentiating between musculoskeletal and non-musculoskeletal causes. It is important to bear in mind that even in the case of a young, outwardly healthy athlete, symptoms experienced in the thorax and abdomen during or after sport may be from sources independent of that activity, such as the appendix, heart, lung, gut or renal areas.

Broadhurst (1987) stated that a patient presenting with chest pain should be regarded as having cardiac cause until proved otherwise. If the cause is non-cardiac, the possibility of referral from the thoracic spine should be considered.

Grieve (1986), in discussing the involvement of the thoracic joints in simulated visceral disease, stated that clinical experience suggests that the incidence of these changes (lesions in the thoracic segments) producing counterfeit visceral symptoms is probably much higher than actual visceral disease. He also stated that the thoracic spine can cause symptoms such as sweating, dyspnoea, reduced respiratory excursion, flushing, pallor, pulse alterations, nausea and vomiting.

McRae (1983) stated that because chest and abdominal pains engender a sense of foreboding in patients, the early classification of simulated disease is important.

It is clear that pain felt in the abdominal region may not be due to a local visceral or musculoskeletal cause, but referred from the lower thoracic spine or upper lumbar spine.

Too often the medical practitioner may focus upon the visceral cause of pain and neglect to consider a musculo-skeletal cause. In contrast the physiotherapist may place too much emphasis upon the mechanical causes of pain.

The following sections discuss possible musculoskeletal and non-musculoskeletal causes for symptoms in the thorax and abdomen.

Musculoskeletal conditions of the thorax and abdomen

Bony injuries

Occasionally, traumatic injuries to the thoracic spine occur, resulting in fracture and fracture dislocation. The mechanics of such an injury are usually due to hyperflexion and compression, producing an anterior wedging of the vertebral body. This may occur anywhere in the spine, but is most common at the thoracolumbar junction (Williams 1976). These major bony injuries usually occur in sports such as motor racing, horse riding and hang gliding. Fractured ribs, however, are common in many sports, particularly those which involve direct contact. Athletes can also fracture ribs from falls, as in diving to field a ball, and in horse racing and equestrian events.

Usually a single rib, or at most two, is fractured following a severe blow to the chest. It is usually associated with a 'winded' sensation. Difficulty of breathing usually follows and deep respiration, sneezing and coughing become painful. Flailing may occur in more extensive injuries.

Radiological examination will confirm a rib fracture and help differentiate it from a soft tissue (usually intercostal muscle) injury. This examination will also detect any complication from a rib fracture, such as damage to the internal mammary artery or the lung, which could cause haemothorax, pneumothorax or penetration of the peri-cardium. A more frequent injury is damage to the intercostal vessels and nerves, which will result in rather marked local swelling and formation of a haematoma (O'Donoghue 1967).

Stress fractures of ribs can also occur after repetitive overuse of the shoulder as in throwing sports, tennis and rowing (Muckle 1971). The upper ribs are those involved, and are found on the dominant side. Local tenderness and chronic pain which has an insidious onset are the main presenting signs and symptoms. However, X-rays can be negative and if a definite diagnosis is thought necessary, a bone scan is more definitive.

Fractured ribs unite to become painless in 4–6 weeks and union is invariable (Cyriax 1957). Various methods of treatment, such as strapping the ribs, have been advocated over the years, but encouraging resting and deep breathing exercises is now the more accepted approach.

The injection of a local anaesthetic under the margin of the fractured rib (an intercostal block) may be considered with severe pain and associated breathing difficulties.

In most cases of rib fracture the author has found that athletes have difficulty with any activity which requires an expansion of the thorax or pull of the trunk muscles for at least 3 weeks following the injury. It is therefore difficult for the athlete to resume running and other forms of training within that time span.

The sternum may be fractured by a severe direct blow. The fracture is usually through the upper portion of the body of the sternum. The sternum may also be dislocated when the body of the sternum is driven forcibly in while the manubrium is held forwards by the rigid first and second ribs so that the upper portion of the body tends to override the lower (O'Donoghue 1967).

As with the fractured rib, the fractured sternum causes immediate loss of breath and, although breathing recovers, pain persists over the fractured area and swelling develops.

The possibility of complications from a fractured sternum should be kept in mind, as they will often develop insidiously over several hours. For this reason the patient should be kept recumbent in hospital and observed for signs of breathing difficulty, impending shock or acceleration of the pulse which may result from haemorrhage into the pleura, pneumothorax or subcutaneous emphysema (O'Donoghue 1967).

Muscular injuries

The muscles of the thorax and abdomen may be injured by overstretching, sudden severe contractions of these muscles or by direct trauma. The most commonly affected are the intercostal muscles and the anterior abdominal wall group.

The intercostal muscles may be strained by rotatory stress of the thorax, vigorous serving in tennis and forceful tackling in football. They are usually injured in conjunction with rib fractures and are in fact a strong contributing factor to the painfulness of rib fractures.

Treatment of the intercostal muscle is by local anaesthetic if necessary in the early acute phase and later the use of ultrasound and transverse frictions. Deep breathing and the thoracic movements of rotation and lateral flexion help restore function. Non-steroidal anti-inflammatory drugs (NSAIDs) may also be of value.

The abdominal muscles can be quite a difficult injury to treat, when we realize the role the abdominals play in everyday activities. Their postural role and role in increasing intraabdominal pressure in such activities as defecation, sneezing and coughing make it difficult to fully rest the injured area.

As well as the common abdominal muscle strains the muscles may rupture in violent movements associated with weightlifting, throwing, gymnastics, rowing, wrestling and pole-vaulting. Strains leading to inflammation can occur in any sporting events, but particularly in strength training, sit-ups, shooting, football, serving and smashing in tennis and badminton (Peterson & Renstrom 1986).

The unusual case of rhabdomyolysis (muscle fibre necrosis) of the rectus abdominis has been reported by Haycock (1986). She cited a West German study by Schmitt et al (1983) of a case where a bodybuilder developed acute abdominal pain one week after vigorous exercise, and suffered muscle fibre necrosis. Haycock (1986) stated that such a possibility must be kept in mind when delayed abdominal wall symptoms are reported following an abdominal strain or blow.

Treatment consists of ultrasound to the tender area, soft tissue techniques including transverse frictions and stretching and strengthening exercises. Again, NSAIDs may be used. The rectus abdominis is best stretched by performing spinal extension standing and in the prone position, as in the McKenzie extension routine for a lumbar disc lesion (McKenzie 1981). The internal oblique is stretched by rotating the trunk in the sitting position away from the painful side, and the external oblique by rotating towards the painful side. Combinations of extension, rotation and lateral flexion can also be experimented with to obtain the best 'stretch'.

Within the limits of pain abdominal muscle strengthening should commence as soon as possible. It should begin as an abdominal-bracing muscle contraction, and progress to full sit-ups, with the hip/knee flexion position and sit-ups with rotation to fully exercise the abdominal muscle group.

A differential diagnosis is necessary to differentiate between lower abdominal muscle strain and an inguinal hernia.

Joint injuries

The sternocostal and sternoclavicular joints together with the costochondral junctions and intervertebral joints may be injured in the thorax. Injury may occur from a direct blow to the articulating bony structures, producing strain into the joints. This is common in Australian Rules football, rugby and to a lesser extent basketball and soccer. Repetitive activities and those involving twisting, such as weightlifting and wrestling may also result in injury (see Ch. 23).

Costochondral junction injuries. There is a high incidence of costochondral tears in wrestling due to the nature of the sport (Estwanick et al 1980). Estwanik et al (1980) explained that if the wrester underneath is flattened, has his or her arms far in front of the head, and applies much force in an attempt to get to his or her knees, the wrestler is vulnerable to the injury. If the longitudinal axis of the body is twisted to its limit as great effort is expended, again the wrestler is susceptible to injury. Other sports which involve similar positions and forces would also subject athletes to this condition. Costochondral separation occurs when a force is applied to the chest, causing the costocartilage to separate from the sternum. The area is very tender and painful on movement and the athlete may also feel a 'slipping out' or snapping sensation. This condition, also called 'slipping rib', may need local anaesthesia, a chest binder and prolonged rest until symptoms disappear (Kulund 1988).

Polyarthritis and Tietze syndrome can also refer pain to the region of the costochondral junction (Corrigan & Maitland 1983).

Tietze syndrome is a painful, tender swelling occurring in one of the upper costochondral junctions. Young adults suffer most commonly from this condition, which is made worse by movements, strain and coughing. The second costochondral junction is involved in over 50% of cases (Corrigan & Maitland 1983).

Radiological examination is normal in Tietze syndrome and biopsy of the costocartilage shows only minor inflammatory changes (Landon & Malpas 1959) with no other pathology.

Treatment of Tietze syndrome, sternocostal joint and sternoclavicular joint strain is done by corticosteroid injection into the affected region, while the athlete rests from pain-provoking activity until the pain and tenderness subsides.

The use of ultrasound and NSAIDs may assist in lowering inflammation, but otherwise no active physical therapy is of value in the author's experience.

The intervertebral joint lesion. The term 'intervertebral joint lesion' (IJL) was used by Boudillon (1982) when describing pain arising from a spinal joint. He classified such a lesion as a joint which was found to be hypomobile and have increased tenderness and associated muscle spasm, all of which could be detected upon palpation.

Intervertebral joint lesions in the thoracic spine may be disc lesions, facet joint lesions or costovertebral lesions. The precise differentiation is always difficult, but certain presenting signs and symptoms are common in each case.

In sport IJLs occur from sudden sharp movements as in serving in tennis or bowling in cricket, or slouching after training or competition. In the author's experience, sitting with an increased kyphosis and protracted scapular as in the slumped, forward reach position is a common precipitating posture for the onset of an IJL. Two common positions are when driving a motor vehicle or when working over a desk. If active sport is undertaken immediately following these poor postures, injury may be more likely to occur (McKenzie 1980).

Cruess and Rennie (1984) claim that thoracic disc herniation is rare with an incidence of 1–6 of every 1000 disc herniations involving the whole spine. When disc herniations occur the most common levels of involvement are at the 11th interspace (25%) with a further 50% at 'the 9th, 10th or 11th interspaces. It is rare to encounter a thoracic disc herniation above the 6th interspace (Cruess & Rennie 1984).

Broadhurst (1987) also stated that disc herniation is rare in the thoracic spine and reports that 1 in 200 occur in this area. He stated that the most common cause of pain originating from the thoracic spine is dysfunction of one or more of the joint articulations, either the costovertebral joints or the apophyseal (facet) joints or both.

This claim is confirmed by the clinical picture of a thoracic IJL, which usually settles much more quickly than the true disc lesion as seen in the lumbar spine. Knowledge of the anatomical features of the thorax with its inherent immobility, narrower disc spaces and less elastic discs (O'Donoghue 1967) adds substance to this theory.

A thoracic IJL usually has a quite sudden onset, often following sudden sharp movements in the sports previously described. Examination reveals restriction of movement

upon rotation of the spine, usually one side more than the other. Less frequently, lateral flexion, flexion and extension are restricted and painful. Deep breathing and coughing will often cause pain.

Dural structures can be compromised with spinal joint injuries. These structures are best tested by the slump test which may produce the pain complained of (see Ch. 33).

Palpation of the painful area often reveals several areas of tenderness. Care must be taken to eliminate the cervical spine as a cause of pain felt in the thoracic spine area. 'Cloward's spots' (Cloward 1959) are referred areas of pain coming from a cervical disc lesion, which may produce local joint and soft tissue tenderness in the thoracic spine even when no injury exists below the seventh cervical spine (see Ch. 21).

Any pain felt above the lower angle of the scapula may be of cervical spine origin. It is therefore important that the cervical spine be thoroughly examined to exclude it as a cause of pain. Pain felt below the angle of the scapula cannot be directly attributed to the cervical spine, based on Cloward's findings (1959).

Referred pain associated with a thoracic spine IJL is common, and can be unilateral or bilateral. Chest pain is a common area of referred pain from the cervical and thoracic spine. A complete picture of the areas of distribution of referred pain as described by Kellegran (1939) is shown in Figure 22.1.

Treatment of an IJL can often bring about a quick recovery. Manipulation is usually the treatment of first choice and use of the supine 'fist' manipulation as described by Stoddard (1974) and Maitland (1986) or the prone 'screw' manipulation as described by Stoddard (1974) can quickly solve the problem.

Mobilization techniques as described by Maitland (1983), using the postero-anterior central vertebral pressure, transverse vertebral pressure and postero-anterior unilateral vertebral pressure may also be used if the presenting condition is severely painful or irritable and the precise pathology is questionable. These techniques are less forceful

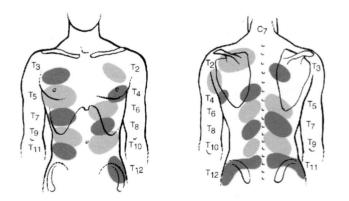

Fig. 22.1 Areas of distribution of referred pain after stimulation of deep joints of the thoracic spine. Source: adapted from Kellegren (1939)

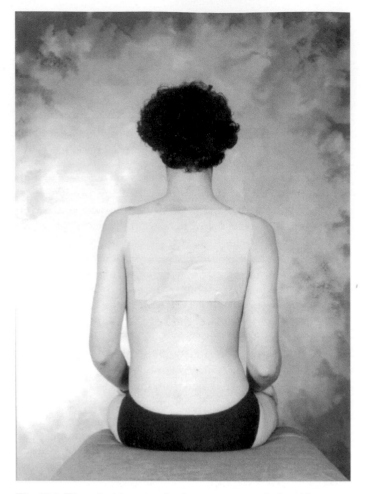

Fig. 22.2 Thoracic spine strapping in correct anatomical position

than manipulation and can be used where care is required, as in the osteoporotic spine.

Maintenance of the improved state following manipulation can be achieved by strapping the area, in its correct anatomical position, for 2–3 days, with care to avoid thoracic spine flexion and flexion combined with shoulder protraction (Fig. 22.2). After removing the supporting strapping repeated extension as described by McKenzie (1981) should be undertaken. Rotation movements can also be introduced.

Ongoing repeated trunk rotation in both sitting and standing and spinal extension lying and standing positions should be practised as a warm-up procedure before all sports. Tennis, bowling in cricket, windsurfing and athletic field events require a thorough warm-up routine for the thoracic spine.

In the author's experience, the role of electrotherapy modalities is limited in the treatment of IJL. Interferential, heat and ultrasound may have a minor role to play as a prelude to manipulation and mobilization.

Soft tissue techniques as described by Stoddard (1974) to relieve muscle spasm before mobilization or manipulation

can make the techniques more effective and allow less force to be used when applying the manipulative thrust.

T4 syndrome. IJL lesions of the thoracic spine may cause the so-called 'T4 syndrome'. The upper thoracic IJL may produce symptoms including pain and parasthesia in the upper limbs and/or head which may be vague and widespread (McGuckin 1986).

The presenting symptoms of the T4 syndrome can vary, but in a series of 90 patients McGuckin (1986) found that the hand was affected in all cases, and the upper limbs and head were less commonly involved.

While the T4 level is always involved in the syndrome, other joints from T2–T7 may be implicated as well (McGuckin 1986) (Fig. 22.3).

Although the cause of T4 syndrome has not been proven the current theories indicate that the proximity of the thoracic ganglion to the costovertebral joints could predispose them to be affected if the joints are swollen or 'sprained'. This causes mechanical irritation and perhaps stimulates sympathetic outflow to the head and upper limb, causing vasoconstriction. On the other hand, the syndrome could be due to irritation of the spinal nerves as they emerge from the intevertebral foramen in this region, through their connections to the sympathetic chain.

McGuckin (1986) stated that the predisposing factors may include unaccustomed lifting, stretching, pushing or exercises as well as trauma such as a fall. Posture also plays a role in the onset of the syndrome, with a slumped posture, a forward-poking chin, increased thoracic kyphosis and protruded shoulder girdle likely to predispose the athlete to the problem. It is therefore highly likely that the athlete, when performing movements which place strain on the thoracic spine in sporting, vocational or recreational activities, may be a candidate for this condition.

Treatment of the syndrome is the same as for the typical IJL with mobilization and manipulation being very effective. Postural correction and thoracic extension exercises are important to maintain improvement following treatment and prevent recurrence (see under 'Scheuermann's disease').

Differentiation must be made to exclude the cervical spine, carpal tunnel and thoracic outlet as a cause of symptoms which may be attributed to the T4 syndrome.

Scheuermann's disease. Scheuermann's disease is the osteochondrosis of the vertebral epiphyses in juveniles. The pathogenesis of the condition has been disputed since Scheuermann postulated the cause as due to aseptic necrosis of the vertebral bodies. Other authors have described the presence of herniated nuclear material within vertebral bodies, and suggested that penetration occurred through altered cartilaginous vertebral plates rather than the ring apophyses, and produced an anomaly in the enchondral ossification leading to an increased kyphosis (Bradford 1985). Cyriax (1957) attributed the cause to an anterior disc lesion which affects the end plate of the vertebrae, leading to erosion of the bone and the resultant wedging seen on radiological investigation.

A review of the literature reveals a strong hereditary predisposition to Scheuermann's disease, although the exact mechanism is unclear.

Some authors, such as Bradford (1985), suggested that mechanical factors are involved, after having encountered a higher incidence in patients subjected to heavy workloads.

The condition is also a common problem in the sporting adolescent. Baker (1988) in his review of the condition concluded that it affects 20–30% of the population with males and females affected equally.

Scheuermann's disease must be suspected in the adolescent, particularly 12–16 year olds, who presents with thoracic spine pain associated with the vertebral deformity of increased thoracic kyphosis. The condition may be present even if there is no discomfort or pain, the only sign being an increased kyphotic curve.

Baker (1988) also stated that the condition can occur in other areas of the spine, with the lumbar and very infrequently the cervical spine being involved.

Radiological evaluation usually reveals three or more wedge-shaped vertebral bodies with at least 5 degrees of wedging and the existence of Schmorl nodes (Nudel 1989).

Many authors including Williams (1976) have found a high incidence of hamstring tightness associated with Scheuermann's disease. This, together with tight lumbar dorsal fascia (Nudel 1989), places excessive strain on the thoracic spine.

As well as rowing and weightlifting sports, excessive and repeated trunk movements such as occur during bowling in cricket, hockey and tennis will aggravate the condition.

As with other conditions of osteochondritis, the adolescent is most at risk during growth spurts. While skeletal development progresses rapidly the soft tissue development does not keep pace, leading to soft tissue tightness and undue strain being placed upon the bony attachment.

While Cyriax (1957) reported successful treatment with manipulation, this author believes a more conservative approach is indicated. The athlete should cease active sport if symptoms are present to allow the growth spurt changes to occur, and then recommence physical activity very gradually. During this period particular attention should be paid to limiting the developing thoracic kyphosis. Limitation of the deformity can only be achieved while the skeleton is immature (Beyeler et al 1979) and therefore stresses the need for early treatment once the increasing kyphosis is noticed.

Although stretching tight muscle groups such as the pectorals, latissimus dorsi and hamstrings is useful, the author believes that thoracic spine extension and postural correction are the main means of improving the condition.

Extension in prone (McKenzie 1981) is the most important exercise to passively stretch the tight structures which are involved in the developing kyphosis. During this exercise the cervical spine should also be hyperextended as this helps extend the upper thoracic region.

Dorsal raise exercises with emphasis upon shoulder retraction are also valuable for increasing muscle tone and strength in the extensor muscle group (Fig. 22.3). Pain should always be the limiting factor with this condition, and should not be caused by exercise.

Postural correction is essential to minimize the increasing thoracic kyphosis. In both sitting and standing postures three manoeuvres should be regularly practised to ensure good postural alignment. These are the creation of a good lumbar lordosis, then the retraction and depression of the scapulae with resultant straightening of the thoracic spine, and finally cervical spine retraction to straighten the cerviothoracic junction. The adolescent should be encouraged to repeat the three manoeuvres regularly and hold the position in a relaxed manner.

Competitive sport should not be participated in during the painful phase of Scheuermann's disease. Such sports as Australian Rules football, rugby, basketball and soccer which may involve body contact must be avoided. Other sports such as tennis, cricket and hockey which involve twisting and sharp sudden thoracic spine movements should also be avoided during the painful phase.

In order to maintain general body fitness and improve the muscle tone of the extensor group of the spine, swimming can be performed providing it is pain free. Cycling is another activity safe to continue as long as care is taken not to spend long periods cycling in the flexed, kyphotic posture. Having the handlebars raised to allow a more upright posture will assist in this regard.

Non-sporting daily activities which are heavy should also be avoided during the active/painful phase of the

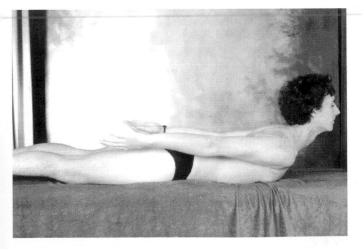

Fig. 22.3 Dorsal raises with scapula retraction

disease. Lifting, repeated bending and twisting activities should be undertaken with care.

Winged scapula

A winged scapula is seen occasionally in athletes. When pushing forwards against resistance with an extended arm, the affected scapula will become 'winged'. This is usually due to a neuritis of the long thoracic nerve causing weakness of the serratus anterior (Cyriax 1957). Following 2–3 weeks constant aching of the scapular region and arm the condition becomes painless and recovery occurs spontaneously in 4–12 months (Cyriax 1957).

Williams (1976) cited an example of an international swimmer who suffered winged scapulae as the result of neuralgic amyotrophy from a viral infection, but recovered fully and won an Olympic medal.

The reader is referred to Chapter 23 for further reading on injuries to the scapular region.

Non-musculoskeletal conditions of the thorax and abdomen

Visceral injuries

Internal or visceral injuries, although rare compared to the total number of sporting injuries, must be recognized and differentiated from the musculoskeletal structures when dealing with pain felt in the thorax and abdomen. All will require an urgent referral for medical assessment and intervention.

Muckle (1971) has classified the following signs and symptoms of visceral injuries which assist in differentiation.

1. Pain:
   a. local
   b. referred (e.g. pain is felt over the tip of the shoulder if blood or pressure irritates the diaphragm)
2. Shock: due to bleeding and subsequent rapid pulse
3. Rigid abdomen: spasm due to peritoneal irritation
4. Vomiting or nausea
5. Blood in urine or bowel motion

More common visceral injuries which should be differentiated from musculoskeletal injuries following severe trauma (such as a kick from a horse or a knock in football) are listed below.

Ruptured spleen. A direct blow to the upper left region of the abdomen occasionally in association with a fracture of the 9th and 10th ribs may result in a rupture of the spleen.

Peterson and Renstrom (1986) stated that an athlete who has had infectious mononucleosis (glandular fever) recently is more at risk. Frelinger (1978) reported 22 cases of injury to the spleen and found that 41% had infectious mononucleosis at the time of injury.

The rupture of the spleen causing bleeding into the abdominal cavity leads to the signs and symptoms mentioned previously. Frelinger (1978) stated that radioisotope scanning, ultrasonography and CAT scanning facilitate diagnosis.

Ruptured liver. A direct blow to the upper right region of the abdomen just below the rib cage can lead to a rupture of the liver. Again, the signs and symptoms mentioned previously will cause suspicion of such an injury.

High speed accidents such as motor racing, skiing or sledding are the most common causes, according to Haycock (1986).

Ruptured kidney. A direct blow to the posterior aspect of the thorax above the pelvic girdle to the right or left of the spine may cause rupture of a kidney. This is a common injury in Australian Rules football, where the footballer is kneed over the kidney while contesting a mark.

A differential diagnosis from bruised muscles and a fracture of the transverse process of the upper lumbar spine must be made. Blood in the urine together with local pain over the site of the kidneys should cause suspicion of a kidney injury.

Any haematuria (blood in the urine), whether from a direct blow to the kidney area or not, must be investigated.

Injuries to the intestine. Trauma over the abdominal region may lead to injury of the intestines. A case study by Vaos et al (1989) highlighted how the small intestine may be injured in a gymnast. Lower abdominal pain and vomiting followed the injury when the gymnast slipped and struck her abdomen on a parallel bar. A 5 cm jejunal tear was found to be the cause of her symptoms when a laparotomy was performed.

Inguinal hernia. As stated earlier, pain in the lower abdominal region may be due to a lesion in the abdominal muscles or to an inguinal hernia. A differentiation needs to be made.

Pain in the lower abdominal/groin area which is caused by exercise, coughing or sneezing may be from an inguinal hernia. Examination should be performed to detect any swelling along the inner half of a line between the pubic tubercle and the anterior superior iliac crest. This swelling (hernia) is due to a protrusion of the abdominal contents through the peritoneum due to a weakness of the muscles and connective tissue layers of the abdominal wall. If a hernia is suspected, a medical opinion should be sought.

Surgical repair is required for an inguinal hernia, with a return to strenuous sport 8–10 weeks later (Peterson & Renstrom 1986).

Neoplasms and inflammatory lesions of the thoracic region

A differentiation must be made between mechanical pain in the thoracic spine and the inflammatory problems which

Chest pain: non-cardiac sources

Thoracic organs
- aorta
- pulmonary artery
- broncho pulmonary tree
- pleura
- mediastinum
- oesophagus
- diaphragm

Musculoskeletal
- cervical spine
- thoracic spine
- thoracic joints
  - sternoclavicular
  - manubriosternal
  - costochondral
  - sternocostal
  - xiphoid
  - scapulothoracic
- ribs
- muscles
- skin

Subdiaphragmatic organs
- stomach
- duodenum
- pancreas
- gall bladder

may occur. MacNab (1978) stated that severe pathological processes involving the vertebrae and intervertebral joints such as infections, neoplasms and metabolic disorders frequently present as pain in the back.

The key factor in suspecting an inflammatory lesion in the thoracic spine is that the athlete complains of constant pain, which is usually worse at rest, particularly while attempting to sleep. The objective examination is often atypical with abnormal movement patterns and there will be no response to treatment.

Benign tumours of the spine mostly affect the under 30 population and malignant tumours affect the over 40 population, their incidence increasing with age (McNab 1978).

A bone scan can be useful to screen for benign tumours such as osteoid osteoma as well as for other tumours or infection.

In the case of herpes zoster (shingles), an acute presentation will be easily differentiated by the presence of small cutaneous vesicles as well as pain in a segmental distribution. Post-herpatic neuralgia should be suspected with patients presenting with pain in a well defined distribution and a history of the condition.

Chest pain

Specific differentiation of chest pain with a cardiac origin or a musculoskeletal origin can be aided by the following analysis. Broadhurst (1987) stated four criteria for chest pain of musculoskeletal origin:

1. Quality: dull ache with exacerbations. Often has experienced similar pain elsewhere
2. Severity: will be variable and relates to posture and activity
3. Location: usually corresponds to the area of true origin except when referred from the thoracic spine
4. Distribution: has a more segmental region of pain especially if pain is referred.

While the thoracic spine is the most common source of non-cardiac chest pain, many other sources must be considered. The box summarizes the full range of possibilities (Broadhurst 1987).

Idiopathic spontaneous pneumothorax

Chest pain associated with difficulty in breathing and referred pain to the tip of the shoulder may be due to an idiopathic spontaneous pneumothorax (ISP).

Pfeiffer and Young (1980) stated that the literature indicates that the specific pathology is a ruptured apical lung bulla and that subpleural bullae occur bilaterally in a significant number of cases. The incidence of bullae seems higher in tall, thin, young, male athletes. In Pfeiffer and Young's study of 203 hospital admissions of idiopathic spontaneous pneumothorax only 6% were related to exercise. They do, however, describe a case study where a jogger sustained a ISP and warn that athletes with a high pain tolerance may not seek medical treatment after an ISP.

Other conditions

Winding

A blow to the abdomen, common in contact sports, can temporarily cause the athlete to 'double up' in discomfort. The athlete usually recovers quickly if he or she is 'winded', but if rapid recovery does not occur, a more serious internal injury must be suspected.

The cause of winding is the result of neurogenic shock due to stimulation of the coeliac (solar) plexus. The abdominal wall becomes rigid and the diaphragm undergoes spasm.

Relaxing the abdominal muscles by loosening restrictive clothing and pumping the legs into the abdomen helps return the circulation and relieve the spasm.

Stitch

Pain in the upper abdominal area is often experienced in athletes, particularly when running. It usually occurs some time after commencing running and may be experienced on either the right or left side. Deep expirations usually increase the pain, while deep inspiration eases the pain. The pain is known as a 'stitch'.

The cause of a stitch is not clearly understood, but Peterson and Renstrom (1986) stated that a purely mechanical effect may trigger it. They state the connective tissue which anchors the abdominal organs bears a much greater load just after a meal, and physical activity at this time could cause strain and minor internal bleeding. Other possible causes are lack of sufficient oxygen to the diaphragm, or pain arising from the internal abdominal organs such as the spleen and the liver as the blood is redistributed.

Cyriax (1957) stated that a stitch may be an ischaemic phenomenon of the diaphragm similar to claudication. Panting leads to pain at the lower costal margin which comes on as the athlete draws breath in, thus stopping full inspiration.

Peterson and Renstrom (1986) made some suggestions on how to avoid stitches. These include avoiding activity for a few hours after meals, running bent over, stopping the activity to allow the stitch to disappear or squeezing a hard object, like a stone, in the hands. The latter remedy, for which the mechanism of improvement is unknown, is found by most athletes to give relief.

Breast injuries

Breast injuries occur in sport to both male and female participants and may be due to a direct blow or from prolonged irritation. Haycock (1987) described how the female breast may be damaged in contact or racquet sports. Most injuries are not dangerous; applying ice immediately to the injured area can minimize damage.

Skin irritation of the nipple occurs in 'runners' nipples' and is caused by the shirt rubbing on the nipples. This may cause bleeding and the possibility of a secondary infection. Haycock (1987) recommended the use of a bandage over the nipple as a good preventive measure. She also suggested the use of a good sports bra to prevent the problem in women.

'Bicyclists' nipples', as described by Haycock (1987), is a condition caused by exposure to cold. It may persist for several days after the ride. For prevention of this superficial frostbite, McRae (1983) recommended the use of wind-breaking jackets and even several layers of newspaper under the jacket.

SUMMARY

The thorax and abdomen are injured less frequently in sport than most other areas of the body. However, when injury occurs it may have serious consequences and be of a life-threatening nature. The examining physiotherapist must be able to differentiate between a simple musculoskeletal injury and signs of a serious visceral injury. Once a clear diagnosis has been made, recovery via the appropriate treatment techniques can occur quite rapidly. This is especially true of pain emanating from the thoracic spine, where the use of manipulative and mobilizing techniques can quickly restore normal function. Postural correction, stretching and strengthening exercises also play an important role in regaining and maintaining good alignment and function.

It is important that the physiotherapist not only possess a good knowledge of the possible causes of thorax and abdominal pain and be able to examine thoroughly, but also possess a good range of manipulative and mobilizing techniques for the effective treatment of sporting injuries.

REFERENCES

Baker K G 1988 Scheuermann's disease: a review. The Australian Journal of Physiotherapy 34:(3)
Beyeler J, Reichmann B, Schneider W, Schweizer A 1979 Thoracic Scheuermann's disease: results of surgical and conservative therapy in patients followed 10 years or more. Orthopade 8:180-183
Boudillon J 1982 Spinal manipulation. Heinemann, London
Bradford D S 1985 The paediatric spine. Thieme, New York
Broadhurst N A 1987 The thoracic spine and its pain syndromes. Australian Family Physician 16(6):738
Chusid J C 1970 Correlative neuroanatomy and functional anatomy, 14th edn. Lange Medical Publications, Los Altos
Cloward R B 1959 Cervical diskography. Annal of Surgery 150:1052
Cooper M 1992 Personal communication
Corrigan B, Maitland G D 1983 Practical orthopaedic medicine. Butterworths, London
Cruess R L, Rennie W R J 1984 Adult orthopaedics. Churchill Livingstone, vol 2
Cyriax J 1957 Textbook of orthopaedic medicine. Cassell & Co, London, vol 1
Estwanik III J J, Bergfeld J A, Collins R H, Hall R 1980 Injuries in interscholistic wrestling. The Physician and Sports Medicine 8(2):111-121
Frelinger D P 1978 The ruptured spleen in college athletes: a preliminary report. American Journal College Health Association 26:217

Grieve G P (ed)1986 Manual therapy of the vertebral column. Churchill Livingstone, Edinburgh
Haycock C E 1986 How I manage abdominal injuries. The Physician and Sports Medicine 14(6):86-89
Haycock C E 1987 How I manage breast problems in athletes. The Physician and Sports Medicine 15(3):89-95
Houston J C, Joiner C L, Trounce J R 1978 A short textbook of medicine, 5th edn. Hodder & Stoughton, London
Kapanji I A 1974 The physiology of joints, vol III. The trunk and vertebral column, 2nd edn. Churchill Livingstone, Edinburgh, p. 132
Kellegren J H 1939 On the distribution of pain arising from deep somatic structures with charts of segmental pain areas. Clinical Science 4
Kulund D N 1988 The injured athlete, 2nd edn. J B Lippincott, Philadelphia
Landon J, Malpas J S 1959 Tietze's syndrome. Aurals of Rheumatic Disease 18:249
Macnab I 1978 Backache. Williams & Wilkins, Baltimore
Maitland G 1986 Vertebral Manipulation, 5th edn. Butterworths, London
McGuckin N 1986 The T4 syndrome—modern manual therapy of the vertebral column. Churchill Livingstone, Edinburgh
McKenzie R A 1980 Treat your own back. Spinal Publications, Lower Hutt

McKenzie R A 1981 The lumbar spine—mechanical diagnosis and therapy. Spinal Publications, Lower Hutt

McRae R 1983 Clinical orthopaedic examination, 2nd edn. Churchill Livingstone, Edinburgh

Minucci A 1987 Palpation of thoracic spine. Manipulative Therapists Association of Australia, Proceedings of Fifth Biennial Conference, Melbourne

Muckle D S 1971 Sports injuries. Oriel Press, Newcastle Upon Tyne

Newland I 1989 Personal communication

Nudel D (ed) 1989 Paediatric sports medicine. PMA Publishing, New York: pp. 169, 183-185

O'Donohue D H 1967 Treatment of injuries in athletes. Saunders, Philadelphia

Peterson L, Renstrom P 1986 Sports injuries—their prevention and treatment. Methuen, Australia

Pfeiffer R P, Young T R 1980 Case report: spontaneous pneumothorax in a jogger. The Physician and Sports Medicine 8(12):65-67

Schmitt H P, Bersch W, Feustel H P 1983 Acute abdominal rhabdomyolysis after body building exercise: is there a 'rectus abdominis syndrome'? Muscle Nerve 6 (March-April):228-232

Stoddard A 1974 Manual of osteopathic technique. Hutchinson, London

Vaos G C, Maridaki M, Eston R C 1989 Case study: unusual intra abdominal injury in a female gymnast. Australian Journal of Science in Sport 21(1):20-21

Warrick R, William P L 1973 Grays anatomy, 33rd edn. Churchill Livingstone, Edinburgh

Williams J G P (ed) 1976 Sports medicine. Edward Arnold, Dublin

Zettenburg C, Anderson G B J, Schultz A B 1987 The activity of individual trunk muscles during heavy physical loading. Spine 12:1035-1040

23. The shoulder complex

Craig Allingham

The shoulder region provides the sports physiotherapist with a great professional challenge. The extreme mobility of the joint with its dependency on muscular function and control means that the value of rehabilitation is perhaps greater than for any other joint in the body. Thus the physiotherapist becomes a prime determinant in the success or otherwise of any treatment and management program, whether it be conservative or surgical in nature.

With such an opportunity to optimize outcomes comes the responsibility of ensuring a current knowledge of shoulder kinesiology, sports biomechanics, assessment tools, treatment options, surgical techniques and rehabilitation protocols. This chapter endeavours to consolidate current research and practice in shoulder physiotherapy for athletes and to present it in such a manner as to maximize clinical applications.

The initial material on anatomy is provided as a review and as an update on recent findings. The sections on biomechanics provide a valuable insight into the actions and stresses that sport imposes on the shoulder and underpins the subsequent discussion of pathomechanics, shoulder pathology, tendinitis, impingement, instability, surgical repair and, of course, physiotherapy management of these conditions.

STRUCTURE AND FUNCTION

Anatomy

Clavicle and scapula

The clavicle provides the mechanism by which the glenohumeral joint, and thereby the arm, is suspended beside the thorax allowing maximal mobility of the upper limb. The s-shape of the clavicle serves to amplify small ranges of motion at the sternoclavicular joint into much larger arcs of movement at the acromion (Kaput 1987). The curving of the bone may also provide improved strength by way of curved stress-bearing trabeculae, similar to those in the femoral neck. Such adaptation is vital because the clavicle must simultaneously support the upper quadrant and transmit forces arriving from the arm to the thorax.

The thin, broad body of the scapula is the opposite to the solid, sinuous clavicle. Broad expanses of scapula provide anchoring for the many muscles attached. The spine of the scapula resembles the clavicle more closely, and provides a strong bony lever about which the large scapular muscles can generate torques to rotate the bone during arm elevation.

Clavicular joints

The medial articulation of the clavicle is deceptive in its apparent simplicity. The sternoclavicular joint is a poorly congruous saddle joint with an intervening intra-articular meniscus (Warwick & Williams 1973). The singular positioning and attachment of this disc allow it to fulfil two functions not usually shared by one structure. First, it acts as a hinge for the clavicle, thereby improving mobility, and second it stabilizes the clavicle to prevent medial dislocation of the clavicle in the event of compression loading (Peat 1986). The costoclavicular ligament further stabilizes the joint by binding the head of the clavicle to the first rib and costal cartilage. The stabilizing mechanisms of this joint are quite effective, as indicated by the frequency of clavicular fractures rather than sternoclavicular subluxations.

Laterally, the clavicle articulates with the acromion process of the scapula. The joint line is curved front to back allowing gliding of the acromion around the end of the clavicle, and is oblique down and medially. This angle tends to force the acromion below the clavicle when a compressive force is applied, resulting in the characteristic 'popped-up' end of the clavicle in acromioclavicular joint separations (Peat 1986).

The ligaments of the acromioclavicular joint are of particular clinical relevance. The joint itself is bridged by a capsule and superior acromioclavicular ligament (Warwick & Williams 1973). This ligament is not strong and permits the glide, hinge and pivot movements that occur at this joint. The primary stability for this joint is provided by the two parts of the coracoclavicular ligament—the trapezoid and conoid components (see Fig. 23.13, p. 369). These two strong bands suspend the scapula from the clavicle and form a fulcrum about which the acromioclavicular joint movements occur.

The trapezoid ligament counteracts the obliquity of the joint line, preventing over-riding of the clavicle. Injury to this ligament (grade 2 or grade 3 acromioclavicular joint sprain) permits the 'step' seen commonly in contact sports. The conoid ligament transmits the rotary force of scapular abduction to the clavicle initiating axial rotation of the clavicle, a vital component of elevation of the arm beyond 100° (Peat 1986).

Glenohumeral joint

The extremely mobile shoulder joint is a complex articulation which receives more comprehensive description elsewhere (Warwick & Williams 1973). This brief discussion will focus on those details of particular structural, biomechanical or clinical relevance.

The glenohumeral joint comprises a mismatched apposition of the head of the humerus and the glenoid fossa of the humerus. The discrepancy in size contributes to mobility but sacrifices intrinsic stability of the joint. The glenoid labrum imparts some expansion of the scapular articular surface by providing a fibrocartilaginous rim projecting laterally to embrace the humeral head (Warwick & Williams 1973). The outer surface of the labrum attaches to the joint capsule, and the inner surface is lined with synovium (Peat 1986). As the head of the humerus rotates the labrum conforms to maintain articular congruity.

The capsule of the joint is thin and generous, allowing separation of the joint surfaces of up to 3 mm if distracted in the loose packed position. This capsule is reinforced by ligaments and by the muscles of the rotator cuff. The passive restraint mechanisms of the glenohumeral joint are primarily anterior as the direction of the glenoid fossa (anterolaterally relative to the thorax) inherently stabilizes the posterior aspect of the joint (Pappas et al 1983). The three glenohumeral ligaments are vital to anterior stability. The superior glenohumeral ligament is important in preventing downward displacement of the humeral head, assisted by the coracohumeral ligament, the supraspinatus and the long head of biceps brachii (Fig. 23.1).

The middle glenohumeral ligament is an important stabilizer in the middle ranges of abduction, and the inferior glenohumeral ligament provides protection in the upper ranges of abduction (Ferrari 1990, O'Connell et al 1990, Peat 1986, Turkel et al 1981). Anterior stability in the resting position is reliant on subscapularis, which (being a dynamic restraint) must be active to be effective.

The inferior glenohumeral ligament consists of two bands (anterior and posterior) between which an axillary pouch lies. This arrangement allows both bands to be active as stabilizers in abduction irrespective of the rotation of the humerus. If the abducted arm is in internal rotation,

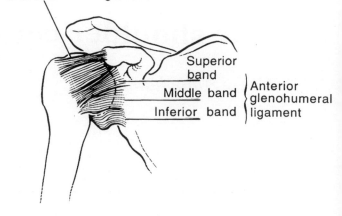

Fig. 23.1 Glenohumeral ligaments—anterosuperior view

the anterior band lies beneath the joint and supports the humeral head, while the posterior band now lies behind the humerus. If the arm is externally rotated, the posterior band moves beneath the humeral head to become its support, and the anterior band moves to lie in front of the joint, taking up its role as the primary anterior constraint (Bowen & Warren 1991, O'Connell et al 1990).

Thus, lesions to the inferior glenohumeral ligament complex will most likely result in a multidirectional instability due to its versatile role.

Glenohumeral musculature includes the large prime movers of the shoulder joint, and the smaller rotator cuff muscles. Of the former group, the deltoid and biceps brachii are the main elevators of the arm, while the pectoralis major, latissimus dorsi and teres major are the main internal rotators and concentric adductors of the arm (Basmajian & de Luca 1985).

The muscles of the rotator cuff are of particular interest to the clinical sports physiotherapist since the activity of these muscles is paramount in joint function or dysfunction. The four cuff muscles (supraspinatus, subscapularis, infraspinatus and teres minor) all arise from the scapula and attach to the tuberosities of the humerus just distal to the anatomical neck. The tendons all merge with the fibres of the joint capsule adding a dynamic component to the restraint mechanisms of the shoulder joint (Peat 1986).

The tendons of the long heads of biceps and triceps brachii arise from the superior and inferior poles, respectively, of the glenoid labrum and contribute to the composition of that structure. The long biceps tendon arises within the joint capsule, but remains extrasynovial by virtue of being invaginated by the synovial membrane of the joint (Kapandji 1970).

The vascular supply to the rotator cuff is derived from the posterior and anterior circumflex humeral arteries and the suprascapular artery supplying the anterior and posterior components. The supraspinatus is supplied from the thoracoacromial artery (Warwick & Williams 1973). The subacromial part of the cuff is considered hypovascular compared with the other components (Rathbun & McNab 1970). This area was described by Codman as the critical portion of the tendon and is now sometimes referred to as 'Codman's zone' (Allman 1985). The hypovascular area includes the supraspinatus, the long head of biceps and the upper portion of the infraspinatus tendons. At rest, these tendons are wrung out by the pressure of the humeral head beneath them (Rathbun & McNab 1970). During abduction, the coracoacromial arch provides additional pressure to these areas, further compromising the circulation, and in abduction and lateral rotation the torsion of the capsule serves to wring out the cuff blood supply (Perry 1983) (Fig. 23.2).

It is thought that this vascular compromise may initially predispose to inflammatory, degenerative changes in the cuff, and later it may slow or interfere with normal tissue repair (Rathbun & McNab 1970).

The articular neurology has been reviewed by Peat (1986) and reported to be rich. The spinal roots supplying the cuff and the articular structures are C5, C6 and C7, with a minor contribution from C4. The ligaments, capsule and synovial capsule are supplied by the axillary, suprascapular, subscapular and musculocutaneous nerves, with the distribution being variable (Peat 1986).

The nerve supply to the elements of the rotator cuff is via the upper and lower subscapular nerves to subscapularis, the suprascapular nerve supplies the supraspinatus and then the infraspinatus, the teres minor receives its supply from the axillary nerve and the biceps brachii from the musculocutaneous nerve with a branch to each belly (Warwick & Williams 1973).

Subacromial joint

The subacromial joint is one of two physiological joints around the shoulder, the other being the scapulothoracic joint (Kapandji 1970, Kaput 1987). These functional zones are described as joints to indicate their importance in contributing to shoulder mobility.

The components of the subacromial joint are the contents of the subacromial space—the superior rotator cuff tendons (supraspinatus and infraspinatus), the long head of biceps tendon and the subacromial bursa. These structures lie beneath the coracoacromial arch which is composed of the acromion, the coracoacromial ligament and the coracoid process. This arch comprises a superior restraint mechanism for upward movement of the humeral head and is necessary because of the lax inferior joint capsule. Interestingly, the shoulder region boasts two ligaments that do not span a joint—the coracoacromial and transverse humeral ligaments. There are three if one includes the 50% occurrence of the spinoglenoid ligament (Black & Lombardo 1990).

The subacromial bursa is one of eight around the shoulder joint (Peat 1986) and is the largest bursa in the body (Codman 1934). It lies not only below the acromion, but extends anteriorly beneath the coracoacromial ligament and distally to lie beneath the deltoid muscle. The undersurface of the bursa lies against the supraspinatus and infraspinatus proximally, and the head of the humerus distally (Warwick & Williams 1973) (Fig. 23.3).

During elevation of the shoulder, the bursa contributes to the smooth passage of the rotator cuff muscles and then the greater tuberosity of the humerus beneath the coracoacromial arch with minimal compression of the enclosed tissues. This 'movement requires fine muscular coordination, laxity of soft tissues and proper rotation of the humerus. Impairment of any of these factors can result in faulty movement, pain and disability' (Cailliet 1966).

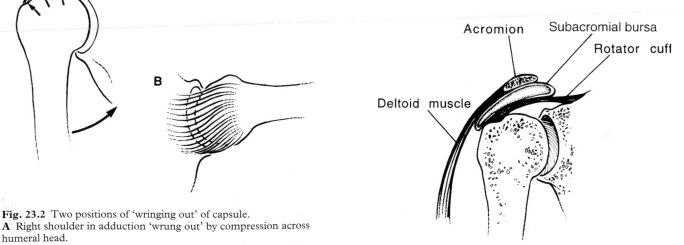

Fig. 23.2 Two positions of 'wringing out' of capsule.
A Right shoulder in adduction 'wrung out' by compression across humeral head.
B Left shoulder in external rotation and abduction 'wrung out' by torsion on cuff

Fig. 23.3 Subacromial joint

Kinesiology

Like the anatomy, the kinesiology of the upper quadrant is well described elsewhere (Basmajian & de Luca 1985, Peat 1986, Perry 1978). All that remains to be done here is to highlight some of the characteristics of shoulder mechanics that have a particular clinical relevance.

Force couples

The complexity of shoulder co-ordination becomes evident when the two pairs of force couples acting around the region are discussed. The more proximal *scapulothoracic force couple* is that acting on scapular motion under the control of the upper and lower fibres of trapezius and the serratus anterior. This coupling rotates the scapula upwards around the thoracic wall, while the levator scapulae and rhomboids balance the unwanted action of these muscles (scapular depression) to stabilize the root of the spine of the scapula about which this rotation occurs (Peat 1986). The *glenohumeral force couple* controls glenohumeral motion and is generated through the actions of the deltoid and the rotator cuff with the upper trapezius actively balancing the downward rotating effect of the deltoid muscle (Peat 1986) (Fig. 23.4).

The scapulothoracic couple is responsible for rotating the scapula upward across the costal surface so as to position the glenoid fossa optimally for arm elevation and function. This movement takes place initially during the range from 30-100° of abduction and occurs about an axis through the root of the spine of the scapula. At around 100°, the costoclavicular ligament prevents further clavicular abduction, so the acromioclavicular joint becomes the centre for further scapular rotation. This permits the root of the spine of the scapula to move laterally. Towards full elevation

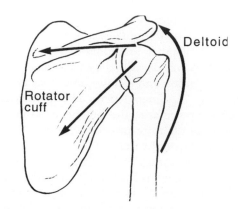

Fig. 23.5 Distal force couple

the trapezoid ligament tautens and locks the acromioclavicular joint, preventing further motion. Terminal abduction is achieved by rotation of the clavicle about its long axis (Peat 1986).

As the scapulothoracic couple repositions the scapula throughout arm elevation, the glenohumeral force couple is also in operation. The short cuff muscles (subscapularis, teres minor, infraspinatus) provide a downward and inward force vector to oppose rotary component of the deltoid (Perry 1978). These two elements act on opposite sides of the centre of rotation of the humeral head as the arm elevates, providing a strong force couple to facilitate that movement (Peat 1986). Calculations of the force summation of the total rotator cuff (all components are active during abduction) show a force line downwards and medially, approximately along the lower third of the subscapularis belly (Perry 1978) (Fig. 23.5).

Note that the distal force couple is acting from a mobile scapula, necessitating continual feedback and adjustment of muscle activity to accommodate changing joint angles and the effect of gravity as the glenoid is repositioned. The synergy and neuromuscular integration of simple elevation is complex and elegant. The demands on this integration are phenomenal when activities, such as tennis serving or overarm throwing are performed.

As well as the rotary component of the glenohumeral force couple, there is a second contribution. The downward force provided by the lower rotator cuff muscles prevents excessive upward migration of the humeral head during elevation. This is further assisted by the actions of the long head of biceps (through its bicipital groove pulley) and the supraspinatus (Peat 1986). In normal function, the head of the humerus is centred on the glenoid during initiation of elevation. This involves a 3 mm superior glide from the dependent position (Peat 1986). Once centred, the head remains so throughout the remaining elevation. Unfortunately, physiotherapists are usually dealing with abnormal function where this dynamic stabilization may not be as effective.

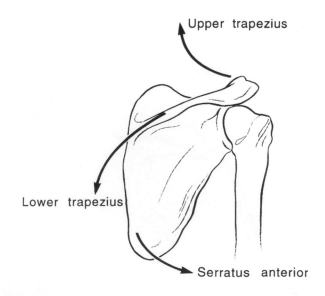

Fig. 23.4 Proximal force couple

Co-contraction of the rotator cuff muscles also produces a compression force, whereby the humeral head is centred in the concavity of the glenoid cavity. This contributes to the stability of the glenohumeral joint (Matsen et al 1991), but is only effective when the muscles are acting in a synchronous manner. Pain, injury or proprioceptive loss can reduce the effectiveness considerably.

Scapulohumeral rhythm

The proportional movement between scapula and humerus has been a subject of discussion for many years (Cailliet 1981, Codman 1934, Kapandji 1970). Peat (1986, p 1862) examined the literature and offered a summary, 'the initial 30° of abduction are essentially the result of glenohumeral motion. From 30° to full arm abduction movement occurs at the scapulothoracic and glenohumeral joints'. He avoided providing a 'normal' value for the ratio of relative movement at each segment, pointing out that various investigators have arrived at different figures. He attributed these differences to variations in the plane of the arc of the elevation between studies, loading on the arm and anatomical variations between subjects.

To a sports physiotherapist, normal scapulohumeral rhythm can often be assessed as that displayed on the non-injured arm, and any variations noted on the injured side are deemed pathological or at least symptoms of dysfunction. It is likely that such a simplistic notion is valid only as an observation, and to place diagnostic weight on it is fraught with danger. However, in combination with other examination results and specific testing of scapulohumeral rhythm under load, unilateral variations become useful in the overall assessment and management of athletes.

For readers still not satisfied, a ratio of approximately 2:1 for glenohumeral to scapulothoracic motion through abduction is considered normal. It is also much more easily estimated than some of the other ratios, for example, 1.35:1 and 2.34:1 (Peat 1986).

Sports biomechanics

The kinesiology of normal elevation is of interest to a sports physiotherapist, but the mechanics of the upper quadrant in sporting activities provides far more stimulating fare.

The three main actions in sport that contribute to overuse injuries have one factor in common, that the arm is placed in elevation and rotation while under heavy loading. These three are overarm throwing, swimming and overhead strokes in racquet sports. Each has been well investigated (Atwater 1979, Beekman & Hay 1988, Costill et al 1992, Fleisig et al 1989, Glousman et al 1988, Jobe et al 1983, 1984, 1986, Moynes et al 1986, Nuber et al 1986, Pappas et al 1985b, Perry 1983) and the important mechanical and pathomechanical features will be discussed in this section.

Throwing

The action of propelling an object, ball or javelin using an overarm throw involves the whole body. An efficient transfer of body momentum starts at the feet with forward body movement, at each successive body segment forces and torques are developed by muscle activity and added to those forces being transferred toward the throwing arm. Finally, the arm accepts the body generated momentum, adds to it, and steers the resultant forces so that the thrown object travels at the desired velocity.

If the throwing action was 100% efficient, all the body momentum would be transferred to the object and the throwing arm would cease movement at the point of release. The body is not that efficient, so the unspent forces must be reabsorbed by the body during the follow-through action. This involves a gradual deceleration of body parts and transfer of momentum back along the kinetic throwing chain.

The action of overarm throwing places the arm in extremes of rotation and horizontal extension in the cocking phase, and abduction in the follow-through. It also necessitates a combination of abduction and lateral rotation, the close packed position of the joint (Peat 1986), under extremes of load. Add to these extremes of range, the explosive nature of throwing and the high forces generated, and one can appreciate the high risk of shoulder injury in throwers.

A more detailed examination of the throwing action is useful to understanding the physiological stress points of the activity. Throwing is usually divided into its component parts for analysis and various reporters use three, four or sometimes five phases. For this discussion the phases of the throw will be divided into cocking, acceleration and follow-through as first described by Tullos and King (1973), with the additional inclusion of release as a fourth phase (Fig. 23.6).

Windup. This is the preparatory phase during which the body is positioned for throwing, and the arm begins its movement toward the cocking position. This phase utilises the large muscle groups of the lower body (quadriceps, gluteals, abdominals) to raise the centre of gravity (front leg lift) and then drive forward off the back leg, converting the potential energy to kinetic energy. The trunk converts

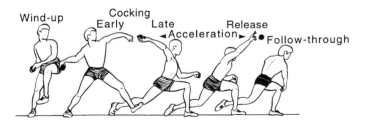

Fig. 23.6 Phases of throwing.
Source: adapted from Glousman et al (1988)

the momentum from forward to rotatory. The arm swings away from the trunk under its own weight, and then is raised into the cocked position of abduction and external rotation. The arm path is down, back then up.

The importance of the windup is that it sets up the body and arm position for the violent act of throwing to follow. Any loss of control, balance or stability of the trunk will reduce the efficient transfer of momentum to the throwing arm which in turn will place increased demands on the shoulder muscles and restraints to control the forces and to contribute more strongly to make up for the deficit. Problems with the windup phase may be a cause of shoulder injury as it strives to supplement and compensate for poor body mechanics or inefficient control.

Cocking. This position involves the throwing arm moving to full external rotation in about 90° of abduction. Cocking is characterized by strong contraction of the external rotators of the shoulder joint in order to store elastic energy in the recoil system. This activity of the posterior deltoid, supra and infraspinatus and the teres minor muscles continues until the explosive medial rotation of the humerus signifies the onset of the acceleration phase. At the end of cocking there is strong activity in the internal rotators as they decelerate the lateral rotation predisposed by the opening of the shoulders as the trunk commences to rotate. This flash of activity is most likely an eccentric contraction which serves to store elastic energy similar to that described by Komi (1988) as a stretch shortening cycle. This eccentric pre-loading increases the power of the subsequent concentric contraction and is a high speed neuromuscular adaption to training.

Late cocking places the glenohumeral capsule (and cuff) in maximum lateral rotation and horizontal extension at around 90° of abduction. In this position the capsule of the joint is under stress from two sources. Firstly, the torsion effect of the rotation wrings the capsule posteriorly further compromising the tenuous vascularity of the upper tendons of the rotator cuff. Secondly, the strong contraction of the posterior fibres of the deltoid lever the head of the humerus anteriorly hard against the anterior labrum and cuff (Perry 1983). Repeated episodes can stretch the anterior shoulder capsule predisposing to hypermobility problems and perhaps anterior instability. The short external rotators of the cuff (teres minor and infraspinatus) must work hard to prevent the humeral head from migrating forward under the force of the deltoid. Weakness or inhibition will reduce this stabilization and increase anterior joint trauma. The muscle activity during the cocking action involves deltoid, supraspinatus, infraspinatus and teres minor and then subscapularis. This is the recruitment sequence reported by Jobe et al (1983), who then notes there is an overlap as they come into play. The late recruitment of subscapularis is interpreted to be a deceleration of the lateral rotation momentum of late cocking just prior to acceleration.

There are several pathomechanical cocking patterns that can be seen in throwers, patterns that deviate from the accepted normal of a smooth up and backward movement of the hand, keeping the hand on top of the ball for as long as possible moving into the position of maximal lateral rotation and 90° of abduction. These patterns are demonstrated by Thurston (1985a, 1985b).

The first deviation is an incorrect roll over, where the thrower shortens the cocking phase by externally rotating the shoulder too early. This exposes the anterior shoulder to injury as the trunk rotates to open the shoulders.

The second anomaly is the thrower who over extends the throwing elbow towards the end of early cocking. The elbow should not get much beyond 45° of flexion or else the arm is late to arrive in the cocked position and the immediate acceleration stresses the rotator cuff. The third variation is the thrower who brings the arm too far backward across the midline of the body, usually through excessive trunk rotation and shoulder extension. The need to rapidly accelerate the arm to catch up with the trunk rotation stresses the shoulder and elbow.

Acceleration consists of the explosive medial rotation and forward translation of the humerus commencing after late cocking and concluding with release of the thrown object. Accompanying the arm movement is a rotation and lateral flexion (ipsilateral or contralateral depending on the style of the thrower) of the trunk. In expert throwers the timing of this phase is remarkably consistent, as it must be to maximize efficient transfer of momentum. The degree of lateral trunk flexion determines the apparent elevation of the arm at release (Pappas et al 1985b). Actually, the shoulder remains around 90° of abduction in all overarm throwing or hitting actions, however the degree and direction of lateral trunk flexion can give the appearance of a side-arm or 3/4 action (Fig. 23.7). 'Submarine' pitchers in baseball laterally flex toward the throwing side so as to pitch upwards at the batter, the arm remains at around 90° of abduction but the illusion is otherwise (Fig. 23.7).

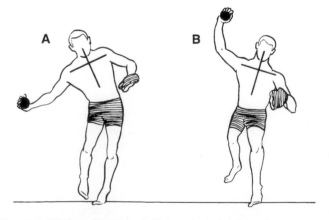

Fig. 23.7 90° throwing angle. **A** 'Submarine' pitching style. **B** 'Normal' pitching style

The angular velocities achieved during expert throwing are extremely high, in the order of 6000-7000° per second (Pappas et al 1985b). The torques generated around the longitudinal axis of the humerus have also been investigated. At late cocking there is a lateral rotation torque of around 17 600 Joules, upon acceleration the torque reverses to an internal rotary force of around 18 900 Joules. Following release of the object, the external rotators decelerate the arm by producing yet another torque reversal of similar magnitude. These three cycles of loading/unloading occur within 1/10 of a second (Gainor et al 1980).

Not surprisingly, as the measured fracture torque for a freshly disected humerus is only 14 900 Joules (Gainor et al 1980), such high rotary forces can fracture the humerus during throwing (this author has witnessed two occurences). It is thought that the extra load capability can occur due to the axial compression of the humeral cortex by those muscles active during the acceleration phase, especially the triceps. Fatigue or poor synergy of axial loading can leave the humerus unbraced and susceptible to fracture in the act of throwing (Gainor et al 1980).

The acceleration phase is powerful but short lived, lasting around 50 ms in expert throwers. As mentioned above, there is a powerful rotation and lateral flexion of the trunk as the humerus is internally rotated during acceleration. This rotation of the trunk produces an opening of the shoulders and contributes to the stretch shortening cycle of the internal rotators as they are activated to accelerate the arm. The latissimus dorsi and pectoralis major produce the medial rotation (Jobe et al 1984) with little activity of the subscapularis (Jobe et al 1983).

During acceleration there is other muscle activity around the shoulder, primarily involved in stabilizing against the powerful forces being transferred and summated. The scapula is firmly fixed against the thorax by the activity of serratus anterior (Jobe et al 1983, Pappas et al 1985b). Meanwhile, the infraspinatus, teres minor and, to a lesser degree, the supraspinatus are active to stabilize the humeral head in the glenoid (Jobe et al 1983, 1984). The downward force of these cuff muscles (discussed above) should assist in minimizing the subacromial impingement that can occur during acceleration. The role of teres major is not yet clear; the work of Basmajian (Basmajian & de Luca 1985) indicates that the muscle is only recruited for medial rotation adduction/extension when working against resistance. Whether the explosive nature of throwing or the inertial resistance of the cocking position is sufficient to recruit this muscle is still unanswered. The EMG investigations by Jobe et al (1983, 1984) and Glousman et al (1988) did not monitor the teres major. More work on this and on the role of trapezius at the scapulothoracic junction is required.

During acceleration, the triceps is active in its role as an elbow extensor. In doing so, it exerts some force across the glenohumeral joint via the attachment its long head to the inferior glenoid tubercle. The extent and significance of this effect has not been investigated.

Release of the ball or other object signifies the end of the acceleration phase. When throwing for maximal power the release point occurs when the arm is parallel with the line of the shoulders, and in 40-60° of lateral rotation (Pappas et al 1985b). When throwing a ball with slower velocity, the release point is more anterior to this coronal plane of the body with the arm in significant horizontal flexion (Pappas et al 1985b).

Follow-through phase commences with release and continues until the unspent forces of the throwing action are dissipated. During this stage there is an active attempt by the body to absorb these unspent forces by transferring the arm and trunk momentum back along the same kinetic chain that generated them.

At the arm, the external rotators, deltoid (middle and posterior) and rotator cuff all are active to decelerate respective components of the follow-through. This effort is provided by eccentric contraction of these muscles once the internal rotators relax upon release of the object. The forces exerted are quite high (Glousman et al 1988) and recruitment must be rapid as the timeframe is brief. This rapid eccentric loading indicates a high stress factor on the tendon structures involved predisposing them to breakdown and the development of tendinitis (Curwin & Stanish 1984). In addition to the glenohumeral deceleration, the serratus anterior is active to control the scapula (Glousman et al 1988) and it is likely that the trapezius is also active in this role.

Forward movement of the arm, medial rotation of the shoulder and protraction of the scapula must all be decelerated. The mechanics of the follow-through will determine whether the attenuation of these forces is performed within the physical and physiological limits of the tissues, or if an injury will occur.

A long, deep follow-through provides time and range of motion for the attenuation of the unspent forces. This is particularly true around the shoulder where the arm should pass down and across the body so that the hand finishes approximately lateral to the contralateral knee. As this is occurring, the trunk continues to flex and rotate and the body weight is shifted onto the leading leg as hip and knee flexion lower the centre of gravity. These actions allow the larger muscles of the trunk, buttocks and thigh to play an active eccentric role in decelerating the body and absorbing momentum as it is transferred caudally from the throwing arm and shoulder girdle. It is appropriate that these large muscle groups be recruited for this purpose rather than using the smaller muscles of the rotator cuff or scapula; after all, they generated the forces in the first instance.

A shallow follow-through reduces the contribution of the larger hip and leg muscles, meaning that more deceleration must be provided by the shoulder girdle muscles. Overstress to these structures will predispose to injury of the external rotators of the shoulder. In order to accomplish a deep follow-through, the athlete must have adequate flexibility in the hip, gluteal and lumbar regions. Tightness in these areas can restrict the follow-through action and place more strain on both the shoulder and the tight pelvic area.

One interesting effect of a deeper follow-through in which the trunk flexes rapidly after release is that as the arm continues forward there is an effective abduction at the glenohumeral joint. As the inertia of the arm tends to continue in the line of the thrown object, the shoulder adductors must become active to decelerate the abducting humerus. Failing to do this will predispose to subacromial impingement. Accordingly, if an athlete with a posterior cuff strain due to shallow follow-through is retrained to deepen the trunk flexion, attention must be paid to the strength of the adductors to prevent an impingement syndrome developing.

Care of the throwing arm

The best care for a thrower's arm is preventive care, the kind of care that will avoid or restrict the development of injury. The following information has evolved from the author's work with international representative baseball, and particularly with Bill Thurston, a leading pitching coach in the USA.

Common causes of sore arms and injuries:
1. Lack of proper stretching and warm-up.
2. Lack of proper conditioning. Not building strength, flexibility, and endurance in a progressive program.
3. Improper pitching/throwing mechanics.
4. Throwing too often or too long, and not allowing sufficient recovery time.
5. Throwing new pitches.

The following principles of care should be applied:
1. Proper conditioning of the throwing arm and the whole body, because correct throwing is a total body activity.
2. Proper stretching program done daily, not just at practice and on game days. Thorough stretching should be done prior to picking up a baseball.
3. Proper warm-up time. This will vary with individuals, and pitchers can usually organize their own timing. The rest of the team should warm-up together. Late comers must always be given time to warm-up.
4. Teach proper pitching mechanics within the limits of individual variation.
5. Develop a training program that builds strength, stamina and flexibility.
6. Allow players an adequate rest and recovery period. Pitchers will vary, so get to know their capacity for recovery.
7. Monitor the workload of pitchers, know what pitches they have thrown, how many, how long since they have thrown and what they have been doing in the bullpen.
8. Reduce the physical stress of learning a new pitch by reducing the speed and distance. There should be no hard throws or snapping until the pitcher has learned the proper arm action and release.
9. A long-sleeved undershirt will absorb perspiration and avoid chilling of the arm while pitching.

10. Between innings all pitchers, and any other player with arm soreness, should keep the arm warm and loose. A jacket and/or light throw will suffice.
11. Sustained hard throwing usually leads to arm soreness. To a degree, this is normal. Players should recognize the difference between the usual dull ache and anything more sinister (e.g. persistent aching pain, or sharp pain). If in doubt, stop throwing and seek treatment.

Care of the arm after pitching:
1. After finishing pitching, complete a warm-down (light throw, light run and stretch). There should be no more throwing once the pitcher has cooled down.
2. Keep the arm warm, put on a jacket and wear it home.
3. Avoid or minimize alcohol consumption, it will increase any inflammation and delay recovery.
4. Day one after pitching should comprise jogging and running, a thorough stretching session, easy tossing (not pitching) with a full range of motion, pitcher's drills (no throwing) and conditioning drills (pick-ups, interval sprints, poles, etc).
5. Each subsequent day introduces more throwing, moving toward full pitching on day four or five depending on the rotation. Weekly games take the pressure off recovery time, but for good quality of recovery a similar program should be used.
6. The routine use of ice on a pitchers arm after an outing is much over-rated. A thorough warm-down and solid workout next day will be much more beneficial. Ice need only be used when:
   • there is an injury
   • there is swelling
   • there is a history of one or the other.
7. Relying on rub-downs, ointments, manipulations or whatever is the lazy pitcher's way of avoiding the responsibility of looking after his or her own arm. Caring for it by developing stamina, strength, flexibility, proper mechanics and common sense about his or her capacity is the best way to become an efficient and safe pitcher.

Racquet sports

The mechanics of an overhead stroke or serve in a racquet sport provide similarities with that of an overarm throw. The most obvious difference is the use of a racquet. The ball is propelled by an impulse force at the racquet face some distance from the arm that is delivering the momentum to the racquet. This enables much more force to be imparted to the ball compared with throwing, or similar forces being imparted for less musculoskeletal effort.

Again, the biomechanics of overhead strokes are divided into phases comparable to those of throwing (Fig. 23.8).

Windup is again a preparatory action where the body and arm is positioned to allow a forceful and accurate serving action. As with throwing, balance, control and a stable trunk/pelvic segment will maximize efficiency of force summation and assist with injury prevention.

Cocking occurs with the backward swing of the racquet which is then cocked by rotating the shoulder externally as the elbow flexes into the so-called 'back-scratch' position. In this action there is much more elbow flexion than with a cocked throwing arm, and less shoulder extension and lateral rotation (Leach 1985). Electromyographic data (Ryu et al 1988, Moynes et al 1986) shows the three most active muscles for this stage to be serratus anterior, supraspinatus and infraspinatus. Biceps brachii is active in flexing the elbow and subscapularis becomes active in the late stage of cocking to decelerate the external rotation momentum and prepare for internal rotation.

The importance of the serratus anterior in stabilizing and positioning the scapula is emphasised by Ryu et al (1988).

Acceleration is an explosive medial rotation of the shoulder and accompanying extension of the elbow. The subscapularis and pectoralis major work intensely to rotate the humerus, assisted by latissumus dorsi. The serratus anterior reaches peak activity in this phase as it controls the scapula (Ryu et al 1988). Infraspinatus is important in stabilizing the humeral head (Moynes et al 1986). The upward movement of the racquet head during acceleration provides a different shoulder momentum compared with throwing. The latter involves throwing the shoulder away from the body, whereas the tennis serve is more a control of the arc movement of the racquet head at the time of impact (Leach 1985).

Follow-through phase involves decelerating not only the arm (as in throwing) but the racquet as well. This obviously has the potential to increase the loading on those posterior glenohumeral muscles and stabilizers, until one takes into account the reactive force of the ball against the racquet face.

This phase involves moderate to high activity in many glenohumeral muscles. Following ball contact, the arm continues to internally rotate as it starts to move across the body. Immediately after contact, the trunk flexes, which results in the shoulder continuing to abduct by virtue of its upward momentum. The latissumus dorsi, subscapularis and pectoralis major are active at this point (Ryu et al 1988), perhaps to decelerate the abduction, thus the internal rotation continues into the follow-through.

The biceps brachii becomes active after ball impact to decelerate the elbow extension and prevent hyper-extension.

At impact there is a reaction force that is equal in magnitude and opposite in direction to the force accelerating the ball. This force assists in decelerating the racquet head, reducing the workload for the posterior muscle groups. The more momentum transferred to the ball, the stronger is this reactive force. If the ball is struck 'sweetly' (i.e. in the centre of percussion of the racquet), more momentum is delivered. If the ball is struck poorly, there remains greater unspent forces in the kinetic system of the player which must then be reabsorbed. This has consequences for skilled versus less skilled players.

The follow-through continues down and across the body with only minor variations due to angling the stroke to impart different spins to the ball. As for throwing, a deep follow-through provides greater safety and efficiency for force dissipation, but must be weighed up against the need to react to the returning ball.

Swimming

Understanding the action of swimming and its effect on the shoulder is vital to the sports physiotherapist, for the swimming injuries that occur in the upper quadrant are intimately related to mechanics and pathomechanics of the stroke movement. Discussions of these movements can be found in Pettrone (1985), Falkel and Murphy (1988), and Falkel (1990), but a far more detailed analysis is provided by Costill et al (1992). The earlier works described the strokes as comprising recovery, catch, and power phases. Costill et al (1992) further dissect the swimming mechanics

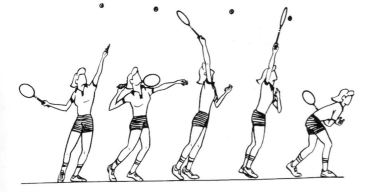

Fig. 23.8 Phases of tennis serve.
Source: adapted from Kirby & Roberts (1985)

and identify component movements within these broad phases. For example, various 'sweeps' of the propulsive (power) phase are described for each stroke.

Perhaps the most profound difference in this nomenclature is in relation to the 'catch' position (catch being the beginning of the propulsive phase). The earlier workers equated hand entry with catch, however Costill et al (1992) describe catch as occurring after hand entry, at the beginning of the first propulsive sweep. This is further discussed in the specific stroke analyses below.

Prior to discussing the four competitive swimming strokes it may be useful to discuss some general aspects of propulsion and resistance in relation to swimming. This material is condensed from Costill et al (1992) and the reader is referred to that text for more detailed information. In fact, the text is highly recommended for readers with an interest in swimmers and their injuries.

In its simplest analysis, the science of swimming is aimed at overcoming the resistance of the water while applying force to the water to gain propulsion. The resistance is due to various types of drag, these are form, wave and frictional drag. Form drag relates to the cross-sectional profile that the swimmer presents to the water as he or she moves through it. The more compact the profile, the less drag. Thus the body should remain as horizontal as possible and maintain a tapered lateral alignment (minimize lateral wiggling). The symmetrical strokes (butterfly and breaststroke) are not affected by this factor.

The second form of drag is wave drag. This is the resistance presented by turbulence at the surface of the water. Bow waves are formed as the head and trunk move through the water and are unavoidable. However the wave drag caused by the arm entering the water is influenced by the amount of turbulence created by the recovery/entry phases. A splashing impact into the water will create excessive turbulence and will resist forward propulsion. Likewise, pushing the back of the hand forward through the water during entry will reduce speed, thus a blade-like entry with the side of the hand is recommended by coaches.

Frictional drag makes up the third of the resistive forces that the swimmer must overcome. This is the friction between the skin and the adjacent layer of water molecules. The more friction that occurs, the more turbulent is the fluid flow past the body thus increasing drag. Research has shown that removal of body hair will significantly reduce frictional drag (Costill et al 1992), confirming the validity of shaving-down that has been practised for some years in elite competitive swimming.

The exact mechanisms making up the propulsive forces in swimming are still not fully understood, but the recent work presented in Costill et al (1992) goes a long way to reducing the uncertainty. Work done by Brown and Counsilman (1971) promoted the theory of propulsion through Bernoulli's theory of differential pressures as water passed the back of the hand (convex surface) more quickly than across the palm of the hand (flat surface) as the hand stroked through the water. This produced a lift force much the same way as an aircraft wing, and provided the propulsive force for the swimmer. This principle was inferred from the diagonal stroking pattern common to all the propulsive phases of competitive swimmers. Costill et al (1992) believe that Bernoulli's theorem is the lesser of two forces providing propulsion. The more important being Newton's third law of motion relating to every action having an equal and opposite reaction. That is, when a swimmer pushes water backwards, the body is accelerated forwards by the reaction force.

Costill et al (1992) go on to explain how the swimmer's hand can then force a greater body of water backwards by occasionally altering the direction of the arm movement in order to seek non-turbulent water against which to push, thus maximizing the reaction force. Accordingly, the propulsive phase of stroke mechanics can then be divided into directional sweeps for the purposes of analysis. These four basic sweeps are outsweep, downsweep, insweep and upsweep, and they will be discussed under each of the stroke descriptions.

Freestyle. Front crawl is the stroke commonly referred to as freestyle. This has come about because swimmers universally adopt this stroke when competing in freestyle events (where the choice of stroke is up to the swimmer). The term freestyle will be used in this text to describe the front crawl stroke.

Freestyle can be divided into the phases of entry and stretch, downsweep and catch, insweep, upsweep, release and recovery (Fig. 23.9) (Costill et al 1992). This contrasts with the earlier divisions of entry, pull and recovery phases (Pettrone 1985, Falkel 1990). These stroke components are summarised in Table 23.1.

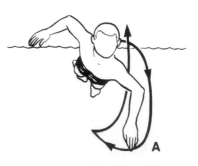
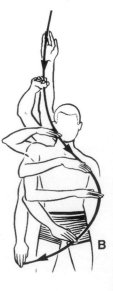

Fig. 23.9. Arm movement during freestyle seen from A the front and B below.
Sources: A adapted from Costill et al (1992); B adapted from Falkel et al (1988)

Table 23.1 Mechanics of freestyle (front crawl)

Phase	Comments
Entry	Palm out. Elbow is flexed then extends during glide
Downsweep	Elbow and shoulder flexion keeping elbow higher than hand (no 'dropped elbow')
Catch	Beginning of propulsive stroke, occurs about one-third of way through the underwater stroke
Insweep	Semicircular movement to bring hand beneath midline of body
Upsweep	Strongest propulsive movement, arm is brought up and outward toward surface of water, force easing as hand passes the thigh
Release	Overlaps with upsweep, palm turns in to thigh, and propulsive force is released
Recovery	Hand comes forward in straight line, with elbow kept high to allow sufficient external rotation of humerus to prevent impingement. Elbow extends and palm turns inward, to allow entry without crossing midline

Source: from Costill et al 1992

The external rotators and posterior deltoid are important muscles throughout the swimming cycle despite their not contributing much to the propulsive sweeps. Their role is to position the arm so that the muscles of propulsion (internal rotators, triceps and biceps) can generate force across a longer and more mechanically advantageous sweep. In addition, they recover the arm and place it in the optimal position for entry. Fatigue weakness or dysfunction of these muscles will increase the likelihood of injury and will reduce performance.

Likewise, fatigue or dysfunction of the humeral head depressors (infraspinatus, teres minor and teres major) during the early pull phase can predispose to impingement by failing to stabilize the humerus in the glenoid and allowing excessive superior migration (Costill et al 1992, Falkel & Murphy 1988). The long head of biceps may also contribute to this stabilization of the humeral head (Nuber et al 1986).

There are several other aspects of the freestyle swimming stroke that deserve mention in relation to mechanics and injury. Body roll during recovery of the arm is important in order to minimize the degree of horizontal extension required to lift the elbow from the water, and to allow sufficient lateral rotation of the humerus to avoid impingement as the arm comes through (Beekman & Hay 1988). The normal range of body roll during swimming is 40-60° from the neutral position in the water (prone). Excessive roll is associated with a midline crossover entry or dropped elbow during downsweep with likely impingment. Insufficient roll places more stress on the shoulder as the required lateral rotation to allow clear passage of the greater tuberosity beneath the acromion is difficult to achieve.

Falkel and Murphy (1988) report that many investigators have attempted to link breathing side with laterality of shoulder injuries in swimmers, but that little consensus is evident. If a swimmer is developing impingement signs on the non-breathing side, it may be due to an imbalance of body roll as the swimmer hyper-rolls when a breath is taken compared with the flatter body position during the recovery of the opposite arm.

Backstroke. Backstroke can also be divided into stroke phases, in this case entry, four sweeps of the power phase, release and recovery (Fig. 23.10). These are summarized in Table 23.2.

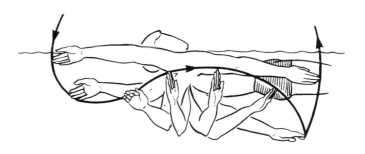

Fig. 23.10 Arm movement pattern during backstroke.
Source: adapted from Costill et al (1992)

Table 23.2 Mechanics of backstroke

Phase	Comments
Entry	Arm enters in fully extended position, with the palm turned outwards
First downsweep	Elbow flexes and hand turns down to achieve *catch* position
First upsweep	From catch, the arm pushes upwards and toward the feet until elbow is at about 90° flexion when the hand is at chest level
Second downsweep	Internal shoulder rotation pushing hand downwards (toward floor of pool), hand keeps wide of thigh and points away from the body. Most powerful
Second upsweep	Wrist is extended and palm turned upwards as hand moves toward surface of water. Force eases as hand passes thigh
Release/recovery	Palm turns inwards, arm reaches high and overhead to entry position with palm outwards

Source: from Costill et al 1992

Breaststroke. Breaststroke has generally been considered less stressful on shoulders than the other strokes, perhaps due to the avoidance of horizontal hyper-extension. However, a recent rule change which now allows swimmers to drop the head beneath the water has negated this advantage, and we may see an increase in shoulder problems with this stroke, or at least lose one of the options for allowing a swimmer with a shoulder injury to continue training using this stroke.

The breaststroke arm action is the less complicated part of the event, the kick motion being more intricate. Nevertheless, the arm stroke comprises several phases, namely

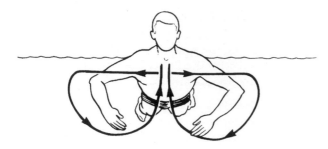

Fig. 23.11 Arm movement pattern during breaststroke.
Source: adapted from Costill et al (1992)

Table 23.3 Mechanics of breaststroke

Phase	Comments
Outsweep	Arms start fully extended forwards, palms then turn outward as the arms sweep laterally to the *catch*. Palms then turn back and downwards
Insweep	The propulsive stage comprising a large curving movement as both shoulders internally rotate and the elbows flex. Hands come together beneath the head or neck as the pressure is *released* for recovery
Recovery	Elbows squeeze in and then extend to project hands forward in the midline of the body to recommence outsweep

Source: from Costill et al 1992

outsweep, insweep and recovery, with the catch occuring during outsweep (Fig. 23.11). These are summarized in Table 23.3.

Butterfly. The butterfly stroke is the second of the symmetrical swimming motions, and the arm stroke is divided into entry, outsweep and catch, insweep, upsweep and release and recovery phases (Table 23.4).

Butterfly involves similar stroke mechanics to freestyle with an overarm recovery, elevated catch position and similar sweeps in the propulsive phase. One obvious difference is that butterfly is bilateral, so body roll is non-existent and the breathing is in the midline during late

Table 23.4 Mechanics of butterfly stroke

Phase	Comments
Entry	Hands enter water about shoulder width apart, thumbs downwards
Outsweep	Hands turn out and back, elbows flex to engage *catch* position. Elbows should be kept high
Insweep	Medial rotation of shoulders bringing hands beneath body as elbows flex to 90°
Upsweep	Hands move out and around the body in preparation for recovery. Palms are pitched out and the force is *released* as they pass the thighs
Recovery	Once out of the water, both arms are circled out, over and forwards. The arms are held flexed throughout, terminal extension of the elbows being achieved just after entry to initiate outsweep

Source: from Costill et al, 1992

power/early recovery phase. The absence of body roll means that the shoulders must accomplish the necessary lateral rotation during the recovery phase while in horizontal extension. Especially during any non-breathing stroke cycles. This predisposes to impingement, and an ability to lift the shoulders clear of the water during recovery should reduce subacromial and anterior joint stress. The power phase involves combined medial rotation and horizontal flexion which can also cause subacromial impingement. Entry position is with the hands about shoulder width apart, thereby avoiding the crossover problems seen in freestyle (Fig. 23.12).

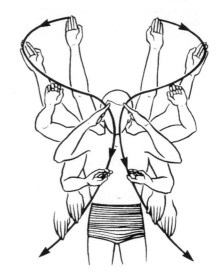

Fig. 23.12 Arm movement pattern during butterfly.
Source: adapted from Falkel et al (1988)

There are two important physiological/functional differences between the overarm actions of throwing or serving, and swimming. First, there is no eccentric muscle activity during the swimming cycle, any deceleration required is provided by the resistance of the water. Second, the power phase of swimming involves the muscles working with reversed origin and insertion, the hand remains virtually stationary pressed against the water as the body is pulled and then pushed past that point. Both these factors are important considerations in the rehabilitation of swimming injuries when one looks at specificity of re-training.

INJURY PATTERNS

Injuries to the shoulder region result from the same two mechanisms as those occurring elsewhere in the body: macrotrauma or repetitive microtrauma. The former generally results from point of shoulder impact injuries to the ground or between competitors, or due to intentional or incidental forces being applied to the outstretched arm.

The over-use injuries are usually due to repetitive, forceful activities frequenting the extremes of range, particularly abduction and lateral rotation.

Trauma

Acromioclavicular joint

The acromioclavicular joint is commonly injured in sports, especially collision sports. Typically the athlete sustains an impact to the point of the shoulder either from another competitor or upon hitting the ground. The angle of the acromioclavicular joint drives the acromion beneath the clavicle with resultant ligamentous damage.

The site and severity of the ligament damage reflects the forces applied at the time of injury (Fig. 23.13). A grade 1 sprain involves disruption of only the capsular ligaments of the acromioclavicular joint. There is sharp local pain on movement or palpation, but no deformity (Falkel & Murphy 1988). Grade 2 injury involves complete capsular disruption and partial tearing of the coracoclavicular ligament. As expected, the pain is more severe, movement is restricted and there is a palpable step at the line of the acromioclavicular joint where the clavicle rides upwards. Total rupture of the coracoclavicular ligament signifies a grade 3 injury. The deformity is easily visible and the pain quite severe, as is the incapacity (Stewart 1985).

Management of the two more severe grades of injury is aimed at achieving optimal realignment and/or functional stability of the acromioclavicular joint. Realignment in the acute stage of injury should ensure the ligamentous repair occurs in a position as close as possible to anatomically correct. This is not difficult in a grade 2 injury as the joint is only slightly subluxed and there are fibres of the coracoclavicular ligament remaining intact to provide a scaffold for repair. A third degree sprain involves dislocation of the acromioclavicular joint. This may be reduced with appropriate strapping or bracing which should be worn day and night for at least 14 days (to allow ligament healing). It is often difficult to prevail upon a patient to comply with this regimen in view of the added restriction to activities of daily living. Alternatively, a surgical fixation may be contemplated depending on the athletes sport, occupation, age and expectations. Each case should be evaluated individually, and options for treatment and likely outcome (functional and cosmetic) discussed with the patient. Larsen (1986) however, found no significant outcome between those who had internal fixation and those who were managed conservatively. When considering surgery, instability in both the anteroposterior and superoinferior directions must be assessed. Stewart (1985) describes a radiographic examination of the superoinferior component by taking a standing X-ray of both shoulders with a 4.5 kg weight suspended passively from each wrist (note, not being held by the athlete) in order to maximize joint separation

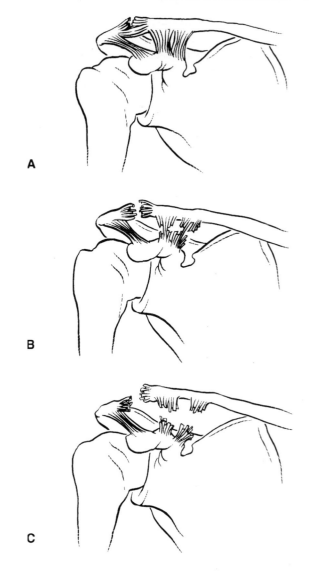

Fig. 23.13 Three degrees of acromioclavicular joint sprain. **A** Grade 1. Tearing of acromioclavicular ligaments. No deformity. **B** Grade 2. Rupture of acromioclavicular ligaments and partial disruption of the coracoclavicular ligament. Mild deformity. **C** Grade 3. Total disruption of both ligament groups

and minimize muscular effort in the upper limb. The decision regarding surgery is discussed more fully on p. 389.

Rotator cuff strain/rupture

Acute strains of the rotator cuff can occur during a fall or wrenching of the arm, or in the event of a strong contraction of the cuff during which the expected transfer of momentum does not eventuate. An example of this latter mechanism would be a mis-hit tennis backhand, or a poorly co-ordinated hard throw. In these cases, it is likely that the cuff had some underlying weakness due to previous injury or repetitive microtrauma (Falkel & Murphy 1988, Simon & Hill 1989).

Complete ruptures of the cuff are possible and tend to occur in the older athletes due to a longer history of use and abuse, this has been described as long ago as 1934 by Codman in his classic treatise on supraspinatus tendon ruptures. Diagnosis is by clinical testing of cuff function and further investigation as indicated. Arthrography is usually conclusive as it demonstrates the contrast medium leaking from the joint through the deficit in the capsule/cuff. Optimal management is early surgical repair followed by progressive rehabilitation and functional retraining. Return to sport is common in athletes with a grade 3 tear providing the surgery is prompt and there is no underlying hypermobility or instability of the joint (Reid et al 1987).

Partial tears (grades 1 and 2) are more common in the sporting population and are generally managed conservatively (Blackburn 1987, Falkel & Murphy 1988). These tears are longitudinal occurring on the undersurface of the cuff, i.e. the intra-articular aspect, and most commonly to the supraspinatus (Falkel & Murphy 1988, Codman 1934). Arthrography does not reveal these partial thickness tears, however arthroscopy can view the inner surface of the cuff and demonstrate the exact site and degree of damage (Simon & Hill 1989).

Investigations of suspected rotator cuff injury are often frustrating, as the site and nature of the tear will determine which of the investigations is likely to be conclusive; but until the tear is identified the appropriate investigation cannot be decided upon. For example, diagnosis of a cuff tear can be made through arthroscopy as both the superior and inferior surfaces of the cuff can be visualized, provided the tear presents at a surface of the tendon. Athrography will confirm a full thickness (complete) tear of the cuff, but will miss a partial tear (McCue et al 1985). An insubstance tear fully contained within the body of the tendon will not be visible on either of these invasive procedures. Diagnostic ultrasonography is an excellent non-invasive tool for confirming the clinical suspicion of a tear, and magnetic resonance imaging provides an excellent tool for visualizing the rotator cuff. Both these latter procedures will detect partial, full thickness and significant within substance tears. However, to be reliable, the ultrasound investigation requires an experienced sonographer and radiologist.

For these reasons it is not unusual for the injured athlete to undergo multiple investigative procedures in an effort to conclusively identify the rotator cuff tear. In such cases the athlete requires counselling and information to ensure that he or she understands the rationale for these expensive and inconvenient tests.

The degree of pain, disability and tenderness generally reflects the severity of a rotator cuff injury. However, it is not unusual for a grade 3 injury to cause less pain at rest or on compression (e.g. affected side lie) than a grade 2, as pressure cannot build within the opened joint space to cause a stretching of the tear. Specific muscle tests for rotator cuff function will be painful and weak, especially the supraspinatus test (p. 400). Impingement tests (p. 400) may be positive due to the swelling and sensitivity of the injured subacromial structures.

Fractures

Scapula. Fractures of the body of the scapula rarely occur in sport as a result of direct trauma, due to the muscle cushioning in the area. The mechanism is usually a fall onto the outstretched arm accompanied by strong serratus anterior activity. Pain and disability result, but little deformity. The injury is characterized by pain on scapular motion, deep inspiration or coughing, resisted activity of scapular muscles and specific tenderness over the site of injury. X-ray confirms the diagnosis. Treatment consists of resting the arm in a sling until pain settles, followed by gentle scapular mobilizing exercises. Strength exercises and faster movements are introduced after three weeks and return to contact sport can occur after five or six weeks. Non-contact sports can be resumed as soon as able. Swimming provides a good fitness maintenance activity during recovery.

Fractures to the glenoid rim of the scapula may accompany glenohumeral dislocations and contribute to subsequent instability. Such an injury usually requires open fixation, possibly in conjunction with a shoulder reconstruction.

'Floating shoulder' results when the neck of the scapula and the acromioclavicular arch are both fractured, or when the arch and the proximal humerus are both fractured. Treatment is surgical to restore integrity and stability.

Avulsion fractures of the coracoid process can occur due to forceful activity of the biceps brachii and the coracobrachialis. Screw fixation or bone suturing is required to restore function.

Clavicle. The most common fracture around the shoulder is that of the clavicle. The mechanism of injury is usually a fall onto the outstretched arm, although direct impact can also be a cause. Clavicular fractures are more common in adolescents (including greenstick fractures), while in adults ligamentous injuries are more likely. The fracture is usually in the middle third of the clavicle, where ligament support is least.

Presentation of a clavicular fracture includes severe pain; the athlete supports the affected arm and tilts his or her head toward that side (easing muscle tension across the clavicle). Deformity is likely, with tenderness and swelling. In some cases, the swelling may mask any bone deformity.

Optimal reduction of the fracture is desirable to maintain the integrity of the thoracic outlet. A figure-of-eight clavicle strap is used to achieve closed reduction and should be worn for at least six weeks. Heavy activity and return to sport should be avoided until point tenderness has disappeared, fracture healing time has been allowed, and/or union is apparent on X-ray.

Humerus. Fractures of the proximal humerus usually occur as a result of a fall onto the arm. It is extremely difficult to differentiate between such a fracture, an acute dislocation or a combined fracture/dislocation, without resorting to X-ray confirmation. Thus, athletes suffering a first time (apparent) glenohumeral dislocation should be managed with caution until a fracture is discounted.

Proximal humeral fractures with minor displacement are managed with a sling and broad bandage for three to four weeks, followed by mobilizing exercises and graduated return to activity. More severe displacements can usually be reduced without surgery but may require some traction to achieve this. Immobilization may last up to six weeks followed by rehabilitation.

Midshaft fractures of the humerus can occur as a result of excessive axial torque being generated along the bone. Indeed, the author has witnessed two humeral fractures occurring in mid-pitch. Diagnosis in such cases is simple, the athlete reports that his or her arm has snapped. Closed reduction is usually possible with up to six weeks of immobilization. Rehabilitation is uneventful except for the mental barrier to forceful throwing. The inhibitive effect of a throwing fracture appears to be extremely potent.

Internal fixation of shaft fractures allows for earlier mobilization of the shoulder and elbow joints. This can reduce joint stiffness and muscle atrophy, making it the treatment of choice for some athletes (e.g. veteran or professional).

Acute glenohumeral dislocations

Direct trauma to the shoulder region or indirect forces applied along the extended arm can dislocate the humeral head beyond the margin of the glenoid. This can occur anteriorly, posteriorly or inferiorly. Primary occurrences should be referred for radiological investigation, with the suspicion of a post-dislocation fracture drawn to the attention of the radiologist. This will increase the likelihood of all relevant views being taken (anterior, lateral, sub-acromial, axillary) and of the films being examined for a Hill-Sachs defect.

Anterior. The anterior dislocation is most often caused by hyper-abduction of the arm when it is in abduction and lateral rotation, usually during a tackle in contact sports, although it can occur in other close proximity sports such as water polo or basketball.

The humeral head can lie in one of two positions, in the case of an anterior dislocation, either subcoracoid or subglenoid. The athlete presents with shoulder pain and lack of movement due to pain. Examination shows an antero-lateral depression and absence of the normal deltoid

Table 23.5   Classification of anterior dislocation lesions

	Group 1	Group 2	Group 3
Capsule tear	yes	yes	yes
Labral lesion	no	partial	detached
Unstable under anaesthesia	no	mildly	grossly
Haemarthrosis	little	mild	large

Source: Baker et al 1990

curve. There is usually a prominence anteriorly. Palpation confirms the malposition of the humeral head.

During the anterior translocation of the humeral head the anterior restraining structures sustain various sites and degrees of damage. Baker et al (1990) classified three distinct patterns of lesion occurring with an initial acute dislocation as evaluated at arthroscopy. This is summarised in Table 23.5.

As the humeral head dislocates anteriorly it may avulse the labrum from the glenoid and slip medially between those two structures, stripping the periosteum from the scapular neck and forming an anterior pouch (Falkel & Murphy 1988, Baker et al 1990). Upon humeral reduction, the pouch remains, leaving a deficit in the anterior restraining mechanisms; this is known as a Bankart lesion (Fig. 23.14).

With such a violent forward slip of the humerus the posterior articular aspect of the humeral head can sustain a compression fracture as it impacts against the anterior rim of the glenoid fossa (Slaughter 1990). The consequent depression in the humeral head is the Hill-Sachs lesion (Fig. 23.14) and provides radiographic support in the diagnosis of anterior dislocation.

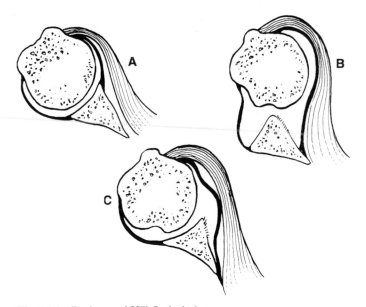

Fig. 23.14 Bankart and Hill-Sachs lesions.
A Normal glenohumeral joint.
B Anterior dislocation with periosteal stripping from neck of scapula and a depression fracture on posterior humeral head.
C Joint is reduced. An anterior pouch remains (Bankart lesion) as does the depression on the humeral head (Hill-Sachs lesion)

The presence of a Bankart lesion can be diagnosed by arthroscopy, CT-arthrogram or magnetic resonance imaging. Suspicion of a labral lesion may be heightened using the tests for anterior instability and labral integrity (see pp. 381–3, 384).

Posterior. Posterior dislocations occur with falling forward onto the outstretched arm, especially with shoulder medial rotation (Falkel & Murphy 1988), or by direct impact against the anterior humeral head. Commonly they occur during epileptic seizures or concurrently with an electric shock injury through the upper limb. The athlete presents with acute pain, a flattening of the anterior aspect of the shoulder with the coracoid becoming prominent, and an inability to externally rotate or abduct the arm. There is also a fullness behind the shoulder. Anteroposterior X-rays may not reveal this dislocation, and a lateral or transscapular view may be required. Management of resultant posterior glenohumeral instability is discussed from p. 390.

Inferior. Inferior dislocations present with pain and dysfunction consistent with a history of trauma. There is a marked flattening or depression of the deltoid contour from the lateral border of the acromion.

Over-use injuries

In clinical practice, the sports physiotherapist will be more often confronted with over-use injuries to the shoulder than with traumatic or post-surgical. The anatomy and biomechanics of the region, combined with the demands placed on it in the pursuit of sport, predispose the shoulder to over-use injuries. Table 23.6 lists the primary and secondary factors involved in over-use shoulder injuries occurring in sport.

It is common practice to discuss shoulder over-use injuries under the primary diagnostic labels of tendinitis, laxity and impingement. However this is a gross over-simplification, as elements of these three conditions do not only co-exist, but are often inter-related. Figure 23.15 illustrates the relationships between the three conditions.

Table 23.6 Primary and secondary predisposing factors toward shoulder over-use injuries in sport

Primary	1.	Extremes of range are used
	2.	High forces are developed
	3.	High repetition rates
Secondary	1.	Impingement beneath coracoacromial arch
	2.	Poor training/conditioning
	3.	Poor technique in sport movement
	4.	Poor vascularity of cuff tendons
	5.	Muscle strength imbalance
	6.	Muscle stamina imbalance
	7.	Hypomobility
	8.	Hypermobility
	9.	Protection of other injured area(s) e.g. elbow or cervical spine
	10.	Interplay of above

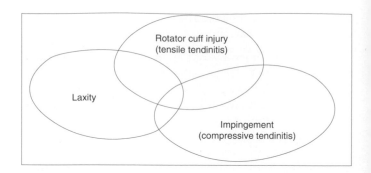

Fig. 23.15 Relationship between shoulder over-use pathologies

Whenever an athlete's condition comes within the circle in Figure 23.15, he or she will likely develop elements of the other two conditions, and with time may present with symptoms of all three.

Injury to the rotator cuff causes pain inhibition to the muscular function, decreasing the co-contraction stabilizing of the humeral head. Thus the joint experiences greater translatory movements and increased stress to the passive restraints, bringing about laxity. This laxity and inhibition allows upward excursion of the humeral head, producing subacromial impingement.

Similarly, primary injury to the labrum or anterior structures increases the demand on the rotator cuff as it strives to stabilize the humeral head. The cuff subsequently deteriorates, becomes dysfunctional and impingement can occur.

Finally, subacromial impingement due to faulty biomechanics will inhibit and injure the rotator cuff. As the cuff shuts down, humeral head control is reduced and the translation stresses the restraint mechanisms, producing laxity.

The individual pathologies will now be described, and strategies for diagnosis and management will be addressed separately. It is important to keep in mind that elements of the three conditions are likely to co-exist in varying proportions: a sort of pathological soup!

Tendinitis

The pathophysiology of tendon lesions has been described fully by Curwin and Stanish (1984) in a text all sports physiotherapists should read. From their work, the concept of utilizing eccentric exercise in tendon rehabilitation was substantiated.

An understanding of tendon structure and function is important when treating tendinitis in athletes, and particularly in their shoulders. The role of a tendon is to transmit the contractile force of the attached muscle to the bone, fascia or other structure into which the tendon is inserted. Thus a tendon is structured to withstand tensile forces applied parallel with the collagen bundles of which it is composed. It withstands compressive or shearing forces less well (Curwin & Stanish 1984). The basic unit of collagen is the tropocollagen molecule, and these molecules are aligned in an overlapping fashion and held together by intramolecular and intermolecular bonds or cross-links. This cross-linking contributes to the strength of the collagen fibres by utilizing a load-sharing arrangement between adjacent molecules.

Under conditions of tensile loading the fibrils of the collagen slide past one another, harnessed by the cross links. If the tensile force strains the fibrils to beyond 8-10% of their resting length some of the cross-links fail; if the force continues to be applied, the remaining cross-links also fail as they cannot tolerate the extra loading necessitated by nearby failure. As this process continues, the tendon becomes damaged and may rupture completely if the force is sufficiently strong (Curwin & Stanish 1984).

Tendinitis occurs when the normal repair of any cross links damaged during activity or injury is repeatedly interrupted by further applications of tensile force beyond the load bearing limit of the injured tendon. In such situations the immature, regenerating cross-links are severed again, and an environment of chronic inflammation becomes established. During the early stages of this process, the damage is microscopic and below the athlete's pain threshold, but repeated aggravation will amplify the size of the lesion until the chemical irritation triggers pain and the athlete becomes aware of a new injury. This irritation arises due to bleeding into the tendon structure when arterioles are damaged by the sliding of unsecured fibrils as the infra-structure of the tendon gives way (Curwin & Stanish 1984). The bleeding initiates the inflammatory response, causing the area to become acidic, proteolytic and irritable.

In the early stage of tendon repair, the immature collagen structure is quite soluble, particularly if the chemical environment becomes acidic. This is precisely what occurs each time the inflammatory reaction is exacerbated. In addition, the cellular migration triggered by inflammation is proteolytic so the collagen fibres and links are doubly susceptible (Curwin & Stanish 1984).

The natural history described above is that of a tensile tendinitis i.e. caused by tensile overloading. However, in the shoulder it is possible to generate tendinitis from compressive or shearing forces as the superior rotator cuff tendons endeavour to pass beneath the coracoacromial arch. It is possible that the damage to a tendon's ultrastructure may be different with a compressive tendinitis, and that this difference may be significant in terms of rehabilitation (Allingham 1988).

Curwin and Stanish (1985) admit that eccentric exercise programs are effective in rehabilitating some tendonitides, but less so with others. Around the shoulder they re-commend that biceps and triceps tendinitis should be exercised eccentrically, but with a supraspinatus tendinitis it is 'not indicated' (Curwin & Stanish 1984).

Eccentric exercise provides an efficient tensile loading of the tendon involved in the movement, and therefore will stimulate adaptions within that tendon to help withstand further tensile loading (see Ch. 10). If a tendinitis has been caused by tensile overload, such a program of rehabilitation is logical. Alternatively, if a tendinitis has arisen through repeated impingement of a tendon, the role of eccentric exercise in a rehabilitation program must be re-evaluated. Accordingly, the following discussion of management of shoulder tendonitides will differentiate between tensile and impingement lesions.

Tensile tendinitis. This type of tendinitis around the shoulder occurs in the tendons of biceps (long head), triceps (long head), pectoralis major, latissimus dorsi, teres major and teres minor. As discussed above, the cause of the condition is a tensile overload with insufficient tissue repair between episodes of microtrauma. Similar conditions can occur in the tendons of supraspinatus and infraspinatus, but these are often implicated in coracoacromial impinge-ment, so will be discussed in the following section. When evaluating the shoulder, these conditions are described by the athlete as gradual onset, progressively interfering with performance (Blazina et al 1973).

Information relating to the various electrotherapy modalities and their effects on tissue repair can be found in Chapter 15.

The role of exercise in managing tendinitis is discussed in general terms in Chapter 10. A summary is presented in Table 23.7.

Stretching is one form of exercise that deserves mention separately, and its application in tendon injury management is discussed in Chapter 10. Applying tension along the muscle-tendon unit by taking that unit to its maximal length is another way of providing the axial stimulation for collagen alignment (Curwin & Stanish, 1984).

Table 23.7 Physiotherapy options for treatment of tendinitis

Aim	Possible methods
1. Identify the causative factors and reduce them	Thorough assessment and firm diagnosis of all related problems
2. Decrease the frequency and intensity of inflammatory responses	Rest from aggravating activities Ice applications
3. Facilitate ground substance proliferation to optimize collagen synthesis	Exercise Ultrasound Laser Heat (superficial or deep)
4. Improve the quality of tissue repair	Exercise Ultrasound/laser Massage Stretching Mobilization
5. Restore normal shoulder posture biomechanics and conditioning	Exercise Mobilization Graded return to activity

Massage for tendinitis is often useful to stimulate circulation, overcome congestion within a tendon or its synovial sheath, reduce or prevent adhesions within or around the tendon, or to manually stretch the musculotendinous unit. Aggressive massage techniques (e.g. transverse or cross-fibre frictions) are often more effective if combined with ice massage immediately afterwards. This is to reduce the inflammatory nature of the technique. As massage is a cutaneous modality, it is most effective for more superficial tendons (see p. 396 for more discussion).

Home programs for stretching, eccentric exercising and mobilizing of the soft tissues and underlying joints can be devised for athletes suffering from shoulder tendinitis. The physiotherapist must ensure that the affected tendon or tendons are identified, the level of irritability respected and the patient educated as to the program to be followed. If this is done, good therapeutic results can be expected from the treatment regime.

In summary, for tensile tendonitides around the shoulder, the therapist must identify the tendon and then treat it using rest from aggravation, electrotherapy modalities, eccentric exercise, massage and functional retraining. At all times, respect for physiological healing times and irritability must be observed.

Impingement. The injury to the superior aspects of the rotator cuff differs in impingement lesions compared with tensile lesions. In the former there is direct compression forces that cause mechanical trauma in addition to any tensile overloading. It is likely that this results in physical damage to the actual collagen structure in addition to the breaking of cross links and associated vascular effects. For this reason, the use of eccentric exercise may not be appropriate in the initial stage of rehabilitation (Allingham 1988).

Impingement syndrome of the shoulder is common in those sports involving frequent, forceful, overhead activity such as baseball, swimming, tennis and gymnastics. Repeated compression of the subacromial contents causes micropockets of damage which eventually summate as the activity is persisted with. The ensuing inflammatory reaction involves vascular congestion and oedema into the tendon or bursa which further reduces the available space beneath the coracoacromial arch. Pain results and interferes with normal biomechanics of the shoulder by causing muscle inhibition (due to pain) and compensatory movements or postures.

The main challenge when managing an impingement lesion of the shoulder is its predisposition toward chronicity. This tendency is due to the three factors just mentioned, combined with the recurring inflammation due to active elevation of the arm.

The key to facilitating tendon repair in an impingement syndrome is to reduce the frequency and intensity of the recurrent inflammatory reaction by avoiding impingement.

Impingement can be avoided by preventing the athlete from raising the arm overhead, or by altering the biomechanics of that movement so impingement is minimized. An example of this occurs in tennis players of high standard where the powerful first serve is dependent on the medial rotation that occurs during the acceleration phase. The arm at this stage is in full elevation, thus the medial rotation drags the greater tuberosity along the acromion and the acromioclavicular ligament through the stroke.

As discussed previously, elevation of the arm involves a coupling of forces around the scapula and across the glenohumeral joint. Activity of the rotator cuff controls the stability of the humeral head as the larger muscles raise the arm. The tendon insertion angle of some of the cuff muscles allows them to contribute a downward force to the humeral head, namely the teres minor, subscapularis and lower infraspinatus (Kapandji 1970). If these muscles are inhibited by pain or weakened due to chronic nursing of a sore shoulder, superior migration of the humeral head will occur to a greater degree, with resultant subacromial impingement increasing. Exercises to retrain and strengthen these more inferiorly placed cuff muscles may well provide better control of the humeral head during daily function, reducing impingement episodes and allowing some progression from inflammation to healing (Allingham 1988). Appropriate rehabilitation is discussed later.

Examination of the shoulder should always include tests for impingement. Two tests have been described in the literature by Neer and Welsh (cited in Moran & Saunders 1987) and by Hawkins and Kennedy (1980). These tests are described in detail and their merits discussed later in this chapter (see p. 385). The two tests described are useful in determining whether subacromial impingement exists. They provide no information as to why it arose, or why it will not get better. A test for dynamic impingement has been described (Allingham 1988) which attempts to relate the impingement to glenohumeral mechanics (dynamic impingement test). This test is also discussed and described in the shoulder examination section.

Impingement syndrome of the shoulder can involve the subacromial bursa rather than the cuff tendons. In these cases, the impingement tests are positive, but resisted testing of the cuff (tensile loading) does not accurately reproduce the symptoms. The aim of treatment remains the same however, to prevent the impingement to allow healing.

Unfortunately, tendinitis around the shoulder does not often slot neatly into one of the two categories—tensile or impingement; commonly there is a combination. For example, a tensile tendinitis of the supraspinatus will involve subsequent swelling predisposing to impingement. In these cases it is imperative to reduce the impingement in order to minimize the inflammatory damage. The tensile rehabilitation of the tendon cannot be effective until the interruptions to repair caused by repeated impingement are under control. Only then is there profit in eccentrically loading the damaged tendon to improve the collagen cross-linking.

Another challenge in managing shoulder tendinitis is the likelihood of more than one tendon being involved. The most common combination is the supraspinatus and long head of biceps due to their proximity and susceptibility to impingement. Usually the two components can be defined during resistance testing and palpation. The principles of management remain the same (control the impingement first, then strengthen the tendon) but are complicated by having to introduce specific eccentric rehabilitation for both tendons.

Excessive superior migration of the humeral head has been noted following ruptures of the supraspinatus due to the decrease in subacromial contents as the tendon retracts (Weiner & McNab 1970). This may not happen in the acute stage due to swelling and bleeding in the area, but has been demonstrated radiographically in chronic cases.

One other contributor to impingement may be hypermobility of the glenohumeral joint. Repeated stretching of the shoulder capsule and cuff, either through violent end-of-range activities (throwing) or with rigorous stretching activities (common in swimmers), can increase the available range of gliding of the humeral head. Lengthening of the inferior capsule and ligaments through such measures can lead to inadequate stabilizing of the humeral head centrally in the glenoid at the upper reaches of abduction, predisposing to impingement (Reid et al 1987, Moynes-Schwab 1990). Athletes with hypermobile shoulder joints rely more on muscular control to fix the humerus, especially under conditions of maximal torque loading: for example, the power phase of the swimming stroke, the explosive phase of acceleration when throwing, or during suspension manoeuvres in gymnastics.

When working with flexibility oriented athletes, the physiotherapist should be aware of this predisposition to shoulder pathology and ensure the conditioning routine includes rotator cuff strength and stabilizing exercises to minimize the risk. Education is required of the athletes and coaches only to achieve sufficient flexibility to enable comfortable completion of the stroke, throw or hit.

Glenohumeral instability

Recognition that the glenohumeral joint is embraced by dynamic and static constraints to translation has brought about the 'circle concept of stability' (Bowen & Warren 1991). Briefly, this evolved from progressive dissections of cadaveric shoulders and suggests that for instability to be present, there must be laxity or dysfunction in two areas of the capsule/cuff. For example, for an excessive anterior translation to occur there must be an anterior stability deficit and a posterior laxity or dysfunction to permit the translation.

Another important consideration is that in the glenohumeral joint, instability and laxity are not the same thing. Laxity is a demonstrable mobility when performing clinical tests involving translation of the humeral head. The presence of laxity is not diagnostic of instability. This latter condition is a symptom that occurs when the humeral head is allowed to translate beyond the comfort and functional capacity of the joint. That is, the laxity is not controlled by the rotator cuff complex. Matsen et al (1991) note that many clinically lax shoulders are asymptomatic, and that the amount of laxity in an unstable group was not significantly different from a control group.

Instability of the glenohumeral joint can arise in one of three ways, traumatically, insidiously or congenitally: colloquially, 'torn loose', 'worn loose' or 'born loose'.

Thomas and Matsen (1989) further delineated two groups for anterior dislocators, the traumatic onset usually having a rupture of the glenohumeral ligaments at the glenoid (Bankart lesion) and/or a detachment of the labrum with a unidirectional instability. Those with atraumatic instability are more prone to multidirectional instability which may be bilateral, however the symptoms may be unilateral due to asymmetrical loading of the shoulder joints for example in throwers. Table 23.8 highlights the properties of the two types of recurrent instability.

A *traumatic instability* is the easier to diagnose chiefly due to the definite onset event. An initial traumatic dislocation may be accompanied with a fracture of the rim of the glenoid or of the proximal humerus and an X-ray should be ordered to ensure such an injury is excluded (see p. 371).

The *insidious onset of instability*, due to repetitive microtrauma of the glenohumeral ligaments and cuff, is common in athletes. Gradual deterioration in the ligamentous constraints and cuff shut-down (inhibition) due to the consequent pain combine to permit increased translation of the humerus on the glenoid. This further compromises the capsuloligamentous restraints and the laxity progresses. Eventually the rotator cuff can no longer control the laxity and symptoms of instability begin. These include pain, weakness and 'dead arm' episodes on maximal activity (Rowe 1985).

Table 23.8 Patterns of recurrent anterior glenohumeral instability

Onset	Characteristics
Traumatic event(s) (TUBS)	Unidirectional Bankart lesion present Surgery usually required
Atraumatic onset	Multidirectional Bilateral Rehabilitation indicated Inferior capsular repair may be required

Source: Thomas & Matsen 1989

'Worn loose' type instability can develop anteriorly, posteriorly or inferiorly, but due to the cuff muscle inhibition and usual continued participation in sport a multidirectional instability often results.

Congenital instability occurs in individuals who inherit a connective tissue disorder in which the collagen matrices have a higher than normal elastin component (eg. Marfan's or Ehlers-Danlos syndromes). Ligament and tendon are thus more extensible and the athlete demonstrates hyperflexibility (Corrigan & Maitland 1983).

Signs of this problem include genu and cubitus recurvatum and the ability to touch one's thumb to the ipsilateral forearm. Indeed, these quick tests are used to screen for the disorder.

Initially these athletes are looked upon as potentially gifted, in that they have great flexibility and are often dubbed 'double jointed'. However, the excessive joint play allowed by the ligaments and capsules can eventually lead to joint damage, unless the secondary (muscular) stabilizers can compensate for the hypermobility. In the shoulder, the laxity can predispose to subluxations, dislocations and impingement due to the mobility of the humeral head.

If one of these hypermobile athletes develops symptoms of shoulder instability, it will tend to be multidirectional and the role of surgery is minor, due to the inadequate collagen bridging in any capsular procedure. Rehabilitation offers the best chance for recovery by improving glenohumeral control and enabling a return to overhead sport. More commonly, however, the athlete must discontinue throwing or racquet sports, and perhaps even swimming and any form of contact sport where incidental trauma is causing episodes of partial or total dislocation. In such cases extensive counselling of the athlete, parents and coach (as appropriate) is necessary to explain the problem and direct him or her to more appropriate activities.

The athlete should also be warned against habitual dislocation or any similar party tricks.

Levator scapula syndrome

This condition typically co-exists with cervical, glenohumeral or scapular dysfunction rather than an over-use condition in its own right. However it does merit some discussion given the importance in overall shoulder mechanics.

Compensatory elevation of the scapula in the symptomatic shoulder as it strives to avoid impingement predisposes the levator scapula to hypertonicity and shortening.

This tightness becomes painful in its own right and presents as tender on palpation. The neural connections of this muscle allow referred pain proximally into the cervical spine and distally into the upper arm. This may not be due to direct neural interference from the levator scapula, but to neural irritation arising from altered posture and mechanics of the scapula and cervical spine.

When managing chronic conditions of the shoulder or neck, the levator scapula should be assessed for length, tone and the presence of tender trigger points. Appropriate treatment may require passive stretching followed by home exercises, massage and myofascial releases, modalities to reduce sensitivity of the intramuscular nociceptors such as ice, laser, heat or a combination. In this way the cycle of pain/spasm/pain can be interrupted, allowing stretching and postural correction to prepare for normalizing of the scapula biomechanics.

Muscle energy techniques or those of reciprocal inhibition and hold/relax, developed as PNF (these two schools of thought have similarities, but were evolved and named by different practitioners), can be quite effective in stretching this muscle and restoring the normal resting tension level. Stretches can be applied through either cervical lateral flexion or by scapular depression, whichever is more comfortable for the athlete and effective in the stretch. A regular home routine of stretches incorporating scapular fixation during contralateral flexion is necessary to undermine the reinforcement of habitual postures or movement.

Neurovascular syndromes and injuries

The shoulder region is host to the major neurovascular bundle passing from the cervical and thoracic spine and the thoracic cavity into the arm. This bundle must navigate the musculoligamentous maze around the shoulder and be sufficiently mobile in its own right to tolerate the angles and forces generated during athletic activities. The low incidence of neurovascular entrapments reflects the efficiency of the anatomical relationships in accomplishing this gambit.

Nevertheless, entrapments of and trauma to the neural structures do occur in the shoulder region and must be considered when evaluating an athlete whose pain characteriztics do not conform with a strictly mechanical interpretation of the symptoms.

Long thoracic nerve Traction injury to the long thoracic nerve as it travels from the brachial plexus to supply serratus anterior can arise when loads are repeatedly carried on the shoulder (e.g. by bushwalkers). The injury can also occur as a single traumatic event if forced depression of the scapula occurs upon falling or being tackled.

Burners Acute traction injury to the brachial plexus and/or cervical nerve roots can occur if the cervical spine is laterally flexed while the opposite scapula is depressed. This can occur if the head and shoulder strike the ground simultaneously, forcing the two movements. This injury is termed a 'burner' or a 'stinger', for such is the sensation reported by the athlete (Vereschagin et al 1991). The sharp burning is felt in the shoulder and there may be some parasthesia into the arm or hand. Any sensory loss or diminishing of deep tendon reflexes is indicative of severe neurological insult (axonotmesis or neurotmesis). However most of the injuries are grade 1, that is a neuropraxia which should resolve fully within two weeks. If symptoms are severe or persist, referral to a neurologist is indicated.

Thoracic outlet syndrome Compromising of the neurovascular bundle as it passes between the clavicle and the first rib can occur for a variety of reasons. Spasm or tightening of the scalenus anterior can impinge or tether the adjacent nerve tissues, a poorly healed clavicular fracture can degenerate and cause osteophytic encroachment, or a space occupying lesion can interfere with the bundle. Any of these can be further complicated with the presence of a cervical rib (Pratt 1986). The symptoms arising from such pathology include referred pain into the arm, vascular

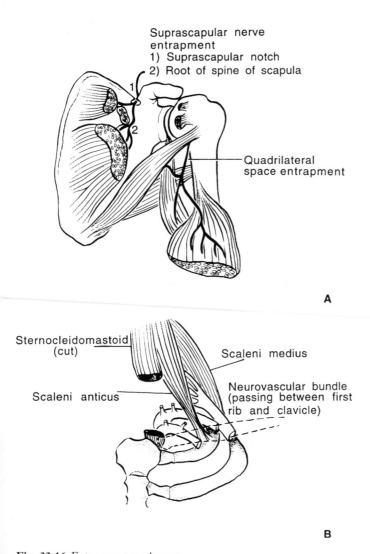

Suprascapular nerve entrapment
1) Suprascapular notch
2) Root of spine of scapula

Quadrilateral space entrapment

A

Sternocleidomastoid (cut)

Scaleni medius

Scaleni anticus

Neurovascular bundle (passing between first rib and clavicle)

B

Fig. 23.16 Entrapment syndromes.
A Suprascapular and quadrilateral entrapments.
B Scaleni nerve entrapment (thoracic outlet syndrome.)

disturbances (swelling, discolouration, coldness), proprioceptive loss, parasthesia and sensorimotor loss. The presence of these should alert the therapist to complete a full neurological evaluation.

Entrapment lesions of the component parts of the brachial plexus can occur at the thoracic outlet or within the cervical spine (Pratt 1986). Impingement and irritation of the neural tissues can produce shoulder pain and muscular dysfunction mimicking glenohumeral joint pathologies. Or more commonly, they occur in conjunction with local mechanical problems. Evaluation and treatment of these lesions is discussed in more detail later in this chapter, and is also covered in the chapter on cervical spine injuries and conditions (see Ch. 21). In addition to cervical pathologies producing shoulder or arm symptoms, dysfunction of the first or second ribs has also been implicated (Griffin & Curtis 1991), (see p. 389).

Suprascapular nerve entrapment The suprascapular nerve can be compromised at two points in its course (Fig. 23.16). At the suprascapular notch where it passes beneath the suprascapular ligament, and at the lateral edge of the spine of the scapula. Damage at the more proximal point will reduce the motor supply to both the supraspinatus and the infraspinatus. Injury at the more distal point will only affect the infraspinatus. The loss is predominantly motor, as the only sensory supply via this nerve is to the posterior shoulder capsule (Pratt 1986).

Quadrilateral space syndrome Quadrilateral space syndrome is a true neurovascular entrapment where both the nerves and blood vessels are compromised as they pass through the space bounded by the humerus laterally, the long head of triceps medially, the teres minor and subscapularis above and the teres major below (more detail of symptoms are described on p. 388). The likely predisposition to injury is compression of the nerve by fibrous bands in the adjacent soft tissues during combined abduction and lateral rotation (the cocking position).

Axillary nerve trauma A common complication of glenohumeral dislocation (or reduction) is trauma to the axillary nerve. This nerve runs a short course and is mobilized by shoulder movement making spontaneous recovery of an axonotmesis or neurotmesis unlikely. Evidence of post-traumatic axillary nerve palsy includes loss of abduction strength, wasting of the deltoid and sensory loss over the deltoid.

While awaiting for recovery, physiotherapy can be utilized to maintain range of motion and monitor strength gains. However, if there is no sign of recovery after three or four months, the athlete should be investigated using nerve conduction techniques and evaluated for surgery.

Daff (1992) recommends exploratory and therapeutic surgery for non-recovering axillary nerve deficit within six months of onset. The procedure will vary from nerve suture, graft or neurolysis depending on the findings on surgery. Nerve grafting is accomplished using the sural nerve.

Other conditions

In addition to traumatic and over-use injuries associated with sport, athletes may develop various other conditions which although not a sports injury, will interfere sufficiently with athletic performance for them to seek assistance from a sports medicine practitioner.

Frozen shoulder Frozen shoulder is a descriptive rather than diagnostic term, however it accurately conveys the nature of the disability. Newnham (1990) notes the three stages of this condition as freezing, frozen and thawing, and the therapy for each is stage-specific.

The exact pathology and aetiology of frozen shoulder is not yet clear. Owens-Burkhart (1987) in her thorough review of the subject arrives at a definition of frozen shoulder as 'glenohumeral stiffness resulting from capsular restrictions' (Owens-Burkhart 1987, p 83). Fibrosis of the capsular structures and loss of intracapsular volume accompanies fibroblastic proliferation and histochemical changes in the connective tissues.

The end result to the athlete is a progressive, insidious onset of shoulder pain, which may radiate into the neck or down to the forearm. The limitations of movement that follow are initially due to pain avoidance, but then as the capsule becomes fibrotic all movements become restricted. The loss of movement is greatest for lateral rotation, then for abduction and medial rotation (Cyriax's capsular pattern, Cyriax 1978). The painful stage can last between two and six months, while the stiff stage continues for an additional four to twelve months (Owens-Burkhart 1987).

The final stage is that of spontaneous resolution, with a gradual return of movement. The degree of return is variable, with many cases having a permanent restriction. This last stage can last for four to eighteen months. It appears that the duration of stages 1 and 3 are often proportional, but not equal (Owens-Burkhart 1987).

The diagnosis of frozen shoulder is often made retrospectively, when mechanical and inflammatory disorders have been excluded and the pattern of symptoms has become established.

Physiotherapy management of frozen shoulder is important, as many researchers conclude that 'exercise is the most useful treatment' (Owens-Burkhart 1987, p 95). However, in stage 1 the primary aim is pain relief to allow some normal use of the limb. Analgesic medication, TENS and intra-articular steroid injections have been found useful, although none will consistently terminate the progression of the condition through its three stages. Active exercise and isometric strength work can be done within the pain and irritability of the joint at this stage.

Once pain abates, active exercises within the available range for mobility, strength and endurance are indicated. Passive mobilizing of the physiological and accessory joint movements can also be undertaken, with the therapist being wary of being too aggressive. Soft tissue mobilization and stretching is also beneficial.

At the early signs of resolution (stage 3) more vigorous mobilizing and muscle stretching can be tolerated, and will bring increases in range. Active strengthening as the movement returns will facilitate safer return to functional activities.

Inflammatory conditions *Ankylosing spondylitis.* Although primarily a disease of the spine, ankylosing spondylitis will sometimes co-present as a spinal/peripheral joint problem (Corrigan & Maitland 1983), with the shoulder being affected. Alternatively, a cervicothoracic presentation could cause referred shoulder pain or interfere with upper quadrant mechanics.

Early detection of this condition will obviously enable appropriate management, it will also reduce the frustration of the therapist with the patient who is not recovering as expected. Suspicions should be aroused in cases when athletes present with an insidious onset, persistent pain for several months, early morning joint stiffness and pain easing with activity. Thorough examination and questioning regarding back pain, especially sacro-iliac pain should be conducted. A history of systemic symptoms of fever, weight loss and general musculoskeletal aching should be asked about.

Suspicion of possible ankylosing spondylitis must be followed up, with referral to the athlete's physician for further investigation and appropriate management. Ongoing active rehabilitation is indicated for this condition, and discussions with the managing physician on this topic should begin.

Rheumatoid arthritis. Rheumatoid arthritis of the shoulder is another of the inflammatory conditions that may present due to limitation of sports activity.

In an acute episode, the shoulder may be swollen, warm and painful on movement and palpation. With more chronic cases, a history of such episodes should be sought. Questioning the athlete regarding other joints, and a family history of rheumatoid conditions can provide valuable clues.

Again, if suspicious, referral to the athlete's physician for examination, radiology and pathology tests is vital. Ongoing active rehabilitation to maximize return to sport or other activity can then be undertaken.

SHOULDER EXAMINATION AND DIAGNOSIS

Examination of the shoulder lends itself very well to the principles systemized by Cyriax (1975). An orderly assessment of posture, movement and specific resisted or tensile testing of the shoulder structures usually makes a diagnosis possible. As our knowledge of shoulder anatomy, physiology and pathology has improved several special tests have been devised for differentiating particular lesions. The general principles of examination are discussed in another chapter, but this section will outline the authors procedure with shoulder examination including special tests and interpretation of findings.

Subjective

The interview stage of assessment is vital to ascertain the mechanism of injury or the causative factors in over-use injuries. Exact site(s) and nature of the athlete's pain must be determined, and the behaviour of that pain in response to training and performing the sporting activity is vitally important. For example, is a thrower's pain during cocking, acceleration or follow-through? Does the swimmer get the shoulder pain on catch, or just afterwards during early power phase? Does the pain on a tennis serve vary with the type of serve? This information may assist in directing the physical examination and in estimating the success of treatment when evaluating functional recovery at a later stage.

A clear understanding of previous injuries, operations and treatment around the shoulder should also be gained during the subjective examination. Current medication, history of steroid infiltrations, relevant changes in training intensity or frequency, changes to technique and occupational activities may all prove relevant when viewed in the light of the subsequent physical examination. Specific questioning about cervical and thoracic spine pain, stiffness or tension should be undertaken to ensure these important regions are not ignored as a source of shoulder and arm pain.

When dealing with impingement syndromes, there are several specific pain patterns which may assist the diagnosis. These are pain when lying on the affected arm, pain on overhead reaching, a painful arc and pain on rapid or unguarded movements. These symptoms are not diagnostic in themselves but certainly raise an impingement syndrome to a high degree of suspicion. Other frequently reported functional restrictions are pain on robing and disrobing or aching after sustained posture work (e.g. writing or typing).

During the subjective examination the physiotherapist should be aware of symptoms that do not appear to be mechanical in nature, for the shoulder is notorious for being the site for referred pain from other sources: not only from the cervical or thoracic spine, but from visceral sources. Corrigan and Maitland (1983) and Cailliet (1966) highlight the possibility of abdominal or thoracic disease causing scapular, shoulder or arm pain. The latter author suggested several patterns of visceral pain referral to the upper quadrant. In summary, these included irritation of the diaphragm producing pain in the upper trapezius, supra-clavicular and superior scapular angle areas; gall bladder disease referring to the point of the right shoulder and to the scapula; and myocardial and aortic disease referring to the left pectoral and axilla area. These pains are usually difficult for the athlete to localize and are not reproduced by musculoskeletal testing of the shoulder structures.

Objective

Once a clear history and pain behaviour cycle has been obtained, a physical examination can begin. The basics of shoulder assessment need not be dwelled upon here, the more useful tests and the overall interpretation is the direction to be taken.

When examining an athlete's shoulder it is important not to seek and find a particular problem which was evident on the basis of the subjective examination. The experienced practitioner will likely find what was sought, but may miss other signs that reflect an underlying causative factor, or a secondary compensatory factor that may prevent adequate resolution of the symptomatic problem.

As the physiotherapist systematically examines the shoulder, many variations of normal posture and function will be noted. None of these variations is diagnostic in its own right and many will prove of little or no pathological significance. Identifying those signs of diagnostic value may not be possible until the entire examination is completed. Only then can the overall pattern of signs, variations and test results be regarded in its entirety in order that a full understanding of posture, pathomechanics and patho-physiology in and around the shoulder is gained.

Wilk (1993) and Andrews (1993) recommend that during the clinical examination screening for instability should precede testing for impingement and muscle testing. This is to allow interpretation of the subsequent tests in respect of any laxity or instability. It also gives the examiner a degree of respect for the shoulder to avoid precipitating a subluxation.

Posture

Posture of the upper quadrant and spine is important when evaluating a shoulder. Variations from normal in the axial skeleton such as scoliosis or kyphosis will have effects on the shoulder mechanics, by altering the plane of the glenohumeral joint, and thus on the movements. For example, a stiff, kyphotic thoracic spine angles the scapula forward so that the acromion terminates elevation while the arm still appears short of the normal 180° (Cailliet 1966). In a swimmer this could predispose to impingement, due to the functional decrease in the subacromial space.

The cervicothoracic posture is of particular significance for two reasons. An excessive kyphosis in this area will affect muscular tension and alignment, which may in turn interfere with shoulder function. It may also affect the cervicobrachial neural tissues which then may be a cause of shoulder pain in their own right.

The posture of the scapula and clavicle are also worthy of note. Asymmetry of scapula or clavicular levels may indicate a scoliosis or tightness of the scapula elevators, provided of course it is the injured arm that demonstrates the elevation. If the resting position of the scapula on the injured side is more protracted, it may indicate weakness or dysfunction of the retractors, or an imbalance between serratus anterior and the rhomboid/middle trapezius combination. Of course, none of this is significant at the time of noting, but may become so later in the examination.

The postural screening should also include observations of the sternoclavicular and acromioclavicular joints. Irregularities in the contours of these joints may prompt further questioning, and should be highlighted for examination of the joint movements.

Contours

Soft tissue contours are a source of information regarding muscle definition, balance, symmetry, atrophy and hypertrophy. Depressions and swellings should be noted in site and degree, and related to the subsequent movement and strength tests. In athletes involved in one arm dominant sports (throwers, tennis players) the more active upper quadrant is usually more hypertrophied than the other side. Symmetry may indicate atrophy or may be due to bilateral gym training or development of a double handed stroke technique. Further questioning may be required.

When assessing muscle bulk it is useful to palpate the thickness of the upper trapezius, the posterior axillary wall and the anterior axillary wall to get a feel of the muscle size, tone and tension. This should be done with the athlete resting the hands on the hips to relax the shoulder girdle and permit axillary palpation.

Active movement and scapulohumeral rhythm

Active movement testing involves a variety of movements while monitoring the quantity and quality of that movement. Movements that are not restricted by pain can be overpressed at the end of range to obtain more information regarding the restraining mechanisms and possible hypermobility.

During active arm elevation, close observation of the scapulohumeral rhythm should be performed. Asymmetry of scapular motion during the ascending and/or descending phase should be noted, as it may prove significant. Variations include early elevation/rotation of the scapula, uneven movement of the scapula once it commences rotating, and sharp movement irregularities of the scapula in the late stage of descending. These variations, and others, may indicate poor scapular control by the stabilizers (trapezius, serratus anterior, rhomboids) which will be

relevant to any rehabilitation program. Free active elevation may not be a sufficient load to induce scapulohumeral asymmetry, so manual resistance should be added from behind, or hand weights added, as the movement is observed. Repetition of the movement (four to six rapid elevation cycles) can induce some fatigue under which subtle departures from normal may become evident. Obvious winging of the scapula may be a pointer to a long thoracic nerve lesion, weakness of the serratus anterior or both. Excessive movement of the scapula laterally at full elevation indicates tightness of the posterior glenohumeral muscles (Moran & Saunders 1987).

If the examiner is suspicious of acromioclavicular or sternoclavicular joint injury, these joints should be palpated for crepitus or irregular quantity or quality of movement as the arm is elevated and lowered.

Elevation of the arm should be tested in three planes, sagittal (flexion), coronal (abduction) and in the plane of the scapula with the overpressure at the end of range continuing in the same plane.

Other shoulder movements to be actively tested are horizontal flexion, internal and lateral rotation beside the trunk and at 90° of abduction (the functional position in sports activities). Be aware that throwers usually demonstrate a predisposition for lateral rotation on their throwing arm. This means they have excessive lateral rotation and less medial rotation compared with their non-throwing arm (Falkel & Murphy 1988).

Horizontal flexion is most useful in testing of the acromioclavicular joint for range and irritation with overpressure. Cervical and thoracic spine movements should also be tested in cases where the subjective examination has aroused the examiner's suspicion of clinical implications in these regions.

Resisted muscle testing

Manual muscle testing around the shoulder provides a useful guide for strength ratios, but its greater value is in the reproduction of the athlete's pain. With a knowledge of basic kinesiology, the sports physiotherapist can test various muscle groups in different positions in order to identify the most likely source of the reproduced pain. If that pain is identical to that experienced during function, that structure is doubly implicated. The other role of manual testing is during screening for neurological deficits at each level of spinal innervation. Thus the deltoid (C-5), biceps (C5-6), triceps (C-7), long finger flexors (C-8) and interossei (T-1) should identify spinal level and proximal brachial plexus motor problems (Falkel & Murphy 1988).

During initial clinical examination the resisted muscle tests should include internal and lateral rotation beside the body, abduction at around 30°, supraspinatus test using the Centinela-empty can position (Blackburn 1987, Falkel

& Murphy 1988), internal and lateral rotation at 90° of elevation in the plane of the scapula, combined shoulder and elbow flexion at about 45° of shoulder flexion, supination of the forearm at 90° of elbow flexion and protraction of the extended arm. (The dynamic impingement test (Allingham 1988) outlined on p. 386 may also be indicated.) Resisted muscle testing in positions of function and/or pain should also be included. Pain in the act of throwing should be tested for in the same position. Swimmers should be evaluated in prone over the side of a plinth, and resistance applied through the appropriate range of the swimming stroke (in supine for backstroke). Reproduction of an athlete's pain within the context of the predisposing movement pattern provides a useful test for subsequent improvement, and illustrates an intelligent appreciation of the athlete's sporting activity. The latter is extremely important when managing sports injuries.

Objective strength testing of the shoulder musculature requires additional equipment. The precision and reproducibility of such testing varies directly with the cost of the equipment used. Cable tensiometers, static dynamometers and isotonic one repetition maximum efforts do provide a quantifiable result. However, computer driven isokinetic dynamometers are the most popular tool for grading the strength, power, endurance, peak torque and work done for the shoulder muscles. Accurate, reproducible values can be obtained for the six or so standard shoulder set-ups on these machines, and variations on the set-ups can test more functional combinations of the artificial linear motions but sacrifice some of the reliability due to less efficient body stabilization. Isokinetic testing allows testing under conditions of movement speed, fatigue and concentric versus eccentric muscle work (see Ch. 17).

Some workers (Vasey et al 1992) have used isokinetic dynamometer results as an indicator of the likely outcome of a conservative rehabilitation program for shoulder instabilities. They concluded that subjects with an external rotation deficit were more likely to respond well to a conservative program. Those with an internal rotation deficit generally had a structural deficit that precluded success without surgical optimization of the joint.

Palpation

The placement of palpation in the assessment procedure is often one of therapist preference. Some practitioners like to palpate early during the assessment, before specific testing of structures, and use this additional information to direct the objective tests. Others prefer to identify positive signs for various structures and then confirm tenderness, swelling and soft tissue tension using palpation. One suggestion is to base the decision on the degree of irritability as perceived during the subjective examination. Probing of extremely sensitive areas prior to testing may lower the pain threshold producing false positive test results. More resilient symptoms should be able to tolerate pre-test palpation.

Once posture, contours, active movement, passive movement, resisted muscle tests and (perhaps) palpation have been completed, testing of specific structures or for specific lesions can be performed. There is quite a range of tests available at the shoulder area, and these are outlined below. Most of the tests described can be followed up in one or more of the source references Falkel and Murphy (1988), Blackburn (1987) and Andrews and Gillogly (1985).

Specific tests

Acromioclavicular joint compression. End-of-range overpressure into horizontal flexion compresses the acromioclavicular joint using leverage afforded by the humerus. The test should reproduce pain on the line of the joint in order to be positive.

Acromioclavicular joint distraction. Instability of the acromioclavicular joint can be demonstrated by applying a downward traction on the arm while palpating the joint line. Reproduction of pain and/or palpable separation of the joint is considered positive.

Anterior apprehension test. Signs of anterior instability of the glenohumeral joint can be elicited using this test. It stresses the capacity of the anterior restraining mechanisms to tolerate forward displacement of the humeral head. Thus it is structurally non-specific, as the anterior labrum, glenohumeral ligament and anterior cuff are all stressed. The manoeuvre consists of passively supporting the arm at 90° of abduction, with the elbow flexed 90°, and then externally rotating the arm. As this is performed, the examiner's thumb applies an anterior directed pressure to the posterior aspect of the humeral head. A positive finding is noted when an avoidance reaction is elicited from the athlete.

This test is used for athletes who have indicated a popping out or giving way of the shoulder, so care must be exercised when simulating the subluxating force. A large hand/small shoulder combination may allow for reinforcement of the anterior shoulder joint by using the fingers of the stabilizing hand on the shoulder. (Fig. 23.17).

Reproduction of pain is a positive sign of anterior joint injury. A full apprehension reaction is a positive sign of anterior instability.

Anterior translation/shoulder 'Lachman's'. Performed in supine with the examiner grasping the humeral head with one hand, and the trapezius/clavicle complex with the other. The more medial hand stabilizes while the other hand applies an anterior translation force much in the manner of the Lachman's test in the knee. The arm being assessed

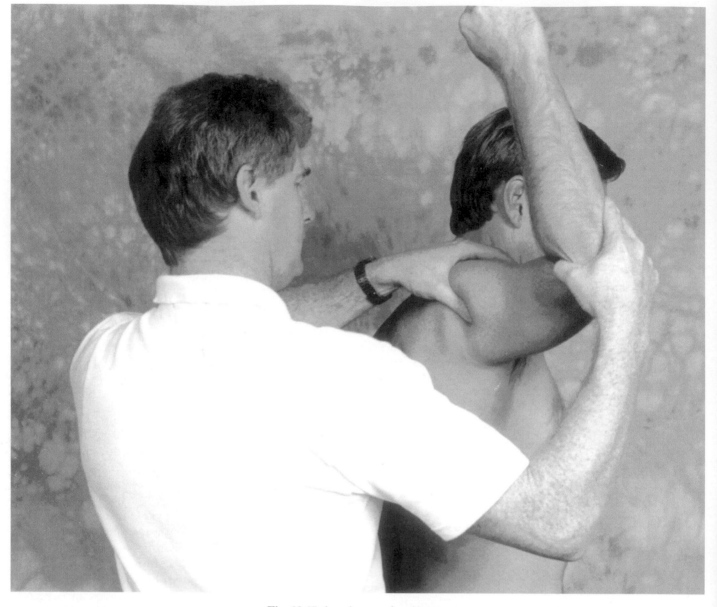

Fig. 23.17 Anterior apprehension test

should be in about 30° of abduction, slight flexion and about 45° of external rotation, with the subject's elbow flexed and the forearm resting on the examiner's more lateral forearm. Comparison with the uninjured side will indicate laxity.

Relocation/containment sign. This is a test for anterior joint pain due to excessive laxity, and may be positive in the absence of apprehension or a lax anterior translation test. This apparent sensitivity to prodromal instability makes it useful for detecting hypermobility-related impingement or anterior capsular conditions (Fig. 23.18).

The test is conducted with the athlete in supine, with the line of the shoulder joint at the edge of the examination table. The examiner takes the athletes arm into a position

of abduction and external rotation of the shoulder to a point that reproduces the athlete's symptomatic pain. This may require some overpressure into horizontal extension also. When the athlete reports reproduction of the pain, the examiner then places his or her free hand on the anterior aspect of the head of the humerus and translates it posteriorly. The athlete is asked what happens to the pain under this force, and again when it is released.

A positive finding occurs when the athlete reports easing of the pain when the humerus is translated posteriorly, and a recurrence when the pressure is released.

There appear to be two views regarding the mechanical effect of this test. One holds that the starting position screws the humeral head into the glenoid fossa as the capsule tightens, and the head then tends to skid in the direction of least resistance, stressing the anterior joint constraints. The second view is that the humeral head translates forwards and compresses the subacromial tissues beneath the anterior end of the coracoacromial arch, reproducing an impingement pain. In common with both views is that the primary finding is one of anterior joint laxity.

Posterior drawer sign. This can be performed sitting or supine. The former is done from behind the athlete with the examiner's stabilizing hand (the opposite from that of the side being tested) buttressed against the body of the scapula and the examiner's elbow locked in extension. The other hand is placed around the head of the humerus so that the pads of the fingers rest on the anterior aspect. This elbow

is also straight. The test movement consists of the examiner posteriorly gliding the head of the humerus by retracting the shoulder girdle on that side. Unless the examiners elbows remain locked in extension, it is difficult to sufficiently draw the humeral head backwards while appreciating the degree of movement available. The test is positive if the glenohumeral joint subluxes, dislocates or at least demonstrates hypermobility compared with the uninjured side.

In supine, the athlete is positioned with the line of the glenohumeral joint at the edge of the examination table, the examiner supporting the arm laterally at an abduction angle not exceeding 90°. The examiner uses anterior manual pressure to glide the humerus posteriorly to its full range. Comparison is made with the opposite side. A positive sign

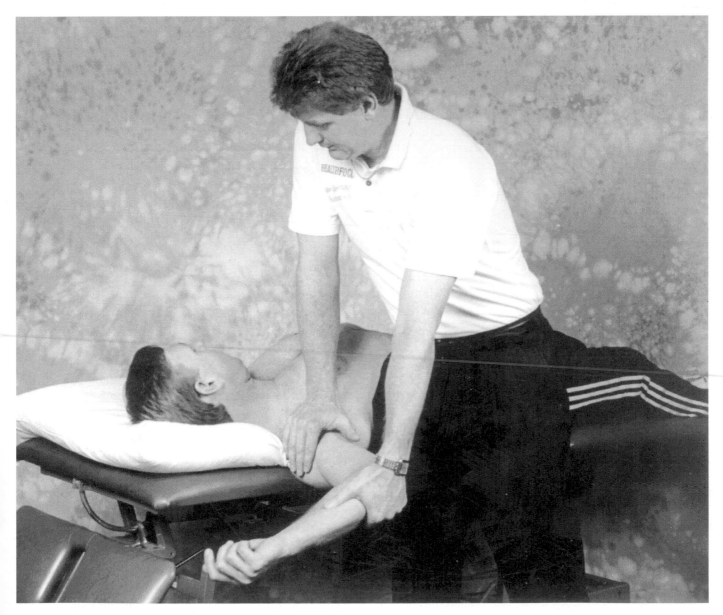

Fig. 23.18 Relocation/containment sign

is as for the sitting test. The supine test allows for convenient testing through a range of abducted positions, the sitting test is a useful quick test which can be followed up in supine if necessary.

Posterior apprehension test. This can also be performed sitting or supine. The examiner takes the athlete's shoulder into a position of 90° flexion, having one hand on the athlete's elbow, and the other placed behind the shoulder joint. The examiner then pushes along the line of the humerus to translate the humeral head posteriorly across the glenoid fossa (Falkel & Murphy 1988).

A positive sign is elicited if the athlete demonstrates apprehension during the manoeuvre. Additional information is gained by the examiner being able to detect the degree of movement as the humeral head fills the hand during the test. The examiner's hand on the posterior joint is also well placed to prevent a posterior subluxation as a result of the test.

Inferior drawer/sulcus test. This test is to assess laxity in an inferior direction. The lower region of the capsule is generous and only restrains the humeral head in the upper ranges of abduction or flexion (Ferrari 1990, Pacelli 1990). The dependent arm is prevented from inferior subluxation by the superior glenohumeral ligament (passively) and the long tendon of biceps (dynamically).

The sulcus test involves a strong downward traction force on the arm while monitoring the superior contour of the shoulder joint. If a significant depression (or sulcus) is evident immediately distal to the acromion, compared with the other side, the test is positive.

Inferior instability occurring in the mid to late range of abduction must be assessed in that range. The athlete is placed supine and the examiner supports the arm while grasping the head of the humerus in both hands. With the body weight stabilizing the scapula, the examiner glides the humeral head inferiorly to the limit of the movement or until apprehension or avoidance by the athlete. Excessive passive glide compared with the other shoulder is a positive test.

Clunk test. A test for the integrity of the anterior glenoid labrum in which the athlete lies supine while the examiner places a hand under the humeral head and grasps the flexed elbow with the other hand. The arm is fully abducted and then the underneath hand pushes the humerus anteriorly while the other passively rotates the humerus. In this manoeuvre the humeral head is forced toward the anterior labrum and then grinds against it, any clunking or grinding is indicative of a tear or partial detachment of the labrum.

Biceps subluxation tests. Three tests have been suggested for testing the integrity of the transverse humeral ligament (Falkel & Murphy 1988). In the first of these the athlete can be sitting or supine with the arm in 90° of abduction and full lateral rotation. The arm is rotated internally while lightly palpating the bicipital tendon, and any popping or snapping of the tendon indicates subluxation.

The second test (Gilcrest's sign) is a more active procedure. The athlete raises a 2 kg hand weight to full elevation with medial rotation and forearm pronation. The arm is then lowered to 90° of abduction while simultaneously externally rotating the humerus and supinating the forearm. Discomfort and/or a palpable snapping of the tendon is considered positive. If the movement is first taught on the unaffected arm, it allows for comparison and ensures immediate correct performance on the injured side.

The third test involves a combination of all the movements generated by the biceps brachii. Falkel and Murphy (1988) cite it as Yergason's test and list it as both a test of the transverse humeral ligament and biceps tendinitis, while Yocum (1983) names it as Speed's test and suggests it is suitable only as a tensile test for bicipital tendinitis. The manoeuvre is identical, and is performed with the examiner simultaneously resisting shoulder flexion, elbow flexion and forearm supination (Fig. 23.19). If looking for tendon subluxation, the biceps tendon should be palpated during this test. If looking for tendinitis, the presence of pain in the bicipital groove area is sufficient for a positive result.

Supraspinatus sign. Devised by Dr Jobe's team at Centinela (California) on the basis of EMG analysis of the rotator cuff, this test virtually isolates the supraspinatus in a tensile test (Jobe & Moynes 1982). Starting in sitting or standing, both the athletes arms are positioned in 90° of abduction, 30° of horizontal flexion and full medial rotation. In this position the supraspinatus is the main support for the suspended arm. Manual resistance to abduction in this position will further stress the supraspinatus, pain on testing indicates a musculotendinous lesion of that muscle.

More recent research by the Jobe team (Townsend et al 1991) electromyographically evaluated a range of common rehabilitation exercises with reference to the glenohumeral muscles. In the course of this project they labelled the movement of humeral elevation in the plane of the scapula as 'scaption'. Their research indicated that scaption with medial rotation (similar to the 'empty-can' test position) was not the strongest activator of the supraspinatus muscle (only producing 74% of maximal muscle tension [MMT]). The honour belonged to the military press (see Fig. 23.30) which produced a peak of 80% of MMT. However, the range at which this peak was achieved was between 0-30°, not at the 90° test position. The anterior and middle deltoid muscles were quite active in the mid-range (72% and 83% respectively) suggesting that an examiner should use clearing tests for the deltoid (e.g. abduction or horizontal extension, both of which favoured the deltoid significantly above the supraspinatus) to ensure the empty-can result reflects the supraspinatus contribution.

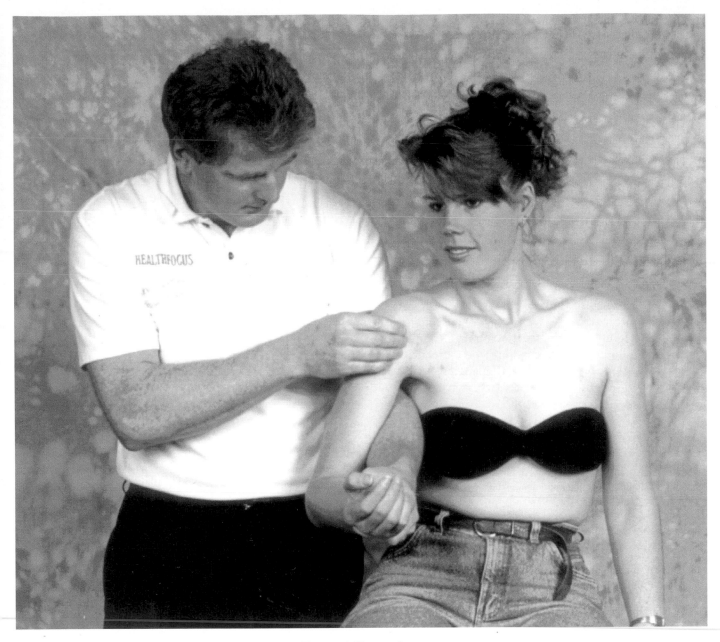

Fig. 23.19 Yergason's test

Impingement tests. Falkel and Murphy (1988) cite four distinct tests for subacromial impingement. Each test attempts to compromise the suprahumeral soft tissues by compressing them against a portion of the coracoacromial arch. Of these four tests, two involve active movement by the athlete, the tests devised by Andrews and Gillogly (1985) and Clancy (Falkel & Murphy 1988). The other two tests are passively conducted by the examiner. By avoiding active muscular elevation or support of the arm by the athlete, reproduction of pain primarily due to a tensile lesion of the rotator cuff can be avoided. For this reason the passive tests should provide a clearer indication of the role of im-

pingement in the reproduction of the athlete's pain. The two tests are described below.

The impingement test devised by Neer and Welsh (cited in Falkel & Murphy 1988, Gerber et al 1985, Moran & Saunders 1987) involves a forced flexion of the humerus jamming the subacromial structures against the anterior third of the acromion process. Reproduction of pain is a positive test, and the test can be confirmed by repeating it following an injection of local anaesthetic and then testing negative.

Hawkins and Kennedy (1980) describe a test for impingement where the examiner positions the athlete's arm at 90° flexion of both shoulder and elbow, and then internally rotates the humerus to drive the greater tuberosity beneath the coracoacromial arch. Reproduction of pain is considered positive.

Both these impingement tests may provoke pain in a normal shoulder if administered too aggressively. Thus it is easy to produce false positive signs of impingement. Careful comparison with the uninjured arm and cautious application and interpretation of the impingement tests should be followed.

The impingement tests are diagnostically non-specific, although Penny and Welsh (1981) intimate that an element of medial rotation in the test may implicate the supraspinatus tendon more so than the bicipital. However, the tests do not identify the structure that is responsible for the pain on impingement, they simply confirm that something in the subacromial space is hypersensitive and thus inflamed. This may be the bursa, a tendon (any or all of biceps, supraspinatus or infraspinatus), the inferior aspect of the acromion or the superior synovial fold of the glenohumeral joint. All these structures are nociceptive. The results of the impingement tests must be correlated with the results of tensile tests, passive movement tests, palpation and history, in order to locate the exact source of the pain and pathology.

The two tests described above are static tests of impingement, their aim being to reproduce pain using an artificial, clinical test. More information on the contribution of glenohumeral mechanics to the impingement is useful when determining optimal management. One test has been described (Allingham 1988) which endeavours to do this. The test is only applicable in athletes who demonstrate a painful arc on active or resisted elevation, and who test positive on one or other of the above static impingement tests.

The dynamic impingement test (Allingham's test) is performed in the painful arc range of elevation in an attempt to relieve the impingement pain by altering the muscle activity.

The athlete elevates the arm to the painful range, and then attempts to adduct against manual resistance provided by the examiner (Fig. 23.20). If the pain is relieved, the test result is positive.

During this manoeuvre, the abductor/flexor muscles are relaxed and the adductor/extensor muscles activated. In so doing, the humeral head is centred inferiorly on the glenoid, increasing the subacromial clearance for the impinged tissues.

In the absence of a positive supraspinatus sign (Centinela test) Allingham's test can indicate the reversibility of the impingement dynamics, and thus the likelihood of success of an adduction based rehabilitation program (see p. 401).

Biceps tendinitis tests. Again there are several tests listed in the literature for this condition, with the best overview presented by Falkel & Murphy (1988). The various tests are outlined below, with the rider that none of them is an independent diagnostic test. Each test may support the diagnosis of tendinitis of the long head of biceps tendon, but must be interpreted in the light of other tests and observations.

Yergason's test. This manoeuvre has been described previously (Fig. 23.19). Pain arising in the anterior aspect of the shoulder during this test may be associated with a biceps tendinitis.

Straight arm raise. Initially reported by Hawkins and Kennedy (1980), this test has the examiner resist isometric shoulder flexion when the elbow is extended. Providing the anterior deltoid is cleared (by testing resisted horizontal flexion across the body), pain in the anterior aspect of the shoulder is positive for biceps tendinitis.

Ludlington's test. The athlete places the hand on the top of the head, and forcefully flexes the elbow against that resistance. Anterior shoulder pain on contraction is positive for biceps tendinitis.

Locking and quadrant tests. Two specific tests of glenohumeral joint mobility in and around the functional range for overhead sports have been described by Maitland (1991). These are the locking position and the quadrant position. Maitland points out that these tests are of particular value when assessing shoulders that demonstrate pain and/or stiffness which cannot be confidently attributed to any specific structural lesion (Corrigan & Maitland 1983). A brief description of these tests follows, further information can be found in the texts cited.

Locking position. From a starting position where the athlete is supine and the examiner standing to the side, the physiotherapist stabilizes the scapula by placing his or her forearm under the athlete, medial to the scapula with the fingers curled over the upper trapezius. The other hand grasps the athlete's flexed elbow in a position of shoulder extension and medial rotation. The test movement sees the physiotherapist take the athlete's arm into abduction and towards a position of full elevation. Movement continues until the humerus reaches a position where it becomes locked. If this position can be achieved easily and without pain, it is considered normal. If not, it indicates glenohumeral joint dysfunction. Note that the locking position seeks to jam the greater tuberosity into the subacromial space and should not be used in cases of irritable impingement syndrome.

Quadrant position. This is a small arc of movement as the arm is released from the locking position on its way to full elevation. The starting position is from the lock as described above, and then the downward pressure on the elbow is eased to allow some anterior movement until lateral rotation becomes possible. Once this occurs the movement

De

Su
sor
the
of t

dec
198
can
Fra
198

dec
resu
Suc
me
hav
is r
Thi
on
wor
pro
succ

sco
and
the
enc
labr
be p
199
surg
and

Soft

Rota

Mos
are
or t
expl
dislc
susta
[
pictu
lesio
seco
acro
Resu
phys
ever
O
cand
anthr

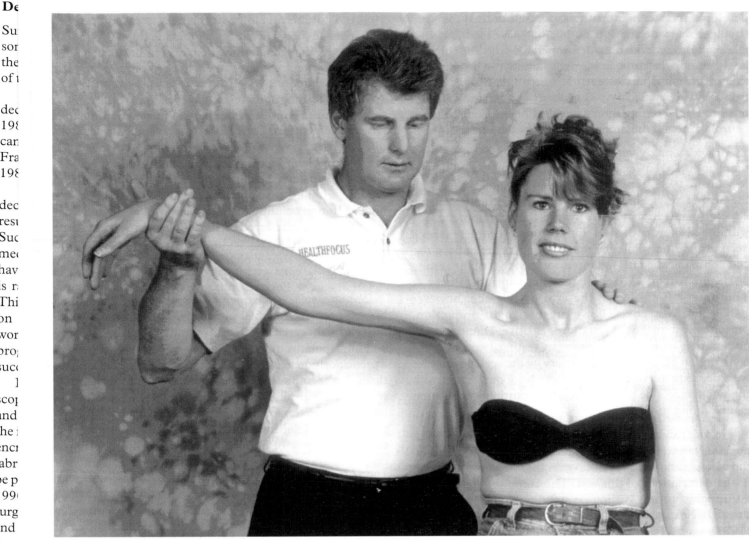

Fig. 23.20 Dynamic impingement test

into abduction continues as does the lateral rotation. The small movement as the glenohumeral joint is 'unlocked' and laterally rotated into abduction is the quadrant position. During this movement the physiotherapist monitors pain and abnormal movement for signs of dysfunction. Over-pressure can be used during the test to elicit signs (Corrigan & Maitland 1983).

Neurovascular tests. It is not uncommon for a mechanical examination of the shoulder to conclude with clouded, confusing or contradictory results, making a specific diagnosis impossible or, at best, tentative. When athletes present with a history suggesting a cervical or thoracic spine contribution to the shoulder pain/dys-function, examination and testing to clear the mechanics of those areas must be performed. In addition, neurological evaluation of strength, sensation and reflexes may be indicated. These examinations are detailed in Chapter 21.

Specific neurovascular tests for shoulder pain and/or dysfunction are indicated in athletes who demonstrate inconclusive mechanical examination results and/or symp-toms such as parasthesia, burning, coldness, muscular weakness or proprioceptive loss. Pratt (1986) provides an excellent description of the various neurovascular en-trapment patterns around the shoulder region and discusses the relevant anatomical relationships. For most of these there are clinical tests available, the results of which may indicate that referral for more comprehensive neurological or vascular assessments is appropriate.

Wing-scapula test. The athlete performs a push-up against a wall while the examiner observes scapula mechanics from behind. Winging of the scapula indicates weakness of the serratus anterior. The weakness may be due to straight muscle weakness or due to dysfunction of the long thoracic nerve. The latter is sometimes a finding in backpackers who advice regarding conservative or surgical management of their instability problem.

Acute anterior glenohumeral subluxation

Trauma to the shoulder can produce instances of anterior subluxation of the glenohumeral joint. The athlete typically reports feeling the joint 'almost popping out' or 'popping out and straight back in again'. Such descriptions of symptoms should alert the physiotherapist to the likelihood of some joint laxity.

Examination usually demonstrates some degree of anterior apprehension, a positive relocation sign and anterior tenderness on the glenohumeral joint line. There may not be a significant passive laxity of the drawer tests evident, due either to muscular guarding or insufficient damage to the constraints.

These episodes are initially quite painful and should be treated with ice, rest, analgesics as necessary, and the arm be kept in a sling for two or three days. They then improve quite rapidly, with the athlete demonstrating almost full range of movement and muscle strength with only minor discomfort often within a week of injury. The athlete (and coach, and parent) then believe the joint is ready to resume sporting participation.

In order to minimize the chance of reinjury, and avoid a worsening of the condition into a frank dislocation, the athlete should be counselled into undertaking a thorough rehabilitation program (pp. 396–404) and avoiding contact sports (or incidental contact sports) for a period of four to six weeks. A gradual return to activity is then continued with the athlete avoiding hard throwing/serving, or tackling situations until competent and pain-free in all other aspects of the sport.

Rotator cuff strains

Acute injuries to the rotator cuff, or acute flare-ups of chronic conditions, require the usual components of the damage control stage of management, namely ice, rest, support and protection. The aim being to relieve pain, alleviate inflammation, reduce repeated irritation and prevent subsequent undesirable tissue shortening (Nitz 1986).

Acute, disabling painful shoulder injuries that do not appear to be a fracture or dislocation should be suspected of being severe rotator cuff tears. Appropriate soft tissue management and support in a sling should be administered, and then the athlete referred on for further investigation of the cuff. Arthrotomography or arthroscopy may be indicated, with an early surgical repair being the treatment of choice, especially for athletes involved in upper quadrant sports of swimming, racquet use, or throwing.

Less severe acute musculotendinous injuries around the shoulder are managed according to the principles of soft tissue treatment (above). As the acute stage of injury resolves, promotion of healing and restoration of function become the priorities. The introduction of heat treatment, muscle stimulation, manual therapy and exercise rehabilitation is accomplished as the athlete's pain and protective guarding diminishes.

Efforts must be made to prevent rotator cuff shutdown. Failure to do this will predispose to the onset of secondary impingement and laxity (see Table 23.6).

Chronic shoulder injuries

Chronic shoulder lesions can usually be attacked more positively from the initial treatment, depending on how recently any reaggravation has occurred. If recently exacerbated, some damage control may be required, otherwise the aims will be to remedy any soft tissue shortening (characterized by loss of physiological and/or accessory ranges of movement), to restore normal posture of the upper quadrant and normal (or better) muscle strength, endurance, flexiblility, balance and synergy.

The management of acute inflammatory exacerbations is discussed in Chapter 10. This chapter is more concerned with the use of exercise therapy and manual therapy when rehabilitating an athletic shoulder injury. These two make up half of the four cornerstones of sports physiotherapy, the other two being electrotherapy and education.

Both manual and exercise therapy are most effective when they are prescribed and dispensed accurately, and on the basis of a thorough assessment. The various techniques and exercises should be used according to what is specifically required by the injured athlete at the time of each consultation or stage of recovery. This necessitates ongoing monitoring of the athletes current capacities and dysfunctions as recovery progresses to ensure that the therapy techniques employed are the most appropriate and therefore fruitful.

Postural retraining

The re-education of an abnormal posture in relation to shoulder lesions is the summation of manual therapy and exercise therapy: the first to help restore the mobility and extensibility of joint, muscle, fascia, neural tissue, etc. so that the desired posture can be achieved comfortably; the latter to train the neurological control, strength and stamina of the muscles to maintain this posture and to superimpose movement. Both these further rely on education of the athlete so that an appreciation of the significance of corrected posture in relation to the long-term treatment goal is instilled.

When embarking on a program of postural re-education, the therapist must first identify those factors that need to be addressed. In the scapular region these include a stiff and/or kyphotic thoracic spine, tightness of the scapula elevators (trapezius and levator scapula) due to persistent hitching of the shoulder when elevating, shortening of the serratus anterior from habitual protraction, and weakness (due increased resting length) of the retractors for the same reason. Across the shoulder joint there may be tightness of the pectoral muscles and latissumus dorsi due to habitual medial rotation, and a co-existing weakness of the external rotators as they are placed beyond their optimal length/tension relationship by the anterior tightness.

Manual therapy techniques (see below) can be used in conjunction with stretching exercises and facilitation techniques to mobilize the tight areas allowing a return toward symmetrical posture. Meanwhile, exercise therapy (see below) can start preparing the weakened or lengthened muscles for the role of postural maintenance.

Manual therapy

The primary role of manual therapy around the shoulder is to reduce soft tissue shortening in order to restore normal ranges of movement (Nitz 1986). A second role is that of joint pain relief. Consideration of whether the restrictive tissue is contractile or inert, and whether the limit is due to pain or stiffness will affect the type and degree of manual therapy to be applied.

Most athletes are not aware of these manual therapy dichotomies, and inevitably present with shoulders displaying elements of pain and stiffness and both muscular and capsular shortening. The astute practitioner must then apportion the culpability for the dysfunction and select techniques accordingly.

The fundamental principles and practice of manual therapy in sports physiotherapy are discussed in Chapter 12. This brief outline will draw attention to shoulder specific aspects of the skills.

Although the range of movement of the shoulder is measured at the glenohumeral joint, contributions to that range are made by the clavicular joints and the scapulothoracic 'articulation'. Restrictions to glenohumeral motion may be due to restrictions of movement in any or all of these joints. Sustained stretching of the restricted glenohumeral movement may slowly free these adjacent joints, but often more satisfactory (and comfortable) progress can be made by passively mobilizing the accessory movements of the sternoclavicular, acromioclavicular and scapulothoracic joints.

Superior-inferior gliding of a tight sternoclavicular joint can mobilize scapula abduction which will, in turn, improve arm elevation. Likewise, anteroposterior gliding of a stiff acromioclavicular joint can improve scapular presentation to allow full arm elevation, horizontal flexion, or medial rotation. These mobilizing techniques are detailed elsewhere (Maitland 1991), and should be continued for as long as those joints are restricted.

The scapulothoracic junction is a soft tissue articulation that requires freedom of movement for normal scapulo-humeral rhythm (Codman 1934). Passive mobilization of the scapula against the thoracic wall in all directions, including rotations, is possible. Examination of active and passive scapular movement will indicate the directions that require mobilizing.

Perhaps the most effective scapula-mobilizing technique is distraction away from the thorax. In this technique the inferior angle and the body of the scapular are lifted away from the rib cage by gripping around the medial border of the scapula (Fig. 23.23). This can be performed in prone or in sidelying. It is important to retract the scapula intially to enable a firm grip to be gained, and to gradually apply the distractive force so as not to stimulate protective spasm of the rhomboids which will loosen the physiotherapist's hold. This technique is often uncomfortable when first applied, but following one or two sustained stretches, the athlete usually reports improvement in pain and movement (Nitz 1986).

Manual therapy for the glenohumeral articulation can be quite effective in facilitating return of lost movement. In athletes, many of the shoulders demonstrate glenohumeral hyper-mobility related problems and mobilizing of the joint in those cases may be counter-productive. Certainly care must be taken to avoid mobilizing to the end of range in the direction of any hyper-mobility. Mobilizing of the clavicular joints and scapula may allow the athlete to achieve or maintain the desired range of motion while relieving the end of range stress on the glenohumeral joint. In other words, judicious mobilizing of restricted proximal elements may allow sharing the flexibility load more evenly along the kinetic chain.

When mobilizing a restricted and irritable glenohumeral joint, the position best tolerated by the athlete is usually

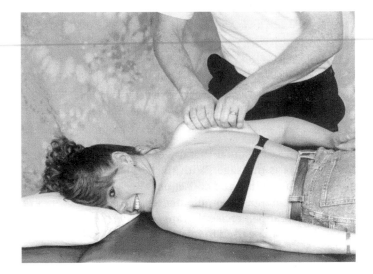

Fig. 23.23 Scapular distraction

One of the most difficult retraining phases of shoulder rehabilitation is the stretch shortening cycle (SCC) as late cocking explodes into acceleration of arm and/or racquet head. At this late stage there is a storing of energy in the series elastic component of the musculotendinous structures (Stanton & Purdam 1989) as the external rotators hold the shoulder while the trunk commences to rotate into the throw. The internal rotators are thus stretched slightly as they respond with an eccentric deceleration of the late cocking stage and then fire as the external rotators relax allowing an explosion into acceleration phase. Exercises to specifically re-educate this transition should be included in the late stage of shoulder rehabilitation (Allingham 1990). This SSC retraining differs from the standard eccentric exercise in that it is a ballistic combination to engage the series elastic component. High speed eccentric exercises usually precede this stage as the rehabilitation program evolves (see Ch. 13).

The eccentric/concentric high speed 'catch and accelerate' cycle described by Komi (1988) should only be commenced when full pain-free range and near normal strength are regained (80-90% of normal). This exercise is started slowly and then increased in speed and power (Fig. 23.31). The training is mainly neurological at this stage as recruitment patterns are learned and refined. The use of weights is not necessary and, if used, should not exceed 1 kg.

The progression toward this SSC retraining is a gradual process during an overall rehabilitation program. Preceding the movement specific SSC exercise should be a series of plyometric exercises first involving bilateral trunk and shoulder muscles, gradually becoming unilateral and finally sport specific.

This exercise is particularly difficult in shoulder rehabilitation as the athlete is exercising in abduction and lateral rotation with a high speed ballistic motion. This is a similar action to that which reproduces most symptoms in shoulder pathology be they instabilities or impingements. The barriers to executing this type of retraining may not necessarily be physical, as the athlete is often apprehensive about approaching skill speeds of execution. Patience and reassurance on the part of the physiotherapist will help maximize the benefits of this late stage rehabilitation.

In addition to the regional strengthening program around the shoulder complex, the athlete should continue, resume or commence a strength, endurance, power training program for the rest of his or her body. Such a program should be specific to the sport and should be planned in conjunction with the athlete's coach or training consultant. Co-operation between the physiotherapist and the coaching staff can ensure that any program will not compromise recovery from the initial injury and that the rehabilitation program can complement the periodization or cycling of the overall coaching pattern (see Chapter 10).

Figure 23.25 outlines a flowchart approach for the exercise rehabilitation of the five types of athletic glenohumeral problems commonly seen in the sports clinic. Following is discussion on each of the components of the chart. The reader will be able to trace the exercise treatment

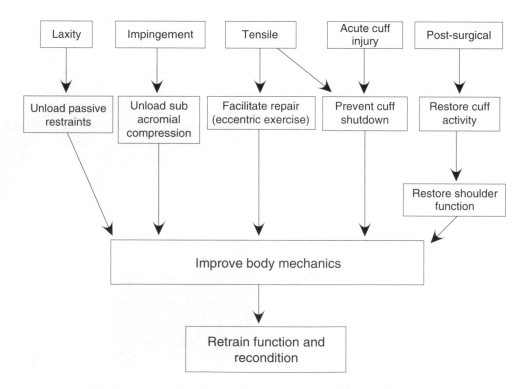

Fig. 23.25 Goals for exercise rehabilitation of common athletic shoulder problems

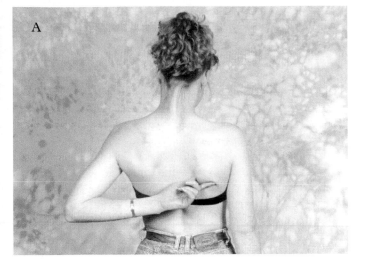

A

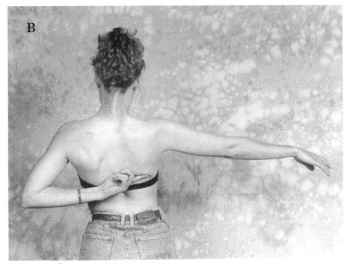

B

Fig. 23.26 A & B Scapular re-education with manual monitoring

resistance in order to co-contract the elements of the rotator cuff as well as the scapular stabilizers has been advocated by Allingham (1990).

A further example involving self-monitoring of scapula postioning is shown in Figure 23.26. Active adduction and depression of the scapula will engage the middle and lower trapezius while simultaneously inhibiting the upper trapezius and the levator scapula. So the hitching muscles of the scapula are suppressed, breaking the compensatory pattern of a disturbed scapulohumeral rhythm while increasing the recruitment of the stabilizers. This exercise can be progressed by adding resistance while maintaining scapular control as shown in Figure 23.27. This manual monitoring of scapula control by the athlete can then be trained and tested by active elevation, sporting patterns and finally faster, ballistic activities.

Improving the muscular control across the glenohumeral joint requires strengthening of the short rotators of the cuff

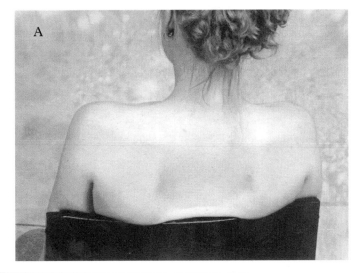

A

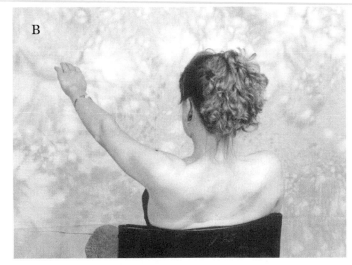

B

Fig. 23.27 A & B Scapular re-education using chair back

progressions from the chart into the text in order to plan a treatment regime for a particular condition or athlete. Remember that many athletes will present with elements of more than one pathology, so do not become fixed on one stream.

Unload passive restraints. To relieve the pathological effects of glenohumeral joint hypermobility or laxity, the injured passive restraints must be relieved of the overloading.

This may be accomplished through exercise by ensuring that the secondary or dynamic restraint mechanisms are functioning efficiently. The rotator cuff muscles must be retrained to effectively centre the humeral head on the glenoid, and to stabilize it during activity. The scapular stabilizers must also be working correctly to enable the cuff muscles to perform their task.

Scapular stabilizing exercises with superimposed glenohumeral co-contraction exercises can facilitate this retraining. The use of glenohumeral adduction against

and integration of that strength into functional patterns of activity. The usual battery of rotator exercises using free weights, pulleys, springs and rubbers is a sound place to start such a program. The initial exercise program should

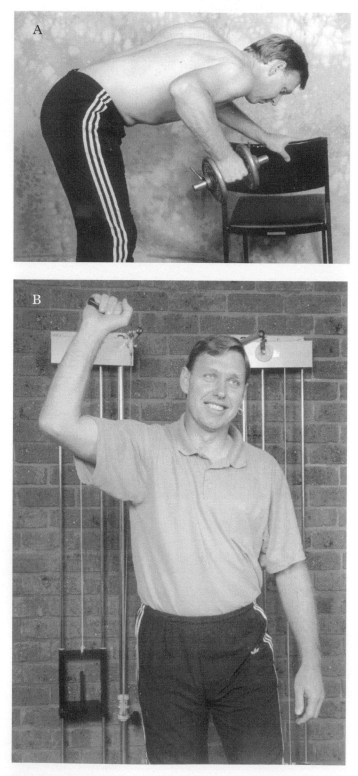

Fig. 23.28 A & B Rotator cuff exercises

avoid positions of instability and impingement, and should avoid reinforcing unwanted patterns of movement (e.g. scapular hitching). As strength and control improve, the arm should be exercised closer to the position of hypermobility so that the cuff muscles become adept at controlling glenohumeral migration in that position. Resistance and speed can be added according to the principles of progressive overload and specificity of training as discussed in Chapter 10. Figures 23.28A and B illustrate exercises appropriate to this strength program.

The direction of hypermobility or instability should give some guidance as to which muscles need retraining. For example, an anterior instability can be assisted by the posterior cuff muscles exerting a centring force on the humeral head, and strengthening of the subscapularis will assist when that muscle bridges the joint anteriorly in mid to late abduction. It is more appropriate to develop this muscular control in the position of instability rather than by the side, but the athlete should approach this position gradually during the strengthening program so to avoid subluxing the joint. Townsend et al (1991) found the most effective exercises for the teres minor and infraspinatus muscles to be lateral rotation in contralateral side lie, and horizontal extension from prone over a bench (Fig. 23.29). The subscapularis was most active during scaption (movement in the plane of the scapula) in medial rotation, the military press (Fig. 23.30), flexion and abduction. It was surprisingly less active during medial rotation in side lie, underlining its importance as a stabilizer during arm activity.

An inferior dislocator will rely on supraspinatus and the long tendon of biceps for dynamic support of the humeral head. Exercises for those muscles should be included in any rehabilitation program as well as the general cuff retraining. Townsend et al (1991) have found scaption exercises and the military press to be effective for supraspinatus.

Manual resisted exercising using proprioceptive neuromuscular facilitation (PNF) is invaluable around the shoulder. The use of reversals to work antagonists and rhythmic stabilizations to promote co-contraction make PNF extremely valuable. This exercise technique can be applied to develop strength, improved recruitment, endurance or flexibility for the shoulder joint and scapula (Knott & Voss 1968) while avoiding positions of instability. These patterns can be repeated at home using rubber tubing exercises.

In the later stage of rehabilitation, the high speed stretch shortening cycle exercises are introduced (Allingham 1990). These are commenced slowly and in a comfortable, supported stable position, usually supine or prone. As the athlete will be exercising in the position of anterior instability some apprehension is likely. Start slowly without weights and monitor the movement for correct execution. In supine, small amplitude lateral rotation under the control of the

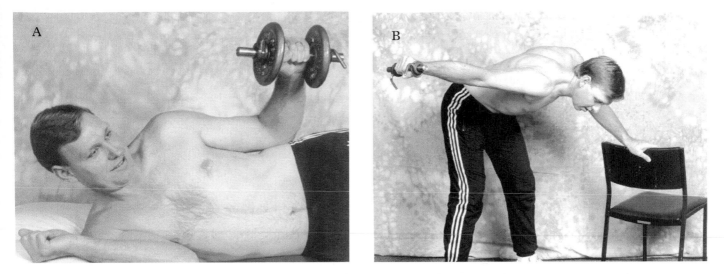

Fig. 23.29 A External rotation. **B** Horizontal abduction in prone

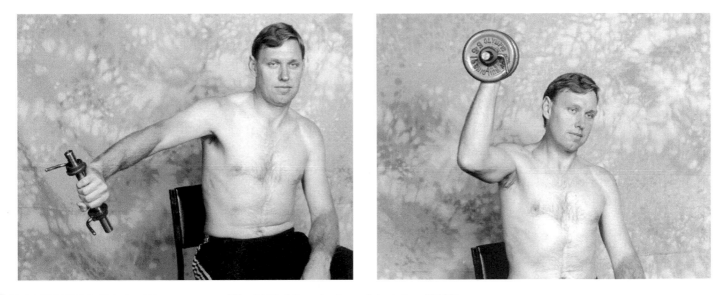

Fig. 23.30 A Scaption in medial rotation. **B** Military press

internal rotators can be performed with the arm dropping back and then being decelerated by the internal rotators in a 'catch-recover' manner (Fig. 23.31). Depth of drop-back (lateral rotation), speed of movement, and number of repetitions can be increased. When control is good, the arm can extend beyond the edge of the plinth, allowing greater movement in a less stable position. Progress to light weights (up to 1 kg) and high repetitions will assist development of endurance and consistency of recruitment patterns.

Unload sub-acromial compression. The aim for impingement symptoms is to reduce the compression on the subacromial contents and, to this end, exercise rehabilitation can prove to be most effective, particularly if the impingement demonstrated a dynamic component on Allingham's test during the assessment (p. 386).

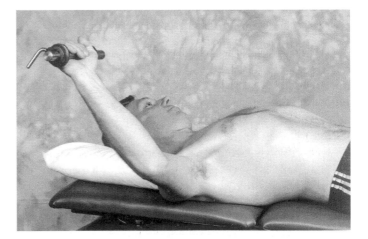

Fig. 23.31 Stretch-shortening exercises—catch

The aim is to reduce the superior migration of the humeral head during elevation of the arm by improving the strength or recruitment of those cuff muscles that exert a downward centring pull. These muscles can be trained using adduction exercises, first inner range and then through range. Isometric adduction with the arm at around 20-30° of abduction can be done using a pillow or rolled blanket. With impingements based on muscular inhibition, rapid improvement in pain-free elevation can be observed following several repetitions of this exercise. The effect is not lasting, and repetition with a home program is required to supplant the old recruitment pattern.

Care must be taken to ensure the athlete does not elevate the scapula as he or she attempts to maximally adduct the shoulder. This extraneous movement is the prime cause of pain when performing this exercise, and can be relieved by asking the athlete to actively depress the scapula throughout the isometric cuff contraction. A second benefit of this depression is reinforcement of the more proximal force couple as the scapula stabilizers are likewise isometrically contracted.

Pulley or rubber exercises can be utilized through impingement range whereby the athlete adducts or extends the shoulder, using the cuff muscles to prevent compromise of the subacromial space. Increases to load and speed follow, and finally progression to functional patterns and intensities. During these stages it is important to monitor the scapulo-thoracic movement and ensure that adequate control of the scapula is possible at all ranges of arm movement and speed. If not, specific scapula stabilizing exercises should be introduced, as mentioned above.

In some cases, the athlete cannot actively control the scapular and/or glenohumeral stabilizers in order to stabilize it during arm activity; or the athlete may be involved in activities that involve repeated elevation of the arm with consequent aggravation of the impingement. It may be necessary to tape these athletes in order to suppress unwanted muscle action and enhance the glenohumeral stabilizers.

Such a taping has been suggested by McConnell (1990, 1992) in which the upper trapezius is taped across its fibres (inhibitory) and the posterior rotator cuff is taped along its fibres (facilitatory). If the tape is to be effective, it will demonstrate this immediately on application; the athlete will report a decrease intensity of the painful arc and/or an increased range of elevation. The taping program need only continue until the active exercise program establishes control of the force couples sufficient to enable pain-free elevation of the arm.

Exercises to stretch the scapular elevators and the pectoral muscles are necessary to ensure normal scapular positioning during shoulder activities. If the athlete's thoracic spine is stiff or excessively kyphotic, exercises should be prescribed accordingly as full elevation of the glenohumeral joint relies on a mobile thoracic region.

The cuff retraining program should continue until the athlete can elevate, throw, swim or perform whatever movement initiated the impingement without reproducing the pain. This indicates that sufficient clearance beneath the acromion has been achieved and retriggering of the inflammatory process preventing resolution is likewise forestalled. Only then can healing of the lesion proceed, irrespective of whether the compression injury is to a tendon or to the bursa.

The role of hypermobility as a predisposing factor for impingement syndromes has been discussed above (p. •••). Thus, early commencement of an adduction program, as outlined above, for hypermobile or unstable shoulders may prevent secondary impingement. Fortunately, the program commences in a position unlikely to complicate the instability.

Prevent rotator cuff shutdown. Any condition that interferes with the normal stabilizing function of the rotator cuff will predispose to further problems (Table 23.6). It is imperative that in cases of impingement, tendinitis or acute cuff strain the rotator cuff be kept active.

To this end, immediate pain-free isometric exercises emphasizing co-contraction of the cuff muscles should be introduced. If pain prevents any activity, then all measures should be directed to alleviating that pain and allowing the exercises to commence. The compressive, centring force of the rotator cuff can be generated using the adduction based program outlined above. Individual exercises into internal or external rotation do not activate both the anterior and posterior cuff components.

When the athlete's pain has settled, isotonic exercises for the shoulder complex can be introduced in order to continue this co-contraction retraining through a range of motion. Resistance can be applied, but should be such to ensure that the movement remains pain-free. Pain during exercise will likely invoke a motor pattern that reinforces the faulty, compensatory pattern.

Facilitate tensile repair. If the cuff lesion is not compressive (i.e. impingement), but is tensile in cause and character, a straight adduction program is not appropriate. It may go some way to relieving impingement of the swollen tendon that is torn or microtraumatized, but it will do nothing to rehabilitate the actual tendon injury. Tensile tendon lesions respond best to tensile exercise programs, especially eccentric exercise programs (Curwin & Stanish 1984). The physiology of this type of exercise is discussed in Chapter 10. Around the shoulder region tensile tendon-itides occur in the tendons of supraspinatus, infraspinatus, teres minor and major, pectoralis major, biceps brachii and triceps brachii. In fact, not much is safe when an overload situation develops.

Following identification of the affected tendon(s) and reproduction of pain on tensile testing (resisted contraction and/or stretching) the initial aim is to suppress or resolve the inflammatory process so that collagen regeneration can occur. Then follows the introduction of an eccentric exercise program to facilitate collagen bonding and alignment

(Curwin & Stanish 1984). Eccentric loading of the tendon is started slowly and at low loading until the tendon demonstrates a tolerance to the force application. Progression of speed and loading is tiered and based on the athletes discomfort during exercise. The program is outlined in Chapter 10.

Devising eccentric exercises for the anterior and posterior shoulder muscles is not difficult. The supraspinatus, however, requires a little more thought. The work of Jobe and Moynes (1982) suggests the ideal position is the Centinela or empty-can position, and this should be reached without using a concentric contraction of the supraspinatus. Starting with the hand by the side, the athlete abducts the arm leading with the thumb (i.e. in lateral rotation), at 90° the arm is inwardly rotated so that the thumb again leads as the shoulder horizontally flexes 30°. Once in this position, the arm again inwardly rotates so that the thumb points downwards, then the arm is lowered in the plane of the scapula, maximizing the contribution of the supraspinatus. This exercise should be performed with normal scapulohumeral rhythm, otherwise compensatory patterns will be reinforced.

Recent EMG studies by Townsend et al (1991) suggest the military press exercise (Fig. 23.30) could be used in the lowermost 30° of range where the supraspinatus is most active. In this case the uninjured arm could be used to assist the concentric elevation, allowing eccentric return unassisted. Scaption with medial rotation (Fig. 23.30) was found to be the best recruiter of supraspinatus through the range 90–120° (Townsend et al 1991).

Restore cuff activity. This applies to post-surgical cases, when due to pain, previous history and apprehension on the part of the athlete, there is little or no appreciable rotator-cuff activity.

Early re-activation of the rotator cuff is vital, but it must be accomplished within the limits of the healing surgical intervention. Consultation with the surgeon regarding early exercise is necessary.

The use of electrical stimulation and biofeedback is helpful in the early stages: as is using distal activity in the upper limb to stimulate proximal co-contraction. For example, tightly squeezing a rubber ball in the hand of the affected arm will initiate a stabilizing contraction in the rotator cuff. Care must be taken to avoid pain which may inhibit the co-contraction pattern.

Active exercise for the scapula, neck, elbow and forearm will also facilitate glenohumeral muscle activity. Attention to correct spinal and upper extremity posture is important, and must be instilled in the athlete.

Isometric cuff exercises, as soon as they are pain-free, will be followed by isotonic work when the period post-surgical of immobilization is completed.

Restore shoulder function. As the limits of surgery are progressively lifted, exercises and activities to restore range of motion, strength and proprioception around the shoulder are introduced.

Through-range exercises are commenced at the earliest opportunity according to the surgeon's protocol or the physiotherapist's judgement, should such responsibility be delegated. Passive mobilizing and assisted-active exercises through the available range are performed as tolerated by the athlete. Avoidance of the appropriate position of previous instability following reconstructive surgery, or positions of impingement following decompressive surgery must be observed for the initial weeks of rehabiliation. Exactly how many weeks will be determined by the type of surgery, extent of surgery, age of the athlete, duration of symptoms, and other factors. Communication with the surgeon is necessary to clarify any questions the physiotherapist may have regarding contraindicated positions or movements.

Strengthening the cuff and prime movers of the scapula and shoulder following surgery is vital in determining the ultimate functional recovery by the athlete. Stability retraining for the two force couples should precede mobility exercises to ensure that the joint is protected once active through-range work is performed. Exercises to improve stability involve active fixation of the scapula during small range movements of the shoulder and arm. The use of mirrors (to allow the athlete to monitor premature elevation of the scapula) or biofeedback on the lower trapezius can be used as learning tools. This proximal control should be developed prior to distal rehabilitation in order to maintain or restore quality of movement.

Strength rehabilitation should follow the guidelines for resistance training discussed in Chapter 10. Loads around 70% of 1RM should be used, but can only be applied when sufficient time for healing has elapsed (at least four to six weeks) and only if proximal stabilizing can be maintained through the range of motion used.

Exercising through the stretch shortening cycle that occurs at the end of the cocking stage of throw or racquet swing should not be attempted until the athlete has full pain-free range of movement and near normal strength return (at least 80% of normal). This exercise is started slowly and then increased in speed and power (see discussion on pp. 398–9).

As the rehabilitation program progresses the elements should be combined into patterns of movement that duplicate or make up the skills that the athlete utilizes in his or her sport. Thus, throwers will build into a throwing action and swimmers into the stroking motions outlined in the biomechanics section. In addition to the patterns, other elements of the relevant sport may be included. For example, using tennis or squash racquets during flexibility and strength exercises, having the thrower grip a baseball during cuff stabilization exercises and getting a swimmer into an appropriate hydrotherapy program as soon as possible.

Improve body mechanics. Many shoulder problems in sport arise from poor body mechanics during execution of athletic activities. Deficiencies in balance, core stability, weight transference, momentum transfer and force summation can overload the upper extremity predisposing to injury. Prevention of reinjury will be greatly enhanced if attention is paid to these factors.

During the rehabilitation program, total body retraining to improve balance, stability of the body core (trunk) during activity of the extremities, sequential movements comprising the sports skills and proprioceptive reactions around the shoulder should all be introduced and practised.

Plyometric exercises for the legs, trunk and then the arm are valuable to develop strength, power, rhythm and confidence. Used in moderation such activities give an excellent return for work invested.

As the athlete becomes proficient with the clinical activities, the skills of the sport should be integrated into the rehabilitation program: initially in a controlled manner, and then progressed to the speed and intensity of the sport itself.

Rehabilitating the arm in isolation will be unrewarding in the long-term, and will not allow the athlete to resume his or her sport at the pre-injury level.

Examples of this evolution are easy to encounter in the shoulder region. Throwing athletes commence a throwing conditioning program which gradually progresses the variables of duration, intensity, frequency, distance, power and accuracy of throwing (Blackburn 1987, Carson 1989, Jenkins & Kegerris 1990). First from a standing start, then from a crow-hop, and finally drills involving chasing the ball, fielding it and throwing in a game simulation. Progression when returning to racquet sports can be done by first having the player free-swing the racquet with a full backswing and follow-through but no power. As comfort indicates, the power is increased and the skill is integrated into a shuttle run drill (simulating across court movement). Such a program can initially avoid the more stressful elements like serving, topspin forehands and backhands. These are added as the player improves and gains insight into how the current level of recovery feels. Finally a ball is introduced and the intensity, duration and frequency of the workouts is increased toward match and tournament tempo.

Players often report an improvement in their tennis/squash/badminton/racquetball game following this program. Phantom stroke play allows for mental rehearsal of perfect shots, and the 'ball' never arrives until the player is in the correct stance and preparatory swing phase. The performance value of this type of practice should not be underestimated and can be used to persuade the player to comply with the program.

Retrain sports function and conditioning. The ultimate goal following shoulder injury and/or surgery is to return the athlete to his or her chosen sport and enable him or her to compete at the highest level possible in view of any residual dysfunction.

A complete body training program incorporating flexibility, strength, power, speed, skill, balance, strategy, etc. should be operative for several weeks before the player is considered ready to return to the competitive arena.

The decision regarding fitness to return to full training and competition should not really be a decision, but more of a stage of the rehabilitation program. The treatment, exercises, mental and physical preparation should have gradually led to the point where the athlete, physiotherapist and coach agree that the next progression is full return.

At this stage the athlete has progressed to a self/coach administered training program similar to the pre-injury status, plus a few extra activities that the physiotherapist may have added to maintain the rehabilitation or prevention theme. Monitoring of the athlete's progress at this stage can provide the physiotherapist with information regarding the success or otherwise of the overall recovery program: not to mention a great deal of satisfaction for a job well done.

SUMMARY

The shoulder complex is an integral part of the biomechanics of many sports. It is particularly of interest to the sports physiotherapist in those sports that involve forceful or repetitious overhead movements, due to the injury patterns that arise.

Some injuries are traumatic, but more commonly overuse syndromes are seen in the clinic. The sections on trauma, diagnosis and acute management will assist the physiotherapist working on site with sports teams, while those on assessment and management of over-use injury will be of more use in clinical practice.

This chapter has outlined shoulder function in the overhead sports and discussed the mechanics of performance and pathology. From this has arisen a rationale for the management of over-use injuries in the athletic shoulder: a system of management based on solutions rather than problems.

Nevertheless, the reader will still encounter the difficult shoulder that appears not to respond to any system of management, but hopefully less frequently.

REFERENCES

Allingham C 1988 Impingement syndrome of the shoulder—assessment and management. In: Current concepts in the management of shoulder region dysfunction. Manipulative Therapists Association of Australia, Sydney, p99-107

Allingham C 1990 Exercise prescription in shoulder rehabilitation. In: The shoulder in focus (Proceedings). Manipulative Physiotherapists Association of Australia, Melbourne, p 21

Allman F 1985 Impingement, biceps and rotator cuff lesions. In: Zarins et al (eds) Injuries to the throwing arm. Saunders, Philadelphia

Andrews J 1993 Instability of the shoulder—pathomechanics and recognition. Course Notes: 11th annual injuries in baseball course, American Sports Medicine Institute, Birmingham, p 189

Andrews J, Carson W 1985 Operative arthroscopy of the shoulder in the throwing athlete. In: Zarins et al (eds) Injuries to the throwing arm. Saunders, Philadelphia

Andrews J, Gillogly S 1985 Physical examination of the shoulder in throwing athletes. In: Zarins et al (eds) Injuries to the throwing arm. Saunders, Philadelphia

Arnheim D 1985 Modern principles of athletic training, 6th edn. Times Mirror/Mosby College, St Louis

Atwater A 1979 Biomechanics of overarm throwing movements and of throwing injuries. Exercise and Sports Science Review 7:43-85

Baker C, Thornberry R 1985 Neurovascular syndromes. In: Zarins et al (eds) Injuries to the throwing arm. Saunders, Philadelphia

Baker C, Uribe J, Whitman C 1990 Arthroscopic evaluation of acute initial anterior shoulder dislocations. American Journal of Sports Medicine 18(1):25-28

Basmajian J, de Luca C 1985 Muscles alive—their function revealed by electromyography, 5th edn. Williams & Wilkins, Baltimore

Beekman K, Hay J 1988 Characteristics of the front crawl techniques of swimmers with shoulder impingement sydrome. Journal of Swimming Research 4(3):15-21

Black K, Lombardo J 1990 Suprascapular nerve injuries with isolated paralysis of the infraspinatus. American Journal of Sports Medicine 18(3):225-228

Blackburn T 1987 Throwing injuries to the shoulder. In: Donatelli (ed) Physical therapy of the shoulder. Churchill Livingstone, New York

Blazina M, Kerlan R, Jobe F, Carter V, Carlson G 1973 Jumper's knee. Orthopedic Clinics of North America 4:669-670

Bokor D 1992 Personal communication

Bowen M, Warren R 1991 Ligamentous control of shoulder stability based on selective cutting and static translation experiments. In: Hawkins R (ed) Basic science and clinical application in the athlete's shoulder. Clinics in Sports Medicine 10(4):757-782

Brown R, Counsilman J 1971 The role of lift in propelling swimmers. In: Cooper J (ed) Biomechanics. Athletic Institute, Chicago

Bryan W, Wild J 1989 Isolated infraspinatus atrophy. American Journal of Sports Medicine 17(1):130-131

Butler D 1991 Mobilisation of the nervous system. Churchill Livingstone, Melbourne

Cailliet R 1966 Shoulder pain. Davis, Philadelphia

Cailliet R 1981 Neck and arm pain, 2nd edn. Davis, Philadelphia

Carson W 1989 Rehabilitation of the throwing shoulder. Clinics in Sports Medicine 8(4):657-689

Codman E 1934 The shoulder. Krieger, Malabar

Corrigan G, Maitland G 1983 Practical orthopaedic medicine. Butterworths, London

Costill D, Maglischo E, Richardson A 1992 Swimming. Blackwell Scientific, Oxford

Coughlin L, Rubinovich M, Johansson J, White B, Greenspoon J 1992 Arthroscopic staple capsulorrhaphy for anterior shoulder instability. American Journal of Sports Medicine 20(3):253-256

Cox J S 1981 The fate of the acromioclavicular joint in athletic injuries. American Journal of Sports Medicine 9(1):50-53

Curwin S, Stanish D 1984 Tendinitis: its etiology and treatment. Collamore Press, Toronto

Cyriax J 1974 Textbook of orthopaedic medicine, Vol 2 Treatment by manipulation, massage and injection, 8th edn. Bailliere Tindall, London

Cyriax J 1975 Textbook of orthopaedic medicine, vol 1 Diagnosis of soft tissue lesions, 6th edn. Bailliere Tindall, London

Daff A, Dalzeil R, Southwick G 1992 Surgical treatment of axillary nerve damage associated with shoulder dislocation. In: Health and sport towards 2000. Proceedings of National Annual Scientific Conference in Sports Medicine, Perth, Australia

Falkel J 1990 Swimming injuries. In: Sanders B (ed) Sports physical therapy. Appleton & Lange, Connecticut

Falkel J, Murphy T, 1988 Shoulder injuries. In: Malone T (ed) Sports injury management. Williams & Wilkins, Baltimore

Ferrari D 1990 Capsular ligaments of the shoulder. Anatomical and functional study of the anterior superior capsule. American Journal of Sports Medicine 18(1):20-24

Fleisig G, Dillman C, Andrews J 1989 Proper mechanics for baseball pitching. Clinical Sports Medicine 1:151-170

Gainor B, Piotrowski G, Puhl J et al 1980 The throw: biomechanics and acute injury. American Journal of Sports Medicine 8:114-118

Gall S 1990 Shoulder injury throws Hershiser a curve. Physican and Sportsmedicine 18(7):15-16

Gerber C, Terrier F, Ganz R 1985 The role of the coracoid process in the chronic impingement syndrome. Journal of Bone and Joint Surgery 67-A:703

Glousman R, Jobe F, Tibone J, Moynes D, Antonelli D, Perry J 1988 Dynamic electromyographic analysis of the throwing shoulder with glenohumeral instability. Journal of Bone and Joint Surgery 70-A(2):220-226

Griffin J, Curtis R 1991 Rib dysfunction in competitive swimmers. Journal of Swimming Research 7(1):29-35

Hawkins R, Hobeika P 1983 Impingement syndrome in the athletic shoulder. Clinics in Sports Medicine 2(2):391-401

Hawkins R, Kennedy J 1980 Impingement syndromes in athletes. American Journal of Sports Medicine 8:151

Howell J, Binder M, Nichols T R, Loeb G 1986 Muscle spindles, Golgi tendon organs and the neural control of skeletal muscle. Journal of the American Ostoepathic Association 86(9):599-602

Janda V 1983a The relationship of shoulder girdle musculature to the aetiology of cervical spine syndromes. In: Proceedings of the International Conference on Manipulative Therapy, Perth, Australia

Janda V 1983b Muscle function testing. Butterworths, London

Jenkins W, Kegerris S 1990 Throwing injuries. In: Sanders B (ed) Sports physical therapy. Appleton & Lange, Connecticut

Jobe F, Moynes D 1982 Delineation of diagnostic criteria and a rehabilitation program for rotator cuff injuries. American Journal of Sports Medicine 10(6):336-339

Jobe F, Moynes D, Tibone J, Perry J 1983 An EMG analysis of the shoulder in throwing—a preliminary report. American Journal of Sports Medicine 11(1):3-5

Jobe F, Moynes D, Tibone J, Perry J 1984 An EMG analysis of the shoulder in pitching—a second report. American Journal of Sports Medicine 12(3):218-220

Jobe F, Mounes D, Antonelli D 1986 Rotator cuff function during a golf swing. American Journal of Sports Medicine 14(5):388-392

Kapandji I 1970 The physiology of the joints, vol 1 Upper limb, 2nd edn. Churchill Livingstone, Edinburgh

Kaput M 1987 Anatomy and biomechanics of the shoulder. In: Donatelli R (ed) Physical therapy of the shoulder. Churchill Livingstone, New York

Kirby R, Roberts J 1985 Introductory biomechanics. Mouvement Publications, New York

Knott M, Voss D 1968 Proprioceptive neuromuscular facilitation, 2nd edn. Harper & Row, New York

Komi P 1988 The musculoskeletal system. In: Dirix A, Knuttgen H & Tittel (eds) The Olympic book of sports medicine. Blackwell, Oxford

Larsen E, Bjerg-Neilsen A, Christensen P 1986 Conservative or surgical treatment of acromioclavicular dislocation. Journal of Bone and Joint Surgery 68-A(4):552-555

Leach R 1985 Tennis serving compared with baseball pitching. In: Zarins et al (eds) Injuries to the throwing arm. Saunders, Philadelphia

MacDonald P, Alexander M, Frejuk J, Johnson G 1988 Comprehensive functional analysis of shoulders following complete acromio-clavicular separation. American Journal of Sports Medicine 16(5):475-480

McConnell J 1990 A new approach to the problem shoulder. In: The shoulder in focus (Proceedings). Manipulative Physiotherapists Association of Australia, Melbourne

McConnell J 1992 Personal communication

McCue R, Gieck J, West J 1985 Throwing injuries to the shoulder. In: Zarins et al (eds) Injuries to the throwing arm. Saunders, Philadelphia

McLaughlin T 1985 Strength/power training for baseball pitchers. In: Zarins et al (eds) Injuries to the throwing arm. Saunders, Philadelphia

Maitland G 1991 Periperal manipulation, 3rd edn. Butterworths, London

Matsen F, Harryman D, Sidles J 1991 Mechanics of glenohumeral instability. In: Hawkins R (ed) Basic science and clinical application in the athlete's shoulder. Clinics in Sports Medicine, 10(4):783-788

Moran C, Saunders S 1987 Examination of the shoulder: a sequential approach. In: Donatelli R (ed) Physical therapy of the shoulder. Churchill Livingstone, New York

Moynes D, Perry J, Antonelli D, Jobe F 1986 Electromyography and motion analysis of the upper extremity in sports. Physical Therapy 66(12):1905-1911

Moynes-Schwab D 1990 Personal communication

Neer C, Foster C 1980 Inferior capsular shift for involuntary inferior multidirectional instability of the shoulder. Journal of Bone and Joint Surgery 62A(6):897-908

Newnham R 1990 Frozen shoulder—adhesive capsulitis: periarthritis. In: The shoulder in focus (Proceedings). Manipulative Physiotherapists Association of Australia, Melbourne, p 20

Nitz A 1986 Physical therapy management of the shoulder. Physical Therapy 66(12):1912-1919

Norwood L 1985 Posterior shoulder instability. In: Zarins et al (eds) Injuries to the throwing arm. Saunders, Philadelphia

Nuber G, Jobe F, Perry J, Moynes D, Antonelli D 1986 Fine wire electromyography of the shoulder during swimming. American Journal of Sports Medicine 14(1):7-11

O'Connell P, Nuber G, Mileski R, Lautenshchlager E 1990 The contribution of the glenohumeral ligaments to anterior stability of the shoulder joint. American Journal of Sports Medicine 18(6):579-584

Owens-Burkhart H 1987 Management of frozen shoulder. In: Donatelli R (ed) Physical therapy of the shoulder. Churchill Livingstone, New York

Pacelli L 1990 Shoulder instability—a new surgical approach. The Physician and Sports Medicine 16(10):103-106

Pappas A, Goss T, Kleinman P 1983 Symptomatic shoulder instability due to lesions of the glenoid labrum. American Journal of Sports Medicine 11(5):279-288

Pappas A, Zawacki R, McCarthy C 1985a Rehabilitation of the pitching shoulder. American Journal of Sports Medicine 13(4):223-235

Pappas A, Zawacki R, Sullivan T 1985b Biomechanics of baseball pitching: a preliminary report. American Journal of Sports Medicine 13(4):216-222

Paulos L, Franklin J 1990 Arthroscopic shoulder decompression development and application. A five year experience. American Journal of Sports Medicine 18(3):235-244

Peat M 1986 Functional anatomy of the shoulder complex. Physical Therapy 66(12):1855-1865

Penny J, Welsh R 1981 Shoulder impingement syndromes in athletes and their surgical management. American Journal of Sports Medicine 9(1):11-15

Perry J 1978 Normal upper extremity kinesiology. Physical Therapy 58(3):265-

Perry J 1983 Anatomy and biomechanics of the shoulder in throwing, swimming, gymnastics and tennis. Clinics in Sports Medicine 2(2):247

Pettrone F 1985 Shoulder problems in swimmers. In: Zarins et al (ed) Injuries to the throwing arm. Saunders, Philadelphia

Pratt N 1986 Neurovascular entrapment in the regions of the shoulder and posterior triangle of the neck. Physical Therapy 66(12):1894-1900

Rathbun J, McNab I 1970 The microvasculature pattern of the rotator cuff. Journal of Bone and Joint Surgery 52-B:540

Redler M, Ruland L, McCue R 1986 Quadrilateral space syndrome in a throwing athlete. American Journal of Sports Medicine 14(6):511-513

Reid D, Saboe L, Burnham R, 1987 Current research of selected shoulder problems. In: Donatelli R (ed) Physical therapy of the shoulder. Churchill Livingstone, New York

Rowe C 1985 Anterior subluxation of the throwing shoulder. In: Zarins et al (eds) Injuries to the throwing arm. Saunders, Philadelphia

Ryu R, McCormick J, Jobe F, Moynes D, Antonelli D 1988 An electromyographic analysis of shoulder function in tennis players. American Journal of Sports Medicine 16(5):481-485

Scarpinato D, Bramhall J, Andrews J 1991 Arthroscopic management of the throwing athlete's shoulder: indications, techniques and results. In: Hawkins R (ed) Basic science and clinical application in the athlete's shoulder. Clinics in Sports Medicine, 10(4):913-927

Simon E, Hill J 1989 Rotator cuff injuries: an update. Journal of Orthopedic and Sports Physical Therapy 10(4):394-398

Slaughter D 1990 Shoulder injuries. In: Sanders B (ed) Sports physical therapy. Appleton & Lange, Connecticut

Smith K 1979 The thoracic outlet syndrome: a protocol of treatment. Journal of Orthopedic and Sports Physical Therapy 1(2):89-99

Stanton P, Purdam C 1989 Hamstring injuries in sprinting—the role of eccentric exercise. Journal of Orthopedic and Sports Physical Therapy 10(9):343-348

Stewart M 1985 The acromioclavicular joint in the throwing arm. In: Zarins et al (eds) Injuries to the throwing arm. Saunders, Philadelphia

Stillman J, Hawkins R 1991 Current concepts and recent advances in the athlete's shoulder. In: Hawkins R (ed) Basic science and clinical application in the athlete's shoulder. Clinics in Sports Medicine 10(4):693-705

Thomas S, Matsen F 1989 An approach to the repair of avulsion of the glenohumeral ligaments in the management of traumatic anterior glenohumeral instability. Journal of Bone and Joint Surgery 71-A(4):506-513

Thurston W 1985a Personal communication

Thurston W 1985b Baseball pitching—the mechanics of correct technique. Dept of Human Movement and Recreation Studies, University of Western Australia, Perth

Tibone J, Sellers R, Tonino 1992 Strength testing after third degree acromio-clavicular dislocations. American Journal of Sports Medicine 20(3):328-331

Townsend H, Jobe F, Pink M, Perry J 1991 Electro-myographic analysis of the glenohumeral muscles during a baseball rehabilitation program. American Journal of Sports Medicine 19(3):264-272

Tullos H, King J 1973 Throwing mechanism in sports. Orthopedic Clinics of North America 4:709-720

Turkel S, Panio M, Marshall J, Girgis F 1981 Stabilizing mechanisms preventing anterior dislocation of the glenohumeral joint. Journal of Bone and Joint Surgery 63-A(8):1208-1217

Vasey A, Watson L, Dalziel R, Wrigley T 1992 Correlation of Cybex findings to shoulder instability to determine likely outcome of conservative program. In: Health and sport towards 2000. Proceedings of National Annual Scientific Conference in Sports Medicine, Perth Australia

Vereshagin K, Wiens J, Fanton G, Dillingham M 1991 Burners: don't overlook or underestimate them. Physician and Sports Medicine 19(9):97-104

Walsh W, Peterson D, Shelton G, Neumann R 1985 Shoulder strength following acromioclavicular injury. American Journal of Sports Medicine 13(3):153-157

Warwick R, Williams P (eds) 1973 Gray's anatomy, 35th edn. Churchill Livingstone, London

Watson M 1989 Rotator cuff impingement syndrome. Journal of Bone and Joint Surgery 71-B(3):361-366

Weiner D, McNab I 1970 Superior migration of the humeral head. Journal of Bone and Joint Surgery 52-B:524

Wells R 1985 Suprascapular nerve entrapment. In:Zarins et al (eds) Injuries to the throwing arm. Saunders, Philadelphia

Wilk K 1993 Principles of rotator cuff rehabilitation: laxity versus rotator cuff disease. Course notes: 11th annual injuries in baseball course, American Sports Medicine Institute, Birmingham, p.191

Yocum L 1983 Assessing the shoulder. Clinics in Sports Medicine 2(2):281-289

24. The elbow complex

Wendy Braybon, John Carlisle, Christopher Briggs

As the link between the arm and forearm, the elbow acts as the mobile segment, enabling effective positioning of the wrist and hand in space without excessive shoulder or trunk movement. It must also tolerate large weightbearing forces transmitted from the hand to more proximal segments. Stability at the elbow complex is due, primarily, to congruency of opposing articular surfaces, with strong ligaments and powerful muscles arranged to resist extraneous movement. In normal daily activities of lifting and carrying the elbow is subject to forces estimated in the vicinity of 0.3–0.5 times body weight (An et al 1984). Sports and activities involving throwing, hitting, punching, hanging or pushing tasks greatly magnify these forces and require the elbow to withstand stresses, often exceeding the tolerance limits of its primary and secondary restraints. These problems are compounded in the young, in which unfused epiphyses are prone to compression and traction injury. The added complications of nerve entrapment and vascular occlusion makes diagnosis of elbow injury difficult.

Examination of the injured elbow requires the physiotherapist to have a sound knowledge of anatomy, biomechanics, pathomechanics, patterns of injury and repair, treatment options and rehabilitation protocols. These topics are covered in this chapter, in which the elbow is subdivided into medial, lateral, anterior and posterior regions for discussion of injury. Injuries that require primarily medical or surgical management have been included in the discussion, to assist the physiotherapist to recognize these entities and aid in their differential diagnosis.

FUNCTIONAL ANATOMY

Developmental anatomy

Traumatic injury to the elbow region is common in childhood and adolescence, and may be associated with damage to ossification centres. Ossification centres are secondary epiphyses, located at the ends of long bones for articulation, and at sites of muscular and ligamentous attachment. They usually appear just before or after birth or in early childhood, and the majority fuse to the shaft of the bone during mid to late adolescence. They are regions of high metabolic activity, and if damaged may result in arrested growth of the bone at that site. At the elbow, epiphyses are found in the distal humerus, proximal radius and proximal ulna. There are four sites in the distal humerus: one in the capitulum and lateral trochlea appears between the first and second years, a centre for the medial trochlea appears in the 9th to 10th year and one for the lateral epicondyle around the 12th year. These three subsequently fuse with the shaft around the 14th year in females, and 16th year in males. An additional centre for the medial epicondyle begins to ossify between the 4th and 6th years. In contrast to the other three, this epiphysis remains separate from the shaft until about 18–20 years of age, when it fuses with the remainder of the bone. Epiphyseal injuries do occur in a small number of adolescent sportspeople (Micheli 1983), however, due to its 'late' union with the distal end of the humerus, the medial epicondylar epiphysis may be misread on X-ray as a fracture.

Articular surfaces

Structurally the elbow joint is a compound, essentially uniaxial joint. Articulation between the humerus and ulna occurs medially and between the humerus and radius laterally. While the shape and configuration of the articular surfaces suggests a typical 'hinge-type' arrangement, small amounts of ulnar rotation and abduction and adduction also occur. The complexity of the articulation, particularly its fibrous capsule and synovial membrane, is increased by the presence of the proximal radio-ulnar joint, which shares with the elbow the one joint cavity. This joint, unlike the shoulder proximally, owes its stability primarily to its bony articular surfaces.

NOTE

The authors wish to thank David Young for his assistance in the preparation of this chapter.

radio-ulnar joint is stabilized by the triceps. Laterally, brachioradialis crosses anterior to the axis of flexion/extension as it descends to the radial styloid process and acts to increase joint compression and stability in all positions of the elbow.

The principal extensor at the joint is triceps. As with biceps, the long head crosses the shoulder and thus has a mechanical advantage in length at the elbow (e.g. for pushing or throwing movements), if the shoulder is simultaneously flexed. The powerful medial and lateral heads arise from the shaft of the humerus, and so are unaffected by shoulder position. Triceps inserts onto the olecranon process and is active not only as a powerful and rapid extensor of the elbow, but also as synergist to biceps, preventing elbow flexion when the biceps is acting as a supinator of the forearm. In addition to their prime-mover roles on the humerus, in which triceps has the greatest work capacity for extension and brachialis for flexion (An et al 1981), both muscles attach to the capsule of the elbow and are responsible for pulling it away from the articular surfaces in flexion and extension respectively.

Anconeus, passing from the lateral collateral ligament to the olecranon process and the annular ligament (Fig. 24.2), is usually considered a muscular extension of triceps across the posterior capsule of the joint. However, others have suggested it both stabilizes the elbow in supination and pronation, and is partly responsible for the ulnar rotation which occurs in the last few degrees of extension. Basmajian and Griffin (1972), in an electromyographic study of anconeus, found only moderate activity in the muscle, and only at the extremes of flexion and extension. They described it as a joint stabilizer. In contrast, Bilodeau et al (1990) assessed EMG activity of anconeus at different maximal voluntary contractions and found it to be active in initiating and maintaining elbow extension and in stabilizing the elbow against varus forces. Maton et al (1980) suggested anconeus may be important in 'braking' slow flexion movements at the elbow, a function performed by triceps during fast movements. Maton et al (1980) further indicate anconeus may have a role to play in enhancing precision movements at this joint and in supplementing the restraining effect of viscoelastic structures. The role ascribed for the triceps, as a phasic muscle braking fast elbow movements, is supported by studies of the muscle fibre characteristics of the muscles of the upper extremity. Both Sjogaard et al (1978) and Johnson et al (1973) report concentrations of fast twitch muscle fibres in triceps ranging from 50–80%. The biceps, in contrast, tends towards a more even distribution of both fibre types.

The pronator teres and supinator cross the elbow obliquely, from the vicinity of the medial and lateral epicondyles to mid-shaft of the radius respectively. Pronator teres, divisible into a superficial head with fibres arising from the medial epicondyle, common flexor origin and intermuscular septum, and a deep head from the ulnar coronoid process, is involved in active or resisted pronation. However, a component of its force also acts across the proximal radio-ulnar joint, helping to maintain contact between the radial head and capitulum. Supinator also has superficial and deep heads, and in addition to fibres from the lateral epicondyle has attachments from the lateral collateral and annular ligaments, and the supinator crest of the ulna. It alone supinates during unresisted movement of the forearm, however against resistance, and when the elbow is flexed, supinator is assisted by the biceps, which is most effective as a supinator at 90° of elbow flexion (Buchanan et al 1989).

In order for the hand to move effectively in sports activities, a stable base is necessary. This base is provided partly by the wrist (although at times it must itself respond to different requirements of the hand) and by the elbow. The majority of muscles which cross the wrist and stabilize it have their origins at the medial and lateral epicondyles of the elbow, therefore the roles these muscles perform are directly affected by their capacity to simultaneously lengthen at one joint while shortening at another. Of chief interest among these are the radial and ulnar flexors and extensors of the carpus. In all racquet sports, particularly in games such as tennis, hockey and cricket, a 'backhand' motion of the forearm and wrist is an integral component of the activity. The muscles requiring a stable base from which to produce resisted extension of the wrist, are those which arise from the vicinity of the lateral epicondyle. Of these, the extensor carpi radialis brevis originates from the lateral epicondyle, although in some cases a tendinous extension may arise proximal to the epicondyle (Briggs & Elliott 1985). While the position of the elbow has little effect on the length of the extensor carpi radialis brevis, pronation of the forearm with flexion at the wrist results in lengthening of the muscle. If additional force is applied to a muscle already undergoing lengthening across two joints, it may be unable to tolerate the additional force and, as a result, shear stresses may develop at the origin. This may lead to inflammation and eventually the muscle can tear ('tennis elbow').

Attempts have been made to quantify threshold strength values beyond which muscle injury may occur and information has surfaced in the sports medicine literature in this area in recent years. Much of the data has been obtained using various forms of isokinetic resistance at variable speeds, although Askew et al (1987) used torque cell dynamometers to measured isometric elbow strength. They found that, in general, dominant extremities are approximately 6% stronger than non-dominant, while mean extension strength is 61% that of flexion, and pronation 86% of supination.

Non-muscular structures susceptible to injury

While pathology associated with throwing activities and racquet sports dominates the sports medicine literature in relation to the elbow, it must be appreciated that other anatomical structures, such as numerous bursae at the periphery, and fat pads within the joint, are also susceptible to injury. Stack (1949) and Bosworth (1955) have alluded to 'tennis elbow' as primarily a bursal problem. One of the author's co-workers has identified a bursal cavity under or within the tendon of the extensor carpi radialis brevis in as many as 50% of surgical cases (Briggs & Elliott 1985). The other well-recognized, although extracapsular, bursa is the subcutaneous olecranon bursa, which is subject to friction injury in a variety of sports.

At the elbow, fat pads are located anteriorly and posteriorly, occupying the coronoid and olecranon fossae when they in turn are not occupied by bone. They possess a nerve supply and when trapped may be a source of joint pain. Their elevation is also a useful radiological guide to the presence of joint inflammation (Miles & Lamont 1989).

Several nerves and one large vessel have important relations to the elbow. In cases of posterior dislocation the median nerve and brachial artery, passing directly anterior to the joint, are susceptible to stretch and tearing. The anterior interosseous nerve, a terminal branch of the median nerve, continues into the anterior compartment of the forearm by passing between two heads of the pronator teres at the distal aspect of the cubital fossa. It is susceptible to compression at this site. Occupying the cubital groove behind the medial epicondyle and passing from the anterior compartment of the arm to the posterior compartment of the forearm is the ulnar nerve. It may be stretched in valgus injury or pulled out of the cubital groove in which it lies, leading to loss of function of the ulnar nerve-innervated muscles of the forearm and hand. Before entering the posterior compartment of the forearm, the posterior interosseous nerve passes between the two heads of the supinator. Compression of this nerve, the so-called 'radial tunnel syndrome', is recognized as one cause of lateral elbow pain (Roles & Maudsley 1972). Although most authors feel 'radial tunnel syndrome' cannot be distinguished from other causes of lateral elbow pain, it is amenable to decompression (Jalovaara & Lindholm 1989). Werner et al (1980) measured intramuscular pressures in supinator and found them to be four times greater during active muscle contraction than at rest. Szabo and Gelberman (1984) indicated that acute nerve compression may occur above a critical threshold pressure of 40–50 mm Hg. This may explain the source of pain and local tenderness in some patients who are resistant to standard physiotherapeutic procedures.

PATHOMECHANICS OF THROWING AT THE ELBOW JOINT

The mechanics of the overarm throw can predispose the athlete to elbow joint injury. Experience shows this occurs particularly in baseball pitchers and javelin throwers. When assessing throwing injuries affecting the elbow, poor throwing mechanics must be suspected as a predisposing factor. The analysis of throwing mechanics must be done by an experienced person with a sound knowledge of the correct technique involved. Initially, pathology occurs on the medial aspect and involves the medial collateral ligament and the flexor/pronator muscle group. It may then spread posteriorly, causing medial and/or lateral olecranon fossa impingement (Andrews & Wilson 1985). Eventually, spurs can develop on the olecranon, progressing to loose bodies in the joint. Yocum (1989) documented cases of athletes in their early teens, who suffered these symptoms and went on to develop major problems, such as osteochondritis dissecans.

Throwing can be divided into four stages: cocking, acceleration, release and follow-through (Tullos & King 1973) (see Ch. 23). The early part of the cocking phase places little pressure on the elbow. However, if the athlete brings the arm across behind the mid-line of the body during this stage, the need to quickly accelerate the arm to match trunk rotation causes valgus stress on the medial joint line. During the acceleration phase, which starts from the point of maximal external rotation of the glenohumeral joint, the trunk and shoulder accelerate at a faster rate than the arm or forearm (Fig. 24.3), applying a valgus stress to the elbow joint (Jobe & Nuber 1986). In the release stage the actions of the elbow extensors and wrist flexors increase the speed of the throw, but also exaggerate medial valgus stress (Reid 1992). Stress is greatest in the presence of faulty technique, and when shoulder abduction drops below 90° (Nirschl 1988).

Excessive valgus stress during the acceleration phase may lead to medial collateral ligament laxity and thus alter the

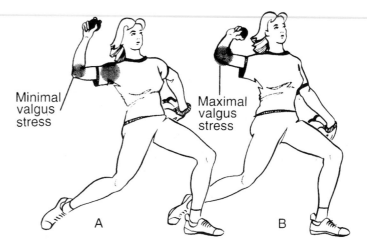

Fig. 24.3 Valgus stress to the medial elbow due to the extremes of the throwing action. (A) start of the acceleration phase; (B) Mid-accelertion phase

axis of movement of the ulna on the humerus, causing impingement of the posteromedial aspect of the olecranon in the proximal portion of the olecranon fossa, and the posterolateral aspect of the olecranon on the distal part of the lateral olecranon fossa. Increased stress at the posterior and posteromedial aspects of the olecranon may lead to chondromalacia, reaction spurs and loose body formation (Andrews & Wilson 1985). Medial joint laxity will result in compression forces at the distal lateral fossa (Fig. 24.4), compression of the radiocapitellar joint and radiohumeral loose bodies (Jobe & Nuber 1986).

During the late stage of acceleration and in the follow-through phase, rapid deceleration occurs at the elbow. This happens sooner at the elbow than the shoulder because of the decreased range of movement at the former joint. If the elbow musculature fails to successfully control deceleration, stress will be placed on the ligamentous and bony components of the elbow to slow the forearm movement (Pappas et al 1985).

Poor throwing technique is also a predisposing factor in medial elbow pain. An example is when a 'curve ball' is pitched in baseball. The commonly accepted theory of pitching a curve ball is that the forearm is supinated, whereas slow motion analysis of the technique actually demonstrates that the forearm pronates, not supinates, immediately after release (Green 1985). Therefore, if pitchers are trying to roll the ball off the middle and ring fingers by supinating the arm in the terminal phase of elbow extension, they are more likely to place excessive stress on medial structures. The pitcher should be encouraged to maintain the natural pronation action, rather than attempting to supinate, when

throwing a curve ball (Green 1985). It must be emphasized here that the curve ball is not recommended for juvenile pitchers as the inherent stresses of the pitch are too great for the immature elbow to tolerate (Hunter 1985).

The throwing athlete's arm undergoes both bony and muscular hypertrophy in adolescents and adults, the former being more susceptible to cortical thickening of the humerus because they are still growing. Flexion contractures are also common (Jobe & Nuber 1986). The muscles most prone to hypertrophy are the flexors of the elbow and wrist. These muscles hypertrophy due to the powerful contraction occurring during the terminal phase of acceleration to maintain speed and strength of a throw or hit, combined with the fact that the elbow never fully extends during the throw. Both pathology and poor biomechanics contribute to the overemphasis of wrist flexor action; the strong concentric action of the wrist flexors causing hypertonicity, associated with inherent shortening. The authors have noted a soft tissue tightening over the anterior aspect of the elbow joint of pitchers, which could be due to the above reasons, or due to microtrauma of the anterior soft tissues, leading to contractures and shortening. Also at risk are the wrist extensors, as they eccentrically control wrist flexion. Increased wrist flexion force, as well as increasing valgus stress over the medial collateral ligament, leads to joint degenerative changes, thus setting up a combination of articular and soft tissue pathology which can obscure the predisposing factors.

Jobe and Nuber (1986) describe how the body's physiological ability to heal itself in overuse injury lags behind the microtrauma caused by the repetitive activity itself. They list four stages of progressive soft tissue degenerative change:

- oedema and inflammation, with round cell infiltration
- immature scar formation
- dense scar tissue with calcific densities
- ossification within the ligamentous tissue, leading to loose bodies and the possibility of complete rupture with application of minimal stress.

These changes present as a gradual progression of pain. As the problem worsens, the pain increases in frequency, taking longer to resolve and becoming more constant as the condition deteriorates. Furthermore, low-grade chronic injury can be exacerbated by periods of high activity, such as competing in a tennis or softball tournament.

The progression of symptoms with activity is demonstrated below, using throwing as an example:

- pain on a hard or mistimed throw
- pain on every throw
- pain on throwing, which takes some time to settle
- pain on throwing, which remains throughout the game
- pain on throwing, which takes time to settle after the game

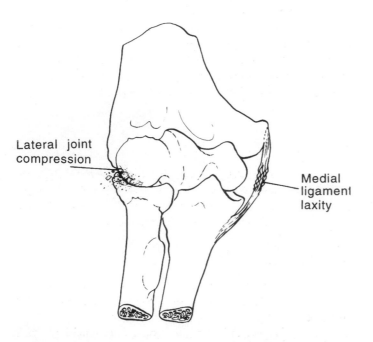

Lateral joint compression

Medial ligament laxity

Fig. 24.4 Medial laxity creates radiocapitellar compression

- pain that makes it very hard to warm up, and does not settle until the next day
- pain does not settle between game and next training session
- pain starts to affect other activities of daily living
- constant pain
- constant pain causing interrupted sleep.

PRINCIPLES OF ASSESSMENT OF THE ELBOW

Elbow injuries are often a secondary dysfunction, related to stiffness or weakness in the shoulder girdle and cervico-thoracic region. Any deficit in the upper quadrant can disrupt the kinetic chain and lead to increased stresses on the elbow joint. For example, a minor restriction of external rotation at the glenohumeral joint may lead to increased valgus stress at the elbow during the act of throwing. Therefore, mobility, muscle balance and strength, as well as structural components of the elbow and forearm, should be included in the assessment.

Examination of the athlete with elbow injury should follow an orderly procedure, as described in Chapter 9. The elbow can be divided into four regions: lateral, medial, anterior and posterior. It lends itself to the assessment style described by Maitland (1986). An orderly assessment of subjective findings, body posture, elbow contours, passive movement, active and resisted movements, palpation, vascular and neurological examination, and joint stability tests will help the physiotherapist assess and manage the lesion. The following discussion is a guide to elbow assessment. Specific tests are described more fully in appropriate sections of this chapter.

Subjective examination

Subjective examination should help to determine the direction and extent of objective assessment. The examination should include careful questioning regarding possible pathology or dysfunction in proximal structures which may refer symptoms to the elbow. In the case of the athlete who presents with severe pain, effusion and altered elbow contours, a full objective assessment will be inappropriate. If the presentation is not severe, or appears to be related to overuse, then careful questioning in relation to the mechanism of injury, aggravating factors, previous injury and treatment, and distribution of symptoms is vital to directing the objective assessment.

A clear understanding of the level of sports participation needs to be determined as a guide to the rehabilitation needs of the athlete. All previous injuries to the region, as well as treatment and surgery to the shoulder, current medication, X-ray findings and history of steroid infiltration, need to be determined. Any changes in training intensity or frequency, in equipment or technique, or even in home or work activities need to be explored as possible contributing factors. As the elbow is also associated with sites of potential neurological compression, it is important to check for distal sensory change as well as muscle weakness. Once the subjective examination is complete the physiotherapist should have a clearer picture of the structures likely to be involved.

Objective examination

The elbow is an easily accessible joint and can therefore be examined in standing, sitting or supine posture. The authors prefer supported supine, as this relaxes the proximal structures as well as the elbow.

Posture

Apart from poor sporting technique, the athlete's sitting and standing posture, when at rest, can also be an aggravating factor which predisposes to elbow pain via neural involvement. A player with increased thoracic kyphosis, decreased mobility of the thoracic joints and decreased strength of both scapular stabilizing and erector spinae muscles, is commonly seen to have an increased cervical lordosis with a classic 'poking chin' posture. The lordosis leads to hyperextension in the mid-cervical region and increased stiffness in the upper and lower cervical joints. Stiffness in the thoracic spine may also lead to referred pain into the arm, as well as directing stress onto other areas of the spine (see Chs 21 and 22).

Elbow contours

Contours at the elbow should be noted for symmetry, muscle balance, swelling, skin condition or bony changes. The more severe fractures and dislocations may be obvious, but this is not always the case. The athlete who engages in games such as tennis will have hypertrophic muscle contours in the dominant arm compared with the other side. Asymmetry, therefore, does not always reflect underlying injury.

Palpation

Palpation may be used to detect joint effusion, soft tissue tension or the site of a lesion. In cases of severe injury, the physiotherapist should palpate with care. In these conditions it should be purely to confirm a diagnosis.

Passive movement

In the acutely injured elbow, where there is risk of underlying fracture or dislocation, passive movement needs to be performed with extreme care. Elbow dislocation and supracondylar fractures can compromise the brachial artery, and flexion may exacerbate this situation.

Normal assessment of full elbow movement will include:

- Flexion—if taken to the full range, compared with the uninjured side and allowing for muscle bulk restrictions, then overpressure may be applied. The next step is to add adduction with pronation, or abduction with supination and gentle overpressure. Overpressure needs to be sensitive to the athlete's pain, while noting the end feel (see Ch. 12).
- Extension—if painfree extension is possible, add the combined movements of supination and abduction, then pronation with adduction, combined with gentle overpressure.
- Supination and pronation—the elbow must be at 90° of flexion and, if necessary, overpressure can be applied.

Abnormalities of the preceding movements (individual or in combination) can alert the examiner to possible articular changes, either as a primary injury (as in olecranon impingement syndrome) or secondary to soft tissue changes (as in lateral epicondylitis or valgus instability).

As well as physiological movements, the elbow complex is associated with accessory movements at the radio-ulnar, radio-capitellar and humero-ulnar articulations. Additional information may be obtained on the condition, or the effectiveness of the treatment, by careful evaluation of the following movements:

- medial and lateral glide of the ulna on the humeral trochlea. The elbow should be positioned at 30° off full extension (Fig. 24.5)
- ulnar distraction with the elbow flexed between 75–90° and the forearm supinated to 30° (Fig. 24.6)
- radial distraction and compression with the elbow flexed to 90° (Fig. 24.7). This can be achieved by ulnar or radial deviation at the wrist

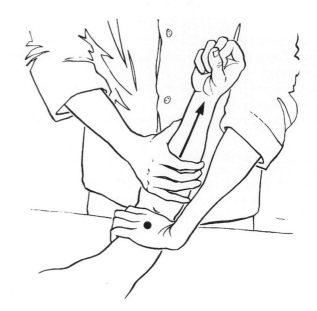

Fig. 24.6 Ulnar distraction with 75–90° elbow flexion and 30° of supination

- anterior and posterior glide of the radial head on the ulna with the elbow flexed to 75–90° and mid-supination of the forearm (Fig. 24.8)
- postero-anterior glide on the olecranon in 90° flexion with gradually increased extension and the glide repeated.

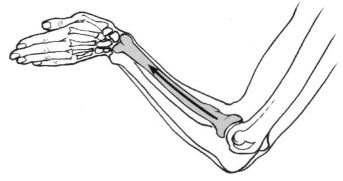

Fig. 24.7 Radial distraction using ulnar deviation of the wrist

Active and resisted movements

Muscle testing at the elbow will include wrist and hand testing, as well as elbow movements. As in muscle testing at all joints, the quantity and quality of the movement needs to be assessed. An indication of the muscles' viability may be seen after repeated activity and/or after resistance is applied. Pain or weakness in itself may not indicate the nature or location of the lesion because of the close proximity of the wrist flexors and extensors to ligaments and capsule of the elbow joint. Before a diagnosis is made these non-contractile structures must also be assessed.

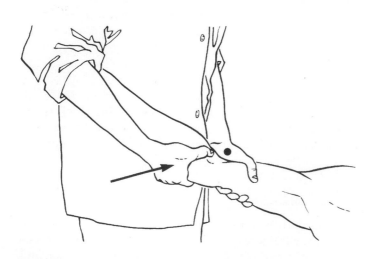

Fig. 24.5 Lateral glide of the ulna. The humerus is stabilised proximally to the elbow

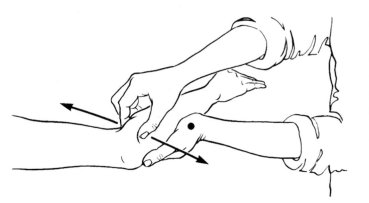

Fig. 24.8 Anterior and posterior glide of the radial head

As neuropathies can occur at the elbow, unexpected movements (at the elbow or wrist), or lack of them, may alert the examiner to possible pathology. For example, wrist extension with radial deviation may indicate the existence of posterior interosseous nerve syndrome.

If the physiotherapist believes objective strength measurement is warranted, use can be made of isokinetic, static and hand-held dynamometers. It is important if attempting to quantify the parameters of strength, power, endurance and peak torque, to appreciate the muscle actions involved as these differ from muscle actions in vivo, as well as the equipment used (see Ch. 17).

Neurovascular assessment

The subjective examination should alert the physiotherapist to the presence of vascular and neurological lesions which may be seen in conjunction with damage to the elbow region. Occlusion of the brachial artery can occur with fractures or dislocations. If suspected, assessment of the distal radial pulse, combined with finger discoloration and decreased sensation should indicate the pathology (see section on Volkmann's ischaemia).

Neurological deficits, due either to sudden injury or chronic entrapment, may be found at the elbow or in the forearm. The reader is directed to the appropriate parts of this chapter for recognition of these.

Joint stability tests

The medial collateral ligament is subject to strong valgus forces in throwing which can result in insidious medial instability, ligamentous tear or avulsion injury (Pappas et al 1985). The lateral collateral ligament is more frequently injured by acute rather than overuse injury, though neither are common. Assessment of each ligament requires the elbow to be placed in 20–30° of flexion to free the olecranon from its fossa and therefore allow movement without a bony block. Hyperextension, compared to the uninjured side, also needs to be determined.

Cervical and thoracic involvement

Pain may be referred to the elbow from the cervical spine. The neurological supply of the elbow and forearm is derived from the C5–C8 nerve roots which leave the spine via the intervertebral foramina between C4/5 and C7/T1 vertebrae inclusive. The nerve root occupies 35–50% of the available space within the intervertebral foramen, and friction or traction at this site may lead to symptoms in both the elbow and forearm (Sunderland 1978).

Bogduk (1983) reviewed published maps of sclerotomes and found that only general conclusions could be made about the sclerotome nerve root distributions. He states that pain may be referred to the arm, forearm and hand from vertebral joints C4/5–T1/2, but no single area is uniquely related to one vertebral segment. Patterns of referred pain are therefore only an approximate guide to the origins of pain. Detailed examination of the vertebral column and thoracic cage is necessary to ascertain the presence of local pain, cervical or thoracic spine pathology (including joint stiffness) or the presence of a cervical rib (Maitlaind 1986).

Stiffness in the lower thoracic spine may alter the biomechanics of throwing, putting stress on the elbow. The thoracic outlet syndrome can also refer pain to the elbow (see Chs 21 and 23).

PRINCIPLES OF MANAGEMENT OF ELBOW INJURIES

Acute management

As described later in this chapter, those injuries which are beyond the realms of acute physiotherapy management require immediate referral to the appropriate medical specialist. The physiotherapy role with these is to ensure no further damage occurs and to make the athlete as comfortable as possible.

The elbow is unique in that it is prone to stiffening after severe injury, and if not mobilized early stiffness may become permanent (Hurley 1990). To complicate matters, the elbow is also prone to myositis ossificans which can develop if it is mobilized into extension too quickly following injury. For this reason, early mobilization is important but continual monitoring and care with stretching the anterior structures is equally relevant.

Post-acute and chronic management

Management of post-acute injuries at the elbow should aim at returning the athlete to sport with an elbow that has been rehabilitated for the required function. The guidelines and treatment techniques found in the section on lateral epicondylitis are appropriate.

If the problem is ligamentous, management will depend on the extent of the injury. Minor ligamentous injury, managed by electrotherapy, muscle re-education, mobilization, soft tissue techniques and sports technique review (if appropriate) will allow a rapid return to sport. If the damage is more extensive and results in joint laxity that cannot be reduced (see section on valgus stress syndrome), then the athlete must be counselled about appropriate ongoing treatment, management of sporting demands, change of position in the team (e.g. in baseball, an outfielder may move to first base for less stressful throwing over a shorter distance) or a complete change of sport.

INJURIES TO THE ELBOW

Lateral elbow injuries

Lateral epicondylitis (tennis elbow)

'Tennis elbow' serves as a blanket term for every condition affecting the lateral compartment of the elbow. Cyriax (1936) collated 26 different lesions ascribed to the condition by 91 authors over a period of 63 years. Despite the many conditions postulated as tennis elbow, it is generally agreed that in most cases the lesion involves the specialized junctional tissue associated with the origin of the common extensor tendon at the lateral humeral epicondyle, specifically the tendinous origin of the extensor carpi radialis brevis. Garden (1961) felt surgery failed in many cases because of inability to expose the deep extensor carpi radialis brevis tendon and the pathological tissue in that area, and stated that this problem would have been clarified had surgeons been more prepared to explore the elbow rather than worry about interference with the joint.

Pathology. According to Wadsworth (1987), the lesion associated with 'tennis elbow' is characterized by superficial or deep macroscopic and microscopic tears at the tendinous origin of the extensor carpi radialis brevis, as well as the periosteum of the lateral epicondyle. He indicated micro-avulsion fractures may be seen, as well as round cell infiltration, scattered foci of fine calcification and scar tissue with marginal areas of cyctic and fibrinoid degeneration. Repair is by immature reparative tissue (Wadsworth 1987). All these findings point to fibre rupture within the tendon. Nirschl (1973) referred to dull greyish oedematous tissue replacing the normal glistening tendon. This tissue often encompassed the entire origin of the extensor carpi radialis brevis tendon to the level of the radial head. Nirschl (1973) found pathological change on the underside of the extensor aponeurosis in approximately 35% of cases. In 20%, calcific exostosis of the lateral humeral epicondyle was present. He reported that if changes do occur in the aponeurosis it is unusual for it to be to an area greater than 50%.

Steiner (1976) commented on the poor blood supply to the lateral epicondyle and how the fibres of tendons attached to the periosteum of the epicondyle are relatively avascular, compared with the muscle. Damage to muscle heals rapidly compared with tendon. Nutrition becomes even further impaired with age-related degenerative changes. In fact, age is described as a dominant factor in much of the literature (Boyd & McLeod 1973, Wadsworth 1987, Nirschl 1988), and partly explains the common occurrence of this condition in 35–50-year-old tennis players.

Due to the intimate association of the extensor carpi radialis brevis muscle to the capsule of the elbow, irritation of free nerve endings in the capsule has been postulated as a cause of joint involvement (Goldie 1964, Coonrad & Hooper 1975). As most chronic sufferers have some joint pathology and loss of normal accessory movements (Maitland 1977), irritation of the ligaments could explain the joint pain, and must be addressed in treatment of both acute and chronic conditions.

Mechanism of injury. Tennis elbow is one of many examples of overuse syndromes caused throughout the body by chronic cyclic activity. 'Overuse is encountered when the body's physiological ability to heal lags behind the microtrauma occurring with the repetitive action' (Jobe & Nuber 1986, p 621). The lower the load the greater the number of cycles needed to produce failure. For most tissues a load limit exists below which an infinite number of cycles will not produce failure. A common factor in all repetitive loading is the occurrence of microtrauma. There are several associated factors:

- Overload, combined with the disadvantaged leverage system caused by the sloping lateral epicondyle, creates a fulcrum effect around the prominent radial head and thus increased tension of the soft tissues in that area, particularly when the forearm is working in the hyperpronated position, i.e. the backhand stroke and volley in tennis (Nirschl 1973).
- Inadequate forearm extensor power and endurance to withstand normal, forceful repetitive moments placed against the forearm flexors (Nirschl 1973).
- Extreme moments of force or repetition, despite reasonable muscle power, endurance and flexibility (Nirschl 1973). Lateral epicondylitis is common among golfers. The action of ulnar deviation, grasping and controlling the small grip of a club, co-contraction during backswing, then impact causes a sudden eccentric overload, placing strain on the lateral extensors and radial deviators of the leading forearm.
- Incidence and recurrence rates increase with age. This is most evident in the over 40s age groups where there is a fourfold increase in prevalence among men and a twofold increase among women (Gruchow & Pelletici 1979).
- A sudden increase of an activity requiring wrist extension on an unconditioned forearm can cause lateral joint pathology. This is well demonstrated by a young badminton player who presents with an acute

lateral epicondylitis following a training clinic. After spending a long period of time perfecting the backhand stroke the athlete cannot grip the racquet the next day because of pain at the lateral epicondyle.

- Poor tennis backhand stroke technique is a common cause of lateral epicondylitis, particularly when the player uses the forearm extensor muscles as a power source instead of the larger muscle groups of the legs and trunk. The forearm extensor muscles should be used purely to fine tune the stroke at the end of the kinetic chain. Bernhang et al (1974) found that most athletes suffering tennis elbow used a leading elbow on the backhand stroke.

- A player who is attempting to topspin on the forehand stroke by using excessive forearm pronation instead of stroking the ball upwards with the racquet may also cause a tugging effect and irritation of the lateral elbow.

- Improper training techniques, using excessive repetitive backhand strokes or overstrengthening of forearm muscles contributing to a large muscle imbalance, will lead to lateral elbow pain.

- Improper equipment and facilities, such as a racquet with the wrong weight or grip size (too large or too small), or incorrect string tension, can contribute to excessive forces at the elbow. Playing with wet tennis balls will also increase the forces generated between racquet and ball.

- Muscle imbalance, where a tournament player with large inflexible forearm extensor muscles is performing a flick of the wrist at the end of the service action to gain greater speed. The lack of flexibility also has a tugging effect on the common extensor origin and thus microtears may occur.

- Sudden onset of lateral epicondylitis occurs with one specific incident, e.g. a mistimed backhand stroke where the forearm extensor power is inadequate to withstand the moments of force being placed on it, thus leading to a tearing. Not all lateral epicondylitis is sport-related, however. The weekend home renovator is as likely to suffer from this condition as the club tennis player. Periods of hammering, painting, bricklaying or chopping wood, are all activities that can lead to development of the problem.

Signs and symptoms.

- Pain: there is localized pain and tenderness, specifically at the origin of the extensor carpi radials brevis just anterior and distal to the lateral epicondyle. There may also be pain and palpable local tenderness in the extensor muscle belly. In severe cases the pain may radiate distally into the forearm, sometimes reaching as far as the wrist, presenting as a constant ache in this region with intermittent bouts of sharp pain when aggravated by activity. The aggravating activity may be minor, such as picking up a tea cup,

but the pain inhibition can be sufficient to cause the cup to be dropped.

- Elbow movement: in more severe cases elbow movements, particularly extension and to a lesser degree end of range flexion, becomes limited. Stiffness is worse on waking in the mornings and gradually reduces during the day. In very severe cases the patient will carry the arm flexed across the body and the range of motion does not improve with activity during the day.

- Effusion: in mild and moderate cases effusion is rarely present, however it may be quite marked in severe cases.

Special tests.

- Grip: testing of grip will reproduce the pain, which will vary depending on the size of the grip and whether the elbow is flexed or fully extended. A smaller grip combined with an extended elbow leads to the greatest pain, as the extensor muscles are contracting with the finger flexors operating in their outer range. This may be progressively tested on the physiotherapist's wrist and then fingers, with the athlete's elbow first flexed and then extended. If the condition is irritable only one grip test with a flexed elbow should be carried out (monitoring for any change in symptoms).

- Resisted extension test: resisted finger extension will reproduce the symptoms. Symptoms may increase when the test is repeated with the arm in full elbow extension, and the forearm in pronation. Resistance of middle finger extension is particularly sensitive because of the insertion of the extensor carpi radialis brevis into the base of the third metacarpal. This test is also applicable for radial nerve neuropathy, but by increasing the tension on the radial nerve (see neuromeningeal assessment of the upper limb) and repeating the test, the physiotherapist can detect variations in the athlete's perception of pain, implicating either the nerve or the tendon (Fig. 24.9).

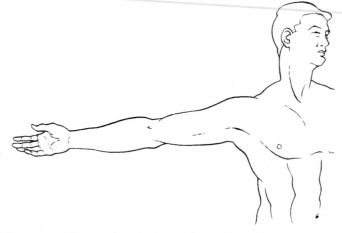

Fig. 24.9 Resist extension of wrist and fingers in modified neuromeningeal stretch position

- Stretch: with the arm in the neutral position, placing the extensor muscles on stretch will often reproduce the symptoms or demonstrate tightness and inflexibility, when compared to the other side (Fig. 24.10).
- Palpation: palpation at the origin of the extensor carpi radials brevis will reproduce very sharp pain, and even in the later stages of rehabilitation tenderness will still be present, although to a lesser degree. The forearm extensor muscle mass may feel very tight with trigger points (Travell & Simons 1983) which when palpated reproduce local or referred pain.

Differential diagnosis. The following conditions can produce lateral elbow pain and need to be excluded from a diagnosis of lateral epicondylitis:

- lateral ligament sprains
- lateral epicondyle avulsion
- radiohumeral bursitis
- lateral epicondyle epiphysis injuries in children
- osteochondritis in children
- cervical and thoracic spine referral
- posterior interosseous nerve syndrome
- neuromeningeal involvement.

Treatment. It is interesting that a condition so easily diagnosed by even the layperson poses such a problem for the professional to treat. This is because, in many cases, only part of the problem is addressed. Epicondylitis is well recognized as a chronic overuse syndrome but is often treated as an acute problem. If treating an athlete with patellar tendinitis, one would not hesitate to examine foot

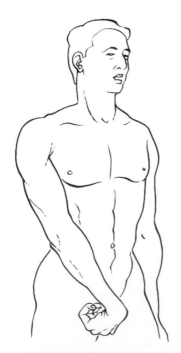

Fig. 24.10 Stretch of the wrist and finger extensors

and hip posture, running style and sports shoes. Therefore, in longstanding epicondylitis, issues such as posture, technique and equipment must be considered and an attempt made to resolve the underlying cause. If this is not done then successful return to play may never be achieved.

Acute epicondylitis

When lateral or medial epicondylitis is the result of one acute injury (e.g. a mistimed stroke or throw) the standard treatment regime of immediate RICE application, electrotherapy, graduated stretching, strengthening and return to play is applied. As with all injuries to a joint, care must be taken to ensure full elbow movement is regained or maintained. Once the acute condition has settled then rehabilitation should incorporate an active exercise regime, with soft tissue stretching and massage. This will most often achieve a successful result, however the timing of return to sport will be determined by the severity of the injury.

Chronic epicondylitis

All factors need to be considered in the management of this condition. It is very important that the athlete understands the cause and nature of chronic epicondylitis and that it will take time and hard work to recover. It is the authors' experience that athletes who do not carry out a prescribed exercise routine do not achieve a good recovery. Priest and Gerberich (1985) found an inverse relationship between the level of success and duration of pain (i.e. the mean duration of pain: 17.3 months, 10.3 months, and 6.3 months correlated respectively with the levels of success: no recovery, moderate recovery and complete recovery). They also found the greater the pain prior to treatment the more likely the chances of a complete recovery. The following are some of the possible treatment modalities that may be employed to treat lateral epicondylitis:

- Passive mobilization techniques: the grade of technique depends on the athlete's condition and whether pain or stiffness is the limiting factor (Maitland 1977) (see Ch. 12):
  - caudad distraction with the elbow in 90° flexion has been found to be a very useful technique to help relieve pain in the irritable condition when extension is limited by pain
  - extension/adduction can be a valuable technique in the treatment of minor joint signs associated with lateral epicondylitis
  - extension/abduction can be beneficial for lateral epicondylitis. However it can be provocative, therefore it is important to monitor the pain response during and after treatment
  - cervical and thoracic mobilization techniques (see Chs 12, 21 and 22).

If the elbow symptoms arise from the cervical and/or thoracic spines, these are the obvious areas to treat. Chronic cases of peripheral pathology in the upper limb may result in proximal tension, which can contribute to neurological and/or vertebral referred pain to the elbow. Therefore areas of the spine must be treated, even if the original condition relates to the elbow. Treatment of the spine may also help, directly or indirectly, to improve faulty upper quadrant biomechanics.

- Massage: when stretch testing of the extensor muscle group is limited by pain or tightness, massage of these muscles may be beneficial in decreasing tightness and therefore relieve the tugging effect occurring at the tendinous origins. Massage may be combined with trigger point therapy which can further relieve tension within the muscle. Both techniques can be easily taught to the athlete as a home routine, and thus reinforce the treatment occurring in the clinic (Travell & Simons 1983).
- Neural mobilization: due to the proximity of nerves to the lateral aspect of the elbow, neural adhesion is, on occasions, associated with soft tissue healing. The appropriate techniques for this problem are soft tissue massage over the course of the nerve, aided by neural stretching (see Ch. 26). This is a useful technique for the low-grade chronic condition which has not responded to local and central mobilizing techniques, or where recovery has plateaued. Home stretching exercises may be carried out, however due to the very sensitive nature of this tissue care must be taken to prevent exacerbation. Strapping of the thoracic spine may be used when the neuromeningeal structures are severly inflamed. Similar to wearing a support for low back and referred leg pain, the strapping unloads the tension on the neuromeningeal structures, and therefore alters the referred pain to the elbow. Once irritibility has decreased, exercises can be introduced to improve postural position.
- Deep frictions: the authors use these in the late stages of treatment, when the objective signs have decreased in number and intensity, but there is still marked tenderness on palpation of the extensor tendon attachment (Cyriax 1975).
- Stretches: stretching of the extensor muscles of the wrist and fingers is achieved by full elbow extension and pronation, then adding wrist and finger flexion to where a strain (no pain) is felt at the lateral elbow and/or along the length of the muscle (Fig. 24.10). In painful conditions this will be achieved by ipsilateral wrist and finger flexor contraction. As the athlete improves, the stretch can be progressed by applying overpressure with the contralateral hand. All stretches should be held for 20–30 seconds with 5 repetitions prior to and after exercising. Stretching of the cervical and thoracic regions (e.g. levator scapulae, upper trapezius, pectoralis major) may also be helpful. In fact, any tissue of the cervical shoulder quadrant that is tight or reinforcing poor posture needs to be stretched.
- Active exercise regime: this plays a key role in the success of the treatment. With manual therapy, if an athlete reports exacerbation following treatment using a mobilization technique, the technique is not immediately discarded but, following reassessment, may be used again but at a lower rate of either grade or duration. The authors recommend a similar approach when prescribing an exercise program. Reassessment of the exercise is important, to consider limiting the range of motion or the number of repetitions should pain be increased following the exercise. In this way, the physiotherapist can maximize the efficiency and effectiveness of exercise.

It is important for both physiotherapist and athlete to understand that one isometric contraction held for 10 seconds 3 times a day can be an effective and positive starting point for an exercise program. The physiotherapist will usually teach an isometric exercise and a static stretch on the first or second treatment, unless the condition is very irritable. The exercises are carried out in the clinic and reassessment of the objective signs allow for modification, if necessary. The athlete is also instructed that the exercises should not reproduce pain. Fatigue is acceptable and there should be no cumulative pain as repetitions are carried out during the day.

When prescribing an exercise program the factors that need to be considered include:

- range of motion (painfree range only)
- number of repetitions
- speed at which the exercise is carried out
- the amount of resistance.

An example of an exercise progression is given below, but the authors emphasize the importance of modifying each program to suit the individual.

Exercise progression.

- Isometric contraction: the elbow is flexed to 90° and the hand of the unaffected arm applies manual resistance over the dorsum of the supinated hand of the injured arm.
- a painfree isometric contraction of the forearm extensors is initiated and held for 5–10 seconds. Repetitions may vary from as few as 1 per hour, to 10 per hour, or 10 repetitions 3 times a day, depending on the physiotherapist's assessment of the irritability of the condition.

Progression may then include:

- forearm pronation as the starting position
- increasing repetitions and then increasing resistance.
- carrying out the above exercise with the elbow in an extended position, starting with a decrease in resistance and repetitions, gradually increasing this as for the flexed elbow.
- active biceps and triceps exercises while holding a weight, so that the forearm muscles are working isometrically as they do when gripping a tennis racquet.
- Active concentric and eccentric exercises: these are introduced as early as pain will allow and may progress in conjunction with the isometric exercises. The forearm is rested on a table with the elbow flexed to 90°, the hand hanging over the edge of the table with the wrist flexed in a relaxed and comfortable position. Concentric extension of the wrist is then carried out until the wrist is in neutral, held for 5 seconds, then slow eccentric work of the extensors lowers the hand back to the relaxed starting position. This procedure may then be increased in range of movement, speed, and resistance. The manner in which the weight is held will also be a progression, e.g. a wide hand grip is harder work for the forearm extensors than an ordinary grip.

Weakness or tightness of other muscle groups may cause greater stress on the elbow region, and specific exercises should also be given for groups of muscles involved in the sport. Particular attention should be paid to the shoulder stabilizing muscles. There are two reasons for this:

- Strengthening the trunk and scapulothoracic muscle groups will help correct the poor posture previously described, and therefore take stress off the neuromeningeal structures.
- Poor mechanics or shoulder pathology places increased stress on the elbow.
- Functional exercises: these may also be commenced as soon as pain allows. A good indication is when the patient can manage a painfree isometric hold when performing resisted elbow exercises. These functional exercises are progressed as follows:
- bouncing a ball on the tennis racquet
- practising tennis strokes without hitting a ball
- gently hitting the ball against a wall for 10 minutes. This may be gradually increased in duration and intensity
- social tennis
- competition tennis.

Return to play should be combined with specific warm-up and cool-down exercises, and icing of the forearm immediately after use. As the athlete has shown a susceptibility to lateral epicondylitis, this needs to be an ongoing routine.

- Counterforce bracing: treatment of lateral epicondylitis may involve the use of counterforce braces. These are non-elastic braces generally secured with velcro straps, designed to place pressure over the muscle bellies of the wrist extensors. Their clinical effectiveness is generally accepted (Nirschl 1973, Burton 1985), and it is proposed their benefit arises from changing the mechanical origin of the extensor muscles at the elbow by effectively supplying a second origin distal to the radial head. This decreases the fulcrum effect of the extensor muscles on the lateral epicondyle, providing a mechanical support for the common extensor origin, reducing further injury and allowing healing of any existing condition. Groppel and Nirschl (1986) state that the gentle compression applied to the musculotendinous region partially decreases muscle expansion during intrinsic contraction and induces tendon movement. This has the effect of decreasing the overall force on the muscle unit and the possibility of further injury.
Groppel and Nirschl (1986) were able to show a reduction of EMG activity in the medial and lateral elbow muscles, as well as reducing angular acceleration of the elbow, while wearing a brace support. Their results imply that wearing a brace, when serving or playing one-handed backhand, provides support for the player. The authors feel that the clinical evidence of pain reduction using these braces is extensive and therefore they are an important part of the treatment for those athletes who cannot (or will not) avoid the causative activities. The physiotherapist must ensure that using this device does not simply mask the symptoms and allow excessive activity, thereby exacerbating the problem. In severe cases this will involve weaning the individual off the brace for all daily activities to only when it is needed for heavy work, repetitive tasks or return to sport.
- Equipment and technique: the tennis backhand stroke and volley are usually the principal causes of lateral extensor injury, where the player is trying to hit the ball using the forearm muscles as the power source, instead of correctly transferring weight from the back to front foot, as well as utilizing the muscles of the posterior shoulder. Often the athlete will use a leading elbow on the backhand stroke. This is a common problem in self-taught athletes (Kamien 1990). Such faulty technique causes the point of impact to occur in front of the forward foot while the wrist and elbow are still moving at the time of impact, thus taking increased stress. This is aggravated further if the ball is mishit, causing increased force on the racquet head and therefore the possibility of extrinsic overload. As a two-handed backhand redistributes the stress to both arms, similar problems do not occur. Kamien (1988)

states that there is no firm evidence of stroke technique being a causative factor in tennis elbow, but clinical results cited by Nirschl (1986), Priest et al (1980), and Gruchow and Pelletici (1979) indicate that it must be addressed in treatment of lateral epicondylitis.

The serve is the one area where the top class player may have problems. Due to an increased forearm muscle mass, there can be a reduction of wrist flexion range, although this situation should not arise if extensor muscle stretches have been carried out. During the serving action the player snaps the wrist into flexion to try to gain extra power. With the backhand grip, which is commonly used for serving, where the arm is already in a pronated position, a sudden stretch placed onto the already stretched extensor muscles can be another cause of extrinsic overload.

A common contributing factor associated with tennis elbow is when an intermediate player decides to add topspin to the forehand stroke. The player starts to roll the racquet over the ball by performing a jerky hyperpronation of the forearm, combined with some wrist flexion. Not surprisingly, the stroke is somewhat of a disappointment and when the player tries again, the signs and symptoms of tennis elbow start to appear. Again, as in the backhand ground stroke, the player must be taught that topspin is achieved by stroking the ball upwards, using transference of weight from the legs and body. It is important that the treating physiotherapist be aware of these problems so they can be discussed, the aggravating factors eliminated and the player referred to a tennis coach to correct faulty technique.

There seems to be no agreement in the literature regarding the type, weight, size of grip and string tension of racquets as aggravating factors. Nirschl (1988) suggests injury is related to heavy and tightly strung racquets and recommends the racquet be strung 30 lb less than the amount stated by the manufacturer. Similarly, there are no consistent findings to suggest that one type of racquet is better than another. Kamien (1988) indicated different types of racquet affect different players. This is confirmed by Carroll (1981) and Gruchow and Pelletici (1979), who found that tennis elbow was unrelated to the type, material or weight of the racquet. Kamien's (1990) review of the current literature makes the following points:

- standard size wood racquets have lower vibration at the racquet head than oversize metal racquets, if the ball is hit off centre.
- the larger sweet-spot in the oversize racquet absorbs vibrations better than a standard size racquet.

However, this must be balanced against:

- when the ball strikes more than 8 cm from the centre, or even hits the frame, the oversized metal racquet has greater frequency and amplitude of vibrations but the lowest dissipation.
- regardless of the racquet material, oversize racquets have a greater potential for producing torque injuries.

Kamien (1990) states there is no proof that vibration is a cause of tennis elbow, though he reports that Carroll (1986) showed an 81% improvement when using a racquet shown by laboratory tests to be effective in reducing off-centre vibration. In advising a racquet change for an athlete with tennis elbow the different combinations of size and material do not allow for flexible decisions. Kamien (1990) recommends a racquet with a 'forgiving nature' (i.e. made of a flexible material) which accomodates an off-centre mishit. Grouchow and Pelletici (1979) showed that changes of both racquet and technique were the most important for improvement in both cases of mild and severe tennis elbow. Priest and Gerberich (1985) found 100% reduction of symptoms by changing stroke technique. The physiotherapist must therefore assess the condition, and the aggravating factors, that produce tennis elbow.

Grip size is considered a possible cause of tennis elbow. Bernhang et al (1974) found that the largest comfortable grip size reduced racquet torque. Murley (1987) states that the greater the grip size, the greater the wrist extension, therefore the less the tension on the wrist and hand extensors. It has been shown that the smaller the grip size, relative to hand size, then the stronger the forearm forces from the racquet (Murley 1987). Nirschl (1988) offers a method of measuring the correct grip size for each player. This is to measure from the proximal palmar crease to the top of the ring finger (Fig. 24.11).

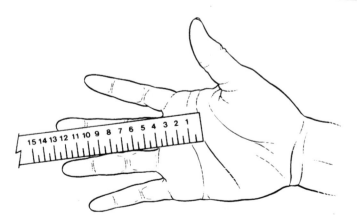

Fig. 24.11 Measure from the lateral side of the ring finger to the proximal palmar crease

The advances being made in different materials, including those for frames, strings and grips, added to the technological advances in racquet design, means that the physiotherapist must keep abreast of the current information, or have ready access to someone who does have this information, to ensure the best treatment of the athlete.

Slow playing surfaces, such as clay, are better suited for players prone to tennis elbow. On faster surfaces, such as cement, grass or artificial turf, ball speed is markedly quicker, placing greater impact loads on the elbow. Heavy duty, hard or even wet tennis balls will cause increased impact force, thereby aggravating or contributing to tennis elbow.

• Anti-inflammatory medication: in the authors' experience, oral non-steroidal anti-inflammatory drugs (NSAIDs) reduce the pain level of both acute and chronic tennis elbow. The obvious benefit— reduction of soft tissue inflammation—allows athletes to increase their rehabilitation program and thus accelerate the healing process. This can also be a trap, however, because of the analgesic effect of the medication, tempting the athletes to increase training before they are ready. Therefore, close professional guidance is necessary on return to play.

The place of cortisone injections in the overall treatment program is a controversial one, but one or two cortisone injections deep to the involved tendon has been shown to be useful and is worth trying in more severe cases (Young 1992). It should be noted that if the injection is placed superficial to the tendon it can lead to significant fat atrophy and vascular changes in the overlying skin, which may be cosmetically disturbing to the patient (Young 1992). Intratendinous injections may be injurious to the healing tissue. Binder and Hazleman (1983) reported 53% improved with ultrasound compared to 89% with steroids, and indicated that while ultrasound is not as effective as steroid injections, the recurrence of symptoms was less frequent with the former. Their paper does not mention other physiotherapy techniques being used, so the apparent limited benefit of ultrasound and the recurrence with steroids is understandable.

When conservative measures have been exhausted, then surgical treatment for tendonitis about the elbow may be indicated.

Indications for surgical treatment. Where athletes have had continuous symptoms for more than 12 months, during which they have undertaken an adequate period of rest (three months), plus a rehabilitative exercise and graduated training program, operative intervention may have a place. Plain X-rays of the soft tissues can be useful in localizing calcification at the centre of the tendonitis. Likewise, ultrasonography has been used to localize areas of degenerative tendon and early calcification. If on radiological views and ultrasonography a significant degenerative tendon or calcification nodule is identified, this may predispose towards early operative intervention (Young 1992).

An athlete who has received multiple cortisone injections in the past, and is not improving under a rehabilitation program, may also be a candidate for surgery. Large volumes of cortisone lying in and around tendon tissues undoubtedly prevent healing and can in fact lead to further chronicity of the problem (Young 1992).

The main indication for surgery, however is unacceptable pain, particularly pain at rest, pain causing sleep disturbance and pain which has inhibited a return to sport, despite an adequate rehabilitative program. If frank tendon fibre failure has occurred, as is obvious on pre-operative ultrasound examination, this indicates a need for surgical intervention (Young 1992).

Radial nerve neuropathy

In some cases of resistant 'tennis elbow' which does not respond to conservative treatment, the pain may be due either to radial tunnel syndrome or posterior interosseous nerve syndrome.

Radial tunnel syndrome

As the radial nerve passes from the arm to the forearm it travels through the radial tunnel in which there are five recognized sites of compression (Posner 1990):

• fibrous bands tethering the nerve to the underlying joint capsule
• a sharp tendinous medial edge of the extensor carpi radialis brevis, which can cause a groove in the nerve with the forearm in full pronation
• the fan of radial recurrent vessels crossing the nerve where it lies in close proximity to the neck of the radius. When these vascular structures dilate with exercise they can cause temporary compression of nearby nerves.
• the 'arcade of Frohse' (Fig. 24.12), a fibrous inverted semicircular arch occurring in the proximal portion of the superficial head of the supinator muscle, can be a potential site of compression. According to Posner (1990) this structure is found in 30% of athletes
• a fibrous band at the distal edge of the supinator muscle.

Signs and symptoms. Many of the signs and symptoms are very similar to those of tennis elbow:

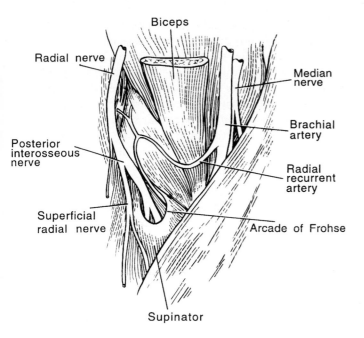

Biceps

Radial nerve

Median nerve

Posterior interosseous nerve

Brachial artery

Radial recurrent artery

Superficial radial nerve

Arcade of Frohse

Supinator

Fig. 24.12 Posterior interosseous nerve and its relationship to the Arcade of Frohse

- pain and tenderness over the lateral epicondyle.
- pain on stretching the extensor muscles and resisted finger extension.
- pain radiating up and down the arm.
- weakness of grip.
- pain caused by resisted middle finger extension.
- occasional superficial radial nerve paraesthesia.
- tenderness over the radial nerve (Roles & Maudsley 1972).

Differentiating features. Tenderness on palpation along the radial nerve, anterior to the radial head, differentiates this syndrome from a 'pure' tennis elbow.

Roles and Maudsley (1972) describe pain at the common extensor origin on resisted middle finger extension as positive for radial tunnel syndrome, as this causes tightening of the extensor carpi radialis brevis muscle, and thus increased pressure on the nerve. They report the test to be painfree within two weeks of surgical release of the radial nerve. However, as previously mentioned, the resisted middle finger test is also diagnostic for tennis elbow but can be differentiated from radial tunnel syndrome by incorporating the upper limb neuromeningeal tension test (see Ch. 26). If radial tunnel syndrome is present then pain levels will change as tension increases on the peripheral nerve.

Resisted forearm supination with the elbow flexed and the forearm in full pronation will reproduce the pain if the nerve is compressed by the supinator muscle (Posner 1990).

Treatment. Rest from all activities affecting the nerve is the initial treatment. The supinator and extensor carpi radialis brevis can be stretched within pain limits, and the stretch ceased immediately if the condition worsens. Recovery may be aided by NSAIDs and massage. If the condition does not resolve in several weeks, or the athlete has recurring problems, surgical decompression may be appropriate (Posner 1990).

Posterior interosseous nerve syndrome

Posterior interosseous nerve syndrome can mimic lateral epicondylitis. The posterior interosseous nerve is purely motor in function and is formed at the bifurcation of the radial nerve, where the motor component passes between the two heads of the supinator muscle (Fig. 24.12). If the arcade of Frohse is present then, as with the radial nerve, the posterior interosseous nerve can become constricted (Posner 1990). Impairment of this nerve may give a unique presentation of wrist extension with radial deviation, combined with MCP joint flexion and interphalangeal extension.

Compression of the posterior interosseous nerve has also been reported in:

- fractures of the proximal end of the radius
- the presence of lipoma or ganglion
- rheumatoid arthritis, causing a proliferative synovitis of the elbow joint
- dislocation of the radial head
- spontaneous paralysis of the nerve following blunt trauma
- hyperextension injuries to the elbow (Sharrard 1966)
- repetitive pronation and supination of the forearm (Mulholland 1966).

Signs and symptoms. The syndrome results in a purely motor deficit, with no sensory change. The patient is still able to extend the wrist, but with radial deviation because of paralysis of the extensor carpi ulnaris. The extensor carpi radialis longus is innervated at a higher level and therefore not usually involved. The extensor carpi radialis brevis is often spared too and therefore a situation of muscle imbalance occurs, resulting in radial deviation.

In the case of complete paralysis of all the digital extensors, the ability to extend the fingers and thumb at the metacarpophalangeal joint is lost. However, extension at the interphalangeal joint is maintained through the action of intrinsic muscles.

Electrodiagnostic testing and EMG examination of the muscles innervated by the posterior interosseous nerve will assist in diagnosis and establishing the extent of compression.

Differential diagnosis. Due to the unique presentation of this condition, the diagnosis is generally clear.

Treatment. If spontaneous recovery has not occurred within 6-8 weeks surgical intervention may be indicated where there are positive EMG signs. The condition can co-exist with tennis elbow, therefore both need to be considered in all cases.

EMG studies show fibrillation in the supinator and compression to the nerve at the proximal end of the muscle. Reproducing these symptoms is an indication of a proximal compression. Some surgeons have been known to routinely decompress the posterior interosseous nerve in all cases of exploration of the common extensor origin. Certainly, in cases of refractory tennis elbow following tendon exploration, this may be a reasonable course of action (Young 1992).

Osteochondritis dissecans

The aetiology of this condition is thought to be by either or both compression of the radial head on the capitulum during the acceleration phase of throwing, or vascular insufficiency in the region (Jobe & Nuber 1986). The condition is most common among children and adolescents participating in racquet or throwing sports. Osteochondrosis is most common in younger athletes (under 12), whereas osteochondritis dissecans is thought to be a later stage, seen in the early teen years (Yocum 1989). Early recognition of the condition is essential because if bony changes occur, they can lead to severe and lifelong consequences of bony overgrowth of the radial head and early osteoarthritis.

Athlete presentation. Athletes with osteochondrosis will present with mild lateral joint line pain and lateral swelling, but generally have full range of elbow movement. The physiotherapist should consider this condition when elbow extension with a valgus stress elicits pain. X-ray findings will confirm the diagnosis.

Osteochondritis dissecans will cause radiocapitellar joint line pain, joint effusion, palpable crepitus, predominantly a flexion contracture and occasional limitation of full flexion. The onset of pain can be insidious, occurring over many years. While the condition is mostly seen in adolescents, adult presentation can occur. Again, X-rays will confirm the diagnosis.

Treatment. This condition has been divided into three groups for the description of treatment:

- group 1: children up to the age of 13 years, with minimal joint changes and symptoms. Treatment involves rest from the aggravating activity. Occasionally, splinting of the elbow may be necessary and only rarely is surgery required. The prognosis in this group is good.
- group 2: 13-year-olds to adulthood, who present with a history of insidious onset of pain combined with repetitive activity. Treatment may involve assessment of the damaged articular cartilage by arthrotomy. Bone grafts and or drilling of the fragment, if it has not become completely detached, may prevent further

cartilage damage and joint surface incongruity. If the damage has not progressed to loose bodies and joint incongruity then the prognosis is good.
- group 3: this group includes adults with a long history of pain, who may have underestimated the seriousness of their condition. By this stage there are loose bodies present, incongruity of articular surfaces and joint erosion. Treatment will involve surgery to remove the loose bodies, and pinning of partially detached fragments. The prognosis for return to throwing or hitting sports is poor (Jobe & Nuber 1986).

Physiotherapy for groups 2 and 3 should be guided by the surgeon's findings and requirements. Generally, supination and pronation can commence 2–3 days post surgery, and active exercises will start at 5–7 days. It is important in the early stages to avoid compression of the lateral joint (McManama et al 1985).

As this condition occurs predominantly in the overactive athlete, a major part of treatment is counselling of parents and coaches on the potential lifelong consequences of the problem.

Lateral condyle fracture

Fractures to the lateral condyle are more common than those to the medial. Athletes, particularly children, are at risk with activities such as gymnastics, riding or cycling in which there is a higher probability of a fall onto the partially extended arm. Generally, the elbow is subject to a varus force, the intensity of which will determine whether the fracture is displaced. If unrecognized, the displaced fracture can cause long-term problems, including ulnar nerve damage (Reid 1992). If the injury is due to a valgus force there may be medial collateral ligament involvement (Watson 1990).

Athlete presentation. On palpation, the patient has pain and effusion over the lateral aspect of the elbow, and with any movement of the elbow and/or wrist. Depending on the extent of the injury, joint deformity may be obvious. This condition should be suspected in children who present with lateral elbow pain following a varus stress to the elbow. They require immediate orthopaedic referral.

Treatment. Closed reduction or internal fixation will depend on the degree of injury and the specialist's preference. The aim is to restore joint articulation congruity and stability. Active movements may start as early as 2-3 weeks for undisplaced fractures, but with special attention to restricting any force that can distract the fracture site.

Lateral epicondyle fractures

Avulsion fractures occur at the lateral epicondyle. The mechanism of injury can be direct contact, as in being hit with a racquet or bat, or having a forceful extension of the wrist suddenly blocked (Hurley 1990). These fractures have a propensity for slow healing or non-union.

Differential diagnosis.

- radiocapitellar incongruity
- radial head fractures
- osteochondritis dissecans
- lateral epicondylitis
- loose bodies
- lateral condyle fracture.

Treatment. For undisplaced fractures simple immobilization is used. As with the medial condyle, the physiotherapist must exercise some degree of caution when initiating stretching and strengthening for the lateral components of the elbow. Early elbow mobilizing should be performed with the wrist in extension. Those fractures managed surgically should be treated as above, under the direction of the surgeon.

Radial head fractures

Radial head fractures are common in the adult sporting population. The most common mechanism of injury is a fall onto the outstretched pronated hand. The extent of the injury can range from a simple undisplaced fracture to a comminuted fracture with associated elbow dislocation.

Athlete presentation. Athletes may present with non-specific elbow pain and effusion, which is often mild. Flexion and extension is usually limited, with pain on palpation over the radial head being the most positive sign, indicating the need for X-ray. Examination of the wrist joint, including X-rays, is important to eliminate possible fracture or displacement (see Ch. 25).

Differential diagnosis:

- lateral epicondylitis
- lateral condyle or epicondyle fracture
- osteochondritis dissecans of the capitulum. Repeated compression of the radiocapitellar joint, generally caused by throwing, can cause incongruity in the joint leading to loose bodies. This may be particularly prevalent in children
- elbow dislocation
- loose bodies within the joint.

Treatment. The condition requires medical evaluation and reduction of the fracture to ensure articular congruity. Treatment of undisplaced fractures requires a short period of immobilization for comfort and protection, with early active exercises for range of motion. The athlete can return to full activity, usually within 3-4 weeks, with pain as a guiding factor (Watson 1990).

Periarticular myositis ossificans is a problem with these injuries, and surgery is advocated within 48 hours (Curtis & Corley 1986). The treatment of more severe fractures is not universally standardized and, despite surgery, there is often poor prognosis for return to competitive throwing. Post-surgery, it is important to obtain good range of elbow movement; however, with more severe injury, limitation of extension, pronation and supination may occur.

MEDIAL ELBOW INJURIES

Medial epicondylitis

The attachment of the common flexors of the wrist and hand is a site of both chronic and acute strain, or even a combination of the two. Constant repetitive overload can cause a tendinitis similar to that of tennis elbow. Acute tears or ruptures may develop due to sudden excessive contraction of the flexors of the wrist and fingers, or when an opponent or a hard object unexpectedly blocks forceful flexion of the wrist.

Chronic onset is more insidious as it involves repetitive activity, leading to microscopic damage to collagen fibres. Initially, the damage is below the athlete's threshold of pain awareness, but with repeated activity it will increase, until bleeding triggers a chemical response, making the athlete aware of the injury (Curwin & Stanish 1984). Even at this stage the athlete will generally continue with the activity, as the pain settles with rest and usually does not inhibit performance.

Medial epicondylitis is common in golfers who continually take divots out of hard ground, resulting in overload to the dominant arm's wrist flexors at the point of impact. Other athletes who require a strong grip (water skiers, gymnasts) or who grip excessively (tennis, squash) are also prone to the condition. It may also occur through excessive training of the wrist and finger flexors.

Athlete presentation. The athlete with a chronic condition will present with gradually increasing medial elbow pain that initially occurs with the action alone, but progresses to pain following sport and, in severe cases, to pain at rest. There is pain on palpation around or just distal to the common flexor origin. Resistance of both wrist and finger flexion is painful, and stretching of these muscles will reproduce pain over the medial elbow. If the injury is acute, occurring as a result of a single incident, causing deformity with a palpable defect and considerable ecchymosis, then a major tear or rupture must be considered (Reid 1992).

Medial epicondylitis can be associated with medial collateral ligament instability as excessive valgus overload during forceful contraction places increased strain on the medial elbow (Tullos & Bryan 1986). The two conditions are often closely related and must be assessed with respect to each other.

Differential diagnosis:

- medial collateral ligament sprain
- medial epicondyle fracture or avulsion
- ulnar nerve entrapment
- medial olecranon fossa impingement

Treatment. Treatment for medial epicondylitis follows the same regime as that for lateral epicondylitis, with emphasis on stretching and strengthening the forearm flexor muscle group. Medial collateral ligament instability and ulnar nerve involvement, if present, must be treated as separate entities. If a major tear or rupture is suspected then an orthopaedic referral is appropriate.

Medial collateral ligament injury (Thrower's elbow)

Despite the fact that the medial collateral ligament is able to withstand normal throwing forces, it is often involved in medial elbow injuries. The acceleration phase of throwing creates large tensile valgus stress on the medial elbow (Fig. 24.13), creating ongoing microtrauma and compromising strength. One episode of valgus overload can be enough to cause a partial tear or rupture (Jobe & Nuber 1986). As the injured ligament fails to fully stabilize the elbow, it can be a predisposing factor in ulnar nerve and flexor muscle injury.

If a complete rupture is suspected then X-ray diagnosis is necessary to rule out avulsion fracture or, in the child or adolescent, epiphyseal separation.

Athlete presentation. The athlete will present with medial joint tenderness and effusion. Tenderness is greater distal to the medial epicondyle. Valgus stress will demonstrate pain and instability, and the stress will need to be applied with the elbow flexed 15–30° to eliminate the stabilizing effect of the olecranon in its humeral fossa. Associated with this injury can be lateral pain due to compression, or ulnar nerve pathology, due to stretching (Jobe & Nuber 1986).

Differential diagnosis:

- medial epicondylitis
- medial epicondyle fracture or avulsion
- ulnar nerve entrapment
- medial olecranon fossa impingement.

Treatment. The initial aim of treatment is to reduce inflammation with electrotherapy and NSAIDs. As the three bands of the anterior portion of the ligament are taut in different parts of elbow movements, all active and passive movement in the first 1–2 weeks should be within the painfree range only. Initially, muscle strengthening is also in painfree range only. A grade I injury will settle in 1–2 weeks, while a grade III tear will require protection from further aggravation for 6 weeks, with return to sport delayed until approximately 3 months post injury.

Final stage rehabilitation. This will follow guidelines similar to those described for lateral epicondylitis, with emphasis placed on the forearm flexor muscle group in a progressive resisted strengthening program. A similar program should be followed for all muscle groups of the arm and shoulder girdle. The program needs to be functional. Once this has been successfully introduced then specific activities, such as throwing, may also be commenced. An example of a throwing program is given below as a guide. It is suggested that the athlete does not progress to the next stage unless he or she is painfree at the time of activity and for 24 hours after. If pain occurs during the activity then it should be reduced to a painfree level then slowly progressed again:

1. High lob, light toss, 15-20 m throwing at 50% of maximum velocity. One set of 10 gradually increasing to 5 sets.
2. Gradually increase by 10 m until normal competitive distance is reached.
3. Repeat exercise but throw straight and flat instead of high lob.
4. Return to 15-20 m throwing at 75% of maximum velocity and gradually progress as for stages 1, 2 and 3.
5. Return to 15-20 m throwing at maximum velocity and gradually progress as for stages 1, 2 and 3.

If there is disruption of the ligament in a throwing athlete, such as a baseball pitcher, then immediate referral to an orthopaedic specialist is advised. Untreated instability of the medial collateral ligament can lead to cessation of the throwing athlete's career.

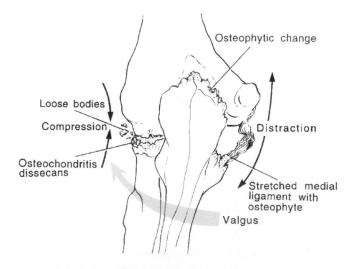

Fig. 24.13 Repetitive valgus stresses associated with throwing produce stretching and instability on the medial side, with shearing forces on the olecranon. The result is growth defects in the young and degenerative changes in the adult.

Valgus extension overload syndrome

This condition occurs predominantly in the throwing arm and is a result of valgus stress on the extending throwing elbow (Fig. 24.13). As the throwing athlete's arm, when combined with cubitus valgus, undergoes bony as well as muscular hypertrophy, this can lead to the formation of an osteophyte butting into the posteromedial aspect of the olecranon fossa. Wilson et al (1983) indicate that when X-rays confirm an osteophyte the only effective treatment is surgery to allow the athlete to return to full function.

Athlete presentation. The athletes complain of posterior elbow pain during the acceleration phase of throwing, with restriction of full elbow extension. They feel they lose control and tire easily. Palpation reveals posterior fossa pain, not necessarily limited to the medial aspect. The medial pain is at the proximal end of the fossa. Full extension may be painful but when a valgus stress is added, pain is both reproduced and increased.

Treatment. Initial treatment to reduce swelling and pain will quickly give way to more active physiotherapy, to encourage and develop functional strength of all elbow and forearm muscles. Any movements or exercises that reproduce posteromedial compression and pain should be avoided. If conservative treatment does not return the athlete to full painfree function in 8–12 weeks, and the diagnosis (aided by X-rays), confirms valgus extension overload syndrome, then surgery is recommended (Andrews & Wilson 1985).

Ulnar nerve neuropathy

Due to the superficial position of the ulnar nerve in the cubital canal, it is the peripheral nerve most susceptible to injury. Injury may be due to direct or indirect trauma.

Direct trauma. Injury may occur if dislocation of the elbow joint or fracture of the humeral condyle occurs. Malunited repair of the fracture, or damage of the epiphyseal plate, can lead to secondary valgus deformity and thus ulnar nerve damage.

Pressure may result from direct ulnar nerve compression due to incorrectly worn or too tight elbow bracing, or by simply resting the flexed elbow on a hard surface. The time it takes to create lasting damage depends on the level of compression.

Indirect trauma. This is seen in throwing and racquet sports, gymnastics and weightlifting. During the act of throwing, the elbow joint is rapidly flexed and extended. If the ulnar collateral ligament has already been damaged, its capacity to resist valgus forces is attenuated and the nerve is more at risk of displacement and relocation during the throwing action. Irritation gradually increases, causing ulnar neuritis (Glousman 1990).

If there are irregularities in the ulnar groove, such as bony spurs, or valgus deformity due to previous damage to the growth plate, the nerve is also susceptible to injury. Subluxation of the nerve from the ulnar groove due to laxity of the ulnar collateral ligament, or trauma, can lead to progressive inflammation.

Cubital tunnel syndrome is the most common cause of neuropathy, where a progressive compression lesion occurs due to:

- osteoarthritis.
- rheumatoid arthritis.
- granulomatous disease.
- ganglions and neoplastic lesions, such as neurilemma (Glousman 1990).

Signs and symptoms:

- pain along the medial joint line of the elbow when throwing.
- clumsiness and heaviness of the hand when throwing.
- pain and paraesthesia down the ulnar aspect of the forearm.
- initial intermittent paraesthesia of the ring and little finger leading to numbness at a later stage.
- weakness of the the ulnar nerve-innervated intrinsic muscles.

Special tests. Palpation over the ulnar nerve as it passes through the cubital tunnel and into the flexor carpi ulnaris reproduces tenderness (Fig. 24.14).

The elbow flexion test (Buehler & Thayer 1986) is also useful. The patient sits with both arms in an anatomical position (elbows fully flexed and wrists fully extended) for a period of 3 mins to provide both compressive and tensile

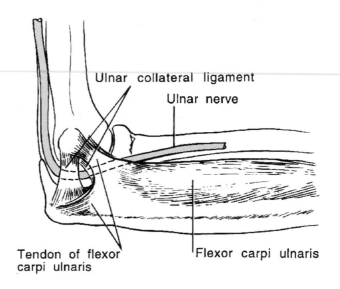

Fig. 24.14 The ulnar nerve as it passes through the cubital tunnel into flexor carpi ulnaris

forces on the nerve. A positive result is the onset of pain and paraesthesia through the ulnar nerve distribution.

Tinel's sign will be positive over the cubital tunnel.

Differential diagnosis:

- entrapment of the nerve within Guyon's canal at the wrist (Berkeley et al 1985)
- thoracic outlet syndrome
- Pancoast's tumour (carcinoma of the apex of the lung)
- systemic conditions, such as diabetes mellitus, alcoholism
- pain referral from the cervical spine
- extrinsic masses, e.g. ganglion or lipoma at the medial joint.

Treatment. Initially, conservative treatment is appropriate. This includes joint mobilization, electrotherapy, soft tissue massage, upper limb neuromeningeal stretches, muscle stretching and re-education, and NSAIDs, with rest from the aggravating factors. If the ulnar neuritis is secondary to ligament instability, it is important that that problem be addressed first.

If conservative treatment is not successful, surgical decompression of the nerve in the cubital tunnel should be performed.

In cases of nerve entrapment syndromes, the decision for operative intervention is usually based on:

- severity of symptoms
- abnormalities on EMG examination
- neurological disturbance in the form of sensory or motor loss in the distribution of the involved nerve (Glousman 1990).

Little leaguer's elbow

The young throwing athlete is subjected to the same stresses as the adult, with the additional risks of epiphyseal injury and overuse stress on immature bone. Throwing a curve ball, plus other breaking pitches, place extra stress over the medial epicondylar epiphysis, the original pathology of little leaguer's elbow. Now the term is used to describe a number of pathological conditions that can occur in the adolescent pitcher (see box).

Mechanism of injury. These various conditions can be attributed to stress applied to the young athlete's elbow during the various stages of the pitching action.

- Cocking phase: there can be considerable stress placed on the medial aspect of the elbow during the later stage of the cocking phase, due to the valgus forces which develop as the hand and forearm trail behind the elbow. Thus the ulnar collateral ligament can be overstretched, leading to traction spurs on the ulnar coronoid process. The flexor muscles may be

---

Classification of pathology in little leaguer's elbow according to anatomical location

Medial: avulsion of the medial ossification centre
strain of the flexor muscles
traction spurs of the ulnar coronoid process
ulnar neuropathy

Lateral: lateral epicondylitis
osteochondral fractures of the capitulum
deformities of the radial head
loose bodies

Posterior: avulsion fractures of the olecranon
olecranon spurs
triceps strain

Anterior: strains or spurs
degenerative joint changes

Source: Hunter (1985)

---

strained and the ulnar nerve stretched and subluxed from its groove.

There may also be lateral compression forces, causing the radial head to impact and deform against the capitulum. Fracture of the capitulum may result, leading to intra-articular loose bodies.

- Acceleration phase: as discussed earlier, the valgus forces occurring at the elbow with acceleration and release can cause proximal medial compression of the olecranon in its fossa, as well as compression of the distal lateral olecranon in its fossa. Lateral compression may result in radiocapitellar damage, while medial distraction will stress the attachments of the medial collateral ligament, causing microtrauma at the epiphyseal plate (Hurley 1990). Additional stress may be due to extreme pronation of the forearm, which places the lateral structures under tension, leading to lateral epicondylitis.
- Follow-through: if hyperextension occurs during this phase it will lead to compression of the olecranon process and spur formation in the olecranon fossa. The high level of activity of the biceps muscle, working eccentrically to slow extension of the arm, may cause it to be strained anteriorly, with damage to the anterior capsule and traction spurs of the coronoid process.

Signs and symptoms:

- Pain: the athlete complains of pain which may have an insidious progression.
- Swelling: initially following the game and then for longer periods.
- Stiffness: this occurs after prolonged periods of throwing, following which there is a progressive decrease in range of motion due to fibrosis of soft tissues and loss of normal contour of the elbow.

- Tenderness: palpation of the involved area reproduces tenderness, which may extend to more than one area.

Special tests. Radiographs are important to detect early bony changes as described above. All overuse injuries in the young athlete should be routinely assessed by X-ray.

Treatment:
- Rest: most cases will respond well with rest from pitching, along with conservative treatment. Avulsion fractures of the medial epicondyle are treated with splinting and rest. However, if rest fails, complete separation of the bony metaphysis may need surgical repair.
Ulnar nerve compression is treated with decompression surgery if rest fails to settle the problem.
- Lateral compartment: degenerative change in this area does not respond well to treatment, and although removal of osteophytes and loose bodies can be carried out, ankylosis of the joint may remain, making it impossible for the child to throw. These children should discontinue throwing sports.
- Epiphyseal changes: if these are evident then the athlete needs to be referred to an orthopaedic specialist.
Education of the athlete, parents and coaches is required to prevent injury and avoid recurrence.

Medial epicondyle fractures

Avulsion of the medial epicondyle from its muscular or ligamentous attachment can be due to massive muscle contraction of the forearm flexors, posterior dislocation of the elbow, a fall on the hand, or repeated valgus stress at the elbow. Throwing is again the causative factor, with repetitive loading causing microtrauma at the epiphyseal plate secondary to distraction forces on the medial aspect of the elbow (Hurley 1990).

Poorly treated medial epicondylar fractures may lead to an inability to throw effectively (Kuland 1982). If the bony fragment has rotated forwards (Fig. 24.15) this alters the medial collateral ligament's function, resulting in valgus instability. This is best assessed radiologically by the 'gravity stress test', where the athlete lies supine, with the shoulder abducted and externally rotated to 90°, and the elbow flexed 15–20° to eliminate the stabilizing effect of the olecranon within its fossa. Simple gravity will open the medial joint, exposing the instability (Kuland 1982, Hurley 1990).

Treatment. The degree of displacement, with any associated instability, will determine the need for surgical intervention, although the current trend is towards surgical fixation even with fragments displaced only 2–3 mm (Hurley 1990). This approach has been found to prevent non-union, or fibrous union, leading to later instability. Surgical intervention is also indicated with:

- ulnar nerve symptoms
- intra-articular joint fragments
- failure of closed reduction
- posterior dislocation of the elbow.

Post surgery, physiotherapists must take care with mobilizing and strengthening the muscles crossing the elbow and forearm. Early active mobilization of the elbow and wrist joints is performed in a painfree range. Wrist extension is accompanied by finger and elbow flexion, to reduce the pull on the medial epicondyle. Gradual resisted exercise can begin at 3–4 weeks but must be within pain tolerance.

ANTERIOR ELBOW INJURIES

Biceps tendinitis

Biceps tendinitis is uncommon at the elbow, but can develop when an athlete uses the elbow flexors while in full or hyperextension, thus placing repetitive (or sudden) overload on anterior soft tissues and particularly the biceps at its insertion.

Signs and symptoms. There may be pain with resisted elbow flexion, stretch and palpation of the biceps tendon. Examination will often show an increased range of elbow extension, which will need to be addressed.

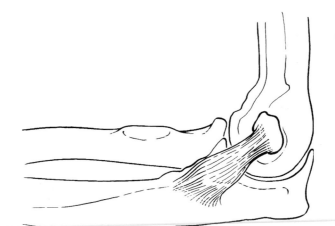

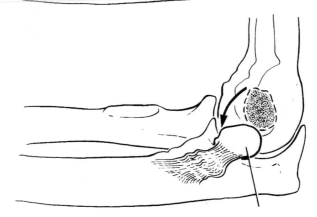

Fig. 24.15 Forward rotation of fractured medial epicondyle fragment

Treatment. Orthosis or strapping may be used in the initial stages to prevent full extension. RICE, soft tissue techniques and electrotherapy are of value in management. Once the lesion settles, a specific strengthening program for the biceps muscle will make it hypertonic, effectively shortening the muscle, while its strength increases. This should improve its natural ability to resist end-range extension via the stretch reflex.

Biceps tendon ruptures

Biceps tendon ruptures at the elbow are rare and may be missed on examination, as haemorrhage can make palpation of the tendon difficult (Reid 1992). If this condition is found or suspected, referral to an orthopaedic specialist is appropriate.

While ruptures of the long head of the biceps are not strictly considered elbow injuries, as the muscle belly retracts a swelling is obvious over the distal portion of the humerus. In older athletes this injury is often due to chronic degeneration of the bicipital tendon in the humeral bicipital groove. An acute traumatic episode of biceps overload is the most common contributing factor in younger athletes. Surgical repair, followed by a rehabilitation program, is appropriate for the latter group. The older athlete rarely experiences any functional impairment due to the rupture, and loss of overall strength is minimal. The reason for surgery in this group is mostly cosmetic.

Median nerve neuropathy

Pronator teres syndrome. As described by Posner (1990) there are four potential sites of compression of the median nerve (in order of frequency):

1. At the pronator teres muscle, where the nerve passes between the superficial head, arising from the medial epicondyle and supracondylar ridge of the humerus, and the deep head, from the medial aspect of the coronoid process of the ulna (Fig. 24.16). A fibrous band may be found on the posterior surface of the superficial head of the muscle, or there may be a band posterior to the nerve, overlying the deep head of the muscle. In some cases the nerve passes deep to the whole muscle.
2. Where the median nerve passes deep to a fibrous arch at the proximal margin of the flexor digitorum superficialis.
3. At the bicipital aponeurosis, where a fibrous membrane spans the flexor muscles and may be abnormally thick.
4. At a proximal fibro-osseus tunnel formed by the supracondylar process of the humerus and the ligament of Struthers, which completes the tunnel as it attaches to the medial epicondyle. The

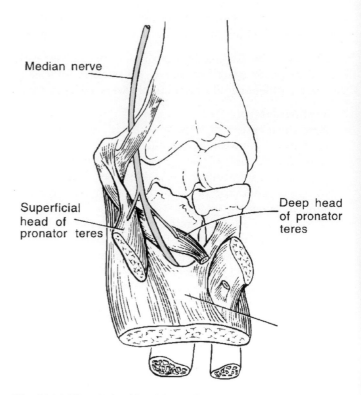

Fig. 24.16 The relationship of the median nerve with pronator teres. Source: adapted from Wadsworth (1987)

supracondylar process is present in less than 1% of the population (Anderson 1983). Trauma and swelling in the region can result in a high median nerve compression.

Signs and symptoms. The athlete complains of pain on the anterior aspect of the arm, which is worse with activity.

Paraesthesia and/or numbness is present in all or part of the median nerve distribution in the hand.

There is weakness of the thenar intrinsic muscles, whereas weakness of the median nerve innervated extrinsic muscles may be more variable.

Special tests. Localized tenderness at the site of compression is an important diagnostic test in nerve compression syndromes (Posner 1990).

Percussion of the area may reproduce pain or paraesthesia in the distal distribution of the nerve.

In pronator teres muscle compression, pain is reproduced with resisted forearm pronation and flexion. The wrist and fingers need to be flexed to relax the flexor digitorum superficialis (Spinner 1980).

In flexor digitorum superficialis muscle compression, pain is often aggravated with resisted flexion of the proximal interphalangeal joint of the middle finger (Spinner 1980).

In bicipital aponeurosis compression, resisted elbow flexion and forearm supination will reproduce the symptoms (Spinner 1980).

In supracondylar process compression, resisted elbow flexion with the elbow flexed at an angle of 120–135° may aggravate the pain. There may also be ischaemic claudication as the brachial artery passes with the nerve through the cubital fossa. If the artery has bifurcated proximal to the process, elbow extension with forearm supination may obliterate the radial and ulnar pulses at the elbow (Posner 1990).

Differential diagnosis. Unlike compression of the median nerve in the carpal tunnel the pain is very rarely nocturnal and patients do not usually wake with pain and paraesthesia. Phalen's wrist flexion test is negative with a pronator syndrome, unlike the positive findings in carpal tunnel compression (Posner 1990).

Treatment. Physiotherapy is not effective in these conditions. A referral should be made to a neurologist.

Anterior interosseous nerve syndrome

This syndrome is characterized by weakness of the flexor pollicus longus, flexor digitorum profundus (lateral two heads) and pronator quadratus. There may also be a mild ache in the proximal forearm that mimics the pronator syndrome, however, as the anterior interosseous nerve is purely motor there will be no sensory change in the hand.

The site of compression of this nerve is usually distal to a fibrous band (when present) deep to the ulnar head of the pronator teres muscle, or deep to the tendon of the flexor digitorum superficialis. In some cases there may be no apparent compression at surgery, however, the nerve is dull and grey and has lost its white glistening appearance (Posner 1990). An enlarged bicipital bursa and thrombosis of the ulnar collateral vessels have also been reported as sites of compression.

Signs and symptoms. The athlete loses the ability to perform the 'pinch test' (opposition of the thumb and index finger) (Fig. 24.17).

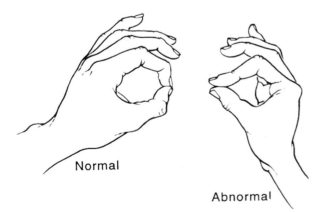

Normal

Abnormal

Fig. 24.17 Pinch test for compression of the anterior interosseous nerve syndrome

There may be variability in the degree of weakness of the muscles. The flexor pollicus longus may display severe weakness, however there may be minimal signs, the only indication being weakness of resisted flexion of the distal interphalangeal joint of the index finger.

Special tests:
- Resisted muscle tests of the flexor pollicus longus and flexor digitorum profundus to the index finger.
- Resisted forearm pronation with the elbow in complete flexion, to neutralize the pronator teres and therefore isolate the action of pronator quadratus.
- Electrodiagnostic testing.

Differential diagnosis:
- No changes of sensation, as in pronator syndrome
- The possibility of tendon ruptures
- Stenosing tenovaginitis of individual muscles.

Treatment:
- Pronator syndrome—surgical decompression
- Anterior interosseous nerve syndrome—initially conservative as spontaneous recovery is common, however, if there is no recovery within 6–8 weeks, surgery may be necessary (Posner 1990).

Surgery is indicated when there are demonstrations of a weak pinch grip, and positive EMG studies.

Supracondylar fractures

These are most commonly seen in children, frequently caused by falls from athletic equipment onto the hand, with the elbow flexed (Apley 1977, Kuland 1982). The usual presentation is posterior displacement of the distal fragment of the humerus. The anteriorly placed neurovascular structures are at risk from compression, and examination of these is vital (Hurley 1990, Kuland 1982, Apley 1977). The radial pulse should be palpated, and the hand observed for signs of neural dysfunction shown by lack of flexion of the distal interphalangeal joint of the thumb and numbness over the tip of the index finger (Reid 1992). If there is any doubt in the examiner's mind, the athlete should be rushed to hospital with the arm splinted in as much extension as possible. The long term consequences of non-recognition is Volkmann's ischaemia (Apley 1977). At no stage should the arm be further flexed as this can occlude the brachial artery.

Athlete presentation. There is an obvious swelling over the distal portion of the humerus, and there may be changes in the contours of the upper arm if swelling is not severe. The athlete's pain will not allow palpation or movement of the region (Apley 1977, Kuland 1982).

Differential diagnosis. Supracondylar fractures have a normal olecranon alignment with respect to the epicondyles, whereas this is distorted in elbow dislocation (Hurley 1990).

Treatment. Medical intervention is required. Physiotherapy for the first 3 weeks will involve only finger, wrist and shoulder movements. When elbow movements are commenced, care should be taken not to mobilize into pain. Long-term elbow stiffness can be a problem and every effort should be made to gain maximum movements quickly and safely within the limits of pain.

Pulled elbow

This is most commonly seen in children of 2–4 years, because of the immature radial head and annular ligament. It occurs as a result of a distraction force with radial rotation, usually the result of swinging the child by the arms. Distraction of the radius causes subluxation or dislocation of the radial head, with associated annular ligament damage (Ogden 1990). The child presents, often in minimal pain, but unwilling to use the arm. Provided there is a clear history of injury with minimal pain, joint effusion or deformity, then reduction by elbow flexion with supination is appropriate. If the reduction does not restore full elbow movement, or if the presentation is unusual, X-rays must be taken. Preventative treatment should include education of the offending adult.

Posterior elbow injuries

Triceps tendinitis

This condition involves microtrauma and inflammation at the insertion of triceps to the olecranon. It is most commonly seen in athletes involved in throwing sports. The athlete presents with localized pain over the triceps insertion, with pain on stretch or resistance to extension.

Treatment. The principles of management of tendinitis apply to this condition (see principles of management), and return to sport should follow a graduated program to enhance strength and endurance, with advice to the athlete to modify training to prevent a recurrence of the condition.

Differential diagnosis. Very occasionally the medial head of triceps will sublux over the medial epicondyle, causing a snapping sensation (Reid 1992). This can result in a triceps tendinitis and is treated with electrotherapy, anti-inflamatories, stretching and strengthening exercises.

Triceps tendon ruptures

A fall on the hand, with the elbow flexed, or strong resistance to the extending elbow can cause rupture of the triceps tendon (Petersen & Renstrom 1983).

Athlete presentation. The athlete presents with elbow pain and an inability to extend the joint. Palpation may reveal a gap within the tendon, and a haematoma may be present. An X-ray is appropriate to exclude any bony

pathology, while ultrasonography or computed tomography will show the soft tissue changes.

As the triceps tendon can sustain strong forces without injury, avulsion injuries will generally occur prior to tendon injury. Where there is tendon rupture, underlying pathology must be suspected (Reid 1992).

Treatment. Full thickness tears will require early surgical intervention to restore the function of the extensor mechanism. Delayed repairs do not always give the same good results (Reid 1992).

Treatment of partial ruptures involve RICE, appropriate electrotherapy and a graduated rehabilitation program, as described for lateral epicondylitis. If throwing is an essential part of the athlete's sport, the guidelines established for medial collateral ligament rehabilitation are appropriate.

Differential diagnosis:

- olecranon fractures
- bursitis.

Elbow dislocation

The most commonly seen dislocation at the elbow is a posterior dislocation, with or without a lateral shift. This is seen more frequently in children than adults, and can be complicated in children by epiphyseal fracture at the site where the ligaments and capsule attach close to the distal epiphysis of the humerus (Ogden 1990). As the force of injury is often large, elbow dislocations can occur in conjunction with medial epicondylar fracture, medial and lateral ligament disruption, capsular tears, biceps and brachialis disruption, radial head fracture, dislocation with a capitellar osteochondral fragment and neurovascular injury (Kuland 1982, Hurley 1990, Berkeley et al 1985, Ogden 1990).

Athlete presentation. Joint deformity and swelling are obvious and the athlete is unable to move the elbow due to pain. The elbow will be difficult to assess because of pain and guarding. Neurological and vascular structures can be compromised and need to be assessed.

Treatment. The joint will require reduction by an orthopaedic specialist. The athlete should not flex the elbow at all prior to reduction, as this may compromise the brachial artery.

Physiotherapy management will depend on whether the joint has undergone open or closed reduction. Athletes with closed reductions can commence early protected range of movement exercises 2–3 days after injury, providing the joint is stable. At this stage, passive stretching to extension is contraindicated due to the risks of myositis ossificans. In most cases extension will return spontaneously, but if this does not occur then gentle passive mobilization and active exercise needs to be introduced at 2–3 weeks. Treatment is progressed slowly, only when the athlete can tolerate increased resistance and range of movement. As the soft tissue damage with elbow dislocation can be extensive, all muscle groups affecting the elbow, wrist and hands need to be included, as well as soft tissue massage to encourage blood supply and reduce adhesions.

Those joints reduced and repaired surgically need to be treated under the guidance of the surgeon, as the knowledge of which structures were repaired will dictate the nature of the rehabilitation program.

In the authors' opinion, protective taping or bracing to reduce extension is recommended on return to sport to protect the elbow and to reassure the athlete.

Olecranon fractures

The most common cause of olecranon fracture is a direct blow to the proximal aspect of the olecranon (Watson 1990, Hurley 1990). To a lesser extent an avulsion fracture of the proximal ulna can be caused by a forceful triceps contraction (Hurley 1990, Apley 1977), although these are more common in pre-adolescent age groups (Hurley 1990). While stress fractures of the olecranon are rare, they have been seen as a result of repetitive strong triceps action (Singer 1985).

Athlete presentation. The athlete presents with posterior elbow pain, a history of a sudden blow or a forceful triceps contraction against a fixed ulna. There is local tenderness and swelling over the olecranon. The athlete has pain with stretch and resistance of triceps, and an inability to straighten the joint (Petersen & Renstrom 1983). X-ray findings will verify the diagnosis.

Differential diagnosis. Olecranon stress fractures are generally seen in pre-adolescents, due to overuse. They have a slow onset and the pain settles with rest, although return to throwing should be delayed for 8–10 weeks.

Traction apophysitis, caused by repetitive triceps contractions on the immature bony insertion, can occur in adolescents. Rest from the harmful activity will usually settle the condition (Hurley 1990).

Treatment. Treatment of these fractures is primarily surgical. Post-operative care should be under the direction of the surgeon and initially aimed at restoration of elbow movement. Strengthening exercises are usually commenced at 8–10 weeks post injury.

Olecranon bursitis

Olecranon bursitis may result from a direct blow or fall onto the elbow. Repetitive rubbing at the point of the elbow can also irritate the bursa, causing a thickening of the bursal wall. Fibrinous or cartilaginous loose bodies may form and be palpable, giving the impression of bone chips within the bursa (Kuland 1982).

Athlete presentation. There is an obvious swelling of the posterior elbow, varying from slight to gross distension. Pain is usual with active and passive elbow movements, with resistance and stretch of triceps, and there is heat in the swollen area.

Treatment. Rest, ice and compression will most often result in a spontaneous recovery. If, however, this is a chronic recurring condition, an infected bursa must be considered. Prompt medical attention is needed to aspirate the bursa, and give antibiotic medication (Petersen & Renstrom 1983, Reid 1992). Failure to do this can lead to the infection spreading throughout the arm. Loose bodies within the bursa, or a thickening of the bursa wall, may cause continued aggravation, even with minor trauma. If this occurs, surgical excision may be required (Petersen & Renstrom 1983).

Olecranon impingement

Olecranon impingement is caused by an extension overload of the tip of the olecranon process in the olecranon fossa. This is a common gymnast's problem (Aronen 1985). The athlete presents with inflammation and pain on full extension, particularly when overpressure is applied. Treatment consists of reducing the causative activity, along with biceps strengthening to resist elbow hyperextension.

Other elbow conditions

The following conditions are briefly mentioned to complete the differential diagnosis of the elbow. If the likelihood of these is suspected, the problem is not responding to treatment, or the signs and symptoms are unusual, medical assessment must be sought.

Myositis ossificans

Myositis ossificans may develop following a direct blow to a muscle, or secondary to severe trauma, such as fractures or dislocation around the elbow, or by early (not necessarily forceful) elbow extension following injury. The brachialis muscle is the most common site for ectopic bone formation. Ossification does not form for approximately 3 weeks, so initial radiographs are negative (Ireland & Andrews 1988).

Signs and symptoms. There is an increase in pain and decrease in range of movement. Palpation of the soft tissue may show a firm mass within the muscle. X-rays should be repeated every 2 weeks if the condition does not improve (Reid 1992).

Treatment. Treatment will include anti-inflammatory medication and rest from all activity (including physiotherapy and electrotherapy). Immediate gentle active movements may be carried out within the painfree available range. As the condition resolves, gentle physiotherapy may be introduced to increase joint range and muscle strength, but must be controlled at all times to avoid recurrence.

Stress fractures of the forearm

While stress fractures of the forearm are uncommon, there have been reports of mid-ulnar stress fractures following overuse in athletes (Curtis & Corley 1986, Tanabe et al 1991). Although they appear more commonly in throwing activities, they have been seen in racquet sports (Tanabe et al 1991). A thorough subjective diagnosis, aided by a bone scan, will confirm the condition.

Volkmann's ischaemia

Volkmann's ischaemia occurs with partial or short periods of full arterial obstruction (as distinct from gangrene, which is a result of long-term arterial obstruction). Nerve tissues can survive 2–4 hours without nutrition and can theoretically regenerate. Muscles may survive 6–8 hours, but if in a compartment (as in the forearm), the ischaemic muscle swelling caused by congestion and metabolic changes can lead to soft tissue necrosis (Apley 1977).

Mechanism of injury. This can be secondary to fracture or dislocation at the elbow where major arteries traversing the region are compromised.

Athlete presentation. In all traumatic injuries of the elbow it is important to assess adjacent nerves and the patency of arteries. If there is any doubt regarding these, a lesion must be assumed and an immediate medical referral made. The athlete may present with pale bluish fingers, absent radial pulse and decreased finger sensation. There may be obvious tension in the forearm and any attempt to straighten the fingers will be painful and resisted. Pain can be severe and if one of the other signs is present then urgent action is required.

Treatment. If splints or bandages are suspected of causing compression they must be removed. Care should be taken not to flex the elbow and if it is already acutely flexed it should be straightened a little. Ice should be applied to the forearm to reduce metabolic needs and the athlete is rushed to hospital.

Complications. Contraction of the forearm muscles will follow ischaemia. The athlete presents with deformity of the forearm and hand, stiffness and weakness, and may have neural changes. These changes can be permanent and close consultation with the athlete's medical practitioner is essential to formulate a realistic rehabilitation program.

Fractures and fracture-dislocations of the elbow and forearm

Fractures of the radius and/or ulna may be found in almost all sports and age groups. They can be caused by a fall onto the arm, or a direct blow (usually on the ulna). While the area of fracture may vary along the shaft of the bone, diagnosis can be relatively easy. The history of injury, site of pain, restriction of movement (especially supination and pronation) and possible deformity, can aid diagnosis. X-rays of the elbow and wrist are essential to differentiate fractures as described below (Watson 1990):

- Monteggia's fracture: a fracture of the proximal third of the ulna and radius with a radial head dislocation.
- Galeazzi's fracture: involves the mid to distal third of the radius with dislocation or subluxation of the distal radio-ulnar joint.
- Essex-Lopresti fracture/dislocation: involves injury to the distal radio-ulnar joint with a fracture of the radial head.

Treatment. All forearm fractures must be referred for medical management, as precise anatomical alignment is essential to return to pre-injury range of movement. Early rehabilitation following immobilization should include active, non-resisted flexion/extension of the elbow and wrist. Supination and pronation must be avoided until there is radiographic evidence of healing (Watson 1990). Once osseous healing has been established, light weights and full rotational movements can begin. With removal of the cast, soft tissue management of the forearm is commenced to ensure reduction of adhesions and scar formation, muscle pliability, improved blood flow and full joint movement.

Rheumatoid arthritis

Rheumatoid arthritis is an uncommon presentation at the elbow but may be suspected if previous diagnosis elsewhere in the body has been made.

Osteoarthritis

Osteoarthritis is usually a result of previous trauma. In its mild form it may go unnoticed, except for a decrease in extension with occasional ulnar nerve palsy (Reid 1992, Apley 1977).

Synovial chondromatosis

Athletes present with pain, reduced movements, catching or locking of the joint.

Haemophilia

The joint surface and synovium is damaged due to recurrent bleeding. The elbow will have reduced range of movement, deformity and X-ray changes.

Pigmented villonodular synovitis

This condition is characterized by repeated episodes of bleeding into the joint.

SUMMARY

As demonstrated throughout this chapter, injury to the elbow joint can be complex with a multistructural pathology. Therefore, a thorough examination, based on sound anatomical and biomechanical knowledge of the entire upper quadrant, is of the utmost importance to achieve the correct diagnosis. Whole body posture should be considered when assessing the stresses placed on the elbow joint during the athlete's sport, as well as daily activities. Treatment will consist of acute management, physiotherapy modalities, muscle re-education and stretches. It should then progress to whole body rehabilitation, followed by functional retraining with specific attention to technique and equipment, supervised by the athlete's physiotherapist and coach working in close co-operation. This will achieve a full recovery and a return to the athlete's previous level of sport.

REFERENCES

Amiss A A, Miller J H 1982 The elbow. Clinics in Rheumatic Diseases (London) 8(3):571–593

An K N, Hui F C, Morrey B F, Linscheid R L, Caho E Y 1981 Muscles across the elbow joint: a biomechanical analysis. Journal of Biomechanics 14(10):659–669

Anderson J E 1983 Grant's atlas of anatomy. Williams & Wilkins, Baltimore, pp. 6–118

Andrews J R, Wilson F 1985 Valgus overload syndrome. In: Zarins B, Andrews J R, Carson W B (eds) Injuries to the throwing arm. W B Saunders, Philadelphia

Apley A G 1977 System of orthopaedics and fractures, 5th edn. Butterworths, London

Aronen J G 1985 Problems of the upper extremity in gymnastics. Clinics in Sports Medicine 4(1):61–71

Askew L J, An K N, Morrey B F, Chao E Y 1987 Isometric muscle strength in normal individuals. Clinical Orthopaedics Sept 222, 261–266

Bartz B, Tillmann B, Schleicher A 1984 Stress in the human elbow joint. II Proximal radio-ulnar joint. Anatomy and Embryology (Berlin) 169(3):309–318

Basmajian J V, Griffin W R Jr 1972 Function of anconeus muscle. An electromyographic study. Journal of Bone and Joint Surgery 54A(8):1712–1714

Berkley M, Bennett J, Woods G 1985 Surgical management of acute and chronic elbow problems. In: Zarins B, Andrews J R, Carson W B (eds) Injuries to the throwing arm. W B Saunders, Philadelphia

Bernhang A M, Dehner W, Fogerty C 1974 Tennis elbow—a biomechanical approach. Journal of Sports Medicine 2:235–260

Bilodeau M, Arsenault A B, Gravel D, Bourbonnais D 1990 The influence of an increase in the level of force on the EMG power spectrum of elbow extensors. European Journal of Applied Physiology 61(5–6):461–466

Binder A I, Hazleman B L 1983 Lateral humeral epicondylitis—a study of natural history and the effect of conservative therapy. British Journal of Rheumatology 22:73–76

Bogduk N 1983 Referred pain from the cervical and thoracic vertebral column. Conference on Manipulative Therapy, Perth WA, pp 198–209

Bosworth D M 1955 The role of the orbicular ligament in tennis elbow. Journal of Bone and Joint Surgery 37A:527–533

Boyd H B, McLeod A C 1973 Tennis elbow. Journal of Bone and Joint Surgery 55A:1183–1187

Briggs C A, Elliott B G 1985 Lateral epicondylitis. A review of structures associated with tennis elbow. Anatomica Clinica 7:149–153

Buchanan T S, Rovai G P, Rymer W Z 1989 Strategies for muscle activation during isometric torque generation at the human elbow. Journal of Neurophysiology 62(6):1201–1212

Buehler M J, Thayer D T 1986 The elbow flexion test. Clinical Orthopaedics and Related Research 233:213–216

Burton A K 1985 Grip strength and forearm straps in tennis elbow. British Journal of Sports Medicine 19(1):37–38

Carroll R 1981 Tennis elbow—incidence in local league players. British Journal of Sports Medicine 15(4):250–256

Coonrad R W, Hooper W R 1975 Tennis elbow, its course, natural history, conservative and surgical management. Journal of Bone and Joint Surgery 53A:117–182

Curtis R J, Corley M D 1986 Fractures and dislocations of the forearm. Clinics in Sports Medicine 5(4):663–680

Curwin S, Stanish D 1984 Tendonitis: its etiology and treatment. Colamore Press, Toronto

Cyriax J H 1936 The pathology and treatment of tennis elbow. Journal of Bone and Joint Surgery 28(4):921–940

Cyriax J H 1975 Textbook of orthopaedic medicine. Bailliere Tindall, London

Fuss F K 1991 The ulnar collateral ligament of the elbow joint. Anatomy, function and biomechanics. Journal of Anatomy 175:203–12

Garden R S 1961 Tennis elbow. Journal of Bone and Joint Surgery 13B:100–106

Gerberich S G, Priest J D 1985 Treatment for lateral epicondylitis: variables related to recovery. British Journal of Sports Medicine 19(4):224–227

Glousman R E 1990 Ulnar nerve problems in the athlete's elbow. Clinics in Sports Medicine 9(2):365–377

Goel V K, Bijlani V 1982 Contact areas in human elbow joints. Journal of Biomechanical Engineering 104(3):169–175

Goldie I 1964 Epicondylitis lateralis humeri. Acta Chirurgica Scandinavica (Suppl 339)

Green C P 1985 The curve ball and the elbow. In: Zarins B, Andrews J R, Carson W B (eds) Injuries to the throwing arm. W B Saunders, Philadelphia

Groppel J L, Nirschl R P 1986 A mechanical and electromyographical analysis of the effects of various joint counterforce braces on the tennis player. American Journal of Sports Medicine 14(3):195-200

Gruchow H W, Pelletici B S 1979 An epidemiologic study of tennis elbow. American Journal of Sports Medicine 7:234–238

Hunter S C 1985 Little leaguer's elbow. In: Zarins B, Andrews J R, Carson W B (eds) Injuries to the throwing arm. W B Saunders, Philadelphia

Hurley J A 1990 Complicated elbow fractures in athletes. Clinics in Sports Medicine 9(1):39–57

Ireland M L, Andrews J R 1988 Shoulder and elbow injuries in the young athlete. Clinics in Sports Medicine 7(5):473–494

Jalovaara P, Lindholm R V 1989 Ultrasonic demonstration of the elbow fat pads. Archives of Orthopaedic and Traumatic Surgery 108(5):243–245

Jobe F W, Nuber G 1986 Throwing injuries of the elbow. Clinics in Sports Medicine 5(4):621–636

Johnson M A, Sideri G, Weightman D, Appleton D 1973 A comparison of fibre size, fibre type contribution and spatial fibre type distribution in normal human muscle and in muscle from cases of spinal muscular atrophy and from other neuromuscular disorders. Journal of Neurological Science 20:345–361

Kamien M 1988 Tennis elbow in long time tennis players. Australian Journal of Science and Medicine in Sport 20(2):19–27

Kamien M 1990 A rational management of tennis elbow. Australian Journal of Sports Medicine 9(3):173–191

Kapandji J A 1982 The physiology of the joints, vol 1. Churchill Livingstone, Melbourne

Kuland D N 1982 The injured athlete. J B Lippincott, Philadelphia

Lee D G 1986 Tennis elbow—a manual therapists perspective. Journal of Orthopaedic Sports Physical Therapy (Baltimore) 8(3):134–142

Maitland G D 1977 Peripheral manipulation, 2nd edn. Butterworths, Sydney

Maitland G D 1986 Vertebral manipulation, 5th edn. Butterworths, Sydney

Maton B, Le-Bozec S, Cnockaert J C 1980 The synergy of elbow extensor musles during dynamic work in man. II Braking of elbow flexion. European Journal of Applied Physiology 44(3):271–278

McManama G B, Micheli L J, Berry M V, Sohn R S 1985 The surgical treatment of osteochondritis of the capitellum. American Journal of Sports Medicine 13(1):11–21

Micheli L J 1983 Overuse injuries in children's sports: the growth factor. Orthopaedic Clinics of North America 14(2):337–360

Miles K A, Lamont A C 1989 Ultrasonic demonstration of the elbow fat pads. Clinic. Radiol. 40(6):602–4

Morrey B F, Chao E Y 1976 Passive motion of the elbow joint. Journal of Bone and Joint Surgery 58A(4):501–508

Morrey B F, An K N 1983 Articular and ligamentous contributions to the stability of the elbow joint. American Journal of Sports Medicine 11(5):315–319

Morrey B F, An K N, Stormont T J 1988 Force transmission through the radial head. Journal of Bone and Joint Surgery 70A(2):250–256

Morrey B F, Tanaka S, An K N 1991 Valgus stability of the elbow. A definition of primary and secondary constraints. Clinical Orthopaedics 265:187–195

Mulholland R C 1966 Non-traumatic progressive paralysis of the posterior interosseous nerve. Journal of Bone and Joint Surgery 48B:781–785

Murley R 1987 Tennis elbow—conservative, surgical and manipulative therapy. British Medical Journal 294:819–840

Nirschl R P 1973 Tennis elbow. Orthopaedic Clinics of North. America 4(3):787

Nirschl R P 1986 Soft tissue injuries about the elbow. Clinics in Sports Medicine 5(4):637–652

Nirschl R P 1988 Prevention and treatment of elbow and shoulder injuries in the tennis player. Clinics in Sports Medicine 7(2):250–256

Norkin C C, Levangie P K 1983 Joint structure and function. A comprehensive analysis. F A Davis, Philadelphia

Ogden J A 1990 Paediatric trauma. In: Tailoukian R J (ed) Mosby Year Book, 2nd edn. Mosby, St Louis

Pappas A M, Zawakki R M, Sullivan T J 1985 Biomechanics of baseball pitching. A preliminary report. American Journal of Sports Medicine 13(4):216-22

Petersen L, Renstrom P 1983 Sports injuries—their prevention and treatment. Methuen, Australia

Posner M A 1990 Compressive neuropathies of the median and radial nerves of the elbow. Clinics in Sports Medicine 9(2):343–63

Priest J D, Braden V, Gerberich S G 1980 The elbow and tennis. Part 2. A study of players with pain. The Physician and Sports Medicine 19(4):224-276

Reid D C 1992 Sports injury assessment and rehabilitation. Churchill Livingstone, New York

Rogers A W 1992 Textbook of Anatomy. Churchill Livingstone, Edinburgh

Roles N C, Maudsley R H 1972 Radial tunnel syndrome: resistant tennis elbow as a nerve entrapment. Journal of Bone and Joint Surgery 54B:499–508

Schwab G H, Bennett J B, Woods G W, Tullos H S 1980 Biomechanics of elbow instability: the role of the medial collateral ligament. Clinical Orthopaedics 146:45–52

Sharrard W J W 1986 Posterior interosseous neuritis. Journal of Bone and Joint Surgery 48B:777–780

Singer J M 1985 Radiographic evaluation of the throwing elbow. In: Zarins B, Andrews J R, Carson W B (eds) Injuries to the throwing arm. W B Saunders, Philadelphia

Sjobjerg J O, Ovesen J, Gundorf C E 1987 The stability of the elbow following excision of the radial head and transection of the annular ligament. An experimental study. Archives of Orthopaedic and Traumatic Surgery (Munchen) 106(4):248–50

Sjogaard G, Houston M E, Nygaard E, Saltin B 1978 Subgrouping of fast twitch muscle fibres in skeletal muscles of man. Histochemistry (Berlin) 58:79–87

Spinner M 1980 Management of nerve compression lesions of the upper extremity. In: Omer G E, Spinner M (eds) Management of peripheral nerve problems. Saunders, Philedalphia

Stack J 1949 Acute and chronic bursitis in the region of the elbow joint. Surgical Clinics of North. America 29:155–162

Steiner C 1976 Tennis elbow. Journal of the Osteopathy Association 75:575

Sunderland S 1978 Nerves and nerve injuries, 2nd edn. Churchill Livingstone, New York

Szabo R M, Gelberman R 1984 Peripheral nerve compression: etiology, critical pressure threshold and clinical assessment. Orthopade (Berlin) 7:1461–1466

Tanabe S, Nakahira J, Bando E, Yamaguchi H, Migamoto H, Yamamoto A 1991 Fatigue fracture of the ulna occurring in pitchers of fast-pitch softball. American Journal of Sports Medicine 19(3):317–321

Travells J G, Simons D G 1983 Myofascial pain and dysfunction—the trigger point manual, vol 1. Williams & Wilkins, Baltimore

Tullos H S, King J W 1973 Throwing mechanisms in sport. Orthopaedic Clinics of North America 4:709–720

Tullos H S, Bryan W J 1986 Functional anatomy of the elbow. In: Zarins B, Andrews J R, Carson W B (eds) Injuries to the throwing arm. W B Saunders, Philadelphia

Wadsworth T A 1987 Tennis elbow: conservative, surgical and manipulative treatment. British Medical Journal 294:621–623

Watson J T 1990 Fractures of the forearm and elbow. Clinics in Sports Medicine 9(1):59–83

Werner C O, Haeffner F, Rosen I 1980 Direct recording of local pressure in the radial tunnel during passive stretch and active contraction of the supinator muscle. Archives of Orthopaedic and Traumatic Surgery (Munchen) 96(4):271–8

Williams P L, Warwick R, Dyson M, Bannister L 1989 Gray's anatomy, 37th edn. Churchill Livingstone, London

Wilson F D, Andrews J R, Blackburn T A, McCluskey G 1983 Valgus extension overload in the pitching elbow. American Journal of Sports Medicine 11(2):83–88

Yocum L A 1989 The diagnosis and non-operative treatment of elbow problems in the athlete. Clinics in Sports Medicine 8(3):439–451

Young D 1992 Personal communication

25. The wrist and hand

Elizabeth Tully, Jane Abbott

Part 1
ANATOMY AND BIOMECHANICS
Elizabeth Tully

The wrist complex consists of the radiocarpal and midcarpal joints, and is closely associated to the distal radioulnar joint. The normal wrist requires both mobility and stability for effective function. It plays a major role in precise positioning of the hand, and in maintaining optimal length for the development of tension in the muscles responsible for grasp and manipulation. During sporting activities which require the use of hand held equipment such as racquets, clubs or bats, the wrist must remain stable in the presence of significant static and dynamic forces. This is also evident in the case of the gymnast, who may land on the hands with the full force of body weight, or suspend, swing, or twist the body while gripping overhead apparatus.

ANATOMY AND BIOMECHANICS

The radiocarpal joint

The radiocarpal joint is formed by the radius and the radioulnar disc proximally, and the scaphoid, lunate and triquetrum distally (Fig. 25.1). The proximal row of carpal bones is joined by the intrinsic interosseus ligaments which are covered by a thin layer of articular cartilage, so that an uninterrupted biconvex articular surface is presented. The distal end of the radius has concave impressions for the scaphoid and lunate, but because of the disc, which is part of the triangular fibrocartilage complex (TFCC), the ulna is not part of the articulation. The radiocarpal joint is enclosed by a somewhat loose but strong capsule which is attached to the dorsal and volar surfaces of the proximal row of carpal bones, sealing the radiocarpal joint into a single unit which does not communicate with other joints.

NOTE

The authors wish to thank Katie Watkin B App Sci (OT) for organising the artwork.

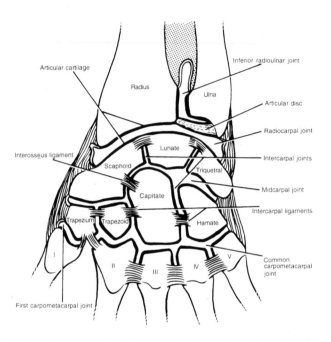

Fig. 25.1 Coronal section through the radiocarpal, midcarpal, and carpometacarpal joints, and the interosseus ligaments of the intercarpal joints. Source: Williams et al (1989)

The scaphoid, which may be damaged by falls on the outstretched hand, or direct impact from the handle of a bat or club, has a tenuous blood supply. 70-80% of the intraosseus blood supply of the scaphoid, including that to the entire proximal pole, comes from branches of the radial artery which enter the dorsal ridge of the bone near the waist. Since most scaphoid fractures occur in the region of the waist, the proximal pole is vulnerable to avascular necrosis (Gelberman & Menon 1980, Gelberman et al 1983a, Gelberman & Gross 1986).

The midcarpal joint

The midcarpal joint consists of the articulation between the scaphoid, lunate and triquetral proximally, and the trapezium, trapezoid, capitate and hamate distally (Fig. 25.1). The joint has a capsule that is continuous with each intercarpal articulation but does not connect to the radiocarpal joint space. The scaphoid, assisted by the wrist ligaments, acts as an intercarpal bridge, providing a stabilizing mechanism between the carpal rows during wrist movement. Without the scaphoid, the central radiolunocapitate link would be very unstable under compression loads and would tend to crumple (Taleisnik 1985).

Ligaments of the wrist complex

In most synovial joints of the body, the function of the ligaments is to give stability to the joint, and to guide and limit the amount of movement which can occur. However, at the wrist, as there are no muscles inserting directly onto the proximal row of carpal bones, the behaviour of individual carpal bones and of the carpus as a whole is produced by interacting contact pressures from bony surfaces, and by ligamentous forces. The wrist ligaments, as well as providing stability to both radiocarpal and midcarpal joints, are capable of inducing bony displacements and transmitting precise loads at a distance (Taleisnik 1985). The flexor carpi ulnaris (FCU) does attach to the pisiform in the proximal row, but passes on to be inserted into the hamate and fifth metacarpal. The function of the pisiform is to act as an anatomical pulley, increasing the moment arm of FCU during activities requiring powerful wrist flexion and ulna deviation.

Loss of integrity of the wrist ligaments associated with bony malalignment and dysfunction of normal wrist mechanics causes considerable disability for the sports person. Most sports injuries follow compressive loading of the wrist in some degree of extension. Rotation of the forearm or of the wrist itself is usually present, and may be combined with radial or ulna deviation. The final injury depends on the magnitude of the force, its point of application and direction, the rate of loading, and the inherent mechanical properties of the individual wrist ligaments (Mayfield 1984, Taleisnik 1992).

The ligamentous system of the wrist can be divided into two major groups (see box): the extrinsic ligaments which course between the radius and the carpal bones (proximal extrinsic ligaments) and between the carpals and metacarpals (distal extrinsic ligaments); and the intrinsic ligaments which originate and insert on the carpal bones (Taleisnik 1985).

The extrinsic ligaments

The proximal extrinsic ligaments play an important role in stabilizing the radiocarpal joint on all sides, and in guiding the excursion of the distal row of carpal bones on the proximal row at the midcarpal joint.

The radial collateral ligament (RCL) arises from the radial styloid, runs volar to the transverse axis of wrist flexion

and extension (Taleisnik 1985) and attaches to the radial side of the waist of the scaphoid (Fig. 25.2). It is fairly lax in the neutral wrist position and only becomes taut in extreme ulnar deviation (Bogumill 1988). It is very elastic, and is the weaker of the two collateral ligaments (Mayfield et al 1979).

The deep volar radiocarpal ligaments are three bands of fibres which pass from the radius to the carpal bones (Fig. 25.2). The radio(scapho)capitate ligament (RSC) passes across the waist of the scaphoid, to which it is attached and gives support, and terminates on the volar aspect of the capitate. This ligament provides the fulcrum around which the scaphoid rotates from a position of dorsiflexion in wrist extension and ulna deviation, to a position of volarflexion during wrist flexion and radial deviation. The radiotriquetral (RT) ligament is a large bundle of almost transverse fibres, comprising the radio-lunate (RL) ligament and the lunotriquetral (LT) ligament. It is the strongest of all the volar radiocarpal ligaments, and acts as a volar sling for the lunate (Mayfield et al 1980, Mayfield 1984). During wrist extension, an interligamentous space (the space of Poirier) develops on the volar aspect of the wrist between the radio(scapho)capitate and radiotriquetral ligaments. This space overlies the capitolunate joint, and with no interosseus ligament binding the lunate to the capitate, it is through this space that dislocations may occur (Mayfield et al 1976).

The radioscapholunate (RSL) ligament consists of short fibres passing from the volar margin of the radius to the scaphoid and lunate bones. Biomechanical studies by Mayfield et al (1979) have verified the weakness and elasticity of the radioscaphoid band, whereas the lunate insertion is

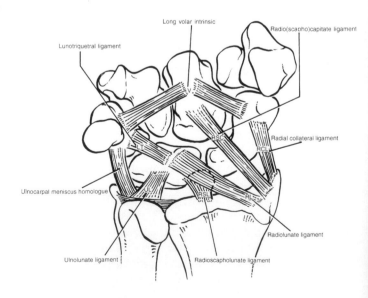

Fig. 25.2 The deep volar extrinsic ligaments of the wrist.
Source: adapted from Taleisnik (1985)

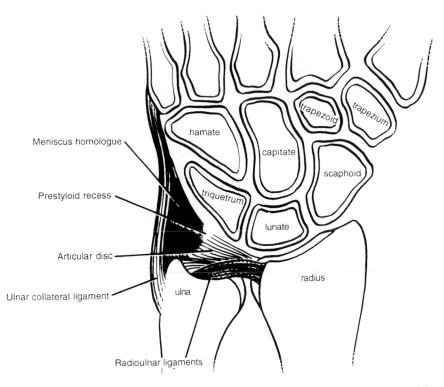

Fig. 25.3 Coronal section through the right wrist and hand (volar aspect) showing the component parts of the triangular fibrocartilage complex.
Source: adapted from Palmer & Werner (1981)

strong (Taleisnik 1985). In full flexion of the scaphoid, the radioscapholunate ligament and the radio(scapho)capitate ligament bind the proximal pole of the scaphoid to the volar margin of the radius, so that it resists dorsal displacement. As the scaphoid rotates into dorsiflexion during wrist extension and ulna deviation, the radioscapholunate ligament provides a restraint to excessive anterior displacement of the proximal scaphoid pole (Taleisnik 1985).

During sporting activities forceful impact loading on the thenar side of the hand causes the wrist to be progressively levered into hyperextension, with ulna deviation and intercarpal supination, which is the same as pronation of the forearm on the carpus (Mayfield et al 1980, Mayfield 1984). This may result in bony injury such as fractures of the distal radius, the radial styloid or the scaphoid, and/or tears to the volar part of the interosseus scapholunate ligament complex and the deep radioscaphoid band which is maximally taut in this position of full wrist extension (Mayfield et al 1980). Tearing of the radio(scapho)capitate ligament may follw since this ligament is maximally taut in wrist extension and ulna deviation and is the weakest link between the radius and the carpus (Mayfield 1980). Alternatively the ligament may stay intact and cause an avulsion fracture of the body of the radial styloid. Similarly the radial collateral ligament may fail or cause an avulsion fracture of the radial styloid tip. Subsequently the scaphoid may sublux dorsally during activities requiring radial deviation flexion and forceful gripping, since the proximal

pole of the bone is no longer tethered to the volar margin of the radius. Altogether, the radial collateral, radio-(scapho)capitate and radioscaphoid ligament provide a weaker link of ligaments between the forearm and the carpus on the radial side of the wrist (Mayfield et al 1979).

On the ulna side of the wrist, the triangular fibrocartilage complex (TFCC) is the major stabilizer of the ulnar carpus and the distal radioulnar joint (Fig. 25.3). It arises from the distal margin of the ulna notch of the radius and courses toward the ulna, inserting into the fovea at the base of the ulna styloid process. From there it flows distally, joined by fibres arising from the ulnar aspect of the ulna styloid, becomes thickened (the meniscus homologue), and inserts into the lunate, triquetrum, hamate, and the base of the fifth metacarpal (Palmer & Werner 1981). The ulna collateral ligament is closely related to the TFCC but it is not actually a distinct fascicle. It is a thickening of the joint capsule in relationship with the overlying sheath of the extensor carpi ulnaris (ECU) muscle (Kauer 1979, 1980, Taleisnik 1985). The dorsal and volar aspects of the horizontal disc portion of the TFCC are thickened to an average of 4–5 mm, and represent the ill-defined anterior and posterior radioulnar ligaments which help limit the range of pronation and supination at the distal radioulnar joint (Palmer & Werner 1981). On the volar aspect of the wrist the TFCC is strongly attached to the lunotriquetral interosseus ligament, and to the triquetrum via the ulnotriquetral ligament. It is also attached to the lunate via

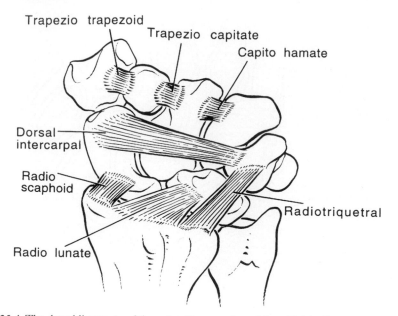

Fig. 25.4 The dorsal ligaments of the wrist. Source: adapted from Taleisnik (1985)

the ulnolunate ligament, with both ligaments extending from the anterior border of the triangular fibrocartilage. The proximal portion of the radiotriquetral ligament and the ulnolunate ligament form an extremely strong triangular ligamentous attachment of the lunate to the forearm (Mayfield et al 1980). Dorsally, the TFCC has a weak attachment to the carpus, except where some of its fibres join the floor of the sheath of the ECU tendon (Palmer & Werner 1981, Palmer 1987).

As well as stabilising the ulna carpus and distal radioulna joint, another major function of the TFCC is to provide a cushion or loadbearing surface at the wrist joint during activities requiring weightbearing on the hands, or pushing objects. Cadaver studies have shown that the radius bears approximately 80% and the ulna 20% of the axial load (Palmer & Werner 1984). Positive ulnar variance, an increase in the length of the ulna in relation to the radius, alters the loadbearing relationship, and in such cases repetitive weightbearing on the hands may be responsible for damage to the central part of the disc and ulnar sided wrist pain. Once degenerative perforation or tears of the TFCC occur lunotriquetral tears may ensue (Taleisnik 1992). Acute tears of the TFCC are rare and degenerative perforations are more common, with the thickness of the central portion of the disc being directly related to ulna variance (Palmer & Werner 1981, Palmer et al 1984). The TFCC receives its blood supply from the ulna artery through its dorsal and palmar radiocarpal branches, and the dorsal and palmar branches of the anterior interosseus artery. Histologic sections of the TFCC reveal vascularity in the outer 15%-20% of the disc, with the rest being avascular (Thiru-Pathi et al 1986).

A decrease in the length of the ulna in relation to the radius (ulna minus) causes increased loads to be borne by the lunate, which is compressed against the distal radius. This may be responsible for initiating the avascular necrosis of this bone seen in Keinboch's disease, and in support of this theory many authors have found negative ulna variance in patients with Keinboch's disease (Gelberman et al 1975, Beckenbaugh et al 1980, Morgan & McCue 1983, Sundberg & Linscheid 1984). It has also suggested that this condition may result from devasculariation of the lunate due to a single traumatic event such as a stress fracture, or avulsion of capsular structures which would include damage to the blood supply leading into the lunate (Lee 1963). However, current opinion is that the cause of avascular necrosis of the lunate may fall into two categories, depending on the mechanism of trauma and the pattern of vascularity. The categories are lunates which have an interruption of palmar nutrient vessels as they enter the bone, and lunates where repeated trauma causes multiple compression type fractures with interruption of the intraosseus blood supply (Gelberman et al 1983b, Gelberman & Szabo 1984, Gelberman & Gross 1986). The latter would be consistent with repetitive minor injuries sustained during sporting activities where the avascular process is secondary to the loss of blood supply to the fractured segments.

The proximal extrinsic ligament on the dorsum of the wrist, the strong dorsal radiocarpal ligament which originates from the dorsal rim of the radius and is inserted into the scaphoid, lunate and triquetrum (Fig. 25.4). It assists in limiting volar flexion of the wrist, and acts to maintain the lunate in apposition to the distal radius. Both the volar and dorsal radiocarpal ligaments are oriented obliquely, passing in an ulnar direction as they pass distally, so that the carpus is passively pulled into pronation and supination by the forearm (Bogumill 1988, Taleisnik 1985).

However, the oblique orientation of these ligaments also renders them vulnerable to injury during activities which require forceful rotation of the wrist itself or the forearm, particularly when the hand is fixed.

The intrinsic ligaments

Three short interosseus ligaments bind the bones of the distal carpal row into one functional unit, with the interosseus ligament between the capitate and the hamate being the strongest (Taleisnik 1985). These ligaments do not usually extend from dorsal to volar capsules, so that the midcarpal joint space may communicate with the carpometacarpal joints (Bogumill 1988).

Three intermediate intrinsic ligaments join the proximal row. The ligaments joining the scaphoid and trapezium consist of volar, dorsal, and lateral bands, which allow the trapezium and trapezoid to ride dorsal to the distal pole of the scaphoid, forcing the scaphoid into flexion during radial deviation of the wrist (Taleisnik 1985). The scapholunate and lunotriquetral ligaments are the most important ligaments where proximal row stability is concerned. The fibres of the scapholunate interosseus ligament run in several directions. On the dorsum of the joint the fibres are thick and short and run transversely (dorsal scapholunate ligament). Within the joint and on the volar aspect (volar scapholunate ligament), the fibres extend obliquely between the two bones, allowing considerable anterior scapholunate gaping during wrist movement (Kauer 1974, Mayfield 1984). During sporting activities where the wrist is loaded in hyperextension, the mobility of the joint allows it to open a little on the volar aspect and some of the load can be dissipated. However if the extension and intercarpal supination force increases, the volar scapholunate ligament may start to tear, followed by the radioscaphoid band and the radio (scapho) capitate ligament, with the result that the scaphoid rotates dorsally on the lunate about a dorsal transverse axis. This rotational instability of the scaphoid constitutes stage one of a condition referred to by Mayfield as 'perilunate instability', in which intercarpal injuries begin at the scapholunate joint. With increased loading force the scaphoid, capitate and triquetrum are progressively dislocated from the lunate. Dislocation of the capitate from the lunate (Stage 2) is always accompanied by failure of the radial collateral ligament or fractures of the radial styloid, and failure of the lunotriquetral and ulno triquetral ligaments accompanies dislocation of the triquetral. Fracture avulsion of the triquetral may also occur. (Stage 3). The final and most severe stage of instability (Stage 4) occurs when the dorsal radiocarpal ligament is torn due to pronation of the forearm on the fixed hand, and the lunate dislocates anteriorly through the space of Poirer, rotating on the hinge provided by the volar radiolunate and ulnolunate ligaments (Mayfield et al 1980, Mayfield 1984).When initial treatment fails to restore carpal alignment following perilunate and lunate

dislocations, late carpal collapse may occur, resulting in intercarpal and radiocarpal arthritis and considerable disability to the sports person (Mayfield et al 1980).

The interosseus lunotriquetral ligament provides a firmer union between the lunate and the triquetral than that which exists between the scaphoid and the lunate (Taleisnik 1985). However, apart from being involved in the sequence of ligamentous tearing resulting in perilunar instability there is enough clinical evidence to suggest that forcible loading on the ulna side of the hand with carpal hyperpronation and radial deviation results in direct injury to the triquetrolunate joint (Reagan et al 1984, Taleisnik 1992).

The long intercarpal ligaments are the deltoid or arcuate ligament, and the dorsal intercarpal ligament. The deltoid ligament forms a V shape which is attached to the volar aspect of the capitate, originating proximally and laterally from the distal pole of the scaphoid, to which it gives support, and medially from the triquetrum (Capitoltriquetral ligament) (Fig. 25.2). Contained within this V is a second V which is attached to the volar aspect of the lunate, and is made up of the radiolunate and ulnolunate ligaments. An important source of blood supply reaches the lunate following these fascicles (Taleisnik 1985). The deltoid ligament is a major stabilizer of the distal carpal row and the double V ligamentous system provides an important linkage between proximal and distal carpal rows during wrist movement (Mayfield 1984, Siegal & Gelberman 1991).

The dorsal intercarpal ligament passes between the scaphoid and the triquetrum, and is thin and ribbon-like (Fig. 25.4). Between the proximal border of this ligament and the dorsal radiolunate band there is an area of weakness situated over the lunocapitate joint, similar to that which exists on the volar aspect of the wrist.

Kinematics of the wrist

The radiocarpal joint is a biaxial ellipsoid joint which permits the primary movements of flexion and extension, and radial and ulnar deviation. These movements may be combined to produce the movement of circumduction.

Wrist extension from the fully flexed position is initiated at the midcarpal joint with the distal carpals sliding on the relatively fixed proximal carpal bones. The triquetral is translated further up the slope of the hamate and the radiolunotriquetral ligament becomes taut. As the radio-(scapho)capitate ligament tightens it creates a sling across the scaphoid, causing the scaphoid and capitate to rotate as a unit into extension/dorsiflexion. The sling effect also causes the lunate to dorsiflex, so that the capitate and lunate remain coaxial as wrist extension proceeds (Weber 1988). The movement is completed at the radiocarpal joint, with the convex surface of the proximal carpal bones sliding in the opposite direction to the movement of the hand. There is lack of consensus among authors regarding the contribution of the radiocarpal and midcarpal joint to the movement, although most agree that the predominance of one joint's contribution to extension is reversed in flexion (Norkin & Levange 1992). The longer dorsal lip and styloid process of the radius limit the range of extension and radial deviation available, and for subjects with ligamentous laxity extension forces may cause the carpus to impinge on the distal radius. The greatest range of motion of the wrist takes place from radial deviation and extension to ulnar deviation and flexion (Taleisnik 1985).

Radial and ulnar deviation occur around an axis passing through the head of the capitate, and the double V ligament system is well placed to control the bony displacements which occur during these movements (Fig. 25.5). During ulnar deviation, the distal row of carpal bones moves in an ulnar direction, until checked by the lateral band of the distal V, while the medial band controls flexion of the capitate. In response to proximal movement of the hamate, the proximal row slides in a radial direction, until limited by the medial band of the proximal V, while the lateral band controls lunate extension (Taleisnik 1988). Radiocarpal motion predominates (Mayfield et al 1976, Youm et al 1978) and the scaphoid and the lunate extend, while the capitate, trapezoid and trapezium flex (Linscheid 1986, Kauer 1986, Taleisnik 1988).

During radial deviation the reverse occurs, with the distal carpal row moving radially on the proximal row until ligamentous and bony structures lock the rows together. Continued force causes the carpal bones to slide in an ulnar direction on the radius and triangular disc. Midcarpal joint motion predominates (Mayfield et al 1976) and both the

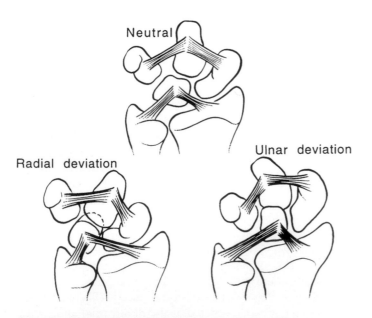

Fig. 25.5 Diagrammatic representation of the double V ligament system on the volar aspect of the wrist. The V shape is only apparent when the wrist is in the neutral position, the orientation changing as the ligamentous bands control the movements of radial and ulnar deviation. Source: adapted from Taleisnik (1985)

scaphoid and lunate flex, while the distal carpal row extends (Linscheid 1986, Kauer 1986, Taleisnik 1988). This 'folding up' movement of the carpal bones allows them to accommodate to the narrowing space between the radial styloid process and the trapezoid, and delays bony impingement at the limit of the movement (Kauer 1986).

The distal radioulnar joint

The distal radioulnar joint is the joint between the convex head of the ulna which is covered with articular cartilage for 270° of its 360°, and the concave sigmoid notch on the distal end of the radius (Palmer 1988). The major stabilizer of this joint is the TFCC, including the ill-defined anterior and posterior radioulnar ligaments. Some stability is also provided by the interosseus membrane and the pronator quadratus muscle which bind the forearm bones firmly together (Palmer & Werner 1981). The extensor retinaculum wraps around the distal ulna to insert on the palmar aspect of the carpus, but having no real attachment to the ulna itself provides little stability for the ulna head. However, the tendon of the ECU lies beneath this retinaculum on the dorsum of the wrist and is held to the distal ulna by its own subsheath, giving some stability to the ulna head and to the distal radioulnar joint (Taleisnik et al 1984, Palmer 1987).

During pronation and supination the forearm rotates around an axis which passes through the radial head proximally and the ulna head distally. In the mid prone position, which is the most commonly used position of the forearm, there is maximal contact of articular surfaces and maximal joint stability. However, a difference in the radius of curvature of the ulna head compared to the sigmoid notch causes the ulna head to move a few degrees posteriorly in pronation, and anteriorly during supination (Ray et al 1951, Rose-Innes 1960, Vesely 1967, Boyes 1970). At the extremes of movement, the ulna head is almost completely uncovered and has little contact with the articulating sigmoid notch, making the joint vulnerable. Forcible twisting of the forearm, or of the wrist itself, may sprain the ligamentous attachments of the distal radioulnar joint, and tears of the TFCC may result in dorsal subluxation or dislocation of the distal ulna with a deformity which is clinically very apparent (Palmer 1987).

During normal pronation the ulna head also moves moves distally in relation to the radius, increasing the effect of a positive ulna variance when weightbearing on the hands. During supination the ulna head moves superiorly (Epner et al 1982, Palmer et al 1982).

POSTURE OF THE HAND

A number of arches have been identified to describe the curved resting posture of the normal hand. The proximal transverse arch is concave anteriorly and is formed by the wedge-shaped carpal bones which are tied together by the flexor retinaculum. The distal transverse arch is formed by the metacarpal heads, held together by the deep transverse ligament of the palm. This arch is also the keystone of the longitudinal arches, which are functional arches fanning out from the wrist, and formed for each finger by the phalanx, metacarpal and corresponding carpal bones. The oblique arches are the functional arches of opposition running between the thumb and each of the fingers (Kapandji 1982).

JOINTS OF THE HAND

Carpometacarpal joints 2-5

The second and third carpometacarpal (CMC) joints are essentially immobile joints which form a rigid middle segment in the hand. Lack of movement at these joints is due to the wedge shape of the bones, causing interlocking of the articulations between the trapezoid, capitate and the second and third metacarpals, and the strong interosseus ligaments binding the adjacent bones together (Kapandji 1982). The rigid middle segment of the hand facilitates a cylindrical power grip by forming a stable floor for the palmar gutter (which runs from the base of the hypothenar eminence to the head of the second metacarpal), and permitting compressive force to be applied to the handle of a racquet or club. The mobile thenar and hypothenar eminences complete the grip by moulding around the handle, while the long finger flexors supply the gripping force.

Limited movement at the second and third carpometacarpal joints also aids the function of the wrist extensors—the extensors carpi radialis longus (ECRL) and brevis (ECRB)—which insert into the base of the second and third metacarpals. During wrist extension, the second and third metacarpals act as a fixed unit with the trapezoid and capitate, enabling the extensors to exert their action on the more proximal midcarpal and radiocarpal joints, and having one less joint over which to shorten can maintain closer to optimal length for the production of tension. Inserted high on the dorsum of the carpal arch the radial wrist extensor muscles have good leverage over these joints.

CMC joints 4 and 5 are plane synovial joints, allowing small movements of flexion (10-20°). The axis for movement of CMC 5 is set obliquely to the long axis of the metacarpal, so that flexion brings the metacarpal a little toward the base of the thumb. In addition, CMC 5 is often described as a saddle joint with 2° of freedom and conjunct rotation (Williams & Warwick 1980, Kapandji 1982). Thus the metacarpal is rotated laterally during flexion, and enhances the cupping or opposition of the ulna side of the hand essential for power grip. Ulna opposition is produced by the hypothenar muscles, abductor digiti minimi (ADM), flexor digiti minimi (FDM), and opponens digiti minimi (ODM).

JOINTS OF THE THUMB

Carpometacarpal joint

The carpometacarpal (CMC) joint is the articulation between the trapezium and first metacarpal. It is a saddle joint with 2° of freedom and a conjunct axial rotation which takes place concurrently with other motions. The fibrous capsule is thick but loose to permit a wide arc of movement, consisting of flexion and extension, abduction and adduction, opposition and reposition. The axis for these movements is oblique because of the position of the joint on the arch of the carpal bones.

The thumb is an essential component of the hand. Without normal function of the thumb the hand is virtually useless. The importance of the thumb is due to its location anterior to the palm, and to the unique movement of opposition. In precision grips, the major feature of this movement is that the thumb moves away from the palm in CMC joint abduction, and maintains a relatively abducted position, while some CMC flexion, adduction and medial conjunct rotation ensure that the sensitive pad or tip of the thumb is opposed to one or several pads of the fingers. The thenar muscles—the abductor pollicus brevis (APB), flexor pollicus brevis (FPB) and opponens pollicus (OP)—are responsible for positioning the thumb, while the extrinsic flexor pollicus longus (FPL) provides the gripping force. In a cylindrical power grip, used for the handles of sporting equipment, once the thumb has been positioned around the object by the thenar muscles the adductor pollicus is recruited to produce powerful flexion and adduction and close the vice. The adductor pollicus with its large moment arm at the CMC is the power muscle of the thumb (Brand 1985).

The conjunct axial rotation occurring during CMC abduction and flexion is due to the geometry of the saddle shape of the articular surfaces and tension in the obliquely directed ligaments. The ligaments of the CMC joint of the thumb are lateral, volar and dorsal. The lateral ligament is a relatively broad band running from the lateral surface of the trapezium to the radial side of the base of the first metacarpal. The volar and dorsal ligaments are oblique bands which run from the volar and dorsal surfaces of the trapezium, and converge on the ulna side of the base of the first metacarpal (Williams & Warwick 1980). During CMC flexion the dorsal oblique ligament tightens and anchors the ulnar side of the base of the first metacarpal while its radial side is still free to move. Thus a medial rotation of the metacarpal occurs during the movement, particularly towards the end of range. The opponens pollicus, inserted lateral to the long axis of the metacarpal and with a good angle of pull on the bone, is well placed to produce an active medial rotation as it contracts to produce CMC flexion and some abduction. The close-packed and most stable position of the CMC joint is in full opposition, which is particularly useful during power grips.

Reposition of the thumb, essential for opening the hand in preparation for grasp, consists mainly of CMC joint extension. During thumb extension/reposition a lateral rotation of the joint occurs, as the ulnar side of the metacarpal becomes anchored by the volar oblique ligament, while the radial side is again free to move. The abductor pollicus brevis (APB) and longus (APL) commence this movement by abducting and extending the CMC joint, and extension is completed by the extensor pollicus brevis (EPB) and longus (EPL).

Metacarpophalangeal joint

The metacarpophalangeal (MCP) joint of the thumb is a condyloid joint with 2° of freedom, flexion and extension and abduction and adduction. The large biconvex metacarpal head articulates with a much smaller concave area on the base of the proximal phalanx, providing little bony stability to the joint. A loose fibrous capsule surrounds the joint. It is strengthened at the sides by the collateral ligaments, and replaced anteriorly by a fibrocartilaginous plate known as the palmar or volar plate (Fig. 25.6). Flexion and extension are the main movements available, with the range of flexion varying in individuals from as little as 30° to as much as 90–100° (Bejjani & Landsmeer 1989). There is little extension available at the joint, since the articular surface does not extend very far posteriorly on the metacarpal head. There is also some axial conjunct rotation of the MCP joint during flexion, which aids opposition of the pad or tip of the thumb toward the fingers. This conjunct rotation is caused by the lateral side of the head of the

metacarpal having a slightly longer antero-posterior curvature than the medial side, so that the lateral side of the joint moves more as the proximal phalanx is pulled anteriorly and distally by the flexor pollicus brevis muscle. Also, the medial collateral ligament is shorter and more readily tightened than the lateral, so that during flexion the displacement of the base of the proximal phalanx is less on the medial side, resulting in a medial rotation of the joint (Kapandji 1982).

The small amount of abduction available serves to augment that produced at the CMC joint, and increases the web span when attempting to grasp a large object. The range of abduction at this joint varies with the width of the metacarpal head, which is flattened in the coronal plane (Kapandji 1982).

The anterior aspect of the MCP joint of the thumb (Fig. 25.7) reveals features which stabilize the joint against hyperextension forces, such as the volar plate with its

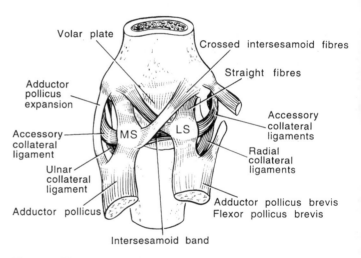

Fig. 25.7 The metacarpophalangeal joint of the thumb, volar aspect. Source: adapted from Kapandji (1982)

attachment to the medial and lateral accessory collateral ligaments, the crossed intersesamoid ligaments (CIL), and the tendons of flexor pollicus brevis and the oblique head of adductor pollicus which insert into the proximal phalanx via the lateral and medial sesamoid bones respectively (Kapandji 1982).

As at the MCP joints of the fingers, the collateral ligaments are taut in flexion and the accessory collateral ligaments are taut in extension, providing the joint with lateral stability in these positions. Contraction of the adductor pollicus provides active stabilization of the MCP joint against forces which tend to abduct the thumb, but the muscle and its aponeurosis do not aid passive stability of the joint (Stener 1985, McCue & Cabrera 1992). The joint is most vulnerable to lateral forces in some degree of flexion, because in extension, resistance to abduction by

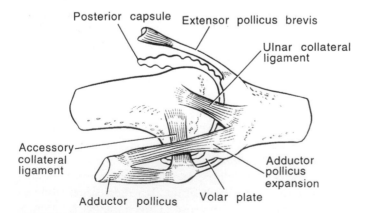

Fig. 25.6 The metacarpophalangeal joint of the thumb, medial aspect. Source: adapted from Kapandji (1982)

the accessory collateral ligament is aided by the volar plate and its attachments (Stener 1985, Nevasier 1992, McCue & Cabrera 1992). However, in a severe abduction extension injury with rupture of both parts of the ulna collateral ligament, the volar plate may be avulsed from its attachments. Instability of the MCP joint in abduction jeopardizes the normal thumb-index pinch essential for normal use of the hand in sport. An additional complication to ulna ligament damage is that the torn end of the ligament may flip out over the expansion of the adductor pollicus to the base of the proximal phalanx, and require surgical repair (Stener lesion).

JOINTS OF THE FINGERS

Metacarpophalangeal joints

The metacarpophalangeal (MCP) joints of the fingers are condyloid joints with 2° of freedom, flexion and extension, and abduction and adduction.

Each articulation consists of a large convex metacarpal head proximally, which articulates with a small concave facet on the base of the proximal phalanx distally. The metacarpal head is covered with articular cartilage for approximately 180° in the sagittal plane, with most of this articular surface lying anteriorly. There is only about 20° of articular surface on the phalanx. Poor mating of surfaces, or joint incongruence, promotes mobility at the MCP joint but provides little stability to the joint during movement.

The fibrous capsule surrounding the MCP joint is loose and is attached closer to the articular margin posteriorly. It is strengthened by the medial and lateral collateral ligaments laterally, and replaced by the volar plate anteriorly (Fig. 25.8a).

The collateral ligaments are cord-like and are attached proximally to the tubercle and adjacent depression on the side of the metacarpal head, posterior to the centre of rotation. From there they pass obliquely downwards and forwards to the lateral aspect of the proximal phalanx. As the joint moves toward flexion the tension in the collateral ligaments increases, reaching a plateau after 45° (Minami et al 1985) (Fig. 25.8b). This is due to the changing radius of curvature of the metacarpal head, causing the distance between the proximal and distal attachments of the ligaments to increase in flexion. Tension in the collateral ligaments in flexion prevents unwanted abduction of the fingers during gripping. During extension the collateral ligaments are loose and permit abduction of the fingers by the interossei, necessary for opening the hand in preparation for grasp (Minami et al 1985).

The palmar or volar plate is a fibrocartilaginous structure attached to the base of the proximal phalanx. The attachment of this plate to the anterior cartilage of the phalanx is formed by a small fibrous band, which acts like a hinge during movement. On each side the volar plate receives

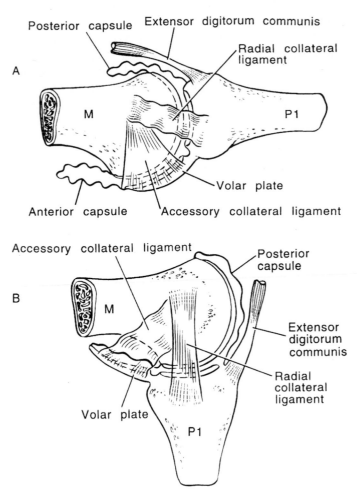

Fig. 25.8 The metacarpophalangeal joint of the finger, lateral view. As the joint moves towards flexion (b) the tension in the collateral ligaments increases. Source: adapted from Kapandji (1982)

the fibres from the accessory collateral ligaments which originate with the cord portion of the collateral ligaments on the metacarpal head. These fibres are loose in flexion, permitting the volar plate to slide along the anterior surface of the metacarpal, facilitated by its flexible membranous proximal portion, and the capsular recess anteriorly (Fig. 25.8b). Thus the volar plate improves the stability of the joint by increasing the amount of articular surface in contact during movement without compromising mobility. The grooved anterior surface of the plate also provides a smooth surface for gliding of the flexor tendons, as well as increasing their moment arm/leverage at the joint. In MCP extension, the accessory collateral ligaments tighten and help prevent MCP hyperextension. As there are no strong check rein ligaments like those found at the proximal interphalangeal (PIP) joints, the lateral bands of the intrinsic muscles provide secondary reinforcement against lateral forces applied to the joint (McCue & Cabrera 1992).

The deep transverse metacarpal ligaments are three short ligaments connecting the palmar/volar plates of the four

MCP joints of the fingers. They bind the metacarpal heads together, and maintain the distal transverse arch of the hand. They are continuous with the palmar interosseus fascia, and blend with the flexor tendon sheaths. They also receive fibres from the distal slips of the palmar aponeurosis, and part of the extensor expansion as it passes forwards on the head of the metacarpal. The interossei pass posterior and the lumbricals, digital vessels and nerves anterior to the deep transverse ligaments (Williams & Warwick 1980).

The range of MCP flexion in the index finger is approximately 90° and increases toward the ulnar side of the hand, with flexion of the little and ring fingers being particularly important for cylindrical power grip. Extension beyond the zero position varies widely among individuals and depends on ligamentous laxity. Abduction and adduction is maximal when the joints are in extension, with the index and little finger having the greatest range and the middle finger being the least mobile. Some axial rotation of the proximal phalanx is available with the MCP joint extended or semi-flexed, due to the laxity of the collateral ligaments in this position. This may be a passive rotation grafted onto the phalanx by the curved shape of the object gripped, or an active rotation produced by an interosseus muscle in association with abduction and adduction (Bejjani & Landsmeer 1989). There is also a conjunct rotation which occurs during MCP flexion due to the asymmetry of the metacarpal heads, and unequal length and tension of the collateral ligaments (Kapandji 1982). In any case, the ability of the phalanx to rotate is useful in approximating the palmar surface of the finger to the surface of a cylindrical handle or curved object to ensure maximal surface contact and sensory feedback, and to produce the best alignment of the finger to facilitate gripping by the long finger flexors.

Interphalangeal joints

The interphalangeal (IP) joints of the hand are inherently different from the MCP joints. The IP joints are hinge joints having 1° of freedom, flexion and extension. The bony shape of the articulating surfaces provides for more lateral stability than that which exists at the MCP joints because the head of the phalanx is pulley-shaped, while the articular base of the distal phalanx has two shallow facets separated by a median ridge, providing a much greater congruence of the opposing articulating surfaces. However, the prime stabilizers of the IP joint are the components of a strong three-sided ligamentous system produced by the collateral ligaments, the accessory collateral ligaments, and the volar plate (Fig. 25.9). The distal attachment of the volar plate to the base of the middle phalanx is quite firm. Proximally the volar plate becomes attenuated centrally as it thickens laterally, where it attaches to the loose areolar tissue of the proximal phalanx forming the two check rein ligaments (McCue & Cabrera 1992). From 0–20° flexion the volar

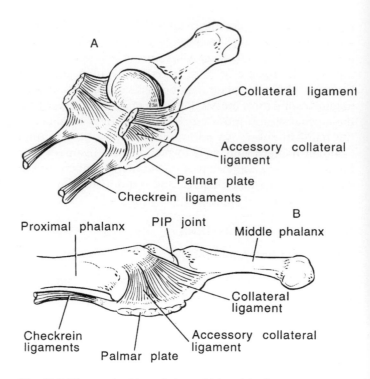

Fig. 25.9 The proximal interphalangeal joint of the fingers. Source: adapted from Bejjani & Landsmeer (1989)

plate and accessory ligaments are taut, stabilizing the joint in extension and preventing hyperextension. In contrast to the MCP joint, the cord-like portion of the collateral ligaments remain taut throughout the entire range of flexion and extension (Kahler and McCue 1992). Proximally these ligaments are attached to the centre of the axis of rotation, and as the head of the phalanx is more spherical than the head of the metacarpal the radius of the head remains fairly constant during finger flexion, producing little change in the length of the ligaments.

The axis of movement for flexion and extension is set obliquely, so that during flexion the fingers move toward the base of the thumb facilitating grasp. Flexion of the proximal interphalangeal (PIP) joint of the index is greater than 90°, and increases toward the ulnar side of the hand with a maximum of about 135° in the little finger. The range of flexion at the distal interphalangeal (DIP) joints is slightly less than 90° and increases slightly from the second to fifth fingers. The PIP has no passive hyperextension, but a small amount occurs at the DIP joint (Kapandji 1982).

Position of safe immobilization

The varying tensions which exist in the ligamentous system in different finger joint positions provide the rationale for the choice of the position of safe immobilization (POSI). In this position the MCP joints are immobilized in at least 45° flexion where the cord-like portion of the collateral ligaments are taut, and the IP joints are immobilized in extension or not more than 15-20° flexion, since the volar plate becomes quite lax in flexion and is prone to becoming contracted if left in this position for long periods.

MUSCLES CONTROLLING FINGER MOVEMENT

Extensor muscles

On the dorsum of the wrist the tendons of the wrist and finger extensors pass through fibro-osseus sheaths that prevent subluxation and act as pulleys (Fig. 25.10). During sporting activities these tendons may be affected by overuse, causing the synovial lining between the tendon and the retinaculum to become inflamed.

On the dorsum of the hand the extensor tendons are relatively thin and wide and vulnerable to injury in this position. They are connected by the juncturae tendinum which diverge from the tendon of the ring finger and connect

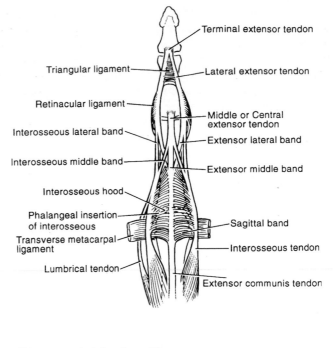

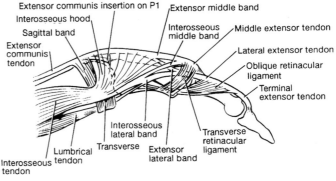

Fig. 25.11 Dorsal and lateral view of the extensor apparatus of the fingers. Source: adapted from Tubiana (1985)

with the long, little and variably the index finger extensor tendons. Laceration of an extensor tendon proximally may be obscured by the contribution of these bands which transfer extension forces to connected fingers (Rosenthal 1990).

In the fingers, the extensor tendons distal to the MCP joints consist of a tendon system, which transmits and imparts motion, and a retinacular system which stabilizes the tendon system (Figs 25.11a, 25.11b). On the dorsum of the MCP joints the broad fibrous hood consists of fibres from the juncturae tendinum, the sagittal bands, and the extensor tendon which has a variable insertion on the base of the proximal phalanx but is not significant for extension of the MCP joint. The sagittal bands are vertically oriented fibres that cover the capsule and the collateral ligaments, and connect the extensor tendons to the volar plate and proximal phalanx on both sides of the joint. It is these sagittal bands which produce extension of the MCP joint.

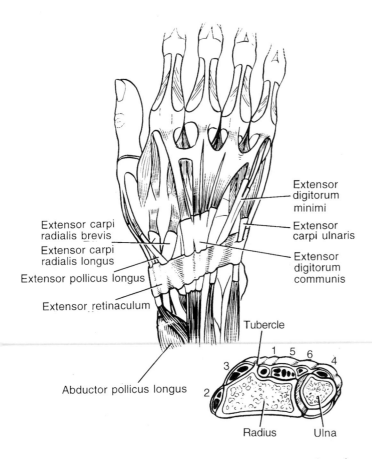

Fig. 25.10 Synovial sheaths occupy the six fibro-osseous tunnels on the dorsum of the wrist deep to the extensor retinaculum. Compartment 1 forms a tunnel for the extensor pollicus longus tendon on the medial side of the dorsal tubercle of the radius. The first radial compartment (2) contains the tendons of APL and EPB. Compartment 3 contains the two major wrist extensors ECRL and ECRB, and compartment (4) houses the ECU tendon. The extensors of the fingers EDC and extensor indicis (EI) occupy compartment 5, and compartment 6 forms a pulley for the tendon of the extensor digiti minimi (EDM). Source: adapted from Boileau Grant (1962)

They also stabilize the extensor tendon on the dorsum of the joint, opposing ulnar displacement forces which are greatest with the MCP joints extended, decrease during the first 60° of flexion, and increase again with greater flexion (Rosenthal 1990). Distal to the sagittal bands the lumbrical and interosseus muscles contribute vertical and distal oblique fibres to the extensor tendons over the proximal phalanx. The vertical fibres assist flexion of the MCP joint and the oblique fibres transmit extensor forces to the PIP and DIP joints. The extensor tendon continues as the central tendon and inserts on the base of the middle phalanx with some medial fibres from the intrinsic tendons. The extensor tendon via the sagittal bands is the only extensor of the MCP joint, and is capable of secondarily extending the IP joints only if hyperextension of the MCP joint is prevented. This is achieved both actively and passively by the interossei and lumbricals which are flexors of the MCP joints and extensors of the IP joints. The conjoined lateral bands represent a continuation of the oblique fibres of the intrinsic tendons with additional lateral fibres from the extensor tendon. The lateral bands continue distally and join over the middle of the distal phalanx to be inserted as a terminal tendon into the base of the distal phalanx. The lateral bands normally lie dorsal to the axis of motion of the PIP joints during extension, and descend to the axis of motion during flexion. Without the shift of the lateral bands the smaller DIP joint would not extend in synchrony with the larger PIP joint due to the difference in radii of both joints (Brand 1985).

The transverse retinacular ligaments consist of fibres which arise from the fibrosseous sheaths of the flexor tendons and the volar plate on the anterior surface of the PIP joints. These fibres course obliquely distally toward the dorsum of the finger lying volar to the lateral bands and covering the insertion of the central tendon and medial fibres of the intrinsic tendons. Their function is to prevent dorsal displacement of the lateral bands and to assist their descent during flexion. They also contribute to axial stability of the PIP joint by limiting unwanted rotations at the joint. The triangular ligament connects the converging lateral bands on the dorsum of the middle phalanx and prevents separation of the bands at this level.

The dorsal plate described by Slattery (1990) is located on the articular surface of the central slip of the extensor tendon overlying the PIP joint. It is a constant structure which is morphologically similar to the patella at the knee joint, and histologically similar to the fibrocartilaginous volar plate at the PIP joint. Its functions appear to include stabilization/centralization of the central extensor tendon, and participation in stabilization of the PIP joint. The collateral ligaments and the volar plate have been described as stabilizers of the lateral and volar aspects of the PIP joint and the dorsal plate completes the picture by providing stability on the dorsal aspect. The articular surface of the dorsal plate is bioconcave with a longitudinal ridge, and this bony shape corresponds exactly to the bicondylar shape of the head of the proximal phalanx. In mechanical terms, the dorsal plate acts as an anatomical pulley in a similar way to the patella. Like the knee joint, the PIP joint flexes to more than 90° and the dorsal plate serves to increase the moment/lever arm for the central extensor of the joint, thus improving the extension torque generated. The dorsal plate also prevents wear to the central extensor tendon as it repetitively flexes and extends over the joint during finger movement, and possibly plays a role in facilitating circulation of synovial fluid (Slattery 1990).

The oblique retinacular ligament arises from the fibrosseus sheath of the flexor tendons on the volar surface of the proximal phalanx. It passes dorsally and distally deep to the transverse retinacular ligament and volar to the axis of the PIP joint. As the ligament approaches the DIP joint, its fibres intermingle with those of the terminal extensor tendon. The ligament passes dorsal to the axis of the DIP joint and is inserted into the base of the distal phalanx, adjacent to the terminal extensor tendon. The oblique retinacular ligament is put under tension by extension of the PIP joint, and passively aids the fully flexed DIP joint to return to mid flexion, assisted by the collateral ligaments and the dorsal capsule. However, only active contraction of the terminal extensor tendon is capable of completing extension of the DIP joint (Rosenthal 1990).

Flexor muscles

All the extrinsic digital flexors pass through the carpal tunnel, where the flexor retinaculum forms a broad restraining pulley at the wrist preventing bowstringing of the flexor tendons. Each finger has a flexor digitorum profundus tendon inserting on the distal phalanx. The counterpart to the thumb is the flexor pollicus longus. The muscle bellies of the flexor profundi to the long, ring and little fingers are often common and interdependent in the forearm, while the muscle belly of the flexor digitorum profundus to the index finger and the flexor pollicus longus each has a separate and identifiable independent muscle belly. Occasionally there is some interdependence between the flexor profundus to the index finger and the flexor pollicus longus (Williams & Warwick 1980). Each of the four fingers also has a flexor digitorum superficialis tendon, which lies superficial to the profundus tendon in the palm. As it passes into the finger it flattens, then splits at the level of the proximal phalanx. Its two flat tails surround the profundus tendon and intersect behind it to insert at the level of the middle phalanx, while the profundus passes through to insert into the base of the distal phalanx. The muscle bellies of the flexor digitorum superficialis tendon lie superficial on the palmar aspect of the forearm and are independent from one another. The flexor digitorum profundus is active during unresisted flexion of the fingers, and is aided by the flexor digitorum superficialis if the wrist is flexed or resistance to flexion increases (Long & Brown 1964, Long 1968). During functional activities, the action of the extrinsic long finger flexors on the interphalangeal joints is balanced by the action of the intrinsic muscles, which by their ability to extend the interphalangeal joints (Backhouse & Catton 1954) enable many different postures of the finger between full flexion and extension to be adopted (Landsmeer & Long 1965, Long 1968).

Flexor tendon pulley system

In each digit, the flexor tendons are surrounded by their synovial sheath and held against the phalanges by a fibrous sheath. As the finger is flexed, the five strong annular pulleys keep the tendons close to the phalanges and prevent bowstringing of the tendons over the joints, which would result an increased tendon excursion at that joint (Bejjani & Landsmeer 1989), and inadequate excursion and subsequent weakness in the more distal joints (Brand 1985). The most critical pulleys are the A2 and A4 pulleys. The three cruciform pulleys (C1, C2, C3) are thinner and more pliable than the annular pulleys, and allow flexibility while still providing support and stability of the fibrous flexor sheath. Within the sheath the blood supply to the tendons is via the vincula which are fed by constant branches of the digital arteries (Fig. 25.12). These branches originate from the digital arteries roughly at the level of the MCP and IP joints (Amadio et al 1992).

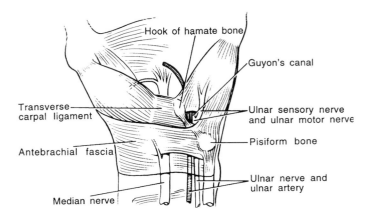

Fig. 25.13 The ulna nerve at the wrist.
Source: adapted from Clark et al (1993)

NERVES OF THE HAND

Median nerve

The wedge-shaped carpal bones tied together by the flexor retinaculum create the carpal tunnel through which the median nerve gains entry into the hand. After passing through the carpal tunnel, the nerve divides into sensory branches, and the recurrent motor nerve to the thenar muscles APB, OP, and the superficial head of FPB. There are also motor branches to the radial two lumbricals from the nerves passing to the index and middle fingers. The sensory nerves supply the palmar aspect and dorsum of the distal phalanx of the thumb, index and middle fingers, and the radial side of the ring finger. The median nerve may be injured following fracture of the distal radius, or the nerve may be compressed by increased volume in the carpal tunnel due to swelling or haematoma, or by being immobilized in an acute flexion posture of the wrist.

Ulna nerve

The ulna nerve is vulnerable to compressive forces at the wrist (Fig. 25.13). It approaches the hand on the lateral side of the flexor carpi ulnaris tendon, and becomes superficial at the wrist, passing in three tunnels into the palm. The first is Guyon's canal, which lies beneath the palmaris brevis muscle and fascia. At this point the nerve gives off deep motor branches to the palmaris brevis, and to the abductor digit minimi (ADM) and superficial branches, including a proper digital nerve to the ulnar side of the little finger, and a common digital nerve to the adjacent sides of the little and ring fingers. The deep branch of the ulna nerve then passes through two more components of the ulna tunnel at the wrist/hand level. The first is the piso hamate tunnel, which lies between the hook of the hamate and the pisiform. Here the nerve may be subject to damage from fractures of the hook of the hamate, which frequently occur as a result of falls, particularly with a tennis

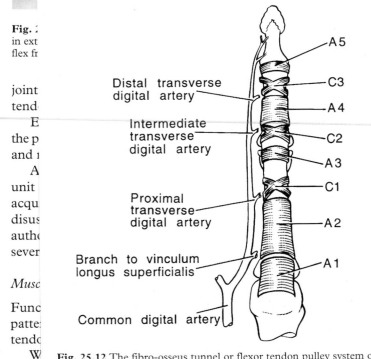

Fig. 25.12 The fibro-osseus tunnel or flexor tendon pulley system on the volar aspect of the fingers. Source: adapted from Van Strien (1990)

will be able to flex the PIP joints while maintaining the DIP extension.

To test for extensor indicis (EI) and extensor digitorum minimi (EDM) ask the athlete to flex the middle and ring fingers into the palm then, while maintaining this flexion, attempt extension of the index and little fingers. By keeping the middle and ring fingers flexed, extensor digitorum communis (EDC) action is eliminated.

Froment's sign tests for the ulnar innervated adductor pollicis. The athlete grips a piece of paper between the thumb and the radial side of the index finger, with the IP joint of the thumb extended. The test is positive when, on resisting the paper being pulled away, the thumb is unstable, moving into the trick movement of thumb IP joint flexion.

Measuring strength

Strength can be measured with a dynamometer and a pinch meter but this is not often necessary. The ability to perform the functional activities of daily living, followed by return to the sport, is a relevant assessment of progression and recovery.

Oedema

Oedema can be measured by noting the finger circumference. However, palpation for pitting oedema and observation of restrictions in range of movement are usually sufficient guides in sports injuries.

Sensory testing

Extensive testing is not often required in sports injuries. Light touch and moving two-point discrimination is assessed when the athlete describes sensory loss and parasthesia or blunt trauma. Tinel's sign is used as an adjunct in diagnosis of compression injuries and neuromas.

The developing field of adverse neural tension is providing exciting new avenues of treating residual pain after forearm and hand injuries. Tension tests have been devised for the median, ulnar and median nerves to diagnose and treat this adverse tension (Butler 1991).

Pathology of the cervical and thoracic spine, elbow and shoulder should always be considered as a source of pain, when regional pathology is uncertain.

Radiography

The wrist has traditionally been difficult to examine, but modern techniques of imaging of the hand have increased the accuracy of diagnosis and treatment of wrist problems. Taleisnek (1985) and Poznanski (1991) discuss X-rays, arthrography and computed tomography. The developing field of wrist arthroscopy can allow injuries to be viewed,

diagnosed and surgically treated with minimally invasive incisions (Whipple & Geissler 1991). Bone scans can be helpful in chronic wrist pain with indeterminate signs.

INJURIES TO THE WRIST AND HAND

Fractures

Distal radius

The common Colles' and Smith's fractures usually occur as a result of a fall on the outstretched hand in field games and contact sports. Resultant radial shortening will predispose the wrist to arthritis and wrist stiffness (Palmer 1988).

In these fractures there is a risk of median nerve compression giving an acute carpal tunnel syndrome and vasomotor disturbance causing a development of Sudeck's atrophy approximately six weeks later. Always check that fingertip sensation and circulation is satisfactory (Frykman & Nelson 1990).

After reduction, either closed or open, a plaster is applied which should leave the MCP joints and the thumb free.

Epiphyseal fractures involving the radial epiphysis are common in children 6-10 years old. Even if there is poor reduction, good functional results are usually achieved unless the epiphyseal plate is damaged, leading to premature closure and subsequent radial shortening (Palmer 1988).

Carpal bones

Scaphoid fracture. This occurs as result of compression of the scaphoid when there is a fall onto the outstretched hand in wrist hyperextension, with additional ulnar or radial stress altering the nature of the fracture (Dobyns & Gabel 1990, Taleisnik 1985). It is most common in the young adult male and is rare in children.

The patient presents with tenderness and swelling in the anatomical snuff-box and a reluctance to move the wrist and thumb. Initial radiographs may not disclose a fracture and the X-ray should be repeated or a bone scan performed if the pain and stiffness do not resolve. In the interim the wrist and thumb are kept well supported, preferably in a plaster extending to, but not including, the distal palmar crease and the thumb IP joint.

Fractures are commonly through the middle third, or waist, of the scaphoid, being classified as horizontal oblique, transverse or vertical oblique. Less frequently seen are fractures of the proximal and distal thirds of the scaphoid.

Stable fractures are treated conservatively, the immobilization time varying from six weeks to six months, depending on radiographic evidence of healing. Green (1988) advises inclusion of the elbow if the fracture is three weeks or later in presenting. Forceful finger exercises and daily activities which place stress across the fracture site, potentially impeding healing, should be avoided but gentle daily use should be encouraged (Taleisnik 1988).

Unstable fractures need to be internally fixed. Non-unions and avascular necrosis are treated with bone graft, arthrodesis or arthroplasty (Taleisnik 1988).

Complications. Fractures of the middle third are often complicated by associated carpal instability and late presentation, leading to non-union. Healing of fractures of the proximal third is compromised by 'the strikingly poor blood supply to the proximal pole' (Taleisnik 1988, p. 835). These factors may give rise to subsequent non-union and avascular necrosis.

Differential diagnosis. de Quervain's disease presents as pain about the scaphoid and distal radius, but has a history of repetition rather than the impact history of scaphoid fracture. Persistent pain, without evidence of scaphoid fracture, could indicate carpal instability. Osteoarthritis of the base of the thumb presents with tenderness along the CMC joint line and not in the anatomical snuff-box. Radial collateral ligament sprain will be positive to ulnar stress test and will have a negative scaphoid investigations.

Lunate fracture. This occurs with a hyperextension force and requires reduction and immobilization (Zemmel 1986).

Lunatomalacia or Keinboch's disease is a collapse of the lunate long after a minor injury or repeated trauma of compression forces. It is seen in gymnastics, karate, volleyball and tennis. The aetiology is uncertain. Some lunate fractures progress to lunatomalacia, and associated primary circulatory changes may be significant. Surgical management is usually required as the natural history is of progressive degeneration (Taleisnik 1985).

Presentation is of persistent wrist pain aggravated by activities. There may be some localized swelling and tenderness dorsal to the lunate, with marked weakness of grip and some loss of wrist movement.

Hook of hamate fracture. This occurs with a direct blow, a fall on the hand or when the sporting equipment being held in the hand strikes the hamate, such as when a golf club hits the ground. The athlete can usually clearly recall the injury-causing incident (Parker et al 1986, Zemel 1986, Culver 1990).

There is a persistent dull ache about the ulnar side of the wrist and hand and tenderness over the tip of the hook and the dorsal/ulnar aspect of the hamate. Wrist flexion and extension increase the pain and there is decreased grip strength.

Oblique and carpal tunnel X-ray views are required to view the hook. If the pain does not settle with conservative measures, surgical removal of the hook is undertaken, followed by rest and return to sport as pain dictates.

Untreated fractures may give rise to subsequent complications of pressure on the ulnar nerve and rupture of the FDP (Parker et al 1986).

Pisiform fractures, subluxations and dislocations. These occur usually with a fall on the outstretched hand with the wrist in dorsiflexion. The athlete complains of pain on passive wrist extension, when the opposing force of the flexor carpi ulnaris (FCU) compresses the pisiform against the triquetral, on active wrist flexion and ulnar deviation when the pisiform is pulled by the FCU, and by passively moving the pisiform from side to side.

Healing should occur when the wrist is splinted in slight volar flexion. If disabling pain persists the pisiform can be excised.

Trapezium fracture. This fracture accounts for less than 5% of all carpal fractures, being caused by a longitudinal force to the abducted thumb, as in falling with a racquet in hand or by a direct blow on the abducted thumb in contact sports (Zemel 1986). Localized swelling and tenderness and weakness of pinch grip are noted immediately after injury. The fracture is confirmed by Bett's and carpal tunnel view X-rays (Taleisnik 1988). Undisplaced fractures require 4–6 weeks immobilization. Displaced fractures are surgically fixed with screws or K-wire.

Joint injuries

Inferior radioulnar joint

Injuries of this joint, usually caused by a fall on the outstetched hand, give painful pronation and supination, intermittent clicking, weakness of grip and local tenderness. If the problem does not resolve in 4-6 weeks with standard soft tissue treatments, arthroscopic examination and repair may be required (Whipple & Geissler 1991). Possible diagnoses include TFCC disruption, ulnar styloid fracture, ulnar length discrepancy and snapping ECU tendon (Bowers 1988, Nathan & Schneider 1991).

Radiocarpal and intercarpal joints

Injuries to these joints, usually as a result of a fall, are potentially disabling, the more severe disruptions, such as scapholunate dissociation, perilunate and trans-scaphoid perilunate dislocations, giving rise to carpal instability and disabling degenerative changes. The injuring forces are not necessarily severe, so even apparently minor injuries should be adequately investigated. Late diagnosis is a common problem (Taleisnik 1985, Green 1988).

On presentation immediately after the injury there is generally moderate swelling over the dorsum of the hand and wrist, in the anatomical snuff-box and distal to the head of the ulnar. The athlete should be able to pinpoint the most painful area.

Careful and thorough palpation by the therapist should be done on the radial and ulnar styloid processes, Lister's tubercle, the distal radioulnar joint, the triangular fibro-cartilage, the anatomical snuff-box, the dorsal scapholunate ligament, the triquetropisiform ligament, and the luno-triquetral ligament to try to reproduce the athlete's pain.

Watson's test for scapholunate instability is performed by moving the athlete's wrist passively into ulnar deviation, then stabilizing the scaphoid anteriorly with the examiner's thumb. The wrist is then passively radially deviated. If dorsal pain is thus elicited, scapholunate dissociation is present, the scaphoid subluxing dorsally. This subluxation may be accompanied by crepitus and may be palpated dorsally by the examiner's fingers (Taleisnik 1985).

Wrist movement is variably limited with episodes of severe catch-type pain. Grip strength is weak. The swelling may increase significantly over the next few days.

X-rays aid in the diagnosis. It is outside the scope of this book to discuss radiographic techniques but the therapist should be aware of the following important signs which are evidence of carpal instability:

• An increased gap between the scaphoid and lunate compared with the other hand (the Terry Thomas sign)
• Palmar tipping of the lunate, known as the 'spilled tea-cup' sign seen in lateral X-ray views
• Palmar flexing of the scaphoid when the wrist is in neutral and an overlap between the proximal and distal carpal rows. (Koman et al 1990, Bond & Berquist 1991, Whipple & Geissler 1991)

Surgical intervention followed by immobilization is frequently required to give the athlete the optimal chance of satisfactory return to sport and to normal daily function (Koman et al 1990).

Differential diagnosis. Osteoarthritis may have an underlying, undiagnosed carpal instability. Rheumatoid arthritis is excluded by blood tests. de Quervain's syndrome is usually able to be excluded by a negative Finkelstein's test (Fig. 25.16).

Treatment of wrist injuries

During periods of immobilization in plaster treatment is directed toward oedema control and regaining and main-taining full range of finger movements.

After the plaster is removed massage the palm, wrist and forearm, seeking out tender areas along joint lines, gently working the MCP joints into hyperextension and stretching the intrinsic muscles. Proceed to frictions along the joint lines of the digits and over the underlying flexor and extensor tendons, facilitating the breakdown of

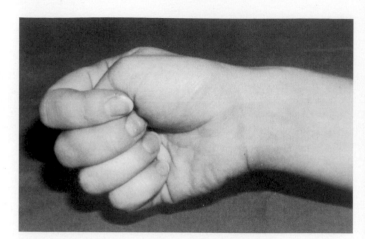

Fig. 25.16 Finkelstein's text for de Quervain's syndrome. The patient is instructed to clench the fingers over the thumb and perform ulnar deviation. If pain is elicited, it is said to be a positive Finkelstein's text. (Source: Katie Watkin)

adhesions acquired at the time of injury or because of immobilization.

Continue all finger exercises, emphasizing thumb opposition to the base of the little finger, a movement that will have been restricted by the plaster. Commence active wrist exercises and functional activities.

Orthotics

Splinting is used in the post-immobilization phase. Palmer (1988) advocates that all distal radial fractures be protected with a prefabricated splint for 2-3 weeks.

The author prefers custom-made thermoplastic splints, which can be remoulded as wrist extension increases. The same splint can then be used for returning to sport (Fig. 25.17).

Tenosynovitis of radial wrist extensors

The tendons and sheaths of ECRL and ECRB are subject to injury in canoeing, rowing and racquet sports, where repeated wrist extension gives rise to inflammation, causing pain, oedema and limitation of movement. This is also known as the intersection syndrome (Froimson 1988, Stern 1990).

Athletes who rapidly increase their workload are susceptible to this overuse syndrome, including both novice and elite athletes. Increases of greater than 10% of the present workload without recovery time are not acceptable (see Ch. 7).

Overuse injury progresses through stages from pain only at the end of the activity with full recovery between training sessions to pain that prevents performance and is present during normal activity (Larkins 1988).

There is pain and a characteristic fusiform swelling 4-6 cm proximal to the wrist on the radial aspect of the dorsal forearm. Repeated wrist extension performed with a closed fist reproduces the pain. Crepitus may be felt on repeated wrist extension, as the tendons move in the sheath.

Differential diagnosis. It is important to differentiate this injury from de Quervain's syndrome where there is a positive Finkelstein's test. A fractured radius is excluded by X-ray.

Treatment. In the early stages, when pain disappears between sessions the athlete may continue to train, but the workload and technique should be reviewed. Ice packs must be used after the activity.

Check that the athlete has a good warm-up routine of jogging and sprinting along the bank or around the court. This uses the large muscles of the legs to increase the blood supply to the muscular system more rapidly than by using the small muscles of the forearm and hand to do the specific action of the sport.

In the more advanced stages immediate total rest is essential. The wrist is supported with a firm figure of eight bandage, a plaster back slab or a volar thermoplastic splint. Ultrasound can be applied daily to the entire musculo-tendinous unit.

Massage is given extensively to the tight and tender muscle bellies in the proximal half of the forearm. It seems reasonable to assume that the elastic muscle unit is liable to shorten as a result of an overuse injury, whereas the inelastic tendon, unless ruptured, will not change its length. The contracted muscle belly exerts a pull on the tendon, lifting it from its optimal position in a bowstring effect. This will accentuate the friction between the tendon and the sheath.

When wrist extension can be performed without crepitus or pain, commence gentle activity with the bandage on. If a splint has been worn, replace it with a bandage. Progress to weaning off the bandage and resuming sport.

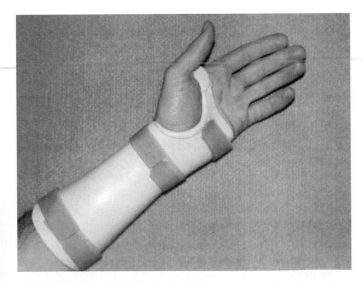

Fig. 25.17 Volar wrist splint to immobilize wrist injuries
Source: Katie Watkin

Minimize the likelihood of recurrence by analysing the athlete's sporting technique, adjusting the equipment and setting out a graduated training program.

De Quervain's syndrome (stenosing tenovaginitis)

This is an inflammation of the tendons and sheath of APL and EPB in the first dorsal compartment of the wrist, with subsequent thickening and stenosis.

It is caused by direct trauma, repetitive lifting, and gripping (usually involving radial deviation with the thumb fixed in the gripping position), in sports such as rowing, table tennis, weight lifting, weight training and contact sports.

There is pain and tenderness over the radial styloid with variable radiation into the forearm, thumb and first web space. A fusiform swelling may be present in the area of the radial styloid. Finkelstein's test is usually positive. The muscle bellies of APL and EPB are tight and tender.

Finkelstein's test. Have the patient place the thumb in the palm, grasp the thumb firmly with fingers, then ulnar deviate the wrist. Pain over the radial styloid is a positive sign (Fig. 25.16).

Differential diagnosis. Tenosynovitis of ECRL and ECRB is excluded with a negative Finkelstein test. Rheumatoid and osteoarthritis can be diagnosed by blood tests and X-ray. Dorsal and volar wrist ganglions have a typical appearance and position. Scaphoid fracture is excluded by X-ray. Neuritis of the superficial branch of the radial nerve will usually have a history of direct trauma to the dorsum of the wrist (Malick & Kasch 1984).

Treatment. The thumb and wrist must be immobilized. A firm bandage in a figure of eight about the wrist and thumb may be sufficient support, but usually a custom-made long opponens splint with the wrist in 15° of extension, the CMC joint in 40° of palmar abduction and the thumb MCP joint in 10° of flexion is necessary. The splint extends to the thumb IP joint. As the fingers remain free there is little interference with daily activities (Fig. 25.18). Ice and ultrasound are applied to the musculotendinous unit.

After 24–48 hours begin massage to the muscle bellies. As pain, local tenderness and swelling subside commence active thumb abduction and reposition exercises within the limits of pain. Also begin Finkelstein stretches. The stretch should be performed gently until the pain is felt, maintained for 15 seconds then relaxed. Repeat 3 or 4 times. Progress by increasing the amount of stretch as pain allows.

Progress to weaning off the splint, combined with increasing light activities, avoiding actions that cause pain. Return to sport is managed with attention to technique and work load and protective splinting or taping (Totten 1990).

Surgical intervention, involving incision of the sheath, is required when conservative methods fail to give lasting

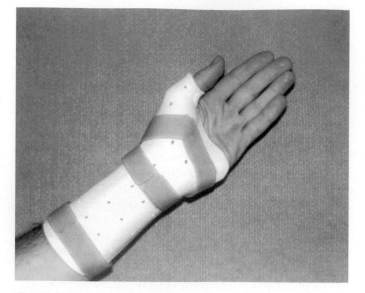

Fig. 25.18 Long opponens splint to immobilize wrist and thumb. Source: Katie Watkin

relief (Kapila 1988). Post-operatively the wrist and thumb are immobilized for 1-21 days then treated as above (Osterman et al 1988).

INJURIES TO THE THUMB

Injury mechanisms and initial management of fractures and sprains/dislocations of the thumb metacarpal and CMC joint respectively require individual discussion but rehabilitation can be dealt with collectively.

Metacarpal fractures

Intra-articular

Bennett's fracture. This is a fracture-dislocation of the base of the metacarpal extending into the carpo-metacarpal joint, with a large dorsal fragment separated from the small volar fragment by the pull of the abductor pollicis longus. It is caused by punching with a clenched fist or direct impact to the base of the thumb. The thumb will be swollen and can appear shortened. Reduction is difficult to achieve and maintain. Internal fixation is usually necessary.

Rolando's fracture. This is a fracture of the base of the metacarpal, sometimes comminuted, with a volar and a dorsal fragment extending into the joint. Reduction is difficult to achieve, so treatment is symptomatic, immobilizing for two weeks to relieve pain, followed by mobilization attempting to remould the joint surfaces.

Extra-articular fractures

These can be transverse or oblique. Treatment is directed at immobilizing the thumb and wrist for four weeks, surgical

intervention being unnecessary unless there is unacceptable shortening of the metacarpal (Brunstrom 1962, Green & Rowland 1975).

Carpometacarpal joint injuries

Sprain

This injury occurs following a stretch beyond normal limits of the joint ligaments. Falling on the outstretched hand, contact with a fast moving ball, or tangling with an opponent are all possible causes. Previous minor trauma may be a predisposing factor.

The patient presents with a painful base of thumb and possible proximal and distal radiation of the pain which is aggravated by active and passive movements of the thumb and wrist. The injury-causing event can be remembered.

There is limitation of opposition and reposition and associated bruising and oedema of the thenar eminence.

Dislocation

This occurs as a result of a longitudinal force on the metacarpal. It is an uncommom injury on its own because the strength of the anterior oblique ligament is such that avulsion of the volar base of the metacarpal occurs, giving a Bennett's fracture-dislocation (see above). Reduction can be achieved but is difficult to maintain, open reduction and internal fixation usually being required. Continuing instability presenting as weakness of grip and persistent pain is a problem.

Differential diagnosis. These injuries must be distinguished from scaphoid, Bennett's and Rolando's fractures by X-ray.

Treatment

To protect the thumb in the initial stages of a sprain, or after removal of plaster, use a 5 cm wide heavy crepe bandage in a figure of eight about the thumb and wrist. The thumb should be in opposition to the index finger and the interphalangeal joint should be left free.

Massage and frictions are given to the thenar eminence, thumb, first web space and hand. The muscle bellies of the extrinsic hand muscles, usually tight as a result of sprain occurring at the time of injury, reinforced by the period of immobilization, require deep massage. Continue for 5-15 minutes, being guided by the patient's response. Aim for reduction in tenderness and stiffness by the end of the session.

- Passive exercise. After massage gently move joints to the limits of passive range. Accessory gliding may also be performed. Corrigan and Maitland (1983) give a detailed description of these techniques.

- Active exercise. Emphasize reposition, opposition and abduction. Reposition is performed with the hand palm-down on a table. Opposition is aimed firstly to the tip, then to the base of the little finger, and finally to the distal palmar crease. Repeat two hourly, or as tolerated. Exercise putty and the light activities of daily living are gradually introduced.

Ultrasound, using underwater technique or a small diameter sound head, can be helpful (Taylor Mullins 1990).

Orthotics. A long opponens splint (Fig. 25.18) gives the best protection for return to sport after Bennett's and Rolando's fractures, but some athletes prefer to compromise with a hand-based splint (Fig. 25.19). Sprains require protection in a splint only until there is full range of movement.

A radiodorsal hand-based splint, extending from the CMC joint to the IP joint, will be sufficient protection for the extra-articular fractures (Fig. 25.19).

Carpometacarpal joint osteoarthritis

This problem occurs in the years after trauma to the joint, or in the middle and later years of life as a result of years of manual work, not necessarily heavy but usually involving repeated pinch grip. It is more common in women than men. Prolonged forceful gripping as in tennis, hockey and rowing may aggravate pre-existing arthritic changes.

There is a dull ache in the base of the thumb, variably spreading into the hand and forearm, with intermittent sharp pain on activity. This activity may be the sport itself, or a simple action like turning a door handle. The sharp pain may cause dropping of the equipment or at least relaxation of the hold, so control of the stroke is reduced. An increase in activity may cause night pain sufficient to disturb sleep.

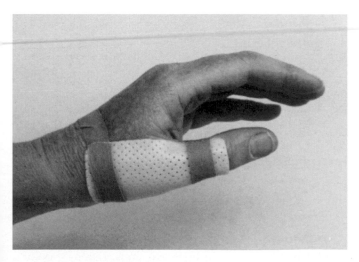

Fig. 25.19 A radio-dorsal hand-based splint, taped into position for protection of extra-articular metacarpal fractures. Radial view

X-rays may show degenerative changes in the joint, the apparent severity of which is not necessarily related to the presenting symptoms.

Clinical assessment is very important. The joint line is tender on palpation, particularly along the anterior aspect, which is often prominent. The part of the thenar eminence adjacent to the joint is tender. If the problem is longstanding, with the pain affecting the way in which the thumb is used, there may be disuse atrophy of the thenar muscles, the grip being weak.

Pain on active and passive movement is present, with the sharp pain experienced on some activities being reproduced by axial compression along the metacarpal. As a general rule, full abduction, midway between opposition and reposition, gives the most active pain, while full reposition gives the most passive pain. This is presumably because the roughened articular surfaces are closely approximated, the difference in active and passive pain being explained by protective muscular actions being present in the former.

Differential diagnosis. Osteoarthritis is distinguished from de Quervain's syndrome by having a negative Finkelstein test and from other bony pathology by X-ray. It is commonly seen in association with carpal tunnel syndrome (Malick & Kasch 1984, Connolly 1980).

Treatment. Commence with frictions to the joint line, concentrating on the most tender areas of the joint. Continue the massage to the thenar eminence, first web space and the intercarpal joints. These adjacent areas are likely to be painful because normal movement patterns have been altered. Resultant soft tissue contraction occurs. Repeat two to three times a day, and before sport participation. Even acute painful joints benefit from gentle frictions.

- Active exercise. Unresisted range of movement exercises are practised twice daily. As the range increases, sport participation will become less painful. Opposition, reposition and abduction are performed separately, then add the combined action of opposition to reposition via full abduction. It is this action that gives the sharp pain in sport and daily use, i.e. the position of open grip used for racquet, bat, and door handles. Add finger exercises if required.
- Ice massage after sport and other pain-provoking activities will reduce next day soreness.
- Joint protection techniques are taught, using the principles of unloading the joint, avoiding detrimental pain and static posture (Leonard 1990).

Orthotics. A short opponens splint (Fig. 25.20) is generally effective in reducing the pain of daily activities. However, if the pain is not relieved, a long opponens splint should be used (Fig. 25.18).

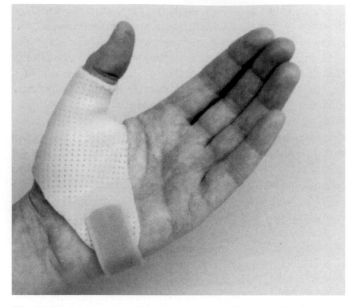

Fig. 25.20 Anterior view of a short opponens splint, used for symptomatic relief of the thumb CMC osteoarthritis. Note the extension of the splint around the ulnar border which further limits CMC joint movement

For sport participation, a soft neoprene support or taping allows an easier grip on equipment than the rigid or semi-rigid thermoplastics, and may give sufficient support. Equipment may need to be padded, and the frequency and duration of participation may need to be reduced.

Metacarpophalangeal joint injuries

Ulnar collateral ligament tear

This injury is known also as skier's or gamekeeper's thumb. It is caused by a fall on the outstretched hand when a radial deviation force is applied to the abducted and extended thumb. Skiers are at risk because the ski poles further force the joint into radial deviation (Dray & Eaton 1988).

There is weakness and pain on pinch and grasp activities. The ulnar aspect of the joint is swollen and tender. The joint is variably unstable to radial stress, depending on the completeness of the rupture, an indication of this being determined by measuring the degree of radial deviation under stress. Greater than 30° is regarded as complete rupture. Plain X-rays should be taken to diagnose accompanying avulsion fractures.

Treatment for an incomplete tear. Rest is supplied by a bandage or short opponens splint, according to the severity of the sprain. Avoid putting stress on the ulnar collateral ligament.

Introduce massage to the first web space, thenar eminence, thumb phalanges and joint lines after the initial pain has subsided.

The exercise program should aim to regain full range of thumb span, thereby reducing long-term splint dependency for sport. Commence with thumb IP joint, finger and wrist movements, progressing to opposition, reposition and abduction, the latter movements ensuring the MCP joint is used in a normal pattern. It is difficult to exercise the MCP joint in isolation.

Orthotics. A lightweight thermoplastic short opponens splint is made for returning to sport. Take care that the splint does not place any radial stress on the joint (Fig. 25.20).

Campbell et al (1992) suggest using a well-padded fibreglass spica cast, applied immediately after the injury is diagnosed, for an immediate return to skiing. Both the thermoplastic splint and the cast can be moulded around a ski pole to allow a good grip of the pole.

Treatment for a complete rupture. This injury is generally thought to require surgical repair because the adductor pollicis aponeurosis is interposed between the ruptured ligament and its insertion Healing of the ligament in its correct anatomical length therefore cannot take place. After surgery the thumb is immobilized in a thumb spica for four weeks. Mobilization then proceeds as for incomplete rupture.

Hyperextension sprain

This sprain is seen in contact sports and ball handling games such as basketball, netball and Australian Rules football when the thumb is forced into hyperextension. The volar plate, the anterior part of the capsule, the muscles of the thenar eminence and FPL are involved.

There is pain on hyperextension of the thumb, and swelling and tenderness about the joint and thenar eminence.

Differential diagnosis. A radial stress test is required to exclude ulnar collateral ligament rupture, although in any hyperextension injury, there may well be some associated damage to the ulnar collateral ligament. An X-ray will exclude a fracture extending into the joint surface.

Treatment. After 24-48 hours massage the joint line and thenar eminence, gently moving the joint into extension. Proceed on to active exercises of opposition and reposition.

Orthotics. A radiodorsal splint is moulded from the interphalangeal joint to the base of the metacarpal, the joint being fixed in 10-20° flexion. The splint must have sufficient depth to protect the joint from lateral stress.

Interphalangeal joint sprain

Interphalangeal joint sprain is treated with rest in a dorsal splint in slight flexion, with active movement commencing as pain subsides.

Differential diagnosis. Damage to the volar plate is treated as for finger volar plate avulsions. Extensor pollicis longus avulsion is detected by an absence of active IP extension and and radiological evidence.

Phalangeal fractures

Proximal phalangeal fracture

The implications of this fracture are not as serious as those of the finger phalanges because of the simpler anatomical arrangements of the thumb, with its two phalanges compared to the three of the other digits. However, fractures extending into the joint surface may need open reduction and internal fixation to preserve length and future function. Treatment is aimed at pain relief with a splint providing protection, followed by regaining movement with frictions and active exercise.

Distal phalangeal fracture

This fracture is treated in the same way as fractures of the distal phalanx of the fingers.

INJURIES TO THE FINGERS

With all finger injuries there is a likelihood of long-term loss of full range movement. It is important to realise the value of splinting in regaining range of finger joint movement after injury. Splints supply a light pressure over a long period to increase range of movement, in contrast to forceful overpressure which causes an increase in pain and oedema and does not achieve an increase in range (Malick 1982, Cannon et al 1985, Fess & Philips 1987) (see Ch. 10).

Fractures

Fractures of the digits occur in sports where the hands are liable to crush, lateral and hyperextension forces, and being caught in equipment and clothing. Boxers and itinerant fighters notoriously suffer fracture of the neck of the fifth metacarpal. In many sports the hands are unprotected but constantly used away from the body, rendering them vulnerable to fracture.

These fractures should be treated with the utmost respect, as overlooking an unstable fracture or incorrectly treating a stable fracture can have long-term disabling effects. The position of safe immobilization (POSI), where the MCP joints are in full flexion and the IP joints in full extension, must be maintained, provided that the healing of the fracture in a good alignment is not compromised. At the same time it is very important to assess associated soft tissue injuries in the digits which, if neglected, may seriously detract from a favourable outcome (Green & Rowland 1975, Boscheinen-Morrin et al 1985, Kapila 1988, O'Brien 1988, Hankin & Peel 1990, Wilson & Carter 1990).

Spiral fractures of the digits involving the joint surfaces have no inherent stability, the two fragments slipping on each other. Similarly, transverse fractures of the shaft of the proximal phalanx shaft are unstable, becoming angulated volarly by the dorsal pull of the central extensor slip and lumbrical on the distal side of the fracture, and the volar pull by the interosseous on the base of the proximal fragment. These unstable fractures require internal fixation.

Complications are bad union with angulation and rotation, tendon adhesions, persistent joint stiffness, infection from open wounds (especially from a human bite), tendon and nerve damage, and stiffness of non-involved digits.

Metacarpal fractures

These fractures often have a diagnostic feature of associated gross oedema of the dorsum of the hand. Stable fractures are protected with a dorsal splint for 1-2 weeks to allow healing.

Fractures of the neck are subject to angulation. This must be assessed for acceptability. The second and third metacarpals can have up to 15° angulation, the fifth metacarpal 50°. These fractures can be reduced by manipulation and maintained by a plaster including the wrist but not the PIP joints.

Open reduction is required when the fracture cannot be reduced by manipulation or a reduction can not be maintained. The fracture is fixed with K-wires or plates and screws, the latter allowing an earlier return to sport. Post-operativly, hand or forearm-based splinting is used for 2-5 weeks (Figs. 25.29a, 25.29b).

Treatment is directed to reduction of oedema in fingers and hand. Wrist movements are commenced as pain allows, followed by gentle active PIP and DIP flexion and extension, intrinsic stretches and MCP flexion and extrinsic extension. It is not uncommon for an extensor lag to develop, a result of the tendon being involved in the area of fracture and subject to adhesion formation. The lag is treated by using a splint to support the MCP joint in full extension, IP joints free, between exercise sessions, or by buddy taping to the adjacent digit for all activities (Green & Rowland 1975, O'Brien 1988) (Fig. 25.21).

Orthotics. Return to sport may be hastened by wearing a padded, light thermoplastic splint, moulded over the dorsum of the hand. Ensure that the distal edge is short of

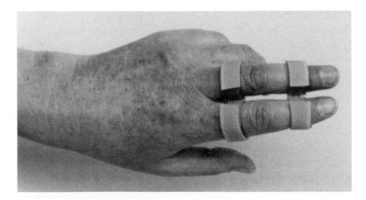

Fig. 25.21 Buddy taping of adjacent fingers using velcro straps

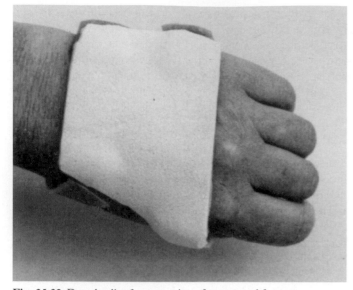

Fig. 25.22 Dorsal splint for protection of metacarpal fractures

the metacarpal heads so that in full flexion of the MCP joints, the splint does not project and endanger other players (Fig. 25.22). The player may use buddy straps for an added feeling of security.

Proximal and middle phalangeal fractures

These fractures can cause loss of PIP joint movement particularly if the fracture is intra-articular, unstable and associated with angulation or rotation. Rotation of a phalangeal fracture is detected clinically by asking the athlete to flex the digits. The tips of the fingers are poorly aligned; one digit may even cross over another.

Undisplaced stable fractures are treated with early active movement as pain permits. Protection of the finger in a dorsal gutter splint, in as near to full extension as possible, is required for 7-10 days, then buddy taping is used. Boscheinen-Morrin et al (1985) suggest a more conservative approach of a forearm based splint, and commencement of active movement at 2-3 weeks.

Unstable and poorly aligned fractures require stabilizing with open reduction and internal fixation. Rotation of a phalangeal fracture is detected clinically when the tips of the fingers are poorly aligned when flexion is attempted, even to the extent that one digit may cross another.

Treatment and orthotics following immobilization is directed towards regaining PIP joint movement as a matter of urgency.

For flexion start with blocked PIP flexion, functional activities and exercising with a silicone-based rubber compound, such as exercise putty.

If flexion progresses slowly, splinting must be implemented. A light pressure over a long time achieves a plastic change, in contrast to a heavy pressure, which can only be tolerated for a short time, giving a temporary elastic change. As a rough guide, there should not be any blanching of the skin when the splint is applied, and the splint should be tolerated for many hours. Intermittent splinting for half-hour periods gives poor results (Brand 1990, Fess 1990).

Forearm-based splints are expensive to make, cumbersome to wear and are used only if unavoidable. Hand-based splints are easily made and are comfortable to wear.

Serial splinting is used to increase flexion up to 60-70°. A splint is made on the dorsal aspect, closely conforming to the finger in the maximum flexion available. The splint should be worn overnight when possible and remoulded into increased flexion every few days.

When flexion is greater than 45°, a strap passing over the dorsum of the finger and around the dorsum of the hand provides a gentle stretch into flexion. The straps are quickly made from velcro or adhesive tape.

Extension can be increased by using a finger-based extension splint. These splints are effective for flexion contractures of 35° or less. The splint is constructed on the volar aspect, extending from the base of the proximal phalanx to the tip of the finger. The splint is made in 0° extension, the dorsal pressure being supplied by a strap or tape over the PIP joint.

Serial splinting for increasing extension is made with plaster, cut into 2 cm strips and wound around the finger. This can be changed every second day.

A dorsal gutter splint, the PIP joint in 20° flexion, gives protection and allows good dexterity when return to sport is permitted.

Distal phalangeal fractures

These may be a crush of the tuft, a longitudinal or transverse fracture of the shaft, or an avulsion fracture of the base, the latter giving rise to a mallet finger deformity.

Management of an undisplaced fracture is rest, in a dorsal or volar splint if necessary for pain relief, followed by active mobilization of the DIP joint and gradual resumption of activity. Displaced transverse and displaced longitudinal intra-articular fractures usually require internal fixation.

Orthotics. Serial dorsal gutter splinting and taping the finger into DIP and PIP flexion are used to regain full DIP flexion. Return to sport may require a light splint, padded for extra impact protection.

Joint injuries

Metacarpophalangeal joints

Metacarpophalangeal joints are likely to sustain injury in contact and ball-handling sports, gymnastics and athletic field events.

Slight sprains. These sprains present with swelling about the dorsum of the joint, flexion and extension being variably limited. The oedema can cause the joint to rest in extension where the collateral ligaments are loose. There is localized tenderness about the joint and diffuse tenderness in the interossei, palm and perhaps the long finger flexor muscle bellies.

Treatment. The joint is rested in the POSI (Figs 25.29a, 25.29b), using a hand-based splint, until pain and oedema subside. Gentle active flexion of the joint is then commenced, followed by extrinsic extension. Buddy taping protects the joint on resumption of activity.

Occasionally an extensor lag develops because of damage to the sagittal bands, which will require splinting in 0° MCP extension, IP joints free, for 3-4 weeks, interspersed with active exercise.

Dorsal subluxation and dislocation. These injuries occur infrequently after a hyperextension force. Clinically dislocation is seen with the MCP joint in extension, the IP joints in slight flexion and the digit centrally deviated. The prominent metacarpal head can be palpated volarly. Subluxation presentation differs only in that the MCP joint lies in 60-80° hyperextension.

Once dorsally dislocated, the joint is irreducible by conservative means because the ruptured volar plate is interposed between the base of the proximal phalanx and the metacarpal head. Attempts to free the volar plate with traction cause the lumbricals and the flexor tendons to be drawn tightly around the metacarpal neck.

A subluxation can be converted into a dislocation by attempting a reduction manoeuvre of traction and hyper-extension. This pulls the proximal portion of the volar plate dorsally, where it becomes interposed as above. The correct technique for reduction is to hold the wrist in flexion then gently apply a distal and volar force to slide the proximal phalanx into a flexed position.

The consequence of attempting to reduce a subluxation by the instinctive reaction of traction on the digit is to convert the situation from one manageable by conservative means, to one that requires open reduction. As a general precaution, it is essential to X-ray before attempting to relocate a joint.

Following reduction the joint is splinted in 30° flexion for two weeks, followed by a dorsal blocking splint preventing the last 10° of flexion for a further two weeks (Dray & Eaton 1988).

Radial collateral ligament sprain. This injury occurs in the ulnar three digits when the flexed finger is forced into ulnar deviation. Shotputters are susceptible to this sprain, an explanation being that under the duress of effort the middle finger moves ulnarly on the shot to aid the ring and little fingers whose combined strength in maintaining flexion is less than that of the thumb and index finger. (If there is loss of active extension refer to extensor tendon subluxation.)

Treatment. The finger or fingers are rested in the POSI in a hand-based splint for 2-3 weeks. Finger flexor strengthening exercises may help the shotputter to correct technique. Buddy taping protects the joint from ulnar stress once activity is resumed.

Proximal interphalangeal joint

Hyperextension stress. This may cause sprain, dorsal subluxation and dislocation, with or without associated fracture involving the joint surface, usually of the middle phalanx.

The injury is seen in ball-handling sports when a ball strikes the end of the finger, in contact sports and in sports where the joint is subjected to repeated extension loading, such as gymnastics and shotput. The injury can cause severe loss of PIP joint function.

The joint is swollen and painful with tenderness along the anterior joint line, often more so about the radial side. This is presumably because the three ulnar digits move into ulnar deviation on weightbearing and on full spanning of the hand. There is a variable loss of flexion and extension.

In severe injuries the joint is unstable, being likely to redislocate on active extension. Alternatively, the joint may rest in a partially dislocated or subluxed position. This should be clinically suspected when it is impossible to perform passive flexion. Any associated collateral ligament damage is apparent on lateral stress after the dislocation is reduced.

X-ray may show avulsion of the volar plate attachment. It is important to note the size of the fragment with respect to the articular surface. If the fracture involves greater than one-third of the articular surface, the joint will be unstable and a surgical opinion should be sought.

Chronic instability progresses to be a swan-neck deformity. The PIP joint rests in hyperextension, and DIP joint in flexion.

Treatment. Sprain (without history of dislocation). Ice massage and Coban bandaging (refer to section on principles of management) are applied, before resting in a dorsal gutter splint in 25° flexion. This is worn continuously, until the pain settles at 1-2 weeks. Then begin active flexion exercises of both the PIP joint and the whole digit. The splint is worn between the two-hourly exercise sessions only progressing to weaning off the splint when there is minimal pain (Fig. 25.23).

Although some therapists favour a more aggressive approach of splinting for 2-3 days only then using a dorsal blocking splint, the author considers the approach that gives minimal pain is to be preferred.

Dislocation/fracture-dislocation. This is an injury of which the severity and the consequences are often overlooked. Treatment is classified according to the stability of the joint. Wilson and Carter (1990) and Boscheinen-

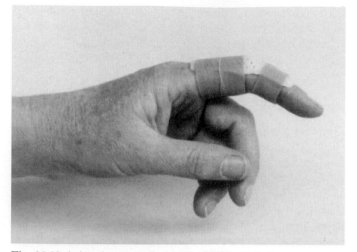

Fig. 25.23 A dorsal gutter splint in 25° of PIP joint flexion

Morrin (1985) set out differing treatment regimes, the former working with a dorsal blocking splint and the latter using the POSI. The author has found the following procedure satisfactory, but some therapists prefer an earlier introduction of the dorsal blocking splint.

Stable joints, with or without fracture, are treated in a dorsal gutter splint in 25-30° of flexion for 1-2 weeks to allow soft tissue healing (Fig. 25.23) The splint is then converted to a dorsal-blocking splint, allowing flexion and limiting extension, by removing the distal tape (Fig. 25.24) (Cannon et al 1985). Over the next 2-3 weeks the splint is opened out into full extension. Passive splinting to regain full extension can be implemented if necessary at 7-8 weeks.

Unstable joints usually require open repair, although the conservative dorsal blocking regime is sometimes recommended. After repair of the volar plate, the joint is immobilized by a K wire for 3 weeks. During this time the DIP joint is exercised. A dorsal blocking splint is used for the next 3 weeks to protect the repair, while encouraging flexion. The splint is gradually opened out into full or nearly full extension by 7 weeks. A severely damaged joint may need flexion-assist splinting. Splinting into extension to overcome any residual flexion deformity should not be implemented before 7 weeks.

Collateral ligament. This sprain occurs with a lateral force in contact and ball-handling sports, often in conjunction with a hyperextension stress.

The joint is swollen and painful. There is limitation of movement. Stress testing under local anaesthesia determines if the ligament is completely ruptured. The finger should be X-rayed to exclude fracture.

Treatment. Incomplete rupture is treated with rest in a dorsal gutter splint in 15-30° of flexion until acute pain subsides, the severity of the injury causing this time to vary from 3 days to 3 weeks. Coban bandage is applied under the splint to reduce the oedema. The splint needs to be

remodelled as oedema subsides, to maintain a close fit. Treatment progresses to active flexion, extension and intrinsic stretching exercises.

The protective splint is discontinued when pain on active movement subsides. Buddy straps are then used to promote constant active use, while preventing further lateral stress. Massage to the extensor muscle bellies in the forearm aids in regaining full flexion.

Complete rupture, often combined with volar plate avulsion, is variably treated with open repair or as for incomplete rupture.

Orthotics. It is essential to protect the joint on return to sport. A dorsal gutter splint, designed by the author, has proved to be satisfactory. The splint is made of 1.6 mm thermoplastic material which has a memory, allowing the material to be stretched thinly without breaking. Stretch the splint thinly over the PIP joint to render it flexible, while extending the splint to half the depth of the digit to prevent lateral and extension stresses.

Taping fingers together is a widely used practice, but is ineffective in preventing hyperextension and limits hand function, especially in athletes requiring a large hand span. e.g. basketballers and netballers.

Distal interphalangeal joint

Volar plate disruption and collateral ligament injuries are rarely seen in the DIP joint. Signs and symptoms are similar to PIP joint injuries, the volar plate disruption being detected by an avulsed fragment of the base of the distal phalanx.

Treatment is as for PIP joint injuries, with both the PIP and DIP joints being included in the splint.

Differential diagnosis. Mallet finger is distinguished by having a loss of active DIP extension, and ruptured FDP by having a loss of active DIP flexion.

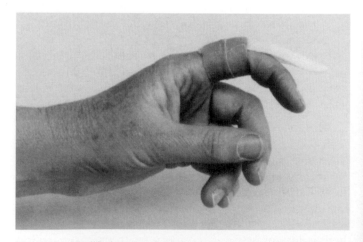

Fig. 25.24 Modified taping of the dorsal gutter splint allows flexion of the affected joint, to minimize stiffness

Tendon injuries

Dislocation of the extensor hood

Injuries to the extensor mechanism at the level of the MCP joint can cause a traumatic dislocation of the extensor digitorum communis hood. Rupture of the sagittal band allows the extensor tendon to migrate medially or laterally to the valley between the metacarpal heads. The most common presentation is a medial subluxation of the middle finger tendon.

The cause is usually an ulnar-directed blow to the flexed MCP joint. The patient presents with a swollen MCP joint and an inability to extend the finger from the flexed position. However, once the joint is passively extended, extension can be maintained because the tendon has been restored to its anatomical position. It is therefore important that the ability to maintain extension not be taken as a positive test for extensor integrity.

Conservative management is successful if the injury is diagnosed and treated within the first few weeks post-trauma. The MCP joint is splinted in neutral, the wrist and PIP joint being left free, for 4 weeks. Hyperextension is contraindicated. Neutral is sufficient to take tension off the healing sagittal band and prolonged hyperextension will allow fibrosis of the collateral ligaments which will restrict the later regaining of flexion. Full active IP flexion should be practised. After 4 weeks gentle MCP flexion is begun, the splint being replaced between exercise sessions for the next 2 weeks. Gradually wean off the splint during the day over the following two weeks. Night splinting is maintained for a further 4 weeks.

Surgical reconstruction is undertaken for late presentations because shortening of soft tissue associated with the sagittal band prevents a strong repair by conservative means (Boscheinen-Morrin et al 1985).

Extensor tendon

Central slip disruption (Boutonniere deformity).
Rupture, avulsion or laceration of the central extensor slip results in a Boutonniere deformity. The finger adopts the posture of flexion of the PIP joint and hyperextension of the DIP joint.

Rupture and avulsion are caused by an acute force into flexion of the PIP joint, with simultaneous active extension of the PIP joint, as occurs in ball-handling sports.

The loss in continuity of the central slip allows stretching of the triangular ligament and a progressive volar displacement of the lateral bands, to the point where the lateral bands sublux volarly to the axis of the PIP joint. They thus become PIP joint flexors and DIP joint extensors. PIP joint flexion is accentuated by the unopposed action of the long flexors (Fig. 25.25).

The patient presents with pain and swelling about the PIP joint after trauma. There may or may not be an initial

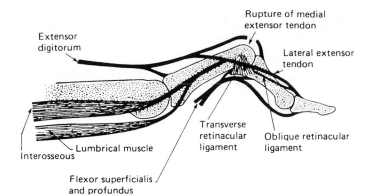

Fig. 25.25 Boutonniere deformity where interruption to the central slip leads to flexion of the PIP joint by flexor digitorum superficialis and the subluxed lateral bands. The oblique retinacular ligaments hyperextend the DIP joint

loss of full extension. Any fracture of the central part of the dorsal base of the middle phalanx necessarily involves the tendon insertion. A large avulsed fragment will require internal fixation.

The therapist must be aware that on initial assessment the complete deformity may not be apparent, but declares itself over days or weeks as the lateral bands sublux. Pain and oedema may also initially prevent passive extension, increasing further the risk of overlooking the tendon absence. Chronic presentation may be that of a PIP flexion deformity.

Differential diagnosis. In both PIP collateral ligament sprain and PIP dorsal dislocation with subsequent volar plate contracture there should be normal DIP mobility.

Treatment. Conservative treatment is used for closed injuries to the tendon and small avulsion fractures. The PIP joint is maintained in full extension for 6 weeks with dorsal, volar or circumferential splinting. The DIP joint must not be included because active and passive flexion of the DIP joint assists in preserving the mobility of the lateral bands, enabling their return to a dorsal disposition, and in stretching the oblique and transverse retinacular ligaments. The splint may be removed for cleaning, but the joint must be supported in full extension at all times (Fig. 25.26).

Surgical repair is undertaken when there is open injury to the tendon. Splinting is maintained for 4-6 weeks, depending on the surgeon's opinion. Commence scar massage when sutures are removed.

After immobilization, flexion of the PIP joint is commenced carefully, the splint being replaced between exercise sessions for decreasing periods over the next 2 weeks. The splint is then maintained at night for a further 2 weeks. If an extensor lag develops, a further period of splinting is indicated (Boscheinen-Morrin et al 1985, Evans 1990).

Orthotics. For return to sport it is advisable that a splint be worn for 10-12 weeks after injury. Wearing the Boutonniere splint may put the DIP joint at risk, so it is

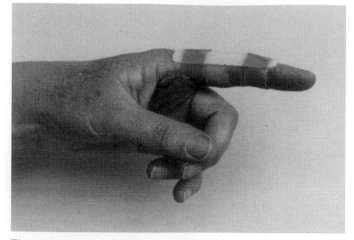

Fig. 25.26 Dorsal splint for Boutonniere deformity

safer to resume contact sports only after recovery of full active extension. Then a dorsal gutter splint, with PIP and DIP joints in slight flexion, gives full protection and satisfactory function.

Terminal slip disruption (Mallet finger deformity). An interruption to the extensor mechanism distal to the PIP joint produces a flexed posture of the DIP joint because of the unopposed action of the FDP. It is universally called Mallet finger (McCue & Wooten 1986).

The mechanism of injury is usually a blow to the end of the extended finger or, less commonly, a crush. It is seen in ball and contact sports. There may be a complete rupture of the tendon or an avulsion fracture at the base of the distal phalanx involving the area of insertion of the extensor tendon. Alternatively, the tendon may be only partially torn or stretched, giving a slight flexion deformity with weak active extension possible. The collateral ligaments, if intact, can support the joint in 45° flexion.

It is important to X-ray these injuries to determine the presence, and if so the size, of an avulsed fragment. If greater than one third of the articular surface is involved, the fragment will require internal fixation.

The injury presents with localized tenderness and swelling over the dorsum of the flexed DIP joint. The joint can be passively extended, although this is variably limited by pain and oedema.

Differential diagnosis. Osteoarthritis of the DIP joints can give the appearance of a flexion deformity, but active extension is present through the available range.

Treatment. In conservative treatment, a Mallet splint is made of thermoplastic material to hold the DIP joint in full extension, leaving the PIP joint free. The joint should not be forced into hyperextension to the extent that skin blanching occurs. The splint may be volar or dorsal. It is useful to alternate the splinting, thus allowing good skin care (see Fig. 25.27).

Commercial splints are available, but it is difficult to achieve a comfortable and effective fit given individual variation in digital contour, oedema and joint flexibility (Malick & Kasch 1984).

The splint is worn continuously for 6-8 weeks, except for cleaning of splint and skin. The joint must be maintained in extension when the splint is off for cleaning. At 6 weeks the splint is removed and the status of the tendon assessed. If the joint can be maintained in extension then weaning off the splint during the day is commenced. The splint should be worn at night for a further 2-4 weeks and during the day when forceful activity is required. If an extensor lag occurs a further 4 weeks of full time splinting should be implemented (Brown Evans 1990).

Surgical treatment involves reducing the fracture, then fixing with a K-wire. The joint is splinted for 6 weeks, after

Fig. 25.27 Dorsal splint for Mallet finger deformity

which time the K-wire is removed and mobilization is as for conservative treatment (Rosenthal 1990).

Swan-neck deformity. A chronic Mallet deformity often leads to a hyperextension deformity of the PIP joint as a result of the changed line of pull of the lateral bands, the combination of the two deformities being called a 'swan-neck' deformity. With the loss of continuity of the terminal tendon the extending forces of the dorsal expansion are concentrated on the central slip and transverse retinacular ligament insertion into the lateral bands (Rosenthal 1990) (see Fig. 25.28).

Splinting is rarely effective in reversing the deformity, only being useful in maintaining the joint temporarily in

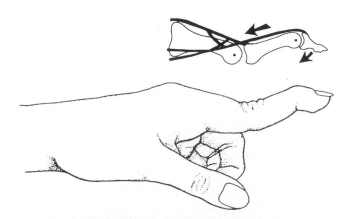

Fig. 25.28 Swan-neck deformity. Source: American Society for Surgery of the Hand (1983)

slight flexion for relief of discomfort. A surgical opinion should be sought if the hyperextension is preventing easy finger flexion.

Differential diagnosis. Other conditions giving rise to swan-neck deformity are volar plate laxity from a hyperextension injury of PIP joint, loss of the flexor digitorum superficialis tendon and rheumatoid arthritis.

Flexor digitorum profundus rupture

Injury to flexor digitorum profundus occurs in contact sports. It is a serious injury, taking 10-12 weeks for the tendon to return to full strength.

The tendon may sustain a closed rupture in the distal half of the digit or be avulsed from the distal phalanx, when the finger is caught in an opponent's clothing. More rarely there may be a laceration, severing the tendon.

The patient presents with pain and oedema about the distal two-thirds of the finger. The diagnostic feature is an absence of active flexion of the DIP joint, while passive flexion is limited only by oedema.

Test for active flexion by blocking the MCP and PIP joints in full extension, then ask the patient to attempt active flexion.

Differential diagnosis. Anterior interosseous nerve syndrome gives loss of index DIP flexion and thumb IP flexion.

Treatment. Following surgical repair the timing of rehabilitation is controversial, very much dependent on the surgeon. Examples are given in the texts by Malick and Kasche (1984) and van Strien (1990). The principles of controlling oedema, maintaining passive range movement, softening the scar tissue, and graduated active range of movement follow, with the expectation of return to full activity in 10 weeks (Wilson & Carter 1990). Inexperienced therapists should discuss the program with a therapist more familiar with this problem.

Other tendon injuries

Injuries to flexor and extensor tendons proximal to the MCP joints by laceration is uncommon in sports injuries. These injuries require surgical repair and a long and carefully timed rehabilitation program, the details of which are outside the scope of this chapter.

General principles of treatment after open repair are to splint the hand so that the repair is protected and there is the range of movement of unaffected joints permitted by the surgeon. Gentle active movement is generally commenced at 3-4 weeks, the splint being maintained between exercise sessions until 6 weeks after repair. Gentle use of the hand then commences. Splinting to regain range of movement involving stretching the repaired tendon should not be used until 7-8 weeks after repair. Normal use is allowed at 8-12 weeks (Malick & Kasch 1984, Boscheinen-Morrin 1985, van Strien 1990).

Those unfamiliar with these injuries should consult with the surgeon and/or experienced therapist prior to commencing rehabilitation.

REGIONAL PROBLEMS

Nerve compression injuries

Peripheral nerves are subject to compression by changes in the dimensions of anatomical tunnels, increase in the contents of tunnels by oedema, direct compression by prolonged pressure from equipment, and by impact pressure.

Carpal tunnel syndrome

Compression of the median nerve in the carpal tunnel is caused by decreased carpal tunnel capacity and/or by an increase of intracarpal pressure, and causes ischaemia of the nerve.

The pressure in the intraneural blood vessels is normally in balance with the pressure in the connective tissue of the endoneurium, but with the increased tissue pressure resulting from the compression the blood vessels' patency decreases, resulting in ischaemia. The problem will worsen at night when there is the additional problem of the normal lower resting blood pressure and an increase in tissue pressure (Omer 1992).

It is most common in women over 50 years of age and occurs with prolonged gripping, wrist hyperextension and contact/fall trauma causing fractures and dislocations to the radius and carpal bones. Problems can arise in sports such as racquet sports, gymnastics, cycling, golf and field games (Eversmann 1988, Kapila 1988).

There is parasthesia and pain in the radial three and a half digits, with variable pain radiation into the arm and remaining digits. The hand may be clumsy and weak. Morning wrist and finger stiffness is present. Wasting of the thenar eminence indicates involvement of the motor branch (Spinner 1978).

Variable relief from the nocturnal symptoms is obtained by hanging the arm over the side of the bed or shaking the hand, actions which presumably increase the resting blood pressure, thus restoring blood supply to the nerve.

The following tests are useful but not necessarily positive.

- Tinel's sign is positive when tapping over the median nerve at the level of the tunnel produces tingling in the relevant digits (Spinner 1978) (see Ch. 10).
- Phalen's sign is positive when symptoms of the syndrome are reproduced when the wrists are held in full flexion for 1 minute.

- Nerve conduction tests of the median nerve give an indication of the severity of the compression.

Acute carpal tunnel symptoms can occur with some carpal and distal radial fracture-dislocations. These injuries must be treated, if unrelieved by elevation, with immediate surgical intervention to prevent permanent nerve damage.

Differential diagnosis. Cervical spine referred pain, anterior interosseous nerve syndrome, ulnar nerve compression at the elbow and wrist and digital nerve neurofibroma are excluded by specific tests for those nerves. The author has observed that osteoarthritis of the base of the thumb is often seen in association with carpal tunnel syndrome.

Treatment. Rest from the provocative activity is essential. A thermoplastic volar wrist splint with the wrist in only a few degrees of extension provides excellent support and facilitates venous drainage. Eversmann (1988) recommends a dorso-ulnar splint to avoid putting any extra pressure on the nerve. The splint is worn continuously until the symptoms subside or surgery is decided upon.

Give massage and ultra-sound to wrist and finger flexor muscle bellies to reduce post-exercise oedema which may be causing increased tension on the tendons.

Tendon gliding exercises are implemented cautiously. These give maximum excursion of the flexor tendons in the tunnel and in relationship to each other, which may assist in reduction of the inflammation (see Ch. 10).

Return to sport should be cautious, monitoring for any return of symptoms. If these occur, reduce training and consider surgical intervention.

Surgical release of the transverse carpal ligament is performed when the symptoms are not relieved by conservative measures.

Post operative management. The wrist is supported by bandaging or use of a volar wrist splint for at least 1 week. When sutures are removed commence massage of scar to reduce the tendency for hypersensitivity to develop. Massage and ultrasound are given to the muscle bellies of the wrist flexors.

Finger and wrist active range of movement is commenced. If there has been atrophy of the thenar muscles attention must be paid to maintaining passive range of movement of the thumb. The MCP joint may need splinting into neutral if a flexion deformity is developing as a result of weakness of abductor pollicis brevis.

Return to sport is gradual, ensuring that extremes of wrist movement are avoided by use of taping or semi-flexible wrist support (Osterman 1988, Baxter-Petralia 1990).

Ulnar nerve neuropathy

This occurs with compression of the ulnar nerve in Guyon's canal. It is seen, for example, in 'cyclists' palsy' where the nerve is compressed between the bony boundaries of the canal and the handlebars (Aulicino 1990).

There is pain about the ulnar side of the hand and parasthesia in the ulnar one and a half digits. Weakness in the ulnar nerve innervated muscles is variably seen. There is local tenderness to pressure over the area of Guyon's canal and a variably positive Tinel's sign.

Differential diagnosis. Compression of the ulnar nerve in the cubital canal has a positive Tinel's sign over the cubital canal and a likely weakness of FDP in the ulnar digits.

Treatment. This is aimed at reducing the compression of the nerve by padding the equipment and padding the hand, around but not on the area of compression. Handlebars are being developed to allow a larger weightbearing area.

Radial nerve neuritis

The superficial (sensory) branch of the radial nerve is likely to give troublesome hypersensitivity after trauma at the wrist level. Paraesthesia and pain spread variably into the dorsal aspects of thumb, first web space and hand. The problem is aggravated by wrist and hand movement and is difficult to relieve. Rest from aggressive wrist movements that provoke the response, followed by attempting graduated return to full activity is the only option (Malick & Kasch 1984). It is a very irritable condition and treatment must proceed with extreme caution.

Digital neurofibroma

Digital nerve compression may lead to formation of a neurofibroma giving pain and paraesthesia in adjacent sides of the affected digits, or one side of a digit, distal to the site of compression (Connolly 1980). It may occur in racquet sports, ten pin bowling, and javelin throwing.

Differential diagnosis. Digital paraesthesia caused by the compression of the median or ulnar nerve has a wider distribution, involving more than the adjacent sides of two digits (Osterman et al 1988, Rettig 1990).

Treatment. Conservative treatment involves rest from sport if pain is severe. Check and pad equipment. Pad the hand, cutting out a window over the affected nerve. Check sporting technique.

Surgery is indicated only if conservative treatment fails.

Anterior interosseous nerve injury

Anterior interosseous nerve injury gives a loss of thumb IP flexion and DIP joint flexion in the index and middle finger. The nerve is subject to injury in the proximal one third of the forearm.

Ganglions

Ganglions are benign tumours of the synovium arising from the joint or tendon sheath. The aetiology is uncertain, but there is a history of repeated strain or trauma in 50% of cases (Kapila 1988).

Common sites for ganglions are the volar aspect of the wrist, the dorsal aspect of the scapholunate joint and over the volar aspect of the MCP joint. These occur in weight-lifting, gymnastics and racquet sports (Connolly 1980 Dobyns & Gabel 1990).

Ganglions may be asymptomatic and/or may disappear spontaneously. Others are aggravated by activity, causing aching in the surrounding area, with consequent decreased range of movement and weakness of grip.

Treatment. This commences with rest from any aggravating activity and/or immobilization in plaster or splint. It is worth trying frictions about the ganglion and surrounding area. If this does not give relief, aspiration or excision may be used.

Aspiration of the ganglion has a 40-60% success rate, with a liklehood of recurrence (Kapila 1988). Surgical excision, with a 95% success rate, is followed by 10 days bandaging/splinting to relieve pain and allow primary healing.

Return to sport should be gradual, especially after excision, taking 6-8 weeks for full recovery. Wrist strapping provides support (Beiersdorf 1979).

Trigger thumb and trigger finger

Trigger thumb and finger is a stenosing tenovaginitis of the flexor tendon. The tendon and/or the tendon pulley is thickened, preventing free gliding of the tendon at the level of the MCP joint. The prolonged gripping of rowing and cycling and the direct trauma of ball sports are likely causes.

The digit clicks and locks during active movement. There is local tenderness and usually a lump can be palpated over the anterior aspect of MCP joint. The lump is more pronounced when the MCP joint is held in extension while active flexion is performed.

Differential diagnosis. Dupuytren's contracture is a fixed flexion contracture of the digit. Boutonniere deformity is a fixed flexion contracture of the PIP joint. PIP joint sprain or dislocation presents as a painful swollen joint, restricted in both flexion and extension.

Associated disorders are osteoarthritis, carpal tunnel syndrome, and rheumatoid arthritis.

Treatment. If the onset follows after a definite recent incident, it is worth resting the thumb IP joint and the PIP joint in a dorsal or circumferential splint for 2-3 weeks to see if the problem resolves. For established triggering surgical release of the pulley is regarded as the optimal treatment (Froimson 1988). It is a simple procedure, allowing an early return to sport as pain allows. Evans et al (1988) offer a conservative approach of splinting, combined with an exercise programme, but results are slow and less reliable.

When the problem is one of minimal locking, associated with an obvious tendonitis with tenderness, redness and crepitus, the hand should be padded, with a piece cut out over the MCP joint, to take direct pressure off the tendon. This may be sufficient to prevent the development of a true trigger finger (Connolly 1980, American Society for Surgery of the Hand 1983).

Reflex sympathetic dystrophy

This condition is not commonly seen in sports injuries, but therapists must always keep this problem in mind, e.g. after Colles fracture, fractures of metacarpals and phalanges and after surgery for carpal tunnel syndrome.

Reflex sympathetic dystrophy (RSD) is caused by an abnormal sympathetic reflex, giving a response to injury that is out of proportion to, and inconsistent with, the injury. Lankford (1990) comments that there is often an associated low pain threshold and unstable personality.

RSD should be suspected if the normal progression of gradual reduction in oedema, pain and stiffness is replaced by an increase in symptoms.

The principal symptom is a burning pain, which can be triggered by light touch, movement, change in external temperature and noise. This pain can be totally disabling, involving the whole limb, or may be such that only a small segment of the hand is involved.

Oedema, seen particularly in the hand, usually accompanies the pain. The skin appears shiny and is usually red, but can appear pale and cyanotic. There may be increased sweating and an increased growth of hair on the forearm and hand.

The MCP joints stiffen into extension and the IP joints into flexion. Osteoporosis and ischaemic contracture develop if the problem is not resolved in 1-3 months.

Hand therapy begins with splinting the hand in POSI, combining it with elevation and gentle massage. A loose fitting glove or bandage may provide additional relief.

Gentle active exercise is performed well within the limits of exacerbating the pain. Passive movements will only increase the pain and oedema.

When progress is slow or symptoms marked, sympatholytic drugs or a sympathetic ganglion block may be used.

Patients make variable and unpredictable progress. Activities of daily living are severely curtailed but they must be encouraged. The patient will need a lot of emotional support to cope with this painful disability (Lankford 1990, Waylett-Rendall 1990).

Other conditions

When examining and treating athletes' hands there are both precautions and differential diagnoses to consider, especially in elderly athletes.

Osteoarthritis

Osteoarthritis in the thumb may be a complicating factor in wrist sprain, carpal tunnel syndrome and de Quervain's syndrome. In chronic osteoarthritis, the presence of marginal osteophytes, known as Herbendon's nodes, on the dorsal aspect of the distal interphalangeal joints, may mimic a mallet finger. Chronic traumatic arthritis of the proximal interphalangeal joints may complicate the assessment and treatment of a recent injury.

Rheumatoid arthritis

Rheumatoid arthritis is distinguished by positive blood tests and X-rays from non-inflammatory joint disorders. It can cause hyperextension (swan-neck) deformity of the PIP joint, which also occurs in volar plate rupture. It frequently gives wrist pain and deformity.

Osteoporosis

Osteoporosis becomes increasingly common in the ageing female, its effects being readily seen in Colles' fracture. Long-term use of corticosteroids for a medical condition can contribute to osteoporosis, therefore care should be exercised when mobilizing and strengthening the hands of athletes taking this medication.

Dupuytren's contracture

Dupuytren's contracture, a progressive contracture of the palmar fascia, may complicate the recovery from an MCP hyperextension sprain.

Muscle wasting of the intrinsics, because of previous inactivity, needs to be distinguished from median and ulnar nerve compression.

Skin integrity and a poor healing rate can be a problem in the elderly.

Elderly athletes with hand injuries need to be reassured that a steady approach to resuming activity will allow an increase in muscle strength, range of movement, joint stability and endurance without an increase in pain (Williams & Sperrin 1976, Grahame 1985, Meier 1990).

PRINCIPLES OF MANAGEMENT

Splinting

'Splints act as a means for delicately controlling, preserving, modifying and affecting motion' (Cannon et al 1985, p. 108). Therapists should combine their knowledge of anatomy, kinesiology, splinting principles and splinting materials to provide a problem solving approach to the individuals' injury restrictions and sport demands.

Low-temperature thermoplastic splints are lightweight and washable and are well accepted by players as minimally interfering with hand function. They have the advantage over plaster and prefabricated splints of being readily altered as required by oedema reduction and changes in range of movement.

Splints should be closely moulded to give good support, but should be flared over bony prominences and at the edges to prevent unwanted pressure.

Splinting to increase range of movement should always be applied with a little pressure over a long time, allowing the collagen to be laid down in the required position, rather than in large forces over a short time, which 'often rupture scar and underlying tissues and set up a vicious cycle of inflammation, further scarring and contracture, which are detrimental rather than beneficial to the recovery of function' (Strickland 1987). Ideally splints to increase joint range should be worn for at least 12 hours per day (Brand 1990, Fess 1990).

Adhesive-backed cushioning is used to line splints where necessary to relieve pressure and to cover the outside of splints to protect other players from harmful impact. The splint must comply with the rules of the sport.

Finger splints are usually fixed on with 1.5 cm. wide strips of non-elastic tape which anchors the splint more firmly than the velcro straps used for wrist splints. Wider tape is used to cover the splint when in competition.

Skin creases provide information on the finished length of splints. The creases must not be occluded if movement is required at the underlying joints. For example, the distal palmar crease must be left free when making volar wrist splints to allow full MCP flexion.

Position of safe immobilization

The position of safe immobilization (POSI) is used for immobilizing the hand after crushes, strains and fractures. It is essential to use this position to prevent the common post-injury contractures of MCP extension and IP flexion in any injury where oedema is preventing reasonably full range of movement. The athlete in danger is one who presents with a swollen dorsum of the hand, the wrist resting in neutral or slight flexion, the digits markedly swollen, the MCP joints resting in neutral and the IP joints resting in flexion.

A splint is made to support the wrist in 30° extension, the MCP joints in maximum flexion and the IP joints in full extension. If the injury is localized to the MCP joint area, a hand-based splint, excluding the wrist may be sufficient (Figs 25.29a, 25.29b) (Malick & Kasch 1984, Boscheinen-Morrin et al 1985, Fess & Philips 1987, Wilson & Carter 1990).

Finger splints are best made on the dorsal surface to leave the volar area free for tactile input (Malick 1982, Fess

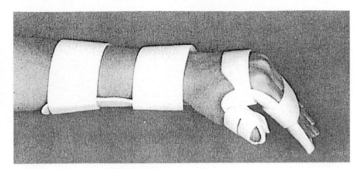

Fig. 25.29a The position of safe mobilization (POSI) forearm based splint. Source: Cannon (1985)

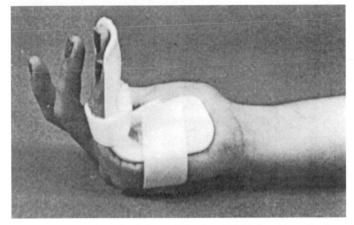

Fig. 25.29b Position of safe immobilization (POSI) hand-based splint. Source: Cannon (1985)

& Philips 1987, Barr & Swan 1988, Hankin & Peel 1990, Press & Wiesner 1990).

Oedema control

Oedema in the fingers and hand is controlled with elevation, compression, positioning, massage and exercise.

Compression is supplied by wrapping with self-adhesive conforming bandage (Coban), or by wearing a tight-fitting glove of cotton or lycra. For the fingers, use a strip of 2 cm wide Coban, wrapped distally to proximally.

Resting the hand in the POSI can have a dramatic effect in reducing oedema. The glove and Coban can be worn in combination with the splint.

Massage, in the form of small circular frictions over all the affected areas, is introduced cautiously in the 24–48 hour post-injury period, avoiding any open wounds and suture lines. It is then performed for 10-15 minutes at treatment sessions and repeated for shorter periods at home. Active exercises are practised after the massage (Malick & Kasch 1984).

Hand exercises

Active exercises are an essential part of regaining range of movement, combined with oedema control and splinting.

The author has reservations about strong passive mobilization. Gentle painfree gliding of accessory movements may be performed (Corrigan & Maitland 1983). However, forceful end pressure to active movements may increase oedema and inflammation, give further scarring and cause pain such that function is decreased. Strickland (1987) makes these observations in reference to forceful splinting but it must be equally applicable to passive mobilization. It is important to treat stiff painful hands gently but firmly to the limit of the pain and movement, such that there is minimal increase in pain after treatment. The athlete should feel that the hand has gained in range of movement and functional ability and feel confident that he/she can continue to progress with the home exercise program.

Assisted active exercises are used when weakness and lack of confidence are hindering progress. The therapist must learn to feel the movement, gently assisting to the limit of the range and encouraging the athlete to work hard to maintain that range.

Exercises

The exercises should be repeated 5-10 times every 1-2 hours. Repetitions should be reduced if there are adverse reactions of oedema and pain.

- Full fist (Fig. 25.30a) and opposition (Fig. 25.30b) should be combined with full extension of the fingers and thumb. This movement from one extreme of range to the other ensures maximum massaging and stretch of the soft tissues.
- The blocking exercises of DIP and PIP flexion (Fig. 25.30c, 25.30d) show up individual muscle weakness, thus demonstrating to the athlete the movements upon which to concentrate.
- The hook grip (Fig. 25.30e) stretches the intrinsic ligaments, which is not achieved with a full fist.
- The emphasis on MCP flexion with IP extension (Fig. 25.30f) reduces the likelihood of perpetuation of extrinsic extensor tightness and the tendency for the MCP joint to rest in neutral. Always aim for MCP flexion before a full fist.

Tendon gliding. When injury involves the FDS and FDP tendons it is useful to note the work of Wehbe (1987) in defining the flexor tendon excursions in the following three different fist exercises.

- The full fist gives maximum profundus excursion.
- The hook grip gives maximal glide between the profundus and superficialis tendons.
- The straight fist, with flexed MCP and PIP joints, and extended DIP joints gives maximum superficialis excursion.

Strengthening techniques. Apart from using graded exercise putty, which is a useful adjunct to the above

A

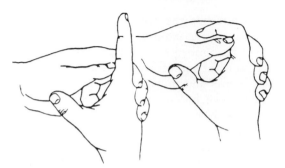

B

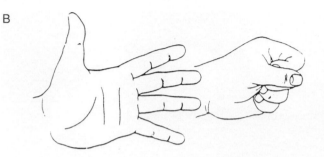

C

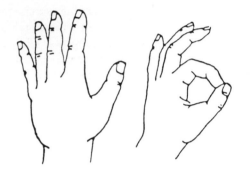

D

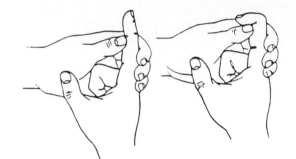

E

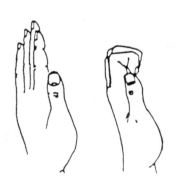

F

Fig. 25.30 Finger and hand exercises

exercises, the author has found that after full range is regained, strength is increased by implementation of daily activities, rather than by any specific exercise equipment.

Functional activities are most important, the hand being used as part of a total movement pattern, instead of the habitual avoidance pattern of injury. Initially it is difficult for the hand to be incorporated back into daily activities but once achieved it means that the hand is being constantly exercised. Check that daily activities such as eating, writing, dressing and opening doors are being performed with the hand and arm in its normal movement pattern and hand dominance.

Exercise putty is a good adjunct to functional activities. It comes in graded resistances and is pleasant to use.

Scar management

Scars have the potential to contract and/or become hypersensitive as they form (Strickland 1987). This phenomena can make return to full function difficult. Sports participants need to be confident about bearing pressure on the scar, for full strength and/or contact to be realized.

Initial treatment is directed at all healed wounds to modify the scar tissue as it matures. This may be sufficient to maintain length and prevent hypersensitivity occurring. The author has found deep transverse friction massage, performed two hourly for 2-3 minutes to be a satisfactory regimen (Stewart 1990). Beware of causing blisters in the early stages. Combine the massage with applications of vitamin E cream to give a good feel to the scar (Miles & Grisby 1990).

If the scar becomes hard and raised some form of prolonged pressure should be applied. Materials developed for treating burn scars are suitable (Johnson 1984, Stewart 1990). Coban (self-adherent conforming bandage) can hold Spenco silicone Gelsheet and Otoform-K (putty-like silicone) pads in place, giving extra pressure. Lycra finger tubes are an easy alternative, but because they are pre-fabricated are not adaptable to increases in circumference occurring during sporting activity.

If the scar becomes hypersensitive, desensitizing is required. Barber (1990) gives detailed instructions for gross hand injuries, the principles of which can be used for sports injuries.

Select five graded textures, e.g. cotton wool ball, gauze square, velvet, loop fastener and hook fastener. Determine the hierarchy of hypersensitivity for the individual. Commencing with the least, rub the scar for 1 minute, then change to the next texture. Continue through all five textures. Repeat as often as can be fitted into the day, e.g. combine with two hourly massage and exercise sessions.

The technique is ineffective on a neuroma established after laceration of a digital nerve. This will need surgical attention or functional adaptation.

SUMMARY

The treatment of hand injuries is a constant challenge, with the rewards of new discoveries likely at every treatment session. The therapist must be inventive and analytical about the presenting problem. A meticulous examination, followed by wide reading and consulting with expert therapists, will give the most accurate diagnosis possible, which in turn provides the basis for treatment.

Traditionally trained therapists must learn new splinting skills, because it is with finely adjusted splinting that the greatest gains in increasing range of movement are to be made when an ordinary exercise program is not sufficient.

Athletes are vitally interested in sharing in the enthusiasm, because the absence from sport resulting from an apparently minor injury is difficult to tolerate. The athletes' frustration must not cause the therapist to compromise his/her opinion on the timing of returning to competition.

REFERENCES

Amadio P, Jaeger S, Hunter J 1992 Nutritional aspects of tendon healing. In: Hunter J, Schneider L, Mackin E, Callahan A (eds) Rehabilitation of the hand: surgery and therapy, 3rd edn. C V Mosby, St Louis, pp 373–378

American Society for Surgery of the Hand 1983 The hand: examination and diagnosis, 2nd edn. Churchill Livingstone, Edinburgh, p 77–78

Aulicino P 1990 Neurovascular injuries in the hands of athletes. Hand Clinics: Hand Injuries in Sports and Performing Arts 6(3):455–466

Aulicino P, DePuy T 1990 Clinical examination of the hand. In: Hunter J, Schneider L, Mackin E, Callahan A (eds) Rehabilitation of the hand, 3rd edn. C V Mosby, St Louis, ch. 4

Backhouse K M, Catton W T 1954 An experimental study of the function of the lumbrical muscles in the human hand. Journal of Anatomy 88:133–141

Barber L 1990 Desensitization of the traumatized hand. In: Hunter J, Schneider L, Mackin E, Callahan A (eds) Rehabilitation of the hand, 3rd edn. C V Mosby, St Louis 56:721–730

Barr N, Swan D 1988 The hand: principles and techniques of splintmaking, 2nd edn. Butterworths, London

Bassett F, Malone T, Gilchrist R 1979 A protective splint of silicone rubber. American Journal of Sports Medicine 7:358–360

Baxter-Petralia P 1990 Therapist's management of carpal tunnel syndrome. In: Hunter J, Schneider L, Mackin E, Callahan A (eds) Rehabilitation of the hand, 3rd edn. C V Mosby, St Louis 48:640–646

Beckenbaugh R D, Shives T C, Dobyns J H 1980 Keinbochs disease and consideration of lunate fractures. Clinical Orthopaedics and Related Research 149:98–106

Beiersdorf 1979 Modern sports strapping and bandaging techniques. Beiersdorf (Australia), Sydney, p. 73

Bejjani F J, Landsmeer J M 1989 Biomechanics of the hand. In: Nordin M, Frankel V H (eds) Basic biomechanics of the musculoskeletal system, 2nd edn. Lea & Febiger, Philadelphia, pp 275–304

Bergfeld J, Weiker G, Andrish J, Hall R 1982 Splint for protection of significant hand and wrist injuries. American Journal of Sports Medicine 10:293–295

Bogumill G P 1988 Anatomy of the wrist. In: Lichtman D M (ed). The wrist and its disorders. W B Saunders, Philadelphia, ch 2, pp 14–26

Bond J, Berquist T 1991 Radiologic evaluation of hand and wrist in motion.IHand Clinics: Imaging of the Hand, vol. 7(1)(Feb): 113–124

Boscheinen-Morrin J, Davey V, Connolly W 1985 The hand: fundamentals of therapy. Butterworths, London

Bowers W 1988 The distal radio-ulnar joint. In: Green D (ed) Operative hand surgery, 2nd edn. Churchill Livingstone, Edinburgh 2(21):939–989

Boyes J H (ed) 1970 Bunnell's surgery of the hand, 5th edn. J B Lippincott, Philadelphia, pp 2–5

Bradley J 1982 The modified silicone rubber playing cast. Physical Therapy and Sports Medicine 10(Nov):68

Brand P 1990 The forces of dynamic splinting: ten questions before applying a dynamic splint to the hand. In: Hunter J, Schneider L, Mackin E, Callahan A (eds) Rehabilitation of the hand, 3rd edn. C V Mosby, St Louis 87:1095–1100

Brand P W 1985 Clinical mechanics of the hand. C V Mosby, St Louis, pp 229–236

Brown Evans R 1990 Therapeutic management of extensor tendon injuries. In: Hunter J, Schneider L, Mackin E, Callahan A (eds) Rehabilitation of the hand, 3rd edn. C V Mosby, St Louis 36:492–511

Butler D 1991 Mobilisation of the nervous system. Churchill Livingstone, Melbourne

Campbell J, Feagin J, King P, Lambert K, Cunningham R 1992 Ulnar collateral ligament injury of the thumb. American Journal of Sports Medicine 20(1):29–30

Cannon M, Foltz R, Koepfer J, Lauck M, Simpson D, Bromley R 1985 Manual of hand splinting. Churchill Livingstone, New York, ch 10

Chase R A 1984 Atlas of hand surgery. W B Saunders, Philadelphia, vol. 2

Clark G L, Shaw Wilgis E F, Aiello B, Eckhaus D, Eddington L V (eds) 1993 Hand rehabilitation, a practical guide. Churchill Livingstone, New York

Connolly W B 1980 A colour atlas of hand conditions. Wolfe Medical Publications, London

Corrigan B, Maitland G D 1983 Practical orthopaedic medicine. Butterworths, London, ch. 8, pp. 87–90

Culver J 1990 Sports-related fractures of the hand and wrist. Clinics in Sports Medicine 9(1)(Jan):85–89

Dobyns J, Gabel G 1990 Gymnasts wrist. Hand Clinics: Hand Injuries in Sports and Performing Arts 6(3):495–49

Doyle J R 1988 Extensor tendons—acute injuries In: Green D (ed) Operative hand surgery, 2nd edn. Churchill Livingstone, Edinburgh 3(52):2045–2072

Dray G, Eaton R 1988 Dislocations and ligament injuries in the digits. In: Green D (ed) Operative hand surgery, 2nd edn. Churchill Livingstone, Edinburgh 1(18):777–811

Epner R A, Bowers W H, Gailford W B 1982 Ulna variance: the effect of wrist positioning and roentgen filming techniques. Journal of Hand Surgery 7:298–305

Evans R 1990 Therapeutic management of extensor tendon injuries. In: Hunter J, Schneider L, Mackin E, Callahan A (eds) Rehabilitation of the hand, 3rd edn. C V Mosby, St Louis 36:492–511

Evans R, Hunter J, Burkhalter W 1988 Conservative management of the trigger finger. Journal of Hand Therapy (2)(Jan-Mar):59–68

Eversmann W 1988 Entrapment and compression neuropathies. In: Green D (ed) Operative hand surgery, 2nd edn. Churchill Livingstone, Edinburgh 2(36):1423–1460

Fess E 1990 Principles and methods of splinting for mobilisation of joints. In: Hunter J, Schneider L, Mackin E, Callahan A (eds) Rehabilitation of the hand, 3rd edn. C V Mosby, St Louis 88:1101–1108

Fess E, Philips C 1987 Hand splinting: principles and methods. C V Mosby, St Louis

Froimson A 1988 Tenosynovitis and tennis elbow. In: Green D (ed) Operative hand surgery, 2nd edn. Churchill Livingstone, Edinburgh 3(53):2117–2127

Frykman G, Nelson E 1990 Fractures and traumatic conditions of the wrist. In: Hunter J, Schneider L, Mackin E, Callahan A (eds) Rehabilitation of the hand, 3rd edn. C V Mosby, St Louis 18:267–283

Gelberman R H, Panagis J, Taleisnik J, Baumgaertner M 1983a The arterial anatomy of the human carpus. Part I. The extraosseus vascularity. Journal of Hand Surgery 8:367–375

Gelberman R H, Panagis J, Taleisnik J, Baumgaertner M 1983b The arterial anatomy of the human carpus. Part II. The intraosseus vascularity. Journal of Hand Surgery 8:375–382

Gelberman R H, Szabo R M 1984 Keinboch's disease. Orthopaedic Clinics of North America 15:355–367

Gelberman R, Gross M 1986 The vascularity of the wrist. Identification of arterial patterns at risk. Clinical Orthopaedics and Related Research 202:40–49

Gelberman R, Menon J 1980 The vascularity of the scaphoid bone. Journal of Hand Surgery 5:508–513

Gelberman R, Salamon P, Jurist J, Posch J 1975 Ulna variance in Keinboch's disease. Journal of Bone and Joint Surgery 57A:674–676

Grahame R 1985 The musculo-skeletal system. Diseases of the joints. In: Brocklehurst J C (ed) Textbook of geriatric medicine and gerontology, 3rd edn. Churchill Livingstone, Edinburgh 39:795–798

Green D 1988 Carpal dislocations and instabilities. In: Green D (ed) Operative hand surgery, 2nd edn. Churchill Livingstone, Edinburgh 2(20):875–938

Green D, Rowland S 1975 Fractures and dislocations in the hand. In: Rockwood C, Green D Fractures. J B Lippincott, Philadelphia 1(6):265–336

Hankin M, Peel S 1990 Sport-related fractures and dislocations in the hand. Hand Clinics: Hand Injuries in Sports and Performing Arts 6(3)(Aug):429–454

Hunter J M, Schneider L H, Mackin E J, Callahan A D (eds) 1990 Rehabilitation of the hand: surgery and therapy, 3rd edn. C V Mosby, St Louis

Johnson C 1984 Physical therapists as scar modifiers. Physical Therapy 64(9)(Sept):1381–1387

Kahler D M, Mc Cue F C 1992 Metacarpophalangeal and proximal interphalangeal joint injuries of the hand including the thumb. Clinics in Sports Medicine 11(1):57–76

Kapandji I A 1982 The physiology of the joints: annotated diagrams of the mechanics of the human joints. Upper limb, 5th edn. Churchill Livingstone, Edinburgh, pp. 168–228

Kapila H 1988 Essential hand surgery. Trans-Australian Publishing, Sydney

Kauer J M G 1974 The interdependence of carpal articulation chains. Acta Anatomica 88:481–501

Kauer J M G 1986 The mechanism of the carpal joint. Clinical Orthopaedics and Related Research 202:16–26

Kettlecamp D, Flatt A, Moulds R 1971 Traumatic dislocation of the long extensor tendon: a clinical, anatomical and bio-mechanical study. Journal of Bone and Joint Surgery 53(A):229

Koman L, Mooney J, Poehling G 1990 Fractures and ligamentous injuries of the wrist. Hand Clinics: Hand Injuries in Sports and Performing Arts 6(3)(Aug):477–491

Landsmeer J M, Long C 1965 The mechanism of finger control based on electromyograms and location analysis. Acta Anatomica 60:330–347

Lankford L 1990 Reflex sympathetic dystrophy. In: Hunter J, Schneider L, Mackin E, Callahan A (eds) Rehabilitation of the hand, 3rd edn. C V Mosby, St Louis 59:763–786

Larkins P 1988 Common running problems. Their assessment, management and prevention. Australian Sports Medicine Federation. Syntex Australia, Canberra, pp. 9–14

Lee M 1963 The interosseus arterial pattern of the carpal lunate bone and its relation to avascular necrosis. Acta Orthopaedica Scandinavica 33:43–45

Leonard J 1990 Joint protection for inflammatory disorders. In: Hunter J, Schneider L, Mackin E, Callahan A (eds) Rehabilitation of the hand, 3rd edn. C V Mosby, St Louis 72:908–911

Linscheid R L 1986 Kinematic considerations of the wrist. Clinical Orthopaedics and Related Research 202:27–39

Long C 1968 Intrinsic extrinsic control of the fingers: Electromyographic studies. Journal of Bone and Joint Surgery 50A:973–984

Long C, Brown M E 1964 Electromyographic kinesiology of the hand: muscles moving the long finger. Journal of Bone and Joint Surgery 46A:1683–1706

Malick M 1982 Manual on dynamic hand splinting with thermoplastic materials. Harmaville Rehabilitation, Pittsburgh

Malick M, Kasch M 1984 Manual on management of specific hand problems, Series 1. Aren Publications, Pittsburgh

Mayfield J K 1984 Patterns of injury to carpal ligaments: a spectrum. Clinical Orthopaedics and Related Research 187:36–42

Mayfield J K, Johnson R P, Kilcoyne R F 1976 The ligaments of the wrist and their functional significance. Anatomical Records 186:417–428

Mayfield J K, Williams W J, Erdman A G, Dahlof W, Wallrech M et al 1979 Biomechanical properties of human carpal ligaments. Orthopaedic Transactions 3:143

Mayfield J, Johnson R, Kilcoyne R 1980 Carpal dislocations: pathomechanics and progressive perilunar instability. Journal of Hand Surgery 5:226–241

McCue F C, Cabrera J M 1992 Common athletic digital joint injuries of the hand. In: Strickland J W, Rettig A C (eds) Hand injuries in athletes. W B Saunders, Philadelphia, pp. 49–94

McCue F, Wooten S L 1986 Closed tendon injuries of the hand in athletics. Clinics in Sports Medicine: Injuries to the Elbow Forearm and Hand (4)(Oct):741–745

Meier R H 1990 Mobility, exercise, muscular problems and rehabilitation. In: Schreir R W (ed) Geriatric medicine. W B Saunders, Philadelphia 32:368–375

Miles W, Grisby L 1990 Remodelling of scar tissue in the burned hand. In: Hunter J, Schneider L, Mackin E, Callahan A (eds) Rehabilitation of the hand, 3rd edn. C V Mosby, St Louis 65:841–857

Minami A, Kai-Nan An, Cooney W, Linscheid R, Chao E Y 1985 Ligament stability of the metacarpophalangeal joint: a biomechanical study. Journal of Hand Surgery 10A:255–264

Morgan R F, McCue F C 1983 Bilateral Keinbochs disease. Journal of Hand Surgery 8:928–932

Nathan R, Schneider L 1991 Classification of distal radioulnar joint disorders. Hand Clinics: Problems of the Distal Radioulnar Joint 7(2)(May):239–247

Nevasier R J 1992 Collateral injuries of the thumb metacarpophalangeal joint. In: Strickland J W, Rettig A C (eds) Hand injuries in athletes. W B Saunders, Philadelphia, pp. 95–106

Norkin C, Levange P K 1992 Joint structure and function: a comprehensive analysis, 2nd edn. F A Davis, Philadelphia, pp. 107–127

O'Brien T 1988 Fractures of the metacarpals amd phalanges In: Green D (ed) Operative hand surgery, 2nd edn. Churchill Livingstone, Edinburgh 1(17):709–775

Omer G 1992 Median nerve compression at the wrist. Hand Clinics: Nerve Compression Syndromes 8(2)(May):317–324

Osterman A, Mascow L, Low D 1988 Soft-tissue injuries of the hand and wrist in racquet sports. Clinic in Sports Medicine 7(2)(Apr):331–348

Palastanga N, Field D, Soames R 1989 Anatomy and human movement: structure and function. Heinemann Medical Books, Oxford, p 249

Palmer A 1988 Fractures of the distal radius. In: Green D (ed) Operative hand surgery, 2nd edn. Churchill Livingstone, Edinburgh 2(22):991–1022

Palmer A K 1987 The distal radioulnar joint: anatomy, biomechanics, and triangular fibrocartilage complex abnormalities. In: Taleisnik J (ed) Hand clinics. W B Saunders, Philadelphia 3:31–40

Palmer A K 1988 The distal radioulnar joint. In: Lichtman D M The wrist and its disorders. W B Saunders, Philadelphia, pp 220–231

Palmer A K, Glisson R R, Werner F W 1982 Ulna variance determination. Journal of Hand Surgery 7:376–379

Palmer A K, Glisson R R, Werner F W 1984 Relationship between ulna variance and triangular fibrocartilage complex thickness. Journal of Hand Surgery 9A:681–683

Palmer A K, Werner F W 1981 The triangular fibrocartilage complex of the wrist: anatomy and function. Journal of Hand Surgery 6:153–162

Palmer A K, Werner F W 1984 Biomechanics of the distal radioulnar joint. Clinical Orthopaedics and Related Research 187:26–34

Parker R, Berkowitz M, Brahms M, Bohl W 1986 Hook of the hamate fractures in athletes. American Journal of Sports Medicine 14(6):517–523

Poznanski A (ed) 1991 Hand Clinics: Imaging of the Hand 7(1)(Feb)

Press J, Wiesner S 1990 Prevention: conditioning and orthotics. Hand Clinics: Hand Injuries in Sports and Performing Arts 6(3)(Aug):383–392

Ray R D, Johnson R J, Jameson R M 1951 Rotation of the forearm. An experimental study of pronation and supination. Journal of Bone and Joint Surgery 33A:993–996

Reagan D, Linscheid R, Dobyns J 1984 Lunotriquetral sprains. Journal of Hand Surgery 9A:502–513

Rettig A 1990 Neurovascular injuries in the wrists and hands of athletes. Clinics in Sports Medicine 9(2)(Apr):389–417

Rose-Innes A P 1960 Anterior dislocation of the ulna at the inferior radioulnar joint. Journal of Bone and Joint Surgery 42B:515–521

Rosenthal E A 1990 The extensor tendons. In: Hunter J M, Schneider L H, Mackin E J, Callahan A D (eds) Rehabilitation of the hand: surgery and therapy, 3rd edn. C V Mosby, St Louis, pp. 458–491

Sarrafian S K, Melamed J L, Goshgarin G M 1977 Study of wrist motion in flexion and extension. Clinical Orthopaedics and Related Research 126:153

Schneider L (ed) 1991 Problems of the distal radio-ulnar joint. Hand Clinics 7(2)(May)

Siegal D B, Gelberman R H 1991 Radial styloidectomy: an anatomical study with special reference to radiocarpal intracapsular ligamentous morphology. Journal of Hand Surgery 16A:40–44

Slattery P G 1990 The dorsal plate of the proximal interphalangeal joint. Journal of Hand Surgery 15B:68–73

Spinner M 1978 Injuries to the major branches of peripheral nerves of the forearm, 2nd edn. W B Saunders, Philadelphia

Stener B 1985 Acute injuries to the metacarpophalangeal joint of the thumb. In: Tubiana R (ed) The hand. W B Saunders, Philadelphia, vol II, pp. 895–903

Stern P 1990 Tendinitis, overuse syndromes and tendon injuries. Hand Clinics: Hand Injuries in Sport and Performing Arts 6(3)(Aug)

Stewart K 1990 Therapist's management of the mutilated hand. In: Hunter J, Schneider L, Mackin E, Callahan A (eds) Rehabilitation of the hand, 3rd edn. C V Mosby, St Louis 16:240–252

Strickland W 1987 Biological basis for hand splinting. In: Fess E, Philips C Hand splinting: principles and methods. C V Mosby, St Louis 2:43–70

Sundberg S, Linscheid R 1984 Keinbochs disease: results of treatment with ulna lengthening. Clinical Orthopaedics and Related Research 187:43–51

Taleisnik J 1985 The wrist. Churchill Livingstone, New York, pp. 8, 13–38, 41

Taleisnik J 1988 Fractures of the carpal bones. In: Green D (ed) Operative hand surgery, 2nd edn. Churchill Livingstone, Edinburgh

Taleisnik J 1988 Current concepts review: carpal instability. Journal of Bone and Joint Surgery 70A:1262–1268

Taleisnik J 1992 Soft tissue injuries of the wrist. In: Strickland J W, Rettig A C (eds) Hand injuries in athletes. W B Saunders, Philadelphia, pp. 107–127

Taleisnik J, Gelberman R, Miller B 1984 The extensor retinaculum of the wrist. Journal of Hand Surgery 9A:495–501

Taylor Mullins P 1990 Use of therapeutic modalities in upper extremity rehabilitation. In: Hunter J, Schneider L, Mackin E, Callahan A (eds) Rehabilitation of the hand, 3rd edn. C V Mosby, St Louis 14:195–219

Thiru-Pathi R G, Ferlic D, Clayton M L, McClure D C 1986 Arterial anatomy of the triangular fibrocartilge complex of the wrist and its surgical significance. Journal of Hand Surgery 11A:258–263

Totten P 1990 Therapist's management of de Quervain's disease. In: Hunter J, Schneider L, Mackin E, Callahan A (eds) Rehabilitation of the hand, 3rd edn. C V Mosby, St Louis 22:308–317

Tubiana R (ed) 1985 The hand. W B Saunders, Philadelphia, vol II

Valentin P 1981 Physiology of extension of the fingers. In: Tubiana P (ed) The hand. W B Saunders, Philadelphia 1(40):389–388

van Strien G 1990 Postoperative management of flexor tendon injuries. In: Hunter J, Schneider L, Mackin E, Callahan A (eds) Rehabilitation of the hand, 3rd edn. C V Mosby, St Louis 30:390–409

Verdan C 1966 Primary and secondary repair of flexor and extensor tendon injuries. In: Flynn J (ed) Hand surgery, 3rd edn. Williams & Wilkins, Baltimore 8:220–275

Vesely D G 1967 The distal radioulnar joint. Clinical Orthopaedics and Related Research 51:75–91

Wadsworth H, Chanmugam A 1980 Electrophysical agents in physiotherapy. Science Press, Australia, ch 5

Waylett-Rendall J 1990 Therapist's management of reflex sympathetic dystrophy. In: Hunter J, Schneider L, Mackin E, Callahan A (eds) Rehabilitation of the hand, 3rd edn. C V Mosby, St Louis 60:787–792

Weber E R 1988 Wrist mechanics and its association with ligamentous instability. In: Lichtman D M (ed) The wrist and its disorders. W B Saunders, Philadelphia, pp. 41–52

Wehbe M 1987 Tendon gliding exercises. American Journal of Occupational Therapy 41(3)(March):64–167

Wheeldon F 1954 Recurrent dislocation of extensor tendons. Journal of Bone and Joint Surgery 36(B):612

Whipple T, Geissler W 1991 Arthroscopic management of the athlete: part ll: triangular fibrocartilage tears. Journal of Hand Therapy 4(1)Apr-Jun:61–63

Williams J, Sperrin P 1976 Sports medicine, 2nd edn. Edward Arnold, London 27:520

Williams P, Warwick R 1980 Grays anatomy. Churchill Livingstone, Edinburgh, pp 471–472, p 1100

Wilson R, Carter S 1990 Management of hand fractures. In: Hunter J, Schneider L, Mackin E, Callahan A (eds) Rehabilitation of the hand, 3rd edn. C V Mosby, St Louis

Wynn Parry C 1973 Rehabilitation of the hand, 3rd edn. Butterworths, London 1:31

Youm Y, McMurtry R Y, Flatt A E, Gillespe T E 1978 Kinematics of the wrist: an experimental study of radioulnar deviation and flexion-extension. Journal of Bone and Joint Surgery 6A:423–431

Zemel N 1986 Fractures and dislocations of the carpal bones. Clinics in Sports Medicine 5(4)(Oct):709–772

Contraindications and/or precautions

- malignancy
- inflammatory conditions
- spinal cord signs
- irritable conditions
- severe unremitting night pain
- nerve-root compression
- recent paraesthesia or anaesthesia
- when active neck movements easily provoke distal symptoms
- reflex sympathetic dystrophy
- unstable shoulder

Care should be taken while performing the test in athletes with an inflammatory process or an 'irritable' condition. The test should be performed in conjunction with other examination procedures of the cervical region (see Ch. 21), upper limb joints and muscles (see Chs 2 and 4) and neurological examination of the upper limbs.

The ULTT produces strain on the BP by a combination of movements involving shoulder girdle depression, shoulder abduction posterior to the coronal plane, external rotation of the shoulder, elbow extension (EE) and forearm supination, followed by wrist and finger extension (WE). In order to further identify a BP or upper limb neural component the limb manoeuvres could be performed with the cervical spine in ipsilateral flexion (ILF) then in contralateral flexion (CLF) (Elvey 1985).

Anatomical studies indicate that upper limb manoeuvres of the test produce strain on the branches of the BP (Ginn 1988, Reid 1987, Wilson et al 1991). Anatomical investigators have also demonstrated that limb manoeuvres of the test with cervical CLF produce greater strain on the C5 to T1 roots of the BP than with cervical ILF (Selvaratnam et al 1989). Therefore, while the limb manoeuvres produce strain on the BP, cervical CLF and ILF would produce a difference in strain on the plexus and thereby identify a BP component in upper limb pain (Selvaratnam 1991).

Elvey (1983) proposed that if there was an abnormal tension or restriction in movement of the BP, limb manoeuvres of the ULTT (e.g. EE and WE with cervical CLF) would increase tension on the BP and thereby reproduce the patient's pain earlier than the total extension pattern with cervical ILF. The range of EE or EE and WE should be evaluated at the point of pain onset (when performed with cervical ILF and CLF) in order to identify a BP component in upper limb pain. The test could also be performed by varying the sequence of limb and cervical manoeuvres in order to identify the potential neural component in upper limb pain.

Elvey (1986a) also postulated that if the patient's upper limb pain could not be reproduced by the test, a BP involvement could be identified on the basis of restriction in the range of upper limb manoeuvres (e.g. EE or EE and WE) with cervical lateral flexion. He suggested that if there were an abnormal tension or restriction in movement of the BP it may limit the total extension range with cervical CLF and thereby assist in identifying a BP involvement. The presence or absence of restriction in movement of manoeuvres of the ULTT should therefore be assessed if the athlete's symptoms are not reproduced by the test.

The contribution of the peripheral upper limb neural structures should be evaluated as well. For instance, if the ULTT was determined to be positive in an athlete with lateral epicondylitis, this may indicate that the pain could be referred from the cervical region or originate from neural structures between the shoulder and elbow region.

The novice performing the test should be cautious in interpreting positive ULTT findings as involvement of the BP since different structures can contribute to the upper limb pain. Indeed, the cervical zygapophyseal joints (Bogduk & Marsland 1988), cervical interspinous ligaments (Kellgren 1939), cervical muscles (Travell & Rinzler 1952), cervical intervertebral discs (Cloward 1959), cervical sympathetic nerves (Middleditch & Jarman 1984), the upper limb muscles, joint structures, arteries and fasciae (Selvaratnam 1991) could also contribute to upper limb pain in an athlete.

Examining the cervical region (see Ch. 21) and upper limb joints and muscles (see Chs 2 and 4) might assist therapists in evaluating if the athlete's upper limb pain has a cervical component or an upper limb component. Anterior palpation of the roots of the brachial plexus and the scalene muscles might reproduce the athlete's upper limb symptoms and thereby assist therapists in identifying the potential cervical component. Care is needed while performing anterior palpation since the phrenic nerve, the vagus nerve and the carotid arteries traverse this region.

While the ULTT produces selective strain on the BP and its peripheral branches, recent anatomical investigations indicate that the manoeuvres of the test may also produce selective strain on the subclavian and axillary vessels, the cervical sympathetic nerves and the cervicothoracic fasciae (Selvaratnam 1991, Selvaratnam et al 1994, Wilson et al 1991). Injury to the subclavian and axillary vessels might produce vascular symptoms in the upper limb (Tullos et al 1972). The vascular contribution may be distinguished from a BP component by examining for the presence of peripheral cyanosis, altered skin temperature and changes in the radial pulse (Kenneally et al 1988). Arterial involvement may be further identified by Doppler investigation and arteriographic studies (Baker & Thornberry 1985) while occlusion of the subclavian vein may be diagnosed by phlebographic studies (McCue et al 1985).

MODIFICATIONS OF THE ULTT

Mark 1 ULTT

It has been found difficult to perform the 'traditional' ULTT (Elvey 1980, 1983) owing to problems with

1

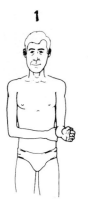

2

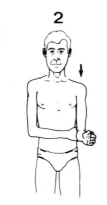

3

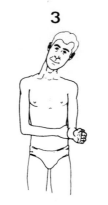

4

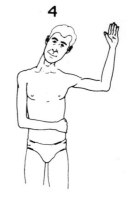

5

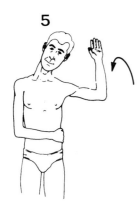

6

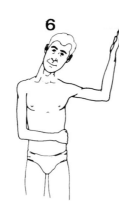

7

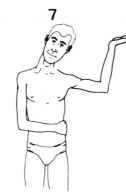

8

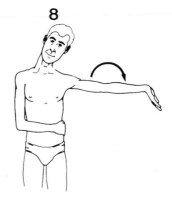

9

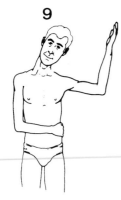

10

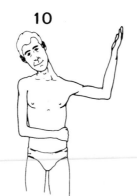

11

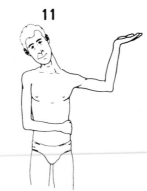

12

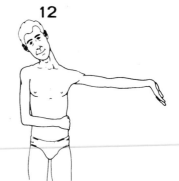

13

1	Starting position
2	Shoulder depression
3	Cervical spine ipsilateral flexion (ILF)
4	Shoulder abduction posterior to the coronal plane
5	Shoulder external rotation with the cervical spine in ILF
6	Forearm supination
7	Wrist and finger extension (forearm supinated and cervical spine in ILF)
8	Elbow extension with the wrist extended and the cervical spine in ILF
9	Elbow returned to 90° flexion (cervical spine in ILF)
10	Cervical spine contralateral flexion (CLF)
11	Wrist and finger extension with the forearm supinated (cervical spine is maintained in CLF)
12	Elbow extension with wrist extended and cervical spine in CLF
13	Elbow returned to 90° flexion and cervical spine in CLF

Fig. 26.1 Steps of the Mark 1 ULTT

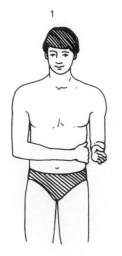

1

Starting position

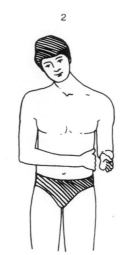

2

Cervical contralateral flexion

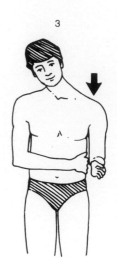

3

Shoulder depression

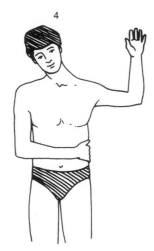

4

Shoulder abduction posterior
to the coronal plane

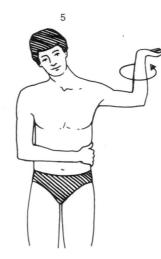

5

Wrist extension and
forearm supination

6

Shoulder external rotation

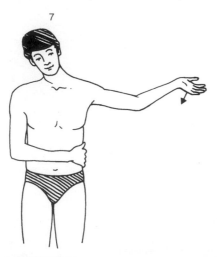

7

Elbow extension

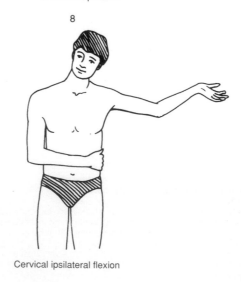

8

Cervical ipsilateral flexion

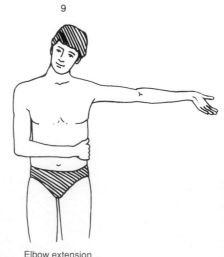

9

Elbow extension
(if pain is reduced on cervical ILF)

Fig. 26.2 Steps of the Mark 11 ULTT

neural component. Due
procedures need to be
assessment of the pain

Management

Day 1

Manual cervical distr
performed in the sup
5 repetitions) since thi
pain on objective exam
the cervical intrathecal
1946) in addition to ot
procedure there was a 3
cervical rotation impro
reproduced with ULTT n
depression and 70° of \

Day 2 (2 days later)

The baseballer reported
that he was still experier
activities. On examinat
changed as at the end of
cervical rotation was mair
at 30° of flexion was repe
objective or subjective si

Treatment was then
cervical spine (Elvey 19
order to mobilize the cerv
intervertebral foramen ar
the irritability of the cond
(Maitland 1986) was perfe
times. Since the objectiv
shoulder girdle depressio
technique; duration 20 s; 3
the anatomical position. F
was reproduced later in th
and right shoulder flexion (1
shoulder depression was p
in 90° flexion) reproduced

Day 3 (1 week later)

The baseballer reported th
activities. Active cervical a
free. The shoulder pain w
abduction (40°) (elbow in 9
girdle depression was rep
day 2. The range of shoulde

Following this, should
duration 20s; 3 repetitions) v
abduction or WE were unal

Elbow extension was th
duration 20s; 3 repetitions)
of abduction (just before p
depressed. The range of pa
to 100°.

measurement of upper limb manoeuvres and errors in measurement (Selvaratnam et al1987, Selvaratnam 1991). In order to reduce the number of variables, the number of angles required for measurement and clinical decision making, a modified ULTT was devised (Selvaratnam 1991). The modified 'Mark 1' ULTT also gives an opportunity to investigate different ways of performing cervical and limb manoeuvres of the traditional ULTT, although in principle the manoeuvres of both tests are the same.

The manoeuvres of the Mark 1 ULTT (Fig. 26.1) are passive shoulder depression, followed by cervical ILF, shoulder abduction posterior to the coronal plane, shoulder external rotation, then forearm supination followed by WE with the elbow maintained in 90° flexion. Next the elbow joint is extended. The limb manoeuvres of the test are performed again with the cervical spine in CLF. In the Mark 1 ULTT the range of EE may be used to determine the involvement of the BP or upper limb neural structures if WE does not reproduce the patient's symptoms.

Mark 11 ULTT

The Mark 11 version of the ULTT (Fig. 26.2) (Fabbri 1988, Selvaratnam et al 1989, Wajswelner et al 1989) was developed since therapists found it difficult to visually estimate the range at which a patient reported arm pain.

All manoeuvres of the Mark 11 ULTT are performed passively to pain onset or change in pain, i.e. reproduction of the athlete's shoulder or upper limb pain. The manoeuvres of the test are performed passively by initially positioning the cervical spine in CLF followed by shoulder girdle depression, shoulder abduction posterior to the coronal plane, WE, forearm supination then shoulder external rotation. Next, the elbow is extended to the point of pain onset. The cervical spine is then positioned in ILF and the athlete's pain response is recorded. A 'positive' test is indicated if limb manoeuvres of the test with cervical CLF reproduce the athlete's pain while cervical ILF reduces the pain. If cervical ILF reduces the athlete's pain, the elbow joint may be extended to further confirm the potential BP or upper limb neural component.

Variations of the ULTT

In order to further identify a BP component or involvement of spinal canal structures the ULTT could be performed on the non-affected arm after performing the test on the symptomatic arm (Kenneally et al 1988, Rubenach 1985). Rubenach (1985) hypothesized that performing the ULTT on the non-affected arm produced lateral displacement of the spinal cord and BP, and thereby could be implicated if the athlete's symptoms were altered.

The ULTT could also be performed in conjunction with single or bilateral SLR (Bell 1987). Any change in the athlete's pain may implicate involvement of the BP and/or spinal canal structures since SLR produces a caudal displacement of the spinal cord and dura and thereby places strain on the roots of the BP (Bell 1987).

The manoeuvres of the ULTT described previously are performed with the forearm in supination and would therefore produce greater strain on the median nerve. The limb manoeuvres of the test could also be performed with the forearm in pronation to produce strain on the radial nerve (Butler 1991, Gross 1989). Forearm pronation may be useful in examining athletes with lateral epicondylitis or posterior forearm pain (Butler 1991, Gross 1989).

The upper limb manoeuvres of the test may also be performed with the shoulder in the quadrant position (Maitland 1977) (Fig. 26.3). This position could assist in evaluating the contribution of the lower roots and lower trunks of the BP or the ulnar nerve. To further evaluate the neural contribution the elbow can be extended with the neck in the anatomical position or with the neck in CLF. If the athlete's pain is not reproduced the wrist and fingers

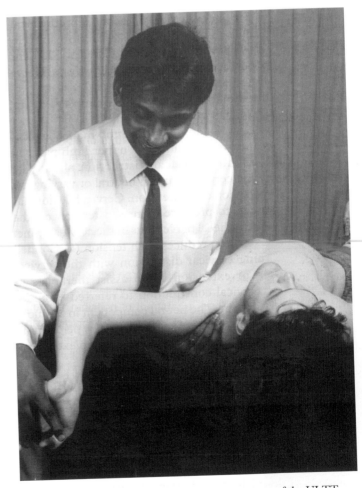

Fig. 26.3 Elbow and wrist extension and manoeuvres of the ULTT performed in the shoulder quadrant position with the cervical spine in contralateral flexion

can be ext(
position cc
radial or u
componen

Modificatio:

The limb n
to consider
presents w:
initially ass(
girdle retra(
These man(
the sitting p(
shoulder gir
C4–C7 nerv
strain produ
external rota
would strain
potential ne
pain. Cervica
shoulder gir
component.

If should(
athlete's sh(
performed to
ILF are thei
volvement. E
formed with t
contribution.

In the acu
the test might
that instance
performed wit
angle of cervic
been demonst
intrathecal and
while cervical
1946). Perfor
spine in flexic
identifying the
and/or upper li
or upper limb p
EE and/or WE

APPLICATIO:

Elvey's pioneer
guidelines on pe
pain perception
upper limb nerv
adopted in mot
noeuvres of the

Passive mo\
mobilize the ner

Wilson S 1989 Strain at the subclavian artery during the brachial plexus tension test. An anatomical study on embalmed cadavers. Unpublished postgraduate thesis. Lincoln School of Health Sciences, La Trobe University, Carlton, Victoria

Wilson S, Selvaratnam P, Briggs C 1991 The strain at the subclavian artery during the brachial plexus tension test. A pilot study in embalmed cadavers. In: Proceedings of the 7th biennial conference of the Manipulative Physiotherapists Association of Australia. Blue Mountains, New South Wales, pp 220-225

Wright I S 1945 The neurovascular syndrome produced by hyperabduction of the arms. American Heart Journal 29(1):1-19

27. The lumbar region

Lance Twomey, James R. Taylor, Charles Flynn

PART 1
ANATOMY AND BIOMECHANICS
Lance Twomey, James R. Taylor

Sporting injuries of the lumbar spine need to be considered against a background of the changes through which the region passes in the life cycle of development, maturation and progressive decline. Just as the nature of the sports enjoyed by individuals changes through life, so do the stresses imposed on the vertebral column, and so also does the column respond differently to such stresses. Sport is no longer the sole province of the young and there are many individuals who participate in active sport well into their eighth and even ninth decades.

The flexibility and biomechanics of the lumbar spine change considerably during life, and differ between the genders during the childbearing years. The female vertebral column is usually shorter, more slender and flexible than the male column of the same age (Taylor & Twomey 1984). Thus, while the vertebral column of an adolescent female has the potential for bending further than that of a male under the influence of an applied load, it is less strong than that of the male counterpart and more liable to fail under a given load.

The musculo-skeletal system demands quite high levels of stress-related activity at every stage through life, and in general responds favourably to the usual stresses of sport. However, (particularly with the elite athlete), the size of the loads may be too large for the musculo-skeletal system to absorb safely, or the repetitive nature of the activity may bring about fatigue strain or fracture. The very nature of competitive sport, together with the extraordinarily strong motivation of many participants, can mean that many athletes, by continually attempting to improve their performance, place themselves at considerable risk of musculo-skeletal damage as a regular part of their sporting activity.

Just as different sports impose different forces on the spine, the size of the forces and the response of the spine to these loads in the highly trained elite athlete will differ significantly from those of the weekend sporting amateur. Thus, a load which is readily absorbed by the forearm of a well trained, elite tennis player may be sufficient to produce tendinous damage in the occasional player.

These factors need to be borne in mind when considering the potentially damaging effects of sport on the lumbar spine. Any physiotherapist considering a spinal sports injury needs to view it in the context of the age, gender, level of participation, expectations and likely physiological response to treatment of the involved athlete.

THE LUMBAR SPINE

The adult vertebral column is a segmented, jointed, flexible rod, which supports the load of the body in the upright posture, protects the spinal cord and spinal nerves, allows very considerable flexibility in all directions, acts as a shock absorber and serves as the axial support for the body. Thus, its task is complex and the demands made on it are often contradictory in nature, i.e. it must be stable and yet allow a large range of motion. The spine achieves these goals by virtue of the complex linkage of its structural elements, the vertebral and motion segments.

The spine's ability to properly serve its functions alters significantly through the phases of its life cycle, associated with changes in its posture, mobility and strength. At birth, the C-shaped column is malleable and extremely flexible. In infancy and early childhood it rapidly develops its series of finely balanced curves (Fig. 27.1). Growth and maturation are thus linked with progressive increases in the strength and stability of the spine, although at the progressive expense of some of its flexibility. Middle age is associated with an increase in minor traumatic and degenerative pathology, which is generally associated with a further progressive decline in the range of all movements, but in some instances may result in an abnormal increased range at one or more segments due to segmental instability. In old age, osteopenia brings about a decrease in bone

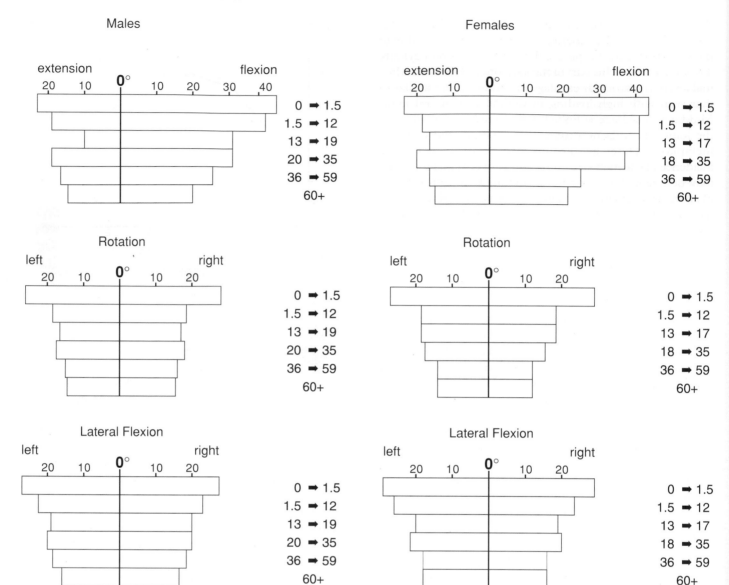

Fig. 27.4 The reduction in the range of movements of the lumbar spine which occurs during the life cycle

Mechanics

The extreme positions of full lumbar flexion and extension are used in quite different ways in Western societies (Twomey & Taylor 1987). Many recreations and occupations may involve a position of full flexion sustained for considerable periods of time, but sustained postures in extension are quite rare. However, there are many activities involving repetitive, intermittent, high velocity movements into full extension, while this is uncommon for flexion.

Sustained loading in flexion and repeated high impact extension movements in adolescent and young subjects may bring about substantial structural changes to the joints and soft tissues of the lumbar spine. Some of these changes may be regarded as part of the normal maturation of the region, although end range loading may also contribute toward pathological change when the stresses and strains at the limits of flexion and extension are excessive (Taylor & Twomey 1986, Twomey & Taylor 1987). Flexion, either of high or low velocity, is progressively braked by the posterior ligaments (supraspinous, interspinous, ligamentum flavum and Z joint capsules), but ceases because of the increasingly strong apposition of the superior and inferior articular facets of the Z joints. Indeed, the restrictive effect of compression of facetal joint surfaces is greater than that of the tension in the posterior ligaments (Twomey & Taylor 1983).

In contrast, full extension is associated with compression of the posterior annulus fibrosis and usually ceases when the inferior facets of the Z joints abut on the laminae of the vertebra below (White & Panjabi 1978). Occasionally in the elderly, due to shortening of the anterior spinal column, the spinous processes 'kiss' (Farfan 1973). The fat pads and loose areolar tissue of the inferior recesses of the two joints (Bogduk & Engel 1984, Lewin 1968) form a buffer between the hard, sharp inferior facets and the solid laminae, and help to attenuate the sudden jarring force of rapid full range extension, a particular feature of some sporting activities. This loading in extension is concentrated in a localized area of each inferior recess, and the loading borne by the lamina at this point (the pars interarticularis) is attested by the sclerosis and thickening of compact bone observed in young adult spines (Fig. 27.5)(Taylor & Twomey 1986). Repetitive, high impact loading as seen in

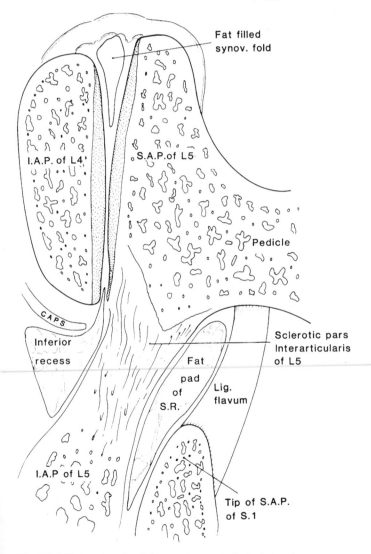

Fig. 27.5 Bone sclerosis of the pars interarticularis region due to repetitive contact of the inferior articular process of the L5–S1 lumbar facet joint
SAP = superior articular process
IAP = inferior articular process
LF = ligamentum flavum
CAP = capsule

some sporting activities may eventually lead to spondylolysis (see below).

Whether the laminae are loaded through the Z facets in sustained flexion, or by high velocity loading in extension, it is the pars interarticularis which transmits these loads. In the adolescent and young adult spine, such activities are associated with a high prevalence of spondylolysis. Such activities as fast bowling, gymnastics and football are linked with a high incidence of spondylolysis. In older subjects, the laminae respond to loading by hypertrophy with the conversion of a triangular spinal canal to a trefoil shape, and thus a risk of developing spinal stenosis (Twomey & Taylor 1987).

Sustained loading

Creep

Creep is defined as the progressive deformation of a structure under constant load by forces which are not large enough to cause permanent damage to the components of the structure (Kazarian 1975, Twomey & Taylor 1982). The lumbar spine is subjected to both axial creep and creep in flexion as a routine part of many daily activities.

Creep in flexion occurs when the spine is loaded in full flexion. This procedure not only squeezes fluid out from the intervertebral discs (IVDs), the articular cartilage of the joints and the spinal ligaments, but it distorts the disc and other soft tissues by redistributing the remaining fluid within them. Creep in flexion is observed as progressive ventral movement further into flexion, so that the end-point of the movement is increased beyond its normal range. The amount of creep in the elderly is greater than in the young and both the creep and the recovery from creep take place over a longer period of time in older subjects (Twomey & Taylor 1982). During this prolonged process the extrusion of fluid from the soft tissues deprives them of a part of their nutrition (Adams & Hutton 1985b). In addition, if the force is maintained for a sufficiently long period, then the 'crimp' in the collagen fibrils is likely to be progressively reduced as the fibrils slowly elongate under the constant pressure (Broom & Marra 1986, Shah et al 1978). If high loads are applied for periods longer than one hour, a large amount of creep is achieved and recovery to the original starting posture (hysteresis) is extremely slow, particularly in the elderly. It takes many hours of rest for the soft tissues to imbibe enough fluid to re-establish their usual shape (i.e. to reach equilibrium) after such sustained flexion loading (Twomey & Taylor 1982).

Motor sports involve creep in flexion, as the drivers sit at the limit of lumbar flexion, under the sustained load of their own torso, accentuated by considerable vibration through the seat. They have little opportunity to move away from this position and may need to sustain it for many hours under racing conditions. The incidence of back pain among racing car drivers is considerable.

The effects of sagittal movements on lumbar joints

Intervertebral discs

The IVDs are always under an external load that changes with posture and activity; it is highest in standing with the lumbar spine flexed, and lowest when recumbent (Nachemson 1960a). The amount of fluid expressed from the IVDs depends both on the size of the external load and the duration of application. Fluid can interchange between the disc and adjacent tissues primarily through the vertebral end-plate. The swelling pressure of the disc arises from the difference between the expansion pressure of the proteoglycans which causes the tissue to imbibe fluid and the tensile forces of the collagen network which limit the swelling (Bayliss et al 1986). This swelling pressure is opposed by external compressive loading of the disc. In this way the disc acts as a pump for fluid and metabolite transfer. Kraemer et al (1985) suggest that under axial load, there is an 11% fluid loss from the annulus fibrosis and an 8% loss from the nucleus pulposus. As previously noted, after a day's activity involving standing, fluid movement back into the discs occurs slowly at rest when recumbent in extension, and more rapidly when the recumbent spine rests in flexion (Tyrrell et al 1985).

Similarly, Adams and Hutton (1985a, 1986) have shown that when lumbar discs are flexed under load, fluid and metabolites are forced out of the anterior, more compressed parts of the discs and squeezed back into the posterior regions. The reverse occurs during extension movements. Thus, IVD nutrition can be significantly increased by the fluid exchanges accompanying reciprocal movements in the sagittal plane. On the other hand, sustained postures at the extremes of a movement range would deprive parts of the discs of their nutrition for long periods of time. It is highly likely that this static situation accelerates age change and degeneration (Frank et al 1984).

High velocity movements to end-range may take parts of the lumbar discs and their attached longitudinal ligaments beyond their normal elastic limits, causing small tears and fissures in the annulus, thereby reducing its capacity to cope with the normal environmental stresses. The discs are particularly vulnerable to these movements after they have been permitted to creep by the prolonged maintenance of a flexed or extended posture. Repeated traumatic episodes to the disc and surrounding bony and ligamentous structures would result in loss of disc tissue, effusion and scarring, and further reduce the ability of the disc to act efficiently as a pump.

Zygapophyseal joints

The anteromedial coronally oriented third of the Z joint articular surfaces is responsible for protecting the IVD from shear forces by load bearing in flexion (Taylor & Twomey 1986). The typical chondromalacia-like age changes seen in this region are those associated with pressure loading. Initially, there is chondrocyte hypertrophy in the mid-zone of the articular cartilage (AC), and increased staining of cells and territorial matrix with haematoxylin. This may progress to vertical splitting of the whole thickness of the AC, which is frequently accompanied by sclerotic changes in the subchondral bone plate. The development of selective wedge-shaped thickening in the anterior part of the adolescent subchondral bone plate of the superior facet, and its continued thickening until middle life, reflect not only greater compressive loading on the anterior part of the facet, but also a greater effect of loading on the concave facet than on the convex surface (Taylor & Twomey 1986). These reactions to the stresses of sustained flexion in the coronal third of the superior articular facets (Fig. 27.6) are frequently accompanied by a different set of changes in the posterior sagittal parts of the joint (Fig. 27.6), particularly in the region of the inferior part of the capsule (the area most under tension during flexion). In middle life and old age, this posterior marginal damage (PMD) may progress to splits in the AC parallel to the subchondral bone plate, stretching and tears in the joint capsule, and the development of osteophytes on the posterior joint margins (Taylor & Twomey 1986).

Similarly, extension brings about changes to the bone, AC and capsule in the region of the inferior recess of the lumbar Z joints (Twomey & Taylor 1987). These changes are evident as hypercalcification and sclerosis of the lamina directly beneath the inferior recess of the joint, and as damage to the joint capsule and AC (Fig. 27.5). Laminal sclerosis may eventually be followed by fracture of the pars interarticularis (spondylolisthesis, as in Fig. 27.7) if the forces transmitted through the inferior facets are excessive or repeated for long enough; PMD is evident as ligamentous tears and stretching of the capsule and fragmentation of the AC.

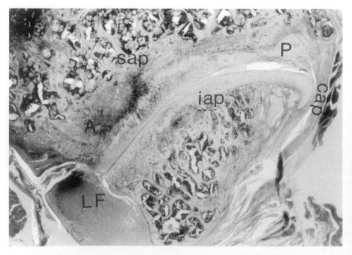

Fig. 27.6 Horizontal section of the L3 facet joint indicating the changes occurring at the anterior **A** and posterior **P** regions of the joint

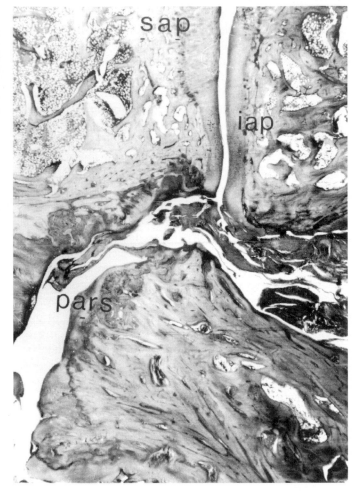

Fig. 27.7 Spondylolisthesis (SP) at the L5–S1 level in a 17-year-old male
SAP = superior articular process
IAP = inferior articular process
PARS = pars interarticularis

The considerable trauma of motor vehicle accidents has been shown to cause considerable damage to the Z joints in the lumbar spine, which are often not seen by conventional radiology (Taylor et al 1990, Twomey et al 1989). The injuries include fractures and infractions of the subchondral bone plate, splitting of articular cartilage and sprains and tearing of the joint capsule. While spinal joint pathology has only been linked with motor vehicle accidents at present, it is possible that severe trauma to the spine associated with sporting activities such as rugby and parachuting may cause similar injuries.

SPINAL INJURIES

Low back pain and dysfunction in athletes

Non-specific low back pain

Low back pain is the most persistent and pernicious musculoskeletal complaint in Western societies (Nachemson 1976). It has been demonstrated that over 80% of all people in 'developed' countries will suffer from backache of sufficient intensity to cause them to seek professional help at least once (Waddell 1987). While in most individuals (95%), this back pain is resolved in 10–21 days, in a small percentage of individuals it persists for very much longer. This 5% of back pain patients constitute 90% of the costs of treatment of low back pain (Ganora 1986, Waddell 1987). These costs include not only the direct cost of treatment, but also the time lost to employment, compensation and considerable suffering for the individuals involved. Athletes are not exempt from these statistics and the incidence of back pain among most athletic groups mirrors that of the population as a whole (Steven & Irvin 1983). However, the general, non-specific back pain which incapacitates members of the general public may be less likely to affect the quality of athletes' performances (Rovere 1987). This is generally considered to be due to the better physical conditioning, muscle strength and motivation of the athletes to continue the physical demands of their chosen sports (Cinque 1989). Since most athletes are well conditioned and fit, often with strong trunk musculature, they are less likely to suffer from the postural back strain or backache which is most prevalent among the general population. Indeed, many of the spinal injuries among trained, fit athletes are directly related to their sport (Steven & Irwin 1983).

Kulund (1988) considers that many athletes develop low back pain because of spending a prolonged amount of time near the limit of lumbar flexion, e.g. while driving a car, or working at some unaccustomed activity such as building. In support of this view, a number of studies have shown that sustained postures at the limit of a joint range are associated with back pain and with an increasing incidence of degenerative change to the discs and facet joints of the lumbar spine (McKenzie 1980, Twomey et al 1988). Occupations and activities which require a sustained load-bearing posture at the limit of flexion are likely to damage the spinal joints and progressively bring about degenerative changes, unless regular opportunities for postural adjustment are encouraged (Twomey & Taylor 1987). Prolonged sitting in full lumbar flexion is potentially hazardous, and emphasizes the need for maintenance of a lordotic lumbar curve as postulated by McKenzie (1980). Athletes need to be aware of the potential dangers associated with sustained lumbar flexion, both in terms of the immediate development of low back pain and in view of the potentially harmful long term effects of the posture (Twomey et al 1988).

Athletes suffer acute mechanical back pain in about the same proportions as do members of the general population (Kulund 1988). However, a greater proportion of them respond favourably to conservative treatment, emphasizing the value of joint motion (Kulund 1988, Rovere 1987). Most athletes recover from acute non-specific low back pain within 10 days, and far fewer athletes than members of the general public progress to chronic, disabling low back pain

(Rovere 1987). Where back pain persists in an athlete for longer than 7–10 days and does not respond fully to conservative treatment, it is likely that there has been substantial damage to either the bony or collagenous components of the lumbar spine.

Contusions to the lumbar spine

Contusions to the lumbar spine are common, particularly in contact sports such as all codes of football. Direct trauma to the large post-vertebral muscle complex is likely to result in haematoma associated with considerable regional swelling and local pain. The dense thoraco-lumbar fascia envelops the back musculature (Bogduk & McIntosh 1984). This can provide an additional complication to the effects of trauma. If there is intramuscular bleeding and swelling within the thoraco-lumbar fascia, a compartment syndrome may develop. This causes considerable pain and muscle spasm and the region is particularly tender to pressure and painful on movement.

Ligamentous damage to either the thoraco-lumbar fascia or to the other posterior ligaments may also result from direct trauma or from injuries which take a joint complex beyond its normal range. Although 'sprain' of the ligaments of the back is not currently a fashionable diagnosis, efforts to achieve maximum performance may mean that collagenous structures are taken beyond their normal limits of movement and thus ligaments may tear (Corrigan & Maitland 1983).

Spondylolysis and spondylolisthesis

The incidence of spondylolysis and spondylolisthesis among sports persons is considerably higher than in the general population (Wiltse et al 1975). Spondylolysis is a mechanical failure of the pars interarticularis of the lamina of a lumbar vertebra, resulting in a fracture (Troup 1977). It is most common at the L5 level, less so at L4 and decreasingly common at higher lumbar levels. The bone failure is clearly mechanical and usually associated, particularly in athletes, with a fatigue fracture, following repetitive loading movements in the region (Cyron & Hutton 1978, Hutton et al 1977, Twomey et al 1988).

Spondylolisthesis refers to an anterior 'slip' or displacement of a vertebral body on the one beneath (most commonly L5 on the sacrum), following bilateral fracture of the pars interarticularis (Wiltse & Winter 1983). The anterior displacement or slip may be assigned a grade of I, II, III or IV to describe slips of one, two, three or four quarters respectively of the superior on the inferior vertebra. It may also be defined as a percentage of the antero-posterior diameter of the top of the lower vertebra (Wiltse & Winter 1983). The slip of the upper vertebra on the lower is usually associated with sagittal rotation or 'roll' of the upper vertebra, usually expressed as a slip angle.

Fracture of the pars interarticularis is not always associated with the slip and roll of spondylolisthesis (Wiltse 1969). Why spondylolysis should become spondylolisthesis in some individuals and not in others is uncertain. However, it has been shown that the slip is more common in young people and that persons who develop spondylolisthesis show considerable posterior wedging of the slipped vertebrae. This is usually at the L5 level, and Sim (1973) showed a significant difference in the L5 wedging index in a matched study which compared 24 cases of spondylolisthesis with the general public (an average index of 0.70 compared to an average of 0.91). Another anatomical feature which may predispose some individuals towards the slip of L5 on the sacrum is rounding of the cranial border of the first sacral vertebrae (Wiltse & Winter, 1983). This rounding of S1 is also a feature of advanced, long standing spondylolisthesis and is increased by the remodelling pressure of the slipped L5 on the anterior margin of the cranial border of S1. Most spondylolisthesis occurs in young adults (under 25 years), perhaps because the increasing collagen content of older intervertebral discs makes them stiffer, reducing the likelihood of forward displacement following spondylolysis.

Many sports activities place considerable stress on the pars interarticularis region of the lumbar spine. Sports such as gymnastics, football (particularly Australian Rules and gridiron), cricket, high jumping and tennis subject the laminae of L5 and L4 to repetitive, high velocity impact and bending activities involving movements in the sagittal plane, with or without rotation. High velocity lumbar extension is stopped as the chisel-shaped inferior articular facets of the vertebrae above are driven hard against the lamina directly below. The constant repetition of this is associated initially with bone sclerosis and hypertrophy and eventually by fatigue fracture (Twomey & Taylor 1988, Yang & King 1984). Very often, the full range extension manoeuvres are followed by full range flexion, e.g. in fast bowling in cricket, where the heel strike of bowling is associated with lumbar extension, while the follow through is linked with lumbar flexion (Elliott et al 1986). Thus, the pars region suffers a severe blow followed by a bending moment, resulting eventually in fatigue fracture (Jayson 1983, Miller et al 1983).

Some sports such as golf involve lumbar rotation, which is blocked by facet apposition on the ipsilateral side. High impact rotary forces, particularly when associated with flexion or extension, also place massive stress on lumbar laminae and may result in a unilateral fracture (Adams & Hutton 1983, Bogduk & Twomey 1991).

It is characteristic of spondylolisthesis that the condition is painless when the athlete rests from the particular activity which stresses the pars interarticularis, but when the activity is resumed the pain returns. Where such an injury is suspected due to recurrent back pain on activity, oblique lumbar X-rays and/or a bone scan with a radioactive isotope will usually show an early stress fracture, should one be present (Sward et al 1990). Similarly, CT scans are useful in determining the nature and location of laminar fractures.

Discogenic back pain

Lumbar intervertebral discs have an excellent nerve supply and may be a potent source of low back pain. The sources of the nerve endings in lumbar discs are the lumbar sinuvertebral nerves, branches of the lumbar ventral rami and the grey rami communicantes (Bogduk & Twomey 1991). However, only the outer layers of the annular envelope receive a nerve supply, so that for a disc to become painful any lesion must directly or indirectly involve the outer third of the annulus. Thus, increased intradiscal pressures following disc damage and swelling can indirectly cause discogenic pain (Bogduk & Twomey 1987).

Damage to the intervertebral discs following trauma as a direct result of sporting activities is well recognized. Repeated minor trauma, which may include an element of sustained compression, as in flexed rotated postures, may give rise to circumferential fissues, usually of the inner annulus, but also in the outer layers of the annulus (Adams & Hutton 1986). Such damage to the outer annulus is likely to involve its nerve supply and thus be a source of back pain. The repetition of high velocity forces, particularly in association with torsional loads, may eventually result in radial tears through the annulus, most usually in the postero-lateral regions of the lumbar discs, and will often sprain the outermost lamellae (Adams & Hutton 1986). Again, since it is only the outer few lamellae which receive a nerve supply, the painful discs are those where the fissures extend into that region (Bogduk & Twomey 1991).

Disc fissures also provide a potential pathway for nuclear herniation under very particular circumstances. In most individuals, after the third decade of life, the nucleus is not sufficiently fluid to allow itself to be expressed under normal circumstances (Crock 1986). True nuclear herniation is a condition of young people, generally up to their mid-20s, and is rarely evident in older persons (Bogduk & Twomey 1991, Crock 1986). Nuclear protrusion through an annular defect can thus occur only in young discs, or in older discs where the nucleus undergoes autolysis and relative lique-faction. One rationale for this proposes a prior fracture of the vertebral end-plate, allowing vertebral blood to seep into the region of the avascular nucleus pulposus. Since the circulating blood has not previously been exposed directly to the nuclear protein (it is entirely avascular through life), it reacts to it as to a foreign body, setting up an auto-immune response. Autolysis and liquefaction of the nucleus may follow, as described in Bogduk and Twomey (1991). Once semi-fluid, the nucleus can be expressed through a radial tear in the annulus and perhaps gain access to the spinal canal in the region of the intervertebral canal.

Thus, disc protrusion and massive disc bulging with nuclear displacement is observed in young athletes only.

Disc bulging, due to annular metaplasia, nuclear degeneration or annular failure, however, is seen in older athletes and is usually associated with repeated minor trauma involving sustained postures, compression and torsion. Such pathology may cause spinal canal stenosis or intervertebral foraminal stenosis, and become an important source of low back pain and dysfunction. Thus, internal disc disruption (Crock 1986) is a potential source of local back pain when it is associated with disc swelling or fissuring of the outer annulus, or the leakage of pain-producing chemicals out of the disc into the surrounding region. Many sporting activities, e.g. football, regularly subject the lumbar spine to considerable trauma, thereby increasing the risk of internal disc damage in participants. Similarly, the stresses involved in a single major traumatic event within a sporting contest may be sufficient to severely damage lumbar discs.

Spinal stenosis

Spinal stenosis in an athlete is usually associated with bulging and/or herniation of lumbar intervertebral discs (Cinque 1989). If disc damage is associated with an already narrow spinal canal, then the risk of spinal stenosis with spinal cord, nerve root or cauda equina pressure is considerable (Porter et al 1980). This damage may be insidious or sudden onset, and prove to be very in-capacitating for the athlete concerned. The athlete may complain of pain, numbness and often bilateral muscle weakness, although not always of low back pain. The most commonly narrowed region of the spine is usually between L2 and L4 (Hall et al 1985). For an excellent account of the surgery and rehabilitation of an elite athlete with spinal stenosis as a direct result of a massive disc lesion at the L4–5 level, the reader is referred to the excellent paper by Cinque (1989).

Computed tomography and myelography seem to be the most useful radiological tools to assist in diagnosis. They are used both to evaluate the size of the spinal canal and the transverse area of the dural sac (Bolendar et al 1985, Schonstrom et al 1985). Pain provocation and elimination techniques, used by experienced back pain physicians, can also be useful in locating the symptomatic level.

SUMMARY

The changing structure of the spine during the life cycle means that it is particularly susceptible to different stresses and trauma at different times. Thus, the maturing spine of children, adolescents and young adults, where full bone strength is still developing, is liable to stress fractures and sponydylolysis and spondylolisthesis. While these conditions have been seen in athletes of all ages, young athletes are particularly vulnerable to repetitive, high bone loading forces (Eisenstein 1980, Twomey & Taylor 1988). Similarly, herniation of the nucleus of the intervertebral disc is more likely to occur in younger athletes, where the semi-fluid nature of the nucleus makes it possible for the nucleus to be forced through a tear in the annulus fibrosis following severe or repeated trauma (Bogduk & Twomey 1991). This is less likely in older athletes, as the nucleus progressively loses its fluid/ gel characteristics and water is lost as the biomechanical structure of the disc changes. However, at all ages discogenic back pain in athletes is a possibility. Discogenic pain may be associated with lesions to the well innervated outer third of the annulus fibrosis, or follow disc swelling.

During middle age, the spine shows increasing evidence of instability or loosening of the mobile segments, as the stiffer and more collagenous elements of the joint complexes are damaged by repeated trauma. Thus, the incidence of retrolisthesis and segmental instability causing back pain increases among middle-aged athletes. In old age, hypertrophic changes to the vertebral margins and facet joints causes bone proliferation and spurs to project into the spinal canal and intervertebral foramina. This causes a reduction in space and an increasing incidence of spinal stenosis. The spinal canal is triangular in shape in young adults, but may become trefoil in old age (Twomey & Taylor 1988).

Clinicians must know the changes the lumbar spine passes through if they are to understand properly the different ways in which it reacts to the stresses of sport through life, and to assess spinal performance and treat the back after injury.

Part 2
CLINICAL APPLICATIONS
Charles Flynn

An injury of the lumbar spine can be a major problem to an athlete. Not only is there the immediate interruption to their training and competition schedule, but there is also the fear that a spinal problem could end their career.

Despite the volumes that have been written on the lumbar spine, there has been comparatively little written on the diagnosis and treatment of lumbar spine problems associated with sporting activity. While the first section of this chapter outlined the anatomy, pathology and biomechanics of the lumbar spine, this section will deal with the clinical findings and management of the conditions that have been described.

ASSESSMENT

The basis of any successful treatment program is an ordered subjective and objective assessment of the athlete's problem (Bourdillon 1982, Grieve 1979, Jull 1986, Maitland 1986). A thorough assessment will not only help the therapist reach an accurate diagnosis but also indicate the types of treatment that may or may not be used in the rehabilitation of the athlete.

Subjective assessment

Starting with a body chart, it is important to map out the exact area of pain or other symptoms (paresthesia, numbness), the type, depth and quality of the pain and, in the case of multiple pains, any relationship between them. The area of pain alone is not a good indicator of the structures involved, as the pain may be due to pathology of any of the lumbosacral nerves, nerve roots (radicular pain) or pathology of most of the musculoskeletal structures of the lumbar spine (somatic pain) (Badgley & Arber 1941, Bogduk & Twomey 1991, Cyriax 1975, Feinstein et al 1954, Kellgren 1939, Mooney & Robertson 1976, Travell & Simons 1983). Visceral structures may also be the source of pain in the lumbar spine area, and this will be discussed later in this section. Somatic referred pain tends to be a deep ache and is usually difficult to localize. Radicular pain tends to be a shooting, lancinating pain that is confined to a narrow band in a dermatomal distribution. The only true indicators of specific nerve root involvement are the presence of a sensory deficit, muscular weakness and/or diminished tendon reflex (Corrigan & Maitland 1983, Last 1984, Moore 1985). Once the area or areas of pain and other symptoms have been clearly outlined, the physiotherapist should have a clear idea of all the structures that could possibly cause the symptoms and be able to undertake the objective assessment with confidence.

Joints other than those of the lumbar spine may be involved in the presentation of low back pain. In particular, the hip and sacroiliac joints should be cleared of being possible sources of the pain. Subjectively it is difficult to differentiate, although in some instances the mechanism of injury will give the physiotherapist a good indication of the structures involved (e.g. a direct blow to the hip joint is likely to cause localized hip problems). Objectively it is imperative to fully examine all possible sources of the symptoms (the detailed examination of the hip and the sacroiliac joint is discussed in Chapter 28). This author has found that the most reliable way to differentially diagnose in this area is to undertake a careful and detailed palpatory examination, reassessing the objective findings after each area has been examined.

The physiotherapist must also consider that pain in the lower thorax and lumbar spine may be non-mechanical in origin. Possible causes include spinal infection or tumour, urinary tract infection, renal disease, peptic ulcer and certain systemic disorders. Generally a purely mechanical problem will be the result of specific trauma or a period of strenuous activity, and will tend to be aggravated by movement and eased by rest. An inflammatory problem such as an infection or tumour is generally of insidious onset, will not be eased by rest, and the pain is often particularly severe during the night. If a visceral structure is involved the symptoms are usually poorly localized and, as with infection, the athlete will often complain of feeling unwell. When a non-mechanical problem is suspected the athlete should be referred to a doctor for further examination as soon as possible. With both spinal infection and tumour an initial radiological examination may be normal, so if either is suspected a bone scan should be ordered.

The subjective assessment should include detailed questioning on the aggravating factors during daily activities as well as during any sporting activity. Where the athlete has been advised to rest from some or all sporting activities, the ability of the athlete to perform daily tasks with or without pain will, subjectively, be the clearest indication of progress. It is also necessary to determine the type and level of sporting involvement as the stresses applied through the lumbar spine will differ not only between sports but also between athletes of varying standards. This information will help the physiotherapist reach a diagnosis and decide which activities should be restricted.

Objective assessment

With assessment of the active movements of the lumbar spine it is of vital importance to look at the quality as well as the range of movement. An athlete may appear to have a good range of, for example, flexion when asked to bend forward and touch his or her toes. This range can often be restricted by asking the athlete to repeat the movement with specific instructions to try to 'curl' or flex the lower back, thus localizing the movement to the lumbar spine as much as possible. If a deviation, list or scoliosis is observed an attempt must be made to correct the deformity and any change in the symptoms noted. If there is a change in the symptoms then the deviation is probably due to the presenting injury and the deviation should diminish as the condition is successfully treated.

With some athletes variations from the normal assessment routines may be needed. For example, in the case of a runner who only develops back pain after a long run the objective assessment may need to be more vigorous than normal. The athlete may need to repeat the test movements quickly or be assessed after sustained positioning (Maitland 1986) or on completion of a long run. Combined movements are invaluable as they are most likely to reproduce the action or position that is causing the symptoms and will allow a more accurate choice of treatment technique to be made. Recognizing regular or irregular patterns of movement will assist not only in predicting treatment results but also the manner in which the symptoms and movement signs may improve (Edwards 1986). Palpation findings are also of vital importance and will be outlined with specific conditions later in this chapter.

While leg length discrepancy is an uncommon cause of low back pain, such anatomical variations may become more important at higher levels of activity and minimal variations that may not be of significance in the general population could be of major importance to an athlete (Sperryn 1983). To compensate for a discrepancy, there is tilting of the pelvis and a compensatory scoliosis in the lumbar spine. This altered mechanism may lead to lumbar spine symptoms. A simple heel raise in the athlete's shoe combined with local treatment for the presenting condition is indicated.

As well as considering the mechanism of the injury, there are other factors that need to be considered. Adequate footwear is of vital importance for any one returning to running after an injury to the lumbar spine. Good heel cushioning will aid shock absorption, reducing the load on the lumbar discs. The running surface is also important, and the athlete should be advised to avoid road running and resume on a flat shock-absorbing surface such as a sporting oval. If the athlete is overweight the increased risk of further injury should be emphasized.

Once a diagnosis has been made it is important to take time to explain to the athlete the exact extent of the injury and how it will affect his or her immediate and, wherever possible, long term sporting career. The treatment program should be outlined and a rough time frame mapped out. It should also be explained that the more serious lumbar spine injuries are very restrictive and almost all forms of exercise will be curtailed. As a result it will be difficult for the athlete to maintain cardiovascular fitness, which will further retard full rehabilitation. In this instance strict guidelines will need to be outlined by the treating physiotherapist to enable the gradual return of peak fitness and the ability to return to competitive sport. Problems become recurrent when the athlete has not allowed sufficient time for the injury to heal or there has inadequate rehabilitation before returning to full activity.

DIAGNOSIS AND MANAGEMENT OF BACK PROBLEMS

On-field treatment of acute low back pain

The severity of an injury will dictate the type of treatment required in the case of acute lumbar spine injuries. Contusions should be treated with ice and, in the case of a severe blow, immediate cessation of sporting activity. The possibility of a fracture as the result of a direct blow or severe trauma should be suspected if there is marked erector spinae muscle spasm and acute pain. In this instance the athlete should have a radiological examination of the lumbar spine as soon as possible. With a severe muscle strain, zygapophyseal joint sprain or possible injury to an intervertebral disc, adhesive tape (Fig. 27.8) can be used for support and pain relief.

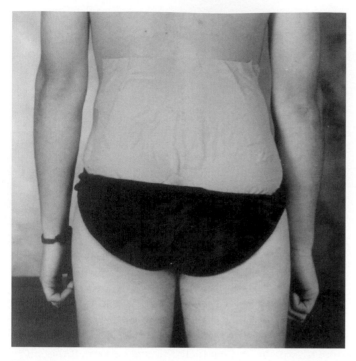

Fig. 27.8 The use of adhesive tape as a temporary support or brace can be a valuable aid in the treatment of acute lumbar spine injury

Non-specific low back pain

Many sporting activities subject the lumbar spine to considerable stress and trauma. While there appears to be little difference between the athletes and the general population, it appears that the tolerance and the ability to overcome backache is greater in the athletic population (Granhed & Morelli 1988, Rovere 1987). As well as the value of increased joint motion this may also be due to greater motivation to improve and better compliance in the athletic population.

There are many causes of backache and some injuries of the lumbar spine will have very definite symptoms that tend to implicate specific structures. Other injuries will have vague or atypical symptoms and it will be difficult to arrive at an exact diagnosis. For example, in a similar pattern to a disc, injury to the zygapophoseal joints may result in localized low back pain, radiating buttock and leg pain and diminished straight leg raise due to hamstring spasm (Dory 1981, Mooney & Robertson 1976). The athlete may also complain of locking and, as in an injury to a disc, will have unilateral distribution of pain making differential diagnosis difficult. This confusion would appear to stem from the fact that different structures in the lumbar spine share a similar segmental innervation (Bogduk & Twomey 1991).

Not all low back pain in athletes is the result of a specific injury and the effects of sustained posture on the lumbar spine have been discussed above (see p. ••). Tightness of the lumbosacral fascia, hamstrings and hip flexors combined with weak paraspinal muscles can also lead to low back pain (Moskwa & Nicholas 1989). The muscle tightness can be easily detected by palpitation and by simple muscle stretches and should be treated with vigorous soft tissue techniques (e.g. cross-fibre stretching) and intensive passive stretching.

LUMBAR SPINE INJURIES IN THE CHILD ATHLETE

By far the largest cause of low back pain in youth sport is overuse or stress-related injuries (Burnett et al 1991, Foster et al 1989). Jackson (1979), in a review of young athletes with low back pain, found that 40% had pars defects and a further 10% had spondylolisthesis. Other causes were symptomatic disc injuries, end-plate fractures, growth plate injuries and neoplasms. Serious pathology, such as a neoplasm, should be suspected in the athlete who presents with an insidious onset and relentless increase of lumbar spine pain that is particularly severe during the night (Adams 1968).

Younger athletes are more likely to have stress fractures and to have congenital predisposition to developing stress fractures than older athletes (Watkins & Dillin 1990). Contributing to this predisposition is the possible lower ratio of muscle and tendon strength to bone length. During the adolescent growth spurt the soft tissue structures are unable to keep up with the bony elements, leading to reduced range of movement, and the growth plate cartilage seems less resistant to repetitive stress than adult bone (Micheli 1979). Also important is the fact that almost half the height of an adult is in the legs whereas in a child it is considerably less than half (Caine & Lindner 1985). These differences become very important when the child or adolescent athlete is asked to repetitively perform activities that were originally devised with the adult frame in mind (e.g. fast bowling in cricket, rowing, gymnastics, wrestling) (Golberg 1989).

Disc injuries are uncommon, but should be immediately recognizable. They tend to occur most often as a result of trauma or a specific overstrain incident (Giroux & Le Clerc 1982). In the acute phase there is generally a pronounced list or deviation with marked limitation of flexion and straight leg raise. The treatment of these injuries is the same as with adult disc injuries, which is described in a later section. Clinically, though, this author has found that juvenile disc injuries can be very troublesome. To allow maximum repair of the annulus, there should be a complete rest from all sporting activity for a minimum of six weeks and then a gradual return to competitive sport over a further six-week period.

Presentation and treatment of specific lumbar spine conditions will not vary significantly from the presenting signs and treatment of the same problems in the adult athlete. However manipulation of pre-adolescent children is inadvisable and this author finds that manipulation of adolescents is rarely indicated. The most important aspect of any treatment program is the education of the athlete, parents and coach. All three parties have to understand the implications that any injury may have on the athlete's chosen sporting activity, and adhere to the guidelines laid down by the treating physiotherapist with regard to rehabilitation. Where incorrect technique is a possible cause of the symptoms then specialist coaching advice (including the use of video equipment) should be sought. Excesses in training should be avoided at all times and there may need to be modifications made to the rules of some sports to ensure that the danger of overuse injuries is minimized. For example, in many underage cricket competitions in Australia, the number of overs (normally less than six) a fast bowler may bowl without a break is strictly controlled.

Ankylosing spondylitis

Ankylosing spondylitis should be considered in any athlete complaining of a gradual onset of back and hip pain or stiffness (particularly prolonged morning stiffness) without a history of trauma. The condition is more common in males and the symptoms usually begin in the late teens to early 20s. Active movements of the thoracic and lumbar spines are usually restricted by stiffness and there is general tenderness and stiffness on palpation. Chest expansion, which should be greater than 2.5 cm (Rovere 1987), is also restricted.

Confirmation of the diagnosis may be made by full blood examination, ESR (usually elevated) and if necessary bone and/or CT scan. In advanced cases, radiological examination will show squaring of the vertebral bodies (in particular the thoracic vertebrae) and fuzziness and eventual obliteration of the sacroiliac joints.

The most important aspect of treating this condition is continued mobility. Sperryn (1983) advocates continued vigorous exercise combined with non-steroidal anti-inflammatory medication. This exercise should include swimming, bike riding as well as general mobilizing and strengthening exercises both in and out of the water (see Ch. 16) To avoid the fixed flexion deformity that is often associated with ankylosing spondylitis, extension exercises should be prescribed and the patient should be encouraged to 'straighten up' against a wall on a daily basis. Excessive sporting activity and body-contact sports should be avoided. The athlete should understand that the condition is a self-help one and thus should be be encouraged to do regular spinal mobilizing exercises and to combine weight-bearing activities with hydrotherapy as often as possible. Other spondyloarthropathies such as psoriasis and Reiter's syndrome may also cause stiffness in the lumbar spine and in this instance can be treated in the same way as ankylosing spondylitis.

Discogenic back pain

Vigorous sporting activities regularly subject the discs of the lumbar spine to considerable trauma, whether it is the continued stress experienced by the forward row in rugby or a single incident such as a fall in gymnastics. The discs are usually injured through rotation and shearing forces (Watkins & Dillin 1990) and are more susceptible to injury if there are bony anomalies such as spina bifida occulta and pars defects (Day et al 1987) or in athletes who have a past history of lumbar spine problems (Guten 1981).

The athlete's presenting symptoms will also vary with the extent and type of damage to the disc. With a minor disc injury the athlete may complain of minimal localized back pain at the initial onset of the symptoms, be able to continue the activity with a gradual increase in pain and stiffness, or experience a gradual increase after cooling down. The more severe the injury, the more debilitating will be the symptoms. Pain and stiffness after long periods of sitting or bending, restriction of flexion and sharp pain with coughing or sneezing, without the presence of leg pain, may also be indicative of localized disc pathology. The symptoms are often eased by rest in either supine or prone, although it may be difficult for the athlete to change positions in bed and there is generally stiffness present in the lumbar spine on rising in the mornings.

The pain associated with disc lesions may be confined to a localized area or may radiate out to include the whole of the lower spine and buttocks. If there is a disc prolapse with nerve root involvement, the pain is usually unilateral and it is important to determine whether the pain is due to nerve root compression or irritation. Although in both cases the leg pain should follow a recognizable dermatomal pattern, only nerve root compression will cause any neurological deficit and it is therefore vital to carry out a full neurological examination of the lower limbs. If a neurological deficit is found, manipulation of that joint is contraindicated because of the danger of further compromising the nerve root involved. Examining the athlete's posture may show a loss of the normal lumbar lordosis coupled with a deviation or scoliosis that is painful to correct, and loss of active movement, paticularly flexion. Straight leg raise is often restricted by posterior thigh pain, hamstring spasm or low back pain.

With upper/mid lumbar problems, the femoral nerve roots may be involved and prone knee flexion can produce the athlete's anterior thigh pain symptoms. To fully investigate the extent of neural tissue involvement, the slump test should be carried out when the acute symptoms have subsided (for the use of slump in assessment and treatment, see Ch. 33). On palpation, there is usually to excessive strain (weightlifting, rowing) or overstretching (fast bowling in cricket). The athlete will usually describe a tearing feeling and some immediate pain that may or may not be debilitating enough to stop activity. On examination there is usually restriction of flexion, localized pain on resisted extension from forward flexion, and pain on palpation.

These injuries usually respond well to local treatment (ultrasound, massage, stretching) but may leave a troublesome fibrous band in the muscle tissue. In this instance deep transverse frictions are most useful in breaking up the adhesions. If the problem remains symptomatic the use of a corticosteroidal injection should be considered (Williams & Sperryn 1976). If the muscle injury has been present for a number of weeks then the joints over which the muscle acts will stiffen and treatment should include mobilization and/or manipulation of those joints.

When discussing muscle injuries of the lumbar spine, it is important to consider the possible presence of trigger points. A trigger point is a localized area of increased sensitivity or irritability in a soft tissue structure that may cause referred pain on palpation (Travell & Simons 1992). Any direct or indirect insult to a muscle which produces pain or spasm may make a trigger point irritable. The muscles most commonly affected are the sacrospinalis, iliocostalis and quadratus lumborum (Mennel 1986). Trigger points are common in athletes with chronic low grade back pain and may persist after recovery from the primary cause of the problem. On examination there may be pain and loss of movement on passive or active stretching of the affected muscle, pain and weakness with resisted movement and a taut, palpable and very painful band within the muscle tissue (Travell & Simons 1992). Common trigger points can be found in the iliocostalis lumborum, around the greater trochanter and the iliac insertion of gluteus medius. Trigger points can be eased by regular, slow, steady stretches of the involved muscles and firm transverse frictions to break up the palpable band (Fig. 27.10). Joint manipulation may also deactivate the trigger spot by restoring normal joint movement or by stretching the muscles while inhibiting protective muscle spasm mediated by the central nervous system (Travell & Simons 1983).

The two major functions of the lumbar muscles are to help maintain the upright position and to help control the descent of the vertebral column in forward flexion and raise it back to the normal position (Bogduk 1986). Any strengthening exercises prescribed should be aimed at improving the efficiency of the muscles with these tasks in mind.

Scheuermann's disease

While normally asymptomatic, Scheuermann's disease can occasionally cause problems in the lumbar spine, particularly in young male athletes (the condition is more

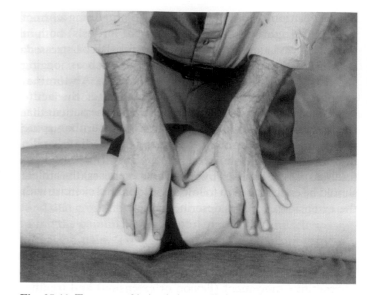

Fig. 27.10 Transverse friction being applied to a trigger point on the gluteal muscle group

prevalent in the thoracic spine and the clinical symptoms and treatment are more extensively outlined in Chapter 22). Frequent findings indicative of the problem are a kyphotic deformity, localized stiffness in the lower thoracic and upper lumbar spines and tight hamstrings (Fisk & Baigent 1981). During the symptomatic period it is important to avoid heavy spinal loading such as weightlifting or body contact sports such as rugby or football. Treatment can be local for pain relief, and stretches of tight anterior musculature and strengthening of posterior musculature are recommended. Swimming should be encouraged and postural maintenance or correction exercises should be prescribed. If heavy sporting activity continues, the vertebral bodies may be left with an irregular shape which will not stand up to heavy weight training or sport and may lead to a future increase in the incidence of lower lumbar spine problems (Stoddard 1983, Sperryn 1983).

Spondylolysis and spondylolisthesis

Spondylolysis and spondylolisthesis are probably the most troublesome and common of the lumbar problems that can affect an athlete. Spondylolysis (and to a lesser extent spondylolisthesis) does not necessarily result in pain or restriction of movement and is more often than not of minimal clinical significance (Jackson 1979, Porter & Hibbert 1984, Semon & Spengler 1981). However, if an athlete under 30 presents with low back pain and has a spondylolisthesis the defect is more likely to be the cause of the athlete's symptoms (Macnab 1977).

There is a strong association with spina bifida occulta and the defect in the pars interarticularis (Fredrickson et al 1984). The defect is thought to be an acquired rather than a congenital lesion (Turner & Bianco 1971, Wertzberger

& Peterson 1980) and is due to fatigue fractures in the pars interarticularis (Caine & Lindner 1985, Wertzberger & Peterson 1980). The breakdown in the pars is due either to a flexion overload, continuous anterior shearing during repetitive extension movement or forced rotation, or a combination of all three forces (Farfan 1976). If spondylolisthesis is present the slip occurs in early childhood or during adolescence unless there has been surgical intervention, trauma or degenerative disc disease (Ciullo & Jackson 1985, McCarroll et al 1986, Wertzberger & Peterson 1980).

Any sport that involves repetitive extension and/or flexion combined with some rotatory movements of the lumbar spine will clearly place the lower lumbar spine at some risk of spondylolysis. At particular risk are child and adolescent athletes involved in activities such as gymnastics and fast bowling in cricket. These athletes will be even more susceptible if they have an incorrect technique or are overtrained. In fast bowlers the defect will occur on the left side in right arm bowlers (Williams & Sperryn 1976) and is just as likely to occur in a bowler with an extension-rotation through to flexion rotation style as one with a front on delivery action (Twomey 1985).

Athletes with symptomatic spondylolysis or spondylolisthesis will often complain of generalized low back ache of diffuse distribution. Leg pain may be present and is usually unilateral, although bilateral dural symptoms can also occur. The symptoms are often aggravated by long periods of standing and eased by sitting. Spondylolithesis should be suspected in an athlete complaining of a gradual onset of low back pain during activities that involve repetitive flexion, extension or rotation of the lumbar spine (Micheli 1979). Where a spondylolisthesis is suspected a standard radiological examination should be carried out, and is the definitive diagnostic tool. In the case of a suspected spondylolysis that is normal on radiological examination, a bone scan should be ordered.

On examination the pain may be produced by the athlete standing on one leg and then guiding the lumbar spine into extension (Ciullo & Jackson 1985, Halpern & Smith 1991). Extension is generally limited by pain or stiffness and will usually reproduce the athlete's symptoms. Flexion may ease the pain and is usually restricted by hamstring tightness. Bilateral hamstring tightness, probably due to constriction of the fifth lumbar nerve root, is common with spondylolisthesis (Barash et al 1970, Jackson 1979, Muckle 1982) and the athlete may walk with an exaggerated lumbar lordosis (Phalen & Dickson 1961, Spencer & Jackson 1983). In severe cases of spondylolisthesis there will be an increase in the lumbar lordosis, bilateral extensor muscle spasm, and a visible slip and skin creases at the site of the slip. A posterior-anterior movement applied to the spinous process immediately above the slip will tend to reproduce the pain and there may be reduced mobility in all levels of the lumbar spine (Pearcy & Shepherd 1985).

The management of spondylolysis and spondylolisthesis is dependent on the relationship between the pathology and the symptoms experienced by the athlete. As stated previously, the condition can be present in asymptomatic individuals so even in the presence of a -lysis or -listhesis, the adjacent discs and zygapophyseal joints must still be considered as potential sources of symptoms. If the condition is thought to be related to the spondylolysis or spondylolisthesis, management will depend on the degree of the athlete's pain and disability. Rest from the aggravating sporting activity may be required. Local treatment can include posterior-anterior mobilizing at the level of the defect or slip to render the available range pain-free, not to increase the overall range of motion (Grace 1985). Therefore vigorous end-range techniques should not be used. Lumbar rotational mobilizing, which can be combined with a hamstring stretch (Fig. 27.11) and cross-fibre stretching of the paraspinal muscles can also be used. Traction may also be of benefit. Manipulation is contraindicated but can be used for hypomobility problems in higher levels.

Lumbosacral corsets and braces offer significant pain relief and support by flattening the lumbar lordosis and thereby reducing the stress on the lumbar spine (Ciullo & Jackson 1985, Stanitski 1982). Any such support should

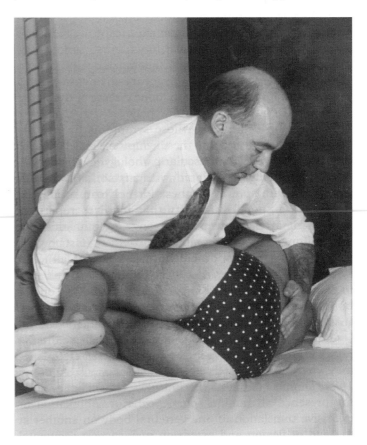

Fig. 27.11 Rotational spondylo-mobilization, combined with hamstring/dural stretching to increase range of flexion when symptomatic with spondylolisthesis

McKenzie R 1980 The lumbar spine. Spinal Publications, Waikanae, New Zealand

McKenzie R A 1981 The lumbar spine, mechanical diagnosis and therapy. Spinal Publications, New Zealand

Mennel J McM 1986 Trigger points in referred spinal pain. In: Grieve G (ed) Modern manual therapy of the vertebral column. Churchill Livingstone, Melbourne

Micheli L J 1979 Low back pain in the adolescent: differential diagnosis. American Journal of Sports Medicine 7:362-364

Miller J A A, Haderspeck K A, Schultz A B 1983 Posterior element loads in lumbar motion segments. Spine 8:(3):331-337

Mooney V, Robertson J 1976 The facet syndrome. Clinical Orthopaedics and Related Research 115:149-156

Moore K 1985 Clinically orientated anatomy, 2nd edn. Williams & Wilkins, Sydney

Moskwa C A, Nicholas J A 1989 Musculoskeletal risk factors in the young athlete. Physician and Sportsmedicine 17(11):49-59

Muckle D S 1982 Associated factors in recurrent groin and hamstring injuries. British Journal of Sports Medicine 16(1):37-39

Nachemson A 1960a Lumbar intradiscal pressure. Acta Orthopaedica Scandinavica, Supplement 43

Nachemson A L 1960b The lumbar spine an orthopaedic challenge. Spine 1(1):59-71

Paris S V 1985 Physical signs of instability. Spine 10(3):277-279

Pearcy M, Shepherd J 1985 Is there instability in spondylolisthesis? Spine 10(2):175-177

Phalen G, Dickson J 1961 Spondylolithesis and tight hamstrings Journal of Bone and Joint Surgery 43A:505-512

Pollock M L, Leggett S H, Graves J E, Jones A, Fulton M, Cirulli J 1989 Effect of resistance training on lumbar extension strength. American Journal of Sports Medicine 17(5):624-629

Porter R W, Hibbert C S 1984 Symptoms associated with lysis of the pars interarticularis. Spine 9(7):755-758

Porter R W, Hibbert C, Wellman P 1980 Backache and the lumbar spinal canal. Spine 5(2):98-105

Rovere G D 1987 Low back pain in athletes. Physician and Sportsmedicine 15(1):105-117

Schneider G 1987 Degenerative lumbar instability. In: Manipulative Therapists Association of Australia Fifth Biennial Conference Proceedings, Melbourne

Schonstrom N S R, Bolender N F, Spencer D M 1985 The pathology of spinal stenosis as seen on CT scans of the lumbar spine. Spine 10:806-811

Semon R L, Spengler D 1981 Significance of lumbar spondylolysis in college football players. Spine 6(2):172-174

Shah J S, Hampson W G J, Jayson M I V 1978 The distribution of surface strain in the cadaveric lumbar spine. Journal of Bone and Joint Surgery 60-B(2):246-251

Sim G P G 1973 Vertebral contour in spondylolisthesis. British Journal of Radiology 46:25-254

Spencer C W, Jackson P W 1983 Back injuries in the athlete. Clinics in Sports Medicine 9(2):419-428

Sperryn P N 1983 Sport and medicine. Butterworths, London

Stanitski C L 1982 Low back pain in young athletes. Physician and Sportsmedicine 10(10):77-91

Steven R, Irwin R 1983 Sports medicine. Prentice Hall, New Jersey

Stoddard A 1983 Manual of osteopathic practice, 2nd edn. Hutchinson, London

Sward L, Hellstrom M, Jacobsson B, Peterson L 1990 Back pain and radiologic changes in the thoraco-lumbar spine of athletes. Spine 15(2):124-129

Taylor J R, Twomey L T 1984 Sexual dimorphism in human vertebral shape: its relation to scoliosis. Journal of Anatomy 138(2):281-286

Taylor J R, Twomey L T 1986 Age changes in lumbar zygapophyseal joints. Observations on structure and function. Spine 11(7): 739-745

Taylor J R, Twomey L T, Corker M 1990 Bone and soft tissue injuries in post-mortem lumbar spines. Paraplegia 28:119-129

Teitz C C, Cook D M 1985 Rehabilitation of neck and low back injuries. Clinics in Sports Medicine 4(3):455-476

Travell J G, Simons D G 1983 Myofascial pain and dysfunction. Williams & Wilkins, Baltimore

Travell J G, Simons D G 1992 Myofascial pain and dysfunction: the Lower Extremities. Williams & Wilkins, Baltimore

Troup J D G 1977 The etiology of spondylolysis. Orthopaedic Clinics of North America 8(1):57-63

Turner R H, Bianco A J 1971 Spondylolysis and spondylolisthesis in children and teenagers. Journal of Bone and Joint Surgery 53–A(7):1298-1306

Twomey L 1985 Fast bowlers and the lumbar spine. In: Proceedings of Manipulative Therapists Association of Australia (Victorian Branch) and Sports Physiotherapy Group (Victorian Branch) Stress injuries in sport: an update. October 19-20, Melbourne

Twomey L T 1981 Age changes in the human lumbar spine. PhD thesis, University of Western Australia

Twomey L T 1991 The effects of severe trauma of the joints of the cervical and lumbar spine and the clinical significance. Sports Health 9(3):6-7

Twomey L T, Taylor J R 1982 Flexion creep deformation, hysteresis in the lumbar vertebral column. Spine 7(2):116-122

Twomey L T, Taylor J R 1983 Sagittal movements of the human lumbar vertebral column: a quantitative study of the role of the posterior vertebral elements. Archives of Physical Medicine and Rehabilitation 64:322-325

Twomey L T, Taylor J R 1985 Age changes in the lumbar intervertebral discs. Acta Orthopaedica Scandinavica 56:496-499

Twomey L T, Taylor J R 1987 Physical therapy of the low back. Churchill Livingstone, Melbourne

Twomey L T, Taylor J R 1988 Age changes in the lumbar spinal and intervertebral canals. Paraplegia 26:238-249

Twomey L T, Taylor J R, Furniss B 1983 Age changes in the bone density and structure of the lumbar vertebral column. Journal of Anatomy 136(1):15-25

Twomey L T, Taylor J R, Oliver M 1988 Sustained flexion loading, rapid extension loading of the lumbar spine. Spine and the physical therapy of related injuries. Physiotherapy Practice 4:129-138

Twomey L T, Taylor J R, Taylor M M 1989 Unsuspected damage to lumbar zygapophyseal (facet) joints after motor vehicle accidents. Medical Journal of Australia 15l:210-217

Tyrrell A R, Reilly T, Troup J D G 1985 Circadian variation in stature and the effects of spinal loading. Spine 10(2):161

Waddell G 1987 A new clinical model for the treatment of low back pain. Spine 12(7):632

Watkins R G, Dillin W H 1990 Lumbar spine injury in the athlete. Clinics in Sports Medicine 9(2):419-448

Wertzberger K L, Peterson H A 1980 Acquired spondylolysis and spondylolisthesis in the young child. Spine 5(5):437-442

White A A, Panjabi M M 1978 The clinical biomechanics of the spine. J B Lippincott, Philadelphia

Williams J G P, Sperryn P N 1976 Sports medicine, 2nd edn. Arnold, London

Wiltse L L 1969 Sponylolisthesis: classification and etiology AAOS. Symposium on the spine. Mosby, 143-167

Wiltse L L, Widell E H, Yuan H A 1975 Chymopapain chemonucleolysis in lumbar disc disease. Journal of the American Medical Association 231:474-479

Wiltse L L, Winter R B 1983 Terminology and measurement of spondylolisthesis. Journal of Bone and Joint Surgery 65-A:768-772

Wright G 1982 Healthy back exercises for the coach and athlete. Sports Coach 6(3):28-30

Yang K H, King A I 1984 Mechanism of facet load transmission as a hypothesis for low back pain. Spine 9(6):557-565

28. The pelvis, hip and thigh

Mary Toomey

Regardless of the sports activity, normal function of the pelvis and hip is a prerequisite for normal athletic performance (Simm & Scott 1986). Injuries affecting the musculoskeletal structures of the pelvis, hip and thigh present the treating practitioner with a complex problem of assessment and management. Generally, thigh injuries have been well documented (Bull 1985, Cibulka 1989, Fox 1986, King & Robertson 1986, Simonet 1987). However, injuries to the pelvis and hip are often more obscure. Consequently, while the signs and symptoms of a range of conditions have been described (Karlin 1986, Medoff 1987, Saudek 1985, Simm & Scott 1986, Waters & Millis 1988), management of these problems has often been less than satisfactory. This may in part be because of a lack of accurate knowledge of the function of the pelvis and hip in sport. Epidemiologic studies of football, soccer and ice-hockey document the involvement of the groin and thigh in 12% of all injuries (Simonet 1987). Injuries may develop as a result of overuse or as a consequence of trauma. Structures affected will include the bony elements (sacrum; ilium, pubis and ischium; femoral head, neck and shaft), the joints (sacroiliac joint, pubic symphysis and the hip joint), and the associated soft tissues (contractile and non-contractile). Consideration should also be given to the possibility of referred pain, originating from more proximal structures, including the lumbar spine and abdominal viscera.

The effective management of the athlete with injuries affecting the pelvis, hip or thigh requires the treating practitioner to have the ability to accurately assess the structures involved, a comprehensive understanding of the function of the affected structures as they relate to the athlete's sport and the possible mechanisms of injury, and an awareness of the implications of the injury to the athlete's performance.

ANATOMY

Pelvis

The pelvis is a unique structure in that it provides a strong and stable base on which both the spine and lower limbs work. In terms of posture and locomotion, the pelvis is designed to support the downward and forward thrust transmitted to it by the weight of the trunk (Simm & Scott 1986). Weightbearing and propulsive forces are also transmitted through the pelvis in a reciprocal direction, as body weight is transferred alternately to each hip joint during gait. The pelvis may be divided into identical halves, each designated as a hemipelvis and each is comprised of three separate bony elements—the ilium, ischium and pubis—which are fused in the adult. Each hemipelvis articulates posteriorly with the sacrum at the sacroiliac joints. The pubic symphysis forms the anterior articulation.

Sacrum

The sacrum is broader anteriorly than posteriorly and wider superiorly than inferiorly. It fits like a wedge or keystone between the paired ilia. Gender differences begin to appear at about puberty. In the adult female the sacrum is shorter and wider than in the male, with a deeper ventral concavity. The pelvic surface of the sacrum also has a more downward inclination than in the male. The sacral articular surface of the sacroiliac joint is shorter in females, but in both males and females it usually extends along the sides of S1 to S3. The sacroiliac joints are generally described as being shaped like a 'C' or an inverted 'L'. The cranial segment is usually shorter and more vertical and the caudal segment longer and more horizontal (Fig. 28.1).

Sacroiliac joints

The sacroiliac joints are generally described as having two components. The small synovial component lies along the bodies of S1 to S3. It is surrounded by the interosseous sacroiliac ligaments which convert the joint into a part syndesmosis. The joint surfaces are irregular, with depressions on the sacral side and elevations on the iliac side. These irregularities appear to be variable both within and between individuals (Alderink 1991). These surfaces provide for a reciprocal fit of the opposing joint components.

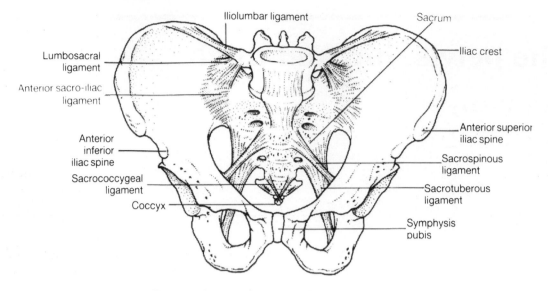

Fig. 28.1 Sacro-iliac ligaments. Source: Rogers (1992)

The nerve supply to the joint is from branches of the obturator (L2, L3, L4) and superior gluteal (L4, L5, and S1) nerves, the dorsal rami of S1 and S2 and from the sacral plexus. This is of importance when considering the concept of referred pain, as these nerves are capable of referring pain from these joints to a wide area, including the groin, buttocks, thighs and even the legs, as these areas share the same segmental nerve supply. The ligaments associated with the sacroiliac joint are listed in the box.

The posterior sacroiliac ligaments are among the strongest in the body, which is indicative of the loads placed on them. The anterior ligaments are weak in contrast. The small movements which occur at the sacroiliac joints may be influenced by lower limb and trunk muscles, but there are no muscles with any direct action over the joint. The piriformis does attach to the sacrum, but has its main action over the hip joint.

The pubic symphasis

The pubic symphasis is formed between the two pubic bones, the articular surfaces of which have a fibro-cartilaginous disc interposed. This disc is reinforced by the superior and arcuate pubic ligaments, as well as the anterior interpubic ligament. Motion occurs vertically, with a shear type displacement of one pubic bone on the other, and in an anterior-posterior rotational direction as one hemipelvis rotates forward on the other in gait. The upper limit of vertical motion of the pubic symphasis is widely accepted as being 2 mm. Rotary movement in both the frontal and sagittal planes is generally less than 1.5°.

The hip joint

The anatomy of the hip joint reflects the requirements of unlimited rotational and angulatory motion in a joint that

must also be able to sustain large forces (Medoff 1987). It is the best example of a ball and socket joint in the body (Saudek

Ligaments of the sacroiliac joint

1. **Ventral sacroiliac ligament**, which is a thickening of the joint capsule. It may resist anterior displacement of the sacral promontory.
2. **Interosseous sacroiliac ligament**, which fills the space above and behind the synovial part of the joint and is the primary constraint against excessive sacroiliac movement. It consists of deep and superficial portions.
3. **Dorsal sacroiliac ligament**, overlying the interosseous ligament. It consists of short cranial and longer caudal fibres. The more caudal dorsal fasiculi, running more obliquely from S3 and S4 to the posterior superior iliac spines, are continuous laterally with slips from the sacrotuberous ligament and medially with the posterior layer of the thoracolumbar fascia (Williams & Warwick 1980). This ligament may resist downward displacement of the sacrum.
4. **Sacrotuberous ligament** blends with the dorsal sacroiliac ligament and arises from the posterior superior iliac spines, the lower sacrum and the upper portion of the coccyx. It inserts onto the ischial tuberosity.
5. **Sacrospinous ligament** lies anterior to the sacrotuberous ligament. It arises from the ischial spine and has a broad attachment to the sacrum and coccyx. Both the sacrotuberous and sacrospinous ligaments indirectly resist anterior tilt of the pelvis, by preventing upward displacement of the sacrum.

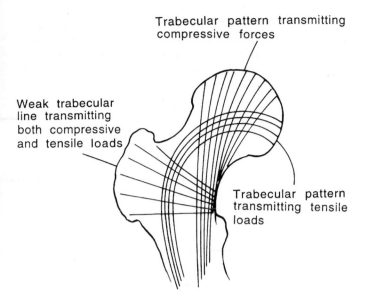

Fig. 28.2 Trabecular patterns around femoral head and neck

1985). The movements available at the hip joint are flexion-extension, abduction-adduction, and internal-external rotation. Accessory movements of caudad and lateral glides also occur, as well as combinations of different movements.

The stability of the joint is in its bony configuration; specifically, the depth of the joint, augmented by the acetabular labrum and the very strong capsular ligaments surrounding the joint.

Inferiorly, the anterior and posterior acetabular walls end before they meet, forming the acetabular notch. The acetabulum projects downward, laterally and forward. The neck of the femur also projects anteriorly.

The trabeculae in the bone of the femoral neck are oriented along lines of stress. The thickest of these extends from the calcar inferiorly to the femoral head superiorly and transmits compressive forces. A smaller trabecular pattern extends from the foveal region across the head and extends along the superior portion of the femoral neck to the greater trochanter. This transmits tensile loads (Simm & Scott 1986). There is also a weak trabecular line extending from the lesser to the greater trochanter, which resists both compressive and tensile loads (Fig. 28.2). These are of some importance when considering stress fractures, as will be discussed later.

In the capsule of the hip joint the fibres generally run longitudinally, parallel with the neck of the femur. A small number also run in a circular direction around the base of the neck of the femur.

The joint capsule is reinforced by the iliofemoral, ischiofemoral and pubofemoral ligaments (Fig. 28.3). The iliopsoas tendon also blends with the anterior capsule, reinforcing it. The capsule is thickest and strongest superiorly, where it is under most load during stance and gait. It is weakest posteriorly. The iliofemoral ligament is one of the strongest in the body and is one of the major contributors to the stability of the hip joint, particularly in

standing. It is divided into two bands, anterior and posterior. The anterior band, by virtue of its attachment along the intertrochanteric line distally and the anterior surface of the body of the ilium proximally, limits extension. The posterior band spirals around the neck of the femur from its proximal attachment along the posterior surface of the body of the ilium to the greater trochanter, and limits internal rotation.

The pubofemoral ligament lies transversely between the body of the pubis and the joint capsule and the more medial fibres of the iliofemoral ligament. Consequently, it is able to limit abduction and external rotation. The ischiofemoral ligament lies posteroinferiorly over the capsule. It is thin and weak.

There are also two ligaments within the hip joint. These are the ligament of the head/ligamentum teres and the transverse acetabular ligament. The ligament of the head arises from the fovea centralis and divides into two bands which attach to the margins of the acetabular notch, along with the transverse acetabular ligament. Mechanically its role is minor, although it is stressed when the leg is abducted in slight flexion. It also has a role in carrying blood vessels to the head of the femur in the young child. This function is probably insignificant by the age of seven (Briggs 1991).

The joint capsule, acetabulum and both surfaces of the acetabular labrum are lined with synovium. Synovium also covers the portion of the femoral neck and head contained within the capsule as well as the ligament of the head and the acetabular fat pad.

The acetabular fat pad fills the acetabular fossa. It acts as a shock absorber in the joint and fills irregularities which are not filled with synovial fluid. The fat pad promotes a better distribution of synovial fluid within the joint (Saudek 1985, Zimmerman 1988).

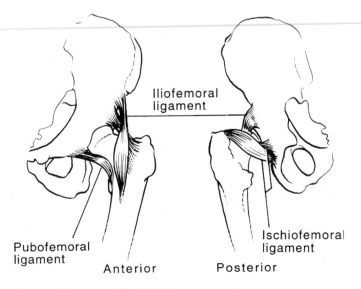

Fig. 28.3 Ligaments of the hip joint

Nerve supply

The sensory nerve supply to the joint capsule is derived from the femoral, obturator and superior gluteal nerves. The posterior aspect of the capsule is supplied by branches of the sciatic nerve, the medial aspect by the articular branch of the obturator nerve and the superolateral aspect by branches of the superior gluteal nerve. The iliofemoral and pubofemoral ligaments are supplied by branches of the femoral nerve. Irritation of any of these nerves can cause hip pain and can refer pain anywhere along the distal distribution of the nerve or its branches (Saudek 1985, Zimmerman 1988).

Blood supply

The hip joint gains its blood supply from the medial and lateral circumflex arteries, branches of either the femoral artery or the profunda femoris artery. These are supplemented by branches of the obturator artery, which are enclosed within the ligamentum teres. The medial and lateral circumflex arteries surround the base of the femoral neck at the level of the joint capsule, and give off branches which enter the hip through the capsule close to the bone. These arteries extend up the femoral neck, between the bone and its synovial lining. The consequences of a compromised blood supply in this area are significant, i.e. avascular necrosis of the femoral head. The greater and lesser trochanters are also supplied by branches of the medial and lateral circumflex arteries.

Bursae

Around the hip joint major bursae can be found between the gluteus maximus tendon and the posterolateral aspect of the greater trochanter, deep to the psoas tendon over the anterior hip joint, and between the tuberosity of the ischium and the overlying hamstring muscle origin. However, it should be noted that there are many more minor bursae, situated at sites of potential soft tissue impingement against bone. These all have the potential to become irritated, particularly as a consequence of overuse irritation.

The femur

The shaft of the femur forms an angle to the neck in two planes. In the adult, because of weightbearing, the angle in the frontal plane, called the angle of inclination, is about 125°. In the transverse plane, the angle is called the angle of anteversion. Normally, the head and neck are externally rotated on the shaft to an angle of about 15-20°. Increases or decreases in this angle can contribute to the development of gait abnormalities and muscle imbalances (Saudek 1985).

Muscles

Examination of the muscles acting about the pelvis, hip and thigh can be difficult. This is because their function may change relative to the position of the pelvis, with respect to the trunk or the lower limbs; with the load to which they are subjected; with the speed of the movement; and because of factors such as lumbar spine dysfunction and degenerative changes affecting the hip joint. As previously stated, the pelvis acts as a stable base on which the trunk above and the legs below move. It allows for co-ordinated muscle action between the lumbar spine and the lower limbs.

When the pelvis is fixed the rectus abdominis, together with bilateral action of the internal and external obliques, produces trunk flexion. The psoas will also act as a trunk flexor when both the pelvis and femur are fixed. Lateral flexion of the trunk is produced by the lateral fibres of the external oblique and the ipsilateral internal oblique. Rotation is produced by action of the external oblique and the contralateral internal oblique.

Muscles acting on the pelvis will also produce anteroposterior pelvic tilt, lateral pelvic tilt and pelvic rotations. Anterior tilt is produced by the combined actions of the hip flexors and the trunk extensors. Posterior pelvic tilt is achieved by action of the trunk flexors combined with the hip extensors. Lateral pelvic tilt occurs with the hip joint of the weightbearing leg acting as a fulcrum. This movement is produced by lateral flexion and rotation of the spine and causes either abduction or adduction of the pelvis over the weightbearing hip. It is controlled by concentric or eccentric action of the contralateral hip abductors. Forward rotation of the pelvis occurs in a transverse plane, about a vertical axis. The weightbearing hip joint again acts as the fulcrum about which movement occurs. The chief extensors of the hip are the gluteus maximus and the ischial portion of the adductor magnus. The gluteus maximus is particularly evident on activities such as stair climbing, running and jumping. The hamstrings contribute to extension, but this is not their primary function. The piriformis and the posterior portion of gluteus medius may also play a role in extension. The iliopsoas and the rectus femoris are the major flexors of the hip, although rectus femoris does not tend to be involved in initiating the movement. The adductors, particularly pectineus, and tensor fascia lata are weak flexors of the hip. The pectineus, in fact, only acts as an adductor when the hip is flexed (Saudek 1985). The tensor fascia lata assists in abduction, but the major abductors of the hip are the gluteus medius and the gluteus minimis. The gluteus medius is also the primary lateral stabilizer of the hip in standing. The hip adductors are divided into anterior and posterior groups. Anteriorly, these are the pectineus, the adductors brevis, longus and magnus and gracilis. Posteriorly, the gluteus maximus, quadratus femoris, obturator externus and the hamstrings assist in adduction.

External rotation of the thigh is produced primarily by gluteus maximus. The piriformis, obturator externus and internus, gemelli and quadratus femoris are also active in external rotation. The iliopsoas has also been shown to be active in external rotation (Hedstrom & Lindgren 1982), but may also act as an internal rotator when the hip joint is in flexion. Internal rotation occurs as a secondary action of several muscles around the hip joint. As the semitendinosis, the semimembranosis and the posterior part of adductor magnus extend the hip, they also act to internally rotate the thigh. The tensor fascia lata, when assisting in flexion of the hip, also acts as an internal rotator. The gracilis internally rotates as it adducts the hip, and the gluteus medius and minimus contribute to internal rotation as they abduct the hip (Saudek 1985).

All the hip flexors are innervated by branches of the femoral nerve. The adductors are innervated by the obturator nerve. The gluteal nerve supplies the abductor muscles and the sciatic nerve innervates the hamstring group. It is worth noting that the long and short heads of the biceps femoris are supplied by different branches of the sciatic nerve. The long head, along with semitendinosis and semimembranosis, is innervated by the tibial branch of the sciatic nerve. The short head takes its nerve supply from the peroneal branch of the sciatic nerve. This may have implications when considering the mechanisms by which hamstring injury develop. The other major hip extensor, the gluteus maximus, is innervated by the inferior gluteal nerve. The muscles of the thigh can be divided into two compartments, separated laterally by the lateral intermuscular septum. The hamstrings group make up the bulk of the posterior compartment and may assist in extension of the hip joint, but they are also active in flexion of the knee and in the control of knee extension during gait.

The iliotibial band, which passes down over the posterolateral aspect of the thigh, has attachment to the tensor fascia lata and the distal expansion of the fascia enveloping gluteus maximus, as well as the lateral intermuscular septum and vastus lateralis distally. It is actually the thickened lateral aspect of the deep fascia of the thigh and, as such, has attachment to the posterior aspect of the sacrum and coccyx, the sacrotuberous ligament and the tuberosity and ramus of the ischium. It also extends medially to have attachment to the inferior ramus, body and superior ramus of the pubis. Above and anteriorly it blends with the inguinal ligament. Laterally it attaches along the entire length of the iliac crest. From the iliac crest it descends as a dense layer over the gluteus medius and envelops the tensor fascia lata and gluteus maximus. The fascia gives partial origin to the tensor fascia lata and gluteus medius and blends with the lateral aspect of the hip joint.

On the lateral aspect of the thigh the fascia is reinforced by tendon fibres from the tensor fascia lata and gluteus maximus. It is this portion that is usually identified as the iliotibial band. Functionally, the medial muscle group, the adductors, can be viewed with the flexors, as they do not lie within a discrete compartment. They are, however, separated from the quadriceps by the medial intermuscular septum. The gracilis and adductors longus, brevis and magnus constitute this group. All are innervated by the

obturator nerve and supplied by the profunda femoris artery.

The anterior thigh musculature consists of the quadriceps group and the sartorius. All of these muscles are supplied by the femoral nerve. The rectus femoris is the only muscle in the quadriceps group with an attachment to the pelvis. The four muscular elements of the quadriceps group fuse into the patellar tendon in a trilaminar fashion. The rectus femoris inserts anteriorly, vastus medialis and lateralis posterior to the rectus and vastus intermedius posterior to this. Some fibres of the rectus femoris extend distally, over the anterior aspect of the patella. The major functions of the anterior thigh musculature are extension of the knee and control of knee flexion, at heel strike, during gait. Specially interesting when considering the function of the anterior thigh musculature is the role of vastus medialis. This muscle has two components: the vastus medialis oblique, which has an oblique orientation of fibres, inserting into the patella tendon at 55–70° from the vertical; and the vastus medialis longus. At its insertion, the fibres of the vastus medialis oblique extend further distally than those of the longus. There is a cleavage line or septum separating the two portions. The two portions of the vastus medialis are supplied by different branches of the femoral nerve, which may be indicative of their separate functional roles. The vastus medialis longus contributes to the extensor function of the anterior thigh musculature, while the vastus medialis oblique maintains the medial stability of the patella and prevents lateral displacement

BIOMECHANICS

An understanding of how the pelvis, hip and thigh function during all forms of locomotion is essential to developing an understanding of how injuries affecting this area may develop in athletes. In the author's experience, this area is particularly prone to overuse injuries, which may have, as one of the predisposing causes, a failure of the normal biomechanics. The therapist is only able to implement strategies to correct biomechanical abnormalities if he or she understands what is required for normal function.

During gait, the primary function of the joints of the pelvis and lower limbs is to provide motion which allows for acceleration of the body in a linear fashion. There is a progressive and integrated motion of various skeletal parts through sagittal and transverse plane rotations. These rotations occur as a consequence of joint movement.

The sacroiliac joint

When considering movement of the sacroiliac joint, it must be remembered that it may function during both open kinetic chain and closed kinetic chain activities. However, the pelvis itself is a closed kinetic chain, i.e. movement of one hemipelvis on the other occurs in a closed loop.

Many reports on sacroiliac motion are based largely on anatomical knowledge and clinical experience (Alderink 1991). This is likely to be due to the difficulty associated with accurately assessing movement at this joint, which appears to be both multidimensional and multiplanar (Colachis et al 1963, Kapandji 1974, Mitchell et al 1979), although some of the work on which these definitions are based is still unverified and has not yet been proven by exhaustive clinical and laboratory testing. Our current understanding of the biomechanics of this region is still quite inadequate, particularly with regard to multi-directional activities, i.e. sports involving twisting and turning. It is possible that sacroiliac motion may be influenced by action of the lower limb muscles, but it is more likely that movement occurs mostly in response to the loads imposed on the joints by body weight and ground reaction forces.

Movement at the sacroiliac joint during gait relates to the anterior-posterior tilting of the pelvis, which is, in effect, rotation of the pelvis in a sagittal plane. Because of the reciprocal nature of gait, anterior-posterior pelvic rotations are likely to involve reciprocal rotations of each hemipelvis. For this to occur, movement must occur at the sacroiliac joints and the pubic symphasis. In gait, the ilium appears to rotate posteriorly during the swing phase and convert to an anterior rotation soon after weightbearing begins, achieving a maximal position of anterior rotation at the end of stance phase.

The sacrum appears to rotate forward about a diagonal axis during weightbearing, reaching maximum displacement at midstance and reversing the process during terminal stance (Alderink 1991). A unified model of sacroiliac joint function has not been developed, but it is generally agreed that movement at the sacroiliac joints is small and consists of sagittal plane rotation and translation of some kind (Alderink 1991).

The pubic symphasis

The pubic symphasis is responsible for the integrity of the pelvic ring. In the mature adult movement of this joint is minimal. A slight torsional movement has been suggested in addition to its known vertical displacement, to accommodate the rotary movement of the ilia in opposing directions on the sacrum. When unilateral weightbearing is needed, the pubic bone on the weightbearing side will move forward in relation to the non-weightbearing side, causing a shear stress at the joint.

The hip joint

The hip joint is inherently stable because of its structure, but mobility is also an important aspect of its function. It has been suggested that the mean motion used during walking by normal men is 15° extension, 37° flexion, 7° abduction, 5° adduction, 4° internal rotation and 9°

external rotation (Saudek 1985). Any loss of normal mobility will mean that at normal and fast walking speeds compensation will occur by:

1. an increased anterior-posterior pelvic tilt
2. an increased horizontal rotation of the pelvis
3. increased knee flexion on that side during stance.

Gait

Running, like walking, is a learned skill. Variations in the velocity of running, jogging and walking cause different gait patterns (Adelaar 1986). The gait cycle is divided into two functional components—stance phase and swing phase. The stance phase is divided into three periods—footstrike, midstance and push-off. Swing phase consists of follow-through, forward swing and foot descent. As the speed of gait is increased, the relative length of the cycle, in terms of time, is decreased. When running, the length of the stance phase decreases: there is no time when both lower limbs are simultaneously in contact with the ground and an intervening airborne phase occurs. To allow a better understanding of the biomechanics of the pelvis, hip and thigh in running at different velocities, it is worth looking first at walking.

In walking there is a rise of approximately 5 cm in the trunk as weight is borne on the stance leg. There is a corresponding shift of the pelvis and trunk to that side by the same amount. There is a downward list of the pelvis toward the swing leg, a movement which is controlled by the abductor muscles of the stance leg. The pelvis undergoes alternating movements of abduction and adduction, about the hip joint of the stance leg, of about 8° (Purdham 1989).

The lower leg, femur and pelvis undergo progressive internal rotation during the swing phase, culminating in magnitude in the stance phase, in full pronation. The total amount of rotation may exceed 35° in fast walking. The direction of rotation continues through the initial contact period, or footstrike. As the body weight moves over the support limb and the transition between footstrike and midstance begins, the subtalar joint begins to supinate and the lower limb begins a progressive external rotation (Root et al 1977). The amount of external rotation is greatest distally.

To better understand muscle action during gait, particularly with increasing speed, it is important to examine the efficiency of eccentric/concentric or stretch/shortening muscle action. Sprint running is one of the most mechanically efficient human skills, because much of the propulsive energy is derived from the elastic recoil of the muscles involved (Purdham 1989). This involves a stretch/shortening sequencing of muscle action which is 20–30% more efficient than purely concentric muscle action (Komi 1973). It is likened to rolling a cube along the ground. Each time a corner hits the ground there will be a reaction force directed vertically and backward. Rolling forward over the edge stores energy, which is released when the next corner hits the ground.

In a similar manner the athlete experiences a horizontal braking and a vertical ground reaction force at footstrike. The extensor muscles at the knee contract eccentrically during impact, opposing the external forces acting on the limb. While the muscle is developing tension it is also lengthening. Because the muscle is already active before the foot contacts the ground, it is capable of storing potential/elastic energy, which can be partly recovered during the subsequent shortening cycle. Eccentric/concentric muscle action, also called the stretch-shortening cycle, where stretch always precedes shortening, is a typical way for muscle to function. The performance of the muscle in the final concentric phase is potentiated/increased over that measured in the purely concentric condition (Komi 1973).

The activity of the gluteus maximus is very similar to the hamstrings at the hip joint. The gluteals and hamstrings perform a large amount of eccentric work in decelerating the thigh during the second half of swing phase, with their activity halting at about 30° of hip flexion. At the same time the hamstrings are working eccentrically to control the rate of extension of the knee. This allows them to store elastic energy and prepares the limb for footstrike, with the hamstrings working across the hip and knee joints. At footstrike the hamstrings and gluteals are already contracting concentrically, which is in part a release of energy stored in the swing phase, to extend the hip and pull the body's centre of gravity over the stance leg. At the same time, the hamstrings are co-contracting with the quadriceps group in stabilizing the knee joint and absorbing the vertically directed forces of 3.5–4.5 times body weight through the stance leg.

It has been shown that the action of the iliacus increases with the speed of running, becoming active immediately after follow through (Mann et al 1986). Follow through can be defined as the late stance and early swing phase of the gait cycle. This muscle, along with the psoas, is a prime flexor of the hip joint, contracting eccentrically in follow through and concentrically in forward swing.

The concept of energy flow across the pelvis during late forward swing as a significant factor in the efficiency of running has been raised (Chapman & Caldwell 1983). That is, as the hip extensors of the stance leg lose their effectiveness toward their inner range, the opposite leg, in its late swing phase, transmits part of its forward momentum to the pelvis and thence to the early swing phase of its counterpart. This is likely to be contributed to by the eccentric contraction of the hip extensors in the late swing phase, slowing the thigh into flexion, as they store energy for the concentric hip extension. This transfer of momentum also involves a deceleration of the forward shank and foot movement, which is in part achieved by eccentric action of the hamstring muscle group acting over the knee. However, this is not really a function of the eccentric muscle action,

but of the energy transfer between segments that it facilitates. As the speed of gait increases the range of hip flexion increases, from 40° in jogging to 80° in sprinting (Mann et al 1986). The range of extension increases from 15° in jogging to 5° hyperextension in running. Hyperextension can be said to define movement of the hip joint into extension range beyond that which would normally be produced by muscle action. That is, the forward momentum of the body forces the joint into an extreme of range. The movement will be limited by the passive joint restraints, i.e. the joint capsule. In sprinting, the range of hip extension actually decreases to 15°. This is likely to be related to the high level of hip extensor/knee flexor activity through footstrike and into mid-support, as the athlete attempts to minimize the braking action at footstrike by pulling the body forward and over the contact point during the initial stage of stance phase (Mann & Sprague 1980). As the length of stance phase decreases with an increasing speed of movement, there will be a more rapid movement of the body over the stance leg and a decreased hip extension time.

The gluteus medius and tensor fascia lata demonstrate little change in speed of action as speed of gait increases, but have been shown to be active for a shorter period (Mann et al 1986). These muscles provide abductor stability to the pelvis just before and just after foot contact. They contract eccentrically during the first stage of weightbearing as the contralateral hip dips, then throughout the remainder of the support phase they contract concentrically.

The tensor fascia lata and piriformis are primary abductors through most of their range (Dostal et al 1986). The gluteus medius is most effective as an abductor in the 0–40° range of hip flexion. After this range is exceeded it becomes more effective as an internal rotator, being the primary internal rotator, along with gluteus minimus, at 90° flexion. The external rotators also work most effectively in the 0–40° range of hip flexion. At greater ranges they work as hip abductors (Dostal et al 1986), although they are much weaker than the gluteals. It is possible that the external rotators act to slow the internal rotation of the femur on the pelvis during stance phase (eccentrically), reversing this during the propulsive phase. Adductor longus activity occurs primarily at toe-off, and continues through recovery phase. This activity decreases with the speed of running, possibly due to the decreased duration of stance phase. It is suggested that its action is to eccentrically control abduction of the pelvis on the femur as the more powerful abductors release their energy, utilizing this energy to assist in flexion of the thigh. The posterior and middle heads of the adductor magnus are thought to play an important role in decelerating hip flexion and forward thrust of the body during locomotion, acting with the hamstrings (Dostal et al 1986).

Electromicrographic studies (Simonson et al 1985) showed that in sprinting, the rectus femoris has two periods of activity. The first occurs immediately following ground contact. As the hip extends and the knee flexes, the muscle stores energy eccentrically. It then releases it concentrically, as it contracts with the other knee extensors to propel the athlete into the next airborne phase. At the end of swing phase the rectus contracts to extend the knee preparatory to footstrike, in conjunction with the vasti. The vasti are activated before footstrike to extend the knee and they preset their tension to absorb the reaction forces on footstrike.

At footstrike in jogging, running and sprinting, hip flexion is initially 50° (Mann et al 1986). In terms of the most effective working ranges for the hip abductors and external rotators this is obviously significant.

During sprinting, the rectus abdominis appears to contract eccentrically bilaterally, to control lumbar lordosis during toe-off, then concentrically to initiate forward flexion of the pelvis and hip. This is important for several reasons. For the body's centre of gravity to follow a smooth, undulating path during gait there must be a change in the relative length of the supporting leg. This is accomplished proximally by pelvic rotation and tilt. Similarly, there is a relative lengthening of the extremity during push-off. It has also been suggested that the initiating force for hip extension, during push-off, commences in the lumbar spine-pelvic unit with the trunk musculature extending the lumbar spine and pelvis (Slocum & Bowerman 1962).

In summary, much of the energy utilized in sprint running is gained from the muscles undergoing a stretch-shortening cycle. Muscles function eccentrically during impact to oppose the external forces that make them stretch (Komi 1973). Because the muscle is already active before the load is applied, it is therefore capable of storing potential (elastic) energy, which can be partly recovered in the subsequent concentric contraction. An important feature of this stretch-shortening phenomenon is that the concentric contraction of the muscle is potentiated over that seen in a purely concentric contraction. The biarthrodial muscles can store elastic energy during the swing phase. The monarthrodial muscles function by presetting their tension prior to ground contact, to achieve a stretch-shortening cycle, with the recovery of energy used to assist propulsion (Simonson et al 1985, Morrison 1970). The EMG activity in selected lower limb muscles, during the running cycle, is most evident before and during the eccentric contraction phase (Komi 1973). There is very little activity during the concentric phase of the stretch-shortening cycle (Mann et al 1986), which would tend to support the concept of the release of stored potential (elastic) energy during running.

At the hip, the energy storage phase occurs at the end of the swing phase. It has been suggested that the central nervous system commands the muscles in such a way that greater activation is timed to take place during that part of the contraction phase, where the load demands are greatest (Komi 1973), i.e. during the period of eccentric activity.

The pelvic bony structure is inherently stable. The pelvis has a small range of movement intrinsically available at each of the sacroiliac joints and the pubic symphasis, which allows for more comfortable and efficient transmission of loads and forces. An understanding of the structure and function of these joints in gait, particularly running, and the muscles which initiate and control the movements, is essential to an understanding of how injuries to the pelvis, hip and thigh may develop in the athlete and what is required for effective rehabilitation.

MECHANISM OF INJURY

It should, by now, be obvious that injury to the pelvis, hip and thigh can be very complex in terms of predisposing factors and mechanisms by which injury, other than that caused by direct trauma, may arise. Consequently, the injury will often be poorly recognised initially and may progress to a more complex, multifaceted problem, which poses real problems in terms of management. This section will deal with developing an understanding of the mechanisms by which injury affecting this area may develop in the athlete.

One study showed that overuse accounted for 82.4% of injuries surveyed affecting the pelvis, and trauma 17.6% (Lloyd-Smith et al 1985). The suggested mechanisms of injury as a consequence of overuse may be related to any or all of the following:

1. musculoskeletal imbalances
2. poor muscular co-ordination
3. inadequate skills
4. inappropriate training drills/schedules
5. fatigue
6. incomplete rehabilitation of previous injury
7. repeated minor trauma, which may or may not have been symptomatic in isolation.

Because of the often insidious onset of symptoms secondary structures may become increasingly affected by the changed mechanics, relative to the initial injury. Analysis of the exact mechanism of injury and which structures are affected becomes increasingly difficult. Evaluation may be easier if the examiner assesses the athlete under the above headings.

MUSCULOSKELETAL IMBALANCES

Any breakdown in the effective function of the lower limbs and pelvic girdle during gait may predispose to injury. Examples of this would include:

1. postural changes due to muscle tightness, specifically the lumbar erector spinae, hip flexors, hip internal rotators, hamstrings and rectus femoris
2. poor co-ordination/early fatigue associated with muscle weakness
3. diminished load bearing capacities of the skeletal structures with these postural changes i.e. hip flexion contracture reducing that joint's ability to deform under load; femoral anteversion affecting foot

placement during gait and potentially diminishing the shock absorbing function of the lower limb

4. leg length discrepancy, which will affect pelvic motion and stride length
5. problems with prolonged or delayed pronation or supination which, by its effect on the function of the foot, will necessarily alter the function of the leg and pelvis, particularly with regard to the range of rotation the limb undergoes and its timing in the gait cycle.

POOR MUSCULAR CO-ORDINATION

Obviously it is difficult to perform a task requiring strength, power, endurance, co-ordination or skill if the muscles required for that activity are functionally impaired by being:

1. weak
2. contracted/shortened
3. elongated/stretched
4. excessively developed or bulky muscle limiting range of movement
5. poorly developed in terms of neuromuscular co-ordination.

Examples of these sorts of problems include:

1. vastus medialis oblique dysfunction
2. 'snapping hip' with a tight psoas tendon
3. loss of the normal quadriceps/hamstrings ratio when there is excessive development of the quadriceps. A normal ratio is generally 60:40 (Hemba 1985).

However, this is not a clear issue and it is possible that the ratio may vary dependent on the speed of the movement and the activity or skill being performed.

INADEQUATE SKILLS

There is a need to look at skills acquisition for the sport being played. It is impossible to appreciate the mechanisms by which an injury may develop if you do not know what the athlete is trying to do and how he or she should be doing it. Skill acquisition involves training the body to adapt to the load being placed on it. It involves neuromuscular learning, which can be assessed by initially examining the basic skills and increasing their complexity until a deficiency is recognized. This should also include an assessment of skills under stress and when the athlete is fatigued. This may also include assessment of pelvic and hip joint motion in running or other sports-specific activities.

INAPPROPRIATE TRAINING DRILLS/SCHEDULES

These would include anything which may overwhelm the body's ability to adapt to new levels of stress, including excessive mileage or a rapid increase in mileage, coupled with an intensive interval training program. Adequate recovery time must be allowed, but the body must not be allowed to cool excessively between repeated intensive workouts. Other common problems include inadequate warm-up and cool-down, faulty stretching and poor running surfaces. For example, cambered running tracks may produce an apparent leg length difference which will decrease the stride length on the shorter leg side and may cause loading problems affecting the musculature around the hip joint. Problems associated with poor equipment could be included. Protective gear, footwear, orthotic devices and clothing are some of the other areas which may need to be considered when assessing the mechanism of injury. For example, inappropriate footwear may exacerbate a problem with the timing of pronation during the stance phase of the gait cycle. This may have the effect of causing an earlier onset of hip internal rotation, thereby altering the mechanics of pelvic-hip function.

FATIGUE

Fatigue affects performance and may predispose to injury both in terms of muscle physiology and gross motor performance. Fatigue may be reflected in a prolonged recovery time at the neuromuscular junctions, which will diminish effective muscle activation, and delayed clearing of metabolites from the working muscle, which will affect the ability of the muscles to generate tension. This may lead to a reduced circulating blood volume, as a consequence of the dehydration which may develop with fatigue. For these and other reasons, fatigue tends to manifest with decreased strength, power, endurance, concentration and gross motor performance/skills, which will increase the risk of injury. This may be one of the mechanisms at work in the development of injuries such as psoas tendinitis, hamstring origin tendinitis and some cases of vastus medialis oblique dysfunction.

INCOMPLETE REHABILITATION

Incomplete rehabilitation inevitably means that the injured athlete has not regained the ability to perform at the expected level of function. Factors which may be important are range of movement, strength (contractile and tensile), power, endurance, flexibility and proprioception. Skill maintenance should also be addressed. The treating therapist must remember to assess the recovery of musculoskeletal functions in terms of the activities or skills the athlete expects to be able to perform. Rehabilitation must continue to a functional level. Failure to do so may indicate an inadequate understanding of what the athlete requires of his or her body in terms of performance. Perhaps the best example of this relates to retraining the stretch-shortening function of the hamstring muscles. The ability to perform a maximal isometric contraction does not necessarily mean that the muscle has developed the neuromuscular co-ordination required to utilize that strength in an eccentric contraction.

REPEATED MINOR TRAUMA

Trauma may not always be significant enough to provoke pain or disability at the time of injury and consequently may not initially impair performance. Conditions which may be classified in this way would include tendinitis (adductor origin, psoas insertion), minor muscle strains (post-exercise soreness) and stress fractures (pubic rami and femoral neck). Deterioration in function may be so gradual as not to be detected until there is a significant problem. Over a period of time it may become difficult to distinguish the original injury, due to the secondary changes which may occur, i.e. muscle weakness (external rotators of the hip secondary to femoral neck stress reactions), contractures (psoas shortening as a consequence of lumbar spine pathologies or dysfunction) and inflammatory irritation of structures removed from the site of original injury due to changed loading patterns.

OTHER CONSIDERATIONS

It should also be remembered that there are non-traumatic causes of hip and pelvic pain. Simm and Scott (1986) state that these may include:

1. Inflammatory conditions:
   a anklyosing spondylitis
   b Reiter's syndrome
   c rheumatoid arthritis

2. Infectious conditions:
   a osteomyelitis
   b septic joint

3. Tumours:
   a Osteoid osteoma
   b metastatic disease

4. Others:
   a referred pain
   b pathologic conditions of the lumbar spine
   c metabolic bone disease with decreased bone density.

Inflammatory conditions

A history of low back, buttock or thigh pain in the young athlete, associated with a prolonged history of low back and hip joint stiffness, should raise suspicion of the possibility of ankylosing spondylitis. There will often be an associated history of a classically inflammatory pattern of morning stiffness, lasting for more than one hour, subsiding through the middle of the day and redeveloping in the evening. Diagnosis can only be confirmed by examination of the human leukocyte antigens (HLA) on blood pathology and by X-ray examination, which will show characteristic sacroiliac joint changes.

Treatment will generally involves both exercise and passive mobilization techniques to limit the development of postural tightness into flexion. Exercises should be directed toward strengthening the posterior trunk musculature and developing of better postural co-contraction between trunk flexors and extensors. Similarly, mobilizing exercises should address the need to maintain a functional range of lumbar spine and hip joint extension. The use of heating modalities and anti-inflammatory medications is valuable in controlling pain and limiting the inflammatory response. Other rheumatological or inflammatory conditions will require similar treatment approaches, but with the emphasis of strengthening and mobilizing being determined by the functional limitations the condition imposes. Accurate diagnosis can only be made by examination of blood pathology and by radiographic evaluation.

Infectious conditions

Chronic pain in the region of the pelvis and hip also warrants investigation for the presence of infection. Diagnosis of infective disorders is made on examining blood pathology, which may show features such as a raised ESR or white cell count. The presence of specific infective organisms may also be noted.

Tumours

The presence of tumours, such as osteoid osteoma in the young athlete or metastatic tumours in athletes of all ages, can be confirmed on X-ray, bone scan, CAT scan or MRI (magnetic resonance imaging). A prolonged history of diffuse low back or pelvic pain, with no specific aggravating movements or activities but which limits performance may suggest the need to check for these possible causes.

ASSESSMENT

The assessment of injuries affecting the pelvis, hip and thigh requires a systematic approach. As usual, the assessment is divided into subjective and objective components.

Subjective assessment

The subjective assessment will provide information regarding the severity and irritability of the condition and the likely structures involved. The areas to be addressed include:

1. Presenting complaint.
2. Location of symptoms. This may help to begin to define the structures causing the symptoms.
3. Onset and duration of symptoms.
4. Nature and behaviour of symptoms. The way in which the symptoms behave may provide information

about irritability and provide clues on activities that require further biomechanical assessment.

5. Past history of similar problems. This may provide information regarding possible biomechanical abnormalities or incomplete rehabilitation of previous injuries.
6. Any previous treatment and results.
7. Relevant other history. This should include information regarding medical conditions (old slipped capital femoral epiphysis, previous hernias, inflammatory conditions etc.).
8. Activities of daily living—work/sport/recreation.

Information in these areas should tell you about the load that the athlete places on the pelvis, hip and thigh. In the case of overuse injuries, the combination of training and competition schedules coupled with a strenuous physical occupation may be the reason for tissue failure, rather than any one isolated activity.

Objective assessment

A logical sequence of assessment of the physical parameters of injury affecting the pelvis, hip or thigh may be designed along the following lines.

Initial observation: posture

1. Gait. Address stride-length differences, antalgic gait, onset of fatigue, joint range of movement, duration of stance phase and any other variations from the normal.
2. Balance. Try to establish if there is equal weightbearing on both limbs. Assess ability to fully weightbear on a single limb.
3. Lumbar spine range of movement. Assessment of the lumbar spine is covered elsewhere in this text, but is included here as a clearing test to exclude the possibility of referred pain.
4. Squat. The squat test should also exclude the knees as a source of thigh pain, but will be useful in assessing the movement of the hip joint under load.
5. Hop; hop and turn to both sides. These are dynamic activities which require strength, power, co-ordination and confidence. They can be useful in assessing the severity of the injury, particularly those affecting the thigh musculature.

Standing: posture

Look for differences in the height of the iliac crests, rotation of one hemipelvis on the other, hip joint posture, knee joint posture, intrinsic lower limb posture (femoral anteversion, tibial varum, forefoot or rearfoot valgum or varus etc.).

Lying supine

1. Palpation of anterior structures, including the anterior superior iliac spine, the iliac crests, the greater trochanters, the pubic tubercles, the inguinal area and the anterior and medial thigh musculature.
2. Leg length measurement, with measurements taken from both the greater trochanters and the anterior superior iliac spines, to exclude apparent leg length differences.
3. Sacroiliac joint compression and distraction. Stressing of these joints should give an indication of whether they are contributing to or causing the athlete's pain.
4. Faber test.
5. Thomas test.
6. Hip quadrant.
7. Hip extension abduction and internal rotation.
8. Straight leg raise: active, passive and resisted movement tests at both the hip and knee joints, to assess strength and flexibility.

Side lying

1. Palpation of lateral and posterior structures, including the sciatic notch, the ischial tuberosity, the greater trochanter and musculature including tensor fascia lata.
2. Active, passive and resisted movement tests.
3. Ober's test.

Prone

1. Palpation of posterior structures, including the posterior iliac spine, the coccyx, sacrum and lumbar spine (see Ch. 27 for detailed assessment), and soft tissues such as the piriformis and gluteus maximus.
2. Active, passive and resisted hip extension, internal and external rotation and knee flexion/extension.
3. Femoral nerve stretch to exclude the possibility of dural irritation in anterior pain affecting the groin or thigh.

Seated

If indicated, slump stretch to exclude dural irritation as a source of posterior pain affecting the buttock or thigh.

Special tests

1. Thomas test. This is used to test the flexibility of the soft tissues anterior to the hip joint, particularly the iliopsoas.
2. Obers test (Fig. 28.4). This test is used to determine the extensibility of the iliotibial band and is discussed in more detail in Chapters 29 and 30. However, the

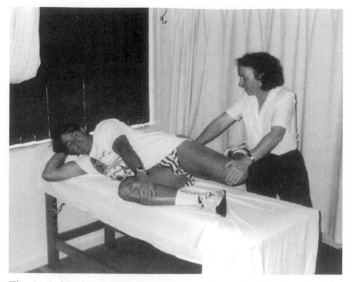

Fig. 28.4 Ober's test. The patient lies on the unaffected side with the hip and knee bent into mid range flexion. The affected leg is moved into a combination of hip extension and adduction, with knee flexion. If tissue tension is normal, the knee of the affected leg should be able to rest on the table. The hip of the unaffected leg is flexed to flatten the lumbar lordosis and thereby stabilize the pelvis

test may not be discriminating enough. The testing position will need to be varied to discriminate between the different muscles which have attachment to the band.

3. Faber test (Fig. 28.5). The flexion, abduction and external rotation test is used to assess the mobility of the hip joint, particularly the anteromedial capsule. The test will also stress the sacroiliac joint on the ipsilateral side.

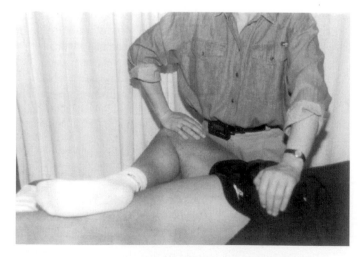

Fig. 28.5 Faber test. The patient lies supine. The affected leg is positioned in hip abduction/external rotation and knee flexion so that the ankle of the affected leg rests on the thigh of the unaffected leg just above the knee. The therapist stabilizes the pelvis by pushing down on the iliac rim on the unaffected side. At the same time, pressure is applied to the medial aspect of the affected knee, increasing the abduction/external rotation stretch at the affected hip

4. Hip quadrant (Fig. 28.6). Combined flexion/adduction with or without compression and/or internal rotation is used to assess the hip joint and related soft tissues, particularly the posterolateral capsule, the posterior musculature and the ligament of the head.
5. Femoral nerve stretch. This stretch is performed in prone. The hip is extended, the knee flexed and the ankle dorsiflexed to assess abnormal tension in the dura investing the nerve roots which constitute the femoral nerve.
6. Slump stretch (see Ch. 33 for detailed discussion).

INJURIES TO THE PELVIS, HIP AND THIGH

Fractures

Pelvic fractures

Pelvic fractures are generally high velocity injuries which occur only under extreme force, and they are not often seen

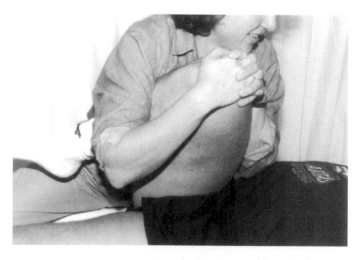

Fig. 28.6 Hip quadrant. Patient lies supine. The affected leg is moved into a combination of hip flexion, adduction and internal rotation with the knee flexed. At the same time, the therapist may apply a compressive force through the joint

in sports. However, they may be seen in sports such as motor racing, equestrian events, skiing and mountain climbing. This author has had personal experience of only one case of pelvic fracture in other sports, which involved a veteran triathlete who sustained an undisplaced fracture of the acetabulum as a result of a high speed fall from his bicycle while on a training ride.

There may be severe complications, such as internal haemorrhage affecting the abdominal and pelvic viscera, or rupture of the bladder or urethra. Management of the bony injury will generally take a lower priority than treatment of the secondary complications. If the fracture does not pass through the pelvic ring, functional stability of the pelvis remains and as long as the injured athlete remains part-weightbearing as pain allows, there should be no long term disability related to altered pelvic mechanics. Fractures which disrupt the pelvic ring generally require fixation to maintain as closely as possible the structural and functional integrity of the pelvis, while the fracture heals.

The differential diagnosis is made by radiographic investigation, although the history should fairly clearly indicate what the likely damage will be. Physiotherapy management will be primarily concerned with maintenance of the musculo-skeletal system, generally at an optimum level within the limitations of the injury. As the injury progresses treatment will develop to include gait re-education, mobility and strength retraining and rehabilitative exercise designed to take the athlete back to a level where he or she can reasonably expect to start training again. Progression of treatment will depend on the state of healing of the fracture, as shown on X-ray examination and on an assessment of the athlete's pain.

Femoral neck fractures

Acute fractures of the femoral neck are more commonly seen in the veteran athlete. They are more common in females than males, probably due to the increased incidence of osteoporosis in the female population after menopause (Saudek 1985, Simm & Scott 1986). Involvement in sport does not appear to affect the frequency with which the injury occurs. The injury tends to occur as a result of trauma, usually a fall, in the older population and relative fitness does not appear to either increase or decrease its incidence.

A fracture can occur in three places:

1. intertrochanteric—between the greater and lesser trochanters
2. subtrochanteric—below the trochanters
3. subcapital—at the junction of the femoral head and neck.

These fractures are often displaced and comminuted. There is a typical presentation of apparent shortening of the leg on the affected side, with the leg falling into an externally rotated position. There is a lot of pain. Diagnosis is confirmed on X-ray. Usual treatment is by open reduction and internal fixation. Subcapital fractures may be best treated by prosthetic replacement of the femoral head, because of the danger of avascular necrosis subsequent to the disruption of the blood supply in what may already be an impaired circulation. It is important that fracture reduction restore the hip to as normal an anatomy as possible so that the biomechanics of gait, particularly running, are maintained and the athlete is not hindered.

Physiotherapy will again be primarily be concerned with the maintenance of the musculoskeletal system, as well as with gait re-education. Again, the progression of treatment will depend on the state of healing of the fracture and on the type of surgical procedure undertaken.

Femoral shaft fractures

Femoral shaft fractures are not often seen in sport. Again, these are usually high velocity injuries. There have been isolated cases reported of spontaneous fracture with no apparent underlying pathology, but these are rare (King & Robertson 1986). There will be immediate pain and collapse, with deformity usually evident at the fracture site. Immediate care should concentrate on supporting the injured limb and managing shock, which can be a problem due to blood loss.

In the long term, the most important thing to remember is that athletes, who have high performance expectations of their bodies, cannot tolerate a significant leg length difference or rotational deformity of the femur, or im-pairment of the very closely related thigh musculature, as this will affect the function of the limb. Its ability to tolerate high performance loading, both within the injured tissue and at the adjacent joints, will be diminished.

The differential diagnosis is again made on X-ray examination, although the history and presentation will be very strong indicators of the injury. Management will vary depending on the type of fracture, its location along the femoral shaft, the amount of displacement, any associated tissue damage and the age of the injured athlete. The personal management preference of the managing physician or surgeon will also obviously determine the course of treatment and rehabilitation. The plethora of different management strategies for fractured shafts of femur is beyond the scope of this chapter. However, as a general principle, physiotherapy management will be concerned with the maintenance of strength and flexibility, within the limitations of the injury of the associated soft tissues and adjacent joints. Further treatment will include gait training, weightbearing activities and resistance training as the state of healing, evidenced by X-ray findings and clinical signs of improvement, progresses.

Stress fractures

Stress fractures can include sacral, femoral neck (transverse/ compression), pubic rami and shaft of femur (Fig. 28.7). They are a common injury presenting to sports injury clinics and may account for as much as 10% of all sports injuries (Matheson et al 1987). Contributing factors to the development of stress fractures are:

1. Repetitive microtrauma/overuse
2. A sudden and rapid increase in training load
3. Poor training surfaces—too hard; cambered, etc.
4. Biomechanical abnormalities
5. Early start of endurance based training in females (pre-menarche).
6. Amennhorea
7. Problems with bone mineralization
8. Dietary problems.

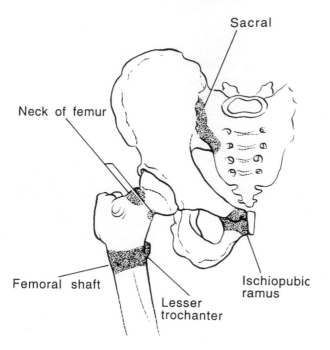

Fig. 28.7 Stress fractures of the regions

In most cases there will be more than one predisposing factor.

Sacral stress fractures are rare. They may, however be seen in distance runners. Pain will usually develop during a run and may be poorly localized to the groin and gluteal region. The pain will eventually prevent further running and may also make walking difficult. The athlete will generally develop an antalgic gait. Hip movement is full range and pain free. There may be tenderness on deep palpation of the sacral and gluteal regions. Sacroiliac joint stress tests may provoke gluteal pain. X-rays will generally be unremarkable. Bone scans, CAT scans and MRI imaging are useful diagnostic tools. Treatment usually involves rest from aggravating activities and protected weightbearing if the symptoms warrant it. The injury usually resolves with no other management, within six weeks (Atwell & Jackson 1991).

Femoral neck stress fractures can develop either as a result of compression or distraction forces. Fractures arising as a consequence of distraction forces will usually appear along the superior cortex of the femoral neck and may relate to either of the tensile load bearing trabecular patterns previously mentioned (Saudek 1985, Simm & Scott 1986, Karlin 1986). Femoral neck stress fractures affecting the inferior cortex will generally develop in response to excessive compressive loads and tend to be located relative to either of the trabecular patterns which transmit compressive loads. These fractures respond well to conservative management. It should be noted that stress fractures in the region of the lesser trochanter are rare (Simm & Scott 1986). They may be suspected in athletes with persistent pain related to the

insertion of iliopsoas and should be confirmed by both a positive X-ray and bone scan.

Transverse femoral neck stress fractures appear at the cortex as a simple crack, which may extend across the neck and ultimately displace. This requires orthopedic referral and possible internal fixation. Femoral neck stress fractures may present with groin pain on weightbearing and during activity, but the pain will eventually be present at rest as the fracture progresses. Clinical findings are minimal, but pain may be reproduced at the extremes of hip rotation. A possible complication of femoral neck stress fractures which should be considered is avascular necrosis. The anatomy of the blood supply to the femoral head, as previously described, may cause the femoral head to be particularly at risk should displacement occur. Pubic rami stress fractures may also produce groin pain, as well as buttock and thigh pain. Diagnosis is confirmed with bone scan, which is positive in 95% of cases. Plain X-rays may take more than three weeks to show diagnostic changes.

Femoral shaft stress fractures are rare and tend to occur at either end of the femoral shaft, such as the femoral neck, which has already been discussed. Stress fractures may, however, be seen in the distal femoral shaft. Typically, these fractures occur in recreational athletes who have undertaken an increase in training load (Fox 1986). The presenting complaint will usually be of a low-grade aching in the distal thigh, with no obvious deformity or suggestion of knee joint pathology. If training is continued, the pain will begin to be felt during normal daily activities. Initial diagnosis may be difficult and not uncommonly these fractures may be presumed to be an iliotibial band friction syndrome (Fox 1986). Treatment with anti-inflammatories will not help the symptoms.

Accurate diagnosis can only be made with the use of bone scans. Standard X-rays may be normal, at least in the early stages. Treatment will generally involve rest from the aggravating activities until the fracture has healed, at which time the athlete can begin a graduated training program with the aim of eventually resuming normal activities.

Femoral shaft stress fractures also occur in the subtrochanteric region. The presenting complaint is usually of anterior or medial thigh pain. Examination and treatment follows the general principles already discussed.

Avulsion injuries

Avulsion injuries are more often seen in the skeletally immature athlete, usually between 14 and 17 years of age. They occur most commonly at the apophysis, where the tenoperiosteal junction is stronger than the unfused growth centre. Common sites for this injury in the area of the pelvis, hip and thigh are:

1. the anterior superior iliac spine (ASIS) at the origin of the sartorius

2. the anterior inferior iliac spine (AIIS) at the origin of the rectus femoris
3. the ischial tuberosity, at the origin of the hamstring group
4. the lesser trochanter at the insertion of iliopsoas.

They occur when the muscle is forcefully stretched beyond its freely available range of movement, or when it meets a sudden, unexpected resistance while contracting forcefully. The working muscle unit is likely to fail at its weakest point. In the skeletally mature athlete this may be the tenoperiosteal or muscle-tendon junctions, but in the younger athlete the unfused growth centre is structurally the weakest link in the bone-tendon-muscle unit. Because of the thick periosteum, significant displacement is uncommon (Simm & Scott 1986). In the case of avulsion injuries affecting the anterior superior or inferior iliac spines, displacement will also be prevented by the overlying musculature. Avulsion injuries are seen more commonly in boys than girls and are seen particularly in sprinting and running sports and in all codes of football.

Ischial tuberosity avulsion injuries may occur in athletes up to 25 years of age, as the ischial apophysis does not unite with the body of the ischium until between 20 and 25 years of age (Simm & Scott 1986). In the running athlete the injury will usually originate in the hamstrings, but the ischial portion of adductor magnus may be avulsed in dance activities, e.g. doing the splits.

Athletes with these injuries present complaining of a sudden onset of pain, with localized swelling, tenderness and limitation of movement over the fracture site. The injury may be mistaken for a muscle strain and X-ray examination is usually undertaken to confirm the diagnosis. Treatment will initially involve rest, ice and elimination of tension and load from the fracture site. Crutches are usually prescribed. Movement exercises are commenced gradually as the pain settles. Resistance training begins when a full pain free range of movement has been regained. Only when there is a full pain free range of movement and normal strength is the athlete allowed to return to sport.

Contusions

Hip pointer

Contusion of the iliac crest, commonly called a hip pointer, is a most debilitating and painful injury. It usually results from a fall against a hard surface, with a lot of force behind the movement. A large collection of blood develops in the subperiosteal space, adjacent to the iliac crest, causing pain as a result of stretching of the periosteum and the resultant pressure on the surrounding, densely innervated tissues. The muscles and soft tissues above the crest are also usually involved, but a hip pointer must be distinguished from a tear of the muscle aponeurosis or an avulsion of the apophysis of the iliac crest (Simm & Scott 1986). In a hip

pointer the local iliac crest pain will generally not be significantly aggravated by contraction of the associated muscles. There is significant local bruising and swelling. The athlete will often have difficulty moving and walking freely because of pain and muscle spasm. X-rays are usually taken to exclude the possibility of a fracture. In the long term this injury is never as serious as a soft tissue haematoma (Bull 1985), primarily because there are less likely to be serious complications.

Treatment usually follows the principles of soft tissue management in the early stage. Specifically, this involves rest, ice and compression. Local physiotherapy modalities are of use in facilitating the body's healing response, i.e. heat, ultrasound, interferential, laser. Anti-inflammatory medication may be prescribed, once it is certain that there is no further bleeding, to facilitate recovery and provide pain relief by limiting the inflammatory response. Exercise to reduce associated muscle spasm and tightness should also be undertaken. Specifically, trunk mobilization and stretching exercises, especially those directed toward contralateral lateral flexion, will be of benefit in restoring full mobility.

In an uncomplicated hip pointer the athlete can usually return to sport within 1–2 weeks, wearing a protective doughnut-type pad to cover the injured area. However, some injuries may take as long as two months to heal to the point where a return to sport is possible.

Haematomas

These injuries commonly affect the thigh musculature, particularly the anterior and lateral compartments. They arise as a result of a collision with a blunt object, often an opponent's knee. Most, while they may be painful, do not significantly interfere with function. However, with a severe blunt force, there may be significant bleeding into the muscle bulk. If the muscle sheath is not disrupted, bleeding into a confined space results, causing significant pain, muscle spasm and limitation of movement. If the swelling is not controlled, secondary damage may develop. This may arise as a result of impaired blood flow because of the increased pressure within the compartment, causing an increased chemical or inflammatory reaction to the initial injury. Local mechanical damage caused by the pressure of the swelling on tissues undamaged in the initial injury may also occur. Other complications which may arise include the possibility of bleeding tracking distally, affecting knee joint function.

Treatment follows the standard principles of soft tissue injury management for the first 48–72 hours. In severe cases crutches can be used to limit use of the injured part and provide further rest. The athlete can begin gentle active and passive stretching within the limits of pain immediately after injury, to limit the secondary effects of the reactive muscle spasm. Tightness which develops after to the initial injury may be the thing which delays a return to sport.

Rehabilitation should be begun as soon as pain allows. The most important consideration should be regaining the full stretch of the injured muscle. The emphasis is on re-establishing the fascial planes and alignment of the muscle fibres (Fox 1986). Stretching also facilitates the breakdown of adhesions, which may form between tissue planes. The athlete should be able to stretch actively, simultaneously flexing the knee and extending the hip. Massage, carefully done, can be of value in assisting in the mechanical breakdown of the haematoma and in limiting the development of adhesions, once the haematoma is no longer developing.

Electrotherapy modalities, which stimulate increased blood flow through the area and facilitate the local cellular response, are of use in encouraging healing. When a functional range of movement has been regained, resistance exercises for strength and endurance can be started, as long as pain is not a problem.

The athlete can usually return to competition when normal muscle flexibility and strength have been regained. There should be a normal agonist/antagonist ratio and strength of all other muscle groups in the affected limb. The athlete may require a protective pad over the original injury to minimize the risk of reinjury.

Myositis ossificans

Myositis ossificans is characterized by the formation of local heterotrophic bone in soft tissues. It may develop as a complication following a direct blunt trauma such as a contact with an opponent's knee, as a consequence of a haematoma, or be iatrogenic in origin. This should not be confused with the ossification that occurs after a sub-periosteal haematoma. In the case of trauma, a soft tissue mass may be evident shortly after injury and calcification may be seen on X-ray at 3-4 weeks. The mass is usually well defined by 6-8 weeks. There is associated heat, swelling and tenderness and frequently, limitation of muscle function due to pain. The lesion usually matures over about 6 months and may then gradually subside. Prolonged problems with pain may be assisted by surgical removal of the lesion, but this is not done for at least 9–12 months after-injury, to allow the lesion to mature.

Treatment usually involves avoiding any potentially aggravating activities and performing a gentle range of movement exercises to prevent the development of contractures. A graduated strengthening program should be begun when pain allows, to prepare the athlete for a return to sport. When the athlete is ready to return to sport, protective padding should be worn, as repeated knocks can exacerbate the condition. The application of physiotherapy modalities and excessive loading with exercise, during the acute stage, may aggravate the condition by increasing of the inflammatory response and osteoblastic activity. It is possible that aggressive physiotherapy, in the case of a severe muscle haematoma, may predispose to the development of myositis ossificans by the same mechanisms.

Groin pain

The term 'groin injury' can describe injury to any of the following muscles: the sartorius, the long head of rectus femoris, any or all of the adductor muscles, the abdominals or the iliopsoas. Groin pain may also present as a symptom of lumbar spine dysfunction, bone and joint lesions, bursitis, osteitis pubis, stress fractures, degenerative changes affecting the hip joint, and occult hernia/conjoint tendon injury

Groin injuries can present as acute or chronic. Acute injuries, such as muscle and musculotendinous strains, should not be difficult to assess and treat, although acute tears of the muscle bellies are extremely rare. Acute injuries affecting the groin area arise as a result of direct or indirect trauma. A sudden overstretch, which most commonly affects the adductor longus, iliopsoas and rectus femoris muscles and their respective tendons, would constitute an indirect trauma. Bone and joint injuries, such as an avulsion fracture or a slipped capital femoral epiphysis, could also be included in this category.

Running sports are most often associated with acute groin strains. There is often a violent external rotation of the thigh while the leg is abducted and the foot planted (Karlin 1986). Diagnosis is usually made by tenderness on local palpation, associated with pain on resisted contraction or stretch of isolated muscles. Elimination of other sources of irritation also has to be undertaken.

Chronic injuries are generally more difficult to evaluate and manage. As the chronicity of groin injuries increases, so does the likelihood of more than one discrete pathological entity occurring. A multifactorial approach to examination and treatment is often required. The majority (85%) of groin problems begin with an acute episode, but there are often additional factors which may mimic or obscure the clinical picture in a refractory 15% of cases (Muckle 1982). Acute groin injuries may become chronic if not effectively treated and managed, as the damaged tissues will have a reduced loadbearing capacity and will be likely to deteriorate further under load. Also, because the damaged tissues cannot function normally, it is likely that the biomechanics of the whole region will be subtly changed, causing relative overload and possibly injury of other structures. It is important for effective treatment, rehabilitation and prevention of further injury, that the mechanism by which the injury developed and the structures involved be identified.

Differential diagnosis of groin pain

When attempting to establish a diagnosis for groin pain the following points should be addressed to gain a good history:

1. Pain distribution (groin, abdomen, scrotum, perineum, back, buttock), which should provide an indication as to whether the pain is referred or local and whether it is mechanical or chemical
2. Burning, which may indicate an inflammatory condition or irritation of a nerve
3. Swelling, which may indicate the presence of a hernia, or a local musculo-tendinous injury
4. Pain on coughing or sneezing which may be diagnostic of a hernia, but which may also indicate a local soft tissue or tendo-periosteal irritation
5. Functional impairment—understanding what it is that the athlete finds difficult to do should provide clues to the location of the injury
6. Training methods, running surface, shoes. Injuries which have an insidious onset may develop as a result of overload, which may be contributed to by any of these factors

Examination

1. Gait. Look for abnormalities of pelvic rotation in the transverse and horizontal planes. There may be differences in stride length or duration of stance phase. Limitation of movement in all directions at the hip joint may also be evident.
2. Biomechanics (leg length, leg alignment, femoral anteversion). All these factors may influence the load under which the muscles and joints in the groin area work and may provide useful diagnostic information.
3. Local anatomy (swelling/tenderness). This should allow further localization of the condition and the structures involved.
4. Active and passive range of movement tests should allow differentiation between joint and soft tissue pathologies.
5. Abdomen, hernias, testes. The physiotherapist should be able to assess the lower abdominal area, with a view to establishing the likelihood of a hernia as the cause of pain. Any suspicions in this area should be referred to a sports physician for assessment.
6. Lumbosacral spine. This should include a full assessment of active and passive (accessory and physiological) movements. Examination of combined movements and accessory movements in the combined movement positions may be of value. Dural tension tests are an important diagnostic tool (see Ch. 33). Examination should not be confined to levels with a direct neural relationship to the groin area, as movement disorders in adjacent or removed areas may precipitate a problem in the area which has direct referral to the groin.
7. General examination. This will usually be carried out by a physician to eliminate any systemic illness.

Investigations for chronic groin pain

1. Plain X-rays—pelvis (A-P lateral and oblique) +/- tomograms of the pubic symphasis:
   a with suspected stress fractures both hips are X-rayed
   b with osteitis pubis and pubic instability, weight bearing views are indicated
   These should be of value when assessing for the possibility of lumbar spine referred pain.

2. Bone scans: particularly useful with stress fractures and osteitis pubis. Angular views are taken to avoid a bladder shadow.
3. Herniography/peritonography: an intraperitoneal injection of a positive contrast medium may reveal a hernia or posterior wall incompetence.
4. Blood pathology: FBE, ESR and rheumatological work-up may be indicated to eliminate systemic disorders.

Classification of chronic groin injuries should include the following.

Tendinitis/tendoperiostitis

Chronic overload can cause microscopic lesions of the musculotendinous unit, resulting in inflammation. These injuries occur when the collagen fibres are stressed beyond their yield point. The adductors, hamstrings and abductors (including tensor fascia lata) appear to be most susceptible to this type of injury (Medoff 1987).

Treatment will generally depend upon the severity of the injury. In mild cases it may be sufficient to reduce the activity level, ice after activity and institute a stretching program to ensure that loss of flexibility secondary to pain inhibition does not occur. In more extreme cases non-steroidal anti-inflammatory medication will generally be prescribed. Massage, particularly frictions applied transversely to the collagen fibre orientation, is useful in breaking down the adhesions which occur secondary to inflammation. There may be a need for complete rest from the predisposing sporting activity or for activity modification, to reduce the irritating load. Stretching is particularly important, both to maintain a functional range of movement and to assist in conditioning the tendon to tolerate the imposed load (see Ch. 13). In the same way, a gradual resumption of sporting activities is necessary, to allow a gradual development of loadbearing capabilities in the tendon. Progression of activity load will generally depend on the previous level of activity being pain free, both during and after the exercise session.

Sacroiliac joint strain

The reciprocal forces imposed on the sacroiliac joint result in a shearing stress which can be quite significant during athletic activity. Faulty mechanics in running will increase the shear stresses and may predispose the athlete to ligamentous strains (Simm & Scott 1986). The pain may not be severe initially, but will increase over 24 hours. The pain will be localized over the hip, buttock, low back and posterior thigh, but may also refer to the groin. There will be a loss of range of movement at the lumbosacral joint and of lumbar flexion range particularly.

Treatment involves rest, modalities to relieve pain, and gentle active and passive mobilization. Abdominal strengthening and mobilizing exercises are often beneficial.

Osteitis pubis

Osteitis pubis occurs in footballers, runners and racewalkers and is especially common in stocky people (Zimmerman 1988). The etiology is unclear and the symptoms vague. The differential diagnosis may include muscle strain, inguinal hernia, anklyosing spondylitis, rheumatoid arthritis, Reiter's syndrome, primary and metastatic tumors (Koch & Jackson 1981), and intrinsic pelvic instability related to pregnancy and childbirth. It may also be called pubic symphysis.

The condition involves an inflammatory reaction affecting the pubic symphysis initially, but possibly extends to include other structures as the condition progresses. It appears likely that the inflammatory reaction develops in response to an overuse irritation affecting the structures involved. Pain is felt in the adductor region, thigh, lower abdomen, perineal and testicular regions. Pain is usually bilateral and worse with exercise. Tenderness can be felt in the adductors, rectus abdominis and the pubic symphysis. Pain often increases with sit-ups and is variable with resisted hip flexion and adduction. There may be a reduction in hip internal rotation. X-rays may show pubic symphysis irregularity, reactive sclerosis, pubic widening, instability on weight bearing (>2 mm vertical shift) or sacroiliac joint changes. There may be increased local uptake on bone scan. Subchondral cystic lesions may develop in response to stress and may become a focal point for infection. At present the best management for osteitis pubis appears to be rest, which may vary from several weeks to several months. Where infection is suspected, it is sometimes recommended that a prolonged course (at least six months) of a broad spectrum antibiotic be undertaken (Dalziel 1992).

Occult hernia/conjoint tendon strain

Inguinal and femoral hernias (herniation of the bowel through the inguinal ring or femoral canal secondary to incompetence of the musculature of the posterior inguinal wall) are common and may cause diffuse groin pain in athletes. These hernias generally tend to occur in younger men, possibly because they still make up the bulk of the sporting population. They can be asymptomatic. Occult hernias are more difficult to understand. Occult hernias are defined as laxity or thinning of the posterior wall of the inguinal canal, with or without bulging of the posterior wall. This defect in the posterior wall has been thought to be in the vicinity of what is sometimes called the conjoint tendon.

The muscle fibres of the transversus abdominis and internal oblique arise from the inguinal ligament and insert into the pubic crest and along the pectineal line. These muscles are said to unite into a common tendinous insertion called the conjoint tendon, although there is debate on whether this tendon actually exists. It is at this point that the defect occurs, possibly due to a conjoint tendon tear posteriorly, where it inserts into the pubic crest and more laterally into the pectineal line, resulting in a weak posterior wall and subsequent bulging (Lovell 1991). It has been suggested that these may in fact be incipient direct inguinal hernias (Lovell & Malycha 1992).

Such an injury could develop as a result of repeated minor trauma or overload, or after a single traumatic incident leading to failure of the musculotendinous unit. Presenting features include a characteristic history of a vague onset of groin pain, initially relieved by rest, but recurring with and aggravated by activity. The pain will recur with exertion, despite prolonged periods of rest. It is often aggravated by coughing, sneezing, doing sit-ups, sprinting or kicking. The pain is unilateral over the lower abdomen and may extend to the upper thigh. There is often local tenderness above the pubic crest (Lovell et al 1990).

Herniography/peritonography is a valuable diagnostic tool in demonstrating these occult hernias and posterior wall incompetence (Zimmerman 1988, Smedberg et al 1985). The defect is not necessarily palpable unless the athlete has recently undertaken activities which provoke the symptoms. It may be asymptomatic at rest. There will generally be a history of failure to respond to rest, medication and physiotherapy.

Treatment of incipient hernias is by surgery. There are various operative procedures which can be carried out. They all involve reinforcement of the posterior inguinal wall. Currently, there is some work being done on repairing these defects laparoscopically, using a mesh patch to reinforce the area of defect. However, open hernia repair is probably still the treatment of choice in athletes. Clinical experience suggests that return to sporting activity, which generally progresses along symptomatic lines, will take between 6–12 weeks after surgery.

Hip joint pathology

Osteoarthritis of the hip may cause groin pain in the athlete. It is the most common painful condition of the hip joint (Saudek 1985). In the athlete it is likely that the degenerative changes affecting the joint may be secondary to damage caused by mechanical disorders, such as a limb length difference affecting stride length and contact time with the supporting surface or prolonged pronation of the foot during the stance phase of gait, which will alter the amount of external rotation occurring at the hip at this time. This will have the effect of reducing the surface area of the hip joint involved in weightbearing. Ageing alone is unlikely to be the sole causative factor. There may be an underlying cause such as previous Perthes disease, a slipped upper femoral epiphysis or dysplastic hip. Overuse may also be implicated. It has been suggested that the repetitive impact loading of cartilage is a primary source of osteoarthritis (Simm & Scott 1986). Symptoms of morning stiffness, pain on weight-bearing, an ache at the end of the day and after activity, early fatigue and night pain are suggestive of this problem. This probably relates to the synovial hyperplasia and synovitis that occur, associated with increased cartilage wear and capsular strain.

The signs and symptoms of which the athlete complains generally relate to the loss of mobility due to capsular irritation. Pain is usually aggravated by attempts to extend, abduct or internally rotate the hip joint. If the condition is long-standing, there will be wasting of the muscles working across the joint and perhaps flexion contractures. X-rays may show narrowing of the joint space, osteophyte formation or loss of the normal joint configuration.

Treatment will initially involve rest from aggravating activities. If the athlete is overweight he or she should consider a weight loss program, to reduce the load on the joint. Exercises for hip joint mobility and strengthening of the associated musculature should be instituted. These can be instituted very effectively by hydrotherapy (see Ch.16 for specific exercise programs). Local treatment modalities, such as heat, are useful in controlling secondary muscle spasm and thereby pain. Passive joint mobilization is of value in restoring the accessory joint movements. Gait re-education, proprioceptive retraining and postural correction or adaptation are perhaps the most important rehabilitative measures which should be undertaken. Operative management, in terms of joint replacement surgery, only becomes an option when the arthritis is severe and the athlete markedly disabled. Generally, the age of the athlete is also a major consideration. The major problem relates to limited prosthetic life expectancy. Whilst it is not uncommon to see prosthetic revisions being done, it is a traumatic procedure with all the inherent risks of major surgery, and is not undertaken lightly. The likelihood of progressive impairment of muscular control of hip joint movement with repeated surgery must also be considered. Return to sporting activities following prosthetic replacement surgery requires careful thought and assessment. The prosthesis would have to show good, solid fixation on X-ray examination. A functional range of movement together with effective muscle control of the hip joint and lower limb are essential. Sports which do not have a repeated high impact load should not be a problem. Lawn bowls, swimming, walking, golf, and so on can generally be resumed with complete safety. Older athletes have returned to playing more vigorous sports, such as tennis, following prosthetic replacement surgery, but each case must be assessed on its own merits in consultation with the managing orthopaedic surgeon. It may be necessary to advise and educate the athlete on the need to modify or alter their sporting involvement. Education and understanding of the nature of the problem are very important.

Acetabular labrum tears

In a hip joint with no other evident pathology, the acetabular labrum may be torn by a rotational or pivoting motion, under load. Athletes with this injury will describe a 'giving way' sensation followed by persisting soreness about the hip (Simm & Scott 1986). They will also often describe a catching pain associated with a twisting motion of the hip, particularly under load. There may be an audible click on passive internal rotation and adduction of the slightly extended hip (Simm & Scott 1986).

Treatment generally involves surgery. In the past this has involved excision of the torn labrum, but recent advances in arthroscopic surgical techniques mean that the defect can now often be repaired.

Pelvic floor myalgia

This syndrome involves tension of the muscles and fascia of the pelvic floor, causing pain. It is not often diagnosed, but is perhaps a poorly recognized component of, or sequel to chronic groin pain and the associated movement disorders. The muscles most frequently involved are the levator ani, coccygeus and piriformis, which form a muscular sling that closes the posterior part of the pelvic outlet. The levator ani and the coccygeus also form the pelvic diaphragm, which is strong enough to support the abdominal contents during running and jumping.

Repeated muscular stress to the pelvis in the athlete causing increased intra-abdominal pressure may cause pelvic floor myalgia. The condition can also develop secondary to lumbosacral, pelvic or hip joint pathology causing pelvic floor irritation (Simm & Scott 1986). Symptoms will include low back and leg pain and, occasionally, discomfort or pain on contraction of the pelvic floor muscles, i.e. painful bowel movements.

If the sacrotuberous and sacrospinous ligaments are also irritated pain will refer to the lumbosacral spine and the sacroiliac joint. Involvement of the piriformis will cause pain in the same distribution as for piriformis syndrome. There may be localized tenderness along the muscle attachments and, when the piriformis is involved, production of pain on internal and external rotation tests.

Treatment should be aimed at pain relief. Heat is a very useful modality. Mobilization of the sacrococcygeal joint can be very effective (Sinaki et al 1977). Pelvic floor relaxation and control exercises can be taught (see Ch. 34). The athlete should also be cautioned to avoid activities or postures that provoke the symptoms. An exercise program to ensure good posture of the lumbosacral spine and pelvis and to address flexibility and strength of the associated soft tissues may be of use in limiting load on the pelvic floor. The pain usually responds quickly to rest and local treatment as previously described.

Spine referral

Evidence of old osteochondritis of the vertebral bodies, a disc lesion at L1 or L2 or a crush fracture at either of these levels can cause a radicular pain that imitates groin strain (Muckle 1982). Similar patterns of referred pain may also arise after to any traumatic or degenerative condition of the posterior vertebral structures at these levels, i.e. facet joints. Such conditions may precipitate nerve root irritation, with distal referral. Lower lumbar spine pathologies may also be implicated. There may be two mechanisms of pain production operating. Firstly, the myotomes and sclerotomes for the groin region take their nerve supply from the lower lumbar and upper sacral levels. Irritation of these nerve roots may cause referral of pain to deep soft tissues in the groin region. Secondly, the postural changes which occur with lumbar spine dysfunction, particularly in the region of the lumbosacral junction, may influence the loading on the musculoskeletal system in the groin area. For example, an alteration in the amount of pelvic tilt secondary to either an increase or decrease in the lumbar lordosis would alter the dynamics of load and force transmission through the pelvis, which may increase the load on the groin structures. Whilst this may not be a true referred pain, it is still a pain which develops secondary to vertebral pathology. Further discussion of this type of pain production is included in Chapter 27.

Soft tissue injury at the hip and thigh

While injury to more proximal structures may refer pain to the hip and thigh, the incidence of direct injuries is the highest in contact sports (King & Robertson 1986). Overuse injuries are also commonly seen in sports with a high training load or with a highly repetitive nature.

Bursitis

There are at least 13 bursae in the hip region, which can become thickened, inflamed and swollen when irritated. Irritation usually develops with repetitive overload. Those most commonly irritated are the ischial, trochanteric and iliopectineal bursae.

Most commonly, the trochanteric bursa, which lies between the tendon of the gluteus maximus and the greater trochanter, will become irritated. It is likely that this irritation will develop as the iliotibial band, into which the gluteus maximus inserts, moves back and forward over the greater trochanter during flexion/extension. If there is any loss of normal flexibility, particularly as the pelvis abducts and adducts on the weightbearing leg during gait, irritation will occur. An imbalance between the abductor and adductor muscles in a runner with a broad pelvis may predispose to trochanteric bursitis (Saudek 1985). Increased supination at heel strike in the runner may result in increased loading on the iliotibial band and the gluteus maximus, predisposing to trochanteric bursitis.

The athlete will present complaining of pain over the lateral hip and thigh. Occasionally there will be radiation down to the knee. Onset is usually insidious. There will be pain on walking, which will be worse with running and with activities such as crossing the legs. There will be an area of increased temperature and tenderness on palpation. Ober's test will generally be positive.

For treatment to be effective, the cause of the irritation must be identified. Treating the symptoms will assist in resolving the pain and disability, but will not prevent a recurrence. Assessment should be made of factors such as gait pattern during running, particularly when fatigued. Posture, flexibility, wear on running shoes, training program and training surface should also be assessed. The athlete may need referral to a podiatrist for assessment regarding orthoses and appropriate footwear. Education regarding training schedules and the format of training sessions may also be appropriate. Local treatment may include ice massage, electrotherapy modalities, stretching of the gluteus maximus, tensor fascia lata and iliotibial band and strengthening of the adductors. In some cases referral for injection of local anaesthetic and corticosteroids is appropriate, to accelerate resolution of the symptoms and allow for earlier rehabilitation.

Ischial bursitis is not seen as often as a consequence of athletic activity. The ischial bursa lies between the tuberosity of the ischium and the gluteus maximus.

Tenderness is localized over the ischial tuberosity and is easily palpated with the hip on the affected side flexed and abducted into a frog-leg position while in prone. Pain radiates into the hamstrings and is aggravated by walking, running and stair climbing. It will also be painful to sit.

Treatment should be directed at resolution of the inflammatory irritation, as for trochanteric bursitis.

Particular attention should be paid to stretching and strengthening the adductors and the hamstrings. Return to training should be graduated and may need to be modified to prevent a recurrence. The iliopectineal bursa lies deep to the tendon of iliopsoas over the anterior aspect of the hip joint. It may become irritated with excessive loading of a tight iliopsoas. Pain will be provoked by resisted contraction of the iliopsoas or by stretching it. There will be tenderness on palpation over the anterior aspect of the hip, in the inguinal area. Referred pain into the anterior thigh and knee sometimes occurs and may result from inflammation causing irritation of the femoral nerve (Saudek 1985). Treatment will follow along the lines previously discussed and should include stretching of the iliopsoas.

Quadriceps strain

The quadriceps group of muscles will usually be at risk of strain while forcefully contracting and meeting a sudden unexpected resistance. The rectus femoris and sartorius are particularly at risk, because of their two joint function. These injuries are commonly seen as a result of kicking in all codes of football. Quadriceps strain may also occur during sudden acceleration. If the muscle is forcefully contracted while the hip is extended and the knee flexed, the rectus femoris will be at risk of strain.

There will be immediate pain, localized to the area of injury, and the athlete will generally describe a sensation of something having torn. In the case of a severe tear, there may be a palpable defect in the rectus immediately after injury. Later the defect will be obscured by swelling and the developing haematoma. Knee flexion and hip extension will be limited by pain and protective muscle spasm. There may be reflex inhibition of quadriceps contraction as a whole.

When the injury has healed there may still be a palpable defect in the rectus. This does not appear to cause any functional problems.

In the acute stage, treatment is the same as for all soft tissue injuries. Rest, ice, compression and elevation are used. If the pain is severe it may be appropriate to use crutches for weight relief. When the acute injury response has settled, the athlete should begin a gentle range of movement work. Local electrotherapy modalities can be used to facilitate healing. Ice can be used effectively to limit muscle spasm both during and after stretching. When pain allows, active quadriceps contraction can be started, usually using isometric contractions. If quadriceps function continues to be inhibited, electrical muscle stimulation can be used.

As muscle function improves through the range, knee flexion/extension exercise can be commenced. Resistance is added and increased depending on the stage of healing and the athlete's level of comfort. Appropriate resistance modalities include riding an exercise bike, using elastic resistance, hydrotherapy, isokinetics and free weights. Functional rehabilitation should be addressed. This encompasses such activities as hill running, graduated sprint programs, swimming with flippers on to increase the water resistance, hopping, bounding, stair running, etc. A progressive return to full training and sport follows, when a full range of pain free motion, with a demonstrable achievement of normal strength (usually assessed isokinetically), is achieved. Assessment of normative values will generally be made by comparison with the uninjured side, unless preinjury data is available.

Correction of the predisposing causes, in other than cases of collision with an external object, will involve assessment and treatment of hamstring flexibility, hip flexion range, gluteus maximus function and perhaps iliopsoas tightness. Factors such as fatigue, weather conditions, the efficiency of the athlete's warm-up and other potentially predisposing factors may also have to be considered. Assessment of running style and of training practices may also be appropriate.

Hamstring strain

Injuries to the hamstrings, particularly at the musculotendinous junctions, are the most common soft tissue injuries in the thigh (Fox 1986, King & Robertson 1986). Sudden, forced change in the musculotendinous length may result in strain or rupture at the junction. In particular, in sprinting, with forceful flexion of the hip and extension of the knee during the swing phase, the hamstrings are placed under extremely high loads in an elongated position. The hamstring group is also placed under considerable load with change of pace, and is prone to injury at this time. This injury appears to have a higher frequency in the older age group and the incidence is also higher in the absence of an adequate warm-up (Fox 1986). Tearing will result in pain, spasm, swelling and inhibition of movement.

With a first degree strain there may be tenderness on palpation, but minimal swelling and no palpable defect. In a second degree strain, there will be partial disruption of the musculotendinous junction. Echymosis develops, leading to increased muscle spasm. In a third degree strain there is marked pain, gross swelling and echymosis, muscle spasm and a palpable defect if examination is carried out early. While there may be almost complete disruption of one of the components of the hamstring group, this is not an injury which is generally amenable to surgical repair. The value of such a procedure is questionable, given that similar situations are produced artificially when anterior cruciate ligament reconstructions are performed using hamstring tendon grafts. Athletes who have undergone this surgery usally make a complete functional recovery, with no apparent problems in their altered hamstring mechanics, if they undergo a comprehensive rehabilitation program.

Treatment is determined by the symptoms. The general principles of management of soft tissue injury, with use of rest, ice, compression and elevation apply. The use of crutches may be indicated for pain relief. Rehabilitation should initially be aimed at maintaining or regaining normal flexibility. Slump stretching techniques may also be of value in accelerating the recovery of Grade 1 hamstring lesions

(Kornberg & Lew 1989). Prevention of secondary muscle shortening should reduce the recovery time, as rehabilitation is not complicated or prolonged by further impairment of hamstring function. Early stretching may also be of benefit in scar tissue formation, as collagen fibres tend to lay down along lines of stress and hence the tensile strength of the developing scar may be increased (see Ch. 3). Strength training begins when pain allows and as the stage of healing dictates. When implementing a strength training program every effort should be made to ensure that the athlete is strengthening through the full functional range of movement and that the strength program is developed along lines which reflect the expected loads and work patterns of the injured athlete. Electrotherapy modalities are useful in facilitating removal of swelling and bruising. Rehabilitation should be aimed at restoring all the component functions required of the hamstring group in the athlete's sport. Care should be taken not to accelerate this process as this may compromise recovery. The demands placed on the injured muscle as the athlete increases the rehabilitation training load should reflect the expected healing times for soft tissue injury and demonstrate an understanding of the capacity of the tissues both to bear load and function in a co-ordinated way while healing. For example, it would generally be expected that a minor, or Grade 1, strain of the hamstring group would require approximately 10 days for the symptoms to subside, but the muscle group may be potentially weaker for up to three weeks. Attention to and evaluation of the athlete's symptoms during rehabilitative exercise should prevent problems. Details regarding expected or normal healing times and the physiology of tissue healing can be found in Chapter 2.

Recurrent hamstring lesions

Apart from a local weakness of the connective tissues which constitute the hamstring muscle group, recurrent hamstring injuries may also develop after a number of removed causes.

Referral of pain from the lumbar spine. Lumbosacral pathologies such as disc bulges at the L4/5 or L5/S1 levels particularly, facet joint arthropathies or spondylosis, may be the source of pain felt in the hamstring group. Irritation of the spinal nerves exiting through the neural foraminae at the affected levels may provoke pain in the distal segmental distribution of that nerve. True hamstring pain may be felt if the affected nerve roots are involved in the motor or sensory supply to the muscle group. Irritation of these nerve roots may provoke local muscular responses such as spasm or a more prolonged, generalized increase in muscle tension.

Meniscal problems at the knee. The hamstrings act as a dynamic stabilizer of the knee. Consequently, incomplete knee excursion due to meniscal tears, degeneration or excision can lead to excessive loading of the hamstrings, especially the biceps femoris, which acts as a dynamic lateral stabilizer, limiting medial rotation of the tibia on the femur and working over the joint compartment most affected by this type of injury. Minor degrees of rotatory instability can also be implicated. Restoration of full knee movement is required.

Adhesion of the lateral popliteal nerve. Following a tear of the lower belly of the biceps femoris, fibrosis and adhesions may develop, trapping the lateral popliteal nerve, causing recurrent painful episodes on stress, i.e. sprinting and hurdling. This should be treated by freeing adhesions.

Abnormal quadriceps power. Unbalanced quadriceps action due to excessive muscle hypertrophy may produce an abnormal force in the hamstrings, particularly when there is a loss of co-ordination due to fatigue. This is potentially a problem in athletes who mix cycling with running, i.e. triathletes. The excessive quadriceps development seen in cyclists may have implications for hamstring injury, if that athlete attempts endurance running events without doing extra work to ensure a good muscle balance.

Dural adhesions. In the area of the lumbosacral nerve roots dural adhesions may also cause pain in the hamstring region. Pain will generally begin with activity and may become severe enough to limit the athlete's ability to continue. Pain may increase suddenly or develop slowly. It will often settle within a day or so of irritation, which should give fairly strong clues aof the precipitating cause. Continued irritation appears to lead to secondary tightness and localized muscular soreness, which may precipitate a true muscle strain. Clinical evidence indicates that loss of mobility or increased sensitivity of the neural tissue and its investments, which traverse from the spine to the lower limbs, may predispose to hamstring lesions (Williamson 1987). Slump stretching is a highly positive indicator of this problem and is covered in detail in Chapter 33.

Disparate growth rates. Another possible cause of the tight calf/tight hamstring presentation may relate to the disparate growth rates of the skeletal and soft tissue structures during puberty. Often, the skeletal growth rate significantly exceeds that of the soft tissues, placing them under considerable tension. They are maintained in a permanently loaded and stretched position, and become tight, fatigued and weak.

Postural variations. If the athlete stands with an increased lumbar lordosis, there will be a concurrent increase in anterior pelvic tilt in the frontal plane. This has the effect of moving the ischial tuberosities further away from the distal attachments of the hamstring group and will generally result in an increase in the resting muscle tension. The muscle will not only be functionally tighter, but it will perhaps be more inclined to fatigue early.

Assessment of this problem must determine whether the postural variation is structural or functional. Functional postural abnormalities require the correction of muscle imbalances, using stretching and strengthening strategies. Structural problems may not fall within the scope of physiotherapy for correction, but should be amenable to adaptive procedures such as technique modification, e.g. an altered stride pattern, which should be undertaken in consultation with a coach, or secondary postural adaptation e.g. orthotics, which would require assessment by a sports podiatrist.

Trigger points. Trigger points generally relate to local areas of specific soft tissue tightness and irritation. They may overlie an irritated nerve or a dysfunctioning joint, or may simply reflect a localized area of overuse secondary to abnormal mechanics or motor nerve irritation. Around the pelvis, hip and thigh, trigger points are commonly found in the soft tissues overlying the sciatic nerve and freeing them with soft tissue mobilization techniques and alternative modalities such as acupuncture has been shown to useful in reducing hamstring pain (Selvaratnum 1992).

Poor running style may also be implicated in the recurrence of hamstring lesions. As previously discussed, the hamstring muscle group work at significantly high speeds with a large eccentric component in running sports. A running style which is poorly co-ordinated or places too large a work requirement on the hamstrings may provoke early fatigue and hence an injury.

The separate nerve supplies of the two heads of the biceps femoris has been suggested as a possible factor in the development of hamstring injury, related to poor timing of muscular contraction. Mistimed contraction of the different parts of the muscle group may mean a reduced capacity to generate effective tension to control the imposed loads on the muscle.

Iliotibial band friction syndromes

Considering the anatomy of the fascia, it would appear that mechanical dysfunction of the pelvis and sacrum could play a role in provoking tightness of the iliotibial band. This may result in a friction type of irritation affecting the iliotibial band as it passes over the bony prominences of the greater trochanter and the lateral femoral condyle. Specifically, this may result from an increased lateral tilt of the pelvis during gait, as a result of a leg length difference, secondary to problems with the mechanics of the foot during gait provoking an increase in lower limb rotation, or as a result of muscle weakness.

Treatment will generally follow the same lines as for tendinitis. Attention must also be paid to assessment and management of any predisposing biomechanical faults to ensure that the problem does not recur.

Piriformis syndrome

The piriformis can be implicated in irritation of the sciatic nerve as it passes through or underneath the muscle. The sciatic nerve passes through the piriformis in about 15% of the population (Calliet 1968). The syndrome occurs more frequently in women then men (Calliet 1968).

Clinical presentation will include complaints of deep localized buttock pain, in the area of the sciatic notch. There may also be pain, tingling or numbness radiating down the leg in a sciatic type of distribution. Assessment must exclude the lumbar spine and sacroiliac joints as possible causes of the pain. Both active, resisted internal rotation and a passive stretch into external rotation will provoke pain, particularly when performed at 90° of hip flexion.

Treatment includes rest, non-steroidal anti-inflammatories, and electrotherapy modalities to aid in resolving the inflammatory irritation. Stretching of the piriformis should be commenced and progressed as pain allows. If the sciatic nerve has become tethered, slump stretching or other neural tensioning techniques may also be appropriate. Massage may also be of value in reducing spasm and in freeing any adhesions which may have developed. Personal experience indicates that, although it may be painful and needs to be done with care, deep frictional massage and myofascial release techniques done at right angles to the muscle fibre orientation can be useful. The athlete should be allowed to return to sport as the symptoms resolve, ensuring that adequate flexibility of the piriformis is maintained.

In some cases, surgical release of the piriformis muscle and any associated adhesions around the sciatic nerve as it passes through the sciatic notch may be undertaken. Postoperatively the athlete will generally be allowed to increase activity and resume training or competition as healing and comfort allow, over a six to eight week period.

DEVELOPMENTAL DISORDERS

Perthes' disease

This condition presents more commonly in boys than girls and is usually evident between the ages of three and twelve. The disease is characterized by avascular necrosis of the femoral head, resulting in a flattened femoral head (Saudek 1985). The child may initially present complaining of knee pain on activity, which progresses to hip and groin pain, with limitation of hip movement, particularly abduction and internal rotation. Onset is usually insidious. The child eventually walks with a protective limp, trying to shorten the weightbearing time on the affected limb. The pain is due to the aseptic avascular necrosis of the femoral head that occurs with the condition, and its associated inflammatory changes. X-ray examination should confirm the diagnosis. Treatment should be aimed at protecting the femoral head through the use of weight-relieving splints and reduction of activity to minimize the load on the femoral head and prevent degeneration or deformity, while it revascularizes and heals. This may require up to a year away from sport.

Physiotherapy will generally be directed toward maintaining the range of movement and strength at the affected hip. However, attention should also be paid to maintaining or improving the strength, flexibility and endurance of the rest of the musculoskeletal system. Exercises in water may be of real value. The physiotherapist should also be able to provide some insight into alternative or adapted physical activities to allow the child some physical stimulation and enjoyment, e.g. swimming, stationary cycling, rowing or paddling.

Slipped capital femoral epiphysis

The exact etiology of this condition is unknown, but the epiphyseal plate of the head of the femur appears especially susceptible to slip before it fuses. It usually becomes evident in the teenage years. Again, it is more common in boys than girls. The slip usually occurs slowly and results in a varus deformity of the lower limb. It can result from direct trauma but sometimes comes on suddenly with no history of injury (Saudek 1985). It is also bilateral in 15–20% of cases, indicating that trauma is not the only cause (Catterall 1972). If the slip is severe enough, the blood supply to the head of the femur may be disrupted and avascular necrosis results. The child usually complains of hip and groin pain, with referral to the knee as the condition develops, which may be mistaken for pain secondary to overuse if there is no history of trauma. Care must be taken with diagnosis. As the slip progresses, the child will develop a Trendelenburg gait. The leg will become externally rotated and abduction and internal rotation will be limited. The diagnosis can only be confirmed on X-ray. Treatment is aimed at preventing further slip by non-weightbearing with or without internal fixation. Non-weightbearing must continue until the epiphysis has healed. Rehabilitation is important for regaining the full range of joint movement, muscle strength and flexibility before returning to sport. It generally follows the same principles of management and progression as for a fracture.

MANAGEMENT OF INJURIES

Because of the variety and complexity of injuries that may occur in this region, it is impossible to give a detailed outline of all physiotherapy treatment strategies within the confines of this text. However, there are some which warrant further discussion.

Treatment of muscle imbalances

There are different approaches to the management of muscle imbalances. Generally, all have merit and using different aspects of each one in a combined approach can be very effective. However, there is every likelihood that treatment will be of no benefit if the athlete does not understand what the physiotherapist is trying to do. Correction of muscle imbalances requires exercises to improve posture, strength and flexibility away from the clinical setting. Education of the athlete has to be an integral part of treatment to correct muscle imbalances.

As a general rule, muscle tightness should be addressed before strengthening (Janda 1983). It is impossible to effectively strengthen a muscle if it does not have an adequate working range. Equally, strength should not be seen as the only aspect of muscle performance requiring rehabilitation. The ability to sustain muscular effort and to continue to produce co-ordinated action involving more than one muscle group must also be addressed.

Guidelines for improving flexibility will be discussed later in this chapter, as will aspects of strength training. What must be considered here is the need to appreciate the balance required in the parameters of musculoskeletal performance (strength, flexibility, endurance, co-ordination, proprioception) for the effective execution of a sports-specific skill.

Correction of dynamic pelvic postural imbalances

Practical experience in the clinical setting has shown that addressing aspects of pelvic postural control, in performing gait-related sporting activities, may be very useful in treating overuse, inflammatory problems in athletes. The pelvis should provide a mobile but stable base on which the lower limbs work, as has been previously stated. Commonly, the author sees athletes with seemingly intractable inflammatory conditions affecting the pelvis and hip (osteitis pubis, adductor origin tendinitis etc.), which have not been helped by standard therapeutic interventions. Very often, retraining pelvic postural dynamic stability has led to a significant reduction in or resolution of symptoms. The following is an example of such a program.

Warm-up

1. Pedalling on an exercise bike or jogging lightly on a rebounder or mini trampoline until the athlete is sweating lightly.

Stretches

1. Active hamstring stretches, pulling the knee to the chest, holding it there and extending the lower leg as far as possible back over the head (Fig. 28.8).
2. Abdominal stretches, using a half push-up type action.
3. Standing hip flexor stretches, taking care to keep the trunk upright (Fig. 28.9).

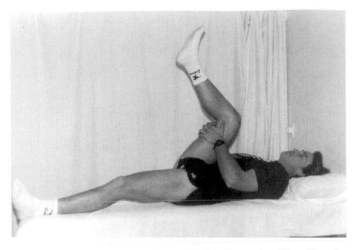

Fig. 28.8 Active hamstring stretches. Patient lies supine. The affected leg is flexed, so that the knee approximates the chest. The patient stabilizes the thigh by hanging on behind the knee, preventing it moving away from the chest. The knee is then actively extended, until hamstring tension limits the range

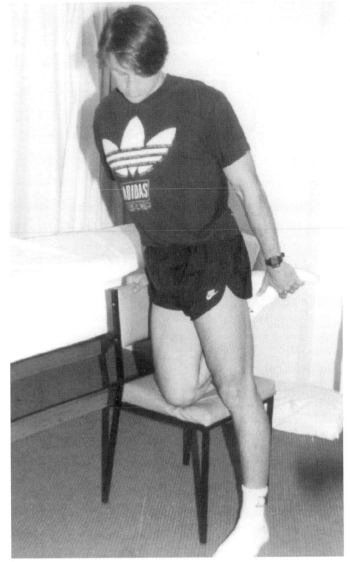

Fig. 28.10 Iliotibial band stretch in knee standing. Patient stands on the unaffected leg with the knee of the affected leg resting on a chair. The body is kept as upright as possible and facing the front. The foot of the affected leg is pulled up behind the opposite buttock and internally rotated. The femur should not be allowed to rotate internally. The pelvis should then be shunted toward the affected side. The stretch is felt in the lower part of the iliotibial band

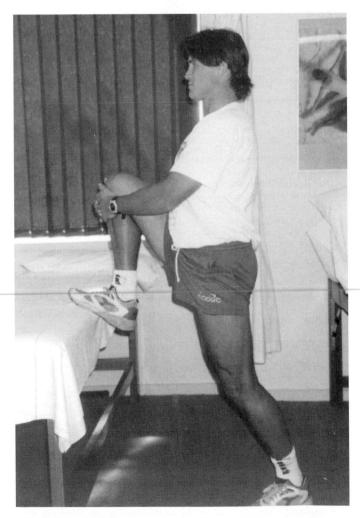

Fig. 28.9 Standing hip flexor stretches. The patient stands on the affected leg. The foot of the unaffected leg is placed flat on a high bench. The body is kept upright. The affected leg is kept as straight as possible with the foot flat. The hips are pushed anteriorly

4. Iliotibial band stretches in kneel-standing, taking care to ensure hip extension and adduction together with knee flexion. At the same time, the lumbar lordosis must be maintained in a neutral posture (Fig. 28.10).
5. Hip adductor stretches. These are generally done in an upright posture as the pelvic posture can be better controlled. The pelvis should be maintained in a neutral posture in terms of anterior/posterior tilt.
6. Hip extensor stretch (Fig. 28.11).
7. Quadriceps stretches.

These first seven stretches are directed at muscles acting around the pelvis and hip, which may have an influence on

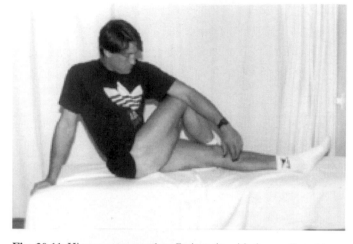

Fig. 28.11 Hip extensor stretches. Patient sits with the unaffected leg straight out in front. The affected leg is bent at both hip and knee, and the foot placed against the outside of the knee on the unaffected leg. The trunk is rotated toward the affected side. The arm on the unaffected side is then placed across the outside of the knee on the affected side. That arm is then used to push the knee across the body further into an adducted position

the posture of the pelvis. They are generally done as passive or sustained stretches as the aim is to increase the resting length of the muscle and thereby alter its pull on the pelvis. The following six stretches, while having an effect on muscle flexibility, are directed more toward joint mobility.

1. Hip joint: flexion, external rotation (Fig. 28.12).
2. Hip joint: extension, internal rotation and abduction (Fig. 28.13).
3. Hip joint: flexion, internal rotation and adduction (Fig. 28.14).
4. Lumbar spine: flexion.
5. Lumbar spine: lateral flexion.
6. Lumbar spine: rotation.

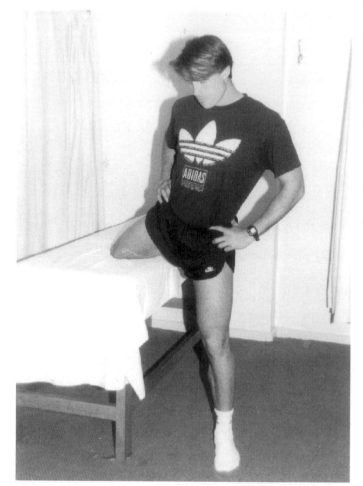

Fig. 28.13 Hip joint extension/internal rotation/abduction. Patient stands on unaffected leg. Trunk is kept upright. Affected leg is placed with the shin resting along a bench. The knee should be behind the hip so the hip is extended. The hand is placed behind the affected hip and a forward pressure applied to increase hip extension. The upper body is rotated toward the unaffected side

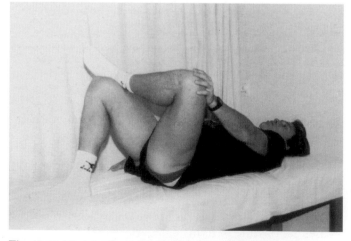

Fig. 28.12 Hip joint flexion/external rotation. Patient lies supine. Unaffected leg is flexed at the hip and knee so that the foot rests flat on the table. The affected leg is positioned so that the outside of the ankle rests on the thigh of the unaffected leg just above the knee. The patient pushes on the medial aspect of the affected knee increasing the external rotation stretch

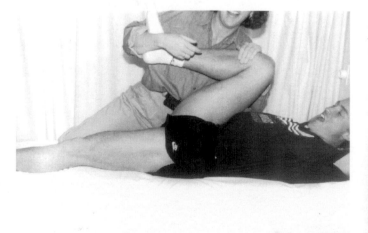

Fig. 28.14 Hip joint flexion/internal rotation/adduction. Patient lies supine. Therapist moves affected leg into full range available flexion. Maintaining flexion, the limb is then moved into adduction. When the limit of range is reached, the foot is then moved outward to rotate the hip internally. The patient is stretched in this position

Lumbar spine extension will already have been addressed when performing abdominal stretches. The joint movement patterns addressed here appear to be those commonly associated with pelvic postural dysfunctions.

Slump stretching should also be addressed, as tightness of the dura centrally may predispose to a postural problem, which musculoskeletal stretching alone will not resolve. Generally, an adapted slump stretch which the athlete can do alone is quite suitable.

Strengthening

Strengthening must address the functional requirements of the athlete. The following is one way in which this can be addressed.

1. Standing on a balance board: single leg/two legs. The emphasis should be on maintaining the pelvis in a

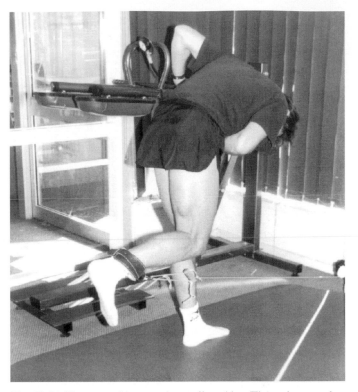

Fig. 28.16 Piston type hip extension—affected leg. The patient stands facing wall pulleys, with the rope attached at the ankle. The patient stands in a forward leaning position. The exercise starts with the affected leg in both hip and knee flexion. The patient kicks the affected leg out backward moving into both hip and knee extension against the resistance of the pulley weights

neutral posture in terms of anterior/posterior tilt. The athlete should perform upper limb activities, e.g. throwing and catching a ball, at the same time to increase the difficulty of the exercise. This should stimulate higher level proprioceptive/postural retraining.

2. Standing on the affected side and using wall pulleys (Fig. 28.15). Straight leg lifts forward, backward and side to side with the resistance attached to the unaffected leg can be done. The athlete should be encouraged to maintain pelvic stability, eliminate lumbar spine movement and isolate the action to the hip joint.

3. Piston type hip extension, again using the wall pulleys (Fig. 28.16), but this time attached to the affected leg. Again the emphasis is on maintaining pelvic postural stability and isolating the movement to the hip joint.

4. Double leg hip extension.

5. Bridging, holding a medicine ball between the knees to increase activity of the adductor muscles in the exercise. The athlete should be taught to rotate the pelvis posteriorly prior to lifting the pelvis off the supporting surface and to try and maintain it in that posture throughout the exercise.

6. Abdominal curl-ups. These are modified sit-ups, which maintain the pelvis in a neutral or posteriorly rotated posture while the exercise is being performed.

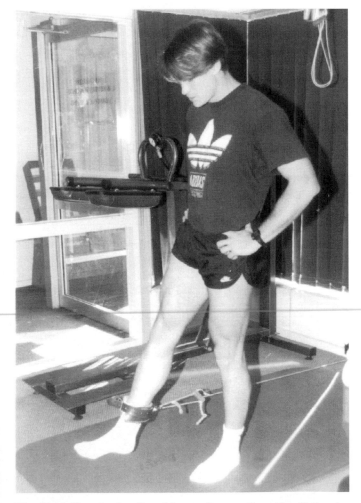

Fig. 28.15 Use of wall pulley while standing on affected leg. Patient is standing on the affected leg. Resistance is attached to the unaffected leg and aims to maintain a stable posture of the pelvis and trunk, over the affected leg, while moving the unaffected leg against resistance. The patient can be positioned so that movement of the unaffected leg can occur in any desired direction, altering the load on the working muscles of the affected leg

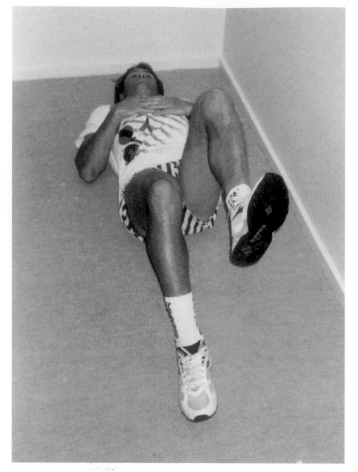

Fig. 28.17 Abdominal stabilization exercise. Patient lies on back. Hand is placed under small of back. Patient pelvic tilts to flatten lumbar spine against hand. This pressure of the back against the hand must be maintained at all times. Hips and knees are flexed at 90°. Keeping knees at 90° heels are lowered to the floor and raised, alternately, until patient is no longer able to maintain lumbar posture

7. Abdominal stabilization program (Fig. 28.17). These exercises encourage the maintenance of a stable lumbar spine and pelvis as the lower limbs move. They are concerned with the functional utilization and application of isolated muscle strength. In particular, these exercises utilize abdominal hollowing and bracing as techniques for achieving co-contraction of the spinal and pelvic support musculature. It is suggested that this co-contraction may prove useful clinically in providing safe and effective support during resistance exercises involving the lower limbs (Richardson et al 1992).

8. Jumping or hopping performed initially on the rebounder but progressing to harder, less compliant surfaces. The emphasis should be on power and getting drive out of the leg, but at the same time maintaining pelvic postural stability.

With all of the strengthening exercises there is generally need for heavy loads or high resistance. Most often, the

emphasis with these exercises will be on improving the functional utilization of muscle strength and, as such, lower loads which are less likely to reduce finer muscle co-ordination are appropriate. Endurance also needs to be addressed as the athlete needs to be able to maintain pelvic postural control even when tired. Lower loads and higher repetitions, perhaps even to fatigue, will address the requirements of speed-endurance training.

Functional exercises

In the pool, the athlete can perform running drills and strengthening exercises. Running drills should be directed to a piston type action at the hip joint, as previously described. As with land based strengthening exercises, the emphasis should be on maintaining pelvic postural stability while the exercise is being performed.

When running drills are commenced, the athlete may initially need to run with an exaggerated motion. This would involve maintaining pelvic postural stability. There may be a need to shorten the stride length and to widen the base of support. As the athlete's proprioceptive awareness improves the running drills can move toward a more normal, functional pattern of movement.

Muscle energy techniques

Muscle energy techniques are particularly useful when treating dysfunction affecting the pelvis, hip or thigh. There is a presumption of a normal range of movement and planes of movement between the three bones of the pelvic girdle. The application of these techniques requires assessment of abnormalities in these patterns. The sacrum and the sacroiliac joints are seen as being the centre around which the pelvis functions. There are two or three horizontal axes around which the sacrum flexes or extends and two diagonal axes around which it rotates (Fig. 28.18) (Stanton 1989). Assessment is directed at evaluating increases in range of movement and 'blocking' around these axes. The therapist

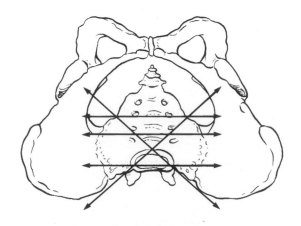

Fig. 28.18 Proposed sacral axis of movement

needs to look at and assess abnormal positions and movements in all planes. Range of movement is assessed in standing, with the standing flexion test being most important as this will generally clearly demonstrate asymmetry of movement.

Assessment in supine lying addresses alignment, functional leg length differences (measured by the medial malleolus position), sacroiliac joint rotation in all planes, differences in pubic symphysis height (viewed from above), and deviations of the anterior superior iliac spines from the midline or vertically.

In prone, the relative levels of the posterior superior iliac spines (PSIS) can be assessed. The sacrotuberous ligament can be palpated and tension differences evaluated from side to side. The sacral sulcus can be palpated by moving medially off the PSIS onto the top of the sacrum and comparing the depth side to side. Most often, pain will occur on the contralateral side if there is a movement block, because there will be a compensatory increased load on that side (Stanton 1989). Abnormal anterior and posterior rotation of either hemipelvis can have an effect on leg length, i.e. anterior rotation of the hemipelvis will increase the downward inclination of the acetabulum, resulting in a functional increase in leg length. Muscle energy techniques use both muscle tensing and relaxation as a means of correcting joint dysfunction which may arise subsequent to a muscle imbalance. The specificity of the contraction appears to be important and it is generally thought that releases, or tensioning techniques, tend to work better than stretches (Stanton 1989).

An example of the use of muscle energy techniques to correct a postural problem can be seen in the correction of a posterior rotation of one hemipelvis. The athlete can be positioned prone with the affected leg hanging over the side of the bed. Starting from a flexed position, the hip is extended until the ASIS starts to rotate forward. A gentle isometric contraction into flexion is performed and held for six seconds. The movement is then progressed until the ASIS starts to rotate again. The procedure is generally repeated three times and the posture then reassessed. Subjectively, the most release appears to follow the second contraction (Stanton 1989).

Retraining eccentric muscle function

When developing rehabilitative exercise programs, it is essential that those programs reflect the specific nature of the muscle or muscle/joint function for the activity to be undertaken. An analysis or understanding of the biomechanics of the pelvis, hip, and thigh in the performance of sporting skills relevant to the injured athlete should provide indicators for the types of muscle function which require retraining. Information on the ranges and direction of movement in which this muscle function is most critical can also be derived.

In respect of two-joint muscles acting across the hip and knee joints, this means that an eccentric retraining program is essential. Their function in a variety of weightbearing, sporting activities often encompasses an eccentric phase, which has been shown by both anecdotal and clinical evidence to be an 'at risk' time. Examples of eccentric retraining exercises would include drop squats for the rectus femoris (Fig. 28.19) and rapid eccentric hamstrings contraction exercises (Stanton & Purdham 1989). Muscle activation is a learned process and concentric or isometric strength programs do not necessarily ensure improvement in eccentric function. However, as eccentric exercise is generally considered to be the most stressful work undertaken by a muscle, it would be logical to ensure that a muscle has regained adequate isometric and concentric strength characteristics before the athlete commences a graded eccentric program. A more complete understanding of these aspects of muscle function can be derived from Chapters 1 and 10.

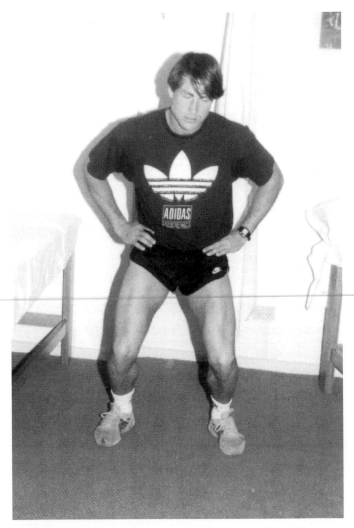

Fig. 28.19 Drop squats. Patient stands with feet shoulder width apart and hands on hips. The patient drops into a half squat position quickly, then brakes the movement, again quickly, using quads. The return to the upright position is slower and more controlled

Stretching

Fundamentally, stretching is aimed at increasing flexibility in order to improve performance. Flexibility may be defined as the possible range of movement at a joint or group of joints. Flexibility is therefore joint or movement-specific. The implementation of a stretching program as part of a rehabilitative progress must take into account this specificity. Consideration must also be given to the neurophysiological basis for stretching.

All postural alignment patterns, all muscle use and development, all human body movement is directed and co-ordinated by the activity of our nervous system. In other words, all movements are based in a neuromuscular control paradigm, therefore stretching is neurally based. In muscle, there are two main types of neuroreceptors which are sensitive to stretch. These are the muscle spindles, which consist of small modified muscle fibres and the Golgi tendon organs. The tendon organs are in series with the extrafusal muscle fibres. The muscle spindles are in parallel with them. Examination of their function shows that basically the tendon organs are responsive to changes in tension and the muscle spindles to changes in length and the rate of such change. Conceptually, therefore, the control of flexibility can be learned and can be changed.

The most common factor limiting flexibility at a joint is the inability of a muscle to stretch to its maximum required length during movement. Possibly the most common cause of injury related to muscle flexibility is the inability of the muscle to control movement adequately through its available range of movement. Stretching therefore should not be concerned only with increasing range of movement, but also with improving muscle co-ordination and control. While controlled stretching techniques e.g. passive, static and PNF, will facilitate the restoration of a limited range of movement to its normal parameters, they may be of no value in retraining the muscle to control the newly available range. Static stretching is performed slowly and carefully and hence does not provoke the stretch reflex. PNF stretching is designed to take optimum advantage of the stretch reflex, the basic premise being that the muscle will maximally relax after a maximal contraction, allowing the muscle to be moved slightly further into range. Ballistic stretching is active stretching, performed at speed and often associated with bouncing movements at the end of range. Passive stretching, which may be used in all the above modes of stretching, implies the absence of participant effort.

All these methods have been shown to cause an increase in flexibility. These changes can be categorized as plastic, permanent changes in muscle length or elastic, shorter term changes. Plastic changes are probably best achieved by sustained holding at the end of range. They may require overpressure from an external agent and probably influence the connective tissue or non-contractile elements of the muscle. Elastic changes perhaps occur as a result of a decrease in muscle tension rather than an increase in muscle length.

From a functional viewpoint, conscious changes in movement patterns, including range of movement, means learning reflected in the ability to make refined discriminations between movements. Stretching-induced increased flexibility is a new movement potential requiring functional practice to allow neuromuscular adaptation or habituation which may be interpreted as learning. It is essential that the newly aquired range of movement becomes functional. The process of creating and learning new movement patterns is necessarily very dynamic. It is only optimally accomplished by methods which integrate and challenge all the functional neuromuscular capacities and therefore utilize all the stretching modalities outlined. In particular, it is essential that ballistic stretching is included as a preferred method of flexibility work, as it represents a functional base for the performance of many movement skills. The term 'ballistic stretching' must, however, be conceptually changed to incorporate the notion of control. It appears logical to suggest controlled practice of available movement potential.

The following is perhaps a useable sequence of stretching procedures to achieve optimal responses in the neuromuscular mechanisms acting at the hip joint. Initially, static or PNF stretching would be performed to produce plastic change in resting muscle length. Strengthening and co-ordination activities would then be incorporated to optimize integration of the new range of movement into useable movement patterns. Ballistic stretching would then be used in order to practise neuromuscular co-ordination at the end of the new range of movement.

When stretching muscles acting across the pelvis, hip or thigh, it is particularly important to ensure that the proximal attachments are adequately stabiluzed. Failure to do so may mean that while a muscle is apparently lengthening over one joint, it may be shortening over another. This is also important when considering ballistic stretching, which should only be undertaken with an emphasis on movement control and learning new, improved patterns of movement.

Isokinetic strength testing

Isokinetic strength testing is widely used as an indicator of recovery following musculotendinous or joint injury. Comparison of results achieved with the uninvolved limb or with the normal population is used as an indicator of having regained normal strength and loadbearing capabilities. It is a useful diagnostic and rehabilitative tool, but is often poorly used. There has been a tendency to equate a favorable isokinetic assessment of muscle function with a capacity for that muscle to undertake a preinjury level of athletic performance. However, this fails to recognize the area of skill acquisition in the performance of sporting activities. The muscle which has been shown on isokinetic evaluation to have regained normal strength will still require a graduated skills retraining program prior to attempting a complete return to sport. Isokinetic evaluation indicating successful recovery of muscle and joint function is best used as an indicator of preparedness to begin a more advanced rehabilitation program or training, which addresses these components of strength, power, endurance and skill as they relate to the particular athlete's sport. Only when the athlete is able to undertake a full training and competition load, with no aggravation of the injury, should full recovery be presumed (see Ch. 17).

Hydrotherapy

Exercise carried out in water has merit, because the load of ground reaction forces on impact is eliminated. However, care should be taken in designing the exercise program. Consideration must be given to the increased load when exercises are performed against the resistance of the water. The appropriate prescription and implementation of hydrotherapy programs for athletic injuries, including those affecting the pelvis, hip and thigh, is covered in Chapter 16.

Strapping

Strapping probably has little therapeutic value around the hip joint except in terms of increasing the athlete's confidence. Because of the multi-axial nature of hip joint movement it is probably not possible to limit joint movement significantly with taping. The compressive element of circumferential taping, as is sometimes used for groin injuries, may limit a muscle's ability to contract, thereby reducing the risk of injury. Strapping to provide biofeedback regarding lumbosacral posture and pelvic postural stability is useful in educating better control of pelvic movement.

Neoprene wetsuits

The use of neoprene wetsuits has gained some popularity in recent times for the management of chronic muscular and musculotendinous strains. The rationale behind this is that the muscle tolerates the load to which it is subjected much better if it is warmer. The wetsuit maintains the soft tissues underneath at a higher temperature by preventing the loss of normal body heat. This appears to have some value in allowing athletes to continue participating in sport if they have only minor musculotendinous injuries. However, care should be taken to monitor the athlete to ensure that the injury is not inadvertently being aggravated. Treatment to assist in the resolution of the injury should also continue.

Protective pads

Protective pads are of value, particularly for the athlete involved in contact sports, in allowing an earlier and safe return to sport following injury, particularly contusions.

Mobilization of accessory movements of the hip joint

The use of a seat belt to assist in the mobilization of the accessory movements of the hip joint, particularly distraction, can be of real value in treating problems where there is an element of capsular tightness or joint impingement (Fig. 28.20). Care must be taken to ensure that the adductor region is well padded with a towel, as the area can be sensitive to pressure from the seat belt.

Massage

Massage is a therapeutic modality which can often be overlooked. It is extremely useful in treating the secondary problems of soft tissue tightness which may develop with overuse or chronic, recurring injuries affecting the groin and thigh particularly. Referral to a therapeutic masseur may be of real value in the overall management of athletes whose injuries come into these categories.

Adapted training programs

The physiotherapist working in the sports area must develop a working knowledge of the biomechanics involved in the performance of sports-specific skills as they relate to the pelvis, hip and thigh. This should then enable the physiotherapist to make informed assessments of the likely mechanisms by which overuse of failure type injuries occur. The therapist can then be of real value in advising the athlete, coach or fitness trainer on what components of the training program are a problem and suggesting possible adaptations.

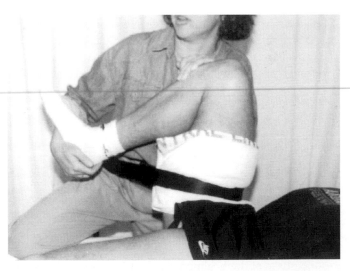

Fig. 28.20 Use of a seat belt to assist accessory mobilization of the hip. Patient lies supine with the hip in mid range flexion, adduction and internal rotation. This position is maintained by the therapist's hand position. A towel is placed over the medial thigh as padding. A seat belt is fastened around the patient's upper thigh and the therapist. A traction force is applied along the line of the neck of the femur by the therapist pushing back against the seat belt while maintaining hip joint posture with the hands

Referral

There are some components of the management of injuries affecting the pelvis, hip and thigh which fall outside the parameters in which physiotherapy alone will assist the athlete in making a full recovery. Physiotherapists must be aware of the role a sports physician, sports podiatrist and therapeutic masseur may play in an effective, comprehensive treatment and rehabilitation program.

GUIDELINES FOR RETURN TO SPORT

The assumption that clinical recovery ensures a safe return to athletic performance is incorrect. Resumption of sporting activity at a preinjury level and prevention of further injuries of the same type may be facilitated by a thorough assessment and treatment program. Both of these should recognise the mechanical implications of the injury to athletic performance and should demonstrate an understanding of the demands imposed on the athlete's body by the sporting activity. This is particularly relevant with regard to overuse injuries, where there will often be an element of pre-existing biomechanical failure. There must be a means of bridging the gap between clinical recovery and return to all levels of sports performance.

Common mistakes in rehabilitation include the following.

1. Rehabilitation is often focused on a single muscle group only. The treating therapist must remember that the injured athlete can carry out a modified training program, on instruction, to maintain fitness and skills within the limitations of the injury. For example, in the running athlete an adapted aerobic training may be carried out on an exercise bike or in the swimming pool. Such a program would need to address the specific requirements of the athlete in terms of activation and utilization of the appropriate energy systems, work/rest recovery ratios, strength and endurance (see also Chs 1 and 2).
2. Rehabilitation is seldom continued until the injured limb is found to be equal to or superior to the uninjured side, when assessing all physical parameters. This may reflect a lack of education of the athlete, who no longer presents for treatment because the pain of the injury has resolved and function appears to be normalizing. This may result from a lack of understanding of pain as a symptom, both of the initial trauma and of the acute and ongoing tissue reaction to injury. Absence of pain does not imply anything other than the completion of one phase of the healing process. It should not be taken as an indicator of the ability of injured or previously injured tissues to withstand load. This problem could perhaps best be addressed by incorporating education about injuries—how they occur—and the mechanisms of recovery, as part of an effective treatment program.
3. Exercises for developing functional proprioception are often forgotten. Proprioceptive retraining must be taken beyond the clinical setting and include activities specific to the athlete's sport.
4. Postural defects and anatomical malalignment, as well as biomechanical imbalances, are frequently neglected.
5. Specific sports skills are often not incorporated in the rehabilitation program. Rehabilitative exercises need to be adapted to and developed for the athlete's specific sport requirements (Roy & Irwin 1983). Absence of pain, associated with regaining a normal range of movement and muscular strength, is usually taken as an indicator of full recovery. However, it should be remembered that the skills that the athlete requires are learned and will be affected by a period of detraining subsequent to injury. At this stage, the athlete is ready to begin a graduated training program, which should become progressively more difficult.

Time should be taken to ensure that movement patterns which may have predisposed to injury in the first place have been assessed and where possible either corrected or adapted to minimize potential aggravation. Similarly, confidence may be a problem and the athlete may require additional counselling and time, particularly if the injury has been long-standing, or severe and has required surgical intervention.

SUMMARY

Injuries to the pelvis, hip and thigh present the treating therapist with a complex problem of assessment, treatment and rehabilitation. The structure and function of the musculoskeletal system in this region requires a comprehensive assessment, which should reflect an understanding of the varied function of different structures relative to posture, activity and load. Effective treatment programs can then be developed and progressed. Successful rehabilitation and return to sport should reflect a comprehensive understanding of the injury and an appreciation of the demands of the athlete's sport, as this will provide the guidelines for progression of exercise. There are no formulae for effective treatment of injuries in this area. However, no treatment can be effective without an understanding of the function of the structures involved. An understanding of biomechanics is essential to the management of injuries affecting the pelvis, hip and thigh.

REFERENCES

Adelaar R S 1986 The practical biomechanics of running. American Journal of Sports Medicine 14(6):497-50

Alderink G J 1991 The sacroiliac joint: review of anatomy and function. Journal of Orthopedic and Sports Physical Therapy 13(2):71-84

Atwell E A, Jackson D W 1991 Stress fractures of the sacrum in runners. The American Journal of Sports Medicine. 19(5):531-533

Briggs Dr C 1991 Melbourne University Medical School Anatomy Department. Personal communication

Bull C R 1985 Soft tissue injury to the hip and thigh. In: Welsh R P, Shephard R J (eds) Current therapy in sports medicine 1985-1986. C V Mosby, Toronto, pp 218-223

Calliet R 1968 Low back pain syndrome, 2nd edn. F A Davis, Philadelphia, pp 23-26

Catterall A 1972 Coxa plana. Modern Trends in Orthopedics 6:122

Chapman A E, Caldwell G E 1983 Factors determining changes in lower limb energy during swing in treadmill running. Journal of Biomechanics 16(1):69-77

Cibulka M T, Rose S J, Delitto D R 1986 Hamstring muscle strain treated by mobilizing the sacroiliac joint. Physical Therapy 66(8):1220-1223

Cibulka M T 1989 Rehabilitation of the pelvis, hip and thigh. Clinics in Sports Medicine 8(4):777-803

Colachis S C, Worden R E, Bechtol C D, Strohm B R 1963 Movement of the sacroiliac joint in the adult male: a preliminary report. Archives of Physical Medicine and Rehabilitation 44:490-498

Dalziel R, 1992 Orthopedic surgeon. Personal communication

Dostal W F, Soderberg G L, Andrews J G 1986 Actions of hip muscles. Physical Therapy 66(3):351-359

Fox J M 1986 Injuries to the thigh. In: Nicholas J A, Hershman E B (eds) The lower extremity and spine in sports medicine. C V Mosby, St Louis, pp 1087-1117

Hedstrom S A, Lindgren L 1982 Acute haematogeneous pelvic osteomyelitis in athletes. American Journal of Sports Medicine 10:44

Hemba G D 1985 Hamstring parity. NSCA Journal 7(3):30-31

Janda V 1983 Muscle function testing. Butterworths, London

Kapandji I A 1974 The physiology of joints, vol 3. Churchill Livingstone, New York

Karlin L I 1986 Injuries to the hip and pelvis in the skeletally immature athlete. In: Nicholas J A, Hershman E B (eds) The lower extremity and spine in sports medicine. C V Mosby, St Louis, pp 1292-1332

King J, Robertson J 1986 Pelvis, hip and thigh injuries. In: Helal B, King J, Grange W (eds) Sports injuries and their treatment. Chapman & Hall, London, pp 345-365

Koch R, Jackson C 1981 Pubic symphysis in runners. American Journal of Sports Medicine 9:62

Komi P V 1973 Measurement of the force-velocity relationship in human muscle under concentric and eccentric contractions. Medicine and Sport: Biomechanics III 8:224-229

Kornberg C, Lew P 1989 The effect of stretching neural structures on grade one hamstring injuries. Journal of Orthopedic and Sports Physical Therapy 10(12):481-487

Lloyd-Smith R, Clement D B, McKenzie D C, Taunton J E 1985 A survey of overuse and traumatic hip and pelvic injuries in athletes. Physician and Sportsmedicine 13 (10):131-137,141

Lovell G, Malycha P, Pieterse S 1990 Biopsy of the conjoint tendon in athletes with chronic groin pain. Australian Journal of Science and Medicine in Sport 22(4):102-103

Lovell G 1991. Personal communication

Lovell G, Malycha P 1992 Inguinal surgery in athletes with chronic groin pain: the sportsman's hernia. Australian and New Zealand Journal of Surgery 62:123-125

Mann R, Sprague P 1980 A kinetic analysis of the ground leg during sprint running. Research Quarterly for Exercise and Sport 51(2):334-348

Mann R A, Moran G T, Dougherty S E, 1986 Comparative electromyography of the lower extremity in jogging, running and sprinting. American Journal of Sports Medicine 14(6):501-510

Matheson G O, Clement DB, McKenzie D C, Taunton J E, Lloyd-Smith D R, MacIntyre J G 1987 Stress fractures in athletes: a study of 320 cases. American Journal of Sports Medicine 15(1):46-58

Medoff R J 1987 Injuries to the hip in athletes. Annals of Sports Medicine 3(2):73-76

Mitchell F L, Moran P S, Pruzzo N A 1979 An evaluation and treatment manual of osteopathic muscle energy procedures. Mitchell, Moran & Pruzzo, Valley Park

Morrison J B 1970 The mechanics of muscle function in locomotion. Journal of Biomechanics 3:431-451

Muckle D S 1982 Associated factors in recurrent groin and hamstring injuries. British Journal of Sports Medicine 16(1):37-39

Purdham C 1989 Physiotherapist, Australian Institute of Sport. Personal communication

Richardson C, Jull G, Toppenberg R, Comerford M 1992 Techniques for active lumbar stabilization: a pilot study. Australian Journal of Physiotherapy 38(2):105-112

Rogers AW 1992 Textbook of Anatomy. Churchill Livingstone, Edinburgh

Root M L, Orien W P, Weed J H 1977 Normal and abnormal function of the foot. Clinical Biomechanics Corporation, Los Angeles

Roy S, Irvin R 1983 Sports medicine. Prentice Hall, London

Saudek C E 1985 The hip. In: Gould J A, Davies G J (eds) 1985 Orthopedic and sports physical therapy, vol 2. Mosby, St Louis pp 365-407

Selvaratnum Dr P 1992 Manipulative physiotherapist and acupuncturist. Personal communication

Simm F H, Scott S G 1986 Injuries of the pelvis and hip in athletes. In: Nicholas J A, Hershman E B (eds) The lower extremity and spine in sports medicine. Mosby, St Louis pp 1119-1169

Simonet W T 1987 Injuries of the thigh and groin. Sideline View 9(2):1-4

Simonsen E B, Thomas L, Klausen K 1985 Activity of mono and bi-articular leg muscles during sprint running. European Journal of Applied Physiology 54:524-532

Sinaki M, Merritt J L, Stillwell G K 1977 Tension myalgia of the pelvic floor. Mayo Clinical Procedures: 717

Slocum D B, Bowerman W 1962 The biomechanics of running. Clinical Orthopedics 23:39-45

Smedberg S G G, Broome A E A, Gullmo A, Roos H 1985 Herniography in athletes with groin pain. American Journal of Surgery 149:378-382

Stanton P 1989 Physiotherapist, Australian Institute of Sport. Muscle Energy Workshop

Stanton P, Purdham C 1989 Hamstring injuries in sprinting—the role of eccentric exercise. Journal of Orthopedic Physiotherapy 10(9):343-349

Waters P M, Millis M B 1988 Hip and pelvic injuries in the young athlete. Clinics in Sports Medicine 7(3):513-526

Williams P L, Warwick R (eds) 1980 Gray's Anatomy. W B Saunders, Philadelphia

Williamson A J 1987 Recurrent hamstring lesions and lower limb tissue mobility. Controversial Issues in Sports Medicine: Proceedings-Australian Sports Medicine Federation National Scientific Conference pp 441-45

Zimmerman G 1988 Groin pain in athletes. Australian Family Physician 17(12):1046-1052

29. The knee

Christopher Briggs, Steven M. Sandor, Michael A. R. Kenihan

PART 1
ANATOMY AND BIOMECHANICS
Christopher Briggs

Owing to its situation between the hip and ankle joints, in the middle of the weight-bearing lower extremity, the knee joint must meet the very exacting static and dynamic requirements which cannot fail to express themselves in the peculiar anatomic construction of this articulation (Steindler 1935, p 239).

The knee joint is the largest and most complex synovial joint in the body. Its presence may be detected by the fourth week of intrauterine development (the 5 mm embryo) and its form is clearly delineated by six weeks. It is normally described as a 'modified hinge joint' in which the primary active movements are flexion and extension; rotation and some abduction/adduction and translatory movements also occur. Situated between the hip and ankle the knee co-operates with both joints in a 'closed kinematic chain', i.e. when supporting body weight in sitting, standing and all locomotor activites. It also acts in an 'open kinematic chain', providing mobility for the foot in space.

On occasions the knee is called upon to sustain extreme loads, representing two to three times body weight (Chen & Black 1980). Unfortunately, opposing articular surfaces show such incongruence that bony stability is inadequate for some activities to which the joint is subjected. At such times it depends instead on a complex arrangement of capsule and ligaments, menisci and musculotendinous structures to maintain normal alignment and stability, and to restrain translation in all planes.

Please note that the description of the knee joint in this chapter relates to the tibiofemoral articulation only. The patellofemoral joint is described in Chapter 30.

ARTICULAR SURFACES

Femur

The femur has two condyles. The lateral condyle is wide and flat, while the medial is narrow, longer and more curved

(Fig. 29.1). Anteriorly the femur possesses a saddle-shaped patellar surface and between the femoral condyles posteriorly is the intercondylar notch or fossa. The lateral condyle is more prominent anteriorly, producing an asymmetry or lipping which resists lateral dislocation of the patella. On the medial aspect of the lateral condyle, within the intercondylar notch, is the anterior femoral notch or groove, which houses the taut anterior cruciate ligament (ACL) in extension. Comparative studies (Straus & Cave 1957, Basmajian 1980) suggest the position of the ACL in this notch is the principal determinant of upright stance (at the knee), and a shallow notch predisposes to instability. Some individuals possess a tight notch, which may lead to excessive wear and tear and eventual shearing of the anterior cruciate ligament under less than normal strain.

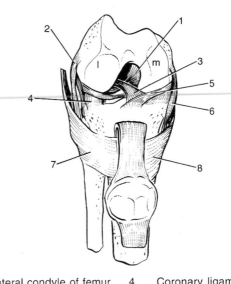

l	Lateral condyle of femur	4	Coronary ligament
m	Medial condyle of femur	5	Medial meniscus
1	Posterior cruciate ligament	6	Medial collateral ligament
2	Lateral collateral ligament	7	Lateral patellar retinaculum
3	Anterior cruciate ligament	8	Medial patellar retinaculum

Fig 29.1 Anterior aspect of knee. The quadriceps tendon has been divided and the patella retracted distally

A feature of the femoral condyles is that while they are convex in the coronal and parasagittal planes, their surfaces show decreasing radii of curvature i.e. they become flatter from anterior to posterior. As a result, the position of the centre of rotation for flexion and extension—referred to as the 'instant centre of rotation' and normally found in the vicinity of the lateral femoral condyle (Frankel et al 1971, Gerber & Matter 1983, Muller 1983)—changes with joint movement. In a normal joint gliding occurs without significant compression or distraction of articular surfaces (Frankel & Nordin 1980). However, even minor changes to articular structures may lead to altered joint biomechanics and dysfunction. Following meniscal or ligamentous damage, for example, the instant centre of rotation can alter dramatically, resulting in increased wear and tear (Fischer & Ferkel 1988).

Tibia

The proximal tibia presents two articular surfaces, the medial and lateral condyles, separated by a midline projection, the tibial eminence, with medial and lateral tubercles or spines. Anterior and posterior to the eminence are the attachments of the menisci and the tibial origins of the cruciate ligaments (Fig. 29.2). With the need to accommodate large rounded condyles, the medial and lateral tibial plateaus should be shaped to maximize congruency. Instead they are only slightly concave, the medial in both the sagittal and frontal planes and the lateral in the frontal plane but convex in the sagittal. The tibial spines may provide stability against medial and lateral translation (Graf 1987).

Capsule

The articular surfaces at the knee are surrounded by an extensive capsule, reinforced on all sides by a combination of ligamentous and tendinous supports. On the femur the capsule attaches to the articular margin, below the level of the epiphyseal line, except in two areas. Posteriorly it is

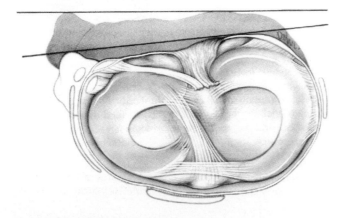

Fig. 29.2 Medial and lateral menisci viewed superiorly. Source: Engle (1991)

attached to the lower limit of the popliteal surface of the femur, and on the lateral condyle it encloses the pit for the popliteus tendon. On the tibia the capsule also follows the articular margin, except where it is attached to the groove for the posterior cruciate ligament posteriorly, and laterally where it continues down over the popliteus tendon to the fibular styloid process. Anteriorly it splits to attach to the margins of the patella. The thickness of the capsule varies at different sites. Below the patella it is thin and is invaginated, along with the synovial membrane, by a large fat pad which lies deep to and then passes both medial and lateral to the patellar tendon. In some areas it is thickened to form capsular ligaments, which together with the extracapsular ligaments form major ligamentous complexes. Deficiencies in the capsule permit communication between the synovial membrane and adjacent bursae, as well as allowing the tendon of popliteus access to the lateral condyle of the femur.

Synovial membrane

The synovial cavity corresponds approximately with the fibrous capsule, except that it invaginates the intercondylar notch, in front of the cruciate ligaments. The synovial membrane at the knee is the most extensive and complex of all the body's synovial joints. It is attached to the articular margin of the femur, then passes around the articular surface of the patella and continues into the suprapatellar pouch or bursa. On the lateral aspect of the femur it is separated from capsule by the tendon of popliteus. On the tibia it extends to the margins of the medial and lateral condyles, and from the posterior aspect of each condyle is reflected forward over the anterior cruciate ligament. The synovium attaches to the superior and inferior aspects of the menisci at their periphery.

The synovial membrane communicates with a number of bursae which, as elsewhere in the body, are located to reduce friction and irritation between skin, ligament, tendon and bone (Fig. 29.3). The suprapatellar or quadriceps bursa extends superiorly a hand's breadth above the joint line, between the quadriceps tendon and the femur. It always communicates with the joint cavity. Others, such as the popliteal and medial gastrocnemius bursa, also communicate directly with the joint (the popliteal bursa often communicates with the superior tibiofibular joint), while the bursa under the medial head of gastrocnemius communicates with the semimembranosus bursa, allowing the latter indirect communication with the joint (McMinn 1990). Many other bursae are associated with the knee but do not communicate with the synovial cavity. The prepatellar bursa is found between skin and the anterior surface of the patella and allows friction-free movement of the skin over the patella during flexion and extension. The superficial infrapatellar bursa lies between the patellar tendon and the overlying skin. Both may become inflamed by direct trauma to the front of the knee ('housemaid's knee') or in prolonged kneeling ('clergyman's knee').

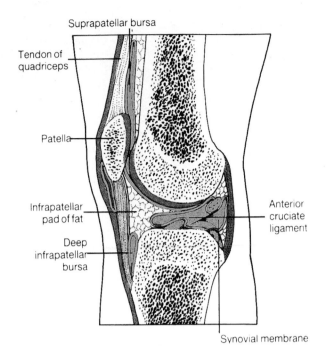

Fig. 29.3 Sagittal section of knee showing extent of synovial cavity. Source: Rogers (1992)

Several small bursae are related to the ligaments, for example between the lateral collateral ligament (LCL) and the tendon of the biceps femoris, and between the LCL and popliteus. A bursa deep to the tibial collateral ligament may be irritated as the ligament glides over the tibia and meniscus (Kerlan & Glousman 1988).

The infrapatellar fold (ligamentum mucosum) extends forwards from the intercondylar notch of the femur (over the anterior cruciate ligament) to the inferior margin of the patella and posterior surface of the patellar tendon, and from there continues both medially and laterally to the upper surface of the tibia as the alar folds. These three folds cover the infrapatellar fat pad and form a flexible 'filler' between patella, tibia and femur which can adapt to variations in the joint space during knee movements. Additional synovial folds, or plicae, may persist in the joints of 20–60% of the population (Hardaker et al 1980). The most common are the suprapatellar and mediopatellar plica. On occasions they become irritated or trapped, and may be a source of joint pain (Hardaker et al 1980).

EXTRA-ARTICULAR LIGAMENTS

The knee joint is inherently unstable. Stability in all planes is provided by a complex of ligaments which reinforce the articular capsule, with further supports provided by the attachments and expansions of the large numbers of muscles which surround the joint on all sides.

Anteriorly the capsule is replaced by the patellar tendon, patella and quadriceps tendon, and is reinforced antero-laterally and anteromedially by expansions of the quadriceps mechanism (Fig. 29.1). These expansions are derived from the vastus lateralis and vastus medialis, and form the medial and lateral patellar retinacula respectively. The lateral is further reinforced by the iliotibial tract, which incorporates fascia derived from the intermuscular septum, which runs between the lateral femoral condyle and 'Gerdy's tubercle' on the tibia (Muller 1983). Posteromedially and postero-laterally the capsule is strengthened by a combination of capsular, ligamentous and tendinous structures, the latter including the insertions of the hamstring muscles. Coronary ligaments (meniscofemoral and meniscotibial) are thicken-ings of the capsule formed at the periphery of both tibia and femur. They loosely attach the two menisci to both bones. It is these which anteriorly form the transverse ligament connecting (in approximately 60% of knees) the anterior margins of the two menisci, allowing them to move in synchrony (Williams et al 1989).

Medial collateral ligament

The principal capsuloligamentous reinforcement medially is the medial collateral ligament (MCL) (Fig. 29.4). Recent editions of anatomy texts (Williams et al 1989, McMinn

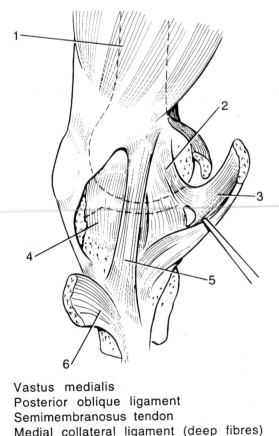

1	Vastus medialis
2	Posterior oblique ligament
3	Semimembranosus tendon
4	Medial collateral ligament (deep fibres)
5	Medial collateral ligament (superficial fibres)
6	Pes anserinus

Fig. 29.4 Medial aspect of knee. Source: adapted from Muller (1983)

1990, Moore 1992) describe this ligament in two parts: superficial and deep. Superficial fibres extend in a broad flat band from the medial femoral epicondyle to the medial aspect of the shaft of the tibia below the 'pes anserinus' (the conjoined insertions of the sartorius, gracilis and semitendinosus). The posterior portion of these is fused to the joint capsule and to the medial meniscus. In extension the superficial part glides forwards and in full extension it is taut, sloping slightly anteriorly. In flexion it slides backwards. Deep fibres, extending from the epicondyle directly to the meniscus, may be referred to as the short internal lateral ligament (McMinn 1990). These deep fibres blend with the superficial part at their femoral attachment, but below this the two are separated by a bursa.

Descriptions of this ligament in the clinical literature differ to varying extents from those in anatomy texts. The accounts of Hughston and Eilers (1973), Warren and Marshall (1979) and Muller (1983) are helpful in formulating an understanding of the region. Muller (1983) includes the MCL as one component of the 'medial capsuloligamentous complex' and organizes it into three layers. Layer 1 (most superficial) consists of fascia extending from the patellar tendon (medial patellar retinaculum) posteriorly to the popliteal fossa, there enveloping the medial hamstring tendons. Layer 2 consists of the MCL which, as it passes posteriorly, becomes more obliquely oriented and joins with the deep capsular ligament (Layer 3) to form the posterior oblique ligament. The meniscus is attached to the posterior oblique ligament by coronary ligaments. The posteromedial aspect of the capsule is reinforced by an expansion from semimembranosus, called the oblique popliteal ligament.

The MCL is the principal restraint to abduction forces; however, because it lies posterior to the axis for flexion/extension it becomes taut as the joint moves into extension, and is tight in the extended knee. Because of its slight anterior alignment in the extended knee, it is capable not just of resisting abduction at the knee but also of restraining anterior sliding of the tibia on the femur, and thereby limiting terminal extension.

Lateral collateral ligament

The lateral collateral ligament (LCL) passes inferiorly as a round cord-like structure from the lateral femoral epicondyle to the head of the fibula (Fig. 29.5). Recent anatomy descriptions (Williams et al 1989, McMinn 1990, Moore 1992) fail to describe any attachment to the lateral meniscus, illustrating the intracapsular tendon of popliteus passing between capsule and the lateral margin of the meniscus. Seebacher et al (1982) suggest, however, the deepest of the lateral capsular layers attach to the lateral meniscus as they form an opening for the popliteal tendon. They describe a layered organization of the 'lateral capsuloligamentous complex' similar to that on the medial

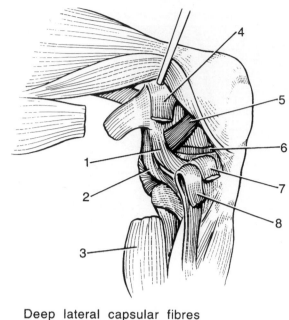

1	Deep lateral capsular fibres
2	Arcuate ligament
3	Lateral head gastocnemius
4 & 7	Lateral collateral ligament (cut ends)
5	Popliteus
6	Lateral meniscus
8	Biceps femoris

Fig. 29.5 Lateral aspect of the knee

aspect. The iliotibial band (ITB) anteriorly and the tendon of biceps and its expansion posteriorly contribute to Layer 1. Layer 2 is formed anteriorly by retinacular fibres from the vastus lateralis with patellofemoral and patellomeniscal ligaments (when present) posteriorly. They describe the 'true' LCL in the third layer, sandwiched between two layers of capsule.

The LCL is positioned to prevent adduction of the leg at the knee, and as it lies posterior to the axis of flexion/extension it also becomes taut on extension and is tight when the knee is in terminal extension. It relaxes in flexion to permit rotation to occur, and when torn, excessive external tibial rotation occurs.

Oblique and arcuate popliteal ligaments

Posteriorly the capsule is thickened in the form of the oblique popliteal and arcuate popliteal ligaments. The oblique popliteal is a fibrous expansion from the semimembranosus which passes posterolaterally and obliquely across the joint to attach to the central part of the posterior capsule. It is perforated by the middle genicular vessels as they run forward into the intercondylar notch to supply the cruciate ligaments. Laterally, the arcuate popliteal ligament arches as a Y-shaped band of fibres from the head of the fibula over the popliteal tendon to attach to the intercondylar area of the tibia and to the lateral epicondyle of the femur. The arcuate popliteal ligament is the principal stabilizer of the posterolateral aspect of the knee, and both ligaments reinforce the posterior capsule, resisting hyperextension. In addition, they may contribute as restraints to other knee motions, such as external tibial rotation with knee flexion and in stabilizing against valgus forces when the joint is in full extension (Indelicato 1988).

INTRA-ARTICULAR LIGAMENTS

The anterior cruciate ligament and the posterior cruciate ligament are the two principal intra-articular ligaments of the knee. They take their names from the position of their attachments on the tibia relative to the tibial eminence. From the tibia they cross in the centre of the joint before attaching to the femur.

Anterior cruciate ligament

The anterior cruciate ligament (ACL) attaches on the tibia to an area anterior to the intercondylar eminence and extends to a smooth impression on the medial aspect of the lateral femoral condyle deep within the anterior femoral notch. Girgis et al (1975) divided the ACL into two bands, a smaller anteromedial and larger posterolateral, taking their names from the relative positions of their tibial origin. Norwood et al (1979), Reiman and Jackson (1987), and Arnoczky and Warren (1988) all divided it into three bundles—anteromedial, intermediate and posterolateral—which twist on each other as they run towards the femur.

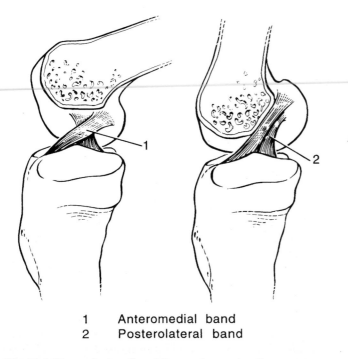

| 1 | Anteromedial band |
| 2 | Posterolateral band |

Fig. 29.6 Two major bundles of the anterior cruciate ligament.

Amiss and Dawkins (1991) suggest that in young knees, where the ACL is surrounded by a thick synovial sheath, there is no easily separable interface between bundles, especially between the intermediate and posterolateral. However, in older specimens, where the synovium is much thinner, three separate bundles are more often obvious. Norwood and Cross (1979) found that the posterolateral bundle is the most vertical and shortest of the three, while the anteromedial bundle is the longest (Fig. 29.6).

The structure and function of the ACL has been the topic of much original anatomical, biomechanical and clinical research (Girgis et al 1975, Kennedy et al 1976, Trent et al 1976, Norwood et al 1979, Butler et al 1980, Grood et al 1981, Clancy et al 1981, Cabaud 1983, Noyes et al 1984, 1986, 1990, Arnoczky & Warren 1988, Amiss & Dawkins 1991). McMinn (1990) notes that the ACL tightens with extension, and indicates its principal role is therefore to provide a pivot around which the medial femoral condyle rotates during the terminal phase of extension. Norwood et al (1979), noting organization of the ligament into separate bundles of fibres, indicate that fibres attaching more anteriorly and medially on the tibia (anteromedial band) tend to originate more proximally and posteriorly on the femur and are taut throughout most of the range of motion. In contrast, fibres which insert towards the posterior aspect of the tibia (posterolateral band) tend to be taut in extension but become lax as the knee flexes. Arnoczky and Warren (1988) support this view and suggest that as the knee is flexed the femoral attachment of the ACL assumes a more horizontal position, causing the anteromedial bundle to tighten and the posterolateral to loosen. In a study of length changes in the ACL, Amiss and Dawkins (1991) indicated that as the posterolateral fibres slacken in flexion, it is the anteromedial bundle which must provide the principal resistance to anterior tibial translation, especially when the knee is flexed to 90°. Amiss and Dawkins (1991) further discuss these relationships from a clinical perspective with the logical suggestion that partial ruptures of the ACL can affect different fibre bundles, depending on the position of the knee at the time of injury. The principal function of the ACL seems therefore to resist anterior translation of the tibia, although it also contributes to stability against varus and valgus loads (Inoue et al 1987). Gollehon et al (1987) noted that internal tibial rotation tends to lengthen the fibres more than external rotation, most obviously at about 30° of flexion, and suggested the ACL also has a role in resisting anterolateral tibial rotation.

Posterior cruciate ligament

The structure and function of the posterior cruciate ligament (PCL) has also received considerable attention in the literature (Kennedy & Gringer 1967, Pournaras et al 1983, Fukubayashi et al 1982, Grood et al 1981). The PCL is slightly longer than the ACL, extending from the tibia posterior to the intercondylar eminence to the lateral aspect of the medial femoral condyle well forward within the intercondylar notch (Fig. 29.7). Similar to the ACL, it consists of anterior and posterior bundles of fibres with variable attachments and orientation (Kennedy et al 1979). Fibres of the PCL which insert anteriorly on the femoral condyle (anterior bundle) tend to be taut in flexion, while those attaching posteriorly (posterior bundle) tend to be taut in extension (Kennedy et al 1979).

Close to the posterior margin of the PCL is the posterior meniscofemoral ligament (Wrisberg's ligament) which passes between the medial condyle of the femur immediately posterior to the attachment of the PCL to attach to the posterior horn of the lateral meniscus (Heller & Langman 1964). An anterior meniscofemoral ligament (Humphrey's ligament) may be present anterior to the PCL, passing between the lateral meniscus and the ACL. Van Dommelen and Fowler (1989) indicate that the meniscofemoral ligaments may be considerably enlarged, as much as one third the size of the PCL or larger.

Butler et al (1980) suggests the PCL is the primary restraint to posterior tibial translation with the knee flexed to 90°. Van Dommelen and Fowler (1989), in a review of the literature on the anatomy and biomechanics of the PCL, support this view and indicated there is an increase in tension in the anterior bundle from 30° of flexion reaching

maximum tension at 90°. Van Dommelen and Fowler (1989) also described increased tension in the PCL with internal tibial rotation and indicated that if the PCL is sectioned there is increased rotational instability in the extended knee.

The menisci

Menisci are wedge-shaped, semilunar discs interposed between tibia and femur (Fig. 29.2). The medial meniscus is characterisically C-shaped, loosely attached to the tibia at its periphery via coronary ligaments, and to the tibial plateau by its horns. The anterior horn is located in the intercondylar region in front of the anterior cruciate ligament, and the posterior horn in the posterior inter-condylar region, between the lateral meniscus and the posterior cruciate ligament. The lateral meniscus has similar attachments to the tibia via coronary ligaments, and to the tibial plateau via anterior and posterior horns, but its horns lie closer together, enclosed within the curvature of the horns of the medial meniscus, giving the lateral meniscus a tight O-shape.

The medial and lateral menisci are unique in size and shape and in terms of the structures that attach to each and which dictate their function. The medial meniscus receives deep fibres of the medial collateral ligament, which attach between its posterior margin and the joint capsule, and posteriorly a fibrous thickening or expansion from semi-membranosus (Kapandji 1982, Levy 1988). These relation-ships, as well as the divergent points of attachment of the anterior and posterior horns, mean that movements of the medial meniscus are relatively restricted. The lateral meniscus is separated from the LCL by the popliteus tendon whose deep fibres, on entering the posterior capsule, have been considered to blend with the posterior margin of the meniscus. This relationship has, however, been disputed by Tria et al (1989). The posterior meniscofemoral ligament (Wrisberg's ligament) attaches the lateral meniscus to the posterior aspect of the medial femoral condyle and the deep fibres of the popliteus. In contrast to the medial meniscus, movements of the lateral are quite free.

Functionally, the menisci divide the knee joint into two compartments. Flexion and extension movements take place above the menisci in the upper compartment of the joint, while rotation takes place below them in the lower compartment (McMinn 1990). During extension, the tibia and menisci glide forward together on the femoral condyles, the lateral with a total range of approximately 12 mm and the medial 6 mm (Kapandji 1982). As the movement progresses the flatter curve of the femoral condyles makes contact with the tibia, opening the menisci out. Meni-scopatellar ligaments (Kapandji 1982) may assist in drawing the anterior horns of the menisci forwards. The net result is the anterior ends of the menisci move forwards and are compressed between the femoral condyles and tibia, while

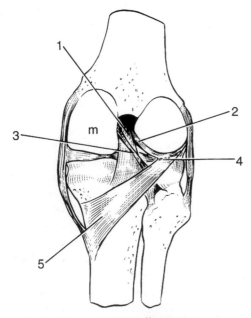

1	Posterior cruciate ligament
2	Anterior meniscofemoral ligament
3	Posterior menisofemoral ligament
4	Attachment from popliteus to posterior horn of lateral meniscus
5	Popliteus

Fig. 29.7 Posterior aspect of the knee. Source: adapted from Indelicato (1988)

their posterior ends show little change in position. In flexion the reverse occurs, with the menisci being compressed posteriorly between femoral condyles and tibia. In flexion, however, movements of the menisci may be assisted by active mechanisms which draw both menisci posteriorly, thereby increasing the surface area for the rolling condyles. The shape of the lateral tibial plateau aids this movement, providing a convex sloping surface down which the lateral meniscus is drawn posteriorly in flexion. In addition, movement of the lateral meniscus is facilitated by the presence of the meniscofemoral ligaments (Fig. 29.2) which during flexion pull the posterior horn of the lateral meniscus anteriorly and medially, increasing congruency between the meniscotibial surface and the lateral femoral condyle.

During rotation the menisci move with the femoral condyles on the upper articular surfaces of the tibia. Acting on a fixed weightbearing knee, the popliteus is responsible for 'unlocking' the knee and externally rotating the femur. Fuss (1989), however, disagrees with this role for the popliteus. He claims popliteus is primarily an extensor at the knee, not a flexor, and the compulsory rotation which accompanies flexion is due not to active contraction of the popliteus but to passive elongation caused by increased tonus. A secondary function attributed to the popliteus has been that of protecting the lateral meniscus, by pulling it out of harm's way over the posterior margin of the lateral condyle as flexion proceeds. However, in a dissection study of forty knee specimens, Tria et al (1989) found no attachment to the meniscus in 82.5% of knees dissected. The fact that the femur externally rotates at the beginning of flexion is indisputable. Although the role of the popliteus in drawing the meniscus posteriorly is open to question, medial movement does occur with tightening of the meniscofemoral ligaments. The semimembranosus, via its expansion to the posterior margin of the medial meniscus, aids its posterior motion. During extension of the knee, elastic recoil allows the menisci to return to their extended position.

The ultrastructural organisation of menisci at the knee is a network of collagen, fibrocartilage and proteoglycans oriented vertically, horizontally and radially in an arcade fashion (Bullough et al 1970). The periphery is particularly dense and capable of withstanding considerable stress, while the junction between central and peripheral parts is often a site of weakness (De Haven 1990). Derived from complete discs embryologically, the medial meniscus covers approximately 30% of the medial plateau while 50% of the lateral plateau is covered by the lateral meniscus (Williams et al 1989). Complete discs may persist, however, usually on the lateral side (discoid lateral meniscus). In the foetus they are fully vascularized, but in the adult only their peripheral portions possess a blood supply which extends along their capsular attachments. Blood vessels are derived from the superior and inferior medial and lateral genicular arteries. These vessels contribute to the formation of a perimeniscal capillary complex (Arnoczky & Warren 1982), although the region of the meniscus adjacent to the popliteus tendon is considered to be avascular. The anterior and posterior horns are supplied by branches from the previously mentioned vessels, with additional important contributions from the middle genicular artery and the synovium.

In addition to a vascular supply the menisci possess a nerve supply. Mechanoreceptors have been localized in the outer two-thirds of the menisci, but the inner third appears to be entirely devoid of nerve endings (Kennedy et al 1982). Zimny et al (1988) report the greatest concentration of nerve fibres and receptors in the meniscal horns and suggest their presence at these sites relates to the need for afferent feedback at the extremes of flexion and extension.

While meniscal-type structures are found at many synovial joints, at the knee 'loadbearing' is now thought to be their most important function (Frankel & Nordin 1980). Other functions attributed to them are that:

- they deepen the tibial plateaus and thereby improve adaptation of opposing articular surfaces. Because they are triangular in cross-section they convert the tibial plateau into a 'socket', thereby increasing joint congruity.
- they spread articular loads across contact areas and increase the surface area from approximately 2 cm^2 to 6 cm^2 (Walker & Erkman 1975). This acts to decrease contact stress, preventing its transmission to the underlying articular cartilage and subchondral bone.
- they assist the ligaments in providing stability, moving across the tibial plateau during flexion and extension to accommodate the changing curvatures of the femoral condyles.
- they assist with shock absorption. The lateral meniscus absorbs most of the load transmitted through the lateral aspect of the knee; while the medial meniscus, relatively smaller in size, absorbs about half the load in the medial compartment. Absence of a meniscus has been shown to increase the load on the underlying cartilage, and to centralize the tibiofemoral contact pressures (Frankel et al 1980).
- they assist with nutrition and with lubrication of the joint.

For further details on the structure and function of menisci the reader is referred to a review, edited by Ewing (1990).

Blood supply

The capsule and joint structures receive their principal blood supply via anastomoses between genicular vessels, derived from the popliteal artery. Maintenance of an adequate blood supply to the cruciate ligaments is considered to be critical in their ability to be repaired and reconstructed (De Haven 1990, Arnoczky et al 1982).

Nerve supply

The capsule of the knee possesses a rich sensory nerve supply, in accordance with Hilton's Law. It is derived posteriorly from articular branches of the posterior division of the obturator nerve, via genicular branches of the tibial and common peroneal nerves and the posterior articular nerve, a branch of the tibial which is often the largest and most consistent nerve supplying the knee (Kennedy et al 1982). Anteriorly it receives branches from the femoral and saphenous nerves. The cruciate ligaments receive their supply via branches of the tibial nerve. Most proprioceptive fibres to the capsule are found in the nerve to the vastus medialis, a branch of the femoral nerve (McMinn 1990).

KNEE FUNCTION

The knee acts as a major weightbearing joint during locomotion. In a normal knee the mechanical axis passes from the centre of the hip to the centre of the knee joint, although it may also pass lateral (genu valgum) or medial (genu varum) to the joint itself. The principal movements at the knee are flexion and extension, combined with rotation in the transverse plane (only possible when the joint is flexed). Slight amounts of abduction and adduction are also possible in the coronal plane, as is anteroposterior translation. However, the magnitude of these side-to-side and anteroposterior displacements varies considerably among individuals, and is generally considered to be the result of joint incongruence and ligament laxity (Torzilli et al 1981, Fukubayashi et al 1982).

Motion in the sagittal plane involves a series of complex movements in which the femoral condyles both roll and glide on the tibial plateaus. The articulating surface of the medial femoral condyle is slightly longer than that of the lateral, even though the bony lateral condyle is the longer of the two. As described in more detail elsewhere (Kapandji 1982, Norkin & Levangie 1992), because of the disproportionate lengths of opposing articular surfaces, during flexion the femoral condyles simultaneously glide forward as they roll backwards. The ratio of rolling to gliding varies throughout the range and between the two condyles. Initial knee flexion is achieved entirely by rolling for 5–10° on the medial side and for about 20° on the lateral side. At this stage the condyles begin to glide, approximately twice as far as they roll, such that by the end of flexion the ratio of gliding to rolling has increased to about 4:1 (Norkin & Levangie 1992). In extension the sequence of movements occurs in reverse.

Motion in the transverse plane (axial rotation) occurs as both conjunct and adjunct rotations. Conjunct rotation takes place as the knee approaches extension and in the initial stages of flexion (the rotation accompanying the beginning of flexion requires contraction of popliteus). During the final few degrees of extension, the lateral femoral condyle is blocked from further gliding by engagement of the anterolateral tibial plateau in the terminal sulcus of the lateral femoral condyle. At this position there is approximately 1 cm of unused weightbearing surface anteriorly and centrally on the longer medial femoral condyle. Additional medial compartment extension is now possible and occurs with the medial femoral condyle gliding until the remaining articular surface is utilized and full extension is achieved. Because the lateral femoral condyle is blocked, preventing additional gliding in the lateral compartment, the femur automatically rotates internally (the tibia externally) approximately 15° to allow the medial compartment motion to occur. As the joint approaches full extension the extra articular surface on the medial condyle is utilized. This combination of extension and conjunct axial rotation is referred to as the 'screw-home mechanism' which allows the joint to undergo terminal internal femoral or external tibial rotation to reach the locked position.

Frankel & Nordia (1980) indicate the maximum passive range of flexion/extension to be 0–140°. They also report 0–45° of external and 0–30° of internal rotation, with maximum rotatory movements occurring at approximately 90° of flexion. Movement in the coronal plane is quite small, and only occurs when the joint is flexed. The ranges of active movements occurring in all planes show considerable individual variation; however, normative data for walking and running may be found in Murray et al (1964) and Perry et al (1977), and in Kettelkamp et al (1970) for transverse and coronal plane movements in level walking and knee movements in household tasks.

Flexion at the knee is produced by the hamstring muscles, assisted by sartorius, gracilis, popliteus and gastrocnemius. In addition, four of these (semitendinosus, semimembranosus, gracilis and popliteus) are considered to medially rotate the knee, while the biceps is normally described as a lateral rotator. Since many of the muscles which cross the knee are two-joint muscles which also cross the hip joint, hip position can influence knee range of motion. Similarly, tight ankle planti- or dorsiflexors may also limit the knee's ability to flex and extend. Only one component of the quadriceps, the rectus femoris, is a two-joint muscle and therefore likely to be limited in its action at the knee by the position of the hip. The remaining vastus muscles are all knee extensors, and their roles, particularly at the patellofemoral joint, have been described in other sections of this book.

One of the major problems posed by the unique anatomy and biomechanics of the knee joint is crediting specific structures with responsibility for stabilization in a certain direction of movement. There seems to be no concensus of opinion on how the various intracapsular and extracapsular ligaments, capsular structures and musculotendinous reinforcements interact to perform this role. Butler et al (1980), Grood et al (1981), Noyes et al (1984, 1986) conducted a series of studies in which supportive structures at the knee were serially sectioned and their function assessed. They designated the role of each structure as a 'primary' or a 'secondary' restraint and in the process elaborated on the limitations to anteroposterior translation and rotation. This work suggests that as the normal limit of motion is reached there are one or more structures that provide the majority of the resistance offered by the joint to that particular motion. These are referred to as primary restraints, and essentially include the intra-articular and extra-articular ligament complexes already described. Should they become stretched or ruptured, there are usually other structures which, although not as well suited to the restraining task as the primary restraints, are often able to give some stability to the knee. These are the secondary restraints.

In many instances the secondary restraints consist of capsule reinforced by active muscular components. For example, semimembranosus, biceps femoris and popliteus all give fibrous contributions to the capsule, and the remaining flexor muscles are intimately related to the joint. The biceps femoris has attachments to the iliotibial band and the lateral patellar retinaculum, suggesting a key lateral stabilizing role for these combined structures (Terry et al 1986). Considering that the short head of the biceps does not cross the hip joint, it would appear to have a unique stabilizing role at the knee. The sartorius, gracilis and semitendinosus attach together on the medial aspect of the tibia, as the pes anserinus, which is ideally placed to stabilize the medial aspect of the joint. Popliteus has been described as a contributor to stability in the first 90° of flexion (Grood et al 1988). Vastus medialis and vastus lateralis both give fibrous expansions to the patella (medial and lateral patellar retinacula) which also reinforce the anteromedial and anterolateral sides of the knee joint. Further evidence that muscles provide active support at the knee joint comes from Herzog and Read (1993). They determined lines of action and moment arms in the sagittal plane of quadriceps and hamstring muscle groups, and suggest these muscle groups are capable of decreasing strain in knee ligaments, depending on the knee joint angle at which forces are applied.

In extension, most of the ligamentous and capsular supports are under tension, the joint is locked and in the close-packed position. As flexion proceeds, many of these structures slacken to varying degrees to permit both translatory and rotatory movements to take place. Butler et al (1980) investigated the relative roles of all potential restraints to anteroposterior motion and found that when experimentally displacing the tibia anteriorly 5 mm, the ACL resisted 87.2% of the displacement at 30° of flexion and 85.15% at 90°. At 90° the relative contributions of the secondary restraints to the remaining 14.9% were, in order, the iliotibial band (24.8%), the mid third of the lateral capsule (20.8%), the superficial MCL (16.3%) and the LCL (12.4%). The anterior and posterior capsules, the PCL and the popliteus tendon provided little or no restraint to anterior displacement. Because all restraining structures become increasingly slack as flexion proceeds, a greater degree of displacement would be necessary at 30° before

both primary and secondary structures would be capable of resisting the motion. Terry et al (1986) suggest that the ITB, through its attachments to the biceps femoris and vastus lateralis muscles, may assist the ACL in preventing posterior displacement of the femur when the tibia is fixed and the joint approaching extension.

Under posterior displacement the PCL was the primary restraint at 30° (96%) and 90° (94.3%) of flexion. At 90° the only secondary restraint that contributed a statistically greater level of the remaining 5.75 (relative to the other ligaments) was the posterolateral capsule, including the popliteus tendon. Lesser contributions were attributed to the superficial MCL, posteromedial capsule, LCL, and the mid third of the medial capsule. The iliotibial band, mid third of the lateral capsule and the ACL provided no restraint to posterior displacement.

Grood et al (1981) reported on the restraints for medial-lateral motion. Under 6 mm of medial displacement the primary restraint at both 5° and 25° of flexion was the superficial MCL, which provided 57.7% and 78.2% respectively of the total. The posterior capsule was the major secondary restraint (17.5%), but its slackening as flexion proceeded to 25° relegated it to minor importance at that flexion angle. The ACL and PCL provided approximately 14% of the restraint in both positions. Lesser contributions from the anterior and medial capsules were evident at both angles. While most authorities agree with Grood et al (1981) that the MCL is the principal restraint to abduction forces, opinion is divided on the relative importance of other structures in resisting valgus stress. Muller (1983) took the view that no single structure on the medial aspect of the knee works alone in resisting valgus stress. Warren et al (1974) suggested the primary restraint to valgus stress on the medial side of the knee is the superficial (anterior) portion of the MCL. Hughston and Eilers (1973) described the posterior oblique ligament, which is functionally distinct from the MCL, as the primary restraint.

For the corresponding 6 mm of lateral displacement, the LCL was the primary restraint at 5° (54.8%) and 35° (69.2%) of flexion. The ACL and PCL were responsible for 22.2% of the total restraint at 5°, and 12.3% at 25°. Smaller contributions at both angles were from the anterior, middle and posterior capsules, the iliotibial band and popliteus. Terry et al (1986) suggests the LCL is significantly aided as a lateral stabilizer by the ITB, although this is not supported by Grood et al (1981). Although the ITB lies anterior to the knee joint axis in extension and posterior to the axis in flexion it is tight regardless of the position of hip or knee (Kaplan 1958), and thus its importance may have been underestimated.

Grood et al (1988) documented the limits to internal rotation when the knee is flexed to 30°. They indicated that the posteromedial and anterolateral structures and the ACL, all working together, provided the main restraint. Sectioning either the ACL or anterolateral structures produced a small increase in rotation, which increased when both were cut. At flexion angles less than 30° the ACL was the dominant restraint, whereas at flexion angles greater than 30° the anterolateral structures dominated while the posteromedial structures became progressively slack.

It is clear that the contributions of ligaments, capsular reinforcements and muscles to the stability of the knee are especially dependent on joint position and the direction and magnitude of the applied force. It also apparent that some structures contribute to stability in several different directions under both normal and abnormal conditions. Some of the differences may be attributable to the nature of experimental conditions used to assess the relative roles of stabilizers at the knee, as well as the unique characteristics of individual joints.

PART 2
CLINICAL APPLICATIONS
Steven M. Sandor and Michael A. R. Kenihan

This section provides guidelines useful in assessment of the knee. It is not intended to be all-encompassing; physiotherapists and physicians can sometimes find assessment difficult and accurate diagnosis is not always possible by clinical examination alone.

The management of the knee in the last ten years, whether it be conservative, operative or post-operative, has taken great steps forward (and occasionally backwards) in order to bring us to optimum care. Even today new knowledge and technology will result in changes in our approach to the treatment of knee injuries.

In the following, the authors discuss the causes of knee injuries, their assessment, diagnosis, management and prognosis.

SUBJECTIVE EXAMINATION

A detailed history is perhaps of greater importance for the knee than for any other joint. The history should look at a number of aspects, including the following:

- pain—onset, area and behaviour
- mechanism of injury or trauma
- swelling
- noises
- giving way
- locking and clicking
- relevant past history.

Pain

The knee is a common site of traumatic, degenerative and inflammatory disorders. The site and nature of pain associated with these conditions is an important diagnostic tool. Injury or trauma to the knee will usually produce pain within the knee itself. When using the site of pain to assist in the diagnosis of the involved structure, the physiotherapist must be aware that the complex neural distribution to the knee can refer pain to variable locations around the joint. Pain felt over the joint line will indicate possible meniscal damage, whereas pain associated with collateral ligament damage may be felt anywhere along the length of the ligament and/or at its bony attachments. Anterior pain may be caused by:

- patellofemoral dysfunction, often seen at the medial side of the distal pole on palpation of the patellar articular cartilage (see section on patellofemoral joint)
- patellar tendinitis at the distal pole of the patella
- fat pad injuries either medial or lateral to the ligamentum patella
- Osgood-Schlatter's disease of the tibial tuberosity
- bursitis anterior or superior to the patella.

Posterior pain may be associated with popliteus tendinitis, hamstring tendinitis, or posterior capsular or ligamentous damage. Posterior pain will often be experienced clinically during knee flexion. While this can also be attributed to compression of torn and swollen soft tissue, it may also be due to a joint effusion being forced posteriorly during this movement. When an athlete describes pain deep inside the knee, the ACL, PCL or articular damage should be suspected.

Articular degenerative change of the tibiofemoral joint gives pain which is often worse when the athlete stands up and starts to walk, or after walking some distance. There is also frequent stiffness in the morning, due to inactivity. Sudden movements, extremes of flexion, extension or twisting can aggravate the condition. Night pain may be experienced with lateral meniscal cysts or degenerative joint disease. Severe unremitting pain will be felt with rheumatoid arthritis and/or associated inflammatory soft tissue disorders.

Pain from hip disease may be referred to the knee, where it elicits a dull aching pain at the joint or in the suprapatellar region. Pain from the hip may radiate down the anterior aspect of the thigh to the knee.

Intervertebral disc prolapse causing L3 or L4 nerve root compression may also elicit pain in the knee. Less obvious lumbar dysfunction or pathology, such as facet joint disease, spinal canal stenosis, inflammatory conditions and tumours can also refer pain to the knee.

Thorough examination of the hip and spine is therefore important to eliminate these areas as sources of knee pain. The examining clinician should be aware of slipped femoral epiphysis in adolescents, or osteoarthritis of the hip in middle-aged patients, as both of these will result in decreased internal rotation of the hip as well as pain in the knee.

Mechanism of injury or trauma

The mechanism of injury is important as it will often provide information helpful in formulating a diagnosis.

Changes of direction, especially involving sudden turns or twisting, can cause excessive strain on cruciate ligaments or menisci due to increased translatory movement of the tibia on the femur, or shearing and compression of the joint surfaces.

Contact with an opponent or object can cause damage. The PCL is often injured by a direct blow to the tibia from the anterior direction. If contact causes abnormal forces to be imparted to the knee, any single or series of structures may be damaged.

Training errors and/or biomechanical problems associated with the lower limb can lead to overuse injuries which may result in the gradual onset of symptoms.

The condition or type of playing surface can cause injury. If the ground is soft, for example wet grass, the foot tends to slide without the boot gripping and can decrease the degree of injury. Synthetic surfaces sometimes cause the player's foot to be 'stuck' on the surface allowing greater rotatory, shearing or compressive forces to be applied to the knee. If the ground is very hard more jarring may occur. Because athletes are able to move faster on hard surfaces collisions between players occur with higher impact forces, often leading to greater injury.

The weather conditions play a role in causing injury. If it is cold and a player is inadequately warmed up, musculotendinous units are susceptible to injury.

The type of footwear may contribute to injury. For example, if athletes use spikes or stops on their boots and these excessively grip the playing surface when pivoting, this will place significant stress on ligamentous structures.

Swelling

When assessing traumatic injuries it is essential to ask specific questions about the swelling.

Immediate swelling may indicate a fracture and/or a full thickness capsular tear.

If the knee becomes swollen quickly (i.e. within 3 to 4 hours) then it is probably a haemarthrosis which in 75% of cases indicates ACL and, less frequently, patella trauma osteochondral or meniscal damage (Renstrom et al 1986).

If swelling is slow in onset, there may be a synovial effusion indicating the synovial membrane has been irritated or extracapsular damage sustained (e.g. MCL, patellofemoral, bursitis, posterior cruciate etc.).

If swelling develops the next day a meniscal lesion should be suspected.

With some ligament ruptures (e.g. PCL, MCL) there may be no evidence of swelling.

Noises

Determine if the athlete heard a noise. A 'pop' or a 'crack' can indicate an ACL injury and this diagnosis will need to be excluded.

Giving way

Athletes commonly describe a feeling of giving way. It may be produced by the patellofemoral joint (PFJ), a torn posterior horn of the medial meniscus (Smillie 1974), a loose body or arthritis. It may also arise from a knee which has rotary instability. The knee gives way without warning when the athlete changes direction with weight on the affected leg, on uneven ground or walking downstairs. This type of instability can occur in athletes who have previously injured their ACL or had corrective surgery. In these cases the person will be playing sport, suddenly change direction and feel their knee collapse. They will describe it as 'I felt the bones move on each other'. This type of giving way is the precipitous type caused by true knee instability.

Instability or giving way may also be caused by inhibition or weakness of the quadriceps mechanism after traumatic injury to capsular ligaments of the patellofemoral joint. Williams and Sperryn (1976) called this 'stable instability', and it is probably due to pain inhibition or loss of proprioceptive feedback.

Locking or clicking

Locking should be viewed as either 'true' or 'apparent'. In 'true' cases it represents a complete block to full extension, usually at about 30° of knee flexion. It can be caused by a loose body or a damaged meniscus, particularly a bucket handle tear. With bucket handle tears it is not uncommon for a locked knee to unlock with a 'clunk'. The knee will then fully extend.

'Apparent' locking implies a knee that is unable to fully extend and on examination has a spongy block to full extension. The pathology in this case may be cruciate damage or internal derangement causing pain inhibition. Again, careful examination is necessary.

Relevant past history

Aspects of past history of injury may include:

- previous or on-going problems with associated structures such as the lumbar spine, hip or feet
- previous knee injury, treatment and outcome
- general health
- medication
- X-rays.

OBJECTIVE EXAMINATION

An acute disabling knee injury should always be X-rayed to exclude fractures, detachments of ligaments with bony fragments or loose bodies. After a full history has been taken the knee is examined and the following procedures followed:

- observation:
  —deformities

—swelling
—muscle wasting
- movements:
—active
—passive
—accessory
- special tests
- palpation
- other joints
- gait assessment.

Observation

In cases of effusion, swelling extends above the patella. The presence of an effusion is assessed by pressing the hands against the areas above and below the patella at the same time as the patella is pressed towards the femur with the thumb of the opposite hand. An alternative way is to empty the normal gutter over the medial compartment of the knee by stroking the fluid out and upwards into the suprapatellar pouch. The other hand from above the knee then moves the swelling inferiorly, where it will be seen to bulge at the medial compartment of the knee.

Deformities to observe include wasting of the quadriceps, the position of the tibia in relation to the femur (particularly with posterior cruciate injuries), and scars from previous surgery.

Movements

Full flexion and extension should be examined both actively and passively. If these movements can be performed to maximum range, the knee should be fully flexed with the tibia internally and externally rotated on the femur. In extension the knee should be moved into a combination of both abduction and adduction.

When assessing movements the physiotherapist should also assess length of the rectus femoris, hamstrings, iliotibial band and hip flexors as these structures, if tight, can contribute to pathology and cause problems on return to sport. In general, decreased ranges of movement indicate some degree of current pathology or previous history of injury.

Rotation of the knee should be assessed with the athlete seated and the knee flexed over the edge of a couch. The normal active range is approximately 40° of external rotation of the tibia and 30° of internal rotation.

Special tests

The following tests should be performed (Table 29.1):

- varus/valgus stress tests
- anterior drawer/posterior drawer and variations
- Lachman test

Table 29.1 Summary of special tests

Test	Structure injured If positive	Comment
Valgus at 30°	MCL	Perform slowly and note the end feel and degree of gapping
Valgus in extension	MCL & PCL +/- posterior joint capsule	Implies more than just MCL damage
Varus at 30°	LCL	Note end feel and degree of gapping
Varus in extension	LCL +/- PCL +/- lateral capsular ligament	Implies more than just LCL damage
Anterior drawer	ACL	Test anteromedial bundle of ACL
• with external tibial rotation	ACL	Be aware of subtleties of the movement and its feel
• with internal tibial rotation	ACL +/- posterolateral capsule of movement	Be aware of resistance to movement as much as degree
Posterior drawer	PCL arcuate complex posterior oblique ligament	Note starting position, otherwise a false anterior drawer can be suspected
Lachman	ACL	Tests posterolateral fibres
Pivot shift	ACL anterolateral instability (anterolateral instability)	Test causes reduction of subluxed tibia on femur Lift by the foot
Posterolateral rotary instability	posterolateral ligament complex	Tibial rotation externally with varus deformity
McMurray's meniscus test		
• valgus stress and external tibial rotation	medial meniscus	Useful in tears of posterior and middle third of meniscus only
• varus stress & internal tibial rotation	lateral meniscus	
Apley's internal rotation	lateral meniscus	Suspect meniscus when compression added to ligament and distraction applied
Apley's external rotation	medial meniscus	
Medial and lateral glides	No specific structure. Just an indication of intra-joint stiffness	May give information about adhesions developing in the stiff knee.

- tests for rotary instability
- McMurray's test and Apley's grind test
- accessory tests
- functional tests.

All athletes should be assessed for 'quadriceps lag' before the other special tests are performed. Quadriceps lag is tested by placing the athlete in a supine position, with the heel resting on a small block allowing the knee to sag into extension. The athlete is asked to lock the knee and lift the heel off the block. If the knee seems to lift before the heel then the athlete is observed to have a lag. This implies a weakness of the quadriceps mechanism.

Vulgus/varus

Valgus or abduction stress test. The abduction stress test should be performed with the knee in extension and at 30° of flexion. The normal knee should be tested first. When examining the right knee the athlete lies supine with the hip slightly abducted. The knee is flexed to 30° and the examiner hugs the athlete's lower leg under their right arm and uses their right hand to steady the lower leg. The examiner's left hand is placed over the lateral aspect of the athlete's knee.

The knee is gently moved into abduction until pain is produced, or gapping of the medial joint line occurs. The degree of gapping must be compared to the normal knee. The test is repeated with the knee straight.

Care should be taken in performing this test as the end feel of the movement is important and if performed too quickly may cause the athlete to contract their muscles and make the test ineffective. In cases of total rupture there will often be no pain.

Implications: If the test is positive with the knee flexed to 30° but negative with the knee straight, it implies injury to the MCL. If the test is positive both at 30° of flexion and in full extension it also implies damage to the posterior joint capsule or posterior cruciate and medial capsular ligaments.

Varus or adduction stress test. The initial position is similar to that for the abduction stress test, but the hands are changed to apply an adduction stress to the knee, where the right hand is placed over the medial aspect of the athlete's knee and the left hand stabilizes the lower leg.

Implications: If this test is positive with the knee flexed to 30° but negative with the knee fully extended, it implies that the lateral collateral ligament (LCL) has been damaged. If it is also positive in extension it implies damage to the posterior cruciate and lateral capsular ligaments. The lateral structures can further be tested in the cross-legged position where the injured leg is crossed over the uninjured in the sitting position. This will gap the lateral joint and makes palpation of the lateral ligament easier (Fig. 29.8).

Anterior and posterior drawer

Anterior drawer. The anterior drawer (A-D) test, if positive, may indicate that the anteromedial band of the ACL has been damaged. The athlete lies supine with the hip flexed to 45° and the knee to 90°. The examiner sits on the dorsum of the foot to stabilize it. The unaffected leg is examined first. The examiner's hands grasp around the

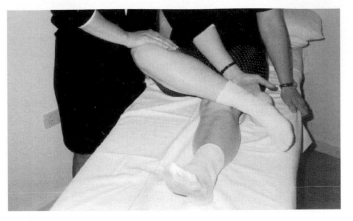

Fig. 29.8 Gapping of lateral ligament in cross leg position

athlete's upper tibia and the fingers are used to palpate the hamstring tendons to ensure they are relaxed. The tibia is gently pulled forwards and the amount of displacement compared to the unaffected leg should be noted, as well as the feel of the displacement. The tibia may come forward to a greater extent on the lateral or medial aspect, or the end feel may not be definite.

When the posterior structures have been damaged, at 90° of knee flexion the tibia will be positioned slightly posteriorly. In these cases the anterior drawer test may only bring the tibial plateau back to its normal resting position, and must not be thought to be a 'positive' anterior drawer test.

Implications: A positive A-D test does not immediately indicate a tear of the ACL. False positive and false negative results may be demonstrated at surgery. The mechanism of this test probably indicates a tear of the medial and lateral capsular ligaments which produce combined anteromedial and anterolateral rotational instability. If the ACL is ruptured the degree of subluxation is increased.

Variations to this test should be performed wih the foot and leg externally rotated to tighten the medial capsular ligaments, and internally rotated to tighten the lateral capsular ligaments. Excessive movement with the anterior drawer test in these cases indicates a rotary instability.

Posterior drawer. If positive, the posterior drawer (P-D) test indicates a tear to the posterior capsular structures and possibly the posterior cruciate ligament. The test should be performed in a similar position to the anterior drawer test, except the tibia is pushed backwards rather than forwards. Again, the clinician should be aware of the end feel and note if the tibia is tending to move backwards more on the lateral or medial side.

In examining the PCL a small block should be placed under the heel to let the knee sag into extension. If this does not elicit pain, the tibia will sit more posteriorly in cases of posterior capsular or posterior cruciate damage. This test will only be effective if the starting position is painfree.

Lachman test

This test is fundamentally an anterior drawer test performed at 10-20° of flexion. If positive, it indicates a tear of the posterolateral fibres of the ACL. It is usually more accurate than the A-D test as the problem of hamstring spasm is all but eliminated. It is also useful in examining an acutely injured knee. The test is performed by the physiotherapist holding the athlete's thigh on the lateral side with one hand, and holding the upper part of the lower leg on the medial side with the other hand. The lower leg is lifted forward. In athletes where the circumference of the thigh is large or the operator has small hands this test is difficult to perform in the way described above. Hence an alternative is illustrated below, where the physiotherapist places their thigh under the athlete's knee and uses one hand to stabilize the thigh from above and the other to pull the tibia forward (Fig. 29.9).

Tests for rotary instability.

Rotary instability of the knee due to ligamentous injury results in an excessive degree of rotation of the tibia on the femur. This occurs most commonly on external rotation, and has been discussed under 'giving way'.

Anterolateral rotary instability. This is an anterior subluxation of the lateral tibial condyle, which also moves into internal rotation on the femur. It is caused by insufficiency of the ACL (Slocum et al 1976). The degree of instability is increased if the lateral capsular ligament is also torn.

It is diagnosed by:

- the anterior drawer test (with internal tibial rotation)—where the lateral tibial plateau can be seen to sublux forward under the lateral femoral condyle.
- the jerk test—performed with the athlete supine, the hip flexed to 45° and the knee at 90°. The examiner grasps the athlete's foot and fully internally rotates the tibia. A valgus stress is applied to the proximal end of the athlete's tibia and fibula. The examiner then

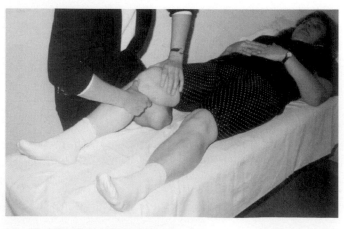

Fig. 29.9 Modified Lachman test

gradually straightens the knee. At about 30° of flexion, the lateral tibial femoral compartment may be seen to suddenly sublux or jerk forward. As the knee is further extended the tibia returns to its former position.

- the pivot shift test—in this test the examiner starts with the knee extended. The knee is pressed into valgus and the lower leg into internal rotation. During passive flexion at 20-30° a forward subluxation of the lateral tibial plateau occurs as the iliotibial band falls backwards over the lateral femoral condyle (Tamea & Henning 1981, Jensen 1990, Back & Warren 1988).

The jerk and pivot shift tests require experience and, with a tense painful knee, are difficult for the inexperienced operator to perform.

Anteromedial rotary instability. This is an anterior subluxation of the medial tibial plateau which moves into external rotation on the femur. It follows a tear of the capsular ligament of the medial joint compartment which is then unable to limit the degree of external rotation of the tibia on the femur. Anteromedial instability is diagnosed in the presence of a positive anterior drawer test, performed while the tibia is held in external rotation.

Posterolateral rotary instability. This is a posterior subluxation of the lateral tibial plateau which rotates externally on the femur. It follows a tear of the posterolateral ligament complex and is diagnosed in the presence of an external rotation—hyperextension test, where the examiner lifts the leg by the foot to produce hyperextension of the knee. The experienced operator may see the tibia rotate externally as the knee develops a varus deformity.

Meniscal tests

McMurray's meniscal test. In McMurray's test the athlete lies supine with the hip and knee flexed at a comfortable range. As the knee is flexed further, internal or external rotation of the tibia is applied. The presence of pain and a palpable 'clunk' is a positive McMurray's test and indicates meniscal injury. However, even if the athlete's pain is reproduced without a 'clunk', there may still be meniscal injury. The test should be applied gently at first, with gradually increasing force of tibial rotation. Adding a valgus or varus stress to the joint while the tibia is undergoing rotation will help to provide a positive response.

Implications: This test is useful for tears in the posterior and middle thirds of the meniscus but not for the anterior third. It is difficult to assess the anterior third of the meniscus. Palpation is the best approach.

Apley's test. The athlete should be prone with the hip extended and the knee flexed to 90°. The examiner may need to place their knee across the back of the athlete's thigh to stabilize it. The lower leg is rotated internally and externally while at the same time applying first a downwards compression, then upwards traction.

Implications: If rotation of the knee with compression produces pain or a click, a tear of the meniscus is likely. Pain on rotation with traction may indicate a ligament sprain.

Another test that may be useful with a meniscal injury is that of hyperflexion of the knee with the athlete prone, then externally and internally rotating the knee while forcing it further into flexion. A painful clicking may be elicited over the joint line in a positive test.

Accessory tests

With the athlete in 'crook' lying, the following tests should be applied:

- lateral tibial glides, where the movement is produced by counterpressure from one hand placed superolaterally on the femur against the other placed inferomedially.
- medial tibial glides, where the movement is produced by counterpressure from one hand placed superomedially on the femur against the other placed inferolaterally.

These accessory tests provide information about the accessory glide of the tibia and femur and, if tighter than the unaffected side, indicate that adhesions in the joint may be limiting the range of movement. They may be used as a treatment technique if the knee is stiff.

Functional tests

Where appropriate, the examination should include a functional assessment. These include walking, squatting, kneeling, sitting, jumping, turning, twisting, cutting and pivoting. This type of assessment will be required more often in cases of chronic instability than in acute injury, and will provide good reassessment guidelines.

Palpation

The knee should be carefully and thoroughly palpated both in flexion and extension. The areas to palpate should include:

- the medial and lateral joint lines (on the lateral side care must be taken to ensure the popliteus tendon is examined)
- the patellar tendon and patellar ligament
- the infrapatellar pad of fat
- the patellar margins, especially the inferior pole
- the fibular head and Gerdy's tubercle
- the pes anserinus area and medial ligament along its length
- the hamstring tendons and popliteal fossa (sometimes best palpated with the athlete prone and knee flexed)
- the tibial tubercle.

Other joints

The lumbar spine may need to be examined for range of movement and pain, noting any change in knee symptoms. Movements of internal rotation, flexion and abduction at the hip should be examined to ensure no referral of pain to the knee. Dural tightness should be assessed as a cause of referred knee pain and should be considered in any differential diagnosis (see Chs 26, 27 and 28).

Gait assessment

The knee should be observed when the athlete is walking in order to assess stride length, relative flexion and extension, degree of genu valgum/varum and the ability to take weight on the affected knee. Gait should be assessed at different speeds and in different directions.

LIGAMENT INJURIES

Medial knee compartment injuries

Medial collateral ligament

The MCL can be damaged in three separate situations. The first is when direct contact occurs from the lateral aspect. The second is in an activity where the foot is fixed on the ground and the athlete creates an excessive valgus force (e.g. in skiing when performing a turn, or catching the edge of the ski in the snow). These injuries tend to involve the posterior portion of the MCL and the posterior oblique ligament. The third is when a fall produces a valgus force on a flexed knee and the knee acts as a fulcrum. It is injured both in isolation and in combination with other ligamentous structures, depending on the direction and magnitude of the force. It will be considered in isolation in this description.

Injury to the MCL can range from minor (Grade I) to total rupture (Grade III). It can involve the superficial ligament or both deep and superficial fibres.

Signs and symptoms. The history is often diagnostic. The athlete will describe a sensation of the knee giving way medially, sometimes with a crack and, often, instant pain on the medial aspect. When there is a crack or pop, injury to the ACL will need to be eliminated.

Unless the joint capsule has been damaged an effusion is unlikely, but the athlete will still find it uncomfortable to flex or fully extend the knee. Palpating the medial ligament may show local swelling or thickening as well as tenderness at the insertion on the medial femoral condyle, on the joint line, or at the wide insertion over the medial upper tibia.

If there is pain on the joint line, the medial meniscus may be damaged and there will usually be an effusion. With an acute injury, McMurray's test for meniscal pathology may be positive even though the actual pathology only involves the MCL. Valgus stressing will be painful. The degree of opening and end feel will help determine the grade of injury. This should be performed at full extension and at 30° of flexion. If the end feel is soft there may be some continuity of the fibres. If absent, the ligament has been ruptured. If there is a hard or firm end feel the ligament is intact. The examiner should beware when performing the test not to aggravate the pathology. The knee should be X-rayed, as is the case with *all* traumatic knee injuries.

Treatment: Grade I. This injury should take 3-4 weeks to treat before a full return to sport. Initially treatment should be aimed at reducing inflammation, RICE (rest, ice, compression, elevation), interferential therapy (IFT) or magnetic field therapy (MFT).

Isometric quadriceps exercises should not be performed between 0-20° of flexion to avoid external rotation of the tibia on the femur which occurs in terminal extension. This movement can stress the healing fibres of the ligament. At 20° of knee flexion the MCL is not under stress and therefore isometric exercise can safely be performed. Hamstring work and hip abduction/adduction exercises should be commenced after the first 48 hours.

After one week, frictional massage and ultrasound can be applied at the point of soreness. Quadriceps exercises may be performed avoiding terminal extension, increasing to full extension over the next two weeks. Avoidance of valgus stress is important and athletes should be cautioned about movement in and out of a car or rolling over in bed. If tenderness persists then local laser treatment can be helpful.

Treatment: Grade II. With a Grade II injury valgus stressing will demonstrate medial opening of the joint but will result in a discernible end-feel. There will be no end feel with a Grade III strain! The authors believe these injuries should be placed in a limited motion (20-60°) brace for four weeks to enable the healing ligament to be protected. Provided these restraints of movement are adhered to, the treatment procedure is the same for Grade I injuries.

Once out of the brace, it may be necessary to assist recovery of range of movement using heat, cycling in the available range and mobilizing techniques into flexion. Mobilization into extension should only be performed if there is a firm block to extension, otherwise it is best to let extension return gradually until six weeks has passed, when it may be necessary to perform some extension mobilization if there is still a restriction to passive extension.

Running can be commenced at six weeks provided quadriceps are at 80% of full strength (as measured on an isokinetic device) and range of extension is full and painless (see Ch. 17). Before returning to sport, a full functional program will be necessary. This program should commence with running followed by lateral running, figure eight manoeuvres, full sprints, and finally a gradual return to skill drills specific to the sport (Fig. 29.10).

Treatment: Grade III. If the injury is isolated then a limited motion brace, as for Grade II injuries, should be

worn at all times for a full six weeks. Careful examination of the knee for ACL damage is necessary to confirm that the injury is an isolated MCL tear.

All exercises for the first three weeks should be performed in the brace. Careful strengthening of quadriceps, abductors and hamstrings can be introduced. The progression should be similar to that for Grades I and II, but full strength must be regained in the quadriceps before return to sport at twelve weeks (isokinetic testing). Return to sport should be gradual, using the functional progression outlined in Grade II treatment above. In the authors' opinion, contact sport should not be performed within three months.

Surgical MCL repairs. Although this is not considered by most as the treatment of choice, some physicians and surgeons believe acute surgical repair should be performed on isolated Grade III tears. The reason for this may be based on personal preference rather than scientific rationale. Usually surgical repair is performed when other structures around the knee have also been damaged. Hence, if it has been decided that a knee which has a torn ACL and MCL is not to be reconstructed, then the MCL only is repaired and the athlete left with an ACL deficient knee. This decision will be made because the athlete has decided not to pursue the type of sports which stress the ACL.

It is important that the primary repair is performed in the first 48 hours and the repair should be isometric (i.e. the repaired tissue is at the same length at all ranges of motion).

Rehabilitation will depend on the surgeon's requirements. The athlete will often have a splint or limited motion cast which is worn for six weeks, as with conservative management. It is possible to resume movement of the knee after two weeks using a limited motion cast, combining limited range isokinetic exercise and soft tissue massage to the scar (Sandor et al 1986). The rehabilitation program should be similar in nature to that for Grade II sprains. In some cases range of movement will be slow, so aggressive treatment to improve range of motion may be necessary after six weeks.

Other considerations: pelligrini steida. This condition consists of the formation of a plaque of calcium or bone along the medial femoral condyle in the vicinity of the adductor tubercle, which is separated from the tibia by a band of radiolucent substance. In some instances it is a reaction to a sprain in which there has been forcible detachment of the MCL or partial avulsion of the adductor magnus tendon.

Where pain is a severe problem, the area of plaque should be removed. In most cases, removal of the plaque will not be necessary since, in time, the condition matures and becomes inert. Physiotherapy treatment should be on a symptomatic basis. Care should be taken with massage as it may aggravate the pain.

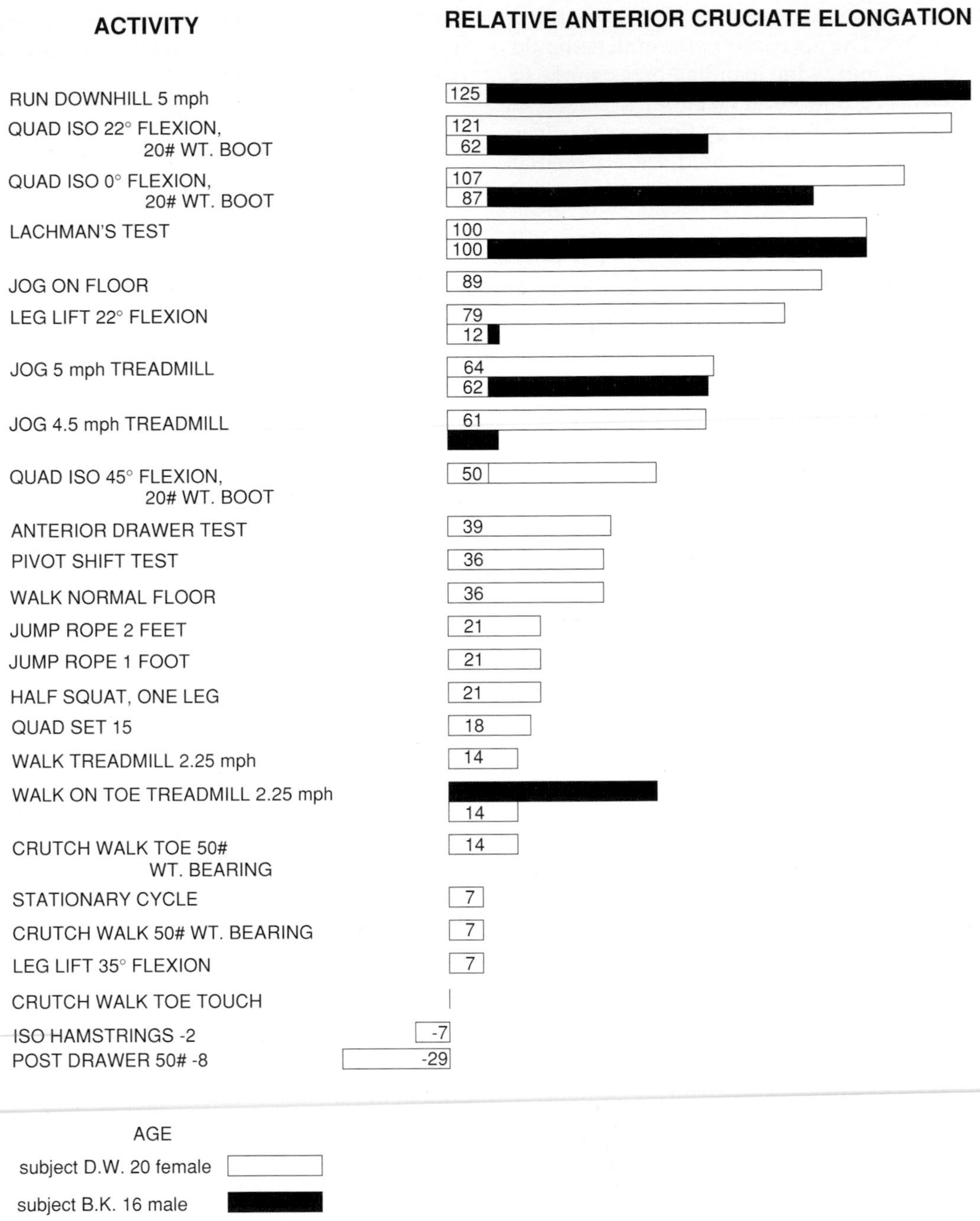

ACTIVITY	RELATIVE ANTERIOR CRUCIATE ELONGATION
RUN DOWNHILL 5 mph	125
QUAD ISO 22° FLEXION, 20# WT. BOOT	121 / 62
QUAD ISO 0° FLEXION, 20# WT. BOOT	107 / 87
LACHMAN'S TEST	100 / 100
JOG ON FLOOR	89
LEG LIFT 22° FLEXION	79 / 12
JOG 5 mph TREADMILL	64 / 62
JOG 4.5 mph TREADMILL	61
QUAD ISO 45° FLEXION, 20# WT. BOOT	50
ANTERIOR DRAWER TEST	39
PIVOT SHIFT TEST	36
WALK NORMAL FLOOR	36
JUMP ROPE 2 FEET	21
JUMP ROPE 1 FOOT	21
HALF SQUAT, ONE LEG	21
QUAD SET 15	18
WALK TREADMILL 2.25 mph	14
WALK ON TOE TREADMILL 2.25 mph	14
CRUTCH WALK TOE 50# WT. BEARING	14
STATIONARY CYCLE	7
CRUTCH WALK 50# WT. BEARING	7
LEG LIFT 35° FLEXION	7
CRUTCH WALK TOE TOUCH	
ISO HAMSTRINGS -2	-7
POST DRAWER 50# -8	-29

AGE

subject D.W. 20 female

subject B.K. 16 male

Fig. 29.10 Relative anterior cruciate elongation. Source: Henning et al
Note: an 80 pound (external load) Lachman test equals 100 units of ACL anteromedial fibre elongation

Athletes involved in any contact sport are at risk, as are snow and water skiers. In the authors' opinion individuals with genu valgum or recurvatum are also at risk.

Coronary ligament

This ligament lies at the anterior aspect of the knee and attaches the anterior horn of the medial meniscus to the front rim of the tibial plateau. It may be damaged by a rotational force, and will present in a similar fashion to a medial meniscus lesion. In this case, there will be minimal effusion and McMurray's test will cause a feeling of stretching, not sharp pain or 'catching'. The joint will not 'lock' and treatment will produce rapid results.

Treatment. Electrotherapy modalities which may be useful are ultrasound, steam packs, IFT, MFT and lasers. Quadriceps exercises, including using isokinetic through range movement, may be performed as long as pain is respected. Cross-frictional massage is useful over the ligament and mobilization into extension can be performed after two to three weeks. During recovery the athlete should be encouraged to cycle and swim, avoiding breaststroke in the first three weeks. The injury will take four to six weeks to heal, but running can commence at three weeks. It is possible for this injury to be associated with a medial meniscal tear and failure to improve would require orthopaedic referral.

Breaststroker's knee

Breaststroker's knee is most likely to be found with the competitive breaststroker, and involves the medial structures of the knee joint, mainly the medial collateral ligament (Hawkins & Kennedy 1974). It is probably caused by repetition of incorrect kicking, although studies have found significant stress on the MCL during the normal breaststroke kick.

In breaststroke swimming, the hips are first abducted with the knees internally rotated. The hips are then actively internally rotated and the knees forcibly extended with a valgus stress placing considerable strain on the medial compartment of the knee. Hence it is important to stretch both hamstrings and hip internal rotators in any treatment program.

Assessment. The swimmer will complain of medial knee soreness while performing the breastroke kicking action. They may also complain of pain walking up stairs and squatting. In these cases the patellofemoral joint should also be assessed as a source of symptoms. On examination, tenderness over the medial joint line, medial coronary ligament pain, swelling in this area and pain on full knee extension helps confirm the diagnosis. McMurray's test may also be painful.

Treatment. Review of training frequency and distance is necessary as well as a full review of kick technique. It may be necessary to discuss these factors with the swimmer's coach. Local treatments such as ice, TENS, ultrasound and laser can help alleviate local tenderness, as can friction massage applied transversely across the ligament. As mentioned above, both hamstrings and internal rotators of the hip need to be stretched.

Other considerations. It may be necessary to stop swimming for a period of two to three months when injured and a break from breaststroke for two months each year is recommended when symptom free.

Predisposing risk factors and sports. Because of anatomical variations, other structures may be stressed (i.e. medial capsule, meniscus or synovium). Risk factors include excessive breaststroke kick, limited hip internal rotation and tight hamstrings. There appears to be a close relationship between frequent knee pain and a number of variables, including the swimmer's age, increasing years of competitive swimming, breaststroke training distance, decreasing warm-up distance, and decreased internal rotation at the hip joint (Rovene & Nichols 1985).

Posterior knee compartment injuries

Posterior capsular region

This is a difficult area of the knee to diagnose accurately. Trauma to the posterior aspect of the knee will often damage a meniscus or the posterior cruciate ligament. In the posteromedial aspect of the knee are fibres from the semimembranosus which support the posterior and posteromedial capsule and attach to the medial meniscus as well as to the tibia. Deep to the medial collateral ligament lie the meniscofemoral and meniscotibial (capsular) ligaments which are attached to the medial meniscus at its periphery. The posterior third of the capsular ligament is referred to as the posterior oblique ligament. It is important in controling posteromedial rotary instability.

Posterolaterally is the arcuate complex which is composed of fibres of the fibular collateral ligament, the popliteus tendon and the arcuate popliteal ligament. The collateral ligaments, the posterior oblique and the arcuate popliteal ligament are important in maintaining the rotatory position of the unloaded tibia and femur relative to one another, although each ligament has an overlapping function. Because of this, it is difficult to analyze the basic structures and their functions at the joint.

Damage to the posterior aspect of the knee is usually caused by a direct force to the anterior aspect of the tibia while the knee is flexed. This forces the tibia backwards on the femur and will damage the PCL and posterior capsule. Complete posterior instability will occur if the PCL, together with the arcuate complex laterally and the posterior oblique ligament medially, are torn. Posterolateral instability occurs with a tear of the arcuate complex and posterior third of the lateral capsule. It leads to posterior subluxation and external rotation of the lateral tibial plateau. Injury to the posterolateral band of the ACL also increases posterior laxity and is caused by a blow to the front of the tibia with the leg externally rotated and planted in a varus position. It is also possible for the posterior compartment to be torn by a hyperextension force, not just a translatory force of the tibia on the femur.

Trauma to the posteromedial or posterolateral compartment may damage the capsule alone or other structures including the PCL, ACL, arcuate complex and posterior oblique ligament. Assessment is difficult and a thorough history of the trauma is required. Clinically, it is possible to test passively for posterolateral instability by performing a test described by Hughston and Norwood (1980). The examiner flexes the knee to 75–90° and the tibia is externally rotated. The examiner then displaces the lateral tibia posteriorly. Subluxation is present with posterolateral capsular injuries. In the active posterolateral drawer test, the knee is positioned at 60–90° of flexion with the tibia externally rotated. Isolated resisted hamstring contractions in this position will further sublux the lateral tibia posteriorly. There is also a reverse pivot shift test (Jokob et al 1981). This is a very difficult test to perform and is not recommended by the authors.

If the damage is capsular only, there will be a loss of both flexion and extension range but the knee will have 50–80% of normal movement. There may be popliteal swelling and restricted gait. Treatment will be as for other soft tissue lesions, with gradually increasing activity as range of motion increases. Resisted knee flexion should be avoided until the late stages of rehabilitation and an early goal is to restore active knee extension range and quadriceps strength. Full recovery will take four to eight weeks.

More serious damage will lead to a knee effusion or haemarthrosis, severe pain, inability to walk and loss of movement. Accurate diagnosis may require arthroscopy and recovery time will be prolonged. Damage to the ACL or PCL will need to be dealt with appropriately. If there is meniscal damage combined with capsular tearing, the meniscus will be sutured or removed at the tear site. The capsule will heal while the knee is recovering from meniscal surgery.

Posterior cruciate ligament

This very strong ligament is usually damaged by a direct blow to the anterior aspect of the upper portion of the tibia. As the tibia is forced posteriorly, the posterior cruciate ligament (PCL) is stretched or ruptured.

Assessment. The acutely injured knee will be swollen and possibly warm. Because both cruciate ligaments are extrasynovial, PCL ruptures do not present as tense haemarthroses unless there are associated collateral ligamentous, meniscal or osteochondral injuries. With the athlete supine and both knees flexed to 90°, the injured knee will appear to sag posteriorly, with a dip in the infrapatellar region (Fig. 29.11). Hughston and Norwood (1980) recognized other findings with acute tears of the PCL. They found a positive abduction or adduction test in full extension, while Grood et al (1988) challenged this finding by saying there was a greater abduction/adduction laxity in a PCL deficient knee when the knee was flexed to 90°. They felt that in flexion, the secondary restraints to posterior tibial translation (the arcuate ligament complex) were more relaxed and that the PCL was best tested in this position. Unless there is significant swelling and muscle spasm, gliding the tibia forwards will demonstrate a glide greater than the uninjured knee. The athlete will complain of pain in the posterior aspect of the knee and will find full flexion difficult. The athlete will be able to weightbear and will not necessarily feel giving way or severe pain. Considerable force is required to damage the PCL, therefore

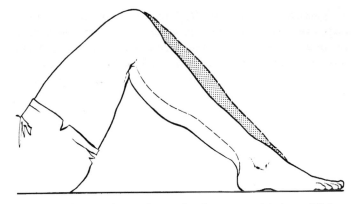

Fig. 29.11 Ruptured posterior cruciate ligament to right knee. With the athlete supine and both knees flexed to 90°, the injured knee will appear to sag posteriorly, with a dip in the infrapatellar region.

X-rays are necessary and the menisci need to be carefully assessed.

Treatment: Grade I. Following a short period of non-weightbearing (NWB), the athlete will have intensive treatment aimed at restoring full range of movement and quadriceps strength. Hamstring strengthening should be avoided, as the pull of the hamstring tendon may aggravate 'healing' PCL tissue or cause capsular damage. Co-contraction work to include hamstring activity is preferred. A return to running can be expected in four to six weeks but it is most important that the correct diagnosis be made early and accurately so that the optimal treatment to assist healing can take place. This lesion is often overlooked and athletes will continue having trouble with forceful kicking or rapid acceleration/deceleration. They will claim that squatting hurts and will have some swelling, but feel capable of participating in sport. Progression should be gradual in the first three weeks. The physiotherapist should aim to regain full flexion and then progress the athlete through strength, proprioceptive and skills work.

Treatment: Grade II. This injury will leave the athlete with some detectable instability both clinically and functionally. Three to six weeks of NWB and bracing is advised to 'settle' the joint before intensive rehabilitation can begin. In the first three to six weeks, treatment should be gentle, emphasizing quadriceps exercises, soft tissue work (including massage and ultrasound to the posterior capsule) and regaining full range of movement. Hamstring and calf stretches should be included. (In the early stage of rehabilitation, quadriceps work should be performed in a manner that does not allow for excessive external rotation in the 0–15° range as this will stress the healing ligament.) After this, full flexion, mobilization, quadriceps strengthening and proprioceptive skills can be pursued. The time span for return to sport is approximately nine to twelve weeks, depending on secondary knee joint damage, the strength of the quadriceps and the type of sport to be played. Isokinetic testing should be used to give an objective strength evaluation late in rehabilitation.

Treatment: Grade III. This is a severe injury which can cause significant joint changes. The knee will be visibly swollen and painful and the athlete will be unable to walk properly. Although this injury will leave the knee joint unstable, it is rarely reconstructed as, in the authors' opinion, long term reviews of this type of surgery have proven it to be unsuccessful. Other reasons for avoiding surgery are that PCL tears are not as symptomatically disabling as ACL instability, and there is less morbidity in PCL lesions. Clancy and Shelbourne (1983) demonstrated the need for acute repair or reconstruction based on patellofemoral and tibiofemoral changes that occur over a period of time. They reported a 90% incidence of medial femoral condylar articular injury in those athletes who had a symptomatic PCL deficient knee for longer than four years. As the secondary stabilizers (ITB, LCL and arcuate complex) lack normal integrity, the tibia drops posteriorly and changes begin in the medial femoral condyle, medial compartment and patellofemoral joint. Parolie and Bergfeld (1986) reported an 80% satisfaction rate among their athletes who were treated non-operatively for an isolated PCL tear. Keller et al (1993) studied a group of forty patients who completed a modified Noyes knee questionnaire. All had isolated PCL tears of approximately six years duration. They found that despite maintaining excellent muscular strength (assessed isokinetically) the patients developed significant symptoms and degenerative changes with increasing interval from injury.

Surgically, Noyes et al (1983) used an arthroscopic approach performed by placing a bone-patellar tendon-bone allograft, through isometrically placed tibial and femoral attachment sites, secured with screw fixation. This procedure requires a specific rehabilitation protocol and its long term results await full analysis. Until recently, however, surgical procedures have not been successful as degenerative changes develop in reconstructed knees that mimic the conservatively treated knee (Bianchi 1983).

The decision to reconstruct an acutely torn PCL depends therefore on the individual situation. It will usually take place in the PCL deficient knee of a car accident victim. If a conservative program has failed, a young person who wishes to pursue heavy work and stressful sports has clearer surgical indications than a person of middle age. If PCL injury is associated with medial or lateral ligament damage, surgery is indicated. However, the PCL must be reconstructed with augmentation unless the knee has a bony avulsion of the PCL that permits anatomic bone-to-bone fixation. The chances of a successful functional recovery in these cases is excellent.

Conservative management. The athlete's management will include non-weightbearing and possibly limited motion bracing for two to six weeks, followed by a graduated program of exercises. As mentioned earlier, the emphasis in rehabilitation will be on regaining full range of motion, quadriceps strength and proprioceptive skills. Depending on the sport, the athlete may be unable to play for three to six months and may have difficulty accelerating, decelerating, squatting, twisting, jumping or kicking, as the secondary stabilizing tissues of the knee may be stretched by the injury. Bracing may be necessary for sport and the athlete should be warned of future degenerative changes that take place in the joint if vigorous sport is attempted. Cycling and swimming, not long-distance running, is recommended to regain cardiovascular fitness. Isokinetic testing should be performed with the goal of achieving 100% quadriceps strength.

Other considerations. In regaining quadriceps strength, caution needs to be directed towards the patellofemoral joint which, due to the altered mechanics of the knee, can become inflamed during normal gait, running or quadriceps retraining. Although quadriceps strength is emphasized in rehabilitation, the final result for the athlete must include optimum co-contraction and proprioceptive skills for the knee. The athlete will also require simultaneous rehabilitation of the hamstring and calf complexes to provide 'total leg' strength.

Bracing. Braces provide functional support but few, if any, are designed to restrain posterior tibial subluxation. It will therefore be necessary to find a brace which gives a feeling of stability to the joint and enhances the athlete's proprioceptive skills. The 'Don Joy' brace and the Australian Hinged Knee brace are recommended. The latter utilizes neoprene material, metallic hinges and velcro attachments superiorly and inferiorly to give the functional support necessary, while the Don Joy relies on a four-point leverage system to minimize tibial displacement.

Posteromedial instability. Severe trauma, perhaps from skiing or a direct blow in football, is required to cause this lesion. In this situation, the medial tibial plateau rotates posteriorly in reference to the femur with medial opening. Structures involved include the MCL, posterior oblique ligament, ACL, medial portion of the posterior capsule and semimembranosus. A hyperextension valgus force can tear these structures, the ACL tearing before the posterior cruciate ligament, which is only mildly stretched. The resulting instability is a sagging backwards of the posteromedial corner of the tibia on the femur with valgus opening. There is disagreement in the orthopaedic world on the existence of this type of instability. This is due to the difficulty in accurately assessing the instability without placing the knee in the close-packed position (i.e. tibia internally rotated on a flexed knee). Unless the PCL is significantly damaged along with posterior capsular tearing, there will not be a 'drop back' in the medial compartment and diagnosis will need to be made based on accurate history, assessment skills and possibly arthroscopy.

Surgery for this instability is rarely presented in the literature, but when mentioned normally involves repair of the posteromedial corner and acute repair of the PCL if that is torn. The athlete is usually introduced to a conservative rehabilitation program, depending on the exact pathology and whether the lesion is acute or chronic. Unfortunately, long term conservative management results are not good. Degenerative changes will develop and functional activities may need to be modified as a result.

Lateral collateral ligament

Injury results from a blow to the medial aspect of the knee causing a hyperextension/varus deformity. It is seen in sports such as football, soccer and skiing. Damage to the LCL is less common than to the MCL. The LCL can be damaged in isolation or in combination with lateral meniscus lesions, superior tibiofibular ligament strains, anterior or posterior cruciate ligament damage and, in severe cases, peroneal nerve injury.

Assessment. As in assessing all acute knee trauma, hand positioning should support the joint so that the athlete can relax adequately. The knee should be given a varus stress both in full extension and in increasing degrees of flexion, asking the athlete where on the knee they can feel the pain. More severe damage to the LCL will result in rotary instability and several tests have been suggested for this pathology (see 'Knee assessment').

Treatment. In Grade I tears the athlete will initially be partial weightbearing and progress to full weightbearing within two weeks. They should wear a supportive bandage and begin quadriceps work immediately. As their range of movement increases, so does their rehabilitation, and full return to sport can be expected in three to four weeks.

Grade II tears will initially require a period of NWB. Return to sport will be four to six weeks. Grade I and II tears of the LCL produce good results after treatment and athletes normally proceed to their normal standard of activity.

Grade III injuries are usually associated with other injuries and may result in posterolateral instability. The tear requires operative repair followed by two to four weeks of non-weightbearing. While NWB the athlete will have the knee either immobilized or in a limited-motion cast. Return to sport may take fourteen to sixteen weeks, once full range of motion, total leg strength and functional skills have been regained.

The treatment of Grade III tears of the LCL progress through three stages:

- maximal protection stage. Over the first four weeks, treatment should include low dosage ultrasound and other pain relieving modalities, massage, hip and ankle strengthening, cycling in the painfree range, painfree quadriceps strengthening and NWB calf work.

- moderate protection stage. Depending on the degree of damage to the ligament, after four to eight weeks knee flexion and extension should approach full range and most of the soreness will be reduced. The athlete will be able to cycle and perform limited range resisted work and will be approaching full weightbearing. Hydrotherapy may begin, but caution is required with resisted hamstring work due to the fact that both the ligament and the lateral hamstrings attach to the fibular head.

- minimal protection stage (after six to eight weeks). Between 6 and 8 weeks, all forms of bracing should be removed and the athlete will be full weightbearing. The goal at this stage will be to restore the quadriceps and hamstrings to normal strength. This can be achieved by using plyometric exercises, isokinetic exercise, free weights and pulleys. Cycling and hydrotherapy become more vigorous and running begins near the end of this stage. Proprioceptive exercise such as balance boards should be included and general flexibility assessed.

If the quadriceps and hamstrings strength are approximately 100% using isokinetic assessment, the athlete should be performing functional/sporting skills. Some athletes may wish to use a knee brace for psychological support. Return to sport is possible when the knee is painfree, has no effusion or patellofemoral pain and is not giving way.

Surgical versus non-surgical approach. As with most knee ligament instabilities, several options exist, although it is acknowledged that reconstruction of this area is difficult (Gollehon et al 1987).

Conservative management needs to be comprehensive and able to provide adequate counterforce to the resultant pathomechanics. Without this muscular and proprioceptive focus, the athlete is likely to face degenerative joint changes, meniscal lesions and patellofemoral dysfunction. Prognosis is not good if there is a physiologically varus knee. The athlete must understand the importance of maintaining muscular strength long-term to get the best results.

Bracing. The brace selected will only be necessary in late rehabilitation of Grade III tears. In this case, the aim is to prevent varus external tibial rotation and hyperextension. Few braces are specifically designed for these needs. The athlete will require a hinged type brace with velcro attachments and, possibly, a patellar cut-out section for further comfort.

Guidelines for treating knee reconstructions

ACL injuries are debilitating and can cut short a promising athlete's career. It must be decided whether operative or non-operative treatment is indicated. Among the factors to be considered are:

- the acuteness of the injury
- other associated lesions involving the knee
- age and level of activity of the athlete
- the degree of instability
- the athlete's ability to comply with the therapeutic program.

The athlete may have an arthroscopy performed, where the cruciate stub is excised or trimmed, or may have a meniscal procedure.

Role of the ACL

The ACL is the primary stabilizer of the knee. It controls the rotation of the tibia on the femur as well as contributing to the control of anterior shear of the tibia on the femur, thereby protecting menisci and articular cartilage. Hence, the aims of any treatment program should be to train the athlete to be aware of and to control these accessory movements as best they can. Functional stability of the knee (Noyes et al 1984) can be achieved essentially by compensation through the neuromuscular system. It will depend on the degree of instability, the sport played, rehabilitation program including hamstring function and proprioception (Giove et al 1983, Noyes et al 1983).

It is important to regain a full, painless range of movement of the injured knee. However, the authors have found in some cases it is better not to stress the joint maximally to regain full extension, as this will allow some fibrosis to occur in the notch and around the ends of the ligament, which subsequently aids stability. Furthermore, the build-up of scar tissue causes part of the ACL to adhere to other joint structures, such as the PCL. The lack of femoral extension can, however, lead to latent PFJ problems.

Mechanism of injury

The ACL is predominantly injured in high velocity, twisting, pivoting sports such as Australian Rules football, American football, soccer, netball, basketball and skiing. A common mechanism is when a player is running and suddenly changes direction, often when accelerating or decelerating. When a player collides with another while weightbearing, various degrees of damage can occur. If a player is pivoting with their leg extended, body rotated and the knee in hyperextension or hit with valgus or varus stress, severe injury may occur.

Individuals with a small intercondylar notch are predisposed to ACL injury, as are those with increased accessory glide of the joint or generalized hypermobility. If the intercondylar notch is small the ACL may be sheared as it passes over the edge of the notch. This may explain why ACL rupture tends to occur in several members of the same family.

Surgical considerations

In order to rehabilitate the knee following reconstructive surgery, the authors believe certain information about the surgery should be understood. Orthopaedic surgeons' protocols vary considerably and, rather than look at numerous surgical procedures, the following information may enable a rehabilitation program to be safely and effectively managed. The physiotherapist should always check with the surgeon concerning constraints, such as when to weightbear or how quickly to progress range of motion. A review of the current literature illustrates certain important factors:

- immobilization has a negative impact on articular cartilage (Akeson 1961, Akeson et al 1968, Akeson et al 1980).
- extension from 30° of flexion to full extension has been shown to increase ACL stress dramatically, thereby jeopardizing surgical grafts (Paulos et al 1981, Arms et al 1984, Daniel et al 1982).
- of the autogenous materials available to surgeons, only a bone-patellar tendon-bone graft is considered to have sufficient strength to allow immediate full passive extension and flexion (Noyes et al 1984, Butler et al 1979).
- grafted structures never reach their pretransplanted strength levels (Oakes 1988).
- increased ACL stress occurs during quadriceps contraction with neutral and internal tibial rotation, where external tibial rotation shows less ACL stress (Renstrom et al 1986).
- with respect to weightbearing, knee stability should be enhanced by tibiofemoral compression, especially at full extension, where the knee is in a close-packed or locked position (Ohkoshi & Yasuda 1989, Shelbourne & Nitz 1990).
- Henning et al (1985) suggest we should be aware of elongation of the ACL which occurs with a variety of different activities (Fig. 29.10).
- operations on the ACL are more likely to be complicated by post-operative arthrofibrosis if the operation is done within two weeks of the injury, especially if the knee is operated on when acutely inflamed and the range of motion restricted (Shelbourne et al 1991).

The above information is important when it comes to determining rehabilitation programs for reconstructed knees. Other information must also be considered.

Type of graft. Is the graft autogenous tissue or synthetic tissue and is it intracapsular or extracapsular?

This information indicates when and how much force may be transmitted to the graft. Synthetic grafts will normally be rehabilitated quite quickly as the tissue does not have to re-establish a blood supply. With autogenous tissue, because of the nature of collagen maturation, most grafts will approach 50% of their previous tensile strength by one year (Oakes 1988). However, Shelbourne and Nitz (1990) found that transplanted tissue remained consistently viable, attaining maximum fibroblast size and number by the sixth post-operative month. It should be known if the operation performed used the patellar tendon, hamstring tendons, iliotibial band or pes insertion.

Arthroscopic versus open operation. These days many reconstructions are performed via the arthroscope, resulting in decreased morbidity because the knee joint itself is less affected. Less swelling and a quicker return of movement are common in these cases, and the patellofemoral joint does not suffer as much stiffness.

Fixation. Has the graft been fixed by staples, by sutures or by other devices? The work of Robertson et al (1986) and Kurosaka et al (1987) examined fixation of bone and soft tissues grafts and showed that placing interference-fit screws between the bone plugs of the graft and the wall of the tunnel, and fixing the soft tissue with a screw and a spike washer, were superior to fixing with staples and sutures.

Casting. Was the knee in a plaster or a brace? Was the knee cast or braced in flexion or in full extension? Was continuous passive motion (CPM) used in hospital and for how long? This information should indicate if flexion or extension will be slow to return to normal. The information is important if the surgeon requires range of motion quickly, especially extension, as neglecting extension can lead to a fixed flexion deformity.

Surgeon's requirement. Is extension allowed to be pushed? Can the quadriceps be worked in the inner range? Is full range of motion by four months a requirement? What about hamstrings emphasis over quadriceps? In the late 1980s and early 1990s there have been three types of operations performed to correct anterior knee instability, especially anterolateral rotary instability, using autogenous tissue. They are:

- Losee anterolateral knee reconstruction
- patellar tendon reconstruction
- hamstring tendon reconstruction.

Pre-operation management

Before knee reconstruction, particularly if the operation is being performed on a chronically unstable knee, it is important to maximize the condition of the athlete's muscles. Where possible, an isokinetic muscle test should be performed and tests for laxity documented. Just prior to surgery the athlete should be educated on what to expect and what exercises to perform in the immediate post-operative period. Appropriate exercises include static quadriceps, straight leg raising and isometric hamstring work.

General physiotherapy treatment guidelines

Treatment initially should be directed towards mobilizing scar tissue and the patellofemoral joint itself. Mobilization also helps to loosen up tight associated structures, such as the popliteal fossa and hamstrings. Massage can help in the early phases. Flexion is often required early, and a good way to assist this is by using an exercise bike in an arc of motion at the limit of flexion, or by using moist heatpacks or a hot spa with gentle active exercises at the limit of range of motion.

Progression will depend on the issues discussed above. Although the authors are loath to present recipes, given the diversity of approaches in surgery and in rehabilition, some guidelines may be of assistance.

When to start weightbearing? Weightbearing is commenced any time within the first four weeks of surgery. Shelbourne and Nitz (1990) permit athletes to begin full weightbearing as soon as possible after a bone-patellar ligament-bone graft, with no detrimental effects.

When to start swimming? Hydrotherapy should be commenced when partial weightbearing is achieved, and can involve hip strengthening and range of movement exercises, partial weightbearing (PWB) or NWB. Kicking with a kickboard can also be performed.

It is important to remember associated muscle groups such as calf, hamstrings, hip abductors and adductors. They will require stretching when tight and general strengthening.

Specific protocols

The following protocols are based on rehabilitation programs developed by physiotherapists in conjunction with surgeons. The protocols serve as guidelines only. Each athlete should progress individually depending upon the type of surgery, assessment of range of motion, pain, presence of swelling or effusion, state of joint surfaces, muscle control, stability and proprioception.

In the authors' opinion, hamstring tendon grafts and the predominantly arthroscopic approaches result in less morbidity. The patellofemoral joint does not lose as much mobility, and normal range of movement returns more quickly. Stability of the grafts will, however, be under close scrutiny as these athletes often return to full sporting participation within six months.

The extracapsular repairs tend to work well on athletes with chronic insufficiency, but require more restraint on movement and exercises to enable the reconstruction to reach it's full post-operative strength. As a result, rehabilitation should take place over six to nine months.

Patellar tendon reconstructions are accepted as the strongest graft, but they cause greater morbidity because of the anterior surgical approach. Sensory difficulties often result. Range of motion is often slow to recover, and the patellofemoral joint remains stiffer to mobilize.

Extracapsular reconstruction

Losee anterolateral knee reconstruction. In this procedure the middle third of the iliotibial band is harvested, placed through a bony tunnel in the lateral femoral condyle and stabilized. It is then reflected through a tunnel created between the lateral capsule and lateral collateral ligament and attached to the proximal lateral tibia. Medial advancement of the medial collateral ligament may be used if there is significant medial ligament laxity (anteromedial rotary instability). This type of reconstruction requires a distinct regime of protection and involves a more conservative rehabilitation (Table 29.2).

Intra-articular patellar tendon reconstruction. In this procedure the middle third of the patellar tendon is used with a piece of the patella attached. It is routed through the tibia, upwards and laterally into the lateral femoral condyle where the bone block is fixed into the tunnel with a screw. The graft should be isometric in all ranges of motion.

Table 29.2 Physiotherapy rehabilitation protocol

Maximum protection phase (0-6 weeks)
- non-weightbearing
- isometric quads at 60° of flexion
- CPM 1-6 weeks
- 0-60° movement in a brace
- patella mobilizing in all directions of movement

Moderate protection phase (6-10 weeks)
- 0-90° range of motion in a brace
- full weightbearing by 10 weeks
- patella mobilizing and gentle static quadriceps with brace on
- walking in the water at 6 weeks, gentle kicking with both legs
- cycling with a high seat

Minimal protection phase (10-26 weeks)
- cease brace at 14 weeks
- co-contraction when standing
- weights for hamstrings, prevent knee falling into full extension
- hamstrings in prone on isokinetic device at 10 weeks
- at 14 weeks commence resisted quadriceps isometrics at 45°-90° of flexion and commence closed kinetic chain exercises for hip flexors, adductors and extensors. Also retrain pes anserinus and semimembranosus to act as internal rotators after anteromedial reconstruction. Closed kinetic chain exercises are appropriate at this stage because they will not cause shearing stresses on the knee joint as they are performed with the knee in a closed packed position.
- review at 6 months with an isokinetic assessment
- maximal hamstring work at 16 weeks

Retraining phase (26-36 weeks)
- full range of motion should be achieved at 26 weeks
- commence resisted quads 20-0°. If quads 75% of the uninjured leg and hamstrings 90%, jogging can commence at 26 weeks. Work on a high hams/quads ratio and a quadriceps equal to 90% at the 9-12 month stage
- at 26 to 30 weeks isokinetic assessment should be performed

---

In this procedure the knee is in full extension with a resting splint and no range of motion restraints (the benefit of this is that in the last 5° of knee extension there is no load on the new graft).

Physiotherapy rehabilitation. There is still no consensus on how much protection the healing reconstruction should actually receive in the first few weeks after surgery. Some surgeons choose to have their athletes full weightbearing with no bracing from day one. Others maintain some external bracing for up to six weeks. In the authors' opinion this issue is one where the physiotherapist should follow the surgeon's advice.

Rehabilitation is commenced, ensuring that full range of extension is obtained. At ranges of 5-30°of knee flexion no loading should occur, hence quadriceps exercise as a straight leg raise is permitted, providing a quadriceps lag does not exist. Emphasis should be on gaining good static quadriceps contraction producing a superior patellar glide. A 'continuous passive motion' (CPM) machine is used from day one to day four when the athlete may be discharged non-weightbearing on crutches, doing static quadriceps and gentle knee flexion in sitting .

0-4 weeks. For the next four weeks, CPM should be used three times per week. Quadriceps are stimulated using a muscle stimulator if necessary, and weightbearing is steadily increased. If a splint is worn it should be phased out as quadriceps control is gained. Wound care and massage should be performed as appropriate, along with patellofemoral joint mobilization. Gait re-education, ensuring extension and quadriceps contraction in stance phase, is necessary.

4- 6 weeks. Active hamstrings 0-90° is performed in prone. Extension should be performed 90-0° passively. An exercise bike is commenced after 4 weeks as comfortable.

At 6 weeks. Closed kinetic chain exercise is commenced in or out of a brace eg. step-ups onto a low box (see Fig. 29.12). Closed kinetic chain exercise controls anterior tibial translation in the pre-loaded knee by the interactive effects of compressive forces and the congruent articular surfaces (Howell et al 1990).

Exercises at 90° flexion for the vastus medialis oblique (VMO) (as described in Ch. 30) should be started.

6-12 weeks. Resisted quadriceps work at 90-60° of flexion can be commenced. No inner range exercises should be performed. Range of movement from full extension to 125° flexion should be expected. Proprioceptive work on a wobble board or mini-trampoline should be included.

12-20 weeks. Jogging in a straight line can be commenced, as long as there are no complications. Hamstring work on an isokinetic device in prone knee flexion over a variety of speeds of movement may be commenced (see velocity spectrum in Ch. 17). Leg press exercises, such as rowing and the stepper (Fig. 29.13) should now be used.

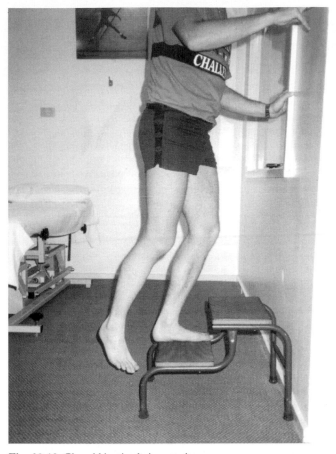

Fig. 29.12 Closed kinetic chain exercise

20-26 weeks. Commence resisted straight leg raise and solo sports such as wall tennis or handball. Increased functional activities, such as skipping, weaving while running and acceleration-deceleration drills can also be introduced.

26-40 weeks. Full isokinetic spectrum training, jumping, twisting, turning and free weights for quadriceps, both as leg extensor and leg press can occur at this stage.

Intra-articular hamstring tendon reconstruction

This procedure uses the semitendinosis and an adductor muscle (usually gracilis). The tendons are harvested and placed through drill holes in the tibia and femur duplicating the anatomical insertion of the ACL and incorporating any of the synovial sheath covering the ACL to aid in its revascularization. A portion of the iliotibial band (ITB) may be used according to the characteristics of the initial injury (e.g. if the surgeon feels that the hamstring tendons harvested are insufficient to stabilize the joint). The ITB is made into a tube and taken from the lateral femoral condyle into the same canal as the other tendons. This creates a double or triple bundle of tissue and hence a reasonably substantial support. A notch arthroplasty may be performed to prevent abrasion occurring in the notch.

Physiotherapy rehabilitation. The aim is to achieve 0-90° of knee flexion in the first two to four weeks post-surgery. Active assisted exercises using the uninjured leg (avoiding hyperextension), leg weights and forceful quadriceps contraction in the last 30° of flexion should commence.

There is an additional two to four weeks protection post-surgery, usually with a brace in a fixed position, if the meniscus is repaired, or with an associated medial or lateral collateral ligament repair.

2-4 weeks. Quadriceps should be exercised isometrically at angles 90-60° of flexion and in sitting with the knee flexed to 80° for VMO (see Ch. 30). Muscle stimulation should be used if there is difficulty initiating quadriceps. Prone knee bending and single leg bridging should occur, as should weaning off crutches (if required post-operatively) and wearing a brace instead. An anti-rotational brace for two to three months after surgery is favoured by some surgeons, but most now favour a light compression bandage only. If crutches are used then partial weightbearing between crutches (Henning et al 1985) can be commenced (at approximately two weeks) following surgery once active assisted terminal extension is achieved.

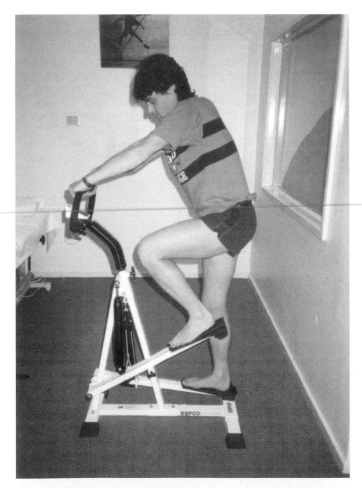

Fig. 29.13 Leg press exercise 'stepper'

4-8 weeks. Wall sits can be commenced from 0–45°. At four weeks early proprioceptive training is started, initially by standing on one leg, then with eyes closed and later with wobble board. Pulley work for abductors, adductors and hip extensors commenced

6-12 weeks. Closed kinetic chain step-ups (Fig. 29.12) and resisted quadriceps work at 90-60° of flexion can be commenced. Bike riding, if range of motion is restricted, can be used at six weeks, but if a notch arthroplasty has been performed, full bike work should be avoided until twelve weeks due to the abrasion sensitivity of the graft.

12-16 weeks. After three months knee extension work can be commenced on an isokinetic device using the anti-shear device (Fig. 29.14). Short arc movements from 90-60° graduating to full range at four months. Single leg squats 45-60° commence.

16-24 weeks. Resisted quadriceps exercise by extension through full range should not be done in the first four months as this has been shown to create significant elongation force in the ACL (Henning et al 1985, Paulos et al 1981). If the surgeon permits, these exercises are commenced at sixteen weeks.

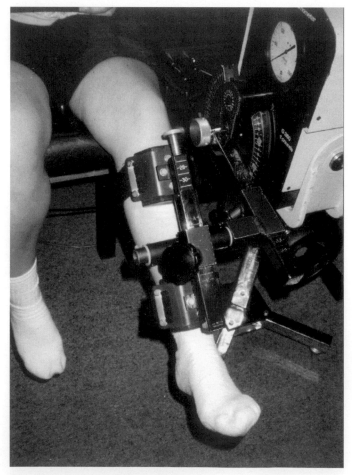

Fig. 29.14 Johnson anti-shear device

24 weeks. Full isokinetic evaluation can be performed between six and nine months, depending on knee stability at that stage (if the surgeon is happy with the clinical stability).

36 weeks. Later rehabilitation should consist of single leg long jump, grapevine running and cutting. This should be repeated with ball control and increased distraction to improve reflex control.

36-52 weeks. High-speed contact sports requiring deceleration, pivot twisting and rapid change of direction are not appropriate until nine to twelve months. However, for professional athletes, if objective isokinetic assessment is at least 90% of the uninjured leg's quadriceps, sports are often performed as early as six months. Tennis, squash and running sports are begun between six and twelve months (Table 29.3).

Direct repair of ACL

Direct repair of the torn ACL is attempted in certain cases. It is recognized that the results of repairs of an intra-substance tear of the ACL with sutures are technically inferior to the results of other operative procedures (Engebretsen et al 1989, Sgaglione et al 1990).

If there has been an avulsion tear of the ligament then the bony fragment is often screwed back into place. Once bony healing is complete (about six weeks) rehabilitation can commence. The knee is usually immobilized and the knee range of motion will be restricted. Hence, use of heat, mobilization of patellofemoral joint and, after eight weeks, extension mobilization of the tibiofemoral joint should be commenced. The quadriceps should be strengthened gradually, with full range isotonic loading taking place at about twelve weeks.

Usually, insubstance ACL tears are not repaired directly but in cases of multiple trauma, e.g. partial dislocation of the knee joint in motor vehicle accidents or extreme sporting trauma, direct repair using suture is attempted. In these cases, immobilization may be lengthy while other structures heal and rehabilitation will be slow. Hence, no restraints are placed on the rehabilitation except by the athlete's pain threshold. All efforts should be made after immobilization has ceased to regain a functional range of motion. If the secondary stabilizing tissues of the knee have been severely damaged extra stability may be given to the repair by autogenous augmentation.

Prosthetic knee ligament reconstruction

Through the 1980s and into the 1990s a number of prosthetic materials were used, including dacron, goretex and carbon fibre. Rehabilitation in knees using these materials is generally faster because no reliance is placed on revascularization when compared with autogenous reconstruction. The failure rate of prosthetic ligaments

Table 29.3   Return to sport guidelines

At the end of rehabilitation and before returning to sport the following points should be noted:
- define which knee movements (e.g. twisting, turning, hopping) occur in the performance of the sport
- progress the activities gradually, building on a functional progression (i.e. walk then run, then twist, then hop etc.)
- ensure all functional activities have been performed at training before return to playing
- ensure both concentric and eccentric quadriceps function are at least 90% when tested on an isokinetic device
- assess the athlete's performance in the field (not just the ability to perform the task but how well it is done) e.g. hop height and length compared with the good leg, weight transference and bearing with high speed change of direction activity, and ability to slow down and accelerate rapidly
- assess the athlete's psychological preparedness e.g. do they feel confident enough to play
- always be sure that the injured tissue has reached the required state of collagen maturation (if surgery has been performed, speak to the surgeon)
- assess whether any of advanced functional activities have created joint soreness, swelling or loss of movement.

remains a problem, however. Fatigue, fretting and wear have resulted in an unacceptably high rate of failure (Olson et al 1988), and the likelihood of the ligament functioning for longer than five years is low. In the authors' opinion, a prosthetic ligament reconstruction is generally performed on a player who does not intend to play high velocity rotational sports for more than another five years.

Physiotherapy guidelines

3-4 days following surgery
- isometric quadriceps and hamstrings
- straight leg raises

2-4 weeks
- hot whirlpool spa, range of movement exercises, such as active assisted flexion (sliding heel to buttock in supine lying), prone knee bending and prone extension with leg lowering over edge of bed
- hip abduction and adduction
- stationary bike
- terminal quadriceps over fulcrum
- leg curls in standing, graduating to greater resistance at six weeks
- isotonic extension exercises with light weights progressing to isokinetic exercises. Gradual return to activities in a functional progression, with full sport at eight to ten weeks.

Conservative physiotherapy management of ACL

Initially, if arthroscopy has been performed, massage to the portals is needed. This will help to desensitize the tender area and subsequently aid regaining full proprioceptive capabilities. The patellofemoral joint should be cared for by mobilization. Taping may be necessary if the symptoms are persistent. As mentioned earlier, tibiofemoral mo-

bilization should not be forced unless it is obvious that pain is due to lack of effective full, passive extension of the knee.

In athletes who present with a positive pivot shift, resisted eccentric tibial external rotation with knee flexion should be commenced immediately. This can be performed with the athlete prone, and resistance provided against the leg as it extends from 90–0° of flexion.

Home exercises should be commenced immediately and include the following:

- bridging
- supine knee extension combined with hip extension
- prone SLR and hamstring curls
- abduction and adduction
- hamstrings and quadriceps co-contraction in standing
- resisted external rotation in knee flexion with rubbers (Fig. 29.15)
- standing knee flexion with hip extension

Strengthening work, especially for the hamstrings, is vital as isometric hamstrings contraction is reported to decrease strain in the ACL (Renstrom et al 1986). If an isokinetic device is available then its use in prone lying is a good idea. It is advisable to use an anti-shear device, which controls shear of the tibia on the femur, by placing two pads proximally and distally on the tibia when forcefully extending the knee. It is used initially only to 20° of knee

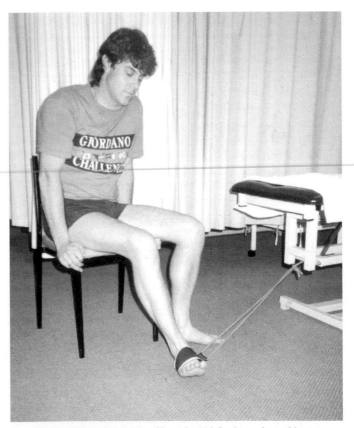

Fig. 29.15   External rotation of knee in 90° flexion using rubber resistance

flexion, gradually increasing to full extension. Lavin and Gross (1990) have shown that tibial translation is less when using the Johnson anti-shear accessory.

Leg press exercises, where the quadriceps are working while the axis of the knee is moving in a translatory motion, are very good exercises as the hamstrings co-contract with the quadriceps (Fig. 29.13).

Proprioception

The athlete should use a wobble board or mini-trampoline, first on two legs with hamstring/quadriceps co-contraction, then on one leg, and ultimately with body rotation on a fixed knee. The degree of difficulty can be increased by the athlete catching a ball while balancing on one leg. Walla et al (1985) have shown that in the ACL deficient knee retraining muscles and altering of technique in those activities involving rapid change in direction, may allow highly motivated people to perform most activities with a decreased risk of injury.

The trampoline is a useful proprioceptive tool. Jumps on one leg can be performed with hamstring/quadriceps co-contraction on landing. This may progress to jumping in the air clockwise and counterclockwise, again landing on the ground. Eventually, jumps can be made from the trampoline to the ground to effect further functional control of the translatory motion of tibia on femur.

Progressions to functional proprioceptive training:

* hop
* jump forward (where control of the forward translation of the tibia is needed)
* jump from height
* standing long jump
* run
* S-bend
* figure-eight
* deceleration to help control the forward translation that occurs in these athletes (Henning et al 1985)
* run downhill
* train with a ball to increase distraction
* plyometric exercises involving jumping onto and off a box or step will help build strength and stamina. With plyometric exercise of this nature the physiotherapist must be careful to assess the patellofemoral joint. Should there be associated problems with this joint the exercise should not be performed.

Other field exercises can include one-leg hops, grapevine running and running with 360° turns. These exercises may be repeated with ball control, or another player applying pressure for the turning manoeuvres. It is important to practise movements that need to be performed in a game (i.e. running backwards, jumping, cutting etc).

The physiotherapist should discuss with the athlete options that may decrease the risk of further ACL injury, such as changing their position on the field of play (e.g. defence to attack), or even changing their chosen sport (e.g. contact or team sport to a non-contact sport).

ACL damage and children

In the authors' opinion ACL deficient knees in children recover spontaneously without surgery. Children appear to have the capacity to develop advanced neuromuscular patterns to compensate for any functional instability.

Conservative vs surgical vs no treatment

With ACL injuries that persistently give way there is no formal rehabilitation, the menisci will eventually sustain damage. As the secondary restraints become overstressed and muscles weaken, articular cartilage lesions develop, leading to a degree of osteoarthritis (Noyes et al 1983).

If the athlete has an ACL deficient knee which does not lead to functional giving way then, in the authors' opinion, there is no evidence to show major deterioration of the joint surfaces. Normally, function can be achieved with a combination of quadriceps and hamstring strengthening, proprioceptive skills, modification of activity and braces (Giove et al 1983)

If the knee is slow to mobilize following reconstruction, particularly into extension, and an athlete has been weightbearing for several months, it is likely the patellofemoral joint will create ongoing problems. If extension is slow to return, the tibiofemoral joint surfaces may develop osteochondral or chondral damage.

Functional ability in any of these cases may be impaired and depends on many factors, including:

* type of reconstruction
* type and length of immobilization
* extent of rehabilitation and when it began
* type of sport played after rehabilitation.

With MCL injuries, if a grade III MCL tear is not repaired, provided it is braced for six weeks with movement allowed from 20-60° then full function is likely to return. If not treated at all severe deficits may occur, particularly when the athlete turns or twists. The knee may give way medially with the likelihood of tears to the medial meniscus or ACL.

PCL ruptures are usually treated with a conservative program of vigorous quadriceps strengthening. If there is severe functional impairment thereafter, surgery is indicated. Joint changes are likely in the long term.

MUSCULOTENDINOUS INJURIES

Iliotibial band

This important stabilizing structure has a role in the running motion and may occasionally become inflamed, usually due to excessive friction of the band pulling across the lateral femoral condyle during knee extension and flexion.

Many surgeons have advocated use of the ITB as an ACL substitute in both extra-articular and intra-articular reconstructive procedures. This is primarily because of its strategic location and dynamic contribution to the knee through the tensor fascia lata and gluteus maximus (Slocum et al 1976). It has several layers: superficial, medial, deep and capsulo-osseous. It attaches to the lateral intermuscular septum, including the vastus lateralis, lateral femoral condyle, lateral capsular ligament, proximal tibia at Gerdy's tubercle and fibula. It also receives an expansion along its capsulo-osseous layer from the short head of the biceps (Terry et al 1986).

The ITB is an important static lateral support of the knee, although it has other roles. In the final 30° of knee extension, it is an active knee extensor. With flexion greater than 30°, the ITB takes the role of flexor or decelerator of knee extension. Beyond 30° of flexion it can exert external rotation on the upper tibia, along with the long and short heads of the biceps femoris.

The ITB is almost always a victim of overuse rather than direct trauma, and athletes usually present for treatment when damage is significant. Minor ITB pathology or inflammation is usually tolerated by athletes, who continue their sport with a tender lateral knee region. The tenderness progressively worsens with exercise however, leading eventually to an inability to continue sport.

Assessment. Stretching the tensor fascia lata and ITB will rarely cause pain over the lateral knee area. It is more likely that the athlete will feel stretching to the lateral thigh and hip (see Ch. 28).

Specific diagnosis is by palpation and elimination of adjacent soft tissue pathologies, commonly to the lateral meniscus. Deep to the ITB there is a bursa which may become inflamed. In acute stages or chronic flare-ups, the athlete may limp into the clinic.

It is difficult to reproduce ITB pain clinically, but in the acute stages the athlete should be examined in side-lying (good side underneath) and then instructed to abduct the hip 30°. The athlete is then instructed to flex and extend the knee. This will reproduce lateral knee pain. Hyper-extension may elicit ITB pain in a nasty flare-up, although this pain may be bursitic in origin as the bursa is compressed against the femoral condyle.

Another test that can confirm the diagnosis is that of flexing the athlete's knee to 90° and placing the examiner's finger over the ITB, just proximal to the lateral femoral epicondyle. The knee is gradually extended and at approximately 30° of flexion, as the ITB crosses over the lateral epicondyle, pain is reproduced.

Treatment. Treatment should be directed towards a stretching program, particularly of the ITB, rectus femoris, vastus lateralis, hamstrings and gluteus maximus. Ice massage and local treatments of TENS and laser should initially be used. Treatment can progress to ultrasound and frictional massage.

In stubborn cases it may be necessary to infiltrate the tender area with local anaesthetic and steroid. Finally, if there is no response, some physicians may recommend a transverse surgical release of the band, proximal to the lateral femoral condyle. This can be done percutaneously or via a 5 cm incision which exposes the band. Its posterior border is then divided transversely at the level of the epicondyle. Recovery from surgery takes approximately six to twelve weeks.

Other considerations. Leg length asymmetry, and hip/lumbar spine pathology or stiffness, muscle tightness and imbalance. The physiotherapist should advise the athlete regarding sport frequency, surfaces (if running) and inclines (if cycling). On return to sport it is strongly recommended there be a slow build-up in intensity and frequency, and the area should be iced following participation. If surgical release is not successful there may be a large bursa between the epicondyle and ITB that requires infiltration or removal.

Differential diagnosis. It is important to eliminate the following alternative diagnoses with this syndrome:

- lateral meniscal injury
- popliteus tendinitis
- patellofemoral pain
- biceps femoris tendinitis.

ITB friction syndrome may be confused with lateral meniscus pathology but in the former McMurray's test will be negative. ITB syndrome is situated more superiorly and anteriorly than popliteus lesions. Patellofemoral pain is more anterior. Biceps femoris lesions will usually be painful with resisted knee flexion. This does not happen with ITB syndrome.

Predisposing risk factors and sports. Excessively worn shoes and varus deformity at the knee, along with prolonged running on a sloping surface (camber on roads), may contribute. A thorough assessment of leg and pelvic biomechanics is necessary as well as correction of foot-related anomalies. Examples include increased lateral tilting of the pelvis and marked subtalar pronation.

Infrapatellar tendinitis

Jumper's knee, or infrapatellar tendinitis, is a strain of the patellar tendon at its insertion into the inferior pole of the patella. The problem occurs predominantly in jumping sports, such as volleyball and basketball, but can be traumatic in origin. The injury often begins insidiously, gradually worsening as participation in sport is continued. By the time the athlete presents, the pathology is often well established, making the condition resistant to treatment.

This places a large emphasis on athlete education. Aggravation is caused by jumping, squatting or step up/step downs.

Assessment. When assessing this condition in the acute stage, a quadriceps contraction will reproduce pain, and palpation is diagnostic. Often the rectus femoris is tight. Occasionally, in severe cases, resisted ankle dorsiflexion will elicit pain. There may be a place for ultrasonography in chronic cases of jumper's knee to determine the extent of damage (Fritschy & Gautard 1988).

Management. This is not just a local inflammatory condition and we must consider strength, flexibility and the biomechanics of the whole limb in determining appropriate management.

Initially, treatment should be directed at decreasing inflammation. Hence ice massage is applied directly to the inferior pole. Magnetic field therapy and local laser treatment can relieve pain and are useful when attempting to keep an athlete competing. Rest has no place in active management, because the athlete with this injury usually plays regularly and rest will only cause atrophy of quadriceps and tightness of all associated muscle groups. In addition, activities can be performed that do not exacerbate the condition, such as controlled functional quadriceps strengthening.

A stretching program for the rectus femoris, hamstrings and iliotibial band should be initiated if painless (Somner 1981). Strength should be assessed functionally and managed with a graded eccentric program incorporating all aspects of the particular sport, hence most work will be weightbearing (Yamaguchi & Zajac 1989). Eccentric exercises, first in lying then in standing (i.e. 1/4 squats followed by step-downs gradually increasing the height of the step).

Running should be commenced (once 1/4 squat is painless) on a mini-trampoline. This should be followed with on-the-spot running then some double leg jumping. Eventually single leg jumping should be attempted.

It should be noted that sometimes biomechanical influences are involved and assessment of the foot and of pelvic control and stability should be made. Taping of the patella inferiorly, or use of an infrapatellar strap, can be beneficial if the condition is slow to respond (Fig. 29.16).

Other considerations. Stubborn cases may require infiltration with steroid. In chronic cases surgical intervention may be warranted.

Differential diagnosis. Infrapatellar tendinitis can be confused with injury to the infrapatellar fat pad. Diagnosis should be made with jumper's knee exhibiting exquisite pain at the inferior pole of the patella. This will not be the case with fat pad syndrome. Also, in the authors' experience, fat pad lesions will be painful on forced passive extension of the knee. Patellofemoral joint pain can masquerade as patellar tendinitis, and patellofemoral joint problems may

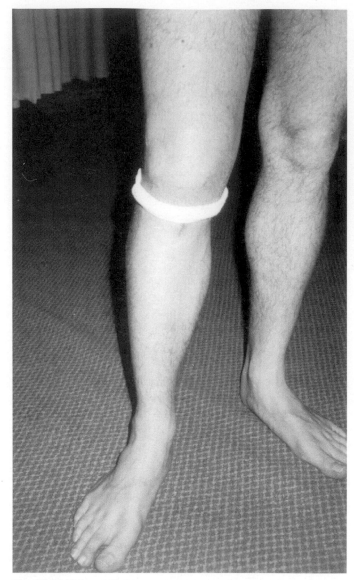

Fig. 29.16 Infra-patellar strap

initiate or contribute to a large number of patellar tendinitis cases.

Predisposing risk factors and sports. Jumper's knee usually develops in sports such as volleyball, basketball and netball. Running uphill is also a risk activity, as is rowing, where excessive stress is placed on the insertion of the patellar tendon. Rehabilitation must be sport-specific and eight to twelve weeks on a conservative rehabilitation program should be allowed before deciding if the treatment is a failure.

Popliteus

The popliteus muscle runs from the posterior surface of the tibia and is attached by its tendon into the lateral surface of the lateral condyle of the femur, just below the epicondyle, and to the posterior margin of the lateral meniscus. It unlocks the knee from the position of full extension by internally rotating the tibia on the femur. The popliteus can be injured at its insertion on the femur or in the belly of the muscle. It is most commonly injured in running sports. The athlete will describe pain on pushing off into a sprint, slowing down, or sometimes when twisting on an extended knee. The muscle is also a decelerator, involved in eccentric control of the knee (with the hamstrings), so an athlete may complain of pain when running downhill.

Assessment. Pain may be reproduced on contraction of the muscle. This is best tested with the athlete lying supine, the hip flexed, abducted and externally rotated and the knee at right angles. The examiner then firmly resists active flexion of the knee with one hand while palpating the tendon just posterior to the LCL with the other. Active knee extension, as well as resisted internal rotation of the tibia on the femur, may be painful.

With the leg in a cross-legged position the tendon's insertion will be exposed and tenderness may be felt just above the lateral joint line, in the posterolateral corner of the knee joint, just posterior to the lateral collateral ligament.

Treatment. In the early stages local electromedical treatment to the popliteal fossa as well as to the lateral insertion is necessary. Later, frictional massage is very useful. Manual techniques of extension mobilization assisted by active extension exercises should be performed. Calf and hamstring stretches are necessary and advisable. Functional exercises, such as practising deceleration and sudden take off manouevres help prepare the injured area for sporting involvement.

Other considerations. Local steroid infiltration can help decrease stubborn tenderness over the insertion.

Differential diagnosis. Popliteus tendinitis can be confused with lateral meniscal injury or iliotibial band syndrome. Careful palpation will help confirm the diagnosis. As mentioned above, popliteus tendinitis elicits tenderness above the lateral joint in the posterolateral corner of the knee joint and in the author's opinion there are some instances of non-specific posterior knee pain.

With a lateral meniscal tear, McMurray's test will be positive and there will be a history of a twisting incident; in degenerative meniscal tears this is not always the case.

Predisposing risk factors and sports. The problem occurs most in track athletes and cross-country runners, although footballers during pre-season training on hard grounds are also susceptible, as are those performing acceleration/deceleration activities. Other athletes at risk are those who are poorly prepared, do repeated deep squats, or have tight hamstrings and calves.

According to Mayfield (1977), of thirty athletes diagnosed with this condition, fifteen gave running or jogging as the cause and six attributed it to extensive walking. There appears to be a strong correlation between popliteus tendinitis and running or walking downhill, although the biomechanical basis is not fully understood. Mayfield (1977) suggests that the popliteus may help retard the lateral femoral condyle from rotating forward off the lateral tibial plateau when moving downhill.

Biceps femoris tendinitis

This inflammatory condition may occur at any part of the biceps femoris tendon. In children the tendon is more likely to be tender near its insertion behind the knee, whereas in adults tenderness is towards the junction of the middle and lower thirds.

Injury may be caused by any sport that requires repetitive knee flexion activities or sustained knee flexion positioning. This includes swimming, running, skiing, cycling and sports which involve running backwards. Downhill running is another aggravating activity, due to the eccentric loading on the biceps tendon.

Assessment. Hamstring flexibility may not be affected, but in severe acute cases crepitus will be detected during active flexion. Resisted knee flexion and palpation will be painful and some thickening may be felt. Full passive knee flexion may be uncomfortable due to compression of inflamed tissue. Squatting may be painful and after prolonged sitting, the athlete may limp for a few steps.

Treatment. Electrotherapy, US, interferential therapy (IFT) and TENS are useful. Anti-inflammatory medication should be used acutely, then gentle massage commenced. The physiotherapist should determine, if possible, why the injury is unilateral. The gluteals and calf muscles require assessment for strength and flexibility. Resisted hamstring work is not recommended in early rehabilitation, but is included in the later stages, especially if the knee has a rotary instability. Stretching of the hamstrings and sometimes slump stretching may be necessary (see Ch. 33).

Other considerations

- This injury can be confused with popliteus inflammation if the pathology is near the insertion of the tendon.
- In some cases the athlete may have bursitis deep to the insertion of the tendon.
- Swimming can aggravate the injury if the kick action is too vigorous.

Differential diagnosis. It is important to eliminate the following alternative diagnoses with this condition:

- superior tibiofibular joint damage
- iliotibial band friction syndrome
- lateral meniscal tear
- biceps femoris bursitis
- lumbar referred pain
- dural tightness.

Quadriceps tendon injury

Any injury to the extensor mechanism of the knee results in rapid loss of quadriceps bulk and strength, especially of the vastus medialis.

The quadriceps tendon may be partially torn or ruptured in sports involving rapid extension against a resistance (e.g. football). It may also tear when falling suddenly if holding a maximum quadriceps contraction and the knee flexes eccentrically (as in skiing). The tear is usually at its insertion to the superior pole of the patella. Inflammatory disorders can occur at this site, usually in the older athlete, and are treated with non-steroid anti-inflammatory drugs (NSAIDs), transverse friction massage and graduated stretching exercises.

Assessment. In partial tears, the quadriceps contraction will be painful and the athlete will be unable to squat, hop, run or resist a strong force while trying to flex the already extended knee. Both partial and complete tears will be painful to palpate, and flexion will be limited.

Diagnosis of a rupture will be made from the athlete's description of a loud 'crack' followed by giving way of the knee and an inability to walk. The suprapatellar area will be swollen and contraction of the quadriceps will be painful and weak. In case of a rupture the knee jerk test will be negative, indicating a loss of integrity of the tendon.

Management. The speed at which the program progresses depends on the degree of pain and nature of the tear. This can be assessed with ultrasound. Partial tears require a graduated physiotherapy program. Initially treatment is directed at tendon healing, pain, swelling reduction and gentle quadriceps activity. Within the first week painfree flexion work is begun, along with massage and partial weightbearing. From two to four weeks the intensity of the quadriceps work, knee flexion activities and deep massage increase. Swimming and cycling will be part of the program, but no speed resisted work should be included until four to six weeks. Eccentric exercise, running, squatting, squat-jumping etc. should begin in six to eight weeks. The athlete must regain full strength and flexibility in the quadriceps and 'explosive' contractile ability.

Following rupture an orthopaedic surgeon may need to repair the lesion. This will be followed by a period of immobilization and graduated rehabilitation. Full return to sport will be achieved in twelve to twenty weeks.

Besides ensuring that the athlete has full flexibility, functional skills and no pain, the physiotherapist may wish to perform a strength and endurance test on isokinetic equipment.

BURSAE

The six main bursae of the knee area are the prepatellar, biceps femoris, infrapatellar, superficial infrapatellar, pes anserinus and semimembranosus bursae. All can become inflamed as a result of overuse or a direct blow. The degree of inflammation will determine the pain and relative loss of function. In most cases, anti-inflammatory medication (AIM), ice and firm compression bandaging will be used to treat the injury. In more severe cases aspiration and corticosteroid infiltration is necessary to hasten recovery. If the bursitis recurs, impeding normal activities, surgical excision may be required.

Prepatellar bursitis

The prepatellar bursa is the most commonly injured bursa at the knee. It lies between the anterior surface of the patella and the skin. When inflamed it is often called 'housemaid's knee', and presents as a superficial swelling on the anterior aspect of the knee. It is caused by falls onto the knee as in volleyball, skiing and football, but can also be created by weightlifting, cycling and rowing where the knee is working with resistance over a long period of time. Patellar tendinitis may give a similar appearance, but the lesion is inferior to the prepatellar bursa.

Infrapatellar bursitis

This bursa lies between the patellar tendon and the infrapatellar fat pad. It is inflamed by activities that require repeated knee flexion/extension against resistance. High jumpers, gymnasts and snowskiers suffer injury to this bursa. It should be differentiated from patellar tendinitis, which is more superficial and swollen when severely inflamed.

Pes anserinus bursitis

The pes anserinus bursa lies between the tibial collateral ligament and its attachment to the tibia and the overlying pes anserinus insertion. It is commonly inflamed by downhill running, direct trauma or repeated knee flexion. Differentiation from MCL pathology may be determined by active stretching or resisted contraction of the 'pes' muscle group (sartorius, gracilis and semitendinosus). A painful response combined with an accurate history provides the diagnosis. Pes anserinus bursitis can present as a complication of osteoarthritis at the knee.

Semimembranosus bursitis

This bursa is found on the medial side of the popliteal fossa between the medial head of the gastrocnemius and semimembranosus tendon. It usually communicates with the knee joint and with another bursa between the gastrocnemius and the posterior capsule of the knee. Swelling is best seen and felt with the knee in extension. In adults swelling commonly results from a synovitis of the knee and in children it may present as a large cystic swelling in the popliteal fossa.

Baker's cyst

A Baker's cyst is a bursitis of the semimembranosus or medial gastrocnemius bursa. Involvement of this bursa causes expansion of its walls, usually posteriorly. It presents as a large soft tumour mass in the popliteal space and is accompanied by an aching pain in the back of the knee. Since the bursa frequently communicates with the knee, swelling may come and go. Baker's cysts may also be associated with degenerative processes at the knee (osteoarthritis and rheumatoid arthritis), as synovial fluid extravasates through the weakened posterior capsule. If the lesion is very large, it may lead to pressure on the tibial nerve or on posterior tibial veins, and create acute distal motor and venous problems.

Treatment may include dissecting out the mass and carefully closing the defect in the knee joint. Physiotherapy management after surgery will involve regaining full knee range of motion and calf-hamstrings flexibility and strength.

Conservative treatment is rarely helpful if the mass is large. If small, avoiding aggravation by rest from sport, local electrotherapy and ice may help. AIMs may also help reduce the size of the swelling.

Biceps femoris bursitis

This bursa lies between the insertion of the biceps tendon and the fibular collateral ligament. It is aggravated by overuse of the hamstring group and presents as a small swelling, made more obvious by resisted knee flexion.

Superficial infrapatellar bursitis

The superficial infrapatellar bursa lies between the tibial tubercle and the skin. Inflammation is produced by overuse of the patellar tendon, although the condition is uncommon. In young people it needs to be differentiated from Osgood-Schlatter's disease, by X-ray examination.

MENISCI

The menisci may be damaged by any activity which involves hyperextension or flexion, or twisting when weightbearing. The hypermobile knee is at risk when snow-skiing. Should the tip of the ski catch in the snow, the ski acts as an extended lever arm and rotates the joint to the point of tearing both meniscus and ligament (usually medial). On the other hand, hypermobility may at times be advantageous, allowing the joint to absorb twisting forces safely.

Athletes with exaggerated genu varum, valgus or recurvatum will have increased torsional stresses through their knee but may never have a problem due to adaptation of the joint. Trauma arises when an unknown or unexpected force is applied which places the 'vulnerable' joint at risk. Other risk factors include shoes that have undersurfaces/spikes which grip excessively to the ground, shoes that slip, wet surfaces, uneven surfaces, heavy tackling sports (gridiron, rugby), jumping and landing (netball, long jumping, Australian Rules) and pivoting (soccer, javelin).

Heavy loadbearing sports, such as weightlifting, place the joint at risk as compressive forces to the posterior aspect of the knee in deep squat positions stress the posterior meniscal surfaces. Technique is vital and over the years athletes develop habits and techniques that allow them to cope with most competitive situations, but it is the unexpected that brings disaster. If not corrected, technique flaws will eventually be exposed under stress, leading to injury. For example, if the hip of a fast bowler in cricket is internally rotated too far on foot strike the torsional forces exerted when releasing the ball may cause a twisting stress at the knee.

Overweight athletes with poor flexibility are at risk unless they avoid maximum effort and body contact. Unknown factors such as congenital discoid meniscus will leave the area vulnerable and a knee that has a previous history of ACL, PCL or MCL tear is likely to sustain meniscal or other joint pathology if rotational forces are applied. As the menisci degenerate they can also develop minor splits which, when combined with the ageing processes of the joint itself, give rise to pain and become limiting for the athlete.

Assessment

There are several types of meniscal tears: radial, longitudinal, flap and horizontal (Fig. 29.17). Menisci may be injured to varying degrees in isolation, or in combination with other knee joint structures.

Medial meniscus

Pain is felt on the medial side of the knee over the joint line. Full flexion or extension is painful, as is turning the foot or tibia outwards while the knee is flexed and weightbearing. In a non-weightbearing position, rotation of the tibia on a flexing/extending knee (McMurray's test) will be painful and perhaps cause a 'clunk' sound. This sound corresponds to a torn flap which has become impinged in the joint, usually in the medial compartment. With a bucket handle tear there will be an effusion and 'locking', or inability to fully flex or extend the knee. 'Giving way' or 'buckling' is often reported by the athlete.

Lateral meniscus

In tears of the lateral meniscus, pain is reproduced when the tibia is internally rotated on an extending knee joint. Although pain may occur at varying points in the full range of flexion and extension, hyperextension and full flexion will increase the pain and there will be soreness on the lateral joint line. Full flexion will be limited due to the intricate connection of the posterolateral horn and the capsule/

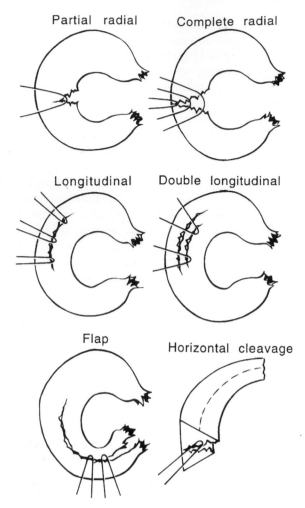

Fig. 29.17 The six most common meniscal tears. The longitudinal tear may extend anteriorly to form a bucket handle tear

arcuate ligament complex. There is normally an effusion following a tear, and the athlete's gait will be affected.

Meniscal lesions are not limited to traumatic tears. Discoid menisci occasionally occur in childhood or adolescence with pain or locking, most commonly in the lateral compartment. Partial meniscectomy may be required to create a more normal cartilage. Cystic degeneration may also take place, again in the lateral compartment. It will present with similar symptoms to a lateral meniscus tear, but there may be no history of trauma. The athlete with this pathology will complain of night pain and localized lateral joint line swelling. If advanced, it will need to be dealt with surgically.

Conservative management

Since the mid 1980s it has been generally acknowledged that preserving meniscal tissue will prevent degenerative joint changes occurring later. There is no doubt about the healing potential of the peripheral meniscus. Studies have documented healing rates as high as 90% in this area

(Cassidy & Shaffer 1982). Other groups of meniscal tears that require no surgery include full thickness tears less than 5 mm long that are stable to surgical probing, radial tears less than 5 mm long, and partial thickness tears that are stable to pivoting and less than 50% complete. Whenever possible, the meniscus should be allowed to heal with varying rest periods prescribed.

Rehabilitation

Medial meniscus

Rehabilitation should be gentle at first, with the goal of reducing swelling and pain. Meniscal lesions may be associated with capsular and medial ligament tears and these tissues will also need to be assessed. If dealing with only a minor medial meniscus lesion, it will be important to regain quadriceps control. The athlete should be non-weight-bearing until the effusion is minimal, flexion over 100° and extension close to zero. Quadriceps work can begin when non-weightbearing. The quadriceps work should be in a painfree range and include exercises such as quadriceps over fulcrum, SLR, prone locking and cycling (Table 29.4).

As walking improves, the quadriceps and hamstring program can be increased. This means that co-contraction work can be included, swimming commenced (no breast-stroke kick), and resisted exercises are generally safe. Caution needs to be shown however performing resisted hamstring work in the early stages of rehabilitation due to the connection with the posterior horn of the meniscus via expansions from semimembranosus (Kapandji 1982, Levy 1988).The use of rubber exercise tubing to do exercises both at home and in the clinic provides varying resistance

Table 29.4   Rehabilitation of meniscal injuries

Initial stage (0-2 weeks)
- straight leg raise
- gentle knee flexion
- calf (non weight bearing) and hip exercises
- quadriceps exercises over a fulcrum
- hamstring exercises in prone or sidelying
- massage, mobilization of the patella if necessary

Middle stage (2-4 weeks)
- cycling, walking
- active exercises for the quadriceps—fulcrum and through range
- hydrotherapy
- submaximal isokinetic work towards 4 weeks
- calf raises
- contralateral resisted leg exercises with rubber tubing while standing on the injured leg to develop co-contraction, proprioceptive exercises, gain full extension and flexion range using mobilization

Late stage (4-6 weeks)
- cycling
- increased isokinetic work
- swimming
- running
- harder proprioceptive work

Functional stage (6-10 weeks)
- sport skills including hard running drills
- isokinetic evaluation

that is simple yet interesting. The physiotherapist should beware of resisted hip adduction work, as this may irritate the medial compartment unless the resistance is applied close to the knee joint.

When the athlete walks confidently, half-squat exercise is painfree and range of movement is close to 100% isokinetic exercise can be pursued through a full range of movement. Prior to this, limited range resistance exercises, isometric and submaximal work can be used on isokinetic equipment. High-speed isokinetic exercise which can shear or inflame the joint surface, and slow-speed isokinetic exercise that can cause excessive joint compression, need to be performed with care until the later stages of rehabilitation.

Towards the end of rehabilitation, harder proprioceptive work should be encouraged. This includes work on the 'spring' wobble board and single leg standing while juggling a ball. Running in a straight line should be possible by this stage and a return to sport acceptable when figure-eight running is painfree. If this level of exercise produces an effusion, a short period of rest from all exercise except cycling and SLR is recommended. An isokinetic assessment may be performed at this stage to objectively assess quadriceps and hamstrings strength. If muscle strength is 90-100% and there are no symptoms, sport can be pursued. The time span for recovery of such a lesion is six to twelve weeks.

Lateral meniscus

The conservative treatment of this lesion is very similar to that for the medial meniscus. In the early part of rehabilitation, efforts should be concentrated on reducing pain and effusion and restoring range of movement. As the joint regains a full range of movement, resisted work may begin and activities such as cycling and swimming can be made more difficult. Treading water is a useful exercise but breaststroke kick should be done with extreme caution. Graded isokinetic work, functional exercises, and proprioceptive work are added as the patient improves and the joint shows no signs of regression. The latter stages of rehabilitation are similar to that of the medial meniscus but the early stages may progress more slowly than for the medial meniscus. By the end of rehabilitation the athlete should be able to fully squat (sometimes slow to return fully) and turn quickly in an outwards direction when running, without experiencing pain.

Partial meniscectomy

Years of clinical evidence documenting articular demise after meniscectomy has converted most orthopaedic surgeons from performing open, complete meniscectomies to partial arthroscopic resection (Di Stefano 1990). Arthroscopy is now a common procedure, and allows rapid post-operative return to sport. Although short term results are good, there is uncertainty about the long term effects. With the removal of

a meniscus, the joint surface is likely to develop long term degenerative changes. Surgery should be deferred if the diagnosis is only suspected and no locking or loss of extension is present. In the elderly, degenerative tears should be removed only if they cause mechanical symptoms, and as much of the meniscus as possible should be preserved.

Following surgery, the athlete will be at home and full weightbearing within forty-eight hours, barring complications. Due to the easier accessibility of the medial meniscus arthroscopically, partial medial meniscectomy is less painful post-operatively than lateral, therefore exercise may begin from day one, with a post-operative bandage in place.

These stages of rehabilitation may be delayed for several weeks if surgery is performed by arthrotomy or if there is a post-operative effusion. The arthroscope portals will be tender post-operatively but this should not prevent normal exercise. The surgeon may give special post-operative instructions but, once again, the physiotherapist needs to arrange a graduated return to activity, and know the complete history of the joint in question. It is possible for professional athletes to return to full function earlier than six to ten weeks due to excellent pre-operative quadriceps strength and accelerated post-operative management (Fig. 29.18). The athlete may, however, inflame the joint in their endeavour to return more quickly to competition.

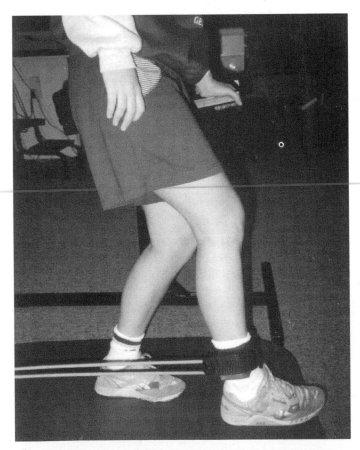

Fig. 29.18 Contralateral resisted leg exercise with weight bearing on injured leg

Meniscal repair

Since the mid 1980s the school of thought is that menisci should be retained because of their role in preventing degenerative changes. Di Stefano (1990) found that partial meniscectomy leads to less severe degenerative changes than complete meniscectomy; the degree of change is directly related to the amount of meniscus removed. There is increasing evidence to show the benefit of retaining meniscal tissue and, in ligamentous instability, its preservation is even more essential.

If the surgeon decides to repair the damaged meniscus, the knee will then be immobilized for four to six weeks in 0-10° extension. Opinion is divided on whether to weightbear (Morgan & Cassells 1986). When the brace or cast is removed, the aim is to regain full range of motion, normal strength and function. This may take a further six to twelve weeks and will initially be slow due to the soft tissue stiffness and likely retropatellar adhesions. Rehabilitation programs should be similar to those for partial meniscectomies. The time frames will be different, however, and there may be some doubt on whether the repair will tolerate more strenuous forms of sport.

Whether or not a repair is undertaken, as opposed to partial removal, depends on advanced arthroscopic skills, experienced assistants, the location of the tear, the length of the tear and the surgeon's ability to reduce and stabilize the meniscus. The athlete's age, work situation and lifestyle also need to be taken into account.

OSTEOCHONDRITIDES

Osteochondral defects and fractures

Osteochondral fractures commonly occur in traumatic situations, often involving violent sporting collisions, leading to compression of the tibiofemoral articulation. Osteochondral defects may also develop as a result of wear and tear associated with overuse, and in acute situations in association with ligament rupture. These defects can occur in young athletes before full bony maturation, or in older athletes as part of normal joint wear and tear.

Assessment. Osteochondral fractures should be considered if the athlete presents with a suspected haemarthrosis. If the knee is hot and has a tense effusion which came on quickly (i.e. within hours of the injury) then it is likely there will be blood in the joint. The knee should be X-rayed and referred to a sports physician for possible orthopaedic opinion. If the defect is large enough it may require surgical fixation, however, if surgery is not performed then the knee is immobilized for a period of three weeks either in POP or resting brace. The duration of immobilization will depend on the size of the defect and whether the joint surfaces have been disrupted.

Treatment. Post-operative treatment will depend on the surgeon. However, it should be directed towards improving range of motion and strength, although if the fracture or defect involves the joint surfaces then care should be taken with exercises that produce compressive and shearing forces. Low resistance exercises, such as light cycling, swimming (with caution that freestyle kicking is not too vigorous), and mid-range quadriceps exercises are appropriate.

Other considerations. Osteochondral defects may occur in chronic cases following previous trauma, when joint integrity has been affected. In these cases erosion of the weightbearing surfaces may cause pain and dysfunction, as well as persistent effusions. They may also require surgical treatment, where the injured area is drilled to promote bleeding and hopefully allow a fibrous covering to form over the area. Athletes must be advised against excessive loadbearing activities, such as long distance running, as this may cause more rapid deterioration of the joint surfaces.

Treatment should be directed towards decreasing swelling and pain, and maintaining quadriceps strength. However, this can be difficult due to the recurring effusion. It is appropriate to prescribe an exercise program in which the joint is worked beyond the painful ranges of motion (e.g. if painful at 45° of knee flexion, then exercises are performed from 0-40° and from 60-90° of flexion).

A management program should be designed to protect the knee joint over the ensuing years. This will include modification of sporting activity and an ongoing exercise program.

Predisposing risk factors and sports. Factors such as previous meniscal removal, collision sports and unstable knees are more prone to articular cartilage damage. Growth plate abnormalities in adolescence may also lead to increased risk of osteochondral damage.

Osteochondritis dissecans

Osteochondritis dissecans is an articular cartilage involvement occuring most frequently at the knee. It is believed to be caused either by ischaemic necrosis or, more commonly, trauma. The pathology consists of separation of a fragment of cartilage from the underlying matrix. The line of separation fills with granulation tissue and, because of poor circulation, the separated fragment necroses. If no defect appears in the articular cartilage at the line of separation then spontaneous healing may occur. On the other hand, if enough of the separated fragment is absorbed to permit it to depress into the crater in the epiphyseal bone, fissuring of the cartilage and ultimate separation may develop. Trauma can subsequently break the fragment loose. It occurs most often in adolescents and young adults.

Damage may be produced as the medial tibial spine impinges against the lateral surface of the medial femoral condyle. This commonly occurs when the leg is in abduction and external rotation with the knee held slightly flexed, as in pivoting on one leg (Corrigan & Maitland 1983). Aitroth

(1971) indicates 85% of cases involve the medial femoral condyle, usually its lateral border. In 15% of cases the lateral femoral condyle is involved, usually on its inferior surface. Furthermore, Aitroth (1971) found that more than 60% of 200 cases were 'better class' athletes and that its incidence parallels the degree of sports participation.

Assessment. This condition may present with discomfort in the joint accompanied by joint effusion. The athlete may describe intermittent locking, but with non-specific joint pain and few localizing symptoms. In all these cases X-ray assessment is essential. Osteochondritis dissecans should be suspected when the probability of meniscal injury is removed and a history of intermittent episodes of locking, clicking, effusion or pain remains, especially in an adolescent athlete. Quadriceps wasting is also a feature of the condition.

Treatment. Treatment extends from conservative in the young (since spontaneous regression will often be seen) to operative excision of the fragment, or internal fixation. Physiotherapy should be directed towards decreasing pain and swelling and maintaining quadriceps strength. Exercises to strengthen the quadriceps should be performed carefully as the joint can be aggravated by excessive resisted exercises, particularly in weightbearing. As a result, straight leg raising and small arc of movement in inner range or mid range will be appropriate. Strapping and bandaging can help if the joint is swollen, and return to sport should be guided by pain and swelling.

It may be necessary for a young athlete to rest from weightbearing sport for several months to see if spontaneous recovery occurs.

Apophysitis of the patellar tubercle (Osgood-Schlatter's disease)

Three manifestations parade as Osgood-Schlatter's disease. One is bursitis of the infrapatellar bursa. The tenderness in this condition is elicited at a point slightly higher than the tibial tubercle and can be treated as a bursitis. The second type of Osgood-Schlatter's is an aseptic necrosis of the tip of the epiphysis for the tibial tubercle, and the third is a true epiphysitis involving the whole epiphysis.

Assessment. Symptoms of the latter two are pain on direct pressure and on active contraction of the quadriceps. Hence the young athlete will complain of pain when landing on the knee, and when squatting or climbing stairs. There will usually be a lump, and X-rays show some separation of the apophysis.

Treatment. Treatment varies according to the pathology and is usually non-surgical unless significant separation has occurred. Conservative treatment involves cutting down the athlete's activities and protecting the tubercle by a volleyballer's knee pad or similar device. It is important to avoid stairs, squats and activities where the knee is flexed. Local treatment will include TENS and IFT, and laser may be useful. Local ice application can relieve acute symptoms.

Before return to sport a gradual build-up of exercises to strengthen the quadriceps is performed, first with SLR (provided it is painless) then with through-range exercise gradually introducing step-up and downs. There should be a gradual return to running, initially on a mini-trampoline progressing to running on grass. Hamstring stretching should be performed to decrease longitudinal stress.

Other considerations. The condition may recur until the apophysis closes. Sometimes immobilization may be necessary to help the condition settle if it is acute and very sore. However, in minor cases and in less demanding sports it is possible for the athlete to continue playing.

Articular cartilage damage

Injuries to the articular cartilage of the knee joint can affect the joint surfaces of the femur, tibia and patella. They may occur as a result of direct impact to the knee joint, or in association with meniscal or ligamentous injury. Any condition that leads to excessive repetitive stress can cause symptoms of cartilage damage. Cartilage damage may be evident as large cracks and defects on the joint surfaces, and continual degeneration. The result can be premature arthritis. It is sometimes difficult, however, to diagnose damage to the articular cartilage on its own because many other injuries (e.g. ligamentous damage) can produce similar symptoms.

Assessment. Swelling occurs due to a recurrent effusion. It is unusual for the joint to be hot. Pain which occurs during extension can mimic a meniscal injury. The injury will often need to be assessed by arthroscope.

Treatment. The quadriceps mechanism should be trained, usually with isometric exercises as through-range exercises can compress and shear the joint leading to irritation of the damaged surfaces. Hence, squats and stepping exercises should be avoided. Use of a neoprene heat retainer can help decrease the aching pain, and provide some compression to decrease the swelling.

Other considerations. Surgery to remove the damaged cartilage may be necessary in the hope that the denuded articular cartilage is replaced by fibrocartilage. A change of sport may decrease the demands on the knee joint (i.e. stop long distance running or high velocity impact sports such as football or netball).

Growth plate fractures

Assessment. Impact against the side of the knee joint in children and adolescents may cause an epiphyseal injury, where a similar impact in an adult may tear the MCL or

ACL. The usual presentation in these cases will be a limp and inability to fully move the joint. Palpation over the suspected site of damage will be painful. There will probably be an effusion.

If an epiphyseal injury is suspected, the knee should be X-rayed and referral to an orthopaedic surgeon arranged because of the risk to impairment of normal growth.

Treatment. If surgical fixation, followed by immobilization of the joint, is required, then treatment will be largely dictated by the surgeon's requirements. Physiotherapy will be directed at a gradual increase in range of movement using heat, massage, patellofemoral mobilization and strengthening of the quadriceps and hamstrings. This occurs firstly through limited arcs of movement. Hydrotherapy will be appropriate to help regain full weightbearing.

ARTHRITIS

The topic of arthritis and its rehabilitation will be confined to osteoarthritis and rheumatoid arthritis. The inflammatory arthritic conditions of subacute gonorrhea, gout, ankylosing spondylitis, ulcerative collitis or psoriasis are rarely seen in the athlete and will not be discussed in this chapter.

Osteoarthritis

Osteoarthritis of the knee is very common in athletes who have suffered earlier knee joint trauma. However, it can also affect those who have never suffered trauma to the knee. In the former group, athletes who have suffered meniscal or ligamentous damage earlier in life are prone to osteoarthritic changes, especially if they continue to pursue vigorous sport. If the knee is unstable, the likelihood of osteoarthritis is even greater. In the case of the athlete with no history of knee trauma, osteoarthritic changes can occur merely due to ageing of the articular surfaces. This process may be hastened if there is knee varus or valgus deformity, poor muscular control or pronated feet, or in specific occupational situations.

It is important to realize that X-rays showing osteoarthritic change may not provide an accurate diagnosis. Osteoarthritis is common in most athletes and in the general population beyond the age of thirty. It should also be realized that osteoarthritic changes vary, as do their symptoms, and therefore rehabilitation should be modified according to the degree of pain, swelling and functional disability.

Assessment. The knee with moderate osteoarthritis will be slightly swollen, warm and lack full extension and flexion. Palpation will reveal synovial thickening on the joint line. There may also be a varus deformity and joint crepitus. The medial compartment is more often affected than the lateral, and the quadriceps (especially VMO) will be wasted, with some patellofemoral pathology. The sufferer may be overweight, and have a limp. An accurate history will be required to determine whether other joint pathology exists, i.e. meniscus, ligament, loose bodies etc. X-rays will usually show medial compartment changes.

Treatment. In osteoarthritis the goal is to improve range of movement, especially in extension, reduce swelling and pain and restore normal function. The referring medical practitioner may prescribe NSAIDs to help settle the joint symptoms.

It is recommended that exercises be done slowly and carefully. Cycling with mild resistance and gentle hydrotherapy are excellent. In the clinic, quadriceps work over a fulcrum and SLR work are recommended. Isometric exercise at different painfree range points is helpful, but weightbearing quadriceps work should be avoided. In all cases, the effect of quadriceps work on the patellofemoral joint should be assessed. Isokinetic exercise is beneficial but needs to be applied at speeds that do not aggravate the joint or surrounding tissues. Its application will depend on the individual athlete.

It is common for the knee to suddenly worsen between treatments. This may not be due to the advised treatment but to the joint's own lack of integrity, especially if already unstable. The physiotherapist should be prepared to 'backpedal' with the exercise prescription and reassure the athlete that some form of regression is common, yet long-term improvement is still possible. It is important to discuss the athlete's lifestyle, hobbies etc. as these may aggravate the symptoms.

The use of a knee brace may help the athlete overcome lifestyle difficulties and allow involvement in non-contact sports (Loomer & Horlick 1991). For example, the 'Generation II brace' provides unicompartment 'unloading'. It uses a poli-axial knee cage made from semi-rigid thermoplastic material, dynamic strapping and two hemispherical domes as hinges. The hinges are hardened high carbon steel which have been teflon coated. Loomer and Horlick (1991) report that knee bracing with a Generation II brace produces statistically significant pain relief in athletes with medial compartment arthritis, although the reasons for the improvement remain unclear.

It is important to remember that the degree of osteoarthritis will vary, as will the degree of pre-existing knee joint pathology. Further, the athlete's joint response may vary from month to month with constant or worsening pathology. It is imperative to tell the athlete that many treatment options exist, that life can be made more pleasant and that their overall health is being considered. The physiotherapist should determine whether these issues have already been dealt with by the referring doctor, as it is important for the athlete to understand their position. In professional sport, it is common for athletes to disregard medical advice and continue playing, despite arthritic change and poor prognosis. They may use braces, AIMs and painkillers to keep playing, and risk premature osteoarthritis. As the practitioner managing their rehabilitation, it is important to explain their position clearly, but also to accept their decision.

Rheumatoid arthritis

This is a painful disease, which in the acute stages will make weightbearing impossible. As a systemic problem rather than a degenerative disease (osteoarthritis), the athlete will be forced to consider lifestyle changes and will have 'flare-ups' that are not predictable. Athletes with this condition will not be able to commit themselves to contact or vigorous sport. Keeping fit by swimming or cycling will be helpful but if recurrences are frequent (e.g. in the teenage years) it is clear that sporting options will need to be assessed. As in osteoarthritis, quadriceps/hamstrings integrity will be vital and at times a comfortable brace will be required for daily activity.

The disease itself gradually erodes the joint surfaces and leads to deformity. Naturally it is difficult to exercise the quadriceps during a flare-up where the joint is warm and painful. At this time, the athlete may also feel quite unwell. The best approach is to immobilize the joint and attempt isometric quadriceps/hamstring exercises. The joint may need bracing and painkillers or AIMs. If necessary, the athlete should be non-weightbearing during a flare-up.

As the flare-up settles and the disease goes into remission, the athlete should gradually attempt hydrotherapy, cycling and through-range exercises. The latter must be prescribed with extreme caution and based on a knowledge of the current joint pathology. The goal of rehabilitation in this case is to regain or retain total leg strength, therefore the hip and ankle regions must not be ignored. Co-contraction work around the knee is helpful but once again weightbearing exercise must be carefully watched. During a remission, and if possible in the early stages after rheumatoid arthritis has been first diagnosed, a modified isokinetic test (either through limited range or at speeds between 90° and 180° per second) provides excellent objective information to keep for future comparisons.

FAT PAD LESIONS

The infrapatellar fat pad is intracapsular but extrasynovial, the synovial membrane being reflected over the lateral margins of the fat pad as the alar ligament. It acts as a mobile cushion and plays an important part in aiding knee movement by changing its shape as it is moved by its alar ligaments. It is commonly damaged by a direct blow to the knee, but can be severely inflamed by hyperextension trauma or direct rubbing by the inferior pole of the patella. The inferior aspect of the patella will be slightly swollen and tender but the knee will have a good range of flexion.

Extension may be very painful at end range. The athlete may even have retinacular structures that are tight inferiorly.

Due to its proximity, its diagnosis may be confused with patellar tendinitis, but the history of trauma or hyperextension will lead the examiner to conclude that the fat pad is damaged. Ultrasound assessment can be used to assess the integrity of the patellar tendon. Damage to the anterior horn of the meniscus also needs to be excluded as a cause of anterior knee pain.

Treatment. Acute treatment will include AIMs, icing and rest. Quadriceps exercises should be avoided and it may be necessary to have the athlete partial weightbearing. From this point, the lesion will settle and ultrasound therapy can be used. As the range of movement increases, so can the exercise program. McConnell (1991) suggests tilting the inferior pole of the patella away from the pad by taping before commencing weightbearing quadriceps work. Quadriceps work performed in inner range must avoid the 'locked back' position (hyperextension) of the knee. It may be necessary to tape the patella as well as the fat pad with the unloading technique (Fig. 29.19).

Adjacent structures which may require a stretching program are the quadriceps, tensor fascia lata and lateral retinaculum. If they are tight they will prevent normal patellar excursion and create additional unwanted forces on the fat pad. As the fat pad settles and VMO strength increases, the aim is to introduce functional exercises that avoid 'locking back'.

Other considerations. On return to running, the athlete must avoid running downhill. During rehabilitation, slow speed isokinetics should be avoided for fear of inflaming the fat pad. Rowing machines and leg press exercises can aggravate the pathology, and forceful resisted

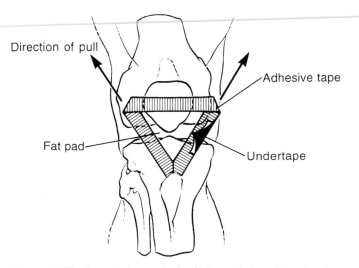

Fig. 29.19 Taping technique to 'unload' fat pad lesion. Directional taping for the patella may not be necessary, depending on clinical assessment

quadriceps work in a sitting position must be performed with caution. Manual glides of the tibia on the femur in an anterior direction will help restore normal extension range but should be avoided until the fat pad irritation has settled.

SUPERIOR TIBIOFIBULAR JOINT

This is a plane synovial joint reinforced by a fibrous capsule, with posterior and anterior ligaments. In 10% of cases it communicates with the knee joint. This joint is often sprained during injury to the lateral collateral ligament. It can also be damaged by trauma to the biceps femoris muscle, which attaches to the head of the fibula. Other contributing factors are severe ankle inversion sprains or fractures of the upper third of the tibia and fibula. Disruption of this joint produces pain over the joint proper. It is a very disabling injury which will affect kicking, jumping and twisting skills.

Assessment. As with all joint sprains, the degree of damage will be classified as Grade I, II or III. In Grade II and III sprains resisted knee flexion will produce posterior glide of the fibula in excess of the unaffected side and simple anteroposterior pressure to the fibula will also demonstrate increased glide. This test is best performed with the knee at 90° of flexion.

Treatment. In all grades of injury some immobilization will initially be necessary. Taping is adequate but care must be taken not to produce excessive pressure over the peroneal nerve. Until the later stages of rehabilitation, quadriceps strengthening should be emphasized. Swimming and hamstring work can begin after approximately three weeks, but the athlete must be warned to avoid strong kick work in the pool as loading the hamstrings may disrupt healing of the capsule and ligament. Surgery is rarely required for Grade III tears, a conservative approach being successful with electrical modalities, strengthening and taping.

PLICAE

Embryologically the synovial membrane at the knee is divided into three compartments; anterior, medial and lateral. During development the partitions where the compartments meet largely disappear, although several remnants remain and become the plicae. Small plicae are frequently seen at arthroscopy, although the medial synovial fold, suprapatellar fold and occasionally a lateral synovial fold are those most commonly identified.

Assessment. Injury to plicae is predominantly overuse in nature. The principal complaint of patients with plicae syndrome will be anteromedial knee pain, at times sharp and of gradual onset. The pain, aggravated by flexion activities and by running, is atypical of patellofemoral pain in that it is usually unilateral and often not aggravated by prolonged sitting.

The medial synovial plica becomes symptomatic when repetitive movement occurs between the articular surfaces of the patella and the femur, with the knee flexed. Symptoms arise when there is chondropathology of the two articular surfaces.

Examination

- Palpation over the medial synovial plica on the medial femoral condyle with the knee flexed to 90° will elicit the athlete's knee pain.
- With the knee extended and relaxed, tenderness is detected in the medial parapatellar region and a sense of rolling a raised tendon structure over the medial femoral condyle is noted.
- Often a retropatellar click is noted in the medial parapatellar region as the knee is passively extended from a position of between 90-70° of flexion. This click often becomes less prominent with active knee extension and usually disappears with resisted extension. The opposite is the case with patellofemoral joint surface irregularity.
- Sometimes pain will be elicited with McMurray's test with external rotation of the tibia.

Treatment. With acute onset of pain, due to synovial irritation, athletes should rest and be prescribed AIMs. Avoidance of aggravating positions is necessary at later stages, and treatment over the medial femoral condyle with the knee flexed using friction massage, ultrasound or laser can help.

The knee should be strengthened with limited arc exercises avoiding painful positions. These exercises should definitely not be performed if they elicit pain, and weight-bearing full-range exercises should be avoided.

Differential diagnosis. As mentioned above, a symptomatic medial patellar plica differs from patellofemoral joint pathology in the following ways:

- it is not aggravated by sitting
- it is usually unilateral
- rarely does an effusion develop
- resisted extension of the flexed knee does not cause pain
- medial taping of the patella can aggravate a symptomatic plica.

The symptomatic plica can also be confused with medial meniscal injury or fat pad syndrome.

Other considerations. It is the authors' impression that no predisposing biomechanics are involved with injury to plicae. However, the condition may be seen with overpronation of the foot, pes cavus or tight or hypermobile patellae. In extreme cases surgery may be necessary. In these cases the fold of synovium is surgically excised, usually arthroscopically.

ARTICULARIS GENU

This muscle is a small but important part of the extensor mechanism, located in the suprapatellar region. Its role is to retract the suprapatellar pouch and maintain it in proper position during knee flexion and extension. The function of the extensor mechanism is disrupted if a suprapatellar or medial plica becomes thickened, scarred or contracted. This prevents the articularis genu from properly retracting this portion of the synovium in the suprapatellar pouch.

The articularis genu is usually damaged by a direct blow, as opposed to overload trauma, and is thus capable of being differentiated from quadriceps tendon lesions. The latter will not be painful with forced extension of the joint, but instead when extension is resisted from 90° flexion. Treatment includes rest, electrical modalities and graduated stretching and strengthening of the quadriceps mechanism. Deep massage to the suprapatellar area and NSAIDs can be helpful if the knee synovium is inflamed in conjunction with the lesion.

FRACTURES OF THE KNEE

The most common fractures of the knee seen in athletes are those to the patella, the head of the fibula, the tibial plateau, the supracondylar region and the tibial spine. Major fractures are infrequently seen in athletes, however, and are readily recognized by the accompanying major disability and by X-ray examination. The physiotherapist should be alert, however, to any associated ligamentous injuries. Fractures of the patella are discussed in Ch. 29.

Avulsion fractures

These fractures can occur when any of the major ligamentous attachments at the knee are severely stressed. Avulsion fracture of the upper tibia is basically an avulsion of the anterior cruciate ligament (tibial spine). Treatment is based on restoration of the ACL to its normal length and function. This is achieved by either a transfixion screw or sutures. Post-surgery, the athlete will require a period of non-weightbearing with limited motion, then a gradual process of mobilizing and strengthening. The rate of progress will be determined by the surgeon. Similar avulsion fractures can occur with the PCL, but we must appreciate that the forces required to cause such a fracture will certainly have secondary effects on adjacent soft tissues. Therefore, rehabilitation should be thorough and begin as soon as the stabilizing procedure of the PCL has some effect.

The medial collateral ligament can be avulsed from its femoral attachment but in these cases it is important to assess the lateral tibial plateau radiologically. Unless the avulsion is very small, reattachment of the MCL and removal of the fragment is necessary. Post-operatively, there will be a period of protection followed by rapid rehabilitation (if the lateral plateau is unaffected).

Fractures of the fibula head

The head of the fibula may be broken by a direct blow. This is usually a comminuted fracture without gross displacement, although the fibular head must always be checked. In fractures of the head of the fibula, the physiotherapist must check the peroneal nerve, lateral collateral ligament of the knee and biceps tendon. If the fracture is below the head, and was caused by a pivoting motion, the ankle joint must also be assessed.

A fracture will normally be treated with immobilization and non-weightbearing for two to four weeks. The athlete then follows a regime of mobilizing the knee and strengthening the quadriceps. Knee flexion exercise must be painfree and involve no resisted hamstring contractions for six weeks. In the later stages of rehabilitation, proprioceptive training will help strengthen the peroneal muscles and a complete return to sport is allowed. Where indicated, the superior tibiofibular joint may need mobilizing.

Supracondylar fractures

Supracondylar fractures are most unusual in sport. The most likely causes are severe falls, as in skiing or cycling, or direct trauma, as in motor car racing. In assessing the knee the physiotherapist should check the anterior and posterior tibial pulses. The knee will be swollen, painful and difficult to move. In cases of displacement, management requires reduction, followed by bed rest and traction. Alternatively, internal fixation and bed rest is required. The fracture takes approximately twelve weeks to unite. Knee movement is avoided for six weeks but static quadriceps, gluteal, ankle and toe exercises can begin much earlier. With internal fixation, mobilization of the knee is commenced much earlier, but there is a danger of reduced knee mobility in these fractures long term.

Femoral condyle fractures

Femoral condyle fractures are usually caused by a fall from a height, where the tibia is driven upwards into the intercondylar notch. A single condyle may be fractured and driven upwards, or both condyles split apart. The knee is swollen, warm and too painful to move. Displaced fractures require aspiration, closed or open reduction and bed rest with traction for six weeks. PWB begins at twelve weeks. Quadriceps and knee flexion exercises begin within the first two weeks. Undisplaced fractures require immobilization in a long leg plaster for eight to twelve weeks but weightbearing is allowed from about four weeks. If reduction is not accurate, osteoarthritis may develop long term.

Fracture-separation of lower femoral epiphysis

In the adolescent athlete the lower femoral epiphysis may be displaced:

- laterally by forced abduction of the straight knee, as when a player falls across the leg or,
- forwards by a hyperextension injury.

On examination, the knee will be swollen, warm and immovable. The pulses in the foot must be checked as the popliteal artery may be obstructed. X-rays will show a displaced triangular fragment of the shaft. The knee must be reduced (closed reduction) and immobilized for six weeks. Range of motion exercise then begins immediately. Long term sporting involvement after this injury is assessed individually. Epiphyseal fractures do not necessarily affect the growth of the bone and they are much less likely to do so if reduction is anatomical and associated with a minimum amount of trauma.

Tibial condyle fractures

A fall from a height or a direct blow may fracture one or both tibial condyles. The most common injury is a fractured lateral condyle caused by a valgus crush 'bumper fracture'. This fracture usually occurs in the 50-60 year age group, when the knee is in extension and valgus (Cohn et al 1990). The lateral tibial condyle is drawn upwards and is smashed by the lateral femoral condyle, which remains intact.

On examination, the knee is swollen, warm, 'doughy', and difficult to lift or bend. X-rays show the fracture. Sometimes the MCL will also be damaged. Management involves either aspiration, traction, reduction and rest in bed; or traction, reduction and plaster. Weightbearing begins at twelve weeks but quadriceps and flexion exercises begin immediately for the athlete confined to bed in traction.

Open reduction is required if good alignment is not possible but the long term results are good. Thorough physiotherapy will be required to prevent long term knee stiffness but some degree of genu valgum is inevitable. The development of osteoarthritis is possible, depending on the degree of articular cartilage damage, and sporting pursuits may need to be modified.

NERVE ENTRAPMENTS OF THE KNEE

There are two nerves near the knee which are prone to entrapment. They are the tibial and the common peroneal nerve. The tibial nerve passes from the upper to the lower angle of the popliteal fossa, bisecting it longitudinally. It can be compressed by trauma to the head of the gastrocnemius, a direct blow to the fossa or aggravation of a Baker's cyst.

In chronically swollen knees or knees that have suffered severe internal derangement, weakening of the posterior capsule occurs and under exertion there may be extravasation of synovial fluid into the fossa. On examination, swelling and possibly a lump will be detected in the fossa. The athlete will be unable to flex the knee fully and prolonged flexion will cause tingling and coldness in the foot as the nerve is compressed.

In severe cases, venous return from the foot will be affected and aspiration of the fossa will be required. If reduction of swelling and symptoms does not occur quickly, orthopaedic intervention may be necessary to repair the posterior capsule of the joint. AIMs should be prescribed initially, along with rest and maintenance of quadriceps strength.

The other nerve entrapment syndrome involves the common peroneal nerve as it passes along the lateral side of the knee and neck of the fibula. Major trauma to the knee involving the lateral ligament, lateral meniscus or superior tibiofibular joint can create an effusion that affects the integrity of the nerve. Symptoms will be those of a neuropraxia and if medication does not reduce the symptoms, decompressive or investigative surgery may be required. Collins et al (1986) reported common peroneal nerve palsy after prolonged ice application to the lateral side of the knee, so this procedure should be approached with caution.

BRACES

There is an extensive range of braces, from simple tubigrip and bandages through to expensive braces such as the Lenox Hill derotation brace. This section does not intend to cover every brace in existence, but to describe some features of braces available in Australia that apply to a particular problem or for use in a specific sport.

It is generally acknowledged that the amount of mechanical stability provided by bracing is somewhat limited, but some athletes find braces useful and often say that a brace makes them feel more secure. This may be due to a brace providing increased sensory afferent awareness and hence better proprioception. It is evident that having an external support makes the athlete more 'aware' of the supported joint and functional ability is enhanced.

Other braces, such as hinged knee braces worn for collateral ligament tears, provide specific mechanical support. Baker et al (1987) demonstrated the support given to the medial collateral ligament by several braces (such as Don Joy, Generation II, Lenox Hill, Pro-Am, Anderson) when specific abduction forces were applied to a cadaveric knee. The derotational or stabilizing role of braces is difficult to prove mechanically, however. In a study of seven functional knee braces similar to those mentioned above, they commented that 'Our subjective results showed that most athletes like to use the braces despite the fact that we could not mechanically show that they were working' (Beck et al 1986).

Many athletes with knee disabilities prefer a type of brace. If this support gives them confidence and they feel it helps, their use should not be questioned.

Knee elastic supports

Other than as an aid to decrease swelling and provide warmth, these supports are mainly of palliative value.

Knee supports

Usually of neoprene, these supports are often tighter than elastic supports and certainly provide more heat. They can be fitted with hinges laterally and medially which can provide limited motion, therefore they become adaptable for use with MCL grade II and III injuries. Another adaptation is to place velcro straps that attach postero-superiorly and cross anteriorly over the upper tibia, restricting the anterior movement of the tibia on the femur.

Functional knee braces

The next group of braces belong to a category that assists ACL deficient knees. Braces such as Don Joy, Lenox Hill, Generation II, Polyaxial and CTi (Carbon Titanium) all claim to be 'derotation' braces. The CTi brace is widely used by motor-cross riders and snow skiers and is very light. It is moulded to the shape of the knee and thigh (from a plaster cast). The Generation II is a semi-rigid thermoplastic and is also moulded from a plaster cast. It is also very light in weight and has a double hinge which approximates the actual hinge action of the knee joint. Straps provide a strut over the tibia to decrease shear forces. This brace can provide stability as well as 'unloading' the joint in osteoarthritic conditions.

The Lenox Hill is the oldest ACL brace available and has proven to be effective. Its straps are elastic and it has sturdy metal supports anteromedially, anterolaterally and inferiorly. It has been available to athletes since the early 1970s and retains popularity in many circles as a derotation brace.

The relative merits of these braces are, however, open to debate. It is sensible to try a less expensive brace first (such as neoprene with hinges) and determine the results. Not all athletes will be prepared to pay approximately $700 to purchase a Don Joy, Lenox Hill, Generation II or CTi. Their decision will be based on financial situation, the level and type of sport they wish to play, the availability of the brace, its weight, colour and comfort. With an ACL deficient knee it is unlikely any brace can provide the support required to prevent the pivot shift manoeuvre, but hinge braces do provide a degree of stability for straight collateral instability.

SUMMARY

The knee joint was the centre of orthopaedic attention during the 1980s. Improved knowledge of collagen repair processes, advances in arthroscopic surgery, the proliferation of assessment and surgical procedures and the specificity of rehabilitation all provided great steps in progress.

It has become all the more important for physiotherapists working in this area to be aware of new trends and research so that their athletes receive the optimum treatment. The knee joint will continue to attract research interest as athletes and practitioners search for precise management. Perhaps, however, it is time to take a 'breather' and more carefully assess our current surgical and rehabilitation regimes before moving on to new territory. The progress made in conservative management has also been staggering, offering athletes the chance to return to sport much more quickly. The early application of exercise post-injury has brought many changes to functional exercise rehabilitation and the use of rehabili-tation equipment. The physiotherapists of the 1990s need to be fully aware of the strengths and weaknesses of each.

Helping the athlete with trauma to the knee joint is both challenging and exciting, as the practitioner's knowledge of assessment, non-surgical and surgical management, and rehabilitation will be tested to the maximum.

REFERENCES

Aitroth P M 1971 Osteochondritis dissecans of the knee. Journal of Bone and Joint Surgery 53B:440

Akeson W H 1961 An experimental study of joint stiffness. Journal of Bone and Joint Surgery 43A:1022

Akeson W H, Amid D, La Violette D 1968 The connective tissue response to immobility: an accelerated aging response. Experimental Gerontology 3:289

Akeson W H, Amiel D, Woo S L 1980 Immobility effects on synovial joints: the pathomechanics of joint contracture. Biorheology 17:95

Amiss A A, Dawkins G P C 1991 Fibre bundle actions related to ligament replacements and injuries. Journal of Bone and Joint Surgery 73B:260-267

Arms S W, Pope M H, Johnson R J, Fischer RA, Arvidsson I, Eriksson E 1984 The biomechanics of ACL rehabilitation and reconstruction. American Journal of Sports Medicne 12:8

Arnoczky S P, Warren R F 1982 Microvasculature of the human meniscus. American Journal of Sports Medicine 10:90-95

Arnoczky S P, Warren R F 1988 Anatomy of the cruciate ligaments. In: Feagin A (ed) The crucial ligaments. Churchill Livingstone, New York, pp 179-195

Baker M, Van Hansuyk E, Bogosian S, Werner F, Mech M, Murphy D 1987 A biomechanical study of the static stabilizing effect of knee braces on medial stability. American Journal of Sports Medicine 15:6

Back B Jr, Warren R 1988 The pivot shift phenomenon: results and description of a modified clinical test for ACL insufficiency. American Journal of Sports Medicine 16:6

Basmajian J V 1980 Grant's method of anatomy. Williams & Wilkins, Baltimore

Beck C, Drez D, Young J, Cannon W D, Stone M 1986 Instrumented testing of functional knee braces. American Journal of Sports Medicine 14(4):256

Bianchi M 1983 Acute tears of the posterior cruciate ligament. Clinical study and results of operative treatment in 27 cases. American Journal of Sports Medicine 11:304-314

Bullough P G, Munuera L, Murphy J, Weinstein A M 1970 The strength of the menisci of the knee as it relates to their fine structure. Journal of Bone and Joint Surgery 52B:264-270

Butler D L, Noyes F R, Grood E S 1979 Mechanical properties of transplants for the ACL. Transactions of the Orthopaedic Research Society 4: 81

Butler D L, Noyes F R, Grood E S 1980 Ligamentous restraints to anterior-posterior drawer in the human knee. A biomechanical study. Journal of Bone and Joint Surgery 62A:259-270

Cabaud H E1983 Biomechanics of the anterior cruciate ligament. Clinical Orthopaedics 172:26-31

Cassidy R E, Shaffer A J 1982 Repair of peripheral meniscus tears. American Journal of Sports Medicine 9:209

Chen E H, Black J 1980 Materials design analysis of the prosthetic anterior cruciate ligament. Journal of Biomedical Materials Research 14:567-586

Clancy W G, Narechania R G, Rosenberg T D, Gmeiner J G, Wisnefski D D 1981 Anterior and posterior cruciate ligament reconstruction in Rhesus monkeys: a histological, microangiographic, and biomechanical analysis. Journal of Bone and Joint Surgery 63A:1270-1284

Clancy W G, Shelbourne K D 1983 Treatment of knee joint instability secondary to rupture of the posterior cruciate ligament. Journal of Bone and Joint Surgery 65A:310

Cohn S A, Solta R F, Bergfield J 1990 Fractures about the knee in sports. Clinics in Sports Medicine 9(1):125-140

Collins K, Storey M, Peterson K 1986 Peroneal nerve palsy after cryotherapy. The Physician and Sports Medicine 14(5):105-108

Corrigan B, Maitland G 1983 Practical orthopaedic medicine. Butterworths, Sydney

Daniel D J, Lawler J, Malcolm L 1982 The quadricep ACL interaction. Orthopaedics Transactions 6:199

De Haven K E 1985 Meniscus repair in the athlete. Clinical Orthopaedics and Related Research 9:31-35

De Haven K E 1990 The role of the meniscus. Articular cartilage and knee joint function. In: Ewing J W (ed) Articular cartilage and knee joint function: basic science and arthroscopy. Raven Press, New York

Di Stefano V J 1990 Function, post-traumatic sequelae and current concepts of knee meniscus injuries: a review. In: Ewing J W (ed) Articular cartilage and knee joint function: basic science and arthroscopy. Raven Press, New York

Engebretsen L, Renum P, Sundalsvoll S 1989 Primary suture of the ACL. A 6 year follow-up of 74 cases. Acta Orthopaedica Scandinavica 60:561-564

Engels R P (ed) 1991 Knee ligament rehabilitation. Churchill Livingstone, New York

Ewing J W (ed) 1990 Articular cartilage and knee joint function: basic science and arthroscopy. Raven Press, New York

Fischer S P, Ferkel R D 1988 Biomechanics of the knee: prosthetic ligament reconstruction of the knee. In: Friedman M J, Ferkel R D (eds) Prosthetic ligament reconstruction of the knee. W B Saunders, Philadelphia

Frankel V H, Burstein A H, Brooks D B 1971 Biomechanics of internal derangement of the knee. Journal of Bone and Joint Surgery 53A:945-962

Frankel V H, Nordin M 1980 Basic biomechanics of the skeletal system. Lea & Febiger, Philadelphia

Fritschy D, Gautard R 1988 Jumper's knee and ultrasonography. American Journal of Sports Medicine 16:6

Fukubayashi T, Torzilli P A, Sherman M F, Warren R F 1982 An in vitro biomechanical evaluation of antero-posterior motion of the knee. Journal of Bone and Joint Surgery 64A:258-264

Fuss F K 1989 An analysis of the popliteus muscle in man, dog, and pig with a reconsideration of the general problems of the muscle. Anatomical Record 225:251-256

Gerber C, Matter P 1983 Biomechanical analysis of the knee after rupture of the anterior cruciate ligament and its primary repair—an instant-center analysis of function. Journal of Bone and Joint Surgery 65B:391-399

Giove T P, Miller S J, Kent B E 1983 Non-operative treatment of the torn ACL. Journal of Bone and Joint Surgery 65A:184

Girgis F G, Marshall J L, Al Monajem A R S 1975 The cruciate ligaments of the knee joint: functional and experimental analysis. Clinical Orthopaedics 106:216-231

Gollehon D L, Torzilli P A, Warren R F 1987 The role of the posterolateral and cruciate ligaments in the stability of the human knee. Journal of Bone and Joint Surgery 69A:233-242

Graf B 1987 Biomechanics of the anterior cruciate ligament. In: Jackson D W, Drez D (eds) The anterior cruciate deficient knee. Mosby, St Louis, pp 55-71

Grood E S, Noyes F R, Butler D L, Suntay W J 1981 Ligamentous and capsular restraints preventing straight medial and lateral laxity in intact human cadaver knees. Journal of Bone and Joint Surgery 63A:1257-1269

Grood E S, Stowers S F, Noyes F R 1988 Limits of movement in the human knee: effect of sectioning the posterior cruciate ligament and posterolateral structures. Journal of Bone and Joint Surgery 70A:88-97

Hardaker W T, Whipple T L, Bassett F H 1980. Diagnosis and treatment of the plicae syndrome of the knee. Journal of Bone and Joint Surgery 62A:221-225

Hawkins J C, Kennedy J 1974 Breaststroker's knee. The Physician and Sports Medicine 2:33-38

Heller L, Langman J 1964 The menisco-femoral ligaments of the human knee. Journal of Bone and Joint Surgery 46B:307-313

Henning C E, Lynch M A, Glick Jr K R 1985 An in vivo strain gauge study of elongation of the ACL. American Journal of Sports Medicine 13:34-39

Herzog W, Read L J 1993 Lines of action and moment arms of the major force-carrying structures crossing the human knee joint. Journal of Anatomy 182:213-230

Howell S M 1990 Anterior tibial translation during a maximal quadriceps contraction—is it clinically significant? American Journal of Sports Medicine 18(6):573-578

Hughston J C, Eilers A F 1973 The role of the posterior oblique ligament in repairs of acute medial (collateral) ligament tears of the knee. Journal of Bone and Joint Surgery 55A:923-940

Hughston J C, Norwood L A 1980 The posterolateral drawer test and external rotation recurvatum test for posterolateral instability of the knee. Clinical Orthopaedics 147:82

Indelicato P L 1988 Injury to the medial capsuloligamentous complex. In: Feagin J A Jr (ed) The crucial ligaments. Churchill Livingstone, New York, pp 197-206

Inoue M, McGurk-Burleson E, Hollis J, Woo S L 1987 Treatment of the medial collateral ligament injury: the importance of the anterior cruciate ligament on the varus-valgus knee laxity. American Journal of Sports Medicine 15(1):15-21

Jensen K 1990 Manual laxity tests for ACL injuries. Journal of Orthopaedic Sports Physical Therapy 11(10):474-481

Jokob R P, Hassler H, Staeubli H 1981 Observations on rotatory instability of the lateral compartment of the knee. Acta Orthopaedica Scandinavica (suppl 191,152:1

Kapandji I A 1982 The physiology of the joints. Vol 2, lower limb. Churchill Livingstone, Edinburgh

Kaplan E B1958 The iliotibial tract. Journal of Bone and Joint Surgery 40A:817-832

Keller P M, Shelbourne D, Mccarroll J, Rettig A 1993 Nonoperatively treated isolated posterior cruciate ligament injuries. American Journal of Sports Medicine 21(1):132-136

Kennedy J C, Gringer R W 1967 The posterior cruciate ligament. Journal of Trauma 7:367-376

Kennedy J C, Hawkins R J, Willis R B, Danylchuck K D 1976 Tension studies of human knee ligaments. Yield point, ultimate failure, and disruption of the cruciate and tibial collateral ligaments. Journal of Bone and Joint Surgery 58A:350-355

Kennedy J C, Roth J H, Walker D M 1979 Posterior cruciate ligament injuries. Orthopaedics Digest 7:19-32

Kennedy J C, Alexander I J, Hayes K C 1982 Nerve supply of the human knee and its functional importance. American Journal of Sports Medicine 16(6):329-335

Kerlan R K, Glousman R E 1988 Tibial collateral ligament bursitis. American Journal of Sports Medicine 16(4):344-346

Kettelkamp D B, Johnson R J, Smidt G L, Chao E Y S, Walker M 1970 An electromyographic study of knee motion in normal gait. Journal of Bone and Joint Surgery 58A:775-790

Kurosaka M, Yoshiya S, Andrish J T 1987 A biomechanical comparison of different surgical techniques of graft fixation in ACL reconstruction. American Journal of Sports Medicine 15:225-229

Lavin R P, Gross M T 1990 Comparison of Johnson anti-shear accessory and standard dynamometer attachment for anterior and posterior tibial translation during isometric muscle contractions. Journal of Orthopaedic Sports Physical Therapy 11:11 May

Levy I M 1988 Posterior meniscal capsuloligamentous complexes of the knee. In: Feagin J A Jr (ed) The crucial ligaments. Churchill Livingstone, New York, pp 207-216

Loomer R, Horlick S 1991 Valgus knee bracing for the osteoarthritic knee. University of British Columbia. Unpublished

Mayfield G W 1977 Popliteus tendon tenosynovitis. American Journal of Sports Medicine 5:1

McConnell J 1991 Fat pad irritation—a mistaken patellar tendinitis. Sport Health 9:4, 7-8

McMinn R M H 1990 Last's anatomy. Regional and applied, 8th edn. Churchill Livingstone, Edinburgh

Moore K L 1992 Clinically oriented anatomy, 3rd edn. Williams & Wilkins, Baltimore

Morgan C D, Cassells S W 1986 Arthroscopic meniscal repair. A safe approach to the posterior horn. Arthroscopy 2(1):3-12

Mow V C, Fithian D C, Kelly M A 1988 Fundamentals of articular cartilage and meniscus biomechanics. In: Ewing J W (ed) Articular cartilage and knee joint function: basic science and arthroscopy. Raven Press, New York

Muller W 1983 The knee: form, function and ligament reconstruction. Springer-Verlag, New York

Murray M P, Drought A B, Kory R C 1964 Walking patterns of normal men. Journal of Bone and Joint Surgery 46A:335-360

Norkin C C, Levangie P K 1992 Joint structure and function. A comprehensive analysis. F A Davis, Philadelphia

Norwood L A, Cross M J 1979 Anterior cruciate ligament—functional anatomy of its bundles in rotatory instability of the knee. American Journal of Sports Medicine 7(1):23-6

Norwood L A, Andrews J R, Meisterling R C, Glancy G L 1979 Acute anterolateral instability of the knee. Journal of Bone and Joint Surgery 61A(5):704-9

Noyes F R, Matthew S D S, Mooar P A, Grood E S 1983 The symptomatic ACL deficient knee. Part II, the results of rehabilitation, activity, modification and counselling. Journal of Bone and Joint Surgery 65A:163

Noyes F R, Butler D L, Grood E S 1984 Biomechanical analysis of human ligament grafts used in knee ligament repairs and reconstructions. Journal of Bone and Joint Surgery 66:344

Noyes F R, Keller C S, Grood E S, Butler D L 1984 Advances in the understanding of knee ligament injury, repair and rehabilitation. Medicine and Science in Sports and Exercise 16:427-443

Noyes F R, Grood E, Stowers S 1986 A biomechnical analysis of knee ligament injuries producing posterolateral subluxation. American Journal of Sports Medicine 14:440

Noyes F R, Grood E S, Butler D L, Paulos L E 1990 Clinical biomechanics of the knee—ligament restraints and functional stability. In: Funk F J (ed) Symposium on the athlete's knee: surgical repair and reconstruction. C V Mosby, St Louis

Oakes B W 1988 Ultrastructural studies on knee joint ligaments: Quantitation of collagen fibre populations in exercised and control rat cruciate ligaments and in human anterior cruciate grafts. In: Buckwalter J, Woo S L-Y (eds) Injury and repair of the musculoskeletal tissues. American Acadamy of Orthopaedic Surgeons, Illinois, section 2, pp 66-82

Ohkoshi Y, Yasuda K 1989 Biomechanical analysis of shear force executed to ACL during half-squat exercise. Orthopaedic Transactions 13:310

Olson E J, Kong J D, Fu F H, Georgescu H I, Mason G C, Evans C H 1988 The biomechanical and histological effects of artificial ligament wear particles: in vitro and in vivo studies. American Journal of Sports Medicine 16:558-570

Parolie J M, Bergfeld J A 1986 Long term results of non-operative treatment of isolated posterior cruciate ligament injuries in the athlete. American Journal of Sports Medicine 14:35

Paulos L, Noyes F R, Grood E, Butler D L 1981 Knee rehabilitation after ACL reconstruction and repair. American Journal of Sports Medicine 9:140

Perry J, Norwood L, House K 1977 Knee posture and biceps and semimembranosus muscle action in running and cutting (an EMG study). Transactions of the 23rd annual meeting, Orthopaedic Research Society 2:258

Pournaras J, Symeonides P P, Karkavelas G 1983 The significance of the posterior cruciate ligament in the stability of the knee: an experimental study with dogs. Journal of Bone and Joint Surgery 65B:204-209

Reiman P R, Jackson D W 1987 Anatomy of the anterior cruciate ligament. In: Jackson D W, Drez D (eds) The anterior cruciate deficient knee. C V Mosby, St Louis, pp 17-26

Renstrom P, Arms S W, Stanwyck T S, Johnson R J, Pope M H 1986 Strain within the ACL during hamstring and quadriceps activity. American Journal of Sports Medicine 14:(1)83-87

Robertson D B, Daniel D M, Biden E 1986 Soft tissue fixation to bone. American Journal of Sports Medicine 14:398-403

Rogers A W 1992 Textbook of anatomy. Churchill Livingstone, Edinburgh

Rovere G D, Nichols A W 1985 Frequency, associated factors and treatment of breaststroker's knee in competitve swimmers. American Journal of Sports Medicine 13(2):99-104

Sandor S M, Hart J A L, Oakes B W 1986 Case study: rehabilitation of a surgically repaired medial collateral knee ligament using a limited motion cast and isokinetic exercise. Journal of Orthopaedic Sports Physical Therapy 7(4):154-158

Seebacher J R, Inglis A E, Marshall D V M, Warren R F 1982 The structure of the posterolateral aspect of the knee. Journal of Bone and Joint Surgery 64A:536-541

Sgaglione N A, Warren R F, Wick I E, Witz T L, Gold D A, Panariello R A 1990 Primary repair with semitendinosus tendon augmentation of acute ACL injuries. American Journal of Sports Medicine 18:64-73

Shelbourne K D, Nitz P 1990 Accelerated rehabilitation following ACL reconstruction. American Journal of Sports Medicine 18:292

Shelbourne K D, Wilckens J H, Mollabashy A, De Carlo M 1991 Arthrofibrosis in acute ACL reconstruction. The effect of timing of reconstruction and rehabilitation. American Journal of Sports Medicine 19:332-336

Slocum D B, James S L, Singer K M 1976 Clinical test for anterolateral rotary instability of the knee. Clinical Orthopaedics 118:63

Smillie I S 1974 Injuries of the knee joint, 5th edn. Churchill Livingstone, Edinburgh

Somner H 1981 Patellar chondropathy and apicitis and muscle imbalances of the lower extremities in competitive sports. Sports Medicine 5:386-394

Steindler A 1935 Mechanics of normal and pathological locomotion in man. Charles C. Thomas, Springfield, Illinois

Straus W L, Cave A J E 1957 Pathology and posture of Neanderthal man. Quarterly Review of Biology 32:348-63

Tamea C, Henning C 1981 Pathomechanics of the pivot shift manoeuver. American Journal of Sports Medicine 9(1)

Terry G C, Hughston J C, Norwood L A 1986 Anatomy of the iliopatellar band and iliotibial tract. American Journal of Sports Medicine 14:39-45

Torzilli P A, Greenberg R L, Insall J 1981 An in vivo biomechanical evaluation of antero-posterior motion of the knee. Journal of Bone and Joint Surgery 63A:960-968

Trent P S, Walker P S, Wolf B 1976 Ligament length patterns, strength, and rotational axes of the knee joint. Clinical Orthopaedics 117:263-270

Tria A J, Johnson C D, Zawadsky J P 1989 The popliteus tendon. Journal of Bone and Joint Surgery 71A(5):714-715

Van Dommelen B A, Fowler P J 1989 Anatomy of the posterior cruciate ligament. A review. American Journal of Sports Medicine 17(1):24-29

Walker P S, Erkman M J 1975 The role of the menisci in force transmission across the knee. Clinical Orthopaedics and Related Research 109:184-192

Walla D J, Albright J P, Mcauley E, Martin R K, Eldridge V, El-Khoury 1985 Hamstring control and the unstable anterior cruciate ligament-deficient knee. American Journal of Sports Medicine 13:34-39

Warren L F, Marshall J L, Girgis F 1974 The prime static stabilizer of the medial side of the knee. Journal of Bone and Joint Surgery 56A:665-674

Warren L F, Marshall J L 1979 The supporting structures and layers on the medial side of the knee. Journal of Bone and Joint Surgery 61A:56-62

Williams J G P, Sperryn P N (eds) 1976 Sports medicine, 2nd edn. Arnold, London

Williams P L, Warwick R, Dyson M, Bannister L H 1989 Gray's anatomy. Churchill Livingstone, Edinburgh

Yamaguchi G, Zajac F 1989 A planar model of the knee joint to characterize the knee extensor mechanism. Journal of Biomechanics 22(1):1-10

Zimny M L, Albright D J, Dabezies E 1988 Mechanoreceptors in the human medial meniscus. Acta Anatomica 133:35-40

30. The patellofemoral complex

Barry Gerrard

The patellofemoral joint has often been described as the most researched small joint in the body, producing pain and disability far out of proportion to its size. Patellofemoral pain is common in all ages of the general population, but even more so among athletes (Dehaven & Lintner 1986, Devereaux & Lachmann 1984). Hording (1983) reported that 10% of Swedish children sought medical advice for patellar pain. Devereaux and Lachmann (1984) found that patellofemoral arthralgia was the complaint in 6% of all patients attending a sports injury clinic, particularly those engaged in athletics and racquet sports. Abnormalities of the patellofemoral joint generally amount to 10% of knees assessed by arthroscopy (Lindberg 1986).

The term 'patellofemoral pain syndrome' (PFPS) can be used to describe the clinical entity of activity induced pain, pain on physical examination of the patellofemoral joint and on at least two of the following: stair climbing, squatting, pseudolocking, and pain or stiffness after prolonged sitting (Lindberg 1986, Malek & Mangine 1981). 'Chondromalacia patella' was an all-embracing term used in the early literature. It is now restricted to those instances where articular cartilaginous degeneration has been shown to be present (Fulkerson & Hungerford 1990).

Various causative factors have been attributed to PFPS. They include poor alignment of the extensor mechanism, poor alignment of the entire lower extremity, and patellar instability (Hughston 1968, Insall et al 1983, Sojbjerg et al 1987, Sommer 1988). Ficat and Hungerford (1977) described the 'excessive lateral pressure syndrome' (ELPS), i.e. a patellar tracking abnormality associated with a tight lateral patellofemoral retinaculum. This may be the result of the action of the malalignment factors listed above, or to the anatomy of the complex and extensive lateral structures of the knee (Ficat & Hungerford 1977, Terry 1989). Merchant (1988), in a detailed classification of patellofemoral disorders, places secondary chondromalacia patellae (i.e. not caused by trauma) under the heading of patellofemoral dysplasias, indicating an aetiology related to malalignment of the lower extremity (Merchant 1988).

ANATOMY

The patella

The form of the largest sessamoid bone in the body is particularly complex. It is shaped like a shield, with the apex pointing distally, and has an anterior and posterior surface and three borders. The articular surface can be divided into medial and lateral facets separated by a central ridge and with an odd medial facet (Fig. 30.1). The patella can be quite small in 'patella parva' and is variable with other aplasias and dysplasias, often occurring without any abnormalities in function (Fulkerson & Hungerford 1990).

While the height and width are nearly constant the thickness of the cartilage and bone varies. The articular cartilage of the patella is thicker than anywhere else in the body. Wiberg (1941), and later additions from Baumgartl (1964), classified the patella into three types:

- type 1, in which the medial and lateral facets are equal
- type 2, (the most common type), where the medial facet is considerably smaller than the lateral facet
- type 3, in which the medial facet is very small and consequently is steeply angled and convex.

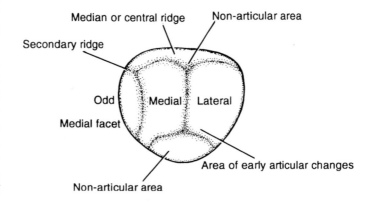

Fig. 30.1 The medial, lateral and odd medial facet of the patella

This shape classification has not been found to correlate either with the presence or site of cartilaginous damage or degeneration (Schulitz et al 1983). However, a type 3 patella with a convex medial facet was found by Weh and Lluer (1987) to increase the degeneration on the odd medial facet and has been strongly implicated in recurrent dislocation of the patella.

The articular surfaces of the femur

The surface of the distal part of the femur articulating with the patella is often called the 'trochlea', the 'patellar facets of the femur', or the 'patellar groove'. It is recognized that the shape of the femoral condyles and the flexion/extension motion of the knee dictate the kinematics or gliding motion of the patella (Van Eijden et al 1986, Lafortune & Cavanagh 1987).

The femoral surface is divided into a medial and lateral facet separated by a shallow groove that distally becomes the intercondylar notch. Both facets are convex in all directions to articulate with the concave medial and lateral facets of the patella respectively. The patellar facets pass down and posteriorly to become the condyles of the femur.

Synovial cavity/membrane

The synovial limits of the patellofemoral joint are essentially those of the anterior knee joint. It covers all the non-articular structures within the fibrous capsule including the suprapatellar pouch, the peripatellar part (the medial and lateral recesses), and the inferior portion (the infra-patellar fat pads).

The suprapatellar pouch has a wide communication with the knee joint and is a good hiding place for loose bodies. They may cause suprapatellar pain on full knee flexion or forceful quadriceps contraction. The pouch is implicated in the formation of anterior femoral erosions, and is separated from the knee joint by the suprapatellar synovial plica (Lafortune & Cavanagh 1987, Rose & Cockshott 1982, Schulitz et al 1983). The thickening of the synovial membrane is not considered to be important in anterior knee pain unless it is large, excessively thickened and continuous with the medial patellar plica. This occurs in 37% of cases (Lafortune & Cavanagh 1987). The supra-patellar plica is a vestigial septum and an embryonic remnant (Jacobson & Flandry 1989, Schulitz et al 1983).

Anterior knee pain, groove formation on the medial femoral condyle, or medial facet chondromalacia of the patella has been correlated with thickened plica. The incidence of medial synovial plicae in painful knees found in the literature varies from 15–55% (Broom & Fulkerson 1986, Fulkerson & Hungerford 1990, Lafortune & Cavanagh 1987, Patel 1986, Schulitz et al 1983).

A thickened plica may produce symptoms that can be mistakenly diagnosed as a torn meniscus or chondromalacia patellae and therefore would need to be differentiated by careful physical examination or arthroscopy (discussed later). However, the clinical importance of synovial plicae in the pain producing situation may well be exaggerated and probably is only relevant in a small percentage of cases where it produces a snapping effect on flexion of the knee.

The infrapatellar plica, commonly called the ligamentum mucosum, passes from the intercondylar notch to the infrapatellar fat pad. This plica has very little clinical significance except that it is often very large and can become irritated (Lafortune & Cavanagh 1987, Schulitz et al 1983).

Capsule

The capsule of the knee anteriorly is continuous on all sides except superiorly where the knee communicates with the suprapatellar bursae. The capsule itself is a very thin structure, with lateral and medial thickenings that form the patellofemoral ligaments, the most common of these being the patellotibial ligaments (Fulkerson & Gossling 1980, Kaplan 1958).

The capsule, thickenings and bands on the lateral side of the knee form a much stronger passive stabilizing force than those of the medial (Fulkerson 1989, Fulkerson & Gossling 1980, Fulkerson & Hungerford 1990).

Muscles affecting the patellofemoral joint

Active stabilization is performed anteriorly by the four main elements of the quadriceps group of muscles, posteriorly by the hamstrings muscles and laterally by the iliotibial tract.

The quadriceps group have been classically identified as three separate layers at their insertion into the superior aspect of the patella. Medially and laterally these three layers reinforce the respective patellofemoral ligaments, to form an active decelerator mechanism with competent static restraints in both a coronal and sagittal plane (Terry 1989).

Vastus medialis

This muscle located on the anteromedial aspect of the thigh arises from the lower portion of the intertrochanteric line, the spiral line, the whole length of the linea aspera, the upper part of the supracondylar line, the tendons of the adductor longus and adductor magnus and the medial intermuscular septum. The majority of fibres of the oblique portion arise from the adductor magnus tendon. The vastus medialis (VM) extends distally towards the supramedial margin of the patella and becomes tendinous on the deep surface of the muscle, a few millimetres before their insertion, into the quadriceps tendon and the medial border of the patella. A few of the superficial fibres are inserted into the tendon of the rectus femoris. Some of the aponeurosis reinforcing the capsule of the knee joint is attached to the medial condyle of the tibia and reinforces the medial patellar retinaculum (Thiranagama 1990, Warwick 1989).

The muscle can be divided into a 'longus' (VML) and 'oblique' (vastus medialis oblique) portion by the presence of a separate tissue plane divided by a cleavage line or fibrofatty plane. The VML muscle fibres are aligned in its proximal portion at 10° and in the distal part at 15–35° to the shaft of the femur. The vastus medialis oblique fibres run obliquely, as their name suggests at 40–70° to the shaft of the femur (Lieb & Perry 1971, Weinstable et al 1989).

The vastus medialis is attached to the adductor magnus tendon although it has been shown that a part of the attachment is deficient in 60% of specimens.

The nerve supply to the vastus medialis is by branches of the posterior division of the femoral nerve which divides after passing under the inguinal ligament. The nerve enters the muscle at the proximal part of the muscle with the nerve trunk descending the medial border of the muscle to where it enters the muscle. The branch to vastus medialis oblique runs either through or superficially over the tissue plane dividing VML from vastus medialis oblique and is present as a separate nerve in 40% of specimens (Gerrard 1990). A further branch to the vastus medialis oblique arising from the saphenous nerve has been isolated by Gunal et al (1992), giving extensive innervation to the vastus medialis oblique. Innervation from this nerve would be disrupted by injury or surgery to the medial side of the knee.

Vastus lateralis

This muscle forming the middle layer of the quadriceps group is a stability synergist acting to provide stability rather than fast movement. Weinstable et al (1989) divided it into a longus and oblique portion. The former fibres insert into the base of the patella at an angle of 12.5° and the latter into the lateral rim of the patella at an angle of 32.4°. The most distal fibres reinforce the lateral retinaculum to form a complex and rigid structure (far stronger than the medial retinaculum) that maintains the lateral alignment of the patella.

Rectus femoris

This long fusiform muscle narrows to a tendon 5–8 cm above the patella, reaching a maximum width of 3–5 cm at its insertion into the superior aspect of the patella. The direction of pull is 7–10° medially in the frontal plane and 3–5° anteriorly in the sagittal plane. Even though the rectus femoris pulls the patella slightly in a medial direction, it is a long and fast-acting muscle that gives little stability to the patellofemoral joint.

Reider et al (1981) found that the rectus component was the only part of the quadriceps whose tendinous fibres continued into the infrapatellar tendon.

Vastus intermedius

These fibres lie in a plane parallel with the anterior aspect of the shaft of the femur. The aponeurotic fibres from the anterior surface of the muscle insert into the superior surface of the patella. They do not continue onto the anterior surface but some fibres blend into those of the vastus medialis and lateralis (Reider et al 1981, Warwick et al 1989).

Articularis genus

This small muscle arising from the anterior surface of the shaft of the femur is attached to the synovial membrane of the knee joint. It is often absent or variable and when present is flat and wispy and ranges from 1.5—3 cm wide (Reider et al 1981, Warwick et al 1989). The main action of this muscle is to pull the synovial membrane out of the way when the knee comes into full extension (see Ch. 29).

Muscle fibre characteristics

Postural muscles such as the quadriceps have a higher content of slow twitch fibres and show more prolonged duration, higher amplitude and lower frequency of contraction than small, short acting muscles such as the intrinsic hand muscles (Vatine et al 1990). Within the quadriceps, the vastus medialis and lateralis are the postural muscles providing active stability to knee mobility and therefore have a higher proportion of type 1 muscle fibres. The rectus femoris is the faster component of the group and has a larger proportion of type 2 fibres (Richardson & Bullock 1986, Richardson & Sims 1991). Atrophy of the vastus medialis to a greater extent than the vastus lateralis is one of the significant signs of patellofemoral pathology. In the treatment program the use of isometric, slow eccentric and concentric exercises are specifically aimed at the stabilizing effect of the type 1 fibres (see section on treatment, later in this chapter). A full description of muscle fibre types and attributes is included in Chapter 2.

Table 30.1 shows the distribution of type 1 (slow twitch) and the distribution of fibre types within the muscle.

Table 30.1 Proportion of fibre types in quadriceps muscles

	type 1 %
Vastus medialis	
• surface	43.7
• deep	61.5
• type 2 fibres: superficial > deep	
Vastus lateralis	
• surface	37.8
• deep	46.9
• type 2 fibres: superficial > deep	
Rectus femoris	
lateral head	
• surface	29.5
• deep	42.0
medial head	42.8
• type 2 fibres: superficial > deep	
• type 2 fibres: lateral head > medial head	

Source: Adapted from Johnson et al (1973).

Iliotibial tract

This thick band, a continuation of the fascia lata, is formed proximally at the level of the greater trochanter by a combination of the tensor fascia lata, gluteus maximus and gluteus medius. It also attaches to the linea aspera of the femur via the lateral intermuscular septum. Distally it separates into the iliotibial tract and the iliopatellar band inserting into Gerdy's tubercle and the tibial tuberosity (Fulkerson & Gossling 1980). According to Terry et al (1986), the functional anatomy of these two bands is complex, with the iliopatellar band influencing knee deceleration and the various layers of the iliotibial tract acting as an anterolateral ligament of the knee. It combines with the vastus lateralis to limit the medial deviation of the patella. Stretching of this band if tight by mobilizing techniques is of considerable importance in the treatment of patellofemoral pain. However, the stretching exercises tend to affect only the proximal muscular attachments rather than the distal thick fascial band portion (Fulkerson & Gossling 1980, Henry 1989, McConnell 1986, Patel 1986, Sahrman & Dixon 1988, Warwick et al 1989).

Intermuscular septa and fascia

There are three intermuscular septa in the thigh that attach to the linea aspera and the corresponding supracondylar line. The lateral septum is thick and strong but the posterior and medial are thin fascial layers on the front and back of the adductor muscles. The fascial covering over the quadriceps muscles is thicker over the vastus lateralis than that over the vastus medialis oblique, vastus medialis or vastus intermedius. This may explain why the muscle atrophy that occurs with knee injuries nearly always seems greater over the vastus medialis oblique (where the muscle bulk is not hidden by fascia) than any other quadriceps muscle. Covering the the vastus medialis oblique the fascia contains a superficial branch of the femoral nerve extending to the capsule of the knee joint. As mentioned before an areolar fascial division has been found to occur between the oblique fibres of the vastus medialis oblique and the predominantly long fibres of the vastus medialis longus (Weinstable et al 1989).

Blood supply

The vascular anatomy demonstrates the relative independence of the patellofemoral joint in that it possesses its own true vascular tree (Fulkerson & Hungerford 1990, p 33). The normal arterial supply to the patella originates from the descending genicular, the lateral circumflex and the popliteal arteries. They supply the superior, medial and lateral superior, the medial and lateral inferior, the anterior genicular arteries and the tibial recurrent artery.

The arterial supply to the condyles of the femur is assured by grid-like webs from the medial and lateral condylar 'cheek' and by branches of the medial genicular artery (from the popliteal artery) through the intercondylar notch. A further branch of a common arterial trunk together with the superior lateral genicular artery supplies the dorsomedial capsule and the dorsal muscles.

The arteries form a subchondral loop with very fine vessels branching off to the condylar articular surface.

Venous drainage

The two principle drainage routes as determined by phlebography are the popliteal vein and the great saphenous vein. The main venous drainage is from the inferior pole of the patella and an accessory system drains the anterior surface.

Increased venous engorgement (thereby producing increased intra-osseous tension) in the patella in the presence of abnormal patellofemoral rhythm and joint overloading has been cited as a cause of pain in the patellofemoral pain syndrome (Waishrod & Treiman 1980). Pain on sustained knee flexion in conjunction with the increased intra-osseous pressure found in chondromalacia patellae has been decreased using a sagittal (longitudinal) osteotomy (Hejgaard & Arnoldi 1984).

Nerve supply

The anterior part of the knee is supplied by the anterior group of afferent articular nerves. The largest of the three articular nerves supplying the quadriceps muscle is the articular branch to the vastus medialis oblique that bifurcates beneath the medial retinaculum to supply a wide area of the medial capsule (Kennedy et al 1982).

The lateral capsule is supplied by the nerve to the vastus lateralis that passes deep to that muscle.

The nerve to the vastus intermedius, consisting of several branches, continues to the suprapatellar pouch and further to the capsule of the knee and the articularis genu muscle.

The infrapatellar branch of the saphenous nerve, itself a branch of the femoral nerve, traverses the medial aspect of the tibia inferior to the joint line to innervate the inferomedial capsule, patellar tendon and the skin overlying the anterior aspect of the knee.

The exact innervation, size and sites of branching of the nerves around the knee is particularly variable (Hejgaard & Arnoldi 1984).

PATELLOFEMORAL BIOMECHANICS AND PATHOMECHANICS

Cartilage-loading, ultrastructure and bone

In the normal state the articular cartilage of the patellofemoral joint is hard, smooth and able to withstand the stresses and strains put on it (see Ch. 3). However, when abnormal alignment and loading factors are imposed on cartilage that is already altered or unable to withstand the increased load, histological changes occur and the condition is called chondromalacia patellae. Chondromalacia patellae is considered by some clinicians to be a distinct clinical entity, but others refer only to cartilaginous changes of softening and fibrillation (Dashefsky 1987, Radin 1983). On arthroscopy, the changes present initially as softening of the hyaline cartilage progressing to a blister and then a 'crabmeat' like appearance. They eventually show as a pitted and cratered articular cartilage that can extend down to subchondral bone. These changes can be explained on a chemical or on a stress-related basis (for further discussion see Chrisman 1986). This stress-related hypothesis has been supported by many authors, but it has also been postulated that the condition may arise from disuse or alteration of load bearing (Fulkerson & Hungerford 1990, Ohno et al 1988). This would affect the stiffness of the underlying bone and the thickness of the cartilage (Akizuki et al 1986, Jurvelin et al 1986). Cartilaginous fibrillation occurs more frequently over stiffer, denser bone, and over prominent orientations of trabecular bone which occurs more frequently over the lateral facet than the medial (Radin 1983). Lesions of the medial surface of the patella do not progress to other surfaces whereas those that start on the lateral facet do progress over the central ridge and are more representative of patellar arthritis rather than chondromalacia patellae (Radin 1983).

Bone density increases in general in chondromalacia patellae, with localized less dense areas, particularly in the area of the central medial facet. The mean bone density beneath degenerated cartilage is similar to that of normal specimens but has a larger range of more and less dense areas (Borkstrom & Goldie 1980).

There is much debate on whether hyaline cartilage heals. Many authors since Hunter in 1743 have reported that it does not but Bentley (1985) showed fibrous metaplasia and cartilage regeneration in early lesions, while Salter et al (1981), with the use of continuous passive movement showed cartilaginous repair with similar composition to hyaline cartilage in young rabbits. Conversely, immobilization has been shown to cause articular damage (see Ch. 2). Healing, when it happens, occurs in small weight-bearing lesions rather than larger or non-weightbearing lesions.

Patellar tracking

The patella has primarily been thought to protect the knee from injury and to increase the efficiency of the quadriceps mechanism. It also protects the patellar tendon from the effects of friction. Fulkerson and Hungerford (1990) also maintain that not only is the patella of aesthetic value but it also transmits compressive loads in a pain free way (in the normal state), to the underlying hyaline cartilage.

The patellofemoral joint functions to increase the efficiency of the extensor mechanism of the knee by:

- increasing the distance of the extensor apparatus from the axis of the knee
- increasing the length of the quadriceps moment arm
- turning the force of the quadriceps directed obliquely, superiorly and slightly laterally into a strictly vertical force (Fulkerson & Hungerford 1990, Kapandji 1987).

The tracking pattern of the patella is mainly a function of the configuration of the femoral condyles and contacting surfaces of the patella, and to a lesser extent the 'Q' angle (see below) and the dynamic balance of the medial and lateral components of the quadriceps mechanism during contraction (Ahmed et al 1989, Lafortune & Cavanagh 1987). If the underlying bony structure and alignment is poor, the prognosis of treatment, particularly conservative treatment, is also likely to be poor. Where the underlying structure is well developed, strategies to affect poor alignment will be more effective and last longer. There is an anatomic predisposition to recurrent dislocation (e.g. a dysplasic femoral trochlear) and 'pathological' patellar tracking starts from the beginning of knee flexion. There is a direct relationship between the vastus lateralis/VM ratio and Q angle in a malalignment group and those with a past history of patellofemoral pain syndrome. There also has shown to be a dominance of the vastus lateralis (Kujala et al 1989, Suzuki et al 1988).

The Q angle

The direction of this quadriceps force produces a measure known as the 'Q' angle—the angle between a line drawn from the anterior superior iliac spine through the centre of the patella and intersecting a line to the tibial tubercle (Insall 1982). The average angle is 15.8 ± 4.5° for females and 11.2 ± 3.0° for men (Horton & Hall 1989). Clinically, above 15° is usually considered to be excessive in men, and 17° in females. This is indicative of severe patellar malalignment and is associated with poor conservative and surgical treatment results. However, the angle measured depends on the position of the subject (Lindberg 1986). Most authors measure the Q angle with the subject supine and the feet together. A more functional method is in standing so that the effect of all structures in the lower limbs is taken into account.

The Q angle is affected by the width of the pelvis, hip rotation, femoral anteversion and the position of the tibial tubercle. The tubercle is affected by tibial rotation which in turn is affected by the position of the foot. It is the effects of these factors that the physiotherapist attempts to alter in conservative treatment.

Patellar alignment

The movement of the patella is controlled by both dynamic and static constraints (Kapandji 1987).

Static constraints are those of the bony configuration of the patella, femur and tibia, the medial and lateral patellofemoral retinaculum, the patellar ligament and the quadriceps tendon.

The dynamic constraints are those of the soft tissues; the quadriceps muscles, mainly the vastus medialis and lateralis and indirectly the hamstrings, adductor magnus and to a lesser extent adductor longus. Added to this list are the effects of the closed kinetic chain above and below the joint that were mentioned before (Table 30.2).

Many authors have considered the patella as a simple pulley, while others have written that the patella moves in a curve concave laterally when the knee is flexed (Ficat &

Table 30.2 List of factors producing poor patellar alignment

Factors	Effect
Static	
Q angle	determines tracking of patella
patella alta (high position), infera (low) parva (small), and dysplasias	alters patellar stability and tracking
genu valgus, varus	alters Q angle
genu recurvatum	irritates the fat pad
femoral trochlear dysplasia	decreases the joint stability
femoral anteversion	increases the Q angle
internal tibial torsion	increases the Q angle
Dynamic	
VMO weakness	allows the VL to pull laterally
gluteal weakness	produces internal rotation during gait
gastrocnemius and soleus tightness	produces premature heel lift and foot pronation
hamstring tightness	causes decreased knee extension and increased knee flexion during gait
iliotibial band and lateral patellofemoral retinacular tightness	causes lateral patellar compression
poor foot posture	alters the Q angle
poor hip control, particularly rotation	allows adduction of the leg during gait with increased Q angle

Hungerford 1977, Fulkerson 1989, Van Eijden et al 1986). Figure 30.2 shows the position of the patella in varying degrees of knee flexion. The patella during knee flexion makes a rolling and gliding motion along the femoral articular surface. When looking distally (at the right knee) the gliding movement is clockwise, in contrast to the rolling movement which is anti-clockwise between 0–90° and clockwise between 90–120° (Van Eijden et al 1986) (Fig. 30.3). Fujikawa et al (1983) also related knee flexion to movements of the patella and found that it rotated laterally by 6.3° (mean) about the anteroposterior axis and medially by 11° (mean) about the supero-inferior axis from

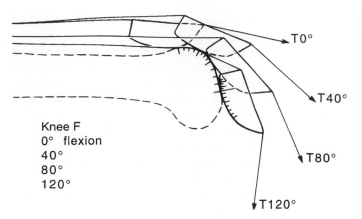

Knee F
0° flexion
40°
80°
120°

T0°

T40°

T80°

T120°

Fig. 30.2 The position of the patella tendon, patella and quadriceps tendon and location of the contact points as a function of the flexion/extension angle. Source: Van Eijden et al (1986)

25–130° of knee flexion. This is the movement limited by a tight lateral retinaculum. Van Eijden et al (1986) consider this movement of the patella to be due to the backward rotation of the patellar ligament relative to the tibial axis. Lafortune and Cavanagh (1987) inserted Steinman pins into patellae and found that in the gait cycle, early adduction of the femur tended to increase the Q angle, whereas its abduction later in the swing phase, combined with the lateral shift of the patella, tended to decrease the Q angle and stretch the medial retinaculum. However, as the study was performed with the subjects walking it did not take into account the reduced abduction phase while running.

Effect of rotation and patellar position

Changing the angle of the tibiofemoral joint increases femoral rotation and alters patellofemoral tracking. Femoral rotation is altered in children with anterior knee pain and an increased Q angle has been recorded with internal

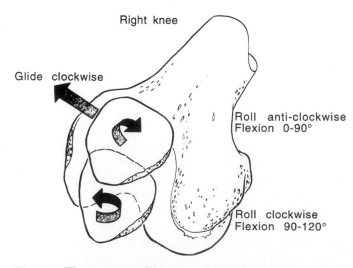

Right knee

Glide clockwise

Roll anti-clockwise
Flexion 0-90°

Roll clockwise
Flexion 90-120°

Fig. 30.3 The movement of the patella during knee flexion. Source: Van Eijden et al (1986)

rotation and pronation of the foot (Fujikawa et al 1983, Olerud & Berg 1984, Sikorski et al 1979).

Maximum quadriceps contraction has not shown a consistent or significant effect on patellar tracking in either control or symptomatic knees. However, the rate of lateral shift of the patella increased on voluntary contraction in symptomatic knees and decreased clinically following surgical realignment in the group of patients whose improvement was satisfactory. In the group of patients whose improvement was not satisfactory the rate of lateral shift was not changed (Sasaki & Yagi 1986). The effects of increasing or decreasing the pull of the different quadriceps components are to increase the pressure on the ipsi or contralateral surfaces respectively and to produce changes in orientation of the patella in the coronal plane.

The medial glide (or shift) of the patella has been measured in young women at 12.3 mm with the knee in full extension (Sahrman & Dixon 1988).

A patient with a hypomobile patella would benefit from stretching of the lateral retinaculum or lateral release whereas a hypermobile patella would not (Lafortune & Cavanagh 1987, Sahrman & Dixon 1988) (see section on treatment below).

The patella shifts 8 mm medially during a complete walking cycle (Lafortune & Cavanagh 1987). The total range of motion of the patella relative to the femur was 21 mm in the anteroposterior and 45 mm in the proximodistal direction. The position of the patella can be altered by taping. This technique is described later in this chapter. Roberts (1989) found a significant increase in lateral patellar displacement of 4.3 mm and lateral patellofemoral angle, of 8° using an isometric radiological technique after medial taping of the patella.

Patellar orientation and mobility

The orientation of the patella during movement of the knee is paramount to the pain free and efficient functioning of the patellofemoral joint. While the Q angle measures the alignment of the lower limb, the A angle measures the relationship of the patella to the tibial tubercle (Fig. 30.4). The A angle has been defined as 'the complement of the angle that is formed by the intersection of the line that bisects the patella longitudinally and the line drawn from the tibial tubercle to the apex of the inferior pole of the patella' (Arno 1990). This measure will be affected by changes in medio-lateral patellar glide and internal-external rotation of the patella. However, it does not measure the other two components of patellar tracking: tilt or the anteroposterior position of the patella. The A angle is significantly increased in patellofemoral pain patients (DiVeta & Vogelbach 1992), but it is not known whether the angle is reduced once the patients are rehabilitated and pain free. The mean A angle in asymptomatic subjects was 12.3° compared to 23.2° for the symptomatic group in one

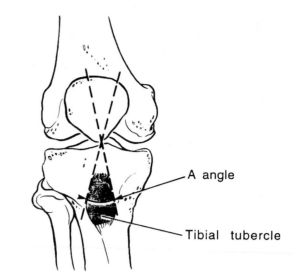

Fig. 30.4 The A angle. Source: Arno (1990)

study and above 35 degrees in another (Arno 1990, DiVeta & Vogelbach 1992).

Gender effects

In the general population females have a higher incidence of patellofemoral pain than males (3:2) except in an athletic population where the numbers are equal. Above 60° of knee flexion, the force between the femoral intercondylar groove and the quadriceps tendon increases linearly with knee flexion. As females have increased knee flexion during the stance phase of walking and as the patellofemoral joint reaction force depends not only on the quadriceps muscle force but also on the degree of knee flexion, it is logical that females develop higher patellofemoral forces than men for the same extending knee forces (Kettelkamp et al 1970, Nisell & Ekholm 1985). The common explanation for females having a higher incidence of patellofemoral symptoms is usually that they have wider hips thereby producing a higher Q angle and an increase in lateral tracking. However, it may simply be due to increased stress in the growing period (Jacobson & Flandry 1989).

Compressive forces

The magnitude of patellofemoral compressive force has been calculated during level walking at 0.5 times body weight (BW), 3.3 BW during stair climbing, 2.6 BW on maximum isometric knee extension, and 7 BW on squatting (Dahlquist et al 1982). The increased load on the patellofemoral joint while climbing stairs, squatting and performing exercises through range in weightbearing could justify concluding in the presence of other factors that patellofemoral pain in adolescents and athletes is primarily due to joint overloading. Pain is rarely seen by itself without any malalignment factors or underlying cartilaginous degeneration. The overloading of the joint by one of these activities may just be the precipitating cause that activates a previously latent problem.

ANTERIOR KNEE PAIN

Patellofemoral pain syndrome (PFPS), patellofemoral instability and patellar tendinitis (PT) are the most common causes of anterior knee pain. It is important to differentiate them from a treatment point of view although each may have components of the other (Table 30.3).

Patellofemoral pain syndrome

The PFPS, or peripatellar tendinitis in Merchant's (1988) classification, which may or may not be a precursor to the excessive lateral compression syndrome (ELPS), will probably not have confirmed chondral damage and therefore not be entitled to be called chondromalacia patellae (Fulkerson & Hungerford 1990). There is often very little connection between minor articular damage and pain. More

advanced degenerative changes are likely to be associated with pain and a worse prognosis.

PFPS is extremely common, occurring in up to 36% of a 14-year-old school population and 25% of knee injuries in a sporting population (Devereaux & Lachmann 1984, Lindberg 1986).

It occurs in adolescents at the time of increased growth and affects girls more than boys, often limiting sporting activity.

In girls it is associated with an increased Q angle, normal lateralization of the patella and decreased activity. Boys with PFPS have a high activity level, normal Q angle and increased lateralization of the patella (i.e. malalignment) (Lindberg 1986). In athletes it affects the sexes equally and is associated with poor alignment, poor training techniques and increased loading of the knee (Dehaven & Lintner 1986). After middle age, more commonly in women, it is associated with the overloading of a degenerate joint. According to Fulkerson and Hungerford (1989), it is due to 'chronic lateral patellar tilt, adaptive lateral retinacular shortening and resultant chronic imbalance of facet loads'.

Symptoms are anterior, posterior (or both) knee pain plus two of the following:

- diffuse ache increasing to sharp on activity
- pain on stairs
- pain on sitting (moviegoer's knee)
- pain on squatting
- crepitus
- giving way
- pseudolocking
- swelling (usually only if associated with instability).

Signs are:

- pain produced on any of the above tests
- signs of malalignment and/or muscle weakness
- absence of tibiofemoral abnormalities that would produce these symptoms
- chronic coexisting conditions that may cause anterior knee pain, e.g. anterior cruciate deficiency.

The treatment of PFPS will be discussed later in this chapter.

Patellar tendinitis or periostitis

The pain occurring in athletes with this condition is very similar to that of PFPS and often occurs simultaneously with it. A prepatellar bursitis and a swollen infrapatellar fat pad can also occur at the same time. Patellar tendinitis is characterized by pain at the inferior angle and border of the patella and there may be accompanying intratendinous pain or swelling (see Ch. 29). This may be seen as a hypo-echoic or black space when viewed with ultrasound. It is debatable whether the presence of a defect is related to the pain. The condition occurs in jumping and aerial activities,

Table 30.3 Clinical signs of PFPS, patellofemoral instability and patellar tendinitis

Signs	PFPS	Instability	PT
Onset	running, stair/step activity particularly eccentric component	any activity	jumping and landing in basketball, netball, volleyball, ballet
Pain	peripatellar and/or posterior, hard to describe	anterior	inferior pole of patella, more localized
Tenderness	peripatella and inferior pole, may not be palpable	antero-medialis	inferior pole, maybe along length of tendon
Crepitus	often present in severe cases	none	none
Giving way	due to quadriceps weakness or pain	yes	not usual
Effusion	occasional but small	yes	unusual, but may be tendinous oedema
Click Clunk	often in older athletes	yes	none
Range of knee	decreased in severe cases	decreased movement	not affected
Patellar mobility	decreased medial glide due to tight lateral retinaculum	increased	normal range unless associated with PFPS
VMO	wasting, VMO/VL imbalance and altered timing	VMO > VL wasting	may have general quadriceps wasting
Effect of activity	pain increases with increasing activity	pain and swelling with activity	pain at start decreases and returns after stopping
Retest sign	stairs, squats, duck waddle	as for PFPS	hopping, jumping, fast squats

particularly in basketball, netball and volleyball players with long and frequent training routines.

The treatment consists of a full assessment of the closed kinetic chain from the hips to the feet and strengthening programs using eccentric and concentric exercises in weightbearing. As it occurs in players with large quadriceps muscle bulk and large peak torque to body weight ratios, emphasis must be given to the quality and timing of the vastus medialis oblique contraction in the early part of the rehabilitation process and activity-specific exercises before the player resumes playing. Stretching of the iliotibial band, hamstring muscles and dura is important. Unlike in PFPS, jogging does not irritate athletes with this condition and can be performed depending on the degree of PFPS also present. According to the degree of PFPS present the treatment may be identical to that of PFPS with modified return to sporting activities once the anterior knee pain has settled down. Activities involving jumping, stopping quickly, cutting and defensive drills will need to be practised with icing of the tendon afterwards to reduce pain and swelling. The use of moist heat, quadriceps and hamstring stretches prior to activity and ice afterwards is important in the return to sport phase.

Electrotherapy does not play a large part in the treatment of this condition except for occasional use of low intensity ultrasound, high frequency galvanic or interferential for pain relief. Electrical muscle stimulation or biofeedback may be used to retrain the selectivity and timing of the vastus medialis oblique. The Chopat strap (infrapatellar strap) or tape worn below the patella alters the pull on the patellar tendon. It often eases the pain and gives protection in the early stages of returning to playing sport.

Quadriceps rupture

An athlete who has severe pain on jumping or landing from a jump and who has swelling, inability to extend the knee and a palpable defect proximal to the patella may have a ruptured quadriceps mechanism. A complete rupture with failure of the extensor mechanism will require open surgical intervention (Schmidt & Henry 1989).

Patellar instability

Merchant (1988) developed a classification of patellofemoral disorders. Three grades were related to patellar instability:

- lateral compression syndrome
- chronic subluxation of the patella
- recurrent dislocation of the patellofemoral joint.

Each class is a progression of the one before and the signs and symptoms of the first grade are not unlike those of PFPS.

Acute and chronic instability occurs usually in the presence of static malalignment factors such as femoral anteversion, femoral groove dysplasia, patella alta and general ligamentous hypermobility. These factors cannot be changed conservatively. However, the dynamic components can be changed.

Acute lateral dislocation of the patella is associated with tearing of the medial retinaculum. The forces involved need not be great and there may also be an osteochondral fracture often with considerable disruption to the articular surface. In children, a sudden contraction of the quadriceps muscle may even produce a transverse avulsion fracture of the lower pole of the patella without any dislocation.

Suzuki et al (1988) (testing patients on stairs using EMG), and Dvir et al (1991) (using isokinetic movement) have both shown a decrease in muscle action at the position in the movement where the knee pain is at its greatest. In an unstable or potentially unstable knee an instability episode is likely to occur when the joint is without the protection of the muscles. Subluxation and dislocation both occur usually where there is internal femoral rotation on a fixed lower leg and foot in external rotation. The physiotherapy treatment for patellar instability in the subacute and chronic stage is essentially the same as for PFPS although increased emphasis is given to muscle retraining particularly in the part of the range where the instability occurs. The treatment results obtained in patients with patellar instability are not as good as those with PFPS. Of the 14% of patellofemoral patients who had instability and who answered a questionnaire 1–5 years after 'successful' treatment, 43% still 'gave way', 38% continued to have swelling and 59% had the same or more crepitus (Gerrard 1990).

Conservative treatment following an acute dislocation will depend on the extent of the damage to the patella, to the surrounding soft tissues and the stability of the joint. Avulsion fractures of the medial surface of the patella occur and the fragments need to be excised if they impinge upon the femoral condyles. In a mild case a bandage may be used to give support and the vastus medialis oblique program started immediately. In a severe case the knee will be immobilized to allow the medial retinaculum to heal for a period of up to 6 weeks, following which there will be a vastus medialis oblique retraining program.

Fractures of the patella

Fractures of the patella can occur as a result of stress, direct or indirect trauma.

Stress fractures are the result of a process of submaximal cyclic loading leading to a point where fatigue failure occurs. Painful bipartite patellae are therefore often confused with slowly forming stress fractures.

Indirect trauma producing a fracture may be as a result of longstanding stress, patellar dislocation (see section on patellar instability), forceful quadriceps contraction or forced flexion of the knee against a contracted quadriceps.

An athlete presenting with an exquisitely tender and painful part of the patella after a forceful action or event must be investigated for a fracture. The athlete may also have muscle atrophy or loss of strength but will rarely have retropatellar crepitus, effusion or swelling. Undisplaced fractures are treated by cylindrical cast immobilization and displaced fractures with open surgical fixation. Athletes presenting with a traumatically induced bipartite patella may heal with a troublesome fibrous non-union if treated with aggressive quadriceps exercises before immobilization. Cast immobilization is indicated for 3–6 weeks before muscle rehabilitation is commenced. Following the removal of the cast a progressive and modified vastus medialis oblique treatment program is commenced (see section on treatment).

A detailed description of patellar fractures is beyond the scope of this book, but is covered by other authors (Smillie 1974, Schmidt & Henry 1989).

Sinding-Larsen-Johansson's disease

A traction osteochondrosis at the inferior pole of the patella may occur and may avulse to form a teardrop ossicle within the tendon. The inferior pole is also the most common site of patellar tendinitis and is usually painful in PFPS as well.

Osgood-Schlatter's disease

This condition is a traction apophysitis of the tibial tubercle that occurs before the secondary ossification centre has closed in adolescents (see also Ch. 29). It results in partial avulsion with repetitive healing and bone accretion. The natural history of this condition is that it is self-limited by ossification and fusion of the tibial tubercle and settles down if the child stops sporting activities. However, this can be rather traumatic to a competitive athlete.

It has been found that the PFPS exercise program using the taping technique to ease the pain and muscle stretches if necessary is an effective treatment program. Just as in PFPS, the lower limb must be assessed for correct alignment, muscle balance and joint proprioception, and if necessary orthotics used to change foot posture. The response is slower than for PFPS but by using this program the child can continue modified sporting activities. Jarring activities and those involving direct contact will need to be modified by wearing shoes with adequate shock absorption properties or braces.

If the pain is severe, localized treatment of ice or ice massage, ultrasound or interferential can be used. Casting is rarely necessary and even then should be limited to 3 weeks and followed up with a stretching and retraining program. A full explanation must be given to the parents, with the assurance that this condition will not permanently affect the knee joint.

EXAMINATION OF THE PATELLOFEMORAL JOINT

Assessment of lower limb mechanics

Treatment of patellofemoral joint involves correcting or altering the effect of those mechanical factors found during the assessment procedure. Any examination of the patellofemoral joint must include the lower limb in standing i.e. the closed kinetic chain, performing those activities that may reproduce pain or malalignment. Tests can also be performed passively in lying (the open kinetic chain). Assessment of the closed kinetic chain takes into account the different synergies involved to allow the whole limb to function correctly. For instance, a full range of hip movement with adequate muscle strength is needed to be able to perform an exercise while standing on one leg.

Note changes and/or pain and compare to the other side but do not overexamine in one session. The tissues of the knee may be very irritable and painful and some tests may be left to a later time (see Ch. 12).

Movement tests

In standing alignment:

- view the genu varus or valgus or recurvatum
- note alignment of pelvis to femur to tibia to feet
- note squinting patella shows femoral anteversion
- note patella height particularly for patella alta
- measure difference in leg length at iliac crests, buttocks and popliteal crease
- note presence and position of oedema
- view or measure muscle atrophy at a consistent distance, e.g. 5–10 cm above the patella
- measure the Q angle with a long-handled goniometer
- note forefoot and rearfoot posture particularly in relation to arches of the feet and position of the calcaneum
- measure calf length because decreased mobility produces premature heel lift and excessive foot pronation during the stance phase.

In walking:

- observe any changes in gait, particularly in the stance phase, i.e. foot pronation, supination, femoral rotation and pelvic stability.

In hopping:

- note hip, knee and foot control
- measure proprioception by watching sway from side to side in one-legged stance and hopping.

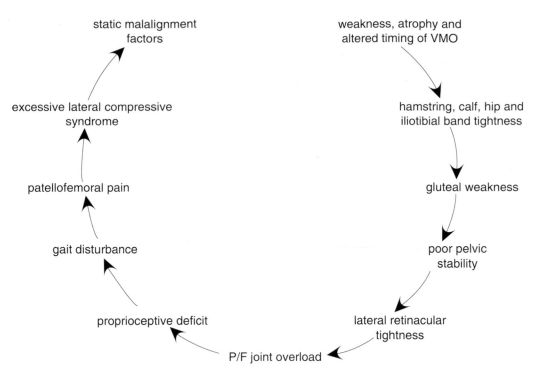

Fig. 30.5 Scheme of factors precipitating patellofermoral pain

On stairs:

- note the quality and pain on stepping up and down, noting eccentric and concentric control and the sideways stability of the knee.

In squatting:

- observe pain and ability to squat on one or two legs or duck waddle
- increase difficulty of activity until enough information or a retesting sign is found.

In the lumbar spine:

- note the presence of symptoms may mean the referral of pain to knee or decreased treatment response.
- test 'quick tests' in standing, i.e. flexion, extension, side flexion, rotation and quadrant. Do not forget the neural tension tests i.e. the slump test, straight leg raise and prone knee bend. (see Ch. 33).

In the hip:

- note the hip can be a source of referred pain to the knee. Flexion, extension, internal and external rotation and the quadrant should display a full pain free range of movement.

In lying:

- measure hamstring length
- test iliotibial band tightness using Ober's test

- measure hip extension in prone lying and gluteal strength on external rotation and abduction
- measure Q angle (if not already tested)
- palpate the lumbar spine for pain, stiffness or muscle spasm
- examine fully the tibiofemoral joint (see Ch. 29)
- note the presence of femoral anteversion and tibial torsion
- test psoas tightness using Thomas's test.

Palpation

To examine the joint, palpate the four directions of movement (cephalad, caudad, medial and lateral) with and without compression for range, pain and glissment. Nipping of the synovial membrane can be avoided by placing the knee in 15° of flexion. Glissment is defined as the sensation of grating bone-on-bone that occurs with cartilage degeneration and is graded 1–3 (1 is mild, 2 moderate and 3 severe). Estimate the range of medial and lateral glide and rotation with the knee in full extension. A tight lateral patellofemoral retinaculum will limit medial glide of the patella and produce anterior tilting of the medial border of the patella. The lateral band may only be tight in the proximal or distal portion producing rotation of the patella on medial glide. Anteroposterior position of the patella, i.e. 'tucking in' of the inferior angle, is also important particularly in relation to the fat pad.

The apprehension test

It is used as an indicator of patellar instability, and performed by laterally gliding the patella with the patient's knee resting in flexion over the therapist's knee. A positive test shows as a very apprehensive look on the patient's face, often with an accompanying exclamation and withdrawal of the limb.

Soft tissue palpation

The border of the patella should be palpated for peripatellar tenderness or synovial thickening, the quadriceps tendon and patellar tendon for defects or pain, the infrapatellar fat pad and the tibial tubercle for swelling or pain. The latter indicates Osgood-Schlatter's disease in adolescents.

Palpation of the medial capsule of the joint may show the thickening of a synovial plica.

Compression of the patella

Compression of the patella with resisted knee extension (Clarke's test) has not been shown to be a reliable test or indicator of a patellofemoral joint cause of anterior knee pain (Gaughwin 1987). However, direct compression is a different test and the information gained regarding the tenderness of the joint is worthwhile.

The patella can be further examined with the patient lying in side flexion and with the knee in varying angles of flexion. However, enough information is usually obtained with the patient supine.

Radiographic examination

For the initial radiographic evaluation an anteroposterior, lateral and skyline view of the patellofemoral joint is sufficient to show the basic structure of the joint. A more complete examination is given by computerized tomography centred on the mid patella at 0°, 30°, 45° and 60°. Radioactive bone scan may be used in the occasional patient to show the presence and severity of patellar arthrosis or the vascularity of an osteochondral fragment. Single photon emission computed tomographic bone scintigraphy (SPECT) can also be useful for osteoarthritis or synovitis, although these conditions can now be seen with magnetic reasonance imaging (Fulkerson & Hungerford 1989). Ultrasound can be used to show tendon defects and synovial plicae. For further reading see Fulkerson and Hungerford (1989).

Differential diagnosis of anterior knee pain

1. Patellar tendinitis or periostitis (Table 30.3).
2. Bursitis. In the acute stage a swollen, boggy and tender bursa is obvious. In the subacute stage the bursa will be thickened and have a history of local irritation. The prepatella, retropatellar tendon, suprapatella and the pes anserinus bursae are the most commonly involved.
3. Plica. Anteromedial knee pain can be caused by a swollen or thickened plical fold. The fold can be palpated and the presence of a painful fold may indicate abnormal patellofemoral mechanics (Fulkerson & Hungerford 1989).
4. Fat pad syndrome. The infrapatellar fat pad can be traumatized directly or by being caught between the tibial plateaus and femoral condyles on knee extension. It can be palpated directly and as it is covered by synovial membrane it is also involved in a general synovitis.
5. Meniscal lesions. PFPS can also cause mild swelling and in the severe cases limitation of movement. The locking of a meniscal lesion can also be confused with the pseudolocking and giving way of PFPS. The pain in a meniscal injury can be localized to the joint line rather than the peripatellar region. Examination of the knee in the flexion/abducted or adducted position combined with internal or external rotation will often show a meniscal lesion.
6. Ligamentous lesions. The presence of an anterior cruciate ligament lesion destabilizes the knee causing pain, swelling, quadriceps weakness and a subsequent alteration in the gait pattern. Anterior knee pain and crepitus occur, particularly in the presence of malalignment. Injury to the medial and lateral collateral ligaments may also precipitate PFPS. Tests for rotary, medial and lateral instability of the knee must be included in the examination of the patellofemoral joint.
7. Osteochondritis disiccans. The symptoms of this condition are pain, locking, intermittent effusion, clicking, giving way, a limp and a tendency to walk with the knee externally rotated. There may be tenderness over the affected femoral condyle and knee extension particularly with internal rotation in the last few degrees (Wilson's sign) is often painful. In the adolescent this condition may be associated with patellofemoral malalignment. An X-ray is mandatory and may also show a loose body.
8. Chondromalacia and arthrosis. A subject may often have asymptomatic chondromalacia. However, a patient may have symptoms, in which case they are more articular than retinacular in nature when compared with PFPS. They also may not fall into the category of a subluxation/instability or a tilt/compression syndrome. These patients will have the same clinical history to that of PFPS but may have a history of trauma or cruciate ligament surgery. They will have symptoms due to increased load on the joint through range particularly on stair climbing, sustained bent knee activities and squatting. If the degenerative changes are as a result of the progression of the tilt/compression syndrome both articular and retinacular symptoms will be present. The most common form is lateral patellofemoral arthrosis following chronic

lateral tilt with or without subluxation. This results in lateral facet erosion. Lateral bicompartmental arthrosis affects both the lateral facet and the lateral tibiofemoral compartment. In other forms of arthrosis the lateral patellofemoral and medial tibiofemoral joints can be involved as well as the medial patellar facet. The medial facet is less commonly involved than the lateral. Cushnaghan et al (1994) found that patellar taping provided short term pain relief in patients with osteoarthritis of the patellofemoral joint. (For a more detailed discussion see Fulkerson and Hungerford (1989).

9. Systemic joint disease. Conditions such as rheumatoid arthritis produce a systemic synovitis in all joints and may affect the patellofemoral joint. The history is of insidious onset, the skin is shiny and often distended and the knee is warm and has a boggy feeling. Rheumatoid arthritis often coexists with malalignment factors and the anterior knee pain can be treated with care once the active disease has gone into remission.

10. Reflex sympathetic dystrophy. This capricious disorder is characterized by excessive pain, oedema, redness and heat in the early stages. In the later stages there may be a hyperaesthesia, decrease in skin temperature and an appearance of cyanosis when cold. The patellofemoral joint may be affected and show all these symptoms as well as joint stiffness, tissue induration and osteoporosis on X-ray. The diagnosis is made on clinical grounds. The response to treatment may be dramatic lasting 1–2 months or may leave the patient with chronic pain and joint stiffness in 1–2 years (Fulkerson & Hungerford 1989).

11. Slipped femoral epiphysis. This condition may cause isolated knee pain and must be considered in all adolescents. Standard x-rays of the hip joint will show the defect. At a later stage knee pain is increased by weight bearing and is accompanied by loss of joint movement. Immediate referral for an orthopedic opinion is essential.

TREATMENT-THE PFPS PROGRAM

The studies on the natural history of PFPS without treatment have been poor but it can be assumed that if all activity is stopped a large proportion of the symptoms will also stop.

It is not known how many children with PFPS already have cartilaginous damage, or who if left untreated will progress to chondromalacia patellae. However, it is unacceptable that these adolescents be prevented from attaining their full athletic potential and be forced to suffer 'growing' pains often for periods longer than 5 years.

Conservative treatment is highly successful, with the proviso that patients with poor alignment of the lower extremity continue a maintenance program of exercises (Dehaven et al 1979, McConnell 1986, Gerrard 1989, Gaffney et al 1991). Conservative treatment is the primary method of treatment with surgery being reserved for those who do not respond. They are often those with severe malalignment factors or joint degeneration.

Successful treatment combines a full biomechanical assessment (see section on examination). Strategies are used to relieve pain and alter the timing and strength of the vastus medialis oblique using isometric, eccentric, concentric and specific activity-related exercises (McConnell 1986). Different measures are used to alter or modify those structures that affect alignment.

Pain

Pain in or around the knee produces reflex inhibition of the surrounding muscles, in particular the vastus medialis. The first priority of an exercise programme is therefore to relieve pain.

Pain relief is best obtained during the treatment program and while playing sport by using the taping technique developed by McConnell (1986) (see Figs 30.6–30.10).

The tape pulls the patella medially 'unloading' the joint and the surrounding soft tissues, allowing for:

- medial glide
- tilt
- rotation
- antero-posterior tilt.

The technique and the direction of pull can be altered to allow for various patellar positions found during the assessment procedure.(see section on examination). A patella with an anteroposterior tilt (with the inferior pole tucked in), can be taped in a more upward direction to bring the inferior pole to a more anterior position. This is the case with a swollen or irritated fat pad.

A non-allergenic tape such as Hypafix (Smith & Nephew) or Fixamul (Beirsdorf) is used to pull the patella medially via the skin. Rigidity is obtained by using a rigid sports tape on top. However, that type of tape will cause a skin irritation if used directly on the skin for a long period of time. The skin should be shaved to decrease pain and irritation. It is important for care to be taken when removing the tape. Once the skin is irritated or broken the tape will need to be angled to avoid the damaged skin. If a large area is damaged, this may not be possible and taping will have to be discontinued until the skin is healed. Unsightly tape residues can be removed with eucalyptus oil, methylated spirits or a tape removing solvent. If used while playing sport the undertape will need to be placed all around the knee as an anchor tape to absorb perspiration and the rigid tape used to pull the patella medially.

The tape is worn all day for the first 2 weeks of the training program but not at night to rest the skin. After

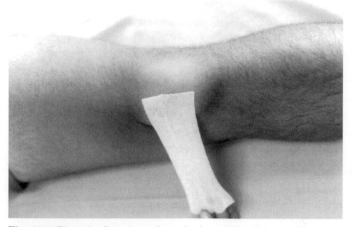

Fig. 30.6 Place the first piece of tape in the middle of the patella and pull the tape medially before attaching it to the skin. The tilt component is controlled by this piece before the tape producing medial glide is attached

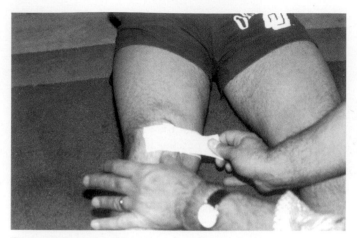

Fig. 30.9 Rotation of the patella (usually internal rotation) is obtained by pulling the tape proximally before fixing it to the skin. Patellar tilt may be controlled better by rotating the patella before affixing the tilt tape

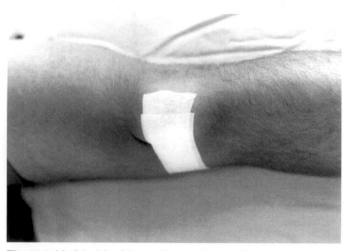

Fig. 30.7 Medial glide of the patella is achieved by fixing the tape to the lateral border and pulling the skin and patella medially before attaching the tape to the skin. The taping action is more effective if the tape is pulled rather than the patellar pushed to produce the medial glide

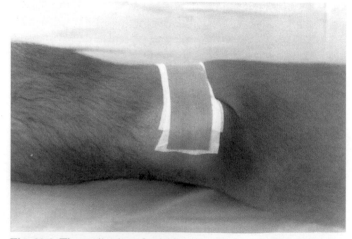

Fig. 30.8 The application of a rigid sports tape over the less allergenic and irritative undertape

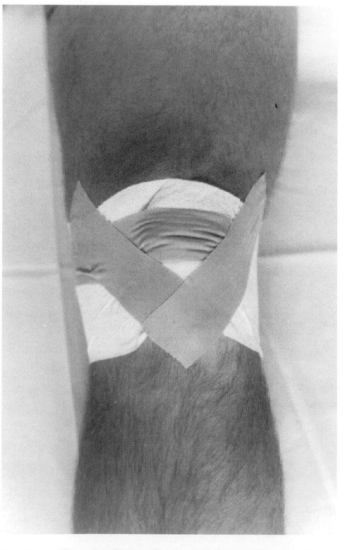

Fig. 30.10 The taping direction can be altered to achieve a reduction in pain. If the inferior pole of the patella appears to be 'digging in', the tape is positioned so that the inferior pole is tilted anteriorly

that the tape is worn only during exercise or while playing sport. Once the pain has gone the tape is no longer necessary although it can be reapplied on a temporary basis if pain reoccurs. In the first few months after the programme, minor and temporary pain may occur with little reason. 'Putting up' with pain or swelling without taping the knee, quickly results in vastus medialis oblique atrophy with the loss of the regained muscle hypertrophy. A maintenance program is therefore necessary.

Other modalities such as non-steroidal anti-inflammatory medications, analgesics and electrotherapy can also be used to ease the pain if the taping does not help.

The exercises have been developed to maximize the effect on the vastus medialis oblique in both a static and active way, taking into account the tissue irritability that is often encountered in PFPS.

A typical exercise program is shown later in this chapter.

Muscle atrophy

One of the components of PFPS is muscle atrophy, particularly of vastus medialis oblique. Pain and swelling have an earlier and possibly greater effect on the vastus medialis oblique than on the vastus lateralis, due to increased reflex inhibition. In the presence of pain and swelling, exercises have little effect on the development of the quadriceps muscles (Spencer et al 1984). Therefore the use of a pain-relieving taping technique enables muscle retraining to be more effective.

Muscle retraining

Patients with PFPS often cannot feel whether the vastus medialis oblique is contracting, particularly isometrically. By pushing the foot forward along the floor very gently and tightening the quadriceps with the knee in 90° of flexion and stopping at the first sign of a vastus lateralis contraction, vastus medialis oblique awareness can be taught (Fig. 30.11). Once the patient can feel the vastus medialis oblique coming in, that same action can be achieved through the flexion and extension range. If the subject finds it difficult biofeedback, or electrical muscle stimulation can be used.

The vastus medialis oblique originates from (among other origins) the tendon of the adductor magnus and is able to pull the patella medially because of the obliquity of the muscle fibres. Therefore to increase that action, the vastus medialis oblique can be taught to contract isometrically with the adductor magnus in the sitting and standing positions and with the hips externally rotated (Figs 30.12, 30.13). Stimulation can be given by touch, electrical muscle stimulation or biofeedback.

Eccentric muscle control during movement is usually poor in PFPS and can be retaught in the stride standing position where a consistent muscle contraction is main-

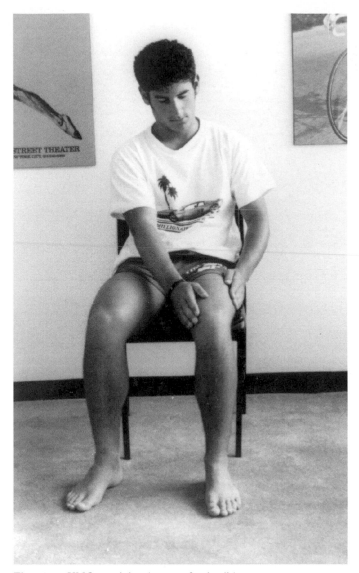

Fig. 30.11 VMO retraining (see text for details)

tained from a fully extended knee position to approximately 70° of knee flexion (Fig. 30.14). A neutral foot posture (neither pronated or supinated) can also be taught as part of this exercise. It would vary in speed, becoming more a lunging action as the patient's skill increased.

Eccentric muscle strength

The eccentric strength of the vastus medialis oblique has been shown to be poor in patients with PFPS (Bennett & Stauber 1986), and therefore strategies have been developed to retrain it, particularly through range and in conjunction with foot control. It is performed in weightbearing as described above and on a step using body weight as a resistance initially (step exercise, Fig. 30.15) and later with extra weight. Eccentric muscle action is used because not only has it been shown to be less painful in PFPS but it develops greater tension within the muscle (Rasch 1974).

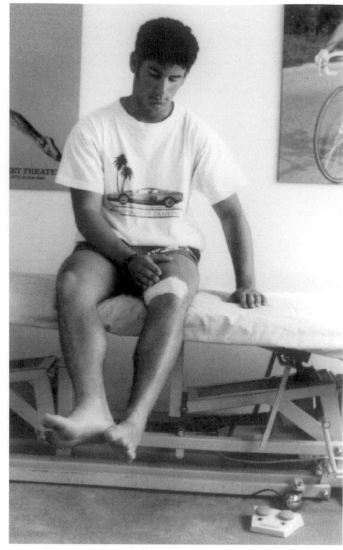

Fig. 30.12 A combined isometric exercise of VMO

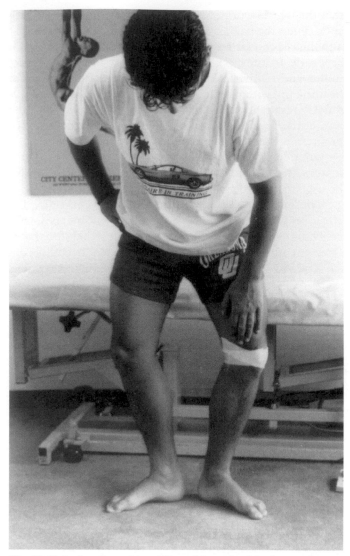

Fig. 30.13 In the plie position, lifting of the arch of the foot teaches foot control while performing an isometric vastus medialis oblique and hip exercise

This enables a greater effect in a shorter time with tissues that are likely to be very irritable. A faster movement is also likely to be less painful (Dvir et al 1991). The concentric portion of the step exercise can be emphasized or not depending on the individual case.

The use of exercises in weightbearing have several advantages. Not only do they strengthen but they involve all the component parts of the limb in a synergy of movement e.g. pelvis, knee and foot in the step exercise. An important component is that of pelvic stability. Each component can be emphasized if necessary and the exercise made 'task-specific'.

Eccentric vs concentric exercise programs

Before the program described above was developed the treatment method of choice used concentric exercises,

electrotherapy, non-steroidal anti-inflammatory drugs and analgesics. Gaffney et al (1991) compared the results using straight leg raising and resisted exercises in the last 30° of range programs instead of eccentric exercises and found that although the results were similar, patients including those with crepitus, responded better to the eccentric program. The younger athlete will undoubtedly respond best to eccentric exercises, with some being pain free within 2–3 weeks (Bennett & Stauber 1986). Sport need only be reduced and not stopped during retraining because the taping technique controls the pain and often swelling, thereby improving patient compliance and the rate of healing. Unfortunately jogging (often the precipitating cause of the pain) should be reduced or discontinued until the joint settles. Older athletes will not respond as well to weightbearing exercises because of increased cartilaginous and joint degeneration. They may benefit from a modified exercise program still using the taping technique and muscle retraining but with less weightbearing and more non-weightbearing bearing straight leg raising exercises. Studies have shown that it is the quadriceps setting component that contracts the vastus medialis oblique rather than the straight leg raising part (Soderberg et al 1987). To maximize the muscle action EMG biofeedback should be used.

Whichever type of exercise is used, all the components of the kinetic chain from the lumbar spine down will need to be assessed and treated if necessary.

Isokinetic exercise program

In general the use of knee extension resisted through range in patients with patellofemoral pain is contraindicated because of the higher patellofemoral compression forces that occur with knee flexion (Whitelaw et al 1989). However, isokinetics can form a valuable part of an integrated exercise program. Quadriceps action can be performed isometrically in the painfree part of the range and progressed to using the pain free range at faster speeds of 180–200°/s. The range of movement frequently used is from 30–0° but Heckmann (1988) advocates using 90–45° because he feels that there is less crepitus in that range (thereby indicating lower compressive forces).

The disadvantage of using isokinetics is that all the components of the quadriceps group are strengthened together, possibly leading to an increase in the imbalance between the vastus lateralis and the vastus medialis oblique. It has also been shown that because the knee extension

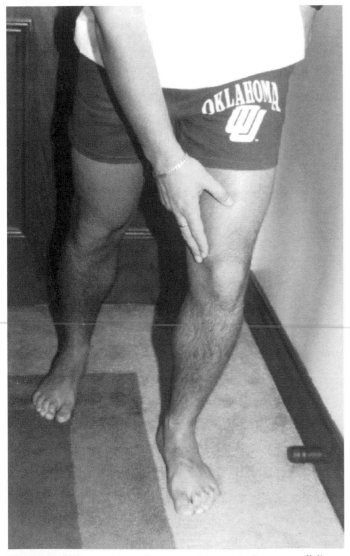

Fig. 30.14 This exercise teaches eccentric control of vastus medialis oblique in conjunction with foot control to keep the foot in a neutral position

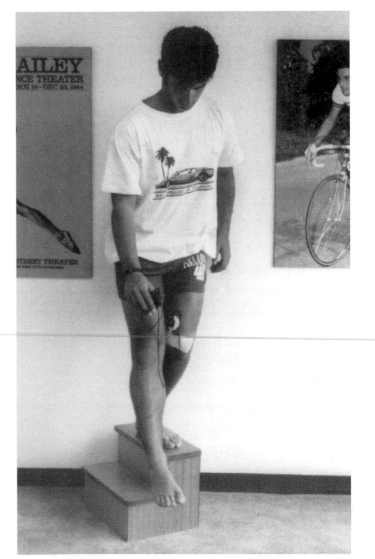

Fig. 30.15 The step exercise strengthens both eccentric and concentric vastus medialis oblique action. It is performed slowly at first, in varying directions (forwards, backwards etc.) and speeds both with and without added resistance

action in sitting is not functional, an increase in isokinetic torque does not necessarily result in an increase on functional activity (Rutherford 1988). However, the use of isokinetics particularly with eccentric action as part of a comprehensive exercise program is worthwhile (Bennett & Stauber 1986).

Functional, task-specific and plyometric exercises

Successful rehabilitation depends not only on muscle strengthening and flexibility but on increased neuro-muscular efficiency and the ability to play without the risk of further injury or reinjury. As soon as the pain level and tissue irritability has decreased and flexibility increased, functional exercises in weightbearing reinforcing the action of the vastus medialis oblique both statically and actively should be used. Progression to low level activities such as swimming, walking, cutting, skipping, cycling, mini-trampolining and low level plyometric exercises will aid the retraining of the type 2 muscle fibres.

Plyometric exercises are those activities which use the eccentric component followed by a rapid change to a concentric component of a muscle action that 'bounce-loads' the muscle. It is the rapid change from eccentric to concentric, or the 'amortization phase', that is important and the exercises are progressed from horizontal to the more difficult vertical activities. Simple exercises utilizing theratubing can be adapted to use these principles. Single leg jumping or bouncing from one side of a line to the other, or backwards and forwards, would progress to jumping over, then onto, off and then on boxes of different heights. Exercises can be made even more functional with the addition of other skills such as catching or hitting a ball while jumping. Electrical muscle stimulation and bio-feedback can be used to reinforce the action of the vastus medialis oblique in that range of movement which might be deficient or painful. It is believed that plyometrics increase proprioception by stimulating the muscle spindle and the Golgi tendon organ. Some authors feel that there is also facilitation of type 1, 2, and 3 mechanoreceptors (Lunden 1985).

Effect of a tibiofemoral lesion on the PFPS program

A patient with PFPS may also have a non-specific tibiofemoral component to the pain. The vastus medialis oblique retraining program will decrease the PFPS, leaving the tibiofemoral component, or in some cases may even relieve it.

Often these patients have a loss of knee extension. This must be mobilized as part of the vastus medialis oblique program even if it is only a small loss found on overpressure of the joint.

Muscle stretches

Flexible and strong muscles acting on and around the knee act to keep it aligned. Conversely, tight structures place an increased and uneven load on the patellofemoral joint and may prevent the joint from settling down.

Hamstrings are best stretched in single long leg sitting with the other leg flexed and externally rotated to produce a sustained stretch. Remember that different positions of the leg may be necessary to stretch all the hamstrings. Neural tightness and immobility may mimic hamstring tightness and can be treated with a straight leg raise or slump technique (see Ch. 33).

The iliotibial band as measured by Ober's test (see Ch. 28), if tight increases the lateral pull on the patella. Stretching is difficult and probably only succeeds in altering the proximal portion. Soft tissue massage or myofascial techniques prior to stretching may soften the distal portion and lateral retinaculum giving a more effective and long-lasting stretch.

Reduced ankle dorsiflexion whether it be due to gastrocnemius or soleus tightness alters the gait cycle at mid stance causing premature heel lift and increased foot pronation. In a simple unpublished retrospective study the author found that in patients with unilateral PFPS, 80% had decreased ankle dorsiflexion on the affected side. The most efficient and long-acting stretch utilizes the reciprocal inhibition produced by bringing in the long toe extensors and then restretching the calf.

Tight quadriceps have not been shown specifically to be involved with PFPS (except in high speed skaters) although any tight muscle group around the knee may cause abnormal stresses. Quadriceps are stretched by knee flexion over the side of the bed while in supine lying or in standing.

Hip stretches and pelvic control

As femoral anteversion is a definite malalignment factor, reduced hip rotation either internally or externally will produce abnormal stresses and will require strategies to correct it. Externally rotating a flexed hip and knee with the patient in prone lying will stretch the hip and retrain the external rotators (Fig. 30.16). External rotation of the hip in standing adds in a compressive component to increase stability and proprioceptive input (Fig. 30.17). Also, the combined exercise in sitting with hips flexed of isometric adduction of the thigh and knee extension strengthens the internal hip rotators and gains increased range of external rotation (see Fig. 30.12 above). It also retrains the synergic action of the adductor magnus and the vastus medialis oblique.

In athletes with PFPS it is often found that they have a lack of pelvic control and/or proprioception sometimes showing up as a Trendelenburg gait or running pattern. More often it is an inability to hold the pelvis level when

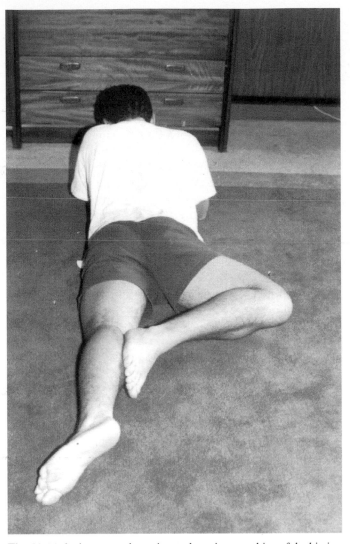

Fig. 30.16 Active external rotation and passive stretching of the hip is achieved by lifting the knee in this prone lying position. This exercise is difficult but important in patients with femoral anteversion

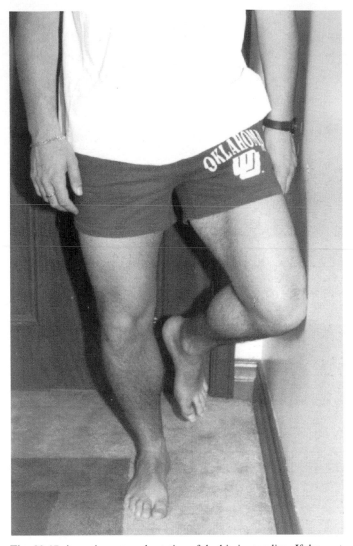

Fig. 30.17 An active external rotation of the hip in standing. If the athlete does not stand straight a trick movement will occur and the movement will not be felt in the hip. Increased proprioception is achieved by compression of the hip in standing

standing on one leg performing exercises. The weakness may only become evident when the athlete tires and shows sign of fatigue. There may be a loss of hip extension, external rotation and weak glutei, not necessarily on the painful side. In the young patient this is probably due to rapid skeletal growth before the soft tissues have time to catch up. In older athletes it may be due to even a minor injury leaving a proprioceptive deficit. Whatever the cause, the remedy is to stretch and strengthen the glutei, hip abductors and adductors using resisted exercises, pelvic stabilization and a balance or wobble board to retrain proprioception.

Lateral retinaculum tightness

Tightness of the lateral retinaculum and associated structures is often present before the onset of any symp-

toms. It is only when there is a precipitating cause such as joint overload or trauma that the symptoms of the excessive lateral compression syndrome appear. Fulkerson (1989) isolated injury to the retinacular nerve as a cause of pain. To mobilize this nerve, deep soft tissue frictions in the region of the lateral part of the lateral femoral condyle prior to stretching of the lateral retinaculum are performed by the patient throughout the day. This is followed by a stretch of the lateral band. The patient can achieve this by performing a grade 4 mobilization technique (small amplitude at the end of range) on the medial border of the patella, thereby tilting the lateral border anteriorly. The patient can easily do this by sitting with the leg in full extension. For the therapist it is more effectively performed in side lying with the knee uppermost and in approximately 90° of flexion or the position where the band is the tightest (Fig. 30.18).

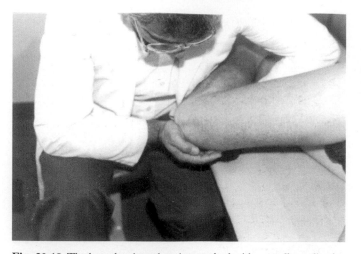

Fig. 30.18 The lateral retinaculum is stretched with a small amplitude mobilisation technique performed slowly at the end of the available range of movement. Medial glide is maintained while the medial border of the patella is moved in an anteroposterior direction to tilt the patella without pain and without increasing patellofemoral compression

Foot posture

The foot acts as a shock absorber and as a lever on which the lower limb can act. In the normal state it has resilience and maintains the lower limb in an optimal position. During the gait cycle at heel strike the foot goes into supination ready to act as a decelerant. As the cycle continues the foot pronates to position the foot for push off. If the foot is not performing that role satisfactorily it can add to poor alignment of the limb above. Rarely is it the sole cause, but the improvement obtained with an orthotic may be enough to alter the pain. In the program described later in this chapter foot control is taught as part of each exercise. Dynamic control of foot position is ideal. However, the structure of the foot in an individual may be so poor that the patient will need a referral to a podiatrist. The patient with gross forefoot or rearfoot pronation or pes planus will not be able to regain enough active control of the foot and will require an orthotic. The use of comfortable shock-absorbent shoes to reduce the jarring effect cannot be emphasized enough in patients with patellofemoral pain. This applies when jogging, running, at work or doing everyday activities (see Ch. 32).

Maintenance

Tissues change according to the stresses and strains put on them. After retraining, athletes, originally with tight muscles and tissues will tend to tighten and revert to their previous state if some form of stretching and exercise program is not continued. The author suggests to his athletes that they continue to perform the eccentric step exercise, the muscle stretches and the balance board before sport and on a daily basis when not playing.

Braces vs taping

There are many different types of braces, including a simple neoprene sleeve with a patellar hole that may or may not have a lateral or C-shaped reinforcement to stabilize the patella. The original Palumbo type brace has an active component designed to pull the patella medially and there are many versions that attempt to do the same. Possibly the simplest and most effective brace is one with a silicon rubber patellar cap and a padded velcro strap. An infrapatellar Chopat strap alters the mechanics of the joint by decreasing the height of the patellar ligament. All braces have the same disadvantages. They are hot, cumbersome, difficult to fit properly, increase the pressure on the popliteal space and lastly but most importantly don't do anything to correct the malalignment problem. Their advantage is that they can remain tighter (but not necessarily more effective) for a longer period of time if fitted properly, and usually don't affect the skin. Taping, on the other hand, is more accurate and effective in the short term but can cause skin reactions if care is not taken. Unfortunately, the most non-allergenic tapes are not rigid and therefore when a longer-term effect is needed a more rigid sports tape is put on top of a less irritative tape (see Fig. 30.8).

TYPICAL 6 WEEK TREATMENT PROGRAM

Note: programs should be designed specifically for each individual and based on their assessment findings

1. Full history.
2. Assessment. Include finding a retest sign.
3. Give the patient a simple explanation of malalignment and use biofeedback and/or electrical muscle stimulation throughout the program to get improved exercise performance and compliance.
4. In sitting:
   a teach isometric vastus medialis oblique control in 90° of knee flexion and after the first week throughout range (5 repetitions, 5/day) (Fig. 30.11).
   b teach frictions to soften lateral p/f retinaculum (if tight) and release retinacular nerve (1 min, 5/day).
   c teach lateral p/f retinaculum stretching (if tight) (1 min, 5/day).
   d teach taping technique with knee in extension (Figs 30.6–30.10).
   The patient repeats the retest sign to show pain relief and wears the tape all day but preferably not at night for 2 weeks, after that only for exercises and sport.
5. Exercise program to be performed twice a day.

1st week

1. Exercise with isometric sitting on table 10 × 10 seconds (Fig. 30.12).
2. Step backwards 10 × 4 seconds down and up (Fig. 30.15).

3. Add in correction of malalignment factors, e.g. calf, hamstring, hip stretches (Figs 30.16, 30.17), gluteal exercises and balance board.

2nd week

1. Check all previous exercises and stretches.
2. Stride standing exercise 20 times.
3. Step sideways (straight down) 10 × 4 s down and up.
4. Continue correction of malalignment factors.

3rd week

1. Change stride exercise to actively striding forwards, twist and hop.
2. Plié 10 × 10 lifts of the arch (Fig. 30.13).
3. Step forward 10 x 4 s down and up and 10 times as fast as possible. Continue for one week and then add 2 repetitions daily until 30 fast and slow steps are performed (Fig. 30.15).

5th week

1. Continue step exercise with increasing resistance, e.g. shoulder bag or weights.
2. Start horizontal plyometric exercises, e.g. fast jumping side to side, back and forwards and forwards and back for 2 minutes.
3. Teach vastus medialis oblique control during performance of functional or sporting activities, e.g. trampolining, golf, skiing.

6th week

1. Continue exercises as necessary.
2. If necessary teach vertical and more complex plyometric exercises. Use theraband or tubing for increased resistance.
3. Explain a maintenance program that continues for at least one year.

Performance may plateau for physical or psychological reasons. To identify physical reasons:

- check progressive steps; motor control may be poor with vastus lateralis dominance
- check muscle tightness
- check lateral band tightness
- check lumbar spine
- check exercise specificity—joint angle and speed.

Psychological reasons may include:

- loss of interest
- focus on wrong cues
- fatigue
- emotions
- lack of physical readiness
- lack of physical aspiration
- misunderstanding directions

- lack of ability to adapt and recognize skills.

For further discussion see Chapter 10.

SURGICAL PROCEDURES AND REHABILITATION

These can be divided into those affecting static or dynamic structures or patellar resurfacing and decompression procedures. Procedures on the static structures are often the first choice because their rehabilitation is usually much faster than that on dynamic structures. The effect is immediately apparent and is based on a mechanical effect rather than relying on the rehabilitation of muscle groups, as do dynamic realignment procedures. Common operative procedures are:

- lateral retinacular release
- distal realignment
- dynamic realignment
- patellar shaving
- patellectomy.

It is not within the scope of this chapter to describe individual operative procedures, but an overview and indications will be given in relation to their post-surgical rehabilitation. For further information see Siegel (1988).

The rate of post-operative rehabilitation will vary according to the operation, the surgeon and most importantly the individual. Accelerated rehabilitation programs are run where it has been shown not to be disadvantageous in the long term. However, the basic principles will apply to all patients.

Lateral retinacular release

Arthroscopic lateral release involves cutting all the lateral structures from the patellar tendon to within the muscle fibres of the vastus lateralis. Good results from this procedure occur only when the strict selection criteria of excessive lateral static pull are observed.

In the post-operative phase usually lasting 2 weeks, the aims are to limit post-operative swelling, reduce pain, start isometric quadriceps control and regain movement. A compression bandage and ice are used to reduce post-surgical haemarthrosis with static quadriceps and ankle exercises to prevent post-operative morbidity. This phase lasts 48–72 hours after which patellar mobilization, active knee flexion and vastus medialis oblique re-education is begun. Electrical muscle stimulation can be used early to facilitate vastus medialis oblique control and ice is used frequently (up to 8 times a day) to control swelling. Partial weightbearing on crutches enables the patient to walk with a normal gait.

Once the pain and swelling have settled the progressive vastus medialis oblique retraining program can be started and increased until the athlete returns to full activity in 2–6 months. Failure of this procedure can be due to:

- a cut which is not extensive enough
- a scar formation that decreases the release effect due to poor patellar mobilization or failure to start knee flexion early
- a severe postoperative haemarthrosis often due to cutting the lateral superior genicular artery. This delays recovery but probably does not affect the outcome
- poor selection criteria.

Distal patellar realignment

In principle, subluxation and dislocation are treated surgically by moving the tibial tubercle medially and changing the Q angle. In the presence of severe degeneration the tubercle will be shifted anteriorly as well. Many different surgical techniques are used but all procedures involve osteomization of the tubercle and the tibia and rehabilitation is limited by post-operative stability and the speed of bone healing. Fixation by screw or staple is subcutaneous and palpable, can cause pain later and may have to be removed. A patella baja (low riding patella) may be produced by the operation and although it may counteract a patella alta (high riding patella), it is also likely to increase the patellofemoral forces through flexion and extension of the knee. Increased patellar rotation and compressive forces may be a side effect of this type of operation.

In the immediate post-operative period the limb will be immobilized for 6 weeks in a cylinder cast, posterior splint or foam hinged cast brace (Heckmann 1988). Isometric quadriceps, ankle, opposite limb and trunk exercises and electrical stimulation are started early. Patellar mobilization with gentle passive movement (with the CPM machine if the tubercle fixation is stable) is started early in the 0–30° range. Partial weightbearing (25%) can be started at 3 weeks as can straight leg raising if there is radiological signs of healing. Full weightbearing is started at the 7–8 week stage depending on pain, swelling and bone healing.

The intermediate and advanced stages of rehabilitation are dependent on pain, swelling and crepitus. They have a strong emphasis on resisted quadriceps setting, straight leg raises, leg presses, cycling and functional activities. It is important to emphasize the proprioceptive and vastus medialis oblique retraining component utilizing the exercises of the PFPS program, biofeedback and electrical stimulation if necessary, throughout the rehabilitation stage. It is extremely difficult to hypertrophy the vastus medialis oblique after this operation, requiring many months of persistent exercise and even then athletes are unlikely to return to their pre-operative level of sport.

Dynamic realignment

Dynamic realignment involves the transfer of muscles or tendons to counteract the lateral tracking and increase the effect of the medial pull of the vastus medialis oblique.

A vastus medialis oblique transfer increases the resting length thereby increasing its pull by reattaching the insertion distally. The main disadvantage of this approach is that it interferes with an already weakened muscle. Another disadvantage is that secure fixation is necessary, often requiring cast bracing that in turn may cause deterioration of an already damaged cartilaginous surface and muscle atrophy. If the reattachment is not distal enough the operation will be ineffective, whereas if it is too distal patellar rotation will occur increasing the patellar chondrosis (Siegel 1988). A lateral patellar release is usually performed simultaneously.

The progress of post-operative care is much slower than that of the procedures described before. For this and the other reasons it is not often performed. For further reading see Siegel (1988).

Patellar shaving

Shaving the damaged and fibrillated articular cartilage was originally hoped to stimulate the production of a smooth and healthy surface. The injured cartilaginous surface has a roughened 'crabmeat' appearance and along with altered lubricant properties is thought to be responsible for crepitus. Unfortunately, shaving produces variable and most often temporary results although the arthroscopic lavage often settles a painful joint. It removes debris that would later loosen and separate from the joint surface. These small articular particles produce synovitis and may lead to the formation of loose bodies.

This operation is usually done in conjunction with other operative procedures. When done by itself the post-operative care involves reducing swelling with ice, compression and elevation. This is immediately followed by active mobilization, quadriceps setting and partial weightbearing on crutches until the pain settles and the patient resumes normal gait. The swelling settles normally by the time the wound heals and it is usually by the 2–3 week stage that the PFPS rehabilitation can be started. It is important that the knee regains full extension at this stage but if it does not, a quadriceps setting exercise and passive mobilization technique will be required as well. The washing out of the knee will reduce the tissue irritability and a previously tried and failed program may become effective afterwards.

Spongialization involves scraping or drilling the articular surface to perforate the subchondral plate. Post-operative histological evaluation indicates that there is sometimes progressive organization of fibrous tissue but that not all areas respond well to provide a functional surface. Post-operative care concentrates on decreasing the haematoma and swelling caused by the procedure and starting early movement to promote orderly tissue repair. Early weight-bearing will depend on individual circumstances but it will take a much longer time for the swelling to resolve, thereby increasing quadriceps atrophy and poor muscle control. Ice, electrotherapy, taping and biofeedback can be used to assist isometric quadriceps exercises until the knee settles. Activities that increase patellofemoral compression should be carefully controlled until the fibrous tissue has had a chance to organize.

Patellectomy

The operation to remove the patella is only likely to occur in patients who have had multiple operations or severe comminuted fractures and who have or are likely to have considerable pain and joint degeneration. It is not within the scope of this book to explore this, save to say that after patellectomy further damage to the articular cartilage occurs related to the amount of pre-existing damage and the passage of time.

GUIDELINES FOR RETURN TO SPORT

There should not be a return to sport unless it can be done with a pain free and stable joint. In the case of PFPS this can be achieved by using the taping technique. One of the best signs of improvement in the patellofemoral joint is whether the vastus medialis oblique has started to hyper-trophy after injury. Until the joint has become pain free and stable the muscle will not recover. A normal vastus medialis oblique is usually a good diagnostic sign that the patellofemoral joint is also normal.

SUMMARY

It is now well accepted that the conservative treatment of patellofemoral pain, malalignment and instability besides being successful should be fully exhausted before any operative procedures are performed. A rehabilitative approach using isometric, concentric and eccentric exercises using a taping technique to relieve pain as developed by McConnell (1986) has been described and has been shown to be effective in more than 85% of cases (McConnell 1986, Gerrard 1989, Watson 1992).

REFERENCES

Ahmed A M, Chan K H, Shi S, Lanzo V 1989 Correlation of patellar tracking motion with the articular surface topography. Transactions of the 35th Orthopaedic Research Society Meeting, Las Vegas, Nevada, p 202

Akizuki S, Mow V C, Muller F, Pita J C, Howell D S, Manicourt D H 1986 Tensile properties of human knee joint cartilage. I. Influence of ionic conditions, weight bearing, and fibrillation on the tensile modulus. Journal of Orthopaedic Research 4(4):379–392

Arno S 1990 The A angle: a quantitative measurement of patella alignment and realignment. Journal of Orthopaedic and Sports Physical Therapy 12:237–242

Baumgartl F 1964 Das kniegelenk. Springer Verlag, Berlin

Bennett J G, Stauber W T 1986 Evaluation and treatment of anterior knee pain using eccentric exercise. Medicine and Science in Sport and Exercise 18(5):526–530

Bentley G 1985 Articular cartilage changes in chondromalacia patellae. Journal of Bone and Joint Surgery 67B(5):769–774

Borkstrom S, Goldie I F 1980 A study of the arterial supply of the patella in the the normal state, in chondromalacia patellae and in osteoarthrosis. Acta Orthopaedica Scandinavica 51:63–70

Broom M J, Fulkerson J P 1986 The plica syndrome: a new perspective. Orthopedic Clinics of North America 17(2):279–281

Chrisman O D 1986 The role of articular cartilage in patellofemoral pain. Orthopaedic Clinics of North America 17(2):231–234

Cushnaghan J, McCarthy C, Dieppe P 1994 Taping the patella medially: a new treatment for osteoarthritis of the knee joint? British Medical Journal 308:753–755

Dahlquist N J, Mayo P, Seedhom B B 1982 Forces during squatting and rising from a deep squat. Engineering in Medicine 11:69–76

Dashefsky J H 1987 Arthroscopic measurement of chondromalacia of patella cartilage using a microminiature pressure transducer. Arthroscopy 3(2):80–85

Dehaven K E, Dolan W A, Mayer P J 1979 Chondromalacia patellae in athletes—clinical presentation and conservative management. The American Journal of Sports Medicine 7(1):5–11

Dehaven K E, Lintner D M 1986 Athletic injuries: comparison by age, sport and gender. American Journal of Sports Medicine 14(3):218–224

Devereaux M D, Lachmann S M 1984 Patellofemoral arthralgia in athletes attending a sports injury clinic. British Journal of Sports Medicine 18(1):18–21

DiVeta J A, Vogelbach W D 1992 The clinical efficiency of the A angle in measuring patellar alignment. Journal of Orthopaedic and Sports Physical Therapy 16(3):136–139

Dvir Z, Halperin N, Shklar A, Robinson D 1991 Quadriceps function and patellofemoral pain syndrome. Part 1: Pain provocation during concentric and eccentric isokinetic activity. Isokinetics and Exercise Science 1(1):26–30

Ficat P R, Hungerford D S 1977 Disorders of the patellofemoral joint. Williams & Wilkins, Baltimore

Fujikawa K, Seedhom B B, Wright V 1983 Biomechanics of the patellofemoral joint. Part 11: A study of the effect of simulated femoro-tibio varus deformity on the congruity the patellofemoral compartment and movement of the patella. Engineering in Medicine 12(1):13–21

Fulkerson J P 1989 Evaluation of the peripatellar soft tissues and retinaculum. Clinics in Sports Medicine 8(2):197–202

Fulkerson J P, Gossling H R 1980 Anatomy of the knee joint lateral retinaculum. Clinical Orthopaedics and Related Research 53:183–188

Fulkerson J P, Hungerford D S 1990 Disorders of the patellofemoral joint. Williams & Wilkins, Baltimore

Gaffney K, Fricker P, Dwyer T 1991 Patellofemoral pain: to tape or not to tape. Proceedings of the 27th National Conference of the Australian Sports Medicine Federation, Canberra

Gaughwin C G 1987 The value of Clarke's sign in diagnosing chondromalacia patella. Proceedings of the 10th International Congress of the World Confederation for Physical Therapy, Sydney 1:404–407

Gerrard B 1987 The McConnell technique-applied science or applied persuasion? Proceedings of the Fifth Biennial Conference, Manipulative Therapists Association of Australia, Melbourne, p 115–122

Gerrard B 1989 The patellofemoral pain syndrome:a clinical trial of the McConnell program. Australian Journal of Physiotherapy 35(2):71–80

31. The leg

Henry Wajswelner

The lower leg is a common region for pain and disability in athletes particularly in track and field, tennis, football, hockey, basketball and netball. As there are no ligamentous structures in this region, injuries involve muscles, tendons and their various attachments to bone as well as the bones themselves, nerves, arteries, and the interosseous membrane. Fractures are sustained due to direct trauma as in football or indirect trauma as in rotational injuries in skiing. Most injuries to the lower leg occur during weightbearing sporting activity especially running. Chronic intrinsic overuse injuries predominate in this region.

Biomechanical alignment, training methods, flexibility, strength and muscle condition, footwear and training surfaces are important predisposing factors. The common patterns of injury to the lower leg include tibial pain or shin soreness (shin splints or medial tibial stress syndrome), compartment syndromes, stress fractures, achilles tendinitis, peritendinitis and rupture, calf muscle strain or tear ('tennis leg'), anterior and posterior tibial tendinitis and teno-synovitis, peroneal tendinitis or muscle strain, nerve entrapment syndromes and vascular insufficiency.

ANATOMY

The tibia is the main weightbearing bone of the leg and its biomechanical characteristics are central to the mechanism of overuse injury in and around the shin area. The smaller and thinner fibula has a minor weightbearing role and helps form the ankle joint but its main role is to provide areas for muscle attachment. The interosseous membrane joins the two bones, dividing the leg into anterior and posterior compartments. The tibia is wider superiorly to accept the weight being transmitted through the femur but becomes progressively narrower to be at its thinnest at the junction of its middle and lower one-third. This is often the site for maximum tenderness with tibial soreness.

The cross-section of the tibia is triangular with its base at the back, its apex forming the sharp anterior border or 'shin' (Fig. 31.1). The fascia enclosing the tibialis anterior muscle is attached along this sharp edge of bone and is a possible site for pain and tenderness due to periostitis. The wide anteromedial surface of the tibia is subcutaneous and is another common site for tenderness. The posteromedial margin of the tibia gives attachment to the soleus muscle and the deep fascia of the leg which continues to enclose the four muscle compartments, namely the anterior, lateral, deep posterior and superficial posterior. This thick membrane which surrounds each compartment plays a major role in compartment syndrome (Fig. 31.2). The postero-medial border of the tibia also gives rise to part of the flexor digitorum longus which can also be a source of tibial pain, in this case due to periostitis at the muscle attachment. Pain along this posteromedial border of the tibia has been reported to account for 60% of all lesions causing leg pain in athletes (Orava & Puranen 1979).

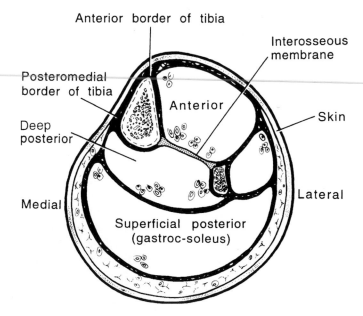

Fig. 31.1 Muscle compartments of the lower leg.
Source: adapted from Oakes (1988)

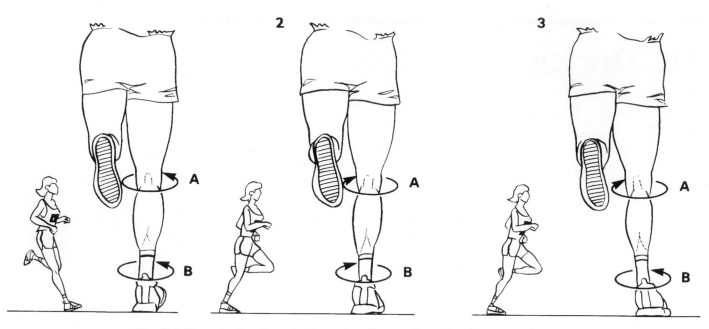

Fig. 31.2 Biomechanics of lower leg in running. Source: adapted from Taunton et al (1984)

Biomechanics

During weightbearing the lower leg sustains both compressive and torsional forces. Subtalar pronation during the stance phase of gait causes the tibia to be internally rotated from below. The screw home mechanism of knee extension causes the tibia to be externally rotated from above. These two forces combine to produce a twisting force on the tibia and fibula in weightbearing (Fig. 31.2). Poor biomechanics or malalignment exaggerates these forces, predisposing the athlete to overuse injuries.

Women tend to be more susceptible to lower leg overuse injuries, shin splints comprising about 20% of women's running injuries, compared with 7% for men (Ellis 1986). Also, according to Ellis (1986), women exhibit more biomechanical features such as increased pronation at the subtalar joint which may lead to overuse injuries of the leg.

Perfect bony alignment in the lower leg and foot is where the rearfoot is perpendicular to the bisection of the leg and the forefoot is perpendicular to the bisection of the rearfoot (McPoil & Brocato 1985). Almost nobody has ideal or 'perfect' osseous alignment. The minor malalignment that most people have normally causes no problems until they begin to participate in weightbearing sporting activities.

The three most common biomechanical malalignments are tibial varus, rearfoot varus and forefoot varus. All cause abnormal pronation at the subtalar joint, which is the combined triplanar motion of forefoot abduction, eversion and dorsiflexion.

According to McPoil and Brocato (1985), 4–6° of pronation is normal in the first 25% of the stance phase, and pronation beyond 6° or if prolonged can be considered abnormal. This means that the foot must roll in, twist and

drop to adapt to the ground, leading to repetitive soft tissue trauma such as traction on the muscles controlling pronation e.g. tibialis posterior, flexor hallucis longus etc.

Abnormal pronation also causes early fatigue, which reduces the shock absorbing capabilities of these muscles that normally help absorb ground reaction forces and causes more shock to be transmitted to the lower leg bones (Viitasalo & Kvist 1983).

Other causes of abnormal pronation include functional or anatomical leg length discrepancy (LLD), loss of flexibility in the soleus, gastrocnemius, hamstrings, hip flexors and iliotibial band (ITB), and weakness of the invertors, hip abductors and lateral rotators and the quadratus lumborum. The effect of a structural LLD is to cause a compensatory overpronation on the longer side, as the leg attempts to make itself shorter. There can also be excessive pronation on the short side, if there is a compensatory toe-out posture (Wallace 1988).

Tight hamstrings, hip flexors, ITB and hip external rotators can also cause toeing out which requires excess pronation to allow forward gait. Tight gastrocnemius and soleus muscles will reduce the available range of dorsiflexion required to walk and run so pronation is increased to compensate, utilizing the dorsiflexion component of the triplanar motion at the subtalar joint (Wallace 1988).

Weakness of the invertors denies the secondary support system of the medial longtitudinal arch. Weak hip rotators, abductors and the quadratus lumborum may lead to a functional LLD due to asymmetrical movements of the pelvis during the gait cycle (Wallace 1988). Where inadequate flexibility and strength are contributing to an excess pronation, control of the malalignment with foot orthoses alone will not resolve the problem (McPoil & Brocato 1985).

From the midstance to the toe-off phase of the gait cycle, the pronation process reverses to allow the foot to become a rigid lever. Supination involves the reverse triplanar movement of forefoot adduction, rearfoot varus and plantarflexion of the foot, resulting in locking of the subtalar and midtarsal joints. Pes cavus, forefoot valgus or a plantarflexed first ray may produce a highly arched or supinated foot type (Nicholas & Hershman 1986) (Fig. 31.3). In contrast to the foot that pronates excessively, the supinated foot or one that does not pronate sufficiently may be responsible for lower leg injury due to a lack of the normal shock absorbing mechanism. It can lead to anterior shin splints (McPoil & Brocato 1985).

The correction of biomechanical malalignments with functional orthotics plays a major role in the management of overuse injuries in the lower leg and will be discussed below.

FRACTURES

Fractures of the tibia and fibula are seen frequently in skiing, usually the result of a rotational force at the boot top level, although their incidence has decreased with improvement in equipment. They are almost universally treated in an

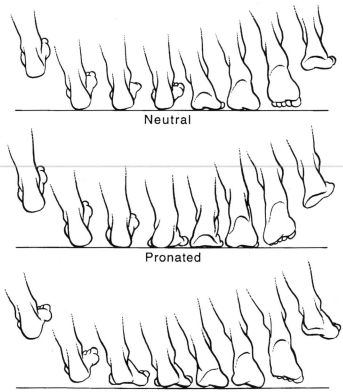

Fig. 31.3 Rear view of three foot types in running.
Source: adapted from Nicholas and Hershman (1986)

ambulatory cast after closed reduction but rehabilitation varies slightly with the method of fixation (Steadman 1986).

Those with closed reduction may begin active strengthening and flexibility exercises at the time of weightbearing. Stationary cycling is increased with increased weightbearing, and active use of the uninjured extremity and upper body should be encouraged in the athlete.

Patients with open fixation can begin mobilization early but must delay weightbearing until 6 weeks, when they can begin to put toe to ground and progress to full weightbearing as X-ray evidence of bony union allows (Steadman 1986).

Lower leg fractures also occur in contact sports such as soccer, especially if there is a blocking contact during the kicking action, direct trauma in tackling, or indirectly if the player's foot is fixed and the body rotates. The use of shinguards should be encouraged to prevent direct contact fractures in the various football codes.

The types of fractures seen in sports depends on a number of factors such as the position of the leg, age and bone density status of the athlete, velocity of injury, presence of protective equipment and duration of impact. A low speed, bending force may produce a simple tranverse fracture of the fibula. High energy, twisting injuries such as in skiing produce a severely comminuted, spiral or 'explosion' fracture of both tibia and fibula with more soft tissue swelling (Steadman 1986).

Treatment of major fractures is the in realm of orthopaedics but minor fractures of the fibula often go unrecognized. Usually misdiagnosed as bruising or muscle strain, the pain fails to settle with soft tissue treatment and there is prolonged tenderness, pain on weightbearing and perhaps pain at night. Once diagnosed, ultrasound over the fracture site should be discontinued. The area may be supported with strapping or a temporary splint, such as an aircast, if there is no instability. Other measures for pain relief may be used such as ice, TENS, magnetic field therapy and laser.

MEDIAL TIBIAL STRESS SYNDROME

The term 'shin splints' has been used to describe various conditions in the lower leg, but it is not an accurate anatomical diagnosis. It is more useful to differentiate between pain of bony, vascular or soft tissue origin.

Friedman (1986) limited shin splints strictly to musculotendinous lesions of the leg. He included lesions of the tibialis anterior, extensor hallucis longus and extensor digitorum as anterior shin splints, which will be described later in this chapter. Lesions involving the posteromedial leg muscles (tibialis posterior, flexor hallucis longus, flexor digitorum longus and soleus) are part of the posterior shin splint syndrome. Because these lesions often involve the periosteum as well, they will be classified as part of what is known as medial tibial stress syndrome (MTSS).

According to Oakes (1988) there are two types of posteromedial tibial pain, both of periosteal origin, but with differing anatomical locations.

The first area of tibial pain described by Oakes is located on the subcutaneous anteromedial surface of the tibia at the junction of its middle and lower one thirds (Fig. 31.4). This area becomes tender on palpation over a wide area and in severe cases may become oedematous, reddened, warm and extremely painful to touch. This usually happens at the start of a competitive season when the athlete attempts too much training on hard training surfaces. The pathological process responsible for the pain is a sterile inflammation of the periosteum, or 'periostitis', due to cyclical overload of the tibia. The tibia actually bends slightly under load, and if this load is repeated often enough, the bone will attempt to remodel itself to adapt and make itself stronger (Oakes 1988). The periosteum starts to lay down new bone in an attempt to thicken the stressed area, but the response is too vigorous and periostitis develops.

The second area described by Oakes is along the middle half of the posteromedial border of the tibia which can be combined with the first area or be a discrete linear pain (Fig. 31.4). According to Oakes (1988) this is the line of attachment of some of the medial fibres of the flexor digitorum longus and of the deep fascia of the leg. The linear pain is thus a 'tenoperiostitis' because muscle

attachments are involved, and this is what is often called MTSS.

Holder and Michael (1985) indicated that the soleus muscle and its investing fascia are implicated in tenoperiostitis at this posteromedial border of the tibia, especially if the heel is pronated. They suggested that this is because the soleus acts as an invertor of the heel and acts eccentrically to control pronation.

The mechanism of injury in tenoperiostitis is traction and stripping from the bony ridges on this border by these soft tissue attachments. There is microtraumatic elevation of the periosteum due to the jerk of the attached muscle and fascia during exercise. Traction is increased if the deep fascia is tight due to increased muscle volume, and often this condition is combined with a mild case of posterior compartment syndrome (Oakes 1988).

According to Friedman (1986) there is vascular resorption of collagen at the tenoperiosteal junction during relative inactivity, such as in the recreational athlete or in the off season. While activity stimulates collagen turnover, newly formed fibres lack strength initially, and the athlete is more susceptible to injury at the beginning of a training period or when activity suddenly increases.

Anterior shin splints

A similar mechanism leads to anterior tibial margin periostitis as the tibialis anterior muscle expands during exercise, causing traction on the periosteal attachment. This was called 'anterior shin splints' by Genuario (1989) and should not be confused with a true anterior compartment syndrome.

This is an overuse syndrome of the tibialis anterior muscle which works in several phases of the running gait cycle. Importantly, this muscle decelerates the foot to prevent foot slap at heel strike and is thus subject to eccentric overload especially on downhill running. It can also be brought on by uphill running, especially if the muscle has to work hard to dorsiflex the foot against tight or over-developed plantarflexors, hard surfaces, changing surfaces or shoes. The tenderness is limited to the lateral aspect of the anterior tibial border, pain being produced by active dorsiflexion and passive plantarflexion.

Predisposing factors

Oakes (1988) listed five predisposing factors that increase the repetitive loading forces on the tibia that may lead to periostitis.

Biomechanical. Viitasalo and Kvist (1983) found that athletes with tibial pain tended to pronate at the subtalar joint more than those without. This was reiterated by Messier and Pittala (1988), who found that athletes with

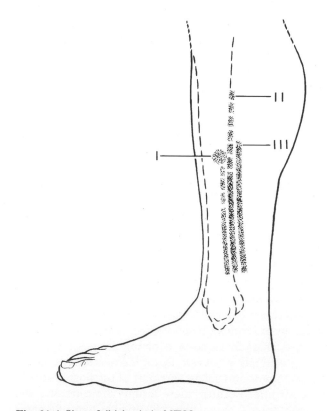

Fig. 31.4 Sites of tibial pain in MTSS.
Source: adapted from Detmer (1986)

shin splints had significantly greater maximum range and velocity of pronation. Delacerda (1982) found that as foot pronation increased, the electromyographic activity of the anterior tibial muscle increased. He suggested that improper alignment in the forefoot (varus) or the rearfoot or functional equinus deformity caused by tightness in the calf/achilles tendon complex is a significant factor in the etiology of tibial pain. This was also stated in studies by Lilletvedt et al (1979) and Gehlsen and Seger (1980).

Ellis (1986) stated that shin splints can plague flat-footed overpronators, but that a too-rigid, highly arched foot underpronates and does not roll sufficiently to absorb the shock of running, leading to periostitis as well. Excess body weight increases the load that must be borne by the lower leg and must also be a contributing factor (see section on biomechanics).

Training methods. As with many other lower leg injuries, MTSS is typically brought on by doing 'too much too soon'. The body has a tremendous ability to adapt to mechanical overload as long as it is given the opportunity to recover adequately from stress.

High intensity, long duration workouts repeated too frequently without allowing for normal physiological adaptation leads to the process of breakdown and failure to recover, injury being the result. Well-conditioned athletes who build up their training gradually have an ability to recover which exceeds the rate of breakdown; the lower leg muscles respond by becoming stronger and attain higher levels of endurance.

A 'hard/easy' or cyclic approach should be adopted for unconditioned athletes or those recovering from previous injury. For example, after 2 weeks of intensive training, the athlete should have a week's rest with a lighter training load and/or substitute less stressful exercise such as cycling or swimming.

Training loads should also be individualized according to the particular athlete's age, ability and level of fitness and performance. Often injuries occur due to athletes attempting to keep up with with their peers when this is beyond their ability.

Training surfaces. During the early 1980s there was a virtual epidemic of tibial pain and stress fractures in women who took up aerobics. These high impact, highly repetitive exercises were at that time done mostly on thinly cushioned concrete floors in poor footwear and with little regard to adequate warm-up and conditioning. Similarly, athletes who introduce track running too suddenly, especially at the start of their competitive season when they are poorly conditioned, will often experience tibial pain. The same goes for hockey players who start playing on artificial surfaces, soccer players on hard grounds and basketballers, netballers, tennis players introduced suddenly to new, harder playing surfaces. Softer surfaces such as sprung wooden floors or rubber underlayed carpet for aerobics, grass or natural trails for running and clay or grass for tennis should be recommended as one strategy for prevention of MTSS.

Muscle dysfunction and inflexibility. Clement (1974) regarded muscle fatigue and resultant disuse atrophy as the major aetiological factor in MTSS in athletes. Weakened anterior and posterior tibial muscles cannot assist in deceleration of the body weight when running and thus allows increased shock to the tibia. He suggested that equal importance be given to regaining muscle strength and endurance as to rest in the treatment of the condition. Oakes (1986) did not see muscle factors as a common cause of increased tibial loading, but stated that a tight gastrocnemius/soleus complex would not allow adequate dorsiflexion and hence create a greater bending force on the tibia. By the same token, athletes with a previous history of ankle ligament injuries may be left with residual loss of range of motion in the ankle joint, particularly dorsiflexion range. This predisposes to overuse injury problems in the lower leg, because normal mechanics are disturbed.

Shoe design. In the early stages of the jogging boom running shoes were little more than sneakers. Technological advances in shoe design have advanced at a tremendous rate since then but along the way there have been certain 'gimmicks' that have undoubtedly contributed to injury. In particular, the very wide heel flares popular in the early 1970s tended to exaggerate any minor biomechanical malalignment problems in runners. The heel flare should be no wider than the width of the ankle.

Shoes without firm heel counters and with inadequate support for the rearfoot cannot control pronation and are thus implicated. Shoes with poor shock absorption are also apt to contribute to the problem; recent research has shown that some popularly used shock absorbing inserts are in fact useless (Lafortune & Maguire 1986). However, midsole materials and built-in shock-absorbing devices are now highly advanced and modern shoe design has gone a long way to reducing tibial impact forces. Very stiff shoes that do not flex sufficently can also cause tibial pain (Lipinski 1987). As many athletes have tight achilles, the heels should be elevated (see section on management of MTSS).

Sport-specific, higher quality sports shoes will reduce the chance of injury. Once the outer sole, which is the most durable part of the shoe, starts to show signs of wear, the midsole has probably lost its shock-absorbing qualities. If the upper is deformed or split in any way, the shoe is probably not providing enough support and should not be used for sport. There is a huge range of shoes now available, and because every athlete has differing needs it is inappropriate to prescribe a particular brand or type of shoe without a thorough history, examination and biomechanical assessment. Advice should be sought from an experienced sports podiatrist who can undertake such an examination and supply orthotics where appropriate.

Diet. Finally, diet has been implicated as a contributory factor by Myburgh et al (1988) who found that shin soreness in a group of 25 men and women was associated with a lower than average dietary intake of calcium.

Pathology of tibial pain

Kues (1990) attempted to describe the pathology of shin splints by critically reviewing previous literature. She reported that studies by Mubarak et al (1982) and D'Ambrosia (1977) failed to show that the pain of posteromedial 'shin splints' was due to increased pressure in the deep posterior compartment.

Puranen (1974) surgically explored the deep posterior compartment of 11 athletes with medial tibial pain and found the crural fascia near its insertion to be tense and thickened, but he did not measure pressure. Surgical release of the fascia gave relief in his series.

Devas (1958) thought that exercise-induced pain along the posteromedial aspect of the tibia was due to stress fractures. He found radiographic evidence such as localized areas of subperiosteal new bone formation in six patients, and incomplete fractures in 10 others. He believed that stress fractures were due to a series of events that eventually led to painful disruption of the medial tibial cortex with little or no X-ray changes.

Roub et al (1979) found that some individuals do indeed have localized changes in the tibial cortex visible as focal, fusiform longitudinal areas of increased radiotracer uptake on bone scans that are not visible on X-rays. Johnell et al (1982) also concluded that shin splints may be due to microfractures in the tibia, which represent the first stage of a stress fracture and are not visible on X-rays.

Kues stated that shin splints may be due to stress fractures of the tibia, but did not view the two syndromes as separate entities as does Oakes (1986) and Jones and James (1987), who recommended the use of bone scans to determine the diagnosis. They pointed out, however, that as healing progresses with stress fractures, the lesion becomes less intense and less localized, giving a fusiform appearance on a bone scan similar to that seen with MTSS.

Kues reported that several authors had hypothesized that shin splints were due to a soft tissue injury, based in either the flexor digitorum longus (FDL), flexor hallucis longus (FHL), soleus or the tibialis posterior (TP). Mills et al (1980) did bone scans and found diffuse linear uptake, different from the focal/fusiform pattern of stress fractures, at what he called the origin of FDL. He stated that these were areas of periosteal tearing.

Holder and Michael (1985) did three phase radionuclide imaging to show that muscle and tendon were not involved because the first two phases (angiogram and blood pool)

were normal. They concluded that the tibia was the source of pain because the third phase of imaging was positive in nine of their 10 athletes, indicating the periosteum had been injured because the uptake was diffuse and linear. They also concluded that this area corresponded to the origin of the soleus.

Kues suggested that several muscles of the lower leg were active during running, and that it seemed unlikely that only one muscle would cause the injury to the periosteum of the tibia.

Kues concluded that biopsies would be required to verify whether the injury was periosteal, but because this was impractical, three phase imaging was useful in determining the pathology associated with shin splints.

Detmer (1986) described three sites of pathology in MTSS. The first was the periosteum itself (Fig. 31.4, Type I). Detmer hypothesized that in chronic cases the periosteum is actually disengaged from the bone either by ballistic avulsion by the powerful muscles or by sufficient subperiosteal haemorrhage or inflammation to lift the periosteum away from the bone (see Fig. 31.4, Type II). He found adipose tissue between the periosteum and the bone at operation, and concluded that once avulsed it cannot heal back onto the bone. This may explain the corrugated texture found at the site of injury in chronic MTSS. Stretching stress of the musculotendinous fibres or posterior compartment investing fascia on the chronically avulsed but innervated periosteum explains the persistent pain, despite normal biopsy findings (Fig. 31.5, Type III).

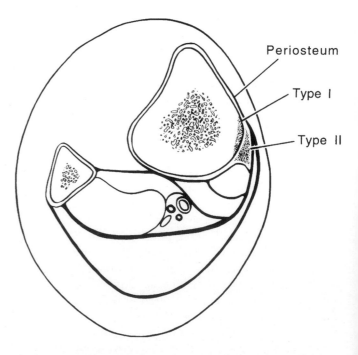

Fig. 31.5 The periosteum is elevated from the tibia with ectopic fat deposited beneath it (type II). Source: adapted from Detmer (1986)

Table 31.1 Differential diagnoses of tibial pain

	Periostitis (MTSS)	Stress fracture	Compartment syndrome	Anterior 'shin splints'	Posteromedial tendinitis
Location	Subcutaneous surface distal 1/3 antero medial tibia	Anywhere on the bone only	In the muscle compartments	Lateral margin of anterior border tibia	Posteromedial margin
Shape	Diffuse	Localized spot or line	Diffuse through muscle belly	Diffuse and linear	Linear and diffuse
Behaviour	Warms up (only if mild) with use and aches afterwards	Gets worse with use, not eased by rest rest	Brought on by use, 'crampy' and eases with	Warms up and aches afterwards	Warms up and aches afterwards
Tenderness to palpation	3–6 cm area exquisitely tender	20–30 mm focal and very tender area with erythema	Only on very deep palpation	May be lumpy along edge of bone	On **muscle** not the bone
Induration	Mild	More (swollen)	None	None	None
X-ray	Negative	Positive after 2–3 weeks	Negative	Negative	Negative
Bone scan	Positive diffuse linear or fusiform uptake	Positive discrete piriform or linear uptake (later may be fusiform)	Negative	Negative	
Compartment pressure testing	Negative	Negative	Positive	Negative	Negative
Night pain	May be if very severe	Yes	No	Not usually	Not usually
Morning stiffness	May be prolonged if severe	May feel better in morning	No	Mild	Mild

Source: from Genuario (1989)

Signs and symptoms

The pain of MTSS typically begins as a dull ache following exercise; which gradually progresses until it begins to hurt during exercise and may start to affect training. Because it is a soft tissue condition, it may actually warm up and ease at the start of training only to return after training and ache for some time afterwards (Table 31.1). The legs may feel stiff in the morning but there is generally no pain at rest or in bed at night, in contrast to stress fracture or osteoid osteoma. Rest overnight often relieves symptoms in the early stages. With continued activity such as running or jumping, pain gets worse and lasts longer. A limp may develop in walking or running. A volleyballer or basketballer will begin to use the unaffected leg for takeoff and landing. When severe there may be pain walking, on stairs and weight-bearing in general.

There may be a well defined but wide area of tenderness, sometimes slightly thickened, palpable. Widespread thickening and scarring is a feature of chronic teno-periostitis, with a lumpy or corrugated texture to the subcutaneous posteromedial tibial border.

Clement (1974) found an increase in the circumference of the affected leg at the level of periosteal induration averaging 0.92 cm plus atrophy of the anterior muscle group and the gastrocnemius averaging 1.46 cm. He postulated that the subperiosteal reaction was caused by a loss of shock absorption due to local muscle fatigue. Resultant disuse atrophy further reduces the shock absorption capabilities.

With continued trauma there is more pain, and the advanced state of the syndrome may progress to a stress fracture.

According to Ellis (1986), the pain of isolated periostitis will virtually preclude running, with pain radiating up the leg at each jarring step. Unlike muscle pain, tendinitis or tenoperiostitis, with warming up it becomes more severe.

Differential diagnosis

Previous classifications of MTSS included stress fracture and compartment syndrome, but for the purposes of clear differentiation, these syndromes should be separated as was recommended by Oakes (1986) and Jones and James (1987). This is best illustrated with the use of a table to compare signs and symptoms, such as that used by Genuario (1989). She included anterior and posterior 'shin splints' as separate entities, i.e. anterior tibial margin periostitis and the linear posteromedial tenoperiostitis described by Oakes (Table 31.1). Tenoperiostitis can also occur laterally, where the peroneal muscles are attached to the fibula.

According to Oakes (1986) accurate diagnosis of tibial pain requires a detailed history, evaluation of workload and state of conditioning, and examination of footwear. Careful palpation to reveal the site and size of area of tenderness will often give the diagnosis without further investigation.

MTSS may be the forerunner to a stress fracture especially if the tenderness is localized, thickened, indurated and exquisitely painful to press with redness and warmth. A tuning fork applied to the area will elicit severe pain, as will ultrasound (Ellis 1986). X-rays will usually be negative for 2–3 weeks unless the beams look directly down the fracture line, which is very difficult to achieve. After this time, callous formation seen on the X-ray is the hallmark of a stress fracture in the absence of a visible line.

However, a bone scan will be positive within 48 hours and a stress fracture will show up initially as a small, focal 'hot spot', and later perhaps as more fusiform in shape (Jones & James 1987). A stress 'reaction' will appear linear but still discrete (Detmer 1986), whilst periostitis will appear diffuse and linear.

The pain of exertional compartment syndrome will be felt over the muscles, not on the tibia. It occurs during running and abates within minutes of stopping (Oakes 1986). It is commonly bilateral. Acute or traumatic compartment syndromes are a separate entity (see section on compartment syndromes).

Chronic muscle or tendinous lesions can mimic MTSS and careful palpation, especially of the calf/achilles complex, will reveal the site of injury (see section on calf muscle injuries).

As in all cases of chronic leg pain, the possibility of a referred component to tibial syndromes from the lumbar spine or more peripherally cannot be overlooked. A thorough history and, where indicated, examination of the neuromeningeal structures that could refer pain to the leg should be perfomed e.g. the slump test (see Ch. 27) and modified SLR.

Popliteal artery entrapment is rare but can occur in athletes (Rudo et al 1982). The symptoms are of claudication or cramping, relieved by rest, due to compression of the popliteal artery if it passes through the medial head of the gastrocnemius muscle. This is confirmed from the history and the fact that the ankle pulses diminish during active calf contraction. Angiography or Doppler flow studies can also be used and the cure is decompressive surgery (see section on politeal artery entrapment).

Other causes of tibial pain include bone tumours, infections, osteoid osteoma and neurovascular malformations (Oakes 1986). In these cases the behaviour of the pain will not be mechanical in nature and severe night pain and systemic signs are likely.

Management of MTSS

Successful management of tibial pain syndromes depends on early and accurate diagnosis and early intervention because they are due to overuse and are progressive in nature. They easily become chronic and rest from overload is an absolute requirement to allow tissues to heal, particularly the periosteum. In those few cases rested early and thus completely resolved, Detmer (1986) speculated that this had occurred because the periosteum had been allowed to heal back firmly to the tibia in type II syndromes. Oakes recommended 2–3 weeks of rest from weightbearing activity, substituting swimming or running in water or cycling to maintain fitness. Running in water can be facilitated with the use of flotation belts and this is now widely used as an adjunct to normal training by elite athletes concerned with reducing tibial impact loading and preventing injury. During this time treatment can commence and predisposing factors should be evaluated and acted upon to speed recovery and prevent recurrence (see Ch. 16).

Biomechanical analysis by a qualified and experienced sports podiatrist should be advised and orthotics may be of assistance where malalignment is suspected to be a contributing factor. In cases where there is minor malalignment, 'soft' or heat moulded orthotics may be sufficient to control abnormal motion or provide extra shock absorption. However, in the author's opinion these materials tend to deform with heavy use. Semi-rigid orthotics, fashioned in a laboratory from a plaster cast of the patient's feet, taken by a podiatrist, provide better control of motion in more severe cases and are more durable for heavy duty wear.

It is vital that the supplier of the orthotics understands the requirements of the athlete and specific training and experience in the manufacture of orthotics for athletes is highly desirable.

Rigid orthotics that are simply too hard to run in lead to poor patient compliance. There is now a large range of sport-specific products that are much more suitable and go a long way to helping cure these and other biomechanically related overuse syndromes.

Dynamic evaluation of running on the track or on a treadmill with videotape analysis is now becoming more widely available and may reveal excessive or prolonged pronation or other evidence of malalignment. The effect of corrective orthotics can readily be assessed in this way.

Overpronation can be managed with firmer, motion-controlling shoes with firm heel counters to control rearfoot motion and/or orthotics. Appropriate footwear is the first step, advice should be sought from a reputable specialist sports shoe store on the correct shoe for individual foot type. The best orthotic cannot do its job in an inadequate shoe, and vice versa. Strengthening of the muscles that control pronation (TP, FHL, FDL, TA) has been advocated (Ellis 1986).

Grant (1990) stated that taping prevents early muscle fatigue and adds some compression to the tibia (Fig. 31.6). The author has used taping of the medial plantar arch to prevent pronation to evaluate if this alters the symptoms and whether motion control would be of use. Neoprene leg sleeves have also been used to add compression and warmth and give some symptomatic relief for tibial pain.

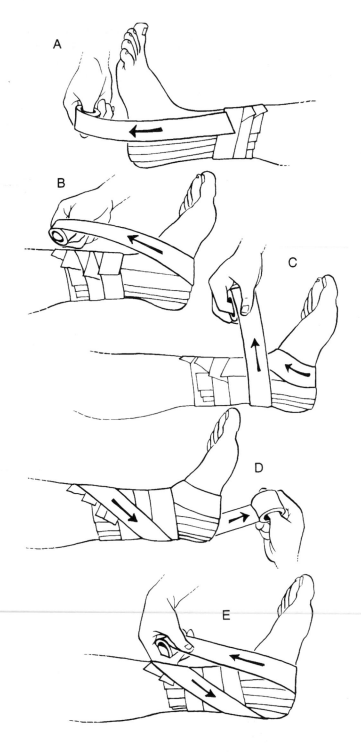

Fig. 31.6 Strapping to limit pronation for tibial pain syndromes. Source: adapted from Grant (1990)

Where there is a problem with inadequate shock absorption, this can be managed with softer slip-lasted rather than board-lasted shoes (which are stiffer). Shoes that are too stiff can be cut where the foot flexes at the metatarsophalangeal joint without affecting the life of the shoe (Lipinski 1987).

Previous trauma to the talocrural and/or the subtalar joints may leave residual stiffness which alters the normal pronation mechanism (see biomechanics section). Under-pronation due to foot type or previous trauma leaving joint motion restriction can be passively mobilized, specifically to encourage pronation or in a more general way, to improve dorsiflexion as described in Chapter 32.

Icing has been widely advocated to reduce pain and inflammation of tibial soreness. In its acute inflammatory stages, ice may be applied as often as hourly for 20 minutes. Ice massage, using the frozen styrofoam cup technique, is localized and very effective.

Non-steroidal anti-inflammatory drugs can also be used to reduce pain and inflammation. Ellis (1986) advocates the use of powdered aspirin in aloe vera gel used externally, and others have used washing soda packs with some success. In the author's experience, electrical modalities for pain relief such as high voltage stimulation, TENS or interferential are of benefit. Low dosage pulsed ultrasound can be used with care to avoid aggravating periosteal pain. Ultrasound is best limited to soft tissue attachments adjacent to the tibia rather than on the bone itself.

Massage is an important way of relieving tension and spasm in adjacent muscles and encouraging circulatory drainage of metabolic waste products. After the acute stage it can be used to directly soften scarred areas, especially in chronic cases where firm massage of the 'lumps' really helps to improve flexibilty and function. This can be very painful so is best done following icing. Portable magnetic field therapy, or stick-on magnets, have been used but there is no scientific information known to the author on its effectiveness. Delacerda (1982) found that iontophoresis with 0.5% hydrocortisone was effective.

Stretching of tight muscles, particularly the gastrocnemius and soleus complex is vital and weightbearing stretches should be taught and performed daily. The anterior muscles should also be stretched if tight, particularly in anterior tibial syndrome, by plantarflexing the ankles and sitting back on the haunches.

These anterior muscles must also be strengthened to redress any muscle imbalance. This is achieved by lifting a weighted paint tin, using therabands or tyre tubes for resistance, or walking on the heels. More complicated equipment, such as hydraulic or isokinetic plantar/dorsiflexion and inversion/eversion systems can be used to test for imbalances and for rehabilitation.

These stretching and strengthening exercises should not be attempted during the acute inflammatory stages of injury and should be done only to the point of fatigue, not pain.

In very resistent cases that are not responding to adequate rest and good conservative therapy, fasciotomy of the deep posterior compartment has been advocated, but its role in the management of MTSS is still uncertain and controversial. Michael and Holder (1985) advocated surgical release of the tight soleus bridge; Detmer (1986) added periosteal cauterization to 'scar' the periosteum back to the bone as he believed it was detached. Jarvinnen et al (1989) reported 78% good to excellent results of fasciotomy under local anaesthetic.

Return to sport should only commence if there is no pain on walking, hopping and jogging on the spot and tenderness to palpation has reduced significantly, although it may never disappear entirely. Initially running should commence slowly and for brief periods on soft surfaces every second day. All predisposing factors must have been addressed and controlled. No speed or track work should be attempted until the athlete has built up some condition and fitness on more yielding surfaces. This should take several weeks using a hard/easy approach with careful and gradual build-up of training intensity.

According to Detmer (1986), type II (periostalgia) will promptly redevelop symptoms on premature return to activity, while if stress fractures do recur, it is usually much later in the rehabilitation phase.

Prevention

Lipinski (1987) outlined several measures for prevention of tibial pain. Specifically, the athlete should avoid sudden changes of training surface, such as from road to track or vice versa. Seasonal athletes should not have a total rest in the off season, which causes a loss of conditioning, but attempt to maintain fitness. They also need to maintain balanced strength and strength in the anterior and posterior muscle groups.

Overworn shoes or shoes with incorrect wear patterns should not be used.

Activities such as skipping and high impact aerobics tend to aggravate tibial pain and probably should also be avoided.

Preseason biomechanical screening and measures instituted early for prevention, such as orthotic therapy and stretching routines, should be considered for high performance athletes, especially in the team sports such as hockey, basketball, netball and football. Self massage of tight muscle bellies will help maintain flexibility, reduce muscle soreness and prevent early fatigue thus lessening the chances of recurrence.

STRESS FRACTURES

Stress fractures are commonly diagnosed in runners following heavy exercise, but occur in other athletes such as basketballers, netballers, tennis players and with activities such as skipping or aerobics. The onset is usually episodic or more sudden than with other lower leg overuse syndromes e.g. after a particular race or game or hard training session, or after a progressively intense training program.

According to Detmer (1986), stress fractures typically occur in well conditioned athletes. This is in contrast to earlier work by Jackson (1978), who suggested that athletes who get stress fractures are usually non-conditioned runners who tend to jog less than 20 miles (21 km) a week and get it from a sudden initiation of an intensive program. The incidence is very high in defence force recruits (Milgrom et al 1986). Women seem to be more susceptible to stress fractures than men (Ellis 1986). Friedman (1986) reported that the tibia and fibula accounted for 45% of all stress fractures in athletes.

The distribution of stress fractures in the tibia was 80% and in the fibula 20% in a study by Hulkko et al (1987) of lower leg stress fractures. 75% of tibial fractures seen in athletes occurred in runners. Radiographs showed 95% of tibial fractures occurred in the posteromedial aspect. In the fibula, 86% were located in the distal third.

The weekly distance run by the injured athletes in this study was significantly shorter for females, for children and for recreational runners compared with competitive runners. The most important aetiological factor was a sudden increase in intensity of training. According to Devas (1970), athletes who overexercise when not in full training are prone to stress fractures.

In another study by Hulkko and Orava (1987) of total body stress fractures in athletes, there were 268 in males and 100 in females. The tibia accounted for 182 and the fibula 44. 72% occurred in runners, who tend to get fractures in the distal third of the fibula or the upper or lower tibia, while ballet dancers tend to sustain fractures in the middle of the tibia in its anterior cortex (Devas 1970).

Stress fractures in the tibia were most common at the junction of the middle and distal thirds and in the proximal metaphysis in a study by Orava (1980) (Fig. 31.7).

According to Friedman (1986), because the tibia bears more weight, it sustains more stress fractures than the fibula. He reported that stress fractures in the distal third of the fibula were common and often confused with peroneal tendinitis. These were 'low risk' fractures, i.e. athletes can usually walk without pain and they heal quickly, although the injury sometimes progresses to complete fracture if ignored. Stress fractures in the proximal fibula are less common. In the posteromedial tibial plateau, they are often confused with medial collateral ligament strain or pes anserinus bursitis. Stress fractures of the anterior tibia just below the tibial tuberosity are often misdiagnosed as patellar tendinitis or malignancy (Friedman 1986). They can also occur in the posterior tibial cortex and be difficult to localize with palpation, being confused with deep calf muscle strain.

Pathology of stress fractures

Old bone is constantly being broken down, and new bone formed in its place. Bone reacts to stress by remodelling itself in an attempt to become stronger (Bates 1985). First it tears itself down by rapid periosteal circumferential resorption of part of the bone matrix that was not strong

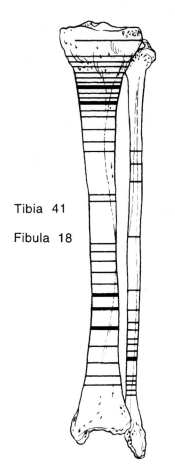

Tibia 41

Fibula 18

Fig. 31.7 Sites of stress fractures in the tibia and fibula. Thick lines indicate sites of higher incidence. Source: adapted from Orava (1980)

enough to cope with the stress demands placed upon it. The body senses this breakdown and works to replace the weakened bone with a stronger matrix. This explains the tibial cortical hypertrophy that is sometimes seen in young distance runners.

During this breakdown period, the bone is vulnerable due to transient weakening of the cortex and if the athlete continues to exercise intensively it may eventually rupture. Thus the stress suffered has exceeded the ability of the bone to remodel itself. The damage may not always proceed to cortical rupture but is a spectrum ranging from simple hypertrophy to fracture or combinations (Bates 1985). An uneven tibial edge is a sign of recurrent new bone formation (Detmer 1986).

Stress fractures on the tension side of a bone are more at risk to go on to delayed union or a complete fracture than those on the compression side. This is common at the anterior tibial cortex and should be suspected in athletes who present with pain and tenderness over the anterior aspect of the mid shaft of the tibia (Rettig et al 1988).

Repeated cyclic tension stress at the site of muscular attachment to bone will induce remodelling. Continued overuse may result in cortical thinning and porosis and eventual fracture. However, this is not the only mechanism

of injury in stress fractures, since tarsal navicular and femoral neck stress fractures occur where there are no muscular attachments, and appear to be related more to stress due to axial load, bending or compression (Markey 1991).

Stanitiski et al (1978) suggested that fatigue of muscles allows excessive force to applied to bone and that stress fractures were due to repeated, rhythmic, muscle-generated insults. Hence muscle fatigue or indeed muscle imbalance as previously described could also be a risk factor for stress fractures specifically. Markey (1991) suggested that as muscles fatigue, their ability to absorb force is diminished and more force is transmitted direcly to bone. Stress fractures hence represented a failure of the muscles first, with bone injury being a secondary event.

Risk factors

Several risk factors, apart from those delineated in Oakes (1986) for tibial pain, have been specifically linked to a higher incidence of stress fractures in the lower leg. Much of this information is derived from research carried out on Israeli army recruits by Giladi et al, who confirmed that a high level of loading of bone was a major etiological factor. They found that smaller values for tibial bone width (Giladi et al 1987a), and a lower area moment of inertia of the tibia (Milgrom et al 1989) were risk factors in tibial stress fractures. They also found the same for increased external rotation values of the hip joint (more than 65°) (Giladi et al 1987b).

Other predisposing factors for stress fractures in the lower leg are more general and apply equally to the syndromes mentioned elsewhere in this chapter i.e. MTSS and compartment syndromes. These include footwear, biomechanical factors, muscle fatigue and imbalance, training distances and training surfaces. However, there have been a number of predisposing factors associated with stress fractures specifically in women involved in repetitive weightbearing exercise such as long distance running, dance and aerobics.

Women and stress fractures

The incidence of stress fractures has been shown to be relatively high in women with athletic amenorrhea; according to some authors (Carbon et al 1990, Myburgh et al 1990). Various hormonal and metabolic factors have been implicated, as well as diet and eating behaviour disorders such as anorexia nervosa (Rigotti et al 1991; see also Chs 34 and 35).

Barrow and Saha (1988) suggested that female distance runners who have a history of irregular or absent menses and who have never used oral contraceptives may be at an increased risk for developing stress fractures. When amenorrheal runners were separated from the very irregular group, an alarming trend was noted in eating behaviour disorders (47%).

The mechanism by which athletic amenorrhea, eating disorders, low body fat levels, calcium, oestrogen, progesterone, low bone density, accelerated bone loss, osteoporosis and stress fractures are related is complex but has been outlined by Highet (1989). Certainly the combination of poor dietary habits and high running mileage seem to be related to injury in females.

The evidence for accelerated bone loss in these young women with hypo-oestrogenaemia is considerable (Linnell et al 1984, Marcus et al 1985, Bourke 1990). Early studies, mostly on trabecular bone in the lumbar vertebrae, showed that amenorrhoeic runners' bone mineral content was significantly reduced, and was only partially reversible with the return of menses. Even those with clinically normal menses may have compromised bone formation, due to reduced progesterone levels (Prior et al 1990).

Further studies have suggested an association between hypo-oestrogenaemia, low body fat, reduced bone density and stress fractures (Highet 1989). However, these phenomena may simply be coincidental and not necessarily sequentially related.

Interestingly, Carbon et al (1990) found that bone mineral density was the same between two matched groups of elite female athletes, nine with stress fractures and nine without, despite the fracture group having significantly less menses per year, significantly lower skinfold values and delayed age of menarche.

This was also the first study to measure bone mineral density in the weightbearing bones of amenorrhoeic athletes (femoral neck). Previous studies had only measured the bone mineral density of the lumbar vertebrae, which have a high proportion of trabecular bone or the radius, while most stress fractures occur in the lower limbs through cortical bone. Carbon et al (1990) concluded that stress fractures in elite female athletes are largely independent of bone mineral density. Markers of bone turnover like urinary pyridium cross-links of collagen for bone resorption may be more relevant than bone density in this context (Uebelhart et al 1990).

However, Myburgh et al (1990) found that in a group of 25 matched athletes with similar training habits, those with stress fractures were more likely to have significantly lower bone density in the femoral neck, lower dietary calcium intake, current menstrual irregularity and lower oral contraceptive use. They also confirmed that gender is a risk factor for stress fractures as well as osteoporosis, suggesting that low calcium intake and/or calcium deprivation could increase the risk of osteoporosis in later life, despite regular exercise.

Signs and symptoms

The classic symptoms caused by a stress fracture begin with a slight ache or nagging pain at the end of activity. With continued sport the pain becomes a more severe focal ache, occurs increasingly earlier in a session and lasts longer afterwards, sometimes disturbing sleep. It does not 'warm up' like soft tissue injuries but continues to worsen with further use, and eventually rest brings no relief (Genuario 1989). It may ease overnight which may encourage the athlete to continue exercising, only to find that the pain returns in a short time and remains even after the activity is stopped, unlike compartment syndrome which starts to ease immediately with rest. If the athlete rests for a week the pain may go completely with ordinary activity but may come on again with return to sport.

On examination there will always be a specific spot on a bone with maximal tenderness, which is very well localized although there may be surrounding soft tissue/periosteal tenderness which is not as severe. The swelling of a bony callous formation may be palpable under the skin, especially with superficial bone such as the distal third of the fibula. The site of a stress fracture will be exquisitely tender on even light palpation. It may also be indurated, or oedematous with local erythema if severe and acute. Springing or bowing the bone by applying pressure away from the painful area will also produce pain at the fracture site (Devas 1970). Percussion may also be positive (Genuario 1989), as is the application of a tuning fork or ultrasound (Ellis 1986).

Diagnosis

The most reliable test is a Technetium bone scan that will reveal a focal 'hot spot' which is the area of greatest turnover of bone, usually of about 20–30 mm diameter (Detmer 1986). Non-focal areas point to impending stress fractures or 'stress reactions' if linear uptake is seen or periostitis that may or may not progress to stress fractures (Chisin et al 1987). In these cases a period of rest should still be advised. Diffuse linear uptake points to medial or anterior tibial stress syndrome as described previously.

Bone pain may precede scintigraphic evidence of a stress fracture (Milgrom et al 1984). Bone scans may need to be repeated especially for persistent and increasing bony pain that exhibits the signs and symptoms described above. MRI and CT can be used to obtain more detail and determine the stage of healing of a stress fracture.

Plain radiographs may show early signs of a stress fracture such as slight loss of bone density followed by a fracture line or callous formation, but these signs may take 2–3 weeks to be visible whereas a bone scan will generally be positive within 48 hours (Bates 1985).

Stress fractures usually only involve one cortex, and can be difficult to see on X-ray. The diagnosis is often only made retrospectively with the late appearance of callous on X-rays and is now often made on clinical grounds.

Evidence of healing of stress fractures can be seen on X-rays as cortical thickening, fluffy or bony callous. Maturing callous will also be heralded by a reduction in pain, swelling and warmth over the injury site (Markey 1990).

See Table 31.1 for an outline of differential diagnosis.

Management of stress fractures

The treatment of stress fractures must involve an initial period of rest from running or impact loading on the lower limbs for a period which varies according to clinical and investigative findings. According to Markey (1990) metaphyseal stress fractures discovered in the healing phase take the least time to heal, while intracortical fractures in the late fracture stage take the longest. He recommended a rest period of 3–8 weeks.

Fibular stress fractures generally are the shortest to heal (Hulkko et al 1987), being at the 3 week end of this spectrum, unless they progress to complete fracture and eventual non-union. Tibial stress fractures should be rested for a minimum of 4 weeks, with a 6–8 week period most often advocated. Tibial fractures in the proximal and distal thirds take longer to heal, with some lasting many months and requiring surgery due to delayed or non-union.

Mid-tibial fractures take the longest to heal with frequent delayed or non-union. The average time for mid-tibial fractures to heal with conservative treatment alone was 8 months in Hulkko et al's study (1987).

During the rest period the athlete should be counselled to alleviate contributory and risk factors. Swimming, pool running with buoyancy vests or belts and cycling are all alternative activities used to maintain fitness and motivation. Ice packs, TENS, high voltage stimulation or interferential can be used for pain relief.

If there is pain weightbearing or if there is a high risk of delayed or non-union (e.g. anterior tibial cortex, medial malleolus), cast immobilization and/or non-weightbearing for 2–3 weeks is used initially. Dickson and Kichline (1987) described the use of an inflatable aircast to give support and relieve pain in partial or full weightbearing to allow more functional management. Some stress fractures develop delayed or non-union tendencies because athletes are too active (Orava & Hulkko 1988), and may require enforced immobilization. Often these athletes become severely depressed when told to rest without adequate counselling and alternative activities. They need to be monitored very strictly to prevent them doing too much weightbearing too soon, as they have the compulsion to keep 'trying it out', thereby delaying their recovery.

Rettig et al (1988) recommended rest and external electrical stimulation for a minimum of 3–6 months in stress fractures of the anterior tibial cortex before considering surgery. The surgery performed on these 'tension' fractures and other cases of delayed or non-union usually involves biopsy and transverse drilling of the hypertrophied cortex or bone grafting (Hulkko et al 1987).

Pulsed electromagnetic field therapy (PEMF) has been used to encourage bone healing in these delayed union stress fractures of the anterior cortex of the tibia with success (Bassett 1984, Rettig et al 1988). PEMF is also being more widely used to encourage faster healing in all stress fractures (see Ch.15).

Return to running or sport should only commence in total absence of symptoms and signs and should be carefully supervised along the lines described previously for tibial pain, keeping in mind that recurrence tends to happen later in the rehabilitation phase than with other lower leg syndromes. Ideally, follow-up X-rays should be taken for objective evidence of healing.

Prevention of stress fractures

Contributory factors, such as those described for tibial soreness, should be systematically addressed to assist prevention of stress fractures. Rationalization of training loads and correction of biomechanical problems are particularly important in terms of prevention.

Nutritional and hormonal factors in females are now also being more widely considered in terms of prevention. In women with hypo-oestrogenaemia, bone loss progresses at approximately 4% per year, with the most loss occurring early after the cessation of menses (Highet 1989). This emphasizes the need for early intervention. Highet suggested that while the role of calcium and oestrogen supplementation in the exercising female remains unclear, an increased calcium intake of up to 1500 mg per day and hormone replacement should be advised.

Myburgh et al (1990) suggested that oral contraceptives appeared to offer some protection, as did an increased calcium intake of more than 120% of RDA (Australian recommended dietary intake is 800 mg). This was necessary to help repair bone microtrauma and offset the increased requirements of athletes with oestrogen deprivation.

Caffeine increases the urinary excretion of calcium in premenopausal women who habitually consume it (Massey & Opryszek 1990), therefore excessive intake should be avoided.

According to Heinrich et al (1990), weight training provides a better stimulus for increasing bone mineral content than does running or swimming, so may be a useful training alternative for both rehabilitation and prevention of stress fractures in the lower leg.

COMPARTMENT SYNDROMES

Many terms have been used to describe effort- or exercise-induced compartment syndromes, such as tibial syndrome, shin splints, exercise ischaemia and myositis. An effort-related compartment syndrome was defined by Martens and Moeyersoons (1990) as a condition in which increased

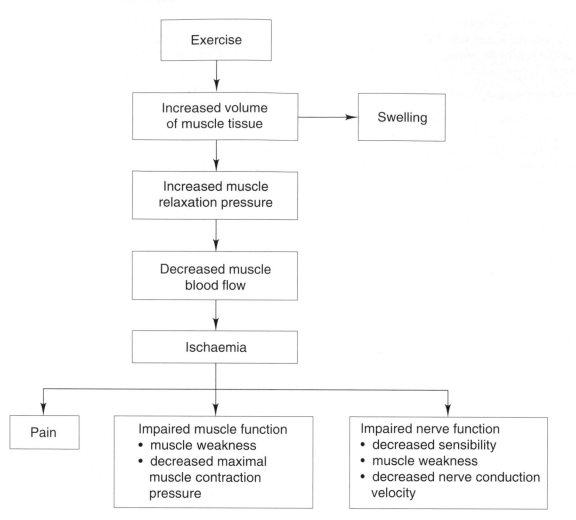

Fig. 31.8 Pathophysiology of chronic compartment syndrome and its relation to symptoms, signs and findings at investigation. Source: adapted from Styf (1989)

intracompartmental pressure induced by effort impedes the blood flow to that compartment, and thus compromises the metabolic demands of tissues within that space (see Fig. 31.8). This may occur wherever there is neurovascular tissue surrounded by a limiting envelope of non-compliant fascia.

Symptoms arise because the increased pressure causes ischaemia of the tissues contained within the compartment, particularly the muscles and nerves. Muscle ischaemia causes pain and nerve ischaemia causes weakness and sensory symptoms in the cutaneous distribution of the nerve.

Chronic or recurrent compartment syndromes are distinguished from the acute by the fact that there are asymptomatic intervals between recurrences and they are reversible, while the acute syndrome is usually due to one incident and is irreversible.

The majority of cases of compartment syndrome occur in the lower leg in the anterior or deep posterior com-

partment but also in the peroneal and superficial posterior compartments. Davey et al (1984) reported isolated exertional compartment syndrome of the tibialis posterior muscle, which they showed was contained in its own osseofascial compartment and which had previously gone unrecognized. Melberg and Styf (1989) could not, however, demonstrate that chronic compartment syndrome in the TP or FDL muscles was a cause for exercise-induced pain in the posteromedial part of the lower leg. Wallenstein and Eriksson (1984) also found normal pressures in the deep posterior compartments of patients with medial tibial syndrome, concluding that it was not a compartment syndrome. They did find increased pressures in the anterior compartment, however.

Pathology

Muscle volume increases with exercise, which leads to increased compartmental pressure. Normal resting intracompartmental pressure is 0–15 mm Hg, measured directly by inserting a 'wick' or 'slit' catheter into the various compartments under a local anaesthetic (Mubarak et al 1976). A non-compliant or 'tight' fascial envelope can cause abnormally high tissue pressure with exercise to the point where it may shut down its own microcirculation, especially if the muscle is hypertrophied. The tissues are thus starved of blood supply and oxygen, the metabolic demands cannot be met and ischaemic pain results. With exercise, pressure may rise to 30–40 mmHg but will return to normal limits within a few minutes. In athletes with a diagnosis of chronic compartment syndrome (CCS), pressure may go up to as high as 80 mmHg with vigorous exercise and remain elevated for 15–30 minutes or longer. The damaging effects of increased tissue pressure are well described (Styf et al 1987, Styf 1989). Figure 31.8 outlines the pathophysiology of CCS and its relation to signs, symptoms and findings on investigation.

It should be emphasised that CCS should be differentiated from ACS which can be a side effect of exertion or a complication of trauma such as contusion, fracture, burn or laceration.

Acute compartment syndromes (ACS)

These can occur due to high energy trauma such as closed comminuted fractures of the tibia and are then easily recognized. The effort-related variety are not as frequently reported as the chronic variety. The syndrome commonly occurs in individuals unaccustomed to strenuous exercise or after a prolonged period of inactivity.

Some patients may have previously suffered from a recurrent syndrome, which, by definition, comes and goes. In this case, however, pain may or may not occur during exercise and the athlete continues on with some stiffness, usually in the anterior shin area. Only some time after completion of the exercise will severe pain, swelling and paralysis become evident. The athlete may wake at night with terrible pain, inability to move the foot, severe local tenderness, redness and heat. Sometimes the symptoms begin during the activity. This usually occurs when athletes push himself themselves beyond the onset of pain.

On examination there is dramatic pain on passive stretch of the affected muscle group, muscle weakness and sensory changes (Friedman 1986). Findings on examination are summarized in Table 31.2.

Straehley and Jones (1986) reported a case of acute exercise-related compartment syndrome (anterior, lateral and superficial posterior) which developed rapidly following a tear of the medial head of the gastrocnemius muscle. There was significant swelling with the right calf 7 cm larger in circumference than the left, reduced sensation to pinprick and light touch in the distribution of the deep peroneal nerve, and pain on active and passive dorsiflexion of the foot. Pressures measured in hospital were 60 mmHg in the anterior compartment, 44 mmHg in the superficial posterior, 50 mmHg in the lateral and 25 mmHg in the deep posterior compartment.

On examination after taking a careful history, therapists should be suspicious of any swelling of the lower leg, severe non-proportional pain, warmth, erythema, taut skin and pain on passive stretch. Peripheral blood flow and distal pulses usually stay normal.

Management of acute compartment syndromes

Acute compartment syndromes are a true surgical emergency due to the impending risk of permanent damage to the muscle and the peripheral nerves contained within each compartment. An athlete who has sustained a direct blow over the anterior tibial compartment, in particular, should be carefully managed and cautioned to avoid ACS. This involves the RICE regime with careful observation for increased swelling and pain, sensation changes or weakness. Athletes should be advised to immediately report any worsening in their condition. If the onset of ACS is suspected, the athlete should be quickly referred for surgery.

Without immediate decompression of the compartment in the form of fasciotomy, the pain will gradually recede over several days but the damage will already have been done. The muscles affected get a hard woody feeling and there may be ischaemic contracture. Voluntary movement will be absent and the affected muscle will be electrically silent, in other words, dead. Thus there is no need to wait

Table 31.2 Findings on acute compartment syndrome examination

Compartment	Sensory ingredient	Muscle weakness	Pain with stretch	Pulses
Anterior	Deep peroneal	Tibialis anterior, extensor hallucis longus, extensor digitorum	Foot and toe flexion	Intact
Lateral	Superficial and deep peroneal	Peroneus longus and peroneus brevis	Foot inversion	Intact
Superficial posterior	Sural	Gastrocnemius and soleus	Foot dorsiflexion	Intact
Deep posterior	Tibial	Tibialis posterior, flexor hallucis longus, flexor digitorum	Toe extension	Intact

Source: from Friedman (1986)

for neurological or ischaemic changes to occur to justify emergency surgery. If fasciotomy is performed early the acute symptoms will disappear and mobility and sensation will be restored. Surgery is often performed when irreversible damage to muscle and nerve has already occurred and results will be disappointing (Martens & Moeyersoons 1990).

Chronic compartment syndromes

Chronic or recurrent compartment syndrome in the lower leg is felt as pain, muscle tightness or swelling, a cramp-like feeling, weakness or numbness during exercise. It usually occurs in running or jumping activities, especially after switching surfaces or rapidly increasing training intensity. The amount of effort required to bring on the symptoms varies between individuals but stays relatively constant for each, i.e. 10–15 mins into a run, a certain number of reps on the track, or a certain type of intense on-court drillwork. The pain is felt over the muscle affected only, not over the tibia, and is frequently bilateral.

Pain will generally force the athlete to stop or at least slow down the activity. In the early stages, as soon as the activity is stopped the symptoms start to abate, usually dissipating within minutes (as compartmental pressures return to normal). If the athlete has continued to exercise despite the pain, the injury begins to take longer to settle and may persist overnight or even into the next day. The mean age of onset is 20 years (Martens & Moeyersoons 1990).

Diagnosis of CCS

In contrast to the acute syndrome, CCS exhibits a marked lack of physical findings with the athlete at rest. Martens and Moeyersoons (1990) did, however, find a 40% incidence of fascial hernias in their group of patients. Physical examination is best performed immediately after vigorous use of the muscles, which should bring on the pain, tenseness and sensitivity to palpation. This can be achieved either by running or resisted ankle exercise on hydraulic or isokinetic equipment.

Direct measurement of intracompartmental pressures with the wick or slit catheter technique confirms the diagnosis of CCS. This should be done at rest first, which may reveal normal readings, but resting pressure in these cases is usually elevated beyond 15 mmHg. Measurements should then be made during and after exercise, with the catheter left in situ. Logan et al (1983) examined anterior tibial compartment pressures in nine subjects running on a treadmill, showing that values were much higher during actual exercise than at rest, and that pressures kept increasing as velocity of running increased. Pressure measurements taken during exercise are, however, un-

reliable, being dependent on the depth of catheter placement and the force of muscle contraction.

A definitive diagnosis of CCS can be made if there is an appropriate history reported, compartmental pressures rise beyond 30–40 mmHg during exercise and remain high or fail to return to normal within 6 minutes (Styf 1988).

Martens and Moeyersoons (1990) suggested the criteria for a positive test finding as follows: resting pressure 15 mmHg or higher, 1 minute post-exercise to be 30 mmHg or higher and 5 minutes post-exercise to be 20 mmHg or higher.

Differential diagnoses includes periostitis or compression lesion of the superficial peroneal nerve in the anterior compartment. This may be caused by fascial defects, muscle herniation, ankle sprain following fasciotomy, or be due to an anomalous course of the nerve, the result being compression of the nerve where it emerges from the lateral compartment (Styf 1989). This is difficult to diagnose, but there may be loss of sensation over the dorsum of the foot, some pain in certain positions of the ankle at rest, fascial defect, positive Tinel's sign, pain on gentle palpation, slight swelling over the anterolateral distal third of the lower leg and positive findings on nerve conduction studies. Eccentric exercise causing delayed muscle soreness, due perhaps to downhill running, gives pain, swelling and tenderness in the anterior compartment but does not tend to recur in the same way as CCS.

Fascial defects may occur in the legs of athletes with CCS due to the increased pressure forcing some muscle to herniate through a weakened area of fascia (Friedman 1986). This may occur in the anterior or lateral compartments. The herniated muscle may be painful due to ischaemia. It is often encountered at the area between these two compartments in the lower third of the leg where they may compress or irritate a branch of the superficial peroneal nerve. Treatment involves decompression with fasciotomy.

Differential diagnoses include stress fractures, DVT, tendinitis or MTSS, referred pain from the lumbosacral spine or other nerve or arterial entrapment syndromes. For alternative explanations of pain in the posteromedial aspect of the lower leg, see section on tibial pain and Table 31.1.

Management of CCS

According to Martens and Moeyersoons (1990), conservative treatment is of no value in CCS and the only alternative to surgery is to quit sports activities or to participate strictly within pain limits or risk an acute compartment syndrome. Hannaford (1988) advocated a trial of conservative therapy including deep massage of the compartments, which was found to be as effective as physiotherapy in the form of ultrasound, interferential, magnetic field therapy and ice. This was especially useful in borderline cases where pressure test findings were equivocal. An unsuccessful 6 week trial of conservative therapy would help in the decision on whether to have surgery.

Fasciotomy of the compartments involved was described by Rorabeck et al (1988). A preoperative pressure measurement is recommended so that all compartments involved may be treated by a surgical release. The results of this surgery are usually good when done with the correct indications i.e. resting pressures in excess of 15 mmHg, elevated post-exercise pressure measurements and delayed normalization (Rorabeck et al 1988). Failure to relieve the symptoms may be due to wrong diagnosis, inadequate release of the involved compartments or fibrous scar formation during healing which starts to act as a new non-compliant fascia. This is due to inadequate rehabilitation.

It was recommended by Rorabeck et al (1988) that special attention be paid to a separate fasciotomy of the tibialis posterior at the time of decompression of the deep posterior compartment. Davey et al (1984) described how this was done through a single lateral approach.

It is imperative for the surgeon to ensure meticulous haemostasis at the time of surgery to prevent the disastrous complication of post-operative haematoma. Fasciotomy is more reliably successful in the anterior compartment than the deep posterior, but if done where indicated, well managed post-operatively and rehabilitated is a reliable, safe, and effective treatment for CCS in the lower leg (Rorabeck et al 1988).

Rehabilitation after surgery

Rehabilitation after surgery is required to prevent recurrence due to fibrous scar tissue formation during healing (Martens & Moeyersoons 1990). Rorabeck et al (1988) recommended that the patient be pushed vigorously to obtain and maintain full range of motion of the ankle and knee joints actively and passively. This is to prevent haematoma formation which could result in scarring near the fasciotomy incision, closing up the released area and causing recurrence of symptoms. However, care should be exercised as there is a distinct risk of wound breakdown if activity is resumed too early.

The post-operative routine generally used consists of active range of motion exercises with weightbearing as tolerated post-operatively. The patients use crutches for the first few days but discontinue as soon as possible. Only when the wound is healed can the athlete begin cycling, swimming and eventually walking progressing gradually to running, every second day at first. Massage and ultrasound over and around the operative site helps regain flexibility. Stretching should be encouraged and a graduated strengthening program should be instituted to allow full recovery of strength and endurance of the involved muscle groups.

ACHILLES TENDINITIS

The well-known vulnerability of the achilles tendon has its origins in ancient Greek mythology. Achilles was the son of Thetis and Peleus, who was one of the Argonauts and a great athlete. Thetis tried to make her children immortal by holding them over a sacred fire, but Peleus interrupted as she was going through this ritual with Achilles. Achilles became the greatest warrior in Greece and was invulnerable except for one heel, by which his mother had held him over the fire. During the Trojan war, Achilles was mortally wounded by an arrow that struck his heel from the bow of Paris, whose hand was guided by Apollo.

Achilles tendon pain is a common cause of disability in athletes. The jogging and fitness boom was probably triggered in 1972 in the United States with Frank Shorter's win in the Olympic marathon. Since then, more people have been exposed to achilles injury than ever before. It occurs mainly in male runners (Williams, 1986) but also in any athlete that performs running or jumping. Taunton et al (1984) reported 78% of runners with achilles injury in their series were males with an average age of 30 years. This may be accounted for by the loss of tendon elasticity in ageing males. The majority of cases are due to overuse but may be precipitated or exacerbated by particular incidents causing acute injuries (see 'Acute tears of the achilles tendon'). In this section, discussion will be limited to tendinitis of the achilles tendon and injury to its surrounding structures.

Anatomy

The gastrocnemius/soleus/achilles tendon complex is a common source of injury, particularly at certain anatomical sites where it is vulnerable. There is an area of constant relative avascularity 2–6 cm above the insertion into the calcaneus (Williams 1986). This is where the achilles tendon is most twisted as it narrows and descends, and the most common site for tendinitis and partial rupture.

The tendon appears to rotate laterally as it descends, beginning 12–15 cm above the insertion, where the soleus begins to contribute fibres to the tendon. The degree of rotation depends on the amount of fusion between the gastrocnemius and soleus portions, which may be variably separated or fused along their length. Minimal rotation is associated with more fusion. This rotation produces a sawing action between the fibres (Taunton et al 1984) potentially causing friction, tearing and damage to micro-vasculature. This often progresses to degenerative change and sometimes rupture, especially in older athletes.

Another common site for rupture in the older age group is the musculotendinous junction of the medial head of the gastrocnemius to the broad gastrocnemius tendon. Here a contractile segment joins a much stiffer non-contractile part.

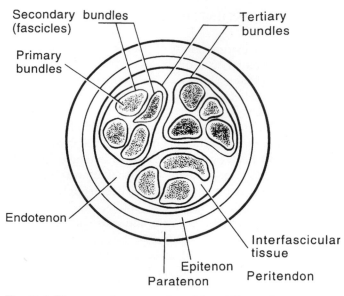

Fig. 31.9 Diagrammatic cross-section of the achilles tendon.
Source: adapted from Smart et al (1980)

With ageing, tendons tend to lose elasticity making this region even more vulnerable. According to Nelen et al (1989), there are three distinct achilles tendon lesions: at the tendon-bone junction, at the musculotendinous junction (see 'Tennis leg'), and 'true' tendinitis 2–6 cm above the insertion.

The insertion af the achilles tendon into the calcaneus is surrounded by two synovial bursae: one between the tendon and the top of the calcaneus in front called the retrocalcaneal bursa; and another behind the tendon separating it from the skin, called the subcutaneous or retroachilles bursa. These structures prevent friction between the tendon and its surrounds, but inflammation and swelling (bursitis) may mimic achilles injury (Maguire & Purdam 1987).

The tendon is enclosed in a fine sheath called the epitenon, which continues into the tendon to surround the fascicles as the endotenon. This in turn is covered by the paratenon, which is a filmy layer of loose areolar tissue containing blood vessels. It acts as an elastic sleeve that allows some sliding movement but maintains tissue continuity. The epitenon and paratenon are collectively known as the peritendon (Fig. 31.9). Where the tendon passes over potential areas of friction or pressure, the peritendon is replaced by a bursa or sheath, but it does not possess a true synovial sheath (Smart et al 1980).

Blood supply to the achilles tendon is from three sources: from the calcaneus distally, from the muscle proximally and from the underlying mesotenon along its length which is the most vital. The mesotenon lies just beneath the tendon and contains a bed of anastomotic vessels derived from branches of the posterior tibial and peroneal arteries (Maguire & Purdam 1987). These vessels then encircle and pass through the paratenon towards the secondary bundles. They branch repeatedly en route before assuming a direction parallel to the fascicles within the endotenon. The capillary plexus does not penetrate the collagen bundles (Smart et al 1980).

Angiographic studies have shown that vasculature is decreased in the area 2–6 cm above the insertion. Smart et al (1980) speculated that this reduced vascularity plays a role in ruptures of the achilles tendon in a similar way to degeneration and rupture of the rotator cuff at its area of reduced vascularity, described by Rathbun and McNab (1970). Tendon vascularity is also reduced in areas of friction, torsion and compression (Curwin & Stanish 1984). This has certain implications for management of achilles tendinitis, every effort should be made so that the achilles is not starved of its blood supply.

Classification

Because the achilles does not have a true synovial sheath, tenosynovitis is not an appropriate classification for injuries involving the tendon sheath. Recognizing this, Maguire and Purdam (1987) agreed with Smart et al (1980) in preferring the term 'peritendinitis' to describe inflammation of the peritendon. Inflammation, swelling, devitalization and disruption of the actual tendon was classified as 'tendinosis' by Smart et al but is commonly called 'tendinitis'. Often both conditions are combined. 'Partial rupture' should be reserved for those cases in which there is evidence of a tear involving a varying number of fibres in the free portion of the tendon and 'total rupture' signifies a complete tear (Smart et al 1980). See Table 31.3 for a method of classification proposed by Williams (1986).

Aetiology of achilles tendinitis

Biomechanical factors

Motion at the subtalar joint affects and is affected by the achilles tendon. Transverse planar movements at this joint twist and untwist the achilles, and inversion and eversion

Table 31.3 Classification of achilles tendon lesions

Type of injury	Subtype of injury
Rupture	Complete
	Partial
	Laceration
Focal degenerative tendonitis	Calcific
	Chondritic
Peritendonitis	Acute
	Chronic
Mixed origin/insertion lesions	Musculotendinous junction
	Insertion
Associated structures	Bursitis
Other mechanisms	Rheumatic
	Metabolic
	Infection

Source: adapted from Williams (1986)

place unequal tensile forces on different parts of the tendon (Maguire & Purdam 1987). Forefoot varus and rearfoot valgus are associated with excessive pronation (Fig. 31.10a).

Clement et al (1984) observed, via slow-motion high speed cinematography, a whipping action or bowstring effect in the achilles caused by prolonged pronation (Fig. 31.10b). They felt that this could potentiate microtears, particularly in the medial aspect of the tendon. Prolonged or excessive pronation makes the tibia to internally rotate, drawing the achilles medially, conflicting with the external rotation force during knee extension as the body weight passes over the foot (Fig. 31.11). This extra twisting force caused by too much pronation is imparted to the achilles tendon and may cause further vascular compromise and subsequent degenerative changes.

Forefoot valgus tends to cause too little pronation, reducing the shock-absorbing capabilities of the foot so that

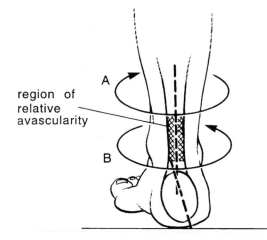

Fig. 31.11 External tibial rotation produced by knee extension. (A) conflicting with internal tibial rotation produced by prolonged pronation (B). Source: adapted from Taunton et al (1984)

the forces must be absorbed abruptly and directly by the supportive structures including the achilles (Smart et al 1980). This is associated with a cavoid-type foot and rearfoot varus with excessive tightness of the achilles complex.

According to Maguire and Purdam (1987), stresses applied to the achilles tendon during sports activities exceed the maximum levels calculated theoretically or under laboratory conditions (Table 31.4). They surmised that the tendon can cope with higher forces when applied rapidly but that biomechanical factors that cause areas of stress concentration in the tendon increase the likelihood of microtears.

Muscular factors

Smart et al (1980) felt that ankle inflexibility due to calf tightness may force more pronation as a compensating mechanism. Clement et al (1984) suggested that fatigue in the calf muscles after days of heavy running depleted glycogen stores in the muscle fibers and this led to increased tendon stress.

Nichols (1989) felt that achilles tendinitis was caused by repetitive eccentric load-induced microtrauma leading to inflammation. According to Maguire and Purdam (1987), the gastrocnemius-soleus complex contracts eccentrically in preparation for heel strike and during the stance phase of running gait to stabilize the lower extremity. It mediates the rate of dorsiflexion of the ankle and flexion

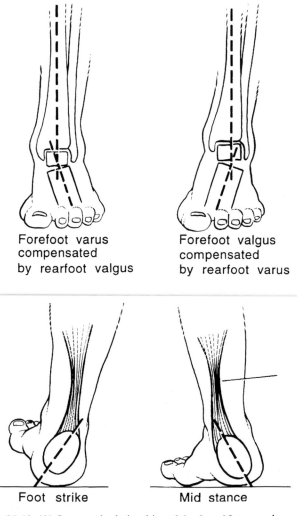

Fig. 31.10 (A) Structural relationships of the foot. Note angular displacements and possible effect on the achilles tendon. (B) Whipping action of achilles tendon produced by overpronation.
Sources: (A) adapted from Smart et al (1980); (B) adapted from Taunton et al (1984)

Table 31.4 Stress in achilles tendon with different activities

Activity	Area (mm2)	Force (N)	Stress (MPa)
Walking	75	1962–2354	26.1–31.4
Running slow	75	3924–5886	52.3–78.5
Running fast	75	8729	117.7
Jumping	75	1962	26.1

Source: from Maguire & Purdam (1987)

of the knee in stance phase and so helps to absorb shock. Work is an important element during running, therefore the calf must be well stretched to allow smooth elastic deformation without premature activation of stretch reflexes that would cause abnormal out-of-phase contraction. They listed three possible mechanisms of acute injury to the achilles tendon:

1. Pushing off with the weightbearing foot while simultaneously extending the knee, common in sprinting, running uphill or lunging forward in court sports
2. Sudden and unexpected dorsiflexion of the ankle, such as slipping on a stair or stepping into a hole, where the heel drops suddenly. The calf muscles are contracted maximally in response to the sudden stretch
3. Violent dorsiflexion while the foot is plantarflexed, such as in jumping and falling. The calf muscles are maximally contracted, and sudden movement leads to a marked stretching of the muscle and particularly the tendon.

Even though the tendon can better cope with high strain rates, it appears that if a force is applied too suddenly perhaps there is not enough time for protective mechanisms, such as muscle relaxation, to occur. More research is needed to explain the interaction between rates of loading and mechanical strain in the achilles tendon (Maguire & Purdam 1987).

Shoe design/footwear factors

Footwear may contribute to achilles tendinitis in a number of ways, usually to do with the shoe heels. A high, poorly padded heel counter or tight boot top or strapping may press and bend the achilles, causing irritation and swelling of the peritendon alone or put pressure on the tendon itself. The offending part of the running shoe should be cut away in this case. Most sports shoes now have a padded notch to accomodate the achilles.

Inadequate heel elevation (flat shoes) may overstretch the tendon between heel strike and toe off by demanding more dorsiflexion than may be available in a tight achilles complex. Athletes who normally wear shoes with heels and suddenly switch to flat sports shoes e.g. tennis, basketball, orienteering or squash shoes, may have shortened tendons and are especially prone. Sports shoes with some heel elevation (wedged between 12–15 mm) and a moderate heel flare are recommended (Taunton et al 1984). The transition from one type of running shoe to another should also be gradual (Smart et al 1980).

Loose-fitting heel counters or those which do not provide enough rearfoot stability to control motion while running may cause achilles problems in the runner who over-pronates. A firm heel counter is required. For runners who

underpronate in particular, the shoe must have excellent shock-absorbing properties. All shoes should be flexible enough to allow bending of the sole readily at the level of the metatarsophalangeal joints. A rigid sole increases the distance from the ankle at which the force is applied at push-off, increasing the force applied to the achilles (Maguire & Purdam 1987). A shoe can be cut at the level of metatarsal heads to make it more flexible (Lipinski 1987).

Training factors

Sudden changes in training habits, surfaces or shoes can often bring on achilles injuries (Nichols 1989, Maguire & Purdam 1987). Clement et al (1984) reported that training errors accounted for 82 out of 109 cases of achilles tendinitis.

Training causes hypertrophy and increased vascularization of active tissues, but inactivity has the reverse effect (Smart et al 1980). With sudden return to training, the diminished blood supply cannot meet the demands of the active tendon, ischaemia, degeneration and rupture being the possible result. These training errors can be summarized:

- changing shoes
- hill running or sprints
- running on a camber or uneven ground
- sudden changes to surfaces with more traction
- surfaces getting harder (seasonal changes)
- inadequate warm-up and stretching/cool-down
- starting a new sport, especially court sports
- sudden increases in mileage/intensity
- recommencing training after long periods of inactivity
- ignoring muscle soreness/tightness.

Other causes of achilles tendinitis/ruptures

A prominant supero-posterior angle of the calcaneum can cause achilles tendinitis due to the compression of the tendon between the bone and the shoe.

Local steroid injections may have been given to alleviate pain and inflammation in achilles tendinitis. However, ruptures are a frequent complication (Smart et al 1980). Steroids given locally or orally tend to diminish the pain, thereby encouraging the athlete to undertake injudicious activity.

Steroids injected directly into the tendon interfere with the healing process, weaken the tendon structurally and are contraindicated within the middle third of the tendon (Curwin & Stanish 1984). Dacruz et al (1988) found that peritendinous injections of steroids were of no benefit in achilles paratendinitis. Smart et al (1980) recommended that if peritendinous steroid injection is used, the patients should refrain from vigorous muscular activity for at least 2 weeks or risk rupture.

Olivieri et al (1987) reported that heel 'enthesopathy' may be, for a long time, the only manifestation of the HLA-

B27 disease process (sero-negative arthritides such as ankylosing spondylitis). Smart et al (1980) also mentioned such diseases as gout, pseudogout and rheumatoid collagenolysis as possible causes of achilles tendinitis.

Pathology

Schepsis and Leach (1987) found several pathological processes seen in surgery of the achilles tendon:

- areas of mucoid or fibrotic degeneration
- partial rupture in the tendon substance
- chronically inflamed sheath
- retrocalcaneal bursitis seemed to be a separate entity with hypertrophy and fibrosis of the bursa (Haglund's syndrome) usually occurring in conjunction with a prominent posterior superior angle of the calcaneus (Fig. 31.12).

Nelen et al (1989) considered the pathology of achilles tendinitis to run in stages. The first stage is confined to the peritendon, which becomes inflamed and thickened and may adhere to the tendon. There may be fluid around the tendon or fibrinous fur, but the tendon itself looks normal. Isolated peritendinitis accounted for 85 of the 143 tendons in their study.

Kvist et al (1987) did a histological and histochemical study of paratendinitis and found marked metabolic changes in the sheath, including increased catabolism and decreased oxygenation of inflamed areas, impairing its gliding function.

The second stage is characterized by degenerative and inflammatory changes in the tendon tissue itself. It may show nodular thickening and a glossy appearance macro-scopically. Histologically there is mucoid or lipoid degeneration, fibroid necrosis and tearing of tendon fibres. There is also a marked proliferation of newly formed capillaries and histiocytes that invade the tendon. Tendinosis does not affect the whole tendon but only parts of it, showing a glossy appearance at the macroscopic level. This was found in 28 of the 143 tendons operated on.

The final stage is macroscopically visible disruption of the tendon either at the periphery or more centrally. Tears were found in 30 of the 143 tendons. This was most notable when local steroids had been used.

History

In the majority of cases in the study of Nelen et al (1989) symptoms started progressively, although some patients noticed a more acute onset, usually traumatic, as described above under 'aetiology'. Partial tears are more likely to have a sudden onset than peritendinitis and focal degeneration, which tend to come on more gradually. Information should be sought on severity, duration, past history and progression of symptoms to help to distinguish between conditions. The patient should be questioned then examined on the mechanism of onset to see if biomechanical, training, muscular, surface, footwear, or systemic factors are responsible (Maguire & Purdam 1987).

Symptoms

Symptoms correlate well with the location and stage of the underlying pathology (Nelen et al 1989). All conditions cause pain as the dominant symptom with inflammation in or about the achilles tendon. It is felt mainly at the area 2-6 cm above

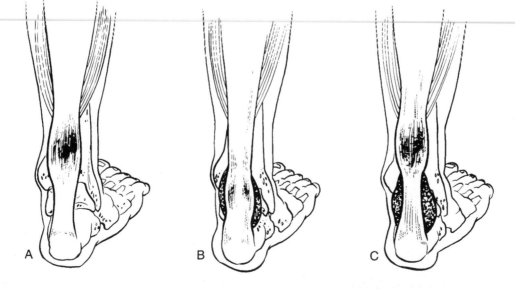

Fig. 31.12 (A) Tendinitis (B) Retrocalcaneal bursitis (C) Combined. Source: adapted from Schepsis and Leach (1987)

the insertion. Initially, the athlete experiences pain only after strenuous exercise e.g. trackwork or hills. In more advanced cases, the pain gradually increases during sports activities, sometimes forcing the athlete to cut down or stop. In some cases there will be pain during normal daily activities, in severe cases there may be pain at rest. The severity of morning stiffness, with the patient having to hobble around unable to put the heel to the ground, is a good guide to the seriousness of the condition (Nelen et al 1989). Prolonged and severe morning stiffness is a sign of chronic or severe inflammation. Sharp or stabbing pains nearly always show partial rupture in surgery (Nelen et al 1989).

Signs

The tendon should be palpated along its entire length to feel for crepitus, nodules, localized pain or diffuse thickening. It should be palpated at rest as well as during the full range of active and passive motion, to see if swelling moves with the tendon or stays static. This is best done with the patient prone, always comparing to the other side (Maguire & Purdam 1987). If the swelling is static but fluctuant this could mean fluid in the paratenon. If it is a hard lump and moves as the tendon moves it is more likely to be a lesion in the tendon itself, such as a partial tear or tendinosis.

Peritendinitis is characterized by a superficial, softer, fluctuant thickening and inflammation of the peritendon, often accompanied by crepitus on movement (Smart et al 1980). The function of the tendon is unaffected, but performance may be limited by pain. Pain is diffuse, increasing with activity.

Tendinosis shows fewer signs and is hard to diagnose clinically, but is characterized by local degeneration often found only by sonography or surgery.

Partial rupture has localized areas of nodular thickening but often no discernible weakness. Strength of the achilles complex can first be tested by asking the patient to stand and rise up onto the toes and adding some resistance on the shoulders if necessary. If this is pain free then jumping, hopping or running on the spot can be used as more functional assessment. Dropping the heel over the edge of a step using body weight can be used to determine if eccentric action is part of the problem (Maguire & Purdam 1987). Often the pain is worse landing from hopping or at the end of eccentric range.

Flexibility should also be assessed in standing by having the athlete lean forward on a support with the heel on the floor and the knee straight to check for gastrocnemius/achilles tightness. Soleus/achilles flexibility should be assessed as well by lunging over the straight foot, which should allow more dorsiflexion because the gastrocnemius is relaxed (Maguire & Purdam 1987). If this is not the case, the soleus component may be tight. Pointing the foot in or out and lunging may elicit the symptoms better.

Cursory biomechanical assessment can be done by observing gait and tibial, rearfoot and forefoot alignment in prone. If poor biomechanical alignment is considered to be a contributory factor, the athlete should be referred to a sports podiatrist for a full assessment and orthotics if necessary.

Diagnosis

In the author's opinion, cases of chronic achilles tendinitis or acute cases where there is a history suggestive of a tear should be referred for medical examination. Ultrasonography facilitates the management of these patients by revealing the presence of partial tears, allowing the assessment of the extent of the damage and giving an indication of prognosis and whether immediate surgical opinion should be sought (Kalebo et al 1992).

Mathieson et al (1988) reported that sonography (ultrasound scans) can differentiate reliably between surgical and conservative cases of achilles injury. Partial ruptures show as thickening whereas tendinitis alone shows no thickening. Maffuli et al (1987) felt that peritendinitis shows up as anteroposterior enlargement on sonography, while tendinitis with rupture shows thickening of the tendon with degenerative nodules.

Laine et al (1987) recommended that sonography should be used as a routine diagnostic aid before any specific treatment is instituted and to monitor progress. Kainberger et al (1990) felt that sonography was valuable in diagnosis of achilles tendon lesions and of surrounding tissues. The major advantages of ultrasonography over MRI are that it is less expensive and quick, giving real time imaging. However, MRI is less operator-dependent, giving a better view of surrounding tissues (Kalebo et al 1992).

Other investigations were listed by Maguire and Purdam (1987) and included: X-rays to exclude bony pathology, bone scans to exclude stress fractures, compartment pressure tests, bursal fluid analysis to exclude crystal arthropathies, uric acid test for gout, blood tests for HLA-B27 and rheumatoid factor, EMG analysis for partial ruptures and xeroradiography and bursography. Surgical examination often reveals devitalized tendon, irregularly orientated collagen fibres, focal or cystic degeneration, streaks of loose, collagen-rich granulation tissue, inflammatory cells, and marked secondary vascular proliferation in the peritendon, invading the tendon in an unorganized fashion (Smart et al 1980).

Differential diagnosis

Calcaneal bone bruises or fractures will have maximal tenderness over the bony site of injury, not the tendon. In plantar fasciitis the pain is localized to the undersurface of the heel.

Retrocalcaneal bursitis is commonly confused with achilles lesions. The edge of a shoe may irritate a prominence on the calcaneus, inflaming the bursa. The pain in this condition can be elicited by forced passive plantarflexion of the ankle, or squeezing the area between the thumb and index finger. It can be confirmed radiologically by the loss of the normally lucent recess in the retrocalcaneal space or a prominence in the calcaneus that may have to be removed. Treatment involves the conservative measures used in achilles tendinitis and usually local injection into the bursa, avoiding the tendon.

In subcutaneous bursitis, exostosis or Haglund's syndrome, the swelling and tenderness are maximal at the tendon insertion with accompanying soft tissue swelling and thickening of the overlying skin.

Rupture of the soleus or medial head of gastrocnemius, tibial stress fractures, tibialis posterior tendinitis and compartment syndromes are differentiated from achilles tendinitis by the site of the lesion on palpation, history, signs and symptoms as described elsewhere in this chapter.

Systemic arthropathies (gout, rheumatoid arthritis, ankylosing spondylitis, sero-negative arthritides etc.) may manifest as achilles tendinitis. The history, signs and symptoms should suggest a strong inflammatory component and there may be other systemic signs of disease. Medical examination may reveal positive pathology test results and diagnosis, but it may be necessary to treat the tendinitis as well as the systemic problem.

Infections should be evident from history with signs of skin trauma, redness, heat or exudate.

Sever's disease is a fairly common syndrome in active chidren or young athletes, especially gymnasts, in the author's experience. It is a traction apophysitis of the separate ossification centre on the calcaneum for the insertion of the achilles and can mimic tendinitis. It is differentiated by the location of maximal tenderness on the heel bone itself and the relative absence of signs in the tendon (see Ch. 32).

Conservative management

Effective treatment involves rest from the aggravating activities. This may involve crutch ambulation or cast immobilization in severe cases, or a temporary heel lift (in both shoes) in milder cases if it allows the athlete to walk comfortably with no limp. This is gradually progressed to full weightbearing, modified activity and alternative training (cycling, swimming, pool running, weights) and finally a carefully graded return to sport. Mileage and intensity of training should be reduced at first with a hard/easy approach to increasing training loads in order to build back tolerance to exercise.

Taping the achilles has been used to facilitate modified training. Indications are to prevent pain on extremes of dorsiflexion or plantarflexion of the ankle. Taping adds support to a weakened achilles, easing some of the pain on stretch, but it should not be relied upon in a competitive situation because of the risk of rupture. Care should be exercised not to irritate the achilles by applying tape too tightly across the back of the lower leg. An open-backed taping method was described by Velasquez (1987).

Recurrence is common after periods of rest, perhaps because the tendon is actually weakened by inactivity, and total rest should be reserved for severe acute cases only. Modified rest including a strengthening and stretching program, measures to control pain and inflammation, and correction of all predisposing factors, such as poor biomechanics and flexibility, is the strategy of choice.

Measures to control inflammation include ice and NSAIDs, the latter being especially useful for morning stiffness.

Physiotherapy can take the form of a number of modalities, including ultrasound, laser therapy, electrical stimulation, TENS, iontophoresis, interferential and magnetic field therapy. In the author's experience, cross-frictional massage is beneficial in reducing pain and improving blood flow, and allows more flexibility by making any tight or scarred tissue more pliable. However, it is best used after the acute inflammation has subsided and in the opinion of this writer, does not help in the long term in cases of severe degeneration or partial rupture. It can certainly be used above and below the site of the lesion combined with other massage techniques to good effect in all cases of achilles pain.

The treatment of peritendinitis and tendinosis or the two combined is basically the same except that in true peritendinitis with crepitus, injections between the sheath and the tendon, not into the tendon itself, have often been used with good results (Maguire & Purdam 1987).

Ultrasound has been used commonly. Purportedly it is absorbed at the tendon/peritendon interface, to disrupt adhesions between the tendon and sheath (Smart et al 1980). Davidson and Taunton (1987) advised caution with ultrasound because it may disturb leukocytes in the traumatized tendon and potentiate the inflammatory response. It has also been used with topical anti-inflammatory agents (phonophoresis) but its long term efficacy in tendinitis has been questioned (Williams 1986).

Magnetic field therapy has demonstrated some success in chronic tendinitis (Maguire & Purdam 1987). This may be due to its beneficial effect on blood supply and collagen deposition. Magnetic strips or foils appear to have similar effects.

Steroid injections into the tendon have largely lost favour due to the weakening effect and the risk of subsequent rupture. However, peritendinous and intrabursal injections, where appropriate, are extremely useful (Maguire & Purdam 1987).

Eccentric program for achilles tendinitis

Stretching and strengthening the weakened achilles is best achieved using an organised 6 week program like that used by Curwin & Stanish (1984). They postulated that eccentric exercise stresses the tendon selectively, citing the fact that eccentric action plays a major role in the mechanisms of injury to the achilles.

Their program consists of a general body warm-up (no running or jumping) gastrocnemius and soleus stretches, then 3×10 repetitions of the eccentric exercise, followed up by more stretching and ice, done once daily. The exercise is best done over the edge of a step, allowing the heel to drop freely, first done slowly on two feet, progressing to faster dropping and adding weights, then finally on the symptomatic foot only. The emphasis in the eccentric exercise is the rapid transition from the downward to the upward motion (see Ch. 13).

There should be mild discomfort in the last set of 10 exercises, as it is necessary for the tendon to be slightly overloaded so that it responds by becoming stronger. The speed of movement and load applied to the tendon are varied keeping this rule in mind. Failure of this regime is usually due to judging the pain incorrectly and going too hard too fast or being too cautious (Fig. 31.13). Patient compliance is a major factor in success of this conservative regime.

Often there will be no appreciable change in symptoms in the first 2–3 weeks but the athlete should be encouraged to be patient and to persevere under the given guidelines. The program must be carefully monitored by the amount of discomfort, which should be mild in the last set of 10 repetitions only and not throughout the whole exercise. Progression can only take place when this discomfort has gone (Maguire & Purdam 1987).

Surgery and rehabilitation

Indications for surgical treatment include failure of an adequate conservative regime and evidence of partial tears seen on sonography (Davidson & Taunton 1987). Recent thinking (Williams 1986) has led to earlier surgical intervention than was previously the case, especially in partial ruptures which are now more easily diagnosed with sonography, where areas of partial rupture show areas of decreased echogenicity. Clinical examination usually reveals nodular and intensely painful thickening, atrophy of the calf muscle, reduced tonus and perhaps increased range if the injury is of long duration. Chronic cases of peritendinitis and/or tendinosis which do not respond to non-operative

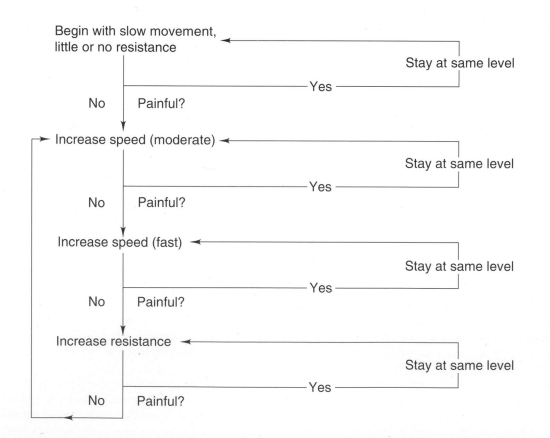

Fig. 31.13 How to gauge progression of eccentric program. Source: adapted from Curwin and Stanish (1984)

treatment may also require surgical intervention. In a study by Davidson and Taunton (1987), 6% of cases did require surgery.

Surgery usually consists of freeing up the tendon and careful excision of all granulation and devitalized tissue. Tendoplasty with the plantaris longus may be required if the rupture is large, and the tendon is sutured side to side (Maguire & Purdam 1987). Schepsis and Leach (1987) reported 87% satisfactory results from surgery in their series. Nelen et al (1989) reported 56% excellent and 28% good results.

Bursography may be required to see if there is a pathological encroachment of the bursa into the achilles with partial rupture in the distal part of the tendon. This may necessitate excision of the posterior tuberosity of the calcaneus, particularly for chronic retrocalcaneal bursitis (Nelen et al 1989). Nelen et al felt that in highly motivated athletes suffering from resistant achilles tendinitis or partial rupture, surgery offers satisfactory results with low morbidity in a high percentage of cases.

Rehabilitation consists of a post-operative regime and gradual return to full activity. A short cast is usually worn for 2–3 weeks with the foot in some plantar flexion. This is replaced by a walking cast with the foot in neutral for a further 3 weeks. Full weightbearing is then permitted with a heel raise and this is retained for the first few months of return to training.

It is also essential to mobilize the operation scar to prevent adhesion formation, using pulsed ultrasound and massage. Attention should also be paid to the proximal muscle belly. Strengthening can commence with light resisted exercise using theraband or surgical tubing and gradually progress to weightbearing, toe raises, isokinetics and eccentrics.

Introduction of high impact stress (sprinting, jumping) should be delayed until all symptoms have abated and a full rehabilitation program including eccentrics has been completed. Schepsis and Leach (1987) emphasized gentle non-painful stretching. Davidson and Taunton (1987) recommended a full return to activity and loading at 18–20 weeks.

Total rupture of the achilles tendon

Total rupture can occur by the same mechanisms as partial ruptures (see above) but often there are previous degenerative changes in the tendon or injections that have weakened it. The patient is immediately disabled with an acute total rupture but often there is an absence of pain initially (Smart et al 1980). The patient may feel that he or she has been shot or struck in the back of the leg and may hear an audible snap. If seen between 6–12 hours after rupture, there is a palpable gap between the torn ends. After 24 hours the gap is filled with haematoma and it becomes harder to feel. The patient may be able to weakly plantarflex the ankle using the secondary plantar flexors but is unable to do so against resistance.

The definitive clinical test is Thompson's calf reflex test (Smart et al 1980) The patient kneels on the couch with the feet over the edge. The examiner should squeeze the two heads of gastrocnemius with one hand to simulate a calf contraction. If the achilles is completely torn, the foot will not move. This is considered to be a specific indicator of total rupture.

A strong natural tendency exists for spontaneous healing of ruptured achilles tendons via infiltration of granulocytes and fibroblasts into the gap between the divided ends, which eventually restores continuity. However, this results in lengthening of the tendon, reducing its functional capacity and leading to calf muscle atrophy. Haggmark et al (1986) found significant atrophy in the calf muscles of non-operatively treated patients with achilles ruptures, while no such differences were found in surgically treated cases at long term follow-up. On the basis of these findings, they recommended that all athletes with achilles tendon ruptures be treated surgically. In non-athletes and older patients, non-operative treatment might be considered, although it will not give as good a result functionally.

Optimum conservative treatment consists of immediate immobilization in an above-knee non-weightbearing cast with the knee in 15–45° of flexion and the ankle in 15–30° of plantar flexion for 4–6 weeks, followed by a below-knee walking cast with the foot in reduced plantar flexion for an additional 4 weeks (Smart et al 1980). Conservative treatment does not require hospitalization and has fewer complications such as infections, skin necrosis and scar adhesions. However, the unknown factor is the degree of retraction of the tendon. Unless the ends are closely approximated, conservative treatment will result in tendon lengthening and impaired function.

Open surgical repair of total rupture is performed with a tourniquet under general anaesthetic. As in partial rupture, devitalized tissue should be removed and the tendon ends approximated, sometimes with a graft. The post-operative routine is the same as for conservative treatment, with a shorter period of immobilization (3 + 3 weeks). Carter et al (1992) advocate early controlled motion with a functional orthosis that allows unrestricted plantarflexion and dorsiflexion to neutral, rather than routine cast immobilization. Toe touch weightbearing is allowed immediately and gradually progressed.

TEARS OF THE GASTROCNEMIUS MUSCLE: 'TENNIS LEG'

This is common in middle-aged tennis players and has been often misdiagnosed as plantaris rupture ('torn monkey muscle'). This usually begins with an acute tearing sensation in the medial calf after exertion or an awkward step or fall. There may again be an audible snap or the sensation of being struck with a tennis ball (Maguire & Purdam 1987). The patient walks with difficulty and has a swollen and tender calf. In the absence of a history of acute injury, referred pain or a deep venous thrombosis should be suspected (see Ch. 27).

With a true muscle injury there may be a palpable defect, usually at the musculotendinous junction of the medial head of gastrocnemius to the proximal tendon, which is the most common site.

Physiotherapy management

Treatment consists of the RICE regime for the first 48 hours and non-weightbearing is advisable until the patient can comfortably bear weight. This is a troublesome condition, easily irritated if pushed to weight bear too early and care should be exercised with early massage and stretching. It is often very painful. Part of the problems in the management of this injury may be due to the fact that it is a grade 3 or complete rupture in an already compromised area in this age group, and thus takes a long time to heal and recover full strength. As the pain decreases, generally after about 1 week, gentle stretching and active exercise can begin. A heel lift and support stocking should be used for about 6 weeks, and the patient should be advised to exercise caution, especially on rising in the morning when the leg is at its stiffest, to avoid reinjury. Recovery is quite a slow and drawn out process; resistant cases are helped by local steroid injection (Maguire & Purdam 1987).

The plantaris muscle rarely tears and the symptoms are similar to those described above, except there is no palpable defect. The patient may complain of pain and swelling around the ankle due to recoil of the tendon (Maguire & Purdam 1987). The lateral head of the gastrocnemius can also tear but this is not as common. Treatment is along similar lines.

SOLEUS

The soleus muscle is usually injured due to overuse especially with running uphill or at an unaccustomed intensity. Delayed muscle soreness is common in the soleus and this causes stiffness and pain that is often associated with trigger points/tight spots in the muscle. Pain in the soleus can occur in combination with other lower leg overuse syndromes such as MTSS and achilles tendinitis.

Tightness can be effectively treated with deep massage, e.g. shifting techniques where the ankle is passively moved while pressure on the sore spot is maintained. Biomechanical analysis and podiatry/orthotics may be required in recurrent cases.

Stretching and strengthening should be performed in knee flexion to isolate the soleus from the gastrocnemius. Stretches can be more effectively done over the edge of a step in some knee flexion or by first dorsiflexing the foot passively on a small incline or step. Strengthening can be achieved by raising up on the toes with resistance applied down over the bent knee, either with a weight hung over the leg or with a weight station type device ('seated calf raise').

Neuromeningeal/referred pain to the soleus area can also occur and mimic soleus muscle strain (see Ch. 27).

ANTERIOR TIBIAL TENDINITIS/ TENOSYNOVITIS

This presents as pain, swelling and stiffness localized to the lower half of the anterolateral shin and is common in racewalkers, who have an exaggerated dorsiflexion at heel strike. It can also be brought on by unaccustomed exercise like jumping or running on a different playing surface or on hills. There may be tenosynovitis of the individual tendons of the tibialis anterior and extensor digitorum longus or extensor hallucis, with crepitus. Each affected tendon is implicated by the appropriate resisted movements. Symptoms do not ease with rest as they do with compartment syndrome, although they are both overuse syndromes with similar aetiologies and are often combined. Total rupture can occur in the older athlete, which will result in a drop foot. The condition can be confused with a neurological lesion such as radiculopathy at L5.

Massage of the bellies and musculotendinous junction areas of the affected muscles is very effective in relieving tension and gaining extra tissue flexibility, which can then be enhanced by gentle stretching techniques, such as sitting on the haunches. Self-massage is a useful way of maintaining these and other muscular conditions at a manageable level between formal treatments (Clews 1990). Rest, ice, compression and other physiotherapy modalities are of benefit and of course biomechanical factors must be addressed to prevent progression and recurrence. Non-weightbearing may be required to adequately rest severe cases of tibialis anterior tendinitis/tenosynovitis.

POSTERIOR TIBIAL TENDINITIS/ TENOSYNOVITIS

This has been partially covered in the section on tibial pain in that it has the same aetiological factors and management as the tenoperiosteal variety of MTSS (e.g. overpronation). The difference is that the symptoms are localized more distally, in the muscle bellies and tendons of the tibialis posterior, flexor digitorum and flexor hallucis longus. Tenderness is definitely localized to the tendons themselves and not the posteromedial border of the tibia.

Pain can be elicited by resisting inversion in plantarflexion. Specific resisted movements of hallux or toe flexion versus inversion may help to implicate an isolated tendon.

There may be fluid accumulation in the synovial sheaths of these tendons, a true tenosynovitis with the accompanying stiffness on moving and possibly crepitus. Symptoms are commonly felt where the tendons pass behind the medial malleolus (see Ch. 32). Acute rupture of the muscle bellies may lead to an isolated acute traumatic compartment syndrome. Differential diagnosis obviously includes MTSS and stress fractures. X-rays or bone scan findings should be negative in tendinitis.

Treatment is along standard lines to ease inflammation and pain such as rest, partial or non-weightbearing for severe pain, ice, ultrasound, interferential or high voltage stims. Correction of biomechanical or other predisposing factors such as muscle belly tightness and inflexibility is vital. Initially, a temporary medial heel wedge can be used. Massage and weightbearing stretches with the ankle in some eversion/pronation are beneficial as the inflammation eases and stiffness remains. Local steroid injection is reserved for recalcitrant cases.

Patients with ankylosing spondylitis can suffer from proliferative tenosynovitis. Chronic cases without a traumatic history may therefore need further investigation.

The tibialis posterior tendon can also rupture. Signs may differ in that there may be less pain and crepitus but more swelling and weakness, and treatment is along similar lines to that described for tendinitis/tenosynovitis.

PERONEAL TENDINITIS

This occurs due to overuse of the peroneal muscles, i.e. repeated eversion as in the breaststroke kick or eccentric inversion from running on a camber. It may be set off by a previous inversion injury to the ankle joint, and is also associated with subluxation of the peroneal tendons over the lateral malleolus or chronic ankle instability (see Ch. 32).

This condition must be carefully distinguished from a stress fracture of the fibula or lateral compartment syndrome by the behaviour and location of the pain and further investigations if necessary. Clinical examination may reveal tenderness localized to the muscle bellies and/or tendons alone, swelling, weakness and pain on resisted eversion and stiffness and pain on passive inversion. Once diagnosed, treatment follows standard lines, with massage again playing a major role. A temporary lateral heel wedge can be utilized. Strapping into eversion with some padding applied to prevent peroneal tendon subluxation can help relieve the condition.

NERVE ENTRAPMENT SYNDROMES IN THE LOWER LEG

Sural nerve

This passes between two heads of the gastrocnemius or through the soleus muscle. It can be entrapped at its point of fascial exit in the lower third of the leg where it gives cutaneous branches to the distal quarter of the leg, the lateral aspect of the heel and the dorsum of the foot. It may be compressed by a tight stocking or skiboot. The nerve is more frequently entrapped behind the lateral malleolus (see Ch. 32).

The symptoms are pain, paraesthesia and sensory changes over the lateral aspect of the foot and ankle. The pain can be reproduced by plantarflexion and inversion of the foot and there may be a positive Tinel's sign.

Treatment involves removal of the offending article of clothing and local anaesthetic/steroid injection.

Deep peroneal nerve

This nerve may be compressed by a space-occupying lesion, constriction or swelling where it emerges with the anterior tibial artery at the midanterior area of the leg. It is mostly entrapped distally in the ankle and foot but may be damaged by tibial fracture.

Symptoms are sensory deficit in the first web space and weakness of the extensor brevis muscle. There may be a positive Tinel's sign. Treatment involves removal of constricting socks or boots, steroid injections or surgical exploration and decompression.

Superficial peroneal nerve

This nerve descends the shaft of the upper fibula and pierces the deep fascia to supply sensation to the distal lateral calf and the dorsum of the foot. Its location makes it vulnerable to compression due to skiboot pressure, direct trauma or fibular fracture. Care should be exercised in applying ice to the area around the head of the fibula where the common peroneal nerve is very superficial. A foot drop can result from freezing of the nerve.

The superficial peroneal nerve can also be entrapped distally by a muscle herniation where there is a weakness in the fascia it pierces. Treatment is along similar lines, i.e. relief of pressure and injection, but neurolysis or fascial release may be needed in very resistant cases.

Deep venous thrombosis (DVT)

This condition has been described as effort-induced in joggers in their 30s and 40s (Harvey 1978), although it is a well-recognized occurrence in sedentary individuals. It often starts as a sharp pain in the calf and the athlete usually tries to ignore it. The pain worsens and there is progressive swelling of the calf. Pain is eased by elevation and aggravated by lowering the leg. On examination there is tenderness to palpation, pain on stretch, heat and ecchymosis, and the calf circumference is increased. Medical referral is indicated and diagnosis confirmed by venography. Treatment of DVT involves rest, elevation and anti-coagulant therapy (heparin). The early recognition and treatment of DVT is vital because of the risk of pulmonary embolism.

Popliteal artery entrapment

This condition should be suspected if there is exercise-related leg pain and the distal pulses are compromised or absent. There is usually an anatomical anomaly in the popliteal fossa that intermittently occludes the artery (Friedman 1986), such as an aberrant gastrocnemius or plantaris muscle insertion or where the artery takes an abnormal course.

Most patients are male and many report bilateral symptoms. These are of claudication, cramping, tightness or fatigue on walking or running, forcing them to stop and rest, which relieves the pain. As the condition progresses there may be pain at rest. The patient may rub the leg or put it in a dependent position. Elevating the leg or cold usually makes the pain worse. If sitting or elevation relieves the pain or if it takes longer than a few minutes to abate, primary disease such as spinal canal stenosis could be the cause (see Ch. 27).

The distance walked before claudication gives some indication of the severity of arterial occlusion. Less than two city blocks indicates significant occlusion (Friedman 1986). On examination the distal pulses are diminished or absent. Active plantar flexion or passive dorsiflexion can further diminish the pulse, but this is also the case in normals. An arteriogram will show the site of occlusion in popliteal artery entrapment syndrome. The treatment is surgical decompression of the artery.

Venous stasis causes posterior calf pain on prolonged standing and is associated with varicose veins and swelling of the ankle and foot. Treatment involves active ankle and calf exercises to encourage venous return. Elastic support stockings, massage and elevation of the legs can also assist. Severe varicose veins may require surgery.

TIBIOFIBULAR SYNOSTITIS

This is calcification of the interosseous membrane from single or repeated injuries such as ankle sprains. It is associated with tearing of the anterior and posterior tibiofibular ligaments and usually the lower third of the membrane, with a widened inferior syndesmosis. It may be triggered by avulsion of the interosseous membrane from its periosteal attachments (Friedman 1986).

Symptoms include a feeling of tightness or spasm in the leg, instability and restricted motion. It may be an incidental finding on X-ray and be asymptomatic. If the disability is severe, however, surgery may be indicated. It is best to defer surgery until active ossification has ceased, confirmed by a normal bone scan, to avoid recurrence.

SUMMARY

Most sporting injuries of the lower leg that are not traumatic involve training errors or biomechanical alignment problems. Differentiation between the various syndromes can be done clinically and is based on history, location and behaviour of symptoms. Where there is doubt, further tests such as bone scans and compartment pressure tests will confirm a diagnosis of stress fracture, MTSS or compartment syndrome. There should be a high suspicion of stress fractures in elite female athletes, especially those with low body fat and amenorrhea.

Examination should include biomechanical assessment, preferably functionally, e.g. on a treadmill. Orthotic therapy plays a major role in management and the services of a podiatrist are often required. Physiotherapy management should include massage, stretching, and correction of muscular and joint restrictions that affect the biomechanics of the foot, ankle and leg linkage system.

With the increased use of sonography and MRI for diagnosis in tendon injuries, the management of achilles tendinitis has become more scientific. The therapist's role in rehabilitation of both conservative and surgical cases is now more defined.

REFERENCES

Barbolini G, Torricelli P, Monetti G, Laudizi L, Gatti G, Sturloni N 1988 Results with high definition sonography in the evaluation of achilles tendon conditions. Italian Journal of Sports Traumatology 10(4):225–234

Barrow G W, Saha S 1988 Menstrual irregularity and stress fractures in collegiate female distance runners. American Journal of Sports Medicine 16(3):209–216

Bassett C A L 1984 The development and application of pulsed electromagnetic fields (PEMFs) for ununited fractures and arthrodeses. Orthopaedic Clinics of North America 15:61–87

Bates P 1985 Shin splints. A literature review. British Journal of Sports Medicine 19(3):132–137

Bourke L 1990 Amenorrhea, low bone density and stress fractures in athletes. What is the dietary connection? Sport Health 8(4):44–47

Carbon R, Sambrook P N, Deakin V, Fricker P, Eisman J A, Maguire K, Yeates M G 1990 Bone density of elite female athletes with stress fractures. Medical Journal of Australia 153:373–376

Carter T R, Fowler P J, Blokker C 1992 Functional postoperative treatment of achilles tendon repair. American Journal of Sports Medicine 20(4):459–462

Chisin R, Milgram C, Giladi M, Stein M, Margulies J, Kashtan H 1987 Clinical signs of nonfocal scintigraphic findings in suspected tibial stress fractures. Clinical Orthopaedics 220:200–205

Clement D B 1974 Tibial stress syndrome in athletes. Journal of Sports Medicine 2(2):81–85

Clement D B, Taunton J E, Smart G W 1984 Achilles tendonitis and peritendonitis: etiology and treatment. American Journal of Sports Medicine 12(3):179–184

Clews W 1990 Sports massage and stretching. Partridge, London

Curwin S, Stanish W D 1984 Tendonitis: its etiology and treatment. Collamore Press, Massachusetts

Dacruz D J, Geeson M, Allen M J, Phair I 1988 Achilles paratendonitis: an evaluation of steroid injection. British Journal of Sports Medicine 12(3)64–65

D'Ambrosia R D, Zelis r F, Chuinard R G 1977 Interstitial pressure measurements in the anterior and posterior compartment in athletes with shin splints. American Journal of Sports Medicine 5:127–131

Davey J R, Rorabeck C H, Fowler P J 1984 The tibialis posterior muscle compartment. An unrecognized cause of exertional compartment syndrome. American Journal of Sports Medicine 12(5):391–397

Davidson R G, Taunton J E 1987 Achilles tendonitis. Medicine and Sports Science 23:71–79

Delacerda F G 1982 Iontophoresis for the treatment of shin splints. Journal of Orthopaedic and Sports Physical Therapy 3(4):183–185

Detmer D E 1986 Chronic shin splints. Classification and management of medial tibial stress syndrome. Sports Medicine 3:436–446

Devas M B 1958 Stress fractures of the tibia or 'shin soreness'. Journal of Bone and Joint Surgery 40B:227–239

Devas M B 1970 Stress fractures in athletes. Journal of the Royal College of General Practitioners 19:34–38

Dickson T B Jr, Kichline P D 1987 Functional management of stress fractures in female athletes using a pneumatic air brace. American Journal of Sports Medicine 15(1):86–89

Ellis J 1986 Shinsplints. Too much too soon. Runner's World 21(3):50–53, 86

Friedman M J 1986 Injuries to the leg in athletes. In: Nicholas J A, Hershman E B (eds) The lower extremity and spine in sports medicine. C V Mosby, St Louis

Gehlsen G M, Seger A 1980 Selected measures of angular displacement, strength, and flexibility in athletes with and without shin splints. Research Quarterly 51:478–485

Genuario S E 1989 Differential diagnosis: exertional compartment syndrome, stress fractures and shin splints. Athletic Training 24(1):31–34

Giladi M, Milgrom C et al 1987a Stress fractures and tibial bone width: a risk factor. Journal of Bone and Joint Surgery 69B(2):326–329

Giladi M, Milgrom C et al 1987b External rotation of the hip. A predictor of risk for stress fractures. Clinical Orthopaedics 216:131–134

Gradisar I 1990 Fracture stabilization and healing. In: Gould J A (ed) Orthopaedic and sports physical therapy. C V Mosby, St Louis

Grant J D 1990 Taping for medial tibial stress syndrome (shin splints). Athletic Training 25(1):53–54

Haggmark T et al 1986 Calf muscle atrophy and muscle function after non-operative vs operative treatment of achilles tendon ruptures. Orthopaedics 9(2):160–164

Hannaford P 1988 Shinsplints revisited. Excel 4:16–19

Harvey J S 1978 Effort thrombosis in the lower extremity in a jogger. American Journal of Sports Medicine 6:400

Heinrich C H, Going S B, Parmenter R W, Perry C D, Boyden T W, Lohman T G 1990 Bone mineral content of cyclically menstruating female resistance and endurance trained athletes. Medicine and Science in Sports and Exercise 22(5):558–563

Highet R 1989 Athletic amenorrhoea. An update on aetiology, complications and management. Sports Medicine 7:82–108

Holder L E, Michael R H 1985 The soleus syndrome a cause of medial tibial stress (shin splints). American Journal of Sports Medicine 13(2):87–94

Hulkko A, Orava S 1987 Stress fractures in athletes. International Journal of Sports Medicine 83:221–226

Hulkko A, Alen M, Orava S 1987 Stress fractures of the lower leg. Scandinavian Journal of Sports Sciences 9(1):1–8

Hunt G 1985 Examination of lower extremity dysfunction. In: Gould J, Davies G (eds) Orthopaedic and sports physical therapy. C V Mosby, St Louis

Jackson D 1978 Shin splints: an update. Physician and Sports Medicine 6:51–56

Jarvinnen M, Aho T, Niittymaki S 1989 Results of the surgical treatment of the medial tibial syndrome in athletes. International Journal of Sports Medicine 10:55–57

Johnell O, Rausing A, Weideberg B, Westlin N 1982 Morphological bone changes in shin splints. Clinical Orthopaedics 167:180–184

Jones D C, James S L 1987 Overuse injuries of the lower extremity: shin splints, iliotibial band friction syndrome, and exertional compartment syndromes. Clinics in Sports Medicine 6(2):273–290

Kainberger F M, Engel A, Barton P, Huebsch P, Neuhold A, Salomowitz E 1990 Injury of the achilles tendon: diagnosis with sonography. American Journal of Roentgenology 155(5):1031–1036

Kalebo P, Allenmark C, Peterson L, Sward L 1992 Diagnostic value of ultrasonography in partial ruptures of the achilles tendon. American Journal of Sports Medicine 20(4):378–381

Kues J 1990 The pathology of shin splints. Journal of Orthopaedic and Sports Physical Therapy 12(3):115–121

Kvist M, Jozsa L, Jarvinen M, Kvist H T 1987 Chronic achilles paratendonitis in athletes: a histological and histochemical study. Pathology (Australia) 19(1):1–11

Kvist M H, Jozsa L, Jarvinen M, Kvist H T 1988 Chronic achilles paratendonitis: an immunohistologic study of fibronectin and fibrinogen. American Journal of Sports Medicine 16(60:616–623

Lafortune M A, Maguire K 1986 Impact loading of the lower limbs during locomotive activities 2. Measurements and results. Abstract 137. Proceedings of 23rd World Congress of Sports Medicine, Brisbane

Laine H R, Harjula A L J, Peltokallio P 1987 Ultrasonography as a differential diagnostic aid in achillodynia. Journal of Ultrasound in Medicine 7(1):351–362

Lilletvedt J, Kreighbaum E, Phillips R L 1979 Analysis of selected alignment of the lower extremity related to the shin splint syndrome. Journal of American Podiatry Association 69:211–212

Linnell S L, Stager J M, Blue P W et al 1984 Bone mineral content and menstrual regularity in female runners. Medicine and Science in Sports and Exercise 16:343–348

Lipinski C 1987 Shin splints rehabilitation and prevention. Australian Runner 4(5):13

Logan J G, Rorabeck C H, Castle G S P 1983 The measurement of dynamic compartment pressure during exercise. American Journal of Sports Medicine 11(4):220–223

Maffuli N, Regine R, Angellilo M, Capasso G, Filice S 1987 Ultrasound diagnosis of achilles tendon pathology in runners. British Journal of Sports Medicine 21(4):158–162

Maguire K, Purdam C 1987 Achilles tendonitis. Proceedings of FISU\CESU Conference Universiade '87, Zagreb, Yugoslavia, pp 278–290

Marcus R, Cann C, Madvig P et al 1985 Menstrual function and bone mass in elite women distance runners: endocrine and metabolic features. Annals of Internal Medicine 102:158–163

Markey K L 1991 Stress fractures. Physiotherapy in Sport 13(3):4–12

Martens M A, Moeyersoons J P 1990 Acute and recurrent effort related compartment syndrome in sports. Sports Medicine 9(1):62–68

Martin A D, Bailey D 1987 Skeletal integrity in amenorrhoeic athletes. Australian Journal of Science and Medicine in Sport 19 (1):3–7

Massey L K, Opryszek A A 1989 No effects of adaptation to dietary caffeine on calcium excretion in young women. Nutrition Research 10(7):741–747

Mathieson J R, Connell D G, Cooperberg P L 1988 Sonography of the achilles tendon and adjacent bursae. American Journal of Roentgenology 151(1):127–131

McPoil T, Brocato R 1985 The foot and ankle: biomechanical evaluation and treatment. In: Gould J, Davies G (eds) Orthopaedic and sports physical therapy. C V Mosby, St Louis

Melberg P, Styf J 1989 Posteromedial pain in the lower leg. American Journal of Sports Medicine 17(6):747–750

Messier S P, Pittala K A 1988 Etiologic factors associated with selected running injuries. Medicine and Science in Sports and Exercise 20(5):501–505

Milgrom C, Chisin R, Giladi M, Stein M, Kashtan H, Margulies J, Atlan H 1984 Negative bone scans in impending tibial stress fractures. American Journal of Sports Medicine 12(6):488–491

Milgrom C, Giladi M, Stein M 1986 Medial tibial pain. A prospective study of its cause among military recruits. Clinical Orthopaedics 213:167–171

Milgrom C, Giladi M, Simkin A 1989 The area moment of inertia of the tibia: a risk factor for stress fractures. Journal of Biomechanics 22(11–12):1243–1248

Mills G Q, Marymont J H, Murphy D A 1980 Bone scan utilization in the differential diagnosis of exercise-induced lower extremity pain. Clinical Orthopaedics 149:207–210

Mubarak S J, Hargens A R, Owen C A, Garetto L P, Akeson W H 1976 The Wick catheter technique for measurement of intramuscular pressure. A new research and clinical tool. Journal of Bone and Joint Surgery 58A:1016–1020

Mubarak S J, Gould R N, Lee Y F, Schmidt D A, Hasrgens A R 1982 The medial tibial stress syndrome (a cause of shin splints). American Journal of Sports Medicine 10:201–205

Myburgh K H, Grobler N, Noakes T D 1988 Factors associated with shin soreness in athletes. Physician and Sports Medicine 16:129–134

Myburgh K, Hutchins J, Fataar A B, Fough S F, Noakes T D 1990 Low bone density as an etiologic factor for stress fractures in athletes. Annals of Internal Medicine 113:754–759

Nelen G, Martens M, Burssons A 1989 Surgical treatment of chronic achilles tendonitis. American Journal of Sports Medicine 17(6):754–759

Nelson M E, Fisher E C, Catsos P D 1986 Diet and bone status in amenorrhoeic athletes. American Journal of Clinical Nutrition 43:910–916

Nicholas J A, Hershman E B (eds) 1986 The lower extremity and spine in sports medicine. C V Mosby, St Louis

Nichols A W 1989 Achilles tendonitis in running athletes. Journal of the American Board of Family Practice 2(3):196–203

Oakes B W 1986 Tibial pain or shin soreness (shin 'splints')—its cause, differential diagnosis and management. In: Draper J (ed) Second report on the national sports research program. Australian Sports Commission, Canberra, pp 47–51

Olivieri B, Gemignani G, Gherardi S, Grass L, Ciompi 1987 Isolated HLA-B27 associated achilles tendonitis. Annals of Rheumatological Disorders 46(8):626–627

Orava S 1980 Stress fractures. British Journal of Sports Medicine 14:40–44

Orava S, Puranen J 1979 Athletes' leg pain. British Journal of Sports Medicine 13:92–97

Orava S, Hulkko A 1988 Delayed unions and nonunions of stress fractures in athletes. American Journal of Sports Medicine 16(4):378–382

Prior J C, Vigna Y M, Schecter M T, Burgess A E 1990 Spinal bone loss and ovulatory disturbances. New England Journal of Medicine 323(18):1221–1227

Puranen J 1974 The medial tibial syndrome: exercise ischaemia in the medial fascial compartment of the leg. Journal of Bone and Joint Surgery 56B:712–715

Rathbun J B, McNab I 1970 The microvascular pattern of the rotator cuff. Journal of Bone and Joint Surgery 52B:540–553

Rettig A C et al 1988 The natural history and treatment of delayed union stress fractures of the anterior cortex of the tibia. American Journal of Sports Medicine 16(3):250–255

Rigotti N A, Nussbaum S E, Herzog D B, Neer R M 1984 Osteoporosis in women with anorexia nervosa. New England Journal of Medicine 311;1601-1606

Rorabeck C H, Fowler P J, Nott L 1988 The results of fasciotomy in the management of chronic exertional compartment syndrome. American Journal of Sports Medicine 16(3):224–227

Roub L W, Gumerman L W, Hanley E N 1979 Bone stress: a radionuclide imaging perspective. Radiology 132:431–438

Rudo N D, Noble H B, Conn J, Flinn W, Yao J S T 1982 Popliteal artery entrapment syndrome in athletes. Physician and Sports Medicine 10(5):105–114

Schepsis A A, Leach R E 1987 Surgical management of achilles tendonitis. American Journal of Sports Medicine 15(4):308–315

Serafin-Krol M, Swiatlowski T 1988 Ultrasonography of the achilles tendon: surgical correlation. Italian Journal of Sports Traumatology 10(3):183–191

Slocum D B 1967 The shin splint syndrome medical aspects and differential diagnosis. American Journal of Surgery 114:875–881

Smart G W, Taunton J E, Clement D B 1980 Achilles tendon disorders in runners—a review. Medicine and Science in Sports and Exercise 12(4):231–243

Smith W, Wynne F, Parette R 1986 Comparative study using four modalities in shin splint treatments. Journal of Orthopaedic and Sports Physical Therapy 8(2):77–80

Stanish W D, Curwin S 1986 Eccentric exercise in chronic tendonitis. Clinical Orthopaedics and Related Research 208:65–68

Stanitiski, McMaster J, Scranton P 1978 On the nature of stress fractures. Journal of Sports Medicine 6(6):391–395

Steadman J R 1986 Skiing injuries. In: Nicholas J, Hershman E (eds) The lower extremity and spine in sports medicine. C V Mosby, St Louis

Straehley D, Jones W W 1986 Acute compartment syndrome (anterior, lateral, and superficial posterior) following tear of the medial head of gastrocnemius muscle. American Journal of Sports Medicine 14(1):96–99

Styf J 1988 Diagnosis of exercise-induced pain in the anterior aspect of the lower leg. The American Journal of Sports Medicine 16(2):165–169

Styf J 1989 Chronic exercise induced pain in the anterior aspect of the lower leg. An overview of diagnosis. Sports Medicine 7:331–339

Styf J, Korner L M, Suurkula M 1987 Intramuscular pressure and muscle blood flow during exercise in chronic compartment syndrome. Journal of Bone and Joint Surgery 69B:301–305

Taunton J, Clement D B, Smart G W 1984 Achilles tendonitis and peritendonitis: etiology and treatment. American Journal of Sports Medicine 12(3):179–184

Uebelhart D, Gineyts E, Chapuy M C, Detmas P D 1990 Urinary excretion of pyridinium crosslinks: a new marker of bone resorption in metabolic bone disease. Bone and Mineral 8:87–96

Velasquez B J 1987 Open-backed ankle tape job. An alternative method for taping achilles tendonitis. Athletic Training 22(4):321–322

Viitasalo T, Kvist M 1983 Some biomechanical aspects of the foot and ankle in athletes with and without shin splints. American Journal of Sports Medicine 11:125–130

Wallace L 1988 Foot pronation and knee pain. In: Mangine R (ed) Physical therapy of the knee. Churchill Livingstone, New York

Wallenstein R, Eriksson E 1984 Intramuscular pressures in exercise-induced lower leg pain. International Journal of Sports Medicine 5:31–35

Williams J G 1986 Achilles tendon lesions in sport. Sports Medicine 3(2):114–135

Williams J G P, Sperryn P N 1976 Sports medicine, 2nd edn. Butler & Tanner, London

32. Foot and ankle

Erica Rundle

Foot and ankle pain and dysfunction are common presentations to physiotherapists working in the field of sports medicine. The vast majority of sports place significant strains on the foot and ankle which function as a unit to provide stability and support in weightbearing while allowing for propulsion. The foot and ankle are designed precisely to meet these demands, however the joints and soft tissues of the region may not withstand the stresses placed on them by the high level athlete who may train and compete to excess, and by the recreational sportsperson who may not have invested in sufficient training. In sport, the foot and ankle may be required to accommodate to a variety of surfaces, maintain propulsion and allow directional changes without faltering. This demands unerring strength, balance and flexibility.

Injuries to the foot and ankle are exceedingly common in normal daily activities, with increasing incidence in sporting activities. Ankle sprains, for example, may be the most common sporting injury. Many authors believe sprains of the ankle to be the injury which most contributes to time lost by athletes (Boruta et al 1990, Nawoczenski et al 1985, Vaes et al 1985, Gungor 1988, Kannus & Renstrom 1991, Ferkel et al 1991, De Carlo & Talbot 1986, Hardaker et al 1985, Gross et al 1987, McCarroll et al 1987, Reid 1992). Physiotherapists must be aware of the propensity for this region of the body to sustain injury. Furthermore, physiotherapists must endeavour to play a role in the prevention of injury and reinjury, and assist the athlete to return to full activity as quickly as possible.

ANATOMY AND BIOMECHANICS

Ankle joint

The ankle is a hinge joint allowing dorsiflexion and plantarflexion movement associated with some accessory gliding. The bony structure is that of a mortice and tenon which gives considerable stability, while the strength of ligaments is necessary to maintain integrity. The mortice is formed by the lateral malleolus, the undersurface of the tibia and the medial malleolus while the talus is the tenon, fitting snugly into the mortice. The ligaments which support the ankle joint are the lateral ligament complex, the medial ligament and the interosseus membrane. The lateral ligament complex can be divided into three components, the anterior talofibular (ATF), calcaneofibular(CF) and posterior talofibular (PTF) ligaments. A fourth component, the lateral talocalcaneal (LTC) ligament, may also be included in the complex (Boruta et al 1990).

The ATF may be considered as a thickening of the anterior joint capsule (Boruta et al 1990), averaging 5 mm in width and 12 mm in length (Ruth 1961). It occupies a position which allows it to assume an orientation perpendicular to the long axis of the tibia when the foot is in equinus, thus enabling it to resist inversion. In the neutral position it is relaxed and closer to the horizontal (Anderson et al 1952).

The CF ligament is more variable in size, position and direction. Ruth (1961) found it to vary from a cordlike structure to a fan shaped band of tissue, with an average width of 6 mm and an angle of 10-45° posteriorly from the long axis of the fibula. It is extracapsular and slightly tense in the neutral position, but in calcaneal supination it assumes a vertical direction which improves its mechanical advantage (Ruth 1961). The ATF is commonly the first ligament to be torn in an inversion injury, and is often associated with a capsular tear. Disruption of the CF may follow the failure of these structures if the inversion force continues to be applied. A significant inversion stress with the ankle in neutral, however, may result in an isolated injury of the CF ligament (Boruta et al 1990).

The PTF ligament connects the posterolateral tubercle of the talus to the medial aspect of the lateral malleolus. It averages 6 mm in width and 9 mm in length, and resists external rotation force in a plantarflexed position (Boruta et al 1990, Ruth 1961).

The medial ligament is strong, flat and fan-shaped with deep and superficial fibres extending from the tip of the medial malleolus to the navicular, sustentaculum tali and the posterior area of the talus. The medial aspect of the ankle is less susceptible to injury but the medial ligament may be injured with an eversion or external rotation force. This may occur in association with a fracture of the lateral malleolus and possibly with disruption of the tibiofibular syndesmosis.

Subtalar joint

The subtalar joint is the articulation of the calcaneus and the talus which form the rearfoot. Movement at the joint is essentially supination and pronation in combination with accessory movement. Pronation occurs with abduction and dorsiflexion, while supination is associated with adduction and plantarflexion. The subtalar joint is sometimes referred to as the universal joint of the foot, as it allows the foot to accommodate to variations in terrain (Parks 1988, Reid 1992, Heil 1992).

Subtalar supination occurs at heel strike to provide a solid foundation for weightbearing. The foot then rapidly moves into pronation with maximum pronation occurring at the end of the footflat phase, allowing the foot to accommodate to the weightbearing surface. Supination of the subtalar joint follows from this point of midstance to toe-off. Supination is essential to provide a rigid lever allowing the foot to push off (Donatelli et al 1988, Heil 1992).

Midtarsal joint

The midtarsal complex consists of the calcaneocuboid and talonavicular joints, and links the subtalar joint and the forefoot. The calcaneocuboid joint is a saddle joint, convex on its transverse surface and concave on its vertical surface, while the talonavicular joint is condyloid, convex on both surfaces to allow the combined motions of supination, adduction and flexion, or pronation, abduction and extension.

The axes in the midtarsal joint are directed such that in inversion they are at an increased angle which restricts movement and locks the joint while tightening the interosseous ligament of the subtalar joint. The foot is then converted into a rigid lever for propulsion. In eversion, the axes are more parallel to allow free movement at the midtarsal joint, or unlocking. This enables the foot to adapt to the underlying surface (Corrigan & Maitland 1983).

Tarsometatarsal joints

The tarsometatarsal joints form part of the transverse arch of the foot. The medial three rays articulate with a corresponding cunieform, while the lateral two articulate with the cuboid. The second to fourth tarsometatarsal joints allow flexion/extension motion whereas the first and fifth metatarsals allow flexion/extension motion together with some rotation (Corrigan & Maitland 1983). The function of the first metatarsal is weightbearing, while allowing the first ray to be flexible. The first metatarsal is usually of greater length than the second metatarsal, which allows it to take increased loads. The second metatarsal is more rigid, because of its articulation with the middle cuneiform. This rigidity provided to the forefoot allows stress to be carried through the second ray. The fifth and second ray both allow mobility, but carry high stresses which may predispose them to possible injury (Sammarco 1989).

Metatarsophalangeal joints

The metatarsophalangeal joints allow flexion/extension motion with a limited amount of side to side motion.

Interphalangeal joints

The interphalangeal joints are hinge joints which have a small but varied range of movement, mainly flexion and extension.

EXAMINATION AND MANAGEMENT PRINCIPLES

Examination of the foot and ankle complex

Examination of an athlete with a suspected disorder of the foot or ankle should follow the principles discussed in Chapter 9, with special reference to the idiosyncrasies of the region. A subjective examination exemplified by the process described by Maitland (1986) is a thorough and structured style which will assist in the performance of a precise objective examination. Specific reference should be made in subjective questioning to aspects peculiar to foot and ankle function. This might include questioning about gait, footwear, running, negotiating stairs, balance or ability to cope with uneven surfaces. Many other aspects peculiar to specific conditions can also be determined by subjective questioning. A thorough history is imperative in examining athletes with a foot or ankle condition, although this may be curtailed in the case of acute trauma.

The foot and ankle are notorious areas for insidious pains of vague origin, and the physiotherapist must always be alert to the possibility of referred pathology. An accurate and thorough history followed by an appropriate objective examination should provide a clear diagnosis. These data may need to be supported by appropriate tests such as X-ray or bone scan. The lumbar spine should not be ignored as a possible cause of vague foot pain and may need to be examined. The presence of systemic disease or sinister pathology must also be considered.

Following complete subjective questioning, an objective examination that has been well thought out and planned is commenced. However straightforward the complaint may seem, it is worthwhile not to draw conclusions too rapidly, or to cease the examination process as soon as a positive sign is found. It may well not be the only or true cause of the problem. Where or when appropriate, the examination should commence with an assessment of the athlete in standing. See Table 32.1 for guidelines of the objective examination.

The aim with the assessment of these functional activities is to reproduce the complaint or to identify an abnormality in function which may be contributing to the complaint. Of course, in the acute severe injury, many of these activities would not be possible and, as with the subjective examination, the objective examination is modified as appropriate. All findings should be recorded and it is helpful to return to these later to assess for change.

After assessment of all aspects of gait, the foot and ankle should be closely examined on the treatment couch. Careful palpation of the area may be revealing and areas of swelling can be assessed. Free active movements can be performed and manual strength tested where appropriate. Isokinetic evaluation of strength may be assessed at a later stage. Neurological examination should be performed when there are neurological symptoms, where there is a suspicion that symptoms are referred from a more proximal source or where there has been trauma possibly associated with peripheral nerve damage.

The next component of the examination is to passively assess the joints and structures of the foot and ankle. It is not necessary to look at all joint movements in the region,

Table 32.1 Objective examination

Standing: Look for:
- Skin condition
- Swelling
- Bruising
- Foot posture

Gait: Look at:
- Step length
- Weightbearing—is it even?
- Pain—if present, where and when?
- Range of movement, especially dorsiflexion
- Balance
- Alterations in foot posture

Progress to:
- Walking on
  -toes
  -heels
  -in inversion
  -in eversion
  -other

If advanced:
- Running
- Hopping
- Stepping
- Duck walking
- Balance with/without visual input
- Reproducing problem sporting activities

but all structures which may be involved should be assessed. Where passive examination is not appropriate, for example in the presence of an acute inflammatory condition or fracture, this may be excluded. It may be possible to perform a useful but restricted examination even with an acute injury but great care must be taken not to aggravate the injury.

Following passive examination, the physiotherapist should be able to ascertain any abnormality in range or function of the joints when compared with the other side. When functional tests were part of the assessment the physiotherapist should re-examine the athlete performing any functional activities which previously reproduced the symptoms to determine if there has been any change. In this way the structures possibly at fault can be methodically tested, and with the knowledge of common pathologies of the foot and ankle in athletes, an accurate diagnosis can be made. Where a precise diagnosis is not reached, it is still possible to ascertain the structure at fault and to determine whether there is a fault of weakness, instability or joint stiffness. It is then possible to commence a program to rectify the problem and return the athlete to sport. The physiotherapist should also remember that the athlete needs to be informed and reassured often during the assessment procedures and ongoing treatment sessions.

Passive assessment and mobilization

Physiotherapists will be greatly assisted in their ability to accurately assess, diagnose and treat conditions and injuries in the foot and ankle if they are skilled in passive or manual assessment. Passive assessment techniques may also form part of the treatment program, since an abnormal joint movement may be improved with passive mobilization of that joint.

The passive movements of the foot and ankle as described by Corrigan and Maitland (1983) should be used as a guide to examination. Table 32.2 lists common inclusions, and figures are included to assist with the assessor's hand placement (Figs 32.1-6).

There are many combinations of passive movements, and it is not usual to perform all of these in one assessment. It is more appropriate to closely examine a region suspected of involvement and to simply eliminate other areas of involvement. The author has noted most of these movements to be performed in a prone position, which may assist the physiotherapist to stabilize the limb and to apply as much force as necessary, particularly where passive assessment treatment of a very stiff foot or ankle is required. There is no fault, however, in performing these tests in an alternative position.

Following passive assessment, the athlete should be reassessed, either by the movement or functional tests which earlier provoked the symptom. A change in these tests of range, quality or pain response may show that the passive

Table 32.2

Ankle
Prone
Dorsiflexion (inversion of the midfoot will 'lock' it, restricting movement to the ankle)
Plantarflexion
Accessory movements including:
    posteroanterior glide
    anteroposterior glide
    rotation
    cephalad (compression)
    caudad (distraction)
Supine/prone
Special tests
    anterior draw
    talar tilt
    Combined accessory/physiological movements
    antero-posterior glide and plantarflexion
    postero-anterior glide and dorsiflexion

Inferior tibio-fibular joint
Prone
caudad—using inversion
cephalad—using eversion
compression
separation—by the use of ankle dorsiflexion

Foot
Subtalar joint
Prone
Inversion, with the ankle fixed in dorsiflexion
Eversion, with the ankle fixed in dorsiflexion

Midtarsal joint
Prone
adduction
abduction
supination
pronation
accessory glides to individual tarsal bones

Tarso-metatarsal joints
Prone
accessory glides
intertarsal glides

Metatarso-phalangeal joints
Prone
flexion
extension
accessory glides

Interphalangeal joints
Prone
flexion
extension
accessory glides

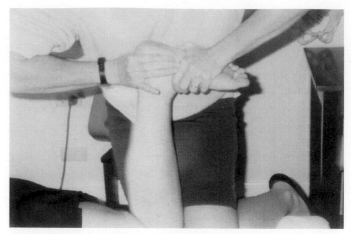

Fig. 32.1 Passive dorsiflexion performed in prone. The examiner grasps the foot proximal to the midtarsal joint and locks it by passively inverting the foot. The calcaneum or heel is held with the other hand. The movement is produced with the proximal hand.

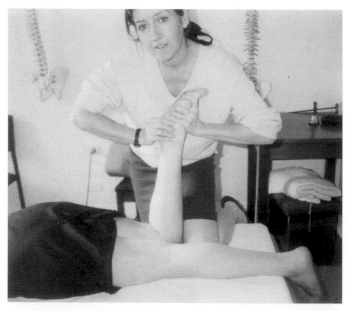

Fig. 32.2 Passive plantarflexion is performed with one hand around the heel, the other placed over the dorsum of the foot.

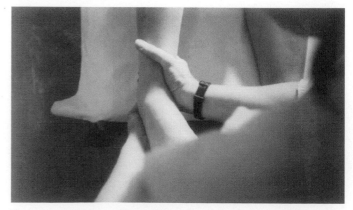

Fig. 32.3 Assessment of talar tilt may be performed in supine or prone with the peroneals relaxed. The examiner stabilizes the tibia medially and grips the calcaneum with the other hand. Care must be taken to ensure that the movement is an inversion of the rearfoot.

movements used in the testing procedure could be appropriate for inclusion in the treatment program.

Management principles of ankle injuries

Acute management

Diagnosis. It is essential to first establish a correct diagnosis before being able to instigate an appropriate treatment regime. Where the physiotherapist is present at the time of an acute injury, observation of the mechanism of injury will greatly assist in the diagnosis. The diagnosis of specific conditions will follow the principles outlined above, and

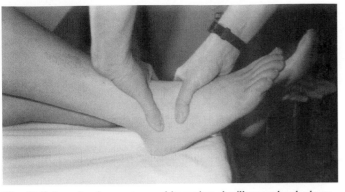

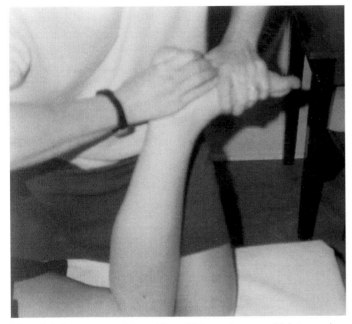

Fig. 32.4 Anterior drawer assessed in supine. A pillow under the knee may be used to allow the foot to relax into slight plantarflexion. The examiner stabilizes the tibia and grasps the dorsum of the foot around the neck of the talus and glides it anteriorly.

Fig. 32.5 Assessment of the midtarsal joint or intertarsal joints requires care in hand positioning. Movement is assessed in prone and care taken to stabilize joints not being assessed.

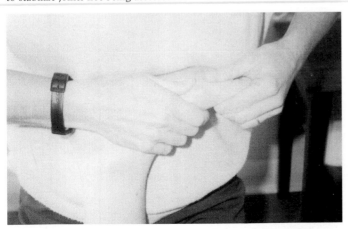

Fig. 32.6 Metatarsophalangeal joints may also be assessed in prone. The examiner localizes the movement with the thumbs on the plantar aspect of the foot proximal and distal to the joint. Physiological movements and glides are assessed.

the need for further diagnostic tests such as X-rays of the acute injury should be considered. Management of specific injuries will be discussed later.

The initial management of injury should include assessment of severity in terms of impairment to circulation. A severe ankle fracture involving dislocation may compromise the circulation of the foot and should be considered a medical emergency. In this case the patient should receive immediate medical assessment where an X-ray can be performed and the ankle dislocation reduced. When the injury is less severe, attention should be given to reduce the acute symptoms of the ankle injury, i.e. to reduce pain and swelling and prevent further injury by suitably protecting the joint.

Treatment. The best method of reducing pain and swelling would be the application of ice with added compression while elevating the limb. The author has found the most effective means of applying ice while minimizing the possibility of ice burn is to use a regimen of 10 minutes on and 10 minutes off, over a 30 minute period. This is repeated up to three times a day where practical over the first three days. Crushed ice is preferable when applying cold therapy and, in the experience of the author, is of much greater benefit than a commercial cold pack. The ice is applied in a damp towel and should completely encase the joint. Compression can be added by bandaging over the pack with a crepe bandage. Icing should be regularly performed 3-4 times a day over the first 48-72 hours after injury.

Between sessions of icing, the athlete should maintain compression over the injured foot and ankle by using a compression bandage or shaped stocking. The compressive bandage is preferable as it will allow some protection of the injured structure if bandaged with the foot in an appropriate protective position. To prevent swelling pooling around the malleoli, foam or felt pads can be cut in a J or U shape to fit around the malleoli under the bandage, thus reinforcing compression to the area (Fig. 32.7). It is also important to keep the athlete non-weightbearing for the first 24-48 hours until the swelling is brought under control. A progression to partial weightbearing and on to full weightbearing is allowed as the joint is reassessed. The athlete is instructed to elevate the limb whenever possible. Athletes should also be warned about the adverse effects of alcohol, which may increase joint swelling in the acute stage.

Further assistance in relieving the area of excessive swelling can be achieved with the use of continuous passive movement (CPM) or a pressure pump, if available.

Once the swelling is controlled a graduated program of early movement can be instigated, commencing with non-weightbearing range of motion activities. Exercises can be performed in a whirlpool or spa to assist reduction of swelling and pain relief. The pool can also be used at this stage for maintenance of aerobic fitness by performing general activities of a non-weightbearing nature.

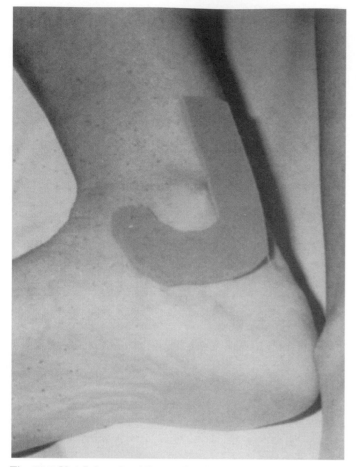

Fig. 32.7 U or J shaped padding used under compression to assist reduction of swelling.

Free active exercise encouraging full range of movement of the ankle and foot are otherwise performed with the foot elevated and should provoke minimal discomfort. Athletes may require encouragement to 'nudge' into some pain in order to regain full range of movement. Where significant ligamentous damage has occurred, movement stressing the injured structure(s) should be avoided initially, although it is possible to incorporate passive mobilization techniques in the acute stage. Gentle passive mobilization of a grade I or II injury will assist to reduce pain and may speed the healing process by improving the joint nutrition and aiding the local circulation (see Ch. 12). For lateral ligament injuries, the direction of mobilization chosen may be into inversion, but gentle techniques for dorsiflexion are also useful. As the injured area will be quite tender, care must be taken with gripping around the ankle and simple physiological movements rather than accessory movements will be easier to perform.

Early post-acute management

When pain reduction and adequate functional range is achieved, partial weightbearing may be commenced.

Exercise may also progress to include sitting and standing activities.

Sitting. In sitting, improvement in the range of plantarflexion and dorsiflexion can be gained by placing the foot flat on a towel on the floor and sliding this forward and back as far as possible without lifting the heel. From the author's experience, this exercise is especially important to regain a range of passive dorsiflexion which cannot be performed actively. Inversion and eversion exercise can also be performed using the towel by keeping the heel in place and sliding the foot in and out. To exercise the intrinsic muscles, the heel is kept still and the toes are used to 'bunch' the towel, drawing it toward the athlete. This exercise can be made more difficult by adding a weight onto the towel. It is very useful to stimulate the circulation when there is significant swelling in the foot after a period of immobilization. A rocker or wobbleboard can also be used effectively in the sitting position to assist the movements of dorsiflexion, plantarflexion, inversion and eversion, while contributing to the re-education of proprioception. Either a multidirectional or bidirectional board may be used (Fig. 32.8).

Standing. Exercise in standing can be commenced as early as tolerated and when safe. It should be noted that if there is an increase in swelling in the foot during exercise the athlete should have regular breaks in which the foot can be elevated for a few minutes. The athlete must perform these exercises in a safe environment as pain and lost proprioception may predispose to loss of balance and injury. Parallel bars are ideal and will allow the athlete to use a rocker board safely either as a mobilizing exercise, or to assist in balance training by attempting to hold the board still in the horizontal position. A lunge exercise in standing is important to regain the range of dorsiflexion (see

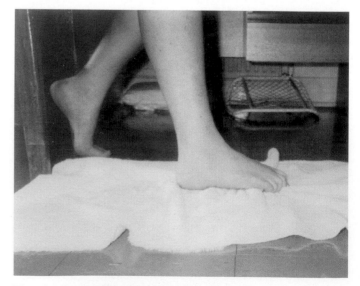

Fig. 32.8 Intrinsic exercises performed sitting

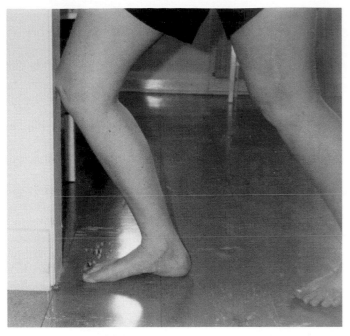

Fig. 32.9 Lunge position

Fig. 32.9). Assessment of the range and quality of this movement is done with the toe of the affected foot placed against an upright or wall, the foot maintained flat on the floor while the knee moves forward to touch the wall. Emphasis must be placed on not allowing the heel to lift. Where it is easy to touch the wall, the toe is gradually moved from the wall until the knee just touches. In order to check progress and to compare with the uninjured leg, a measurement can be made from the toe to the wall or the knee to the wall. As an exercise, the movement can be performed away from the wall although the feedback of the achievement made in range as demonstrated in that position can be encouraging.

Gym exercise. Other useful exercises in the early stages include work on the exercise bike, walking on a trampett with support, toe raising, toe walking in the rails and elastic resisted exercise to strengthen ankle muscles. Recently designed equipment consisting of a foot plate over a balance apparatus controlled by elastic resistance simulates a skiing action, but can also be adapted to perform other re-educative exercises. As the rehabilitation phase progresses, this can be a useful tool to provide variety and is popular with athletes.

Passive mobilization. As athletes are able to tolerate increased weightbearing, they will also be able to gradually tolerate increased grades and amounts of passive mobilization. It is still important to respect the healing ligamentous structures, but mobilization of the ankle complex will help to reduce pain and to regain range of movement at the talocrural and subtalar joints.

At this stage the ankle area should not be as acutely tender and it will be easier to position the hands around the area to perform the technique. Dorsiflexion is commonly restricted and this may improve with a physiological dorsiflexion mobilization, an anteroposterior glide of the talus or a combination of both movements. The grade of movement used will depend on the athletes level of pain and the resistance within the joint. Care must be taken not to overstress the healing ligaments. Plantarflexion may also be restricted and similar techniques can be incorporated to improve this or whichever movement is found to be restricted.

Post-acute management

When full weightbearing is commenced, exercises can be progressed by performing them without support. The rocker board can be used away from support when balance permits and can be progressed by altering visual cues, throwing balls, or standing on the affected leg alone. When the use of a rocker board at home is not possible, athletes can progress by balancing on the affected leg while reading or performing other simple activities. They can also attempt to balance with the eyes shut to remove any visual cues or practise balancing on varying surfaces.

If loss of range of movement is an ongoing problem, more aggressive exercise is required to effectively mobilize the foot and ankle. This may include more vigorous lunging and adding a rocking motion to the movement, rather than performing a straight stretch. Dorsiflexion may also be improved by squatting exercises, descending steps, stretching over the edge of a step and calf stretches. Impaired plantarflexion can be improved by toe-raising or toe-walking and passively stretching the ankle by sitting back onto the heels from a kneeling position.

Passive mobilization is an essential adjunct to treatment for the athlete where loss of range of movement continues to be an ongoing problem. To complement the increased vigour of exercise, stronger mobilizing techniques performed further into resistance or range may be necessary. Such techniques might include accessory movements at the limit of the available physiological movement, for example an anteroposterior glide in the maximum amount of dorsiflexion available. Where mobilizing techniques are incorporated specifically to regain range in very stiff joints, some pain may occur with this treatment. Physiotherapists can assist athletes to tolerate this kind of treatment by providing appropriate explanations and by assisting in subsequent pain reduction by using an easing-off technique or electrotherapy (refer to techniques section). At this stage in management, it is important to have accurately assessed each joint in the foot and ankle complex to determine where there is limitation of movement and which appropriate mobilization technique might be used to restore a normal range and improve function.

More advanced strengthening programs may include resisted activities using commercially graded elastic material to provide resistance, or isokinetics can incorporated for more specific strengthening. This may be particularly appropriate after reconstruction or repair of ankle ligaments, but may only be introduced when the surgeon's post-operative protocol allows.

When the pathology and pain permits, and the athlete has adequate balance, activities such as jogging, jumping, hopping and skipping may be commenced. In the gym environment, these activities may be performed without the security of tape, but for exercise in the field it may be wise to tape the ankle to prevent further injury. Jogging can be commenced on the trampett and the athlete can incorporate jumping and hopping on it as confidence, strength and balance allow. This can be progressed to jumping from the trampett on two feet onto a mat placed on to the ground. When this is performed satisfactorily, the athlete can practise jumping off onto the good leg, and then the injured leg as confidence allows. Hopping can be performed on the mat, and skipping with a rope may be gradually introduced. Exercise in the pool and swimming may also be commenced at this stage.

Graduated return to sport

In preparing the athlete for return to sport, an exercise program must be designed to educate the injured joint and surrounding musculature to respond to the types of stresses that the particular sport may offer. For example, in most codes of football the player needs to have great agility and speed, while the Australian Rules footballer also needs the spring of a basketballer with the confidence and stability in the ankle to land safely. The gymnast or dancer cannot afford to compromise on range of movement and must regain maximum range while retaining strength, stability and balance. A catcher in baseball requires full dorsiflexion, as does a sprinter. Other athletes may be able to sacrifice a small portion of their range for the sake of stability. The physiotherapist must understand the specific requirements of the athlete in order to determine these needs (see Ch. 10).

When the athlete has progressed sufficiently to return to exercise in the field, this should be gradually introduced, first with short jogs, slowly increasing the distance and freqauency as tolerated. The athlete should ensure that there is good light and an even and forgiving surface. Taping the ankle is usually advised and supportive shoes are imperative. If the ankle or foot pain tends to be aggravated or if there is swelling after activity, it may be wise to ice after jogging and possibly restrict this exercise to every second day. As athletes progress, they may add some 'run throughs' where short sprints are incorporated through a longer slow run. This can be performed over several laps around an oval and enables a steady build up of fitness both for the ankle and the cardiovascular system.

Further progression can include the commencement of running around cones on the field, changing direction to the call of an assistant, and alternating running forwards and backwards. The physiotherapist should determine the requirements for the athlete's particular sport and include aspects of those requirements into the program. For example, for a gymnast it may be appropriate to commence basic exercise on a beam placed on the ground. The dancer can progress simple barre work from the pool to the gym, while athletes involved in ball sports need to incorporate the use of a ball into their program.

Discussion with the treating medical practitioner, the athlete and the coach will determine the appropriate time for return to full sport. Athletes must be able to perform all requirements of their sport safely in a controlled environment without showing any aggravation of their condition before such consideration can be given. If possible, an initial return to only a portion of the game, competition at a lower level or taking on a less demanding role within a team may assist the athlete to regain confidence and prevent reinjury.

Management principles of foot injuries

The general management of injuries to the foot is similar to that of the ankle and many of the principles of management already mentioned apply to the athlete who has sustained a foot injury.

Acute management

Foot injuries can be quite painful and associated with significant swelling. Ice and elevation, together with compression, are therefore essential elements in acute management. Crutches may also be necessary in the early stages to prevent excessive swelling. The joints of the foot are prone to stiffness and early movement should be encouraged. Exercise in elevation should include all movements of the ankle, subtalar and midtarsal joints as well as toe movements. Massage to assist in the reduction of swelling is very helpful, and early gentle mobilizing techniques may also assist in reduction of swelling and in regaining a normal range of movement. Pulsed ultrasound progressing to continuous ultrasound may be used, as may interferential therapy which the author has found to be valuable in reducing swelling. This should not, however, be introduced until 48 hours or so after injury (see Ch. 15). Gentle passive mobilization techniques may also be incorporated to assist in the reduction of pain and swelling (see Ch. 12).

Early post-acute management

Treatment at this stage follows the principles of treatment of the ankle. Injury to the foot and subsequent swelling and immobilization may affect both the foot and the ankle joint. Exercise is introduced early, commencing in sitting with a towel or rocker board, with emphasis on the movements of the small joints of the foot and toes. Rolling a ball or jar under the foot will help to regain foot mobility, particularly in the midtarsal and metatarsophalangeal joints. Picking up objects with the toes or scrunching the towel with the toes can assist in regaining movement and strength in the toes. Foot posture can be corrected in the sitting position by encouraging the athlete to raise and lower the longitudinal arch of the foot while maintaining the heel and transverse arch in contact with the floor. This is an appropriate exercise for any conditions of the foot where there has been disruption or a loss of the normal foot posture. Where control of the intrinsic muscle is very poor, faradic stimulation with a foot bath may help.

Mobilization techniques are an essential adjunct to rehabilitation and can be incorporated with great care into a treatment program as early as the acute stage. Stronger mobilizing techniques may then be incorporated as necessary. As with the management of ankle injuries, the grade and direction of mobilization is dependent on the desired outcome. There are many small joints in the foot which may become stiff and will respond well to mobilization, either by using an accessory glide or as incorporated into a physiological technique.

The chronically stiff foot responds well to quite vigorous mobilization, which in combination with an extensive exercise program will achieve a faster progression and better result.

Post-acute management

Exercise now needs to be progressed as with injuries to the ankle. The emphasis is on exercise in weightbearing, or in progressing to more functional and sports-specific activities. The physiotherapist must treat each athlete as an individual and determine the predisposing factors to the presenting disorder and the best way to manage it and prevent recurrence. For example, it is necessary to accurately diagnose existing levels of stiffness, weakness and instability. Presence of ongoing inflammation must be identified and a further period of rest or limitation of training instigated.

Where there is still considerable stiffness in the foot, it is useful to incorporate walking and jogging on the trampett, rocker board activities and walking on a variety of uneven surfaces. Mobilization techniques of increased strength are necessary in combination with this increased vigour of exercise. Where there is considerable foot deformity with loss of strength and resultant instability, taping or orthotics may be required to allow a return to full activity.

Care must also be taken to recall the actual cause of the initial injury or complaint and take steps to prevent a similar occurrence on return to sport.

ANKLE INJURIES

Ankle sprains are common sporting injuries, but there are many other injuries which can occur in the region which must be readily recognized and treated appropriately.

Lateral ligament injuries

Knowledge of the structure and function of the lateral ligament complex enables accurate assessment of the joint and assists the determination of the severity and subsequent implication of an injury.

With an inversion stress to the plantarflexed ankle, the first structure to tear is the lateral joint capsule, followed by the anterior talofibular ligament. After a complete tear of the ATF, the calcaneofibular ligament will be stressed to result in a complete or partial tear. The posterior talofibular ligament, because of its position, is rarely torn (Boruta et al 1990).

Injuries to the complex can be graded by severity, where a grade I injury produces mild stretching and no instability, grade II is a partial but incomplete tear with mild instability, and grade III is a complete tear of the ATF and CF ligaments with gross laxity and instability (Boruta et al 1990).

Diagnosis. The athlete will describe an injury involving a plantarflexion, inversion stress to the joint. This may have occurred on landing from a jump, when changing direction, or when an uneven weightbearing surface has been involved. Less commonly, an injury to the CF ligament may have occurred when an inversion stress has been applied with the ankle in the neutral or dorsiflexed position.

The athlete may hear or feel a pop and, depending on the severity of the injury, will develop swelling and difficulty in weightbearing. Correlation between the amount of swelling and the severity of the injury is not consistent. Caution should be taken with the ankle which displays immediate and gross swelling because the possibility of a fracture or ligament disruption is increased. X-ray examination is necessary when a fracture is suspected, but radiology may not always assist in determining the extent of ligament damage (Boruta et al 1990). The key, therefore, to accurate diagnosis is physical examination of the athlete and an accurate history of the injury. Knowledge of the structure and function of the bands of the lateral ligament complex permits a manual assessment of integrity if the athlete's level of pain or degree of swelling permits. It should be noted that where there is an extensive injury with a torn ligament, a grade III tear, pain may be less severe than with a minor injury. Care must be taken not to underestimate the level of damage sustained. The presence of an associated medical malleolus fracture should also be considered.

The anterior drawer test is a method of assessing the integrity of the anterior talofibular ligament (Black et al

1978, Gungor 1988, Aradi et al 1988, Boruta et al 1990, Karlsson et al 1988) and may be the key test for ankle instability as it provides information about the integrity of both the anterior talofibular and calcaneofibular ligaments. The test requires an anterior movement of the talus in relation to the tibia. A positive or abnormal result is judged by comparison with the amount of movement elicited in the non-injured ankle. Occasionally a 'clunk' or a suction dimple at the lateral aspect of the ankle may be noted during the test. The clunk is probably simply a result of the excess movement, while the suction dimple is thought to indicate a tear in the joint capsule at that site (Aradi et al 1988).

The anterior drawer can be performed in a supine, prone or sitting positon but the emphasis must be on correct hand position to grip around the neck of the talus to pull it anteriorly while stabilizing the tibia. When performed accurately the test provides stress in a direction which should be resisted by the intact anterior talofibular ligament.

The talar tilt (stress) test has been advocated to assist in diagnosis of ligament disruption. This test is to passively invert the rearfoot, producing an angle between the tibial plafond and the dome of the talus (Boruta et al 1990). There is disagreement on what constitutes a positive talar tilt angle. An absolute figure of the degree of tilt which should be considered as the upper limit of normal has been proposed (Freeman 1965), but identification of a range which might be considered normal when compared with the ipsilateral angle as determined by X-ray and findings at surgery has not been achieved (Rubin & Witten 1960). The test is still commonly performed manually, or at X-ray with analgesia or local anaesthetic as required, and may help to determine the diagnosis and the degree of injury.

This test of passive supination of the calcaneum to effectively stress the CF ligament, if combined with plantarflexion, may also stress the ATF ligament. It can be performed with the patient supine, sitting or in prone with the knee flexed to 90°. Although the latter is preferred by the author, any position is satisfactory if the tibia is sufficiently stabilized to ensure that the movement assessed is indeed supination of the calcaneum.

Arthrography has also been promoted as a useful tool for the diagnosis of ankle ligament injuries (Boruta et al 1990, Black et al 1978). This should be performed within 24 hours if possible, but definitely within five days of injury to provide an accurate diagnosis. The ankle joint is injected with contrast material followed by radiology to assess leakage of this contrast from the joint capsule. As the anterior talofibular ligament is closely related to the joint capsule, injury to this ligament in association with capsular damage will allow the contrast material to leak antero-laterally. The calcaneofibular ligament in turn is closely related to the sheath of the peroneal tendons and injury to this ligament may be associated with injury to the peroneal sheath, allowing leakage of contrast material into the sheath

with arthrography of the ankle. As such a leakage indicates a tear of the calcaneofibular ligament and therefore a tear of the anterior talofibular ligament, injection of the peroneal sheath with contrast may be a simpler and equally effective means of evaluating double ligament injuries than ankle joint arthrography as such (Black et al 1978).

Sinus tarsi syndrome

The sinus tarsi is a bony canal formed by the articulation of the talus and the calcaneum. The canal is occupied by the interosseus talocalcaneal and cervical ligaments and can be injured following an inversion or twisting injury to the ankle.

Diagnosis

The athlete will complain of lateral foot pain just anterior to the ankle. Palpation over the sinus will reproduce pain. The condition may occur in association with a lateral ligament injury or may occur in isolation. It is important to identify the presence of the syndrome, because if the condition is treated as a lateral ligament injury alone it will not respond. Where the diagnosis is not clear, injection of local anaesthetic directly into the sinus may assist a positive diagnosis if the symptoms are relieved.

Differential diagnosis

If the diagnosis is unclear, an X-ray or bone scan may be necessary to assess for the presence of osteoarthritis or stress fracture.

Treatment

Local physiotherapy including ultrasound, frictions, stretches and mobilization of the subtalar joint may provide relief. Where conservative treatment has failed, the athlete may be referred for a steroid injection or surgical excision of the inflamed tissue from the sinus if an injection is unsuccessful (Quirk 1993).

Syndesmodic ankle sprains

Syndesmodic sprains occur with an injury to the interosseous membrane together with either or both the anterior talofibular ligament and the posterior tibiofibular ligament. This can occur as the result of an external rotation force or possibly a hyperdorsiflexion injury. Boytim et al (1991) reviewed athletes who had sustained syndesmodic ankle sprains and compared them with a similar group of athletes with lateral ligament injuries. They estimated that such sprains may occur in 10% of ankle injuries and that these probably result from a moderate force.

Syndesmotic sprains were diagnosed when there was tenderness over the damaged ligaments or the interrosseous membrane and when anterolateral pain proximal to the ankle joint was experienced when the ankle was passively externally rotated while in neutral dorsiflexion/plantar-flexion. X-ray examination in their study was often normal and did not provide a definitive diagnosis, but later examination was noted to occasionally reveal calcification of the interrosseous membrane. The inclusion of specific abduction stress views may have been more enlightening as the possibility of injury to the syndesmosis would be suspected where there was significant injury to the medial ligament. Boytim et al (1991) did not address this possible association.

Athletes who sustain syndesmotic sprains have a serious ankle injury and may be slow to gain complete recovery. They must be diagnosed at an early stage and appropriate treatment instigated. Treatment may include the use of bracing or immobilization in the early stages, with careful attention to the recovery of the range of dorsiflexion, tibiofibular glide and re-education of push-off during gait.

Medial ligament injuries

Isolated medial ligament injuries are uncommon, but may be severe and associated with a slow recovery. A pure eversion stress to the ankle may result in a medial ligament sprain, but the strength of that ligament and the protection provided by the length of the lateral malleolus help to account for the rareness of this injury. When there is a combination of some rotary force and an eversion stress, the ligament may be damaged. This may be in conjunction with injury to the tibiofibular syndesmosis. A severe injury may also involve a fracture of the lateral malleolus or, where an external rotation force is present, a high fracture at the neck of the fibula. It is important to bear this in mind when assessing a suspected medial ligament injury, and X-rays to include the neck of the fibula should be performed.

Due to the force of injury which results in a medial ligament injury, and the possible associated structural damage, the extent of bruising, swelling and discomfort may be considerable. Treatment will be similar to that for a severe lateral ligament injury.

Differential diagnosis of ligament injuries

Fractures. In more severe injuries it will be necessary to consider the possibility of an associated malleolar fracture, a high fibular fracture which may occur in association with a medial ligament injury from an external rotation injury, or a fracture at the base of the fifth metatarsal following avulsion of the peroneus brevis tendon. X-ray examination and close palpation of the area will generally be sufficient to allow a definite diagnosis.

The dome or neck of the talus may occasionally sustain a small chip fracture or osteochondral fracture. This will usually be apparent on plain X-ray, or with the assistance of CT scanning or MR imaging. These fractures will be discussed later.

Tendon injuries. Injuries to tendons around the ankle are assessed by careful examination and palpation. The close association of the peroneal sheath to the calcaneofibular ligament should be kept in mind when assessing for involvment of this structure and its tendons when a lateral ligament injury has occurred. Peroneal tendon dislocation is an uncommon but extremely painful injury, which must be excluded. Description of this injury will follow.

Treatment of ankle ligament injuries

Grade I and II ligament injuries

Once diagnosis has been established and the severity of the injury determined, the primary objective in the acute stage is to reduce pain and swelling and to protect the joint from further damage. Early application of ice and compression is essential and advice regarding elevation of the limb must be given to assist a fast recovery. Management follows those principles of treatment for all acute ankle injuries.

A grade I injury is generally effectively managed with the support of a bandage or taping, and only a very short period of restricted weightbearing with crutches or a stick may be necessary.

A grade II injury requires more support and restriction of weightbearing as the joint is potentially more unstable, and there will be more significant swelling and pain. Strapping, together with bandaging and the support of crutches, may suffice, with extreme care required in taping on the skin when the ankle is very swollen. When the athlete is in considerable discomfort, a below-knee plaster or back-slab may assist in the initial reduction of swelling and pain in the acute stage while providing protection to the joint as soft tissue repair commences. The athlete can remain in this plaster for up to two weeks, when active exercise should commence.

In the post-acute and rehabilitation phases, treatment would follow a plan as outlined under management of ankle injuries. Attention should be paid to ongoing protection of the joint, with taping of the joint where appropriate and the inclusion of proprioceptive exercises reflecting the demands of the athlete's sport.

Grade III lateral ligament injuries

The treatment of lateral ligament injuries at the ankle is an area for constant debate in an effort to establish the most appropriate form of treatment. The most contentious issue is the treatment of the grade III injury where the joint is considered to be unstable.

Kannus and Renstrom (1991) reviewed 12 prospective randomized studies presented in the literature which specifically examined treatment of grade III injuries in the acute stage. They were unable to conclude that there was a single most appropriate form of treatment for this condition. Unfortunately many studies had shortcomings and could not be reproduced due to differences in patient populations, variation in surgical techniques and inconsistent methods for assessing a good functional result.

Ruth (1961) presented a series of 235 ankle injuries, of which 45 had surgical repair followed by immobilization in plaster for 6 weeks, while 190 were treated conservatively with a below-knee cast for 6 weeks. He found that there was a 90% return to normal function in the operated group whereas in the non-operated group only 50% attained this level. Of those who were followed up after two years, patient allocation and comparison was inconsistent.

Evans et al (1984) also compared the effects of surgical repair of acutely ruptured ligaments with management in a plaster cast, but their results showed an improved outcome in the conservatively treated group at long-term follow-up. Freeman (1965) studied the long-term outcome of three forms of treatment: surgical repair, immobilization, and mobilization with ankle strapping. His results were interesting, with 58% of patients treated by mobilization, 53% of patients treated by immobilization and only 25% of surgically repaired patients becoming symptom free. Their recommendation, therefore, was that the treatment of choice for most, if not all, ruptures of the lateral ligament should be active mobilization.

Boruta et al (1990) reviewed the literature and recommended a short period of immobilization and protected weightbearing for 3-6 weeks, depending on the patient's progress, and suggested that surgical repair was inappropriate in the majority of cases. Kannus and Renstrom (1991) recommended a treatment regimen of active mobilization, as they believed that the long-term prognosis for patients was good if not excellent irrespective of the the initial treatment.

This plethora of conflicting studies can be particularly confusing to all involved in the assessment and treatment of athletes who sustain an acute lateral ligament tear. However, the primary concern is to accurately diagnose the injury and decide on a treatment plan as soon as possible. Where surgery is considered, early consultation is necessary as it should be performed as soon as possible. When surgery is not considered, appropriate conservative management can then be instigated. It may be fair to say that most surgeons would prescribe a short period of immobilization to assist the reduction of pain and swelling, followed by active mobilization and physiotherapy. However, when faced with the elite athlete or professional sportsperson who has sustained such an injury, the temptation may be to attempt surgical repair in the hope that it may effect a better long-term result despite the evidence to the contrary. The ideal solution for each individual case may be difficult to judge.

Whichever option is chosen, physiotherapy will be essential in the rehabilitation of athletes to their preinjury level of activity. A description of the types of treatment regimens utilized is described under principles of management.

Treatment of medial ligament injuries

Physiotherapy management of the athlete with a medial ligament injury is similar to that for a lateral ligament injury, but protection of the medial ligament in the acute stage requires a different application and style of bandaging or taping. It is usually sufficient to support the ankle in a neutral position rather than to attempt to hold the foot in inversion which may leave the lateral supporting structures vulnerable. Lateral pain and bruising may be caused by compression forces in an eversion injury and this should be differentiated from actual damage to the lateral ligament or fibular fracture. Where neither is present the emphasis is on ensuring that it is the medial side of the joint that is protected.

The severity of ligamentous and associated injuries will determine the need for a period of immobilization. Instability caused by disruption of the tibiofibular diastasis or fracture of the lateral malleolus will require rigid immobilization, either with plaster alone or open reduction, internal fixation and plaster.

In the post-acute and rehabilitation phases, treatment should aim at regaining range of movement, strengthening and re-education of proprioception. Progress may be slower for the athlete with a medial ligament injury, but with appropriate treatment and where there are no associated fractures or disruption to the diastasis, the long-term prognosis should be good.

Long-term complications of ankle injuries

Ankle sprains are notorious for providing ongoing complications and for their propensity to recur. Complications may be in part due to initial misdiagnosis or an underestimation of the severity of the injury.

Athletes may complain of ongoing pain, continued swelling, feelings of instability and stiffness (Bosien et al 1955, Harrington 1979, Freeman et al 1965, Freeman 1965, Anderson et al 1952). Impingement syndromes, peroneal nerve injury and peroneal tendon subluxation or dislocation may complicate the recovery from ankle sprain.

An ankle which has not regained full range of movement after injury will probably continue to have ongoing problems with pain and reinjury not only at the ankle, but may also produce problems in more proximal structures. The ankle needs to have a return of full dorsiflexion range to permit running and other sporting manoeuvres without subjecting adjacent structures to undue stress. Injured ligaments need to regain strength and sufficient mobility to support the joint on return to activity. This requires a rehabilitation program which will strengthen the ligaments by placing controlled stresses on the joint during exercise, and include mobilization of the ankle and subtalar joints to ensure that normal range of movement is regained.

Bosien et al (1955) followed a series of 133 ankle sprains over a period of 27 months and found residual symptoms in 33%, while 36% of the group was noted not to have sustained a recurrent injury to the same ankle. Objective changes in range of joint movement and muscle weakness were found in 60% of cases. Although their testing procedures for muscle strength are not now considered technically current, they felt they had determined a statistically significant incidence of peroneal muscle weakness. Freeman et al (1965) also describe a high incidence of a tendency for the ankle to 'give way' post-injury and suggested that this was due to motor unco-ordination following articular deafferentation. They hypothesized that the initial injury caused damage to nerve endings as well as to the ligament and capsule, and that this defect may be permanent. Anderson et al (1952) also noted the presence of long-term problems following ankle sprains and associated this with anteroposterior instability of the talus in the ankle mortise which may occur with rupture of the anterior talofibular ligament alone.

As discussed in more recent studies, however, accurate diagnosis and early instigation of the appropriate treatment would help to minimize long-term problems. DeCarlo and Talbot (1986) investigated ankle joint proprioception following injection of Xylocaine into the anterior talofibular ligaments of normal subjects. Although their study was not conclusive, their results showed a trend which would support the argument that it is possible to retrain proprioceptive deficits in athletes who have sustained an ankle injury.

McCarroll et al (1987) reported on a group of soccer players who presented with ongoing pain, swelling, locking and recurring sprains. Despite what was considered appropriate conservative treatment, no significant improvement was gained. Arthroscopy was performed on each of these athletes and in all cases a small band of tissue was found between the talus and the fibula in an anterolateral position. Although described as a meniscoid-like lesion, this tissue was thought to result from synovial thickening or inflammatory infiltrate, or to derive from a portion of the torn anterior talofibular ligament. The hypothesis that this meniscoid-like tissue contributed to the athletes' ongoing complaints was supported by the relief gained following its removal.

Arthroscopy may be worth considering when there is an ongoing specific complaint of catching or locking.

Syndromes such as this are addressed as impingement syndromes, and the athletes studied by McCarroll et al (1987) may well have suffered from anterolateral impingement syndromes.

Direct peroneal nerve damage is an uncommon complication of ankle sprain and may result in a temporary or permanent foot drop. More commonly an interference of the normal mechanisms of the peroneal nerve may occur following an inversion injury to the ankle (Butler 1991). This may be due to stretching of the nerve during injury or as a result of compromise to the nerve interface due to bleeding, oedema or scar tissue around the site of injury. The peroneal nerve may normally move 5-8 mm during full inversion (Reid 1992), but if the nerve is tethered and its movement restricted due to scarring or adhesions following such an injury, ongoing pain and dysfunction may ensue. Ankle rehabilitation should address this issue and including mobilizing the peroneal nerve in the treatment regimen may be worthwhile either by direct stretching or mobilization of the nerve at the site of entrapment or compromise. A useful method of stretching is to apply a plantarflexion/inversion stress during a straight leg raise. Care must be taken and the stretch should not be forceful (Butler 1991, Butler & Gifford 1989).

Chronic ankle instability

Physiotherapists are well aware of the problems relating to recurring injury to the ankle, particularly where there has been damage to the lateral ligament complex sufficient to cause joint instability. When there is ongoing instability within the joint which does not respond to conservative treatment, athletes may develop signs and symptoms of degenerative arthritis (Harrington 1979). When there is clinical instability, a reconstruction to restore the lateral stability may be indicated to avoid the delayed complication of osteoarthritis. Reconstruction will commonly involve the use of the peroneus brevis tendon in an Evans (Evans 1953) or modified Evans procedure which attempts to provide a replacement for the ATF ligament.

Observation of athletes following such a reconstruction has led some surgeons to the view that this procedure fails to provide functional stability and that an improved method of reconstruction to more closely replicate the damaged or torn ligament is required (Westh 1993, Dalziel 1993). This is particularly important to the athlete who will find it difficult to return to sport when the ankle reconstruction has provided stability at the cost of mobility. Alternative operative procedures such as a dynamic version of the Evans procedure have become popular. This involves the use of the peroneus brevis tendon which is resected from its passage behind the lateral malleolus and brought anteriorly through a soft tissue tunnel rather than a bony tunnel. This modified procedure is not as restrictive as the Evans procedure and should allow the athlete to regain full range of subtalar motion while stabilizing the ankle (Westh 1993).

Management of the ankle after reconstruction

Guidelines from the surgeon must be adhered to as the management of each case may differ depending on the surgical technique employed. An ankle reconstruction must allow the athlete to regain a high level of function post surgery and rehabilitation. The techniques utilized by the surgeon may differ slightly but the post-operative guidelines and timetable for rehabilitation will be similar to that noted below.

Early post-operative stage
- Athlete remains as an in-patient for 1-3 days.

Period of immobilization
- Temporary plaster for 1 week, stitches removed at 1 week.
- Fibreglass weightbearing cast for 4-6 weeks.
- Lace-up brace to restrict inversion and eversion for a period of time determined by the surgeon.

Physiotherapy
- During immobilization, maintaining range and strength of unaffected joints.
- Post-immobilization, principles of treatment as with any ankle injury while following surgeon's guidelines.
- Dorsiflexion/plantarflexion only at 6 weeks.
- Inversion/eversion commenced at 8 weeks.
- Proprioception and stretching activities commence at 8-10 weeks. Strengthening program including eccentric gradually increased.
- Running and specific skill training at 3 months
- Return to sport at 3-6 months.

In the management of the reconstructed ankle, it is essential to regain strength, proprioception and range of movement of the ankle and subtalar joints. It must be remembered, however, that the purpose of the surgery is to restore stability. The physiotherapist must not be overzealous with rehabilitation and thus jeopardize the reconstruction.

IMPINGEMENT SYNDROMES AROUND THE ANKLE

Anterior impingement syndrome

Sports which demand a full range of ankle dorsiflexion or plantarflexion may contribute to the development of an anterior impingement as the result of different mechanical forces. Catching in baseball, the demiplie in ballet, track and field sports or landing from a jump in Australian Rules football may all result in continued forced dorsiflexion and possible trauma to the anterior margins of the talus or tibia.

This trauma may produce scar tissue or stimulate the development of an exostosis at the anterior margin of the joint. Alternatively, forced plantarflexion in sports such as soccer where repetitive plantarflexion is required with kicking may also result in ongoing traction forces applied to the anterior capsule of the joint (Hardaker 1989, Hughs 1992). Exostoses will most commonly occur at the tibial margin of the joint.

In an anterior impingement syndrome, full dorsiflexion will be limited and painful due to the impingement of scar tissue or impingement of anterior joint structures by the exostosis.

Diagnosis

The initial symptom which would raise suspicion of the syndrome is a difficulty in assuming the fully dorsiflexed position required for the sport. This may be accompanied by poorly localized anterior ankle pain and later by anterior tenderness and swelling. Athletes with such symptoms whose sports require force at the extremes of ankle plantarflexion or dorsiflexion should be suspected of experiencing an impingement syndrome.

An exostosis may be felt by careful palpation with the ankle plantarflexed. Passively dorsiflexing the ankle, squatting or lunging may be painful and restricted. The restriction will be experienced as an anterior rather than posterior restriction such as an achilles stretch might produce. X-ray using a lateral view may reveal the exostoses. Lateral films of the ankle in a dorsiflexed weightbearing position may be necessary in some cases (Hardaker 1989, Hughs 1992).

Differential diagnosis

Restriction of ankle range of movement as a result of osteoarthritis or following a lateral ligament injury should be excluded. Talar dome fractures, osteochondritis dissecans, stress fractures of the neck of the talus and anterolateral compression syndromes may also present in a similar manner and should be excluded (Hughs 1992).

Treatment

Conservative management may include the use of a slight heel raise, restriction of activities requiring extreme dorsiflexion, icing and electrotherapy, passive mobilization techniques at the ankle joint and non-steroidal anti-inflammatory drugs (NSAIDs). Mobilization of dorsiflexion, anteroposterior glides of the talus or a combination of the two may gently stretch any scar tissue which has developed. Mobilization of plantarflexion may also be useful to stretch the anterior joint capsule and to help to dissipate scar tissue which will gain an improvement in the dorsiflexion range. Gentle frictions over the anterior capsule may also assist in reducing the scar tissue. The higher level athlete or dancer can be encouraged to continue a vigorous exercise program in the pool while resting from training.

Where conservative management fails, the option of surgery is considered. This involves excision of the exostosis, which can be performed arthroscopically (Hawkins 1988). Where athletes continue to stress their ankles, the condition is highly likely to recur within 3-4 years (Hardaker 1989, Hardaker et al 1985).

Posterior impingement syndrome

Often termed 'dancer's heel', this impingement occurs where the ankle is repetitively plantarflexed such as in demipointe and pointe in ballet or kicking in football, thus producing pain from the compression of structures at the posterior aspect of the ankle. In this case, the repetitive plantarflexion produces posterior ankle trauma as a result

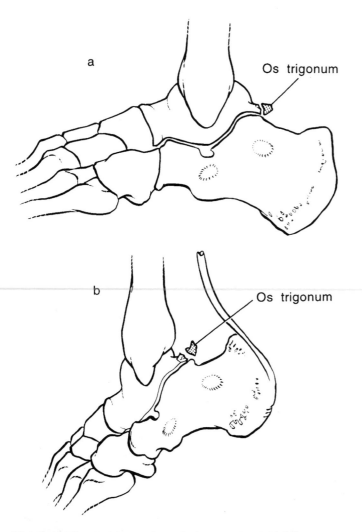

Fig. 32.10 The os trigonum shown in (a) neutral and (b) full plantarflexion.

of compressive forces rather than an anterior trauma as a result of traction forces. In extreme plantarflexion an impingement may be caused by an os trigonum (a prominent posterior tubercle of the talus), or the posterior process of the os calcis. The os trigonum is a small rounded process which may be present as a separate entity when the ossicle has failed to fuse. It is thought to be present in 8-13% of the population and is usually asymptomatic (Fig. 32.10a). With the forced action of plantarflexion, soft tissue structures may be compressed by the prominent posterior aspect of the os calcis causing inflammation, swelling and fibrosis (Fig. 32.10b) (Hughs 1992, Hardaker 1989, Hardaker et al 1985, Brodsky & Khalil 1987).

Diagnosis

The athlete will present with tenderness, swelling and occasionally crepitus in the posterolateral aspect of the ankle. Pain may be reproduced on plantarflexion but posterior pain may also be present on dorsiflexion. X-ray, bone scan and the use of local anaesthetic into the incriminated area may assist the diagnosis.

Differential diagnosis

The presence of achilles, peroneal or flexor hallucis longus tendonitis, retrocalcaneal bursitis, loose bodies and fractures must be excluded. There may be a degree of tendonitis present in association but careful localization of tenderness should clarify the structures involved.

Treatment

This is similar to that outline for anterior impingement syndrome, but the movement which is restricted is plantarflexion. Gentle mobilization of plantarflexion may assist, but care must be taken not to simply exacerbate the impingement. A posteroanterior glide of the talus may be of use, as may stretching into dorsiflexion. Where a conservative approach fails, surgery to excise the os trigonum and possibly release the sheath of the flexor hallucis longus, assisted by a month of rest, may resolve the symptoms.

Anterolateral impingement syndrome

Ferkel et al (1991) described a syndrome in athletes following lateral ligament injuries similar to the ongoing pain and recurrent sprains which McCarroll et al (1987) found in a group of soccer players. Ferkel et al (1991) found that athletes were presenting with chronic anterolateral ankle pain associated with a feeling of giving way or weakness, which they labelled as an anterolateral impingement.

Diagnosis

Impingement of this nature will present after an inversion injury in the post-acute or chronic stage. There may be local tenderness and swelling. X-ray may be of no value but MRI may reveal an increase in the soft tissue present in the lateral gutter. This gutter is an area bordered by the talus medially and the fibula laterally, running under the talofibular ligament posteriorly and the tibiofibular ligament anteriorly (Fig. 32.11). Following an inversion injury, this gutter may be the site for hypertrophy of damaged soft tissue. Arthroscopy may be used both as a diagnostic tool and to provide access for treatment.

Differential diagnosis

Chronic ankle instability, osteochondral lesions of the talus, peroneal subluxation or tendinitis, tarsal coalition, anterior impingement and degenerative joint disease may all mimic some of these symptoms and need to be excluded.

Treatment

As McCarroll et al (1987) found, the ultimate diagnosis and treatment can be performed with the arthroscope which allows the surgeon to debride the hypertrophic soft tissue (Ferkel et al 1991). This is followed by a period of rest and graduated return to sport after 6 weeks. Conservative treatment as outlined in anterior and posterior impingements can be trialled initially but may be found to be of little value. Where arthroscopic debridement has been performed, it may be wise to protect the joint for a longer period and continue touch weightbearing for a period of 8

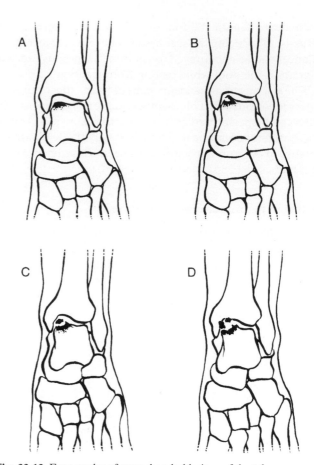

Fig. 32.12 Four grades of osteochondral lesions of the talus.
Grade I: a small area of subchondral compression
Grade II: a partially detached fragment
Grade III: a completely detached fragment remaining in position
Grade IV: a fragment that is loose to the joint. Adapted from Canale & Belding (1980)

weeks to encourage regeneration of good quality fibro-cartilage (Hawkins 1988).

OSTEOCHONDRAL LESIONS OF THE TALUS

Osteochondral lesions, transchondral talar dome fractures and osteochondritis diseccans of the talus are all terms used to describe lesions of the talar dome. There are few cases of primary osteochondritis diseccans (as in the knee); the majority of cases result from trauma. Various authors have investigated the phenomenon and reported that up to 98% of lateral talar dome lesions and 70% of medial talar dome lesions were directly related to trauma (Flick & Gould 1985, Canale & Belding 1980, Alexander & Lichtman 1980). The injury itself can be classified into stages, where in stage I there is a small area of subchondral compression, in stage II there is a partially detached fragment, in stage III the fragment is completely detached but remains in position and in stage IV the fragment is loose within the joint (Fig. 32.12) (Canale & Belding 1980). Flick and Gould (1985) report that the lateral dome lesions probably occur with inversion injuries to the

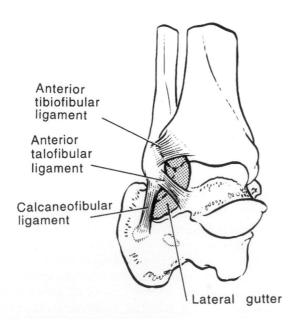

Anterior tibiofibular ligament

Anterior talofibular ligament

Calcaneofibular ligament

Lateral gutter

Fig. 32.11 Position of the lateral gutter. Adapted from Ferkel et al (1991)

ankle where the ankle is dorsiflexed, while medial dome lesions occur with a plantarflexion, external rotation force.

Diagnosis

The condition is often misdiagnosed as a pure ankle sprain, and it may not be until symptoms persist for some months that further investigation may reveal the correct pathology. Such a condition should be suspected and investigated where there has been a history of a severe inversion injury (Flick & Gould 1985) and there are ongoing symptoms of pain, swelling, locking, catching, crepitus, stiffness or giving way.

Investigations include X-ray, perhaps in varying degrees of inversion or plantarflexion, tomography, MRI, CT, bonescan and arthroscopy (Alexander & Lichtman 1980, Sartoris et al 1990).

Differential diagnosis

Impingement syndromes, ankle ligament injuries, stress fractures of the neck of the talus and degenerative joint disease all need to be excluded.

Treatment

As most studies have revealed that a delay in surgical intervention does not appear to affect the long-term results, it is recommended that conservative treatment be trialled in stage I and II injuries. This would include a period of non-weightbearing in a cast, brace or compression bandage for 6 weeks, or in some cases active exercise and electro-therapy with restricted weightbearing. If symptoms persist after a trial of conservative treatment, surgical excision and curettage of the lesion should be carried out (Canale & Belding 1980). Flick and Gould (1985) recommend surgery for all stage IV lesions, with trials of conservative treatment for stages I to III, while Alexander and Lichtman (1980), who studied a population of young fit service personnel, recommended surgical intervention in all patients of athletic inclination who demonstrated ligament instability. Fol-lowing surgery, the patient will be restricted to a period of non-weightbearing of at least 6 weeks during which time active exercise is encouraged.

TENDON INJURIES AROUND THE ANKLE

The tibialis posterior is the most deeply placed muscle of the flexor group, originating from the posterior tibia and interosseus membrane and lying directly behind the posteromedial border of the tibia which it follows to the tip of the medial malleous. It becomes tendinous in the lower quarter of the leg and distally its tendon runs directly to the tuberosity of the navicular into which it inserts, sending additional slips to the tarsal bones. The muscle is active during midstance to prevent the foot from everting past the neutral position (Alexander 1990).

In the action of toe raise, the tibialis posterior is activated first to lock the rearfoot and provide a rigid structure for the manoeuvre while activation of the gastrocnemius completes the procedure (Johnson & Strom 1989). The tibialis posterior is essential to allow toe raising while maintaining the foot in inversion and this may be shown to be weak or painful in the presence of pathology or impossible in the case of rupture of the tendon.

Tenosynovitis of the tibialis posterior tendon

This condition will involve the tendon just posterior or inferior to the medial malleolus. It may occur after local injury, as a result of overuse, in conjunction with in-appropriate footwear or as a complication of pes planus.

Diagnosis

The tendon is subject to inflammation in sports and activities involving toe raising, jumping or propulsion from a toe raised position. Vulnerable athletes include those involved in track and field events, ballet dancers, basket-ballers and footballers.

An accurate history must be obtained and assessment of foot posture and gait performed.

Examination should reveal tenderness localized over the course of the tendon while pain may be noted on resisted inversion, adduction and slight dorsiflexion. The tendon may be passively stretched by everting the foot while palpating posterior to the medial malleolus for crepitus and tenderness. Alternatively, in standing stretching of the tendon in a lunge position where the knee is flexed but the foot remains in contact with the ground, there may be some pain. Swelling along the course of the tendon adjacent to the medial malleolus may also assist the diagnosis.

If the condition progresses, signs may become more obvious as the tendon becomes more elongated and the rearfoot more mobile. Viewing the foot posture in weight-bearing will show the rearfoot to be more pronated with the foot in abduction. If the tendon ruptures, there may be less pain, but the dysfunction and deformity will be more obvious. Despite this, rupture of the tibialis posterior tendon is unfortunately often missed or misdiagnosed. Where doubt of the diagnosis remains, X-ray or MRI may be of some assistance (Sartoris et al 1990).

Differential diagnosis

The presence of rheumatoid arthritis or seronegative spondyloarthropathies needs to be excluded. Tarsal coalition, spastic flat feet, tarsal tunnel syndrome, Achilles tendonitis or rupture and simple ankle sprain should also be excluded. Referred pain from the lumbar spine or involvement of the dura should also be considered in the assessment of foot and ankle pain.

Treatment

Treatment of tendinitis may consist of rest, ice and NSAIDs in the acute stage. If the condition is particularly severe, restricted weightbearing with crutches for up to 3 weeks may be appropriate. Assessment of the causative factors by careful examination and history will assist in modifying contributing factors.

Ultrasound, laser therapy and gentle stretching may also be of assistance with the inclusion of some heating prior to stretching as the condition becomes less acute (Reid 1992, Frieder et al 1988). Return to training should be dependent on the subjective and objective response to treatment and rest. When crepitus and swelling have subsided and there is no pain on palpation, stretch or toe raise, the athlete may begin light running. This should be limited to work on a good track with corrective footwear and the use of orthotics as prescribed. Initially training sessions should be followed by icing for 10-15 minutes. Stretches must be performed pre and post-training in a 'lunge' type position. Exercise in a swimming pool should be encouraged to maintain fitness in the recuperative period, but care should be taken as the kick involved with freestyle or breaststroke may sometimes aggravate the condition.

In the chronic case where conservative treatment is deemed to have failed, surgery may be considered. Where the surgeon discovers the pathology to be that of a peritendonitis, the treatment is to open the tendon sheath along its entire length with the exception of a 1 cm pulley behind the medial malleolus. A synovectomy is performed and the tendon debrided if appropriate or 'debulked' if it appears particularly enlarged. Small tears may be sutured. Post-operatively the athlete will be rested in a weightbearing cast for 3 weeks. If the injury is particularly severe, the tendon may be substituted by the flexor digitorum longus via tendon transfer without a great sacrifice of function (Johnson & Strom 1989).

Flexor hallucis longus tendinitis

This is a condition mainly occurring in classical ballet dancers where a position of extreme plantarflexion is required, the flexor hallucis longus acting as a primary stabilizer of the medial foot and ankle. Prolonged stress to the tendon can cause inflammation and partial tears. Predisposition to this injury can occur with the dancer who has a distally placed muscular belly of the flexor hallucis longus which allows it to impact into the entrance of its fibro-osseous canal (Hardaker 1989, Hardaker et al 1985).

Poor technique in dancers may also contribute to the problem. Allowing the foot to roll in during demipointe or fullpointe will further stretch the tendon and contribute to the pathology. If the condition is allowed to progress, nodules may form within the tendon substance which may impact at the entrance to the tendon's fibro-osseous canal or cause tethering within the sheath, producing a triggering of the great toe or a functional hallux rigidus (Hardaker 1989, Hardaker et al 1985).

Diagnosis

This condition should be suspected when a dancer presents with a history of pain and swelling posterior to the medial malleolus. Crepitus and pain over the tendon sheath may be felt while flexing and extending the great toe. Pain may also be reproduced on toe raise or with resisted flexion of the great toe.

Differential diagnosis

Tibialis posterior tenosynovitis and true hallux rigidus should be excluded.

Treatment

Treatment for any tenosynovitis will follow similar principles in which rest, ice, NSAIDs, and electrotherapy may be useful. With dancers, it is necessary to restrict the practice of demipointe and fullpointe until the condition settles. The dancer may continue to practise these activities and other barre exercises in the pool.

In severe cases, surgical release of the tendon followed by a short period of immobilization is indicated.

Tenosynovitis of the peroneal tendons

This condition most often affects the peroneus longus alone, but can affect both the peroneus longus and brevis simultaneously. Resultant swelling will fill the space behind the lateral malleolus and may be noted along the length of the tendon. Tenderness can be found on palpation and will help to identify the tendon involved. The insertions of the two tendons are quite separate: the peroneus brevis to the base of the fifth metatarsal and peroneus longus posterior to it running to the plantar aspect of the foot through a groove in the cuboid to insert into the plantar aspect of the base of the first metatarsal (Alexander 1990). The condition can be aggravated by an increase in activity which requires the strong action of the peroneals and is commonly described, for example, in figure skaters (McLennan 1980). It may also occur in association with other pathologies such as a cuboid syndrome.

Diagnosis

This is usually clear when athletes present with a history of swelling, pain and possibly crepitus. They will describe a pattern of activity which may have predisposed them to the condition. This might include an increase in training or activity involving directional changes in running, training on a slope or camber, change of footwear, or an initial minor sprain of the ankle. Examination will demonstrate signs localized to the peroneal tendons with palpation, while stretch into plantarflexion, adduction and inversion (peroneus brevis) or dorsiflexion, adduction and inversion (peroneus longus) may be restricted and painful. Resisted activity of the peroneals will also produce pain, either in resisted eversion (peroneus brevis predominantly) or in toe raising (peroneus longus predominantly).

Stenosing peroneal tenosynovitis has been described as a condition of inflammation of the peroneal tendons in which a 'snapping' sensation on ankle movement may be described. This is most probably caused by thickening or restriction within the tendon sheath (Andersen 1987).

Differential diagnosis

Careful examination and an accurate history should exclude isolated lateral ligament injuries, cuboid syndrome, subluxing or dislocating peroneal tendons or achilles tendonitis.

The peroneal muscles and tendons may be injured in association with a lateral ligament injury and, as previously mentioned, this may be evident on arthrography. Inflammation, pain and stenosis within the tendon sheath are possible results if not adequately addressed in the acute stages.

Treatment

The mode of treatment in this condition is as outlined for tibialis posterior tendonitis. The principles of rest, correction of predisposing or contributing factors, ice, stretches, NSAIDs and electrotherapy are all considered. Where mechanical correction at the foot is necessary, the athlete should be assessed for orthotics. In the case of stenosing peroneal tenosynovitis, as with chronic tenosynovitis, surgery to release the tendon sheath and debridement of the tendon may be considered.

Subluxation and dislocation of the peroneal tendons

This painful condition most commonly occurs following an inversion injury. Certain anatomical variations around the peroneal groove may predispose to its occurrence, and the condition may therefore be bilateral. Both tendons may be involved, although the peroneus brevis may be more commonly at fault due to its more anterior placement behind the lateral malleous. The athlete may describe a popping or snapping sensation associated with swelling and tenderness posterior to the fibular malleolus. The specific sporting endeavours most likely to cause the condition are ice skating, skiing and soccer.

Diagnosis

The usual mechanism of the dislocation is a sudden forceful and passive dorsiflexion of the inverted foot against contraction of the peroneals. The athlete may have a history of a inversion injury to that ankle in the past. Spontaneous relocation will often occur after an episode of dislocation. Athletes may complain of a sensation that the tendons are 'slipping' out, or dislocating, and may be able to demonstrate this. Palpation of the site will be tender. Pain is present when manual reproduction of the mechanism of injury, that is resisted dorsiflexion and inversion, is performed. Care should be taken with this manoeuvre as it may cause the tendons to dislocate or sublux with a distinct 'pop'. This sign can be difficult to elicit and is not required for a definitive diagnosis. X-ray may reveal a small avulsion fracture at the lateral edge of the malleolus (McLennan 1980).

Differential diagnosis

It is important to determine that the tendons are in fact subluxing or dislocating and to differentiate this from a tendonitis or stenosing tenosynovitis.

Treatment

Conservative treatment is again the initial choice. In the acute stage, the ankle is strapped, incorporating padding posterior and inferior to the lateral malleolus. Nonweightbearing for 3 weeks is suggested. McLennan (1980) found this to be successful in 88% of cases he reviewed. With athletes who have been shown to dislocate, the need for surgical intervention may be evident and the surgical procedure would be a reconstruction of the retinaculum or deepening of the groove. Surgery is followed by a period of approximately 6 weeks non-weightbearing in a cast followed by 6 months of ankle taping and intensive therapy to strengthen and re-educate the ankle in a fashion similar to that following a lateral ligament injury.

Extensor tendinitis

The extensor tendons over the anterior aspect of the ankle can be subject to inflammation as a result of inappropriate footwear or excessively tight laces. With an increase in sporting activity, consequent overuse of the tibialis anterior in particular may be associated with inflammation around the tendon. The tibialis anterior is the prime antigravity muscle of the foot, controlling foot slap at heel strike with its strong eccentric action.

Diagnosis

This should be straightforward when the athlete complains of localized pain and tenderness. There may be associated swelling. The pain may be reproduced on resisted contraction or stretching of the tendons at fault. The site of pain and the lack of crepitus will assist in differentiation from tenosynovitis which would occur within the tendon sheaths.

Treatment

To determine where the problem lies, the athlete must be questioned as to a change in training routines or footwear. Appropriate management may be as simple as altering the method of tying the laces (i.e. looser, with the bow on the side or using elastic laces) or may call for more significant changes to training, including an eccentric strengthening program of the affected muscle group (see Ch. 10).

HEEL PAIN

Heel pain in the athlete can be a challenging diagnosis. It may derive from local conditions or from a referred source.

Local syndromes and conditions which commonly cause pain in and around the heel include plantar fasciitis, stress fractures, retrocalcaneal disorders and fat pad syndrome.

Due to the large number of local and referred or systemic causes of heel pain, the differential diagnosis is complex. Referred or systemic causes must always be considered when addressing the problem of heel pain in the athlete.

Differential diagnosis

The location and nature of the heel pain will help to determine the exact diagnosis, as will careful questioning about factors provoking the pain and about activities or circumstances which may have contributed to the onset.

Physiotherapists should be alert to the systemic disorders which may present with heel pain and the initial questioning of the athlete must address this possibility. For example, where symptoms are bilateral, inflammatory conditions such as ankylosing spondylitis and psoriatic arthritis must be considered. Further investigation may be necessary if suspicion is aroused by a description of early morning stiffness, deterioration in general health, tiredness or a recent viral infection. Reiter's disease, an inflammatory disease which may occur as a sequel to a venereal infection, can cause asymmetric intense synovitis peripherally, often resulting in a painful heel. Approximately 33% of sufferers will also present with sacroiliitis, and this finding will alert the astute examiner. It would then be necessary to refer to a medical practitioner for further investigation.

The presence of referred pain of spinal origin should also be considered, and examination of the spine should be included when appropriate. Tibial nerve entrapment in the posterior tarsal tunnel may also give rise to symptoms resembling plantar fasciitis and the inclusion of a sensitizing dorsiflexion/eversion component to a straight leg raise test may assist the differential diagnosis (Butler 1991).

When the diagnosis is not clear despite an extensive subjective and objective examination, it may be necessary to consider the possibility of a local tumour. Although rare in the calcaneum, heel pain which is vague, not responding to treatment and causing night pain should be investigated with X-ray and bone scan. The examiner might also consider osteomyelitis as a cause of the symptoms and these investigations will help to identify it if present.

Synovitis of the subtalar joint or hypomobility of the joint should also be considered as they can affect the mechanics of the area, resulting in referred pain to the heel or midtarsal region (Corrigan & Maitland 1983, Harbison 1987).

Plantar fasciitis

The syndrome of plantar fasciitis has also been described as the painful heel syndrome, subcalcaneal pain, medial arch sprain, stone bruise, calcaneal periostitis and calcaneodynia (Leach et al 1986). Lutter (1986) found that plantar fasciitis was aggravated by running or jogging in 76% of athetes studied. 52% were deemed to overpronate, while 42% were considered to have pes cavus. The plantar fascia spans the arch of the foot and runs from the medial tubercle of the calcaneus to blend distally with the soft tissues of the metatarsophalangeal (MTP) joint complex, anchoring into the phalangeal bases. Relaxation of the fascia in stance allows the foot to accommodate to variable surfaces, while in toe-off extension of the MTP joints allows the 'windlass' effect to provide a rigid base for the foot (Reid 1992). While the flat or pronated foot may predispose an individual to plantar fasciitis by allowing stresses to transfer to the fascia, it is also suggested that the rigid cavus foot through decreased accommodation to surfaces in stance phase may be less able to absorb ground reaction forces, thus also stressing the plantar fascia (Leach et al 1986, Lutter 1986).

Diagnosis

Athletes will present with pain at the attachment of the fascia to the medial tubercle of the calcaneum. The pain will often be most severe with the first few steps in the morning. Athletes may also describe increased pain on commencing athletic activity, but this may settle to some extent and they will be able to work through the pain. Walking, running, sprinting, hill running and jumping will all exacerbate the pain (Leach et al 1986, Harbison 1987). To lessen the stress on the fascia, athletes may attempt to walk or run in a supinated posture (Leach et al 1986).

Palpation will reveal tenderness at the insertion of the fascia into the calcaneum and pain may radiate distally along the medial border of the foot. There may be some swelling or the presence of a nodule within the fascia. Active toe raise or passive dorsiflexion may reproduce the symptoms. X-rays may reveal the presence of a calcaneal spur, but this is also known to be a common asymptomatic incidental finding. Spurs are thought to occur as a result of traction. They may in some cases contribute to the symptoms but are not the main cause.

Treatment

Conservative treatment will include a period of rest. The athlete should rest from running or at least curtail sprinting, hill running and jumping. Aerobic fitness can be maintained by exercise in the pool or cycling. Stretching the plantar fascia regularly, particularly before and after activity, is essential. This can be done in a lunge position with the toes dorsiflexed against a wall, or passively by self manual stretching incorporating toe extension while in a cross-legged sitting position. Electrotherapy modalities such as ultrasound may be of use, and electrogalvanic stimulation is often prescribed or recommended. While galvanic stimulation is useful when muscle weakness is a primary problem and assistance to gain active contraction is necessary, it may not assist in treatment when the primary problem is one of mechanics unrelated to muscle weakness.

Active exercises to strengthen the intrinsic muscles and to assist in the correction of foot posture are useful. These may include sitting with a towel under the foot and 'bunching' the towel with the toes, progressing to add a small weight on the towel. Actively attempting to increase the height of the arch while keeping the heel and the first MTP joint still and in contact with the supporting surface will assist in strengthening and re-educating foot posture. This exercise can be progressed to be performed in standing. Rolling the foot over a jar and using the toes to pick up small objects are also useful early exercises to be done in sitting. Walking, bouncing, jogging and jumping on a trampett are more advanced strengthening, re-educative, functional exercises. The rocker board can also be employed in a strengthening program.

A shoe pad or cup for the heel (Seder 1987) can assist in pain relief. When the heel is very sensitive to touch and aggravated by compression rather than traction on the fascia, a doughnut shaped piece of felt or other material can be used to relieve pressure on the painful spot. Taping on the plantar surface of the foot can also help (Fig. 32.17). The method of application is to tape from the level of the MTP joints around behind the heel, back under the foot to the opposite side. The taping is from medial to lateral, then lateral to medial and so on to provide support to the arch (Kosmahl & Kosmahl 1987).

When an acute injury begins to settle, the athlete can be advised on a gradual return to sport. If the pain is severe and conservative treatment has failed, consideration may be given to local injection with corticosteroid (Harbison 1987) or to surgery in which the fascia may be stripped or the spur excised (Leach et al 1986). The role of the spur in the painful heel may need to be carefully explained to athletes who may believe that it is a simple problem which could easily be rectified by surgical removal of the spur. They need to be aware that the spur has probably occurred as a result of their condition and may be contributing only in a minor way to the pain.

Sever's disease

This condition is a traction apophysitis similar to Osgood-Schlatter's disease in the knee. It occurs at the calcaneal apophysis usually from the ages of 10-15 years, is more common in boys and may be associated with repetitive jumping.

Diagnosis

This is difficult as X-ray findings may be equivocal, however the condition should be considered in young athletes who present with heel pain, particularly if they have been involved in jumping sports such as gymnastics, Australian rules football or basketball. The use of flimsy or inappropriate shoes may also be a contributing factor.

Treatment

The most important aspect of treatment is rest and prescription of appropriate footwear. Training should be decreased substantially and all jumping avoided until the symptoms have settled completely.

Calcaneal ethesiopathy

Repetitive microtrauma at the attachment of the achilles tendon can cause the development of a spur extending from the calcaneum into the tendon. This disorder may be associated with a varus deformity of the rearfoot. The athlete will complain of local pain and tenderness, which can be exacerbated by shoes which exert pressure over the tendo achilles attachment.

Diagnosis

The spur can be visualized on X-ray and may be tender to touch. There may be no swelling unless there is associated bursitis or achilles tendonitis. Due to the local trauma there may be pain on stretching the achilles tendon or with jumping or toe raising on the affected leg.

Treatment

Initially a period of rest and local treatment of ice or ultrasound may be of help. NSAIDs can be trialled. Extreme care should be taken if steroid injection is considered because of the proximity of the achilles tendon. Padding may assist in reducing pressure to the area. A felt pad cut into a U shape and applied to the heel will divert the pressure away from the painful area.

In chronic cases where pain and incapacity are considerable, excision of the exostosis may be successful.

Pump bump

This condition is similar to that of calcaneal ethesiopathy, but is descriptive of the presence of the bony enlargement with associated inflammation of the overlying bursa.

The posterosuperior lateral portion of the calcaneum may be particularly prominent in some individuals through congenital variation, or may be acquired after trauma or from pressure of footwear.

Diagnosis

As with calcaneal ethesiopathy, the athlete will complain of local tenderness especially with the added pressure of footwear. There will be associated swelling which may be quite pronounced, and the skin over the area may be red. The condition may be unilateral or bilateral.

Treatment

Treatment should follow that outlined for calcaneal ethesiopathy with careful attention to the use of appropriate sporting and leisure shoes with padding to reduce pressure over the painful area.

Retrocalcaneal bursitis

When this bursa becomes inflamed, there will be symmetrical swelling at the heel around the distal portion of the achilles tendon. There may be an associated exostosis ('pump bump'). The bursitis is usually related to repetitive trauma or inappropriate footwear.

The athlete will complain of local heel pain, which may occur without the added pressure of shoes. When inflamation is substantial, there may be pronounced pain and associated heat and redness.

Diagnosis

The finding of palpable symmetrical swelling will implicate the bursa while achilles tendonitis can be differentiated by pain and tenderness 3-4 cm proximal to the insertion of the tendon, commonly with the presence of crepitus.

Treatment

The principles of treatment are similar to those for calcaneal ethesiopathy and pump bump. Correct footwear, padding,

rest, ice and other local treatment may produce relief. NSAIDs and injection may also be considered.

Fat pad syndromes

The heel pad is a particularly precise structure consisting of fat columns in vertical alignment, controlled by elastic tissue. The structure is like honeycomb, and can withstand great stress but, once severely damaged, may lose its original properties (Miller 1982).

Injury to the fat pad may damage the septa of fibrous tissue responsible for providing a type of hydraulic pressure within the fat columns. If injured, the septa lose their shape and the columns of fat bulge laterally and lose their ability to cushion the heel effectively.

Athletes who participate in an excessive amount of jumping, running or gymnastics may be particularly at risk of injury. Overweight, underweight or middle-aged athletes are at greater risk because of the increased stress on the heel with obesity, and a less resilient heel pad in the underweight or middle-aged athlete. Training on hard surfaces with poor shoes and training on uneven ground or increased hill work may also be predisposing factors and the middle to long distance runner is therefore vulnerable. Overlarge shoe size can aggravate the condition by allowing sheering forces to the heel, and the appropriate shoe size as well as style must be examined.

A single traumatic incident such as jarring the heel or landing from a jump onto the heel can damage the fat pad and result in a severe injury with a long time to full recovery. The fat pad can also be injured in association with an ankle or calcaneal fracture.

Diagnosis

Adequate history and localization of tenderness will assist in diagnosis. The localization of the painful area should avoid confusion with conditions of retrocalcaneal pain or plantar fasciitis. Consideration must be given to the possibility of calcaneal stress fracture, and radiography performed if necessary.

Hopping, heel walking or pounding the calcaneum may also reproduce the athlete's pain.

Treatment

Rest from the aggravating activity and from running should be instigated. NSAIDs and electrotherapy may be of some use. Correction of inappropriate footwear is essential. Taping the heel in a basketweave style can offer some support to the fat pad to prevent bulging, and may offer symptomatic relief.

Assessment for orthotics may be worthwhile if this treatment does not offer sufficient relief. Simple orthotic treatment would usually consist of a heel cup.

The fat pad is notoriously slow to improve from injury and many months of rest may be necessary for what the athlete may have initially thought to be a simple bruised heel.

CONDITIONS OF THE MIDFOOT

Tarsal coalition

Tarsal coalition is the result of restricted movement between two or more of the bones of the rearfoot. This is caused by a congenital fibrous, cartilaginous or bony union between the adjacent involved joints, usually at the calcaneonavicular or talocalcaneal areas, and less commonly at the talonavicular area (Percy & Mann 1988). Recent studies suggest that the condition is much more common than had been previously recognized as it may often be asymptomatic. Snyder et al (1981) found 65% of ankle sprains occurring in athletics showed some degree of calcaneal navicular coalition.

The presentation generally occurs during the athlete's second decade. The athlete will complain of mild pain deep in the subtalar joint and of foot stiffness. Symptoms will be exacerbated by activity and relieved by rest. Exercise involving activity over rough ground or twisting and turning will be particularly aggravating (Mosier & Asher 1984).

Young athletes will commonly present with an acute ankle sprain or a history of repeated ankle sprains. The subtalar joint acts as a shock absorber of ground reaction forces while allowing inversion and eversion. This function is lost in athletes with coalition, thus predisposing them to injury. As the coalition restricts motion in the rearfoot, forceful motion beyond the restricted range may result in ligamentous injuries to the ankle (Snyder et al 1981).

Diagnosis

The diagnosis is based on a history of recurrent ankle sprains, loss of subtalar motion on examination, persistent pain in the foot or ankle and positive findings on X-ray, tomograms or CT (Morgan & Crawford 1986). The coalition may be familial and is often bilateral.

Palpation over the area of the middle talocalcaneal facet just distal to the medial malleolus may produce tenderness. The rearfoot may be valgus in weightbearing, and there may be associated flat feet (Mosier & Asher 1984).

Differential diagnosis

Inflammatory disease, simple ankle sprain, osteochondral lesions of the talus and simple flat feet should be excluded.

Treatment

Initial treatment with rest, orthoses or a cast can be attempted and may provide relief. However, the adolescent athlete who continues to be active in sport may suffer ongoing pain and ankle sprains. Surgery should be con-sidered in these cases or where conservative management has failed. The procedure is to locate and excise the bar, but this must be performed while the athlete is still in early adolescence. In the older athlete with significant dysfunction and considerable pain, a triple arthrodesis may be the only surgical option (Mosier & Asher 1984).

After excision of the bar the athlete will be rested in a short cast, usually for 2 weeks, then allowed to commence active movements, but with restriction of weightbearing for 6 weeks.

Spastic flat feet

The presence of tarsal coalition may be accompanied by the presence of peroneal muscle spasm and there may be shortening of the achilles tendon. Spasm can occur in an intermittent pattern aggravated by activity, or it may be more persistent and prevent correction of the foot deformity (Harris & Beath 1948).

The presence of peroneal spasm can pose some difficulties in treating the young athlete who presents with a tarsal coalition. After surgery, it will be essential to re-educate the peroneals and this should be successful when the spasm is intermittent or present only in weightbearing or in response to pain.

Cuboid syndrome

Athletes who present with lateral instep or lateral arch pain, particularly those involved in running sports, may have experienced subluxation of the cuboid. This is caused by a sprain of the ligaments or capsule of the calcaneocuboid or metatarsal-cuboid joint, allowing a positional change between the cuboid and calcaneum. The stability of the cuboid is partly ruled by the position of the rearfoot whereby overpronation of the foot during gait allows the cuboid and the lateral column to dorsiflex, evert and abduct in relation to the rearfoot. This can lead to a sprain of the supporting ligaments of the cuboid, allowing the foot to become unstable. Pain on weightbearing will ensue (Parks 1988).

Diagnosis

Athletes presenting with this syndrome will describe a dull deep pain at the lateral aspect of the foot, but may also describe severe sharp pain if involved in twisting or unguarded movements. Pain will be precipitated by running, particularly on hard surfaces and in unsupportive shoes. Pain is relieved in non-weightbearing unless there is significant inflammation. Initial weightbearing in the morning may be very painful as the soft tissue structures around the cuboid are subject to initial overstretching.

On examination there will be pain on the dorsal aspect of the foot over the cuboid and its joint lines. Range of movement should be full, but weightbearing will elicit the pain. Walking on the toes may relieve this pain as it will allow the foot to supinate.

Differential diagnosis

There may be associated tendonitis of the peroneals as they struggle to support the foot, but this should not be confused with the primary diagnosis. Ankle sprain, sinus tarsi syndrome and stress fracture should be excluded.

Treatment

The subluxation of the cuboid needs to be reduced, and this is best done with the athlete lying prone (Fig. 32.13). The foot is held in plantarflexion with the fingers on the dorsum and the thumbs over the plantar aspect of the cuboid. Gentle movements to massage the arch of the foot will assist relaxation, while the foot is forced into plantarflexion with thumbs applying further pressure over the cuboid. Subluxation back to the correct position should provide a palpable result. The accompanying click with this manoeuvre has been suggested to be the resumption of the peroneus longus tendon into its groove under the cuboid, the assumption being that it has been displaced from this position as the cuboid subluxed (Parks 1988). Immediate relief on weightbearing should be noted. In the acute stages, pain relief can be assisted by icing, ultrasound and supportive taping under the cuboid. A small heel lift may assist by reducing the effect of the achilles tendon which tends to pull the foot into pronation, and will allow the foot to supinate, thus reducing the subluxing force on the cuboid.

Prevention of a recurrence is assisted by the use of a small felt pad under the cuboid on the plantar surface, prescribed orthotics to resist pronation, appropriate

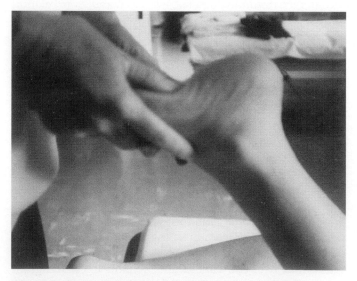

Fig. 32.13 Hand position for reduction of a subluxed cuboid.

footwear and restriction of running on hard surfaces. Addressing abnormal foot mechanics which have predisposed the athlete to the condition is essential, and an appropriate exercise routine should be installed together with the use of permanent orthotics and revision of training programs.

Osteochondritis of the navicular

Also referred to as Kohler's disease, this is a rare condition which presents in children, usually between the ages of three and 8. The diagnosis is worth considering in the very young athlete who presents with a limp and pain in the midtarsal region.

Diagnosis

There may be some swelling and tenderness over the navicular. X-ray will show sclerosis and a squashed appearance of the navicular.

Treatment

The disease is generally self-limiting, but a short period of protection may be necessary for pain relief. This may include a below-knee plaster for up to 6 weeks, or simply an arch support in the shoe. Long-term degenerative problems are a possibility, but are not usual (Corrigan & Maitland 1983).

FRACTURES IN THE FOOT

Stress fractures

Stress fractures can occur in any bone of the foot, but most commonly involve the second or third metatarsals. This predilection is probably due to the relative immobility of those rays (Hardaker et al 1985). These fractures occur mostly in adults, usually in response to the commencement of physical activity or after a significant increase in the athlete's training program. These bones are subject to considerable stress in weightbearing and to forces from attaching musculature. If the inherent strength of the bone is exceeded by these forces, a fracture will occur (Quirk 1987a, Quirk 1993).

Several factors may contribute to these stress fractures, including poor technique in a sporting activity, overtraining, inappropriate footwear, exercising on poor surfaces, the presence of foot abnormalities or foot surgery (Quirk 1987a, Hontas et al 1986).

Diagnosis

Athletes will complain of vague pain associated with activity and, as the condition progresses, will note that the pain occurs earlier in the activity. Progression may see pain beginning to occur at rest. Examination generally does not reveal loss of range of movement in adjacent joints, and all active movements are usually pain free. More strenuous activity such as hopping or jumping may reproduce pain, but in early stages may still be pain free. Palpation over the affected bone may be tender and warm in the more advanced stages, and callus formation may be felt if remodelling is occurring. Palpation over the area in the early stages may be unrevealing.

X-rays are appropriate, but may be negative in the early stages. Bone scan is considered the definitive diagnostic tool, but the use of CT scan and MRI is becoming more popular.

Differential diagnosis

This is dependent on the site of the stress fracture, but care must be taken when there is a complaint of vague pain. There should always be a suspicion of fracture, but the possibility of tumour must also be considered and investigated with diagnostic procedures such as plain X-ray, bone scan, CT scan or MRI.

Referred pain from the lumbar spine and the presence of inflammatory disease should also be considered and investigated. Differentiation in these cases will be assisted by the athlete's history and localization of the pain.

Treatment

Rest is essential. This may need to be emphasized regularly with the high level athlete who may be tempted to resume activity too early. A period of non-weightbearing may be introduced, or it may be sufficient to simply refrain from the specific causative activity. The treatment of choice depends on the site of the fracture.

Navicular stress fractures

Stress fractures of the navicular are now thought more common than previously reported (Hunter 1981, Khan 1992). They result most often from sports involving sprinting, jumping or hurdling.

The athlete will complain of pain during activity but this will often settle quickly with rest. Diagnosis is assisted by a careful history and by a finding of tenderness to palpation directly over the navicular at the point of fracture. Suspicion of a stress fracture would call for radiological investigation. Bone scan is thought to be the most revealing diagnostic modality while plain X-ray, as with most stress fractures, may be of little value in the acute stages. Khan (1992) recommends CT scanning for athletes with a positive bone scan to confirm and evaluate the fracture. He feels this provides a better understanding of the position and state of the fracture.

Navicular fractures are notoriously slow to unite due to the relatively avascular central portion of the bone (Torg et

al 1982). It is therefore important to diagnose the fracture early and promptly instigate correct treatment. The treatment of choice is to rest the athlete in a non-weight-bearing cast for 6 weeks. The cast is then removed and the tender spot on the navicular reassessed. If the area remains tender, the cast should be reapplied for a further 2 weeks. Thereafter, a graduated return to activity is encouraged, provided that the fracture is showing signs of progressing union. If the navicular remains tender and CT scan does not indicate that the fracture is uniting, a bone graft or the use of electrical stimulation may be considered.

Predisposing factors to navicular stress fractures include tarsal coalition, overpronation or restricted ankle dorsiflexion. If present, these factors should be addressed in the post-immobilization period (Khan 1992).

Metatarsal stress fractures

Runners develop these fractures in the metatarsal neck, while dancers tend to develop a fracture in the proximal shaft. As with other stress fractures the onset is insidious, but a complaint of pain with activity and tenderness to palpation are diagnostic clues. A correlation has been suggested between the length of the first metatarsal and the incidence of metatarsal stress fractures, the implication being that a short first metatarsal would predispose the athlete to the injury. However, Drez et al (1980) were unable to substantiate this theory. Predisposing factors for the condition include abnormal foot mechanics, and poor footwear and training patterns.

When there is a positive diagnosis conformed by bone scan, the treatment of choice is rest.

Stress fractures of the fifth metatarsal

Stress fractures of the fifth metatarsal are complicated by their tendency to non-union. Fractures of this bone are usually the result of jumping or twisting forces but can also occur as the result of weightbearing stress. The fracture may be associated with prodromal symptoms over the lateral aspect of the foot prior to the presenting acute injury, and this may be a clue for diagnosis or even an early warning sign in the athlete presenting with lateral foot pain (Acker & Drez 1986).

Treatment of the acute fracture by conservative means in a non-weightbearing cast is recommended, while operative treatment needs to be considered in the case of established delayed union (Lehman et al 1987).

Stress fractures of the talus

These are uncommon and involve the neck of the talus. They occur most frequently in runners, usually in association with abnormal foot mechanics where the calcaneum everts during heel strike to create a fulcrum effect at the talar neck (Hontas et al 1986). Apart from a period of rest, treatment should include assessment and correction of the abnormal mechanics.

Fractures of the base of the fifth metatarsal

Spiral fractures

A spiral fracture of the fifth metatarsal may occur as the result of a severe inversion injury.

Diagnosis

A fracture should be suspected following a severe inversion injury where there is pain and swelling over the fifth metatarsal. There may also be deformity if the fracture is displaced. X-ray will reveal a fracture.

Treatment

Below-knee plaster is applied for 6 weeks, followed by graduated return to full weightbearing. Intensive physiotherapy to regain full range of ankle and foot movement may be necessary, particularly if there has been associated ligamentous damage at the ankle.

Transverse fractures

Fractures at the neck of the metatarsal have been discussed as stress fractures. Transverse fractures may also occur as the result of trauma unrelated to repetitive stress, and again may follow an inversion injury or may occur on landing from a jump.

Diagnosis

When a fracture is suspected, X-rays should be taken to confirm the diagnosis.

Treatment

The potential for non-union in the transverse fracture is greater than in the spiral fracture, and consequently the period of immobilization will be longer. The athlete may be in a weightbearing cast for 8 weeks, but this period may be extended up to 12 weeks if union is delayed. Open reduction and internal fixation may be considered in an attempt to speed the recovery phase.

Following immobilization, physiotherapy will be essential to restore ankle and foot range of movement, strength and proprioception. An orthosis or strapping to protect the foot from inversion forces may be of help during the rehabilitation phase.

Avulsion fractures

The pull of the peroneus brevis tendon may cause an avulsion fracture of the fifth metatarsal in an inversion injury.

Diagnosis

Such a fracture should be considered if there is localized pain over the area following such an injury. X-rays should be performed to demonstrate the presence of the fracture and determine whether it is displaced or non-displaced.

Treatment

If the fragment is not displaced, simple strapping or bandaging may be all that is required until the symptoms settle. This is followed by physiotherapy as with an ankle sprain. If the fragment is displaced, it may require a period of immobilization in plaster.

DISEASES AND CONDITIONS OF THE METATARSALS AND SESAMOIDS

Iselin's disease

Traction apophysitis occurring at the base of the fifth metatarsal was described by Iselin and the disease takes his name (Lehman et al 1986). It is a condition of young athletes who will present with a tender prominence over the proximal portion of the fifth metatarsal and pain on weightbearing. The pain occurs initially after activity but progresses to occur during sport. Repetitive action of the peroneus brevis at the insertional apophysis produces a stress reaction which is the basis of the disease.

Diagnosis

Iselin's disease is diagnosed in the young athlete presenting with tenderness over the peroneus brevis muscle attachment. There may be pain on restricted eversion and pain on passive inversion. There may also be evidence of peroneal muscle spasm. The condition is more common in those participating in ballet, roller skating, jumping or twisting and turning sports. X-ray or bone scan will assist in the diagnosis (Lehman et al 1986).

Differential diagnosis

Tumour, infection and stress fractures can be ruled out with the aid of X-ray and bone scan. Spastic flat feet, tarsal coalition, peroneal tendonitis and ankle sprains need to be excluded.

Treatment

Rest from the exacerbating activities, relief from weightbearing with crutches and casting or taping to reduce the pull of the peroneus brevis are all considered, depending on the severity of the symptoms (Lehman et al 1986). Local therapy with ice, electrotherapy, exercise, stretches and proprioception exercises may all be incorporated into a graduated program for returning to sport.

Freiberg's disease

Freiberg's disease is an osteochondritis occurring as a result of avascular necrosis of the head of the second and, rarely, the third metatarsal. Onset of the disease is in adolescence, and may be related to overuse producing stress at the metatarsaphalangeal joint. Occasionally a fragment will loosen and produce an osteochondritis desiccans.

Diagnosis

The disease may be asymptomatic or the young athlete may present with pain, swelling and tenderness over the site. Pain is increased on weightbearing or when standing on the toes. X-ray will show collapse and flattening of the metatarsal head. As the symptoms settle, the X-ray changes may be unaltered and degenerative changes may follow some years later.

Treatment

Acute management will include rest and simple orthotics to relieve stress at the affected joint. In advanced cases surgical intervention may be necessary to remove loose bodies or to debride the metatarsal head.

Metatarsalgia

Generalized pain of a non-specific origin over the area of the metatarsals may be described as metatarsalgia. Pain under the metatarsal heads may be caused by mechanical faults within the foot or by trauma. Interdigital neuroma may also cause pain in the area and is described with entrapment neuropathies.

Increased pressure over the metatarsal heads may occur particularly with the cavus foot, or in runners who land on their toes, or when there has been significant trauma from repetitive jumping in poor footwear. The underlying bursa may become inflamed, while calluses and corns may develop under the metatarsal heads.

Metatarsalgia in older athletes may be related to lax transverse ligaments and can be aggravated by obesity, a valgus heel, hammer toes or pes planus.

Treatment

Reducing the load on the metatarsals by correction of footwear is important; the use of orthotics may assist as will a period of rest. Ultrasound can provide some symptomatic relief and NSAIDs may be used.

Sesamoids

The function of the sesamoids is to increase the power of metatarsophalangeal flexion and to act as shock absorbers to disperse impact forces on the metatarsal head. Due to their relationship with the flexor hallucis longus tendon, they are able to offer that tendon some protection (Richardson 1987).

Sesamoiditis

The sesamoids are most commonly injured in long distance runners, but injuries may occur in athletes who play racquet sports, basketball, volleyball, football and soccer. Plantarflexed first metatarsals, restricted dorsiflexion of the first metatarsophalangeal joint and excessive pronation may all contribute to the development of pain related to the sesamoids (Lillich & Baxter 1986).

Diagnosis

The athlete will present with a history of several weeks of poorly localized pain around the metatarsophalangeal joint. Careful palpation should precisely localize tenderness over the sesamoid. Redness or swelling may occur in advanced cases. Passive dorsiflexion of the metatarsophalangeal joint may be painful and restricted (Lillich & Baxter 1986). X-ray of the area will assist the diagnosis by excluding osteochondritis, chondromalacia, degenerative arthritis and fracture.

Treatment

Where the condition is considered to be pure sesamoiditis, treatment will include rest, moulded shoe inserts, local electrotherapy and gentle mobilization of the metatarsophalangeal joint to regain extension as the inflammation settles.

Osteochondritis

This condition is revealed on radiological examination which will show a mottled appearance to the bones. It is a process involving necrosis and repair of the bone as a result of repetitive microtrauma which may eventually result in fragmentation and collapse (Richardson 1987).

Stress fractures

Stress fractures of the sesamoids may be an advanced stage of osteochondritis. Care should be taken when evaluating radiological findings to differentiate fracture from bipartate bones, which are not uncommon (Reid 1992, Axe & Ray 1988).

Bursitis

The presence of localized swelling, erythema and tenderness on pinching the bursa from side to side rather than with direct pressure to the sesamoid indicates the presence of a bursitis (Richardson 1987).

Chondromalacia

The medial sesamoid may develop chondromalacia which produces pain specifically on weightbearing.

Differential diagnosis

All conditions of the sesamoids should be carefully examined manually and with X-ray and possibly bone scan to determine the precise pathology. Conditions such as flexor hallucis longus tendonitis, gout, inflammatory disease, osteoarthritis and synovitis should be ruled out.

Treatment

Treatment for these conditions of the sesamoids usually consists of rest, occasionally in a cast. NSAIDs and local injections of steroids may be used in the case of bursitis. Local therapy such as ice, mobilization and electrotherapy can be trialled. Foot mechanics should be assessed and appropriate adjustments and orthotics prescribed if necessary.

Excision of the involved sesamoid may be considered where there is a displaced fracture, or an undisplaced fracture which has failed to respond to conservative treatment in a cast for 12 weeks, sesamoiditis or osteochondritis persisting over a period of 6 months, recurrent protracted bursitis or osteomyelitis. At 2 weeks post-surgery, active and passive mobilization is commenced, including weightbearing activities. Return to full sport is usually permitted after 6 weeks if symptoms permit (Richardson 1987).

INJURIES TO THE METATARSOPHALANGEAL JOINTS

Turf toe

Playing sport on artificial surfaces with lightweight shoes has been associated with an increased incidence of injuries to the first metatarsophalangeal (MTP) joint. Rather than allowing some 'give' between the playing surface and the athlete's foot, the shoe tends to grip the surface, forcing hyperextension of the first MTP as propulsion or an external force pushes the athlete forward while the toe remains jammed (Fig. 32.14). The commonly occurring injury is that termed 'turf toe' which describes an acute sprain of the first MTP joint as a result of such a hyperextension injury. Turf toe is particularly common in American football where Rodeo et al (1989) found that 45% of the footballers studied had incurred such an injury during their career.

The MTP joint is supported by a fibrocartilaginous plate on its plantar surface, and by the flexor hallucis brevis and adductor hallucis. These structures may suffer damage in a severe injury. The resulting sprain may be graded in

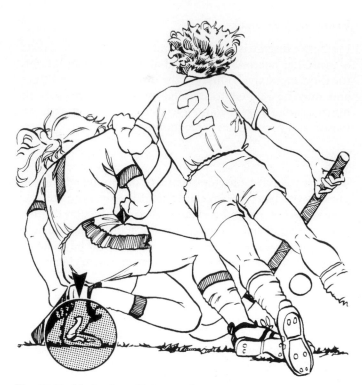

Fig. 32.14 Mechanism of injury, turf toe.

severity from I to III as with ankle sprains, depending on the structures damaged (Clanton et al 1986).

Diagnosis

The athlete will present with a history of a hyperextension injury and the joint will be red and swollen. Palpation over the plantar aspect will be particularly tender and passive dorsiflexion will be painful. Severe injuries may avulse the volar plate and injure the sesamoids. Plain X-ray may be negative if there is no associated fracture (Clanton et al 1986).

Differential diagnosis

Gout may present with similar signs and symptoms, and should be considered although there is usually no history of trauma. MTP dislocation, fracture of the metatarsal or phalanx and sesamoid stress fractures should also be excluded (Clanton et al 1986).

Treatment

In the acute stage, ice, strapping or bandage and NSAIDs are all useful. To relieve the stress of dorsiflexion, the toe can be carefully taped to hold it in a neutral position. It can also be taped to the adjacent toe for further relief. As the acute stage passes, electrotherapy, passive mobilization of the joint and gentle exercise should accompany a graduated return to sport. To provide ongoing protection and to help prevent further injury, a rigid shoe insert can be used inside the regular sports shoe or a shoe, with a slightly stiffer sole may be sufficient (Rodeo et al 1989, Sammarco 1988).

Subluxation of the metatarsophalangeal joint

As a chronic injury, this is most common in middle-aged runners, often at the second MTP joint. Manual examination can reproduce the subluxation which may be extremely painful due to traction on the interdigital nerve. The injury can occur acutely in a severe turf toe.

Treatment to reduce pain and inflammation may be of only limited value. Orthotics and taping, together with modification of activities, may reduce the symptoms (Lillich & Baxter 1986).

Hallux rigidus

Loss of range of movement of the MTP joint of the first toe may result from degenerative changes within that joint. There is particular loss of dorsiflexion which can begin to interfere with sport and even with walking, as the symptoms progress. Hallux rigidus may be a long-term complication of turf toe, but can also commonly predispose to such an injury.

Hallux rigidus may be more likely to occur in individuals who have a long second metatarsal (Morton's toe) and can follow repeated minor trauma to the joint. It may be related to the presence of osteochondritis or may occur simply as a case of primary osteoarthritis (Reid 1992).

Diagnosis

Hallux rigidus is characterized by pain over the joint, associated with a limited range of movement. This will create difficulty in standing on the toes, jumping, running, descending steps and squatting. Examination may reveal local inflammation and swelling if recent trauma has aggravated the condition and loss of range of movement, particularly in dorsiflexion, will be noted. In severe cases, the toe may become fixed in some degree of plantarflexion.

Differential diagnosis

The conditions to be excluded will be as those in turf toe, while turf toe itself also needs to be considered.

Treatment

Local therapy including ice, electrotherapy and exercise are all of use. Passive mobilization techniques should also be instigated to reduce pain and to increase a pain free range of movement. In especially severe cases, orthotics may be useful and surgical intervention may be considered. If the joint is debrided, it will be essential to provide a vigorous post-operative physiotherapy program to regain range and strength and to reduce pain. Other operative techniques which might be considered include osteotomy, arthroplasty and arthrodesis.

Hallux valgus

This term is used to describe the deformity of the MTP of the first toe where the toe deviates into a lateral position. The condition tends result from wearing tight footwear, particularly with high heels, and may be associated with a pronated foot and tight achilles tendon.

Treatment

Avoidance of inappropriate footwear is essential, and intrinsic muscle exercises, taping, orthotics to control pronation and padding can also be of some help. Surgery can be required if the deformity and the symptoms are severe. Surgical options include release of the adductor hallucis, excision of the bunion or capsular plication. Advanced cases may require osteotomy, arthroplasty or fusion where there is a significant primus varus.

TOE INJURIES AND DEFORMITIES

Toe sprains and fractures

Stubbing the toe, kicking and other sporting endeavours may result in a toe sprain or fracture. These can be quite painful, but there is not a lot to offer with treatment except rest, relief of weightbearing and attention to treatment of the acute inflammatory response. This might include ice, contrast baths, NSAIDs, and splinting or taping.

Toe deformities

Athletes commonly present with toe deformities as such, or in association with other conditions being treated. Apparently simple early toe deformities can cause extreme discomfort which in turn may alter the athletes' normal mechanics as they attempt to relieve the pressure from a painful toe. This in turn can cause or contribute to pain elsewhere in the foot or leg. More severe toe deformities or complaints can lead to broken skin, which in turn may allow infection to develop. The athlete may lose valuable training time or be unfit for competition.

Claw toe

This describes a deformity of flexion at both the proximal interphalangeal (PIP) and distal interphalangeal (DIP) joints with the MTP flexed or neutral. The main associated complaint with this deformity will be callus and pain over the dorsum of the PIP. The development of a claw toe may be due to incorrectly fitted footwear.

Hammer toe

The deformity in this case is PIP flexion and DIP extension. The MTP is neutral or extended. Again, the dorsum of the PIP will become painful and develop a callus.

Mallet toe

The mallet toe has a neutral or extended PIP joint and a flexed DIP with the MTP joint in neutral. This may result from a traumatic episode avulsing the long extensor tendon origin.

Treatment

Where the deformity is not fixed, passive mobilization to regain and retain range is instigated. This will include stretching flexor tendons at home and joint stretches and mobilization by the physiotherapist. Both casual and sporting shoes must be well-fitting. Attention from the podiatrist to developed callus and plantar keratomas will relieve some symptoms. The athlete must take particular care with hygiene of the feet to prevent infection where there is abrasion of the skin.

If deformities become fixed and the symptoms are severe, surgery may be considered.

SKIN CONDITIONS OF THE FOOT

As with toe deformities, skin conditions may be noted incidentally when the athlete is being assessed or treated for another foot or ankle condition. It is important to identify particular conditions which may be infection to prevent the condition from being passed to other athletes.

Blisters

Blisters may be the most commonly seen painful condition. They are often caused by pressure or friction of shoes that are too tight. Relief may be gained from pricking the blister, but this should only be done under sterile conditions. Padding around the blister rather than directly over it can help to relieve the pressure from the blister itself. Athletes who are particularly prone to blisters may find it useful to wear a half-stocking under their shoe or boot, while petroleum jelly over the stocking will further reduce the friction.

Callus

Callus can result from chronic friction. Correction of the posture causing the friction may be possible but it may be necessary for the podiatrist and ultimately the orthopaedic surgeon to provide treatment if the callus and the causative deformity are particularly severe.

Corns

Corns are thick hardened responses to pressure or friction, with an inwardly facing apex. Pressure can be reduced from the area with special pads (Fig. 32.15), and the podiatrist may need to pare down the callus.

Warts

Warts on the plantar surface of the foot will probably be self-limiting. Techniques to 'burn' the wart can be used, but may be uncomfortable.

Infection

Tinea pedis is a common fungal infection which can be quite painful. It will usually present between the toes and will respond to the use of an antifungal agent. Care must be taken with foot hygiene and the toes should be carefully dried after washing.

Yeast infections such as candida albicans will affect a similar area and should also respond to topical agents (Carruthers 1987).

ENTRAPMENT NEUROPATHIES

Tarsal tunnel syndrome

There are two tarsal tunnel syndromes and, although both are rare, it is important to be familiar with their presentation to assist with early diagnosis.

Posterior tarsal tunnel syndrome

This syndrome develops when the distal portion of the posterior tibial nerve is entrapped at the level of the medial

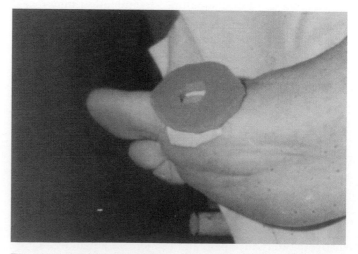

Fig. 32.15 Painful areas of callus or blisters can be protected by the use of a foam 'doughnut' around the blister or prominent area.

malleolus. The main feature is an unpleasant burning pain in the sole of the foot. The condition is characterized by increased pain after a day's activity and nocturnal pain is often present.

The floor of the tarsal tunnel is formed by the talus and calcaneum together with the tibialis posterior, flexor digitorum longus and flexor hallucis longus, while the roof is made up by the flexor retinaculum. Due to the inelastic composition of the tunnel, any degree of inflammation or scarring could allow compression to the posterior tibial nerve. The lateral plantar nerve component is more commonly affected than the medial component (Jackson & Haglund 1991, Dawson et al 1983).

Factors which can contribute to the syndrome include a forced plantarflexion or eversion injury, fracture, arthritic or inflammatory conditions, abnormal foot mechanics and plantar fasciitis (Jackson & Haglund 1991).

Diagnosis

The characteristic pain may occur at night. There may be fatigue of the foot or weakness of the toe flexors and trophic changes at the toes. Pain may be reproduced on forced dorsiflexion and eversion and there may be palpable swelling around the medial malleolus. Sensory changes at an early stage may include loss of two point discrimination and there may be a positive Tinel's sign where tapping over the nerve causes tingling over its distal distribution. Weakness of the intrinsic muscles may be present but is difficult to asses (Jackson & Haglund 1991). Electrodiagnostic studies may be helpful.

Differential diagnosis

Plantar fasciitis, inflammatory diseases, interdigital neuromas, peripheral neuropathies and referred pain from the lumbar spine may be difficult to differentiate from tarsal tunnel syndrome. The characteristic pain of this syndrome, together with its nocturnal tendency, will assist the differentiation.

Treatment

It is important first to determine the aetiology of the condition in the athlete. Any apparent degree of fault in the mechanics of the foot needs to be corrected. The problem may be overpronation and exercises to correct this, together with the use of orthotics, may help. Local therapy including ice or ultrasound could also be trialled. Inflammation may be slow to resolve with conservative treatment and therefore sufficient time should be allowed to assess its benefit.

Local steroid injection or NSAIDs may also be considered to produce relief.

Where conservative treatment has failed, surgery to release the flexor retinaculum may be performed (Jackson & Haglund 1991, Dawson et al 1983).

Anterior tarsal tunnel syndrome

This is an entrapment of the deep peroneal nerve as it runs below the dense superficial fascia of the ankle.

Diagnosis

The symptoms are numbness or paraesthesia in the first dorsal webspace, with occasional tightness and aching over the dorsum of the foot. As the nerve innervates the extensor digitorum brevis, the normal bulk of the muscle belly may be lost (Dawson et al 1983).

Differential diagnosis

Referred pain from the lumbar spine should be excluded, as should more vague foot pain such as that of metatarsalgia.

Treatment

Orthotics may be helpful, or steroid injection may be attempted. Surgery may also be considered.

Morton's neuroma

This is a painful swelling at the bifurcation of one of the digital branches of the plantar nerves. The swelling occurs at the bifurcation of the nerve as it lies between the two adjacent metatarsal heads, the most common site being between the third and fourth metatarsal heads. The neuroma tends to be compressed between the metatarsal heads.

This condition is quite common and occurs four times as often in women as in men, and may often be bilateral.

Contributing factors include tight shoes, certain foot deformities such as pes cavus, local trauma, damage from the mechanical effect of the flexor digitorum locally or the presence of a ganglion or bursa in the region which may cause swelling and pressure on the nerve (Quirk 1987b, Gauthier 1979).

Diagnosis

The athlete will describe a sharp pain, usually at the base of the third and fourth toes which may radiate into those toes with occasional proximal radiation. The pain is described as burning or like an electric shock and is elicited on weightbearing, particularly in tight shoes. There may be numbness or hyperaesthesia.

Palpation will reproduce the pain, particularly if the metatarsal heads are compressed together (Quirk 1987b, Dawson et al 1983).

Differential diagnosis

Pain from a prominent metatarsal head will be felt directly under the metatarsal head rather than between the adjacent heads. Stress fractures may be excluded with the objective examination or with a bone scan if necessary.

Treatment

If the condition is not too chronic, relief may be gained from loose shoes, low heels and orthotics. Where abnormal neural tension in the tibial nerve is present, the condition may benefit from an intermetatarsal glide mobilization with the plantar nerves on tension, or in combination with a slump or straight leg raise stretch. Surgical excision of the neuroma may be necessary if relief is not gained with conservative measures.

TAPING AND ORTHOSES

Taping around the foot and ankle using a non-elastic material such as zinc oxide tape is effective prophylactically, but can also be a useful treatment adjunct when used to modify postures and reduce stress on painful structures. Examples have already given where taping may be used therapeutically. These methods will now be outlined, together with some routine prophylactic styles.

Taping procedure

Inappropriate taping, inadequate precautions and poor taping techniques can cause further injury or significant skin reactions. Before taping the athlete should be questioned about any history of inflammatory or infectious skin conditions or known allergies to taping materials. When there is uncertainty, it is useful to perform a patch test with the taping material to be used.

Prior to applying the tape, ensure the skin is clean and dry. Shaving may sensitize the skin and when it is necessary, shaving should be done on the day before taping. The area may be wiped with benzoin tincture to assist adhesion of the tape. An underwrap material may be applied under the tape if the skin is considered sensitive, although this will decrease its effectiveness.

The foot and ankle are placed in the required position so that the tape can be laid on rather than attempting to achieve this by pulling on the tape. Pulling the tape on the skin in this manner will cause the tape to cut into the skin. Tearing the tape during the procedure can be awkward and it is preferable to cut correct lengths of tape and place them within reach before commencement.

Care must be taken not to completely circle the calf or foot with tape as this may compromise the circulation. Particular care must be taken in the area of the achilles tendon and base of the fifth metatarsal. Complete the taping by ensuring that there are no gaps of skin left exposed which may permit pockets of swelling to form, or which may allow the edge of the tape to dig in. This is easily done with short pieces of tape laid over exposed areas of skin. The heel pad need not be enclosed in tape. The athlete should find the finished tape comfortable and firm but not too tight. Encouragement to walk in the tape for a few minutes will help to gauge its effect and to ensure that the circulation is not impaired.

Tape should be removed by cutting with snub-nose scissors, lifting off small sections gently and pulling the tape back parrallel to the skin surface. An adhesive removal agent may be used. It is unwise to wet the tape prior to removal, as this can damage the skin.

Prophylactic ankle taping

Stirrups

An anchor strap is first placed at approximately the junction of the lower third and upper two thirds of the tibia, taking care to angle the tape so that it does not fully encircle the calf. Three to four stirrups can then be applied, laid down the medial aspect from the anchor, under the heel and pulled firmly up to the anchor laterally while the foot is held in dorsiflexion and eversion. Again, take care not to pull the tape on the skin, but to apply it firmly to the skin while the ankle is held in the correct position. In applying a number of stirrups, they can be fanned out to give broader support over the lateral aspect. At the completion of the stirrups, apply another anchor tape over the top.

Figure six/figure eight taping

To give further support to the anterior talofibular ligament and anterior capsule, figure six or eight taping, usually placed over two to three stirrups, can be effective. A figure six tape is laid down on the medial aspect as with a stirrup, but is taken under the midfoot and over the anterior aspect of the foot to cross back over the medial strip. A figure eight strap is similar but, rather than commencing medially, the strap is commenced laterally, running over the front of the ankle before being pulled up laterally as with a figure six. Three or more figure six or eight straps may be used.

Heel lock

This is a useful technique to finally stabilize the taping and to give support to the medial ligament, fibulocalcaneal ligament and the subtalar joint. It is commenced over the medial instep, runs over the front of the ankle then behind the ankle, and crosses at the front of the ankle to come up on the lateral aspect of the heel and finish over the front of the ankle. One or two heel locks are used.

Medial ligament injuries

These less common injuries can be protected with taping. Stirrups, figure six or eight taping and heel locks can be effective, but usually the aim would be to hold the foot in neutral rather than to attempt to invert it. The direction of the figure sixes or eights may be changed if necessary to supply adequate support, but a better method may be to alternate the direction with each tape so that the foot is held securely in neutral.

Completing ankle taping

At completion of any taping, check there are no areas allowing for pressure or biting into the skin. This can be minimized by applying small strips of tape over what has been applied to fill in any uncovered areas of skin (Fig. 32.16).

Foot and toe taping

Metatarsalgia

In minor cases, relief may be obtained by using a small oval foam pad taped into place over the region of the metatarsal heads (transverse arch).

Plantar fasciitis

Apply an anchor tape across the metatarsal heads on the plantar aspect. Run pieces of 2.5 cm tape from the medial aspect of that anchor, under the foot, behind the heel, then under the sole to the lateral aspect of the anchor tape. Starting

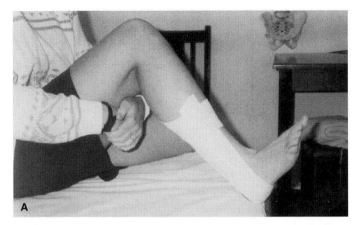

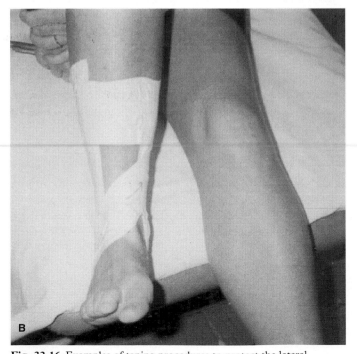

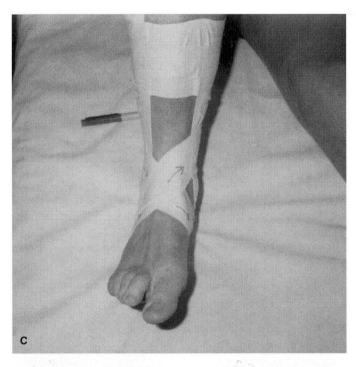

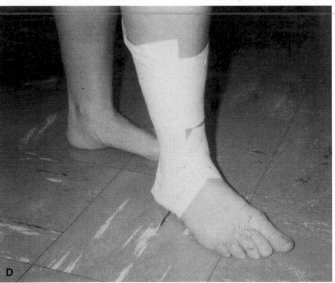

Fig. 32.16 Examples of taping procedures to protect the lateral ligament complex.
(a) Stirrups
(b) Figure six
(c) Figure eight
(d) Heel lock

and finishing aspects can be alternated and up to four pieces used. The tape is finished with stirrups running over the dorsum of the foot under the sole to finish up the medial aspect of the ankle, as with a stirrup tape (Fig. 32.17). This can be repeated three or four times. Again, it may be necessary to fill in any gaps with pieces of tape.

Cuboid syndrome

The cuboid and lateral aspect of the foot can be supported with tape placed under the lateral aspect of the sole of the foot, pulled up firmly over the lateral aspect of the cuboid and finished over the dorsum of the foot.

Turf toe

An anchor tape is applied over the metatarsal region. Strips of tape are then taken from the anchor and looped over the proximal phalanx from the plantar aspect, crossing under the toe and returned to the anchor (Fig. 32.18). This prevents hyperextension of the toe. Care should be taken not to perform this on a swollen toe (Sammarco 1988).

Toe injuries

As in the hand, other minor injuries of the toe can be managed by buddy strapping where the toes are taped together distally and proximally to the interphalangeal joint.

Posterior impingement syndrome/anterior ankle strain

Where restriction of plantar flexion is required, two anchor straps are placed, one over the foot and the other above the ankle. The foot is allowed to rest in a relaxed position and longitudinal strips are run between the anchors, fanning

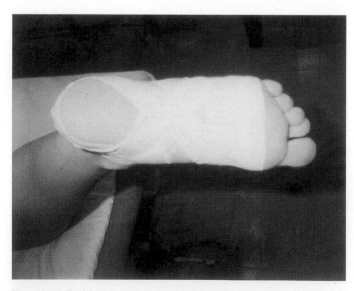

Fig. 32.17 Positioning and direction of tape used for athletes with plantar fasciitis.

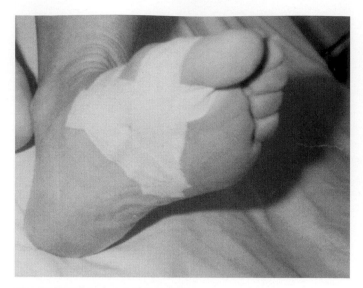

Fig. 32.18 Taping method in turf toe.

out to medial and lateral aspects of the anchors and crossing at the front of the ankle. Pieces of tape are placed across the strips to prevent swelling or cutting in from the tape edges.

Anterior impingement syndrome

A similar method of taping can be used to restrict dorsiflexion by taping over the posterior aspect between anchors with the athlete lying in prone. This method may also be useful as a support for a calf strain or achilles tendon injury. It may, however, be simpler to use a small heel raise in the shoe.

Taping can be a very useful tool in the management of athletes with foot and ankle injuries. The disadvantages in relation to cost and to skin sensitivities must be considered, however, and the use of supportive bracing should also be considered as an alternative.

Braces and orthotics

Braces or orthoses are becoming more popular in the management of an injured ankle. When used in place of plaster to protect an injured ankle and after a procedure such as an ankle reconstruction, an orthosis can provide the athlete with the appropriate support which is light, durable, comfortable and, in general, moderately priced.

Orthoses are of use in the rehabilitation phase as an alternative to taping. An orthosis can give the ankle joint comparable or better support than that provided by taping, particularly in restricting inversion post exercise (Gross et al 1987). Another advantage of the orthosis is that it can be applied by the unskilled athlete, whereas taping an ankle requires considerable skill. The athlete who is sensitive to tape will find an orthosis invaluable, and in the long term the cost can be comparable to continued use of tape. Taping has been shown to be less effective than orthoses in controlling inversion after exercise (Gross et al 1987), and this may be the result of tape loosening on warm or moist skin. When tape is used, it must be reapplied after a period of exercise. An orthosis, however, will be effective over long periods of sport.

There are various orthoses available. Most are light and fit comfortably in the shoe without restricting mobility. The initial cost may appear high, but is justified if the product is durable. Fitting and selecting an appropriate orthosis is essential and the physiotherapist should assist the athlete to make the correct choice of size and style.

The choice between orthosis and tape is a decision which should be made by the athlete and the physiotherapist. Although orthoses have some advantages over taping, some athletes find it difficult to become accustomed to wearing them and the initial cost may be deterring. Tape applied expertly and regularly can be very effective and provide protection for individual needs. For this reason, the author prefers its use in some cases to provide absolute security for the complex injury. Physiotherapists should be flexible and assist athletes to make the correct choice for their particular circumstances.

For the inexperienced physiotherapist, referral to a sports podiatrist for othotic assessment and fitting may be a preferred option.

SUMMARY

The foot and ankle is a complex region for the physiotherapist to diagnose and treat. The ankle is the most frequently injured joint in athletes and the region is subject to diverse injuries. The importance of accurate diagnosis has been discussed and a method for assessing the athlete with foot or ankle pathology outlined.

Physiotherapists involved in the assessment and treatment of athletes must be familiar with the many conditions and diseases which may cause local symptoms in the foot and ankle.

Rehabilitation of the athlete may be very rewarding. This is certainly true in the case of an athlete presenting with dysfunction as a result of foot and ankle injuries. After instigating appropriate management in the acute stage of an injury, there must be a thorough program outlined to cater for the athlete's specific requirements, which must be identified. The physiotherapist must be familiar with the particular demands of that athlete's sport and training program, and should develop communication between the athlete, coach and medical team to ensure a co-ordinated approach to common goals.

The aim of the physiotherapist should be to return the athlete to the highest level of function in the shortest possible time.

REFERENCES

Acker J H, Drez D 1986 Nonoperative treatment of stress fractures of the proximal shaft of the fifth metatarsal (Jones' fracture). Foot and Ankle 7(3):152-155

Alexander A H, Lichtman D M 1980 Surgical treatment of transchondral talar-dome fractures (osteochondritis dissecans). Journal of Bone and Joint Surgery 62A:646-652

Alexander I J 1990 The foot. Examination and diagnosis. Churchill Livingstone, New York

Andersen E 1987 Stenosing peroneal tenosynovitis symptomatically simulating ankle instability. American Journal of Sports Medicine 15(3):258-259

Anderson K J, Lecocq J F, Lecocq E A 1952 Recurrent anterior subluxation of the ankle joint. Journal of Bone and Joint Surgery 34A:853-860

Aradi A J, Wong J, Walsh M 1988 The dimple sign of a ruptured lateral ligament of the ankle: brief report. Journal of Bone and Joint Surgery 70B (2):327-328

Axe M J, Ray RL 1988 Orthotic treatment of sesamoid pain. American Journal of Sports Medicine 16(4):411-416

Black H M, Bland R L, Eichelberger M R 1978 An improved technique for the evaluation of ligamentous injury in severe ankle sprains. American Journal of Sports Medicine 6(5):276-282

Boruta P M, Bishop J O, Braly W G, Tullos H S 1990 Acute lateral ankle ligament injuries: a literature review. Foot and Ankle 11(2):107-113

Bosien W R, Staples O S, Russell S W 1955 Residual disability following acute ankle sprains. Journal of Bone and Joint Surgery 37A(6):1237-1243

Boytim M J, Fischer D A, Neuman L 1991 Syndesmotic ankle sprains. American Journal of Sports Medicine 19(3):294-298

Brodsky A E, Khalil M D 1987 Talar compression syndrome Foot and Ankle 7(6):338-344

Butler D 1991 Mobilisation of the nervous system. Churchill Livingstone, Melbourne

Butler D, Gifford L 1989 The concept of abnormal mechanical tension in the nervous system. Physiotherapy 75(11):622-636

Canale S T, Belding R H 1980 Osteochondral lesions of the talus. Journal of Bone and Joint Surgery 62A:97-102

Carruthers R. 1987 Painful skin conditions of the foot. Australian Family Physician 16(8):1098-1099

Clanton T O, Butler J E, Eggert A 1986 Injuries to the metatarsophalangeal joint in athletes. Foot and Ankle 7(3):162-176

Corrigan B, MAITLAND GD 1983 Practical orthopaedic medicine. Butterworths, London

Dalziel, R. 1993 Personal communication, Melbourne

Dawson D M, Hallett M, Millender L H 1983 Entrapment neuropathies. Little, Brown, Boston

DeCarlo M S, Talbot R W 1986 Evaluation of ankle joint proprioception following injection of the anterior talofibular ligament. Journal of Orthopaedic and Sports Physical Therapy 8(2):70-76

Donatelli R, Hurlbert C, Conaway D, St Pierre R 1988 Biomechanical foot orthotics: a retrospective study. Journal of Orthopaedic and Sports Physical Therapy 10(6):205-211

Drez D, Young J C, Johnston R D, Parker W D 1980 Metatarsal stress fractures. American Journal of Sports Medicine 8(2):123-125

Evans D L 1953 Recurrent instability of the ankle: a method of surgical treatment. Procedings of the Royal Society of Medicine 46:343-344

Evans G A, Hardcastle P, Frenyo A D 1984 Acute rupture of the lateral ligament of the ankle: to suture or not to suture? Journal of Bone and Joint Surgery 66B(2):209-212

Ferkel R D, Karzel R P, Del Pizzo W, Friedman M J, Fischer SP 1991 Arthroscopic treatment of anterolateral impingement of the ankle. American Journal of Sports Medicine 19(5):440-446

Flick A B, Gould N 1985 Osteochondritis dissecans of the talus (transchondral fractures of the talus): review of the literature and new surgical approach for medial dome lesions. Foot and Ankle 5(4):165-185

Freeman M A R 1965 Instability of the foot after injuries to the lateral ligament of the ankle. Journal of Bone and Joint Surgery 47B(4):669-677

Freeman M A R, Dean M R E, Hanham I W F 1965 The etiology and prevention of functional instability of the foot. Journal of Bone and Joint Surgery 47B(4):678-685

Frieder S, Weisberg J, Fleming B, Stanek A 1988 A pilot study: the therapeutic effect of ultrasound following partial rupture of achilles tendons in male rats. Journal of Orthopaedic and Sports Physical Therapy 10(2):39-46

Gauthier G 1979 Thomas Morton's disease: a nerve entrapment syndrome. A new surgical technique. Clinical Orthopaedics and Related Research 142:90-92

Gross M T, Bradshaw M K, Ventry L C, Weller K H 1987 Comparison of support provided by ankle taping and semirigid orthosis. Journal of Orthopaedic Sports and Physical Therapy 9(1):33-39

Gungor T 1988 A test for ankle instability: brief report. Journal of Bone and Joint Surgery 70B(3):487

Harbison S 1987 Plantar fasciitis. Australian Family Physician 16(8):113-115

Hardaker W T 1989 Foot and ankle injuries in classical ballet dancers. Orthopaedic Clinics of North America 20(4):621-627

Hardaker W T, Margello S, Goldner J L 1985 Foot and ankle injuries in theatrical dancers. Foot and ankle 6(2):59-69

Harrington K D 1979 Degenerative arthritis of the ankle secondary to long-standing lateral ligament instability. Journal of Bone and Joint Surgery 61A(3):354-361

Harris R I, Beath T 1948 Hypermobile flat-foot with short tendo achillis. Journal of Bone and Joint Surgery 30A:116-138

Hawkins R B 1988 Arthroscopic treatment of sports-related anterior osteophytes in the ankle. Foot and Ankle 9(2):87-90

Heil B 1992 Lower limb biomechanics related to running injuries. Physiotherapy 78(6):400-412

Hontas M J, Haddad R J, Schlesinger L C 1986 Conditions of the talus in runners. American Journal of Sports Medicine 14(6):486-490

Hughs A 1992 Footballer's ankle. Sport Health 10(2):16-17

Hunter L Y 1981 Stress fracture of the tarsal navicular: more frequent than we realize? American Journal of Sports Medicine 9(4):217-219

Jackson D L, Haglund B 1991 Tarsal tunnel syndrome in athletes. Case report and literature review. American Journal of Sports Medicine 19(1):61-65

Johnson K A, Strom D E 1989 Tibialis posterior tendon dysfunction. Clinical Orthopaedics 239:196-207

Kannus P, Renstrom P 1991 Treatment for acute tears of the lateral ligamnets of the ankle. Journal of Bone and Joint Surgery 73A(2):305-312

Karlsson J, Bergsten T, Lansinger O, Peterson L 1988 Lateral instability of the ankle treated by the Evans procedure. A long-term clinical and radiological follow-up. Journal of Bone and Joint Surgery 70B(3):476-480

Khan K 1992 Personal communication, Melbourne

Kosmahl E M, Kosmahl H E 1987 Painful plantar heel, plantar fasciitis, and calcaneal spur: etiology and treatment. Journal of Orthopaedic and Sports Physical Therapy 9(1):17-24

Leach R E, Seavey M S, Salter D K 1986 Results of surgery in athletes with plantar fasciitis. Foot and Ankle 7(3):156-161

Lehman R C, Gregg J R, Torg E 1986 Iselin's disease. American Journal of Sports Medicine 14(6):494-496

Lehman R C, Torg J S, Pavlov H, DeLee J C 1987 Fractures of the base of the fifth metatarsal distal to the tuberosity: a review. Foot and Ankle 7(4):245-252

Lillich J S, Baxter D E 1986 Common forefoot problems in runners. Foot and Ankle 7(3):145-151

Lutter L D 1986 Surgical decisions in athletes' subcalcaneal pain. American Journal of Sports Medicine 14(6):481-485

Maitland G D 1986 Vertebral manipulation, 5th edn. Butterworths, London

McCarroll J R, Schrader J W, Shelbourne K D, Rettig A C, Bisesi M A et al 1987 Meniscoid lesions of the ankle in soccer players. American Journal of Sports Medicine 15(3):255-257

McLennan J G 1980 Treatment of acute and chronic luxations of the peroneal tendons. American Journal of Sports Medicine 8(6):432-436

Miller E W 1982 The heel pad. American Journal of Sports Medicine 10(1):19-21

Morgan R C, Crawford A H 1986 Surgical management of tarsal coalition in adolescent athletes. Foot and Ankle 7(3):183-193

Mosier K M, Asher M 1984 Tarsal coalitions and peroneal spastic flat foot: a review. Journal of Bone and Joint Surgery 66A:976-984

Nawoczenski D A, Owen M J, Ecker M L, Altman B, Epler M 1985 Objective evaluation of peroneal response to sudden inversion stress. Journal of Orthopaedic Sports and Physical Therapy 7(3):107-109

Parks R M 1988 Biomechanics ofthe foot and lower extremity. In: Appenzeller O (ed) Sports medicine, fitness, training, injuries, 3rd edn. Urban and Schwarzenberg, Baltimore

Percy E C, Mann D L 1988 Tarsal coalition: a review of the literature and presentation of 13 cases. Foot and Ankle 9(1):40-44

Quirk R 1987a Stress fractures of the foot. Australian Family Physician 16(8):1101-1102

Quirk R 1987b Morton's neuroma. Australian Family Physician 16(8):1117-1120

Quirk R 1992 Personal communication, Melbourne

Quirk R 1993 Sporting injuries of the foot and ankle. Modern medicine of Australia 36(4):124-134

Reid D C 1992 Sports injury assessment and rehabilitation. Churchill Livingstone, New York

Richardson E G 1987 Injuries to the hallucal sesamoids in the athlete. Foot and Ankle 7(4):229-244

Rodeo S A, O'Brien S A, Warren R F, Barnes R, Wickiewicz T L 1989 Turf toe: diagnosis and treatment. Physician and Sports Medicine 17(4):133-147

Rubin G, Witten M 1960 The talar-tilt angle and the fibular collateral ligaments. Journal of Bone and Joint Surgery 42A:311-326

Ruth C J 1961 The surgical treatment of injuries of the fibular collateral ligaments of the ankle. Journal of Bone and Joint Surgery 43A(2):229-239

Sammarco G J 1988 How I manage turf toe. Physician and Sports Medicine 16(9):113-118

Sammarco G J 1989 Injuries to the foot. In: D'Ambrosia R D, Drez D (eds) Prevention and treatment of running injuries. Slack, New Jersey

Sartoris D J, Mink J H, Kerr R 1990 The foot and ankle. In: Mink J H, Deutsch A L (eds) MRI of the musculoskeletal system: a teaching file. Ravin Press, New York

Seder J I 1987 How I manage heel spur syndrome. Physician and Sports Medicine 15(2):83-85

Snyder R B, Lipscomb B, Johnston R K 1981 The relationship of tarsal coalitions to ankle sprains in athletes. American Journal of Sports Medicine 9(5):313-317

Torg J S, Pavlov H, Cooley L H, Bryant M H, Arnoczky S P, Bergfeld J, Hunter L Y 1982 Stress fractures of the tarsal navicular. A restrospective review of twenty-one cases. Journal of Bone and Joint Surgery 64A (5):700-712

Vaes P, DeBoeck H, Handelberg F, Opdecam P 1985 Comparative radiological study on the influence of ankle joint strapping and taping on ankle stability. Journal of Orthopaedic and Sports Physical Therapy 7(3):110-114

Westh R 1993 Personal communication. Melbourne

APPENDIX: PODIATRIC CONSIDERATIONS
JASON AGOSTA

NORMAL BIOMECHANICS

For the detection of abnormal biomechanics it is essential to have an understanding of normal biomechanics. Neutral static stance, the neutral position and range of motion of joints, and the normal biomechanics of walking and running will be considered.

The neutral position of the foot is when the subtalar joint is neither pronated nor supinated and the midtarsal joint (talonavicular and calcaneocuboid joints) is pronated (Fig. 32.19). The forefoot is perpendicular to the calcaneal

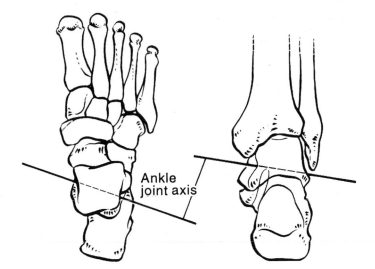

Fig. 32.20 The ankle joint and axis of motion. Source: adapted from Root et al (1977)

bisection and the ankle joint is neither dorsiflexed nor plantarflexed. The bisection of the tibia is perpendicular to the supporting surface. The knee is extended and the hips are not externally or internally rotated, and not flexed or extended. With both feet in neutral position the anterior superior iliac spines are level and the pelvis is slightly tilted anteriorly.

Range of motion of joints in neutral position

Ankle joint range of motion normally consists of 10-15° of dorsiflexion and 45° of plantarflexion (Fig. 32.20). When the foot is perpendicular to the leg the ankle joint is in a neutral position. Normally there is little frontal or transverse plane motion available at the ankle joint. However, when plantarflexing at the ankle joint there is some adduction and when dorsiflexing there is some abduction. For normal locomotion approximately 10° of dorsiflexion is the range required (Root et al 1977).

Supination and pronation of the foot occurs at the subtalar joint (talocalcaneal) (Fig. 32.21). Supination consists of calcaneal inversion, midtarsal adduction and talocrural plantarflexion. Pronation consists of calcaneal eversion, midtarsal abduction and talocrural dorsiflexion. Inversion of the calcaneus is approximately 20° and twice that of eversion, which is approximately 10° (Root et al 1977).

Two joints comprise the midtarsal joint: the talonavicular joint and the calcaneocuboid joint. There are two axes of motion, the longitudinal and oblique axes (Fig. 32.22). The longitudinal axis consists of a small range of inversion and eversion of the forefoot. The oblique axis has a large range of motion including dorsiflexion and abduction (with pronation) and plantarflexion and adduction (with supination). For every degree of abduction there is 1° of dorsiflexion and for every

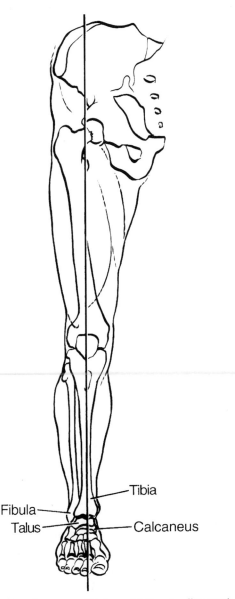

Fig. 32.19 Neutral static stance with the weightbearing line passing through the anterior iliac spine, patella and second metatarsal. Relationship of forefoot, rearfoot and leg in neutral position. Source: adapted from Donatelli (1990) and Subotnick (1989)

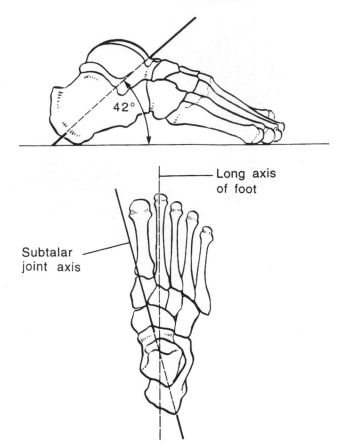

Fig. 32.21 The subtalar joint and axis of motion.
Source: adapted from Root et al (1977)

degree of adduction there is 1° of plantarflexion. Midtarsal joint range of motion is dependent on subtalar joint position. Midtarsal joint range of motion increases with pronation of the subtalar joint and decreases with supination of the subtalar joint (Root et al 1977).

The first metatarsal and first (medial) cunieform make up the first ray of the foot. The first ray dorsiflexes with an equal amount of inversion and plantarflexes with an equal amount of eversion. The neutral position is the midpoint of the total range of motion. Approximately 20° of motion is the normal total range of the first ray of the foot (Root et al 1977).

The second metatarsal and second (intermediate) cunieform make up the second ray. The third metatarsal and third (lateral) cunieform make up the third ray. The fourth metatarsal alone makes up the fourth ray of the foot. The second, third and fourth rays move only in plantarflexion and dorsiflexion. The fifth metatarsal alone makes up the fifth ray. The fifth ray dorsiflexes and plantarflexes with pronation and supination respectively. The midpoint of the total range of motion of the fifth ray is the neutral position.

Dorsiflexion of the first metatarsophalangeal joint is the important motion and is necessary for toe off. Approxi-

mately 65-70° of motion is the normal range motion. Abduction and adduction is evident but appears to have no functional significance (Root et al 1977).

Normal biomechanics of the foot and ankle during walking

From heel strike to forefoot contact the ankle joint plantarflexes. The ankle joint then dorsiflexes as the body and lower limb move forward over the foot during midstance. The ankle plantarflexes again from heel off to toe off.

At heel strike the subtalar joint is slightly supinated and therefore the heel is slightly inverted. The subtalar joint pronates and the leg internally rotates during contact phase. Ideally the heel is only slightly everted. In the normal functioning foot pronation does not occur past the contact period.

At the beginning of midstance, the subtalar joint supinates and the leg externally rotates. As the subtalar joint moves from a pronated position, the heel moves from an everted position to a more vertical position as the subtalar joint approaches neutral. The subtalar joint continues to supinate during midstance and the heel becomes inverted. During the propulsion phase, the subtalar joint continues

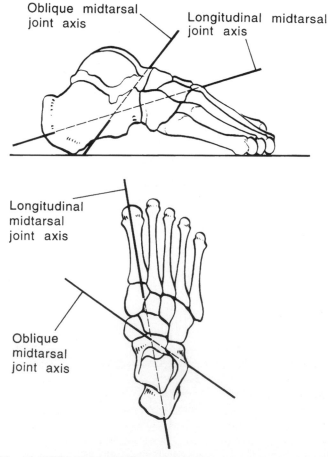

Fig. 32.22 The midtarsal joint axes of motion.
Source: adapted from Root et al (1977)

to supinate until just prior to toe off and the tibia continues to externally rotate.

At heel strike the forefoot is inverted around the long axis of the midtarsal joint. As the forefoot is loaded the subtalar joint is pronating and the heel is everting. Ground reaction forces pronate and lock the midtarsal joint around the long axis. As the subtalar joint supinates for propulsion, the midtarsal joint remains pronated.

The first ray may dorsiflex and invert as the forefoot contacts the ground and the subtalar joint pronates. If midtarsal joint inversion around the long axis is sufficient to compensate for the rearfoot eversion, the first ray may not dorsiflex. Inadequate midtarsal inversion would allow ground reaction forces to dorsiflex and invert the first ray. The first ray will dorsiflex and invert if the subtalar joint excessively pronates. This may predispose to injuries around the first MPJ region.

Normal biomechanics of the foot and ankle during running

The major difference between walking and running is that, when running, the alternate placement of one foot in front of the other is separated by periods when neither foot is in contact with the ground. The foot maintains similar motions in running as walking but variations do occur. The foot functions in a heel-toe manner in slower running. As running speed increases to striding, the foot may strike with the heel and forefoot simultaneously prior to toe off, or may strike with the forefoot initially and the heel then lower to the surface prior to toe off. During sprinting, weightbearing is on the forefoot from contact to toe off, although the heel may lower to the ground at midstance (Fig. 32.23)(Subotnick 1989).

Angle and base of gait in walking and running.

The angle between the longitudinal bisection of the foot and the line of progression is the angle of gait. Ideally the angle of gait should be approximately 10° abducted from the line of progression. An angle of gait greater than this 10° is described as an abducted gait. The angle of gait is determined by hip rotations and tibial torsion position.

The distance between the medial aspect of the heels is the base of gait. Approximately 2–3 cm is regarded as a normal base of gait (Subotnick 1989).

Changes from normal angle and base of gait may be due to compensation for an abnormality or due to structural abnormalities. For example, a wide base of gait may be necessary to increase stability on the side of a short limb. The angle and base of gait decreases as speed increases from walking to running. The angle of gait approaches zero while running and the strike of the feet is on the line of progression. This allows more efficient locomotion as the natural deviation of the centre of gravity is limited as the lower limbs move beneath the body.

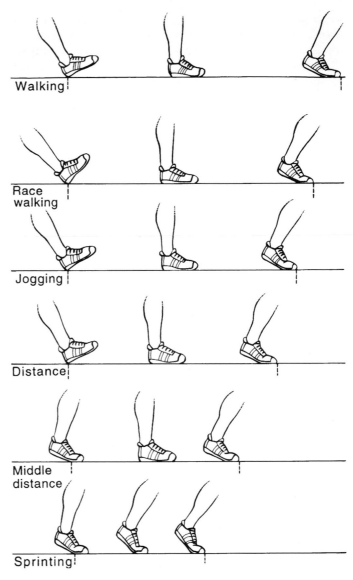

Fig. 32.23 The stance phases of walking, running and sprinting compared with one another. Source: adapted from Subotnick (1989)

ABNORMAL BIOMECHANICS OF THE FOOT AND ANKLE

To understand the relationship between abnormal biomechanics and injury, identifying variations in an athlete's gait is important. Whenever possible the athlete should be observed running. Any change in rotations of the lower limbs and feet in walking or running may be seen from an anterior or posterior position. Stride position and length, as well as anteroposterior posture, may be observed from a side-on position.

Abnormal pronation

Pronation of the foot occurs at the subtalar joint. Abnormal pronation of the foot occurs when pronation is excessive or when pronation occurs during the wrong phase of gait. An excessively pronated foot will cause excessive internal rotation of the lower limb during walking and running (Subotnick 1989). Because of this, joint and plantar ligaments and the plantar musculature of the foot and lower limb are subject to greater demands.

The medial aspect of the foot is subject to greater ground reaction forces with excessive pronation because of the greater medial loading to the foot. This may contribute to the development of first MPJ pathology including hallux valgus and exostoses. Sesamoid pain is also commonly associated with excessive pronation. Due to the shearing stresses on the skin with the pronated foot, callus build up of the skin is common. Interdigital neuroma is common in the pronated foot and is due to metatarsal hypermobility (Subotnick 1989).

Excessive pronation causes the medial longitudinal arch to flatten and lower, straining the plantar fascia and plantar musculature. This straining is accentuated when the foot remains pronated through the propulsive phase.

The pronated foot is often associated with stress fractures. In the pronated foot the uneven distribution of weight across the forefoot and the excessive movement of the metatarsals may contribute to metatarsal fractures. With greater loading of the first ray in the pronated position, stress fractures of the sesamoids may occur. As the foot excessively pronates, the talus plantarflexes and adducts, compressing the navicular and thus possibly contributing to the development of navicular stress fracture. As the navicular is the keystone of the medial longitudinal arch, it is subject to compression with lowering and flattening of the foot. Excessive pronation may lead to stress fractures of the tibia as the musculature of the leg becomes increasingly fatigued and the tibia is subject to greater shock.

In the foot that continually pronates throughout propulsive phase of gait, the peroneal muscles will have to contract harder and longer in an attempt to stabilize the medial and lateral columns of the foot. Chronic overloading may result in stress fracture of the fibula.

Abnormal supination

Abnormal supination of the subtalar joint may occur, to compensate for structural foot abnormalities, as a result of weakness of antagonist pronating musculature, such as peroneals, or as a result of spasm or tightness of the supinating musculature, e.g. gastrocnemius-soleus complex and the deep compartment muscles of the leg. The supinated foot functions in a rigid manner resulting in poor shock absorption, as there is often a range of pronation giving motion in the foot. The poor attenuation of impact may lead to the development of stress fractures such as stress fractures of the metatarsals, calcaneus, tibia and femur (Subotnick 1989).

Functioning of the foot in excessive supination may contribute to lateral instability of the foot and ankle. An increase in the incidence of sprains of the ankle and the foot may result. Excessive supination can occur with inadequately treated inversion injuries, causing a reduced range of movement of the subtalar joint. Often a structural anomaly of the forefoot in a valgus position is evident in the excessively supinated foot. There may be also the tendency to develop increased lateral stress on the lower limb. The iliotibial band becomes tighter and may contribute to a bursitis at the femoral epicondyle (Subotnick 1989).

Ankle equinus

Ankle equinus is where there is less than 10° of dorsiflexion at the ankle joint. Ten degrees of dorsiflexion is necessary for the tibia to rotate over the foot during stance phase without the foot compensating (Fig. 32.24). Ankle equinus

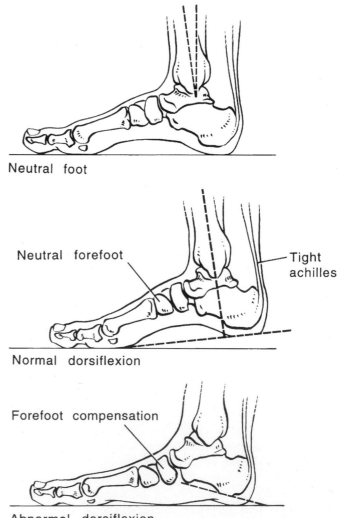

Neutral foot

Neutral forefoot — Tight achilles

Normal dorsiflexion

Forefoot compensation

Abnormal dorsiflexion

Fig. 32.24 Ankle equinus deformity. (a) normal dorsiflexion (b) abnormal dorsiflexion. Source: adapted from Subotnick (1989)

may be caused by a bony restriction of the ankle joint or be due to tight or shortened gastrocnemius or soleus muscles. Limited ankle joint dorsiflexion is compensated for by subtalar joint pronation as the dorsiflexion component of pronation is utilized. The midtarsal joint may also collapse as the dorsiflexion component of the oblique axis may be utilized. Some athletes may present with a bouncy gait due to early heel lift caused by the restricted ankle range of motion. The forefoot is prematurely loaded, predisposing to metatarsal, plantar fascia and toe injuries. Ankle equinus also contributes to achilles and medial shin pain problems as the foot may sometimes eccentrically lower to the ground following forefoot or midfoot strike (Donatelli 1990).

Abnormal function of the foot is commonly caused by intrinsic structural anomalies of the foot. Assessment of the foot in a neutral position may reveal any forefoot or rearfoot relationship assymetry. Figures 32.25 a-h show common anomalies and subsequent compensated positions adopted by the foot and ankle complex.

Plantarflexed first ray

The first ray may often be plantarflexed in regard to the other metatarsals. Compensation occurs with supination around the long axis of the midtarsal joint and the subtalar joint similar to forefoot valgus.

CORRECTION OF LOWER LIMB BIOMECHANICS

In correcting lower limb biomechanics the use of orthotics with appropriate footwear and the correction of abnormal pelvic mechanics is important.

Orthotics

Shoe orthotics are placed in shoes and are designed to correct abnormal lower limb alignment and mechanics. Excessive subtalar and midtarsal joint movements that occur to compensate for other structural anomalies may be controlled. For example, excessive foot pronation compensating for any of the above structural anomalies may be restored to normal foot function with the use of appropriate orthotic control. Structural anomalies (e.g. forefoot varus) are not altered but supported, and orthotics should not be considered as the only means of controlling abnormal movement. The practitioner must consider footwear, surfaces and the influence of tightness and/or weakness of musculature. To achieve optimal foot function, appropriate orthotics are not used alone but in conjunction with appropriate footwear for the individual.

The type of orthotic used depends on the weight of the athlete, type of footwear, sporting activity participated in, extent of abnormal motion and foot type. Orthotics may differ in rigidity and may be casted or non-casted.

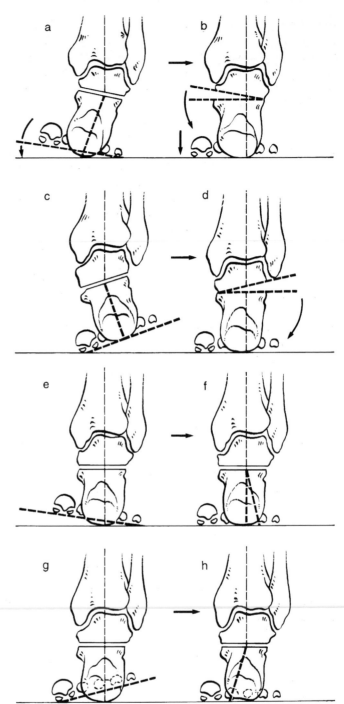

Fig. 32.25 (a)-(h) show common anomalies and subsequent compensated positions adopted by the foot and ankle complex. Source: adapted from Subotnick (1989)
(a) Rearfoot in varus and subtalar joint in neutral
(b) The subtalar joint pronates excessively so the foot can contact the ground for stance
(c) The rearfoot in valgus
(d) The midtarsal and subtalar joints supinate to compensate
(e) The forefoot is inverted on the rearfoot at the midtarsal joint
(f) The subtalar joint pronates excessively for the foot to control ground for stance
(g) The forefoot is everted on the rearfoot at the midtarsal joint
(h) The midtarsal joint supinates around the long axis but this is often insufficient to compensate so the subtalar joint supinates

Non-casted orthotics

Non-casted orthotics are often preformed devices that provide support for the arches and soft tissues of the foot. There is no accurate posting of the orthotic to change the forefoot or rearfoot, but support is given by adhering wedges under the forefoot and/or rearfoot and filling the medial aspect of the device with felt or foams of different densities. Disadvantages of the non-casted orthotics, which are usually flexible, include poor durability and inaccurate control. Athletes who would be subject to less stress may be more suited to the flexible type of insoles. The non-casted orthotics are most helpful in indicating how well an athlete adapts to any change in control of his or her biomechanics. Therefore they are often used initially as a trial in treating problems. Non-casted orthotics do not provide control where there is maximal subtalar joint pronation. Subjects with excessive supinating problems and lateral instability are difficult to support with flexible orthotics. Generally, people who have extensive abnormal biomechanics with large ranges of motions do not respond well to small changes that are achieved with the flexible orthotics. Non-casted orthotics may include the use of different materials such as ethyl-vinyl acetate (EVA), cork, rubber and plasterzote.

Casted orthotics

To change the foot mechanics significantly where there is excessive pronation and supination, an athlete may be prescribed casted orthotics after the examination of an athlete's biomechanics. Measurements are often taken of the lower limbs and feet usually in resting and neutral calcaneal stance positions. A plaster impression of the foot is taken with the foot in neutral subtalar joint position. From the plaster impressions of the feet, solid plaster models of the feet are made by filling the impressions. The solid models are then modified with additions to restore the foot to the required position. For example, in the case of an abducted and/or a rearfoot varus foot type the foot may be excessively pronated at the subtalar joint and there may be considerable midtarsal joint collapse as the medial longitudinal arch of the foot flattens to allow the foot to contact the surface. Casted orthotics may be prescribed to provide optimal control of the abnormal pronation. In sports of multidirectional movement such as netball, tennis and football, achieving optimal positioning of the feet with rigid casted orthotics may be difficult as the athlete may not tolerate the plantar foot pressure that may be applied to the foot as the foot pronates and supinates to compensate for changing body positions. Often athletes in multidirectional sports will require a flexible non-casted orthotic for the sporting activity. Common materials used in the manufacturing of rigid casted orthotics include polypropelene of different densities, and EVA foams of different densities.

Biomechanical assessment must be performed to prescribe the correct type of orthotic and how much control with the orthotic is required. An examination may include the assessment of hip joint range of motion, the alignment of the lower limbs, ankle joint range of motion, subtalar joint and midtarsal joint range of motion, forefoot/rearfoot relationship. Observing athletes while participating in their activity is useful and often important as the extent of abnormal movement during activity is not reflected in measurements taken in stance. The amount of movement that may be observed while running is often much greater than in walking. Video analysis of an athlete running is often the most useful tool in prescribing orthotics and determining the level of control required. This is also the best means of reviewing the function of the orthotic (Brukner & Khan 1993).

For the practitioner reviewing an athlete with orthotics, observing the athlete with video may not always be convenient. Often the practitioner must assess the function of the feet with and without orthotics and relate this to the ideal foot position. In the clinic, the practitioner may observe and evaluate the amount of control in the orthotic as compared to the foot position while standing and walking. Where there is excessive abnormal pronation, the orthotic may be prescribed so that it has a significant amount of rearfoot inversion. This is often the only way of providing optimal control in cases with large degrees of pronation (Blake & Ferguson 1991). Cases with only small or moderate degrees of abnormal movement may be prescribed orthotics with support through the arch and forefoot (Blake & Ferguson 1991).

FOOTWEAR

Depending on the sport participated in, athletic footwear demands vary considerably. Correct footwear for particular activities should be worn.

Running shoes

Running shoes have become complex, sophisticated and often very specialized. For the runner there is a wide range of shoes available. Shoes most suited to the athlete must fit the foot type and function of the individual. The assessment of an individual's foot type and function is essential in advising athletes regarding footwear.

Foot function may be affected by several features of a shoe. The heel counter is the upper rear part of the shoe and should be firm to assist in rearfoot stability. Forefoot flexibility must be adequate to allow easy motion of the foot flexing during propulsion. The most important feature of the shoe is the midsole which is between the upper and outsole. Midsoles are usually made of ethylvinyl-acetate (EVA) or polyurethane (PU). The midsole should be of moderate density. Midsoles which are too soft contribute to excessive mobility. Runners requiring control of excessive motion should use a midsole of dual density, harder on the medial aspect of the shoe (Nigg 1985).

Impact forces vary, in that maximal forces occur at a later stage in the soft shoes than in to harder midsoled shoes. Maximal impact forces have been shown to be lower in shoes of harder midsole density due to greater perception of the surface beneath the foot (Robbins & Gouw 1991). Flaring of the midsole of a shoe should be avoided as this promotes rapid and excessive pronation of the foot. With lateral flaring of the shoes pronatory forces are increased as the point of foot contact is at a greater distance from the calcaneus (Nigg 1985, Subotnick 1989). The negative aspect of lateral flaring outweighs the advantage of decreased impact forces.

The last construction is an important feature of the running shoe. Last construction is where the upper of the shoe is joined to the midsole. Shoes are slip lasted where the upper of the shoe is sewn together and glued directly to the sole. This promotes shoe flexibility but has less stability. Combination lasting is where the rear of the upper is glued to a fibre board in order to promote stability while the front of the shoe is slip lasted to maintain forefoot flexibility.

The shape of a shoe may also influence the movement of the foot. A pronated foot will have more medial support in a straight lasted shoe and will have little control in a curved shoe. A supinated foot is usually more suited to curved footwear. The last shape may be straight, curved or slightly curved. A supinated foot in straight shoes may override the upper of the shoe on the lateral side. This runner may complain that these shoes feel heavy and bulky with excessive weight medially.

The wear pattern on the sole of a shoe can be indicative of foot function. Normally there should be some lateral wearing at the heel area representing lateral heel strike. There should be wearing in the centre of the shoe at the forefoot region and wear just lateral to the centre of the shoe at the toe region representing supination at toe off. Excessive wear at the lateral aspect of the sole of the shoe does not represent a supinated foot type, but an excessive lateral heel strike that may be due to an abducted gait and/or varus alignment. Excessive wear on the medial side of the shoe at the forefoot and toe off regions represents a pronated foot type.

Generally, running footwear may only have a lifetime of 1000-1500 km of running. This is due to the compression of the midsole material from impact and the consistent flexing of the shoe particularly at the forefoot.

Running spikes

The poor design of running spikes is a contributing factor to foot and lower limb injuries. Running spikes are generally lightweight and flexible providing little support of the foot. Most running spikes are designed so that the spike plate is plantar grade in relation to the heel. Thus, when running on a flat surface, the heel lift is therefore 'negative' with regard to the front of the shoe, giving the effect of a negative heel. When running in spikes, the athlete strikes the ground on the forefoot and midfoot and the heel may lower to the ground. As the body weight moves over the foot, the foot lowers to the ground with less stability and greater eccentric load due to the negative heel. Because of the limited lift of the heel, the calf muscles are forced to work harder and longer to plantarflex the foot for propulsion. Because of this, the development of achilles tendon and calf injuries, and shin pain in runners is common with the use of spikes. The spikes may be modified to provide more stability by increasing the heel lift and balancing the shoe.

Multidirectional footwear

Shoes that are often known as cross-trainers are made for activities that are multidirectional such as tennis, basketball and aerobics. They should have strong heel counters and preferably at least be mid-cut in the depth of the upper part of the shoe. The flexibility at the forefoot should be as adequate as in many running shoes. Many cross-trainer type shoes are stiff at the forefoot region. Shoes for the above type of activities are usually more flat in the midsole so as not to contribute to lateral instability. The higher the midsole of the shoe, the more lateral instability.

Football boots

Football boots require all the features of a running shoe in addition to features that allow kicking and changing of direction on soft surfaces. Many types of football boots provide inadequate support for the foot and lower limb. Common inadequate structural features found in football boots include soft heel counters reducing rearfoot support, narrow soles decreasing stability and causing blistering, the curved shape and shallow uppers causing reduced stability, rigid soles limiting forefoot flexibility, negative heel lift contributing to achilles, calf and shin pain problems, and the placement of cleats and stops in causing plantar pressure areas and reduced forefoot flexibility. There should be adequate depth in the upper, a rigid heel counter, sufficient forefoot flexibilty, a wide sole, slightly curved in shape, heel lifted adequately and the cleats or stops placed to allow forefoot flexibility.

Ski boots

There have been considerable changes in ski boot design since the days of leather ski boots. Generally, ski boots have become stiffer. A stiff ski boot does not allow adequate compensatory movement at the foot and places additional stress on the bones and joints of the lower limb. More advanced skiers require stiff ski boots. Ski boots need to be fitted carefully as stiff boots may irritate bony prominences. Ski boots should be fitted individually and boots are available which allow moulding to the shape of the skier's foot. Orthotics can be used in ski boots to correct biomechanical anomalies.

While skiing, control is maintained by pronating the foot to edge the downhill ski into the slope. Skiers with biomechanical anomalies (e.g. forefoot varus) will use their available range of the foot pronation to maintain the foot in a flat position within the boot. As a result, to maintain efficient edge control the skier has to internally rotate at the hip and adopt a valgus position of the lower limb. This may contribute to fatigue and inefficient skiing. The excessive foot pronation may be restored to a neutral position, corrected with orthotics. The degree of control that an orthotic may provide is limited by boot fit. Additional control may be gained by wedging and canting the underside of the boot on the ski, although this may affect the releasing of bindings (Subotnick 1989).

Surfaces

During walking and running, the body is subject to repetitive high forces of short duration. Maximal impact forces during walking have been shown to approach twice body weight, during running 3-4 times bodyweight and during jumping 5-12 times bodyweight (Subotnick 1989).

Surfaces change the forces that the body is subject to. Maximal impact forces have been shown to vary slightly between hard and soft surfaces. The rate of increase in the initial impact forces is lower on soft surfaces. This indicates that the softer surfaces, such as grass, may reduce susceptibility to impact related injuries as the load is applied more slowly to the body (Cavanagh & La Fortune 1980).

REFERENCES

Blake R L, Ferguson H 1991 Foot orthoses for the severe flatfoot in sports. Journal of the American Podiatric Medical Association 81(10):549-555

Brukner P, Khan K 1993 Clinical sports medicine. McGraw Hill, Sydney

Cavanagh P R, La Fortune M M 1980 Ground reactive forces in distance running. Journal of Biomechanics 13:397

Donatelli R 1990 The biomechanics of the foot and ankle. F A Davis, Philadelphia

Nigg B M 1985 Biomechanics, load analysis and sports injuries in the lower extremities. Sports Medicine 2:367-379

Robbins S E, Gouw G J 1991 Athletic footwear: unsafe due to perceptual illusions. Medicine and Science in Sports and Exercise 23 (2):217-224

Root M L, Orien W P, Weed J H 1977 Normal and abnormal biomechanics of the foot. Clinical Biomechanics, Los Angeles

Subotnick S I 1989 Sports medicine of the lower extremity. Churchill Livingstone, New York

33. The slump test

Paul C. Lew, Jenny Keating

The slump test combines cervical/trunk flexion, straight leg raise (SLR) and ankle dorsiflexion. The test is performed with the subject sitting on the edge of a bench, hands clasped behind back, with the thighs fully supported (Fig. 33.1A). The trunk is slumped into flexion (Fig. 33.1B) and this position is firmly maintained by manual pressure applied downwards through the subject's shoulders (Fig. 33.1C). The subject is then instructed to fully flex the cervical spine. This cervical flexion is manually maintained by the chin or stabilizing hand of the examiner (Fig. 33.1D). The knee of the limb to be assessed is then extended maximally. If possible the ankle is fully dorsiflexed. This lower limb position is then maintained manually (Fig. 33.1E). At any point during this sequence of movements, should the pain for which the subject has sought treatment be reproduced, that posture is held by the examiner. The cervical spine alone is then allowed to extend (Fig. 33.1F). Should the pain change with cervical extension alone, while maintaining the position of the rest of the body, it can be concluded that something which moves when the cervical spine moves is implicated in the cause of the pain. If the available range of knee extension significantly increases when the cervical spine is extended, it can be concluded that some structure which is affected both by cervical extension and knee extension is limiting the subject's mobility. The slump test is usually performed first on one lower limb, then the other, and then with simultaneous bilateral knee extension/ankle dorsiflexion.

The slump test is thought to assess the mobility of pain sensitive structures within the vertebral canal (Maitland 1985). These are the spinal cord, dura, nerve roots, ligaments and posterior annulus fibrosis. Since the spinal cord and its attachments are tensioned via stretch to peripheral nerves, the test must also assess the mobility of some peripheral nerves and nerve roots.

Anatomical studies have examined dural and spinal cord movement within the vertebral canal in response to cervical flexion and SLR, although the slump test itself has not been the subject of such studies.

There is general agreement by anatomists that cervical flexion increases the tension in the dura and spinal cord (Adams & Logue 1971, Breig 1960, O'Connell 1946, Reid 1958, Smith 1956). Some researchers report that SLR also increases tension in the spinal cord (Louis 1981, O'Connell 1943, Smith 1956). Almost all agree that SLR increases the tension at least in the lower lumbar and sacral nerve roots (Breig & Troup 1979, Goddard & Reid 1965, Louis 1981, O'Connell 1943, Smith 1956). Therefore SLR combined with cervical flexion should increase the tension in the spinal cord more than either technique performed in isolation. The slump test, by adding trunk flexion to SLR and cervical flexion, should theoretically increase the tension in the spinal cord further. The degree and direction of movement of the spinal cord within the vertebral canal as a consequence of this tension increase has not been established. It seems likely that the sequencing of the slump test components and the nature of the individual's spinal cord mobility will determine the resultant cord movement.

Anatomical considerations therefore support Maitland's (1979) clinical impression that the slump test is more likely to reproduce a subject's symptoms than SLR combined with cervical flexion. Massey's (1982) clinical study provides additional support for Maitland's observations. Her study showed that the slump test more frequently reproduced the symptoms of low back pain (LBP) than the other traditional tension tests of passive neck flexion, forward flexion, SLR and SLR with dorsiflexion.

There is reason to feel confident that symptoms produced by the slump test are clinically reproducible. Massey (1982) has demonstrated that the slump test has high inter-therapist test-retest reliability. This test-retest reliability was reinforced and expanded in a clinical setting by Phillips et al (1989).

There is a sound theoretical basis to the belief that the slump test assesses neural mobility and the test will be discussed in relation to this premise. However, it must be clarified that as yet we have no definitive evidence to support or contradict this. Non-neural structures (e.g. deep fascia, muscles) may behave in a similar way to that proposed for neural structures in response to the slump. On the basis of current anatomical research, we can say with some con-

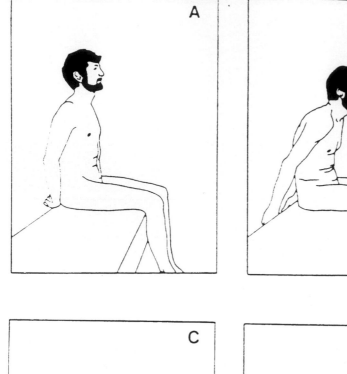

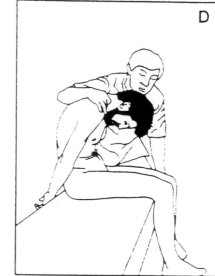

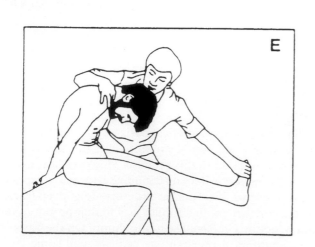

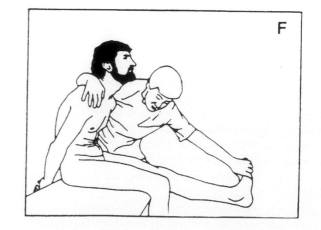

Fig. 33.1 The six steps of the slump test
(a) Step 1   (b) Step 2
(c) Step 3   (d) Step 4
(e) Step 5   (f) Step 6

fidence that if the test reproduces pain in the lower limb which changes with cervical movement, the pain is probably due to either stretch or compression of the posterior dura or nerve roots (Kuslich et al 1991).

While we may be unable to diagnose with certainty the structure which is painful or limits full range during slump testing, this does not diminish the usefulness of the slump for detecting or treating the movement responsible for symptoms. When the clinician is confident that no sinister pathology exists and that the problem is related to restricted mobility, it is appropriate to treat signs and symptoms despite uncertainty regarding which of several possible diagnoses is correct. It is often true in clinical practice that the most confident diagnosis is made when the most helpful treatment is identified. When symptoms are reproduced by the slump test the clinician may consider using the slump as a treatment technique. For the clinician to decide when such a course of treatment is appropriate, it is advisable to first observe movements which consistently reproduce the subject's symptoms, noting the range of available movement and the subjective report of the amount of pain produced. Comparison of these activities before and immediately following use of the slump and between treatment sessions will enable the clinician to confirm whether clinical reproduction of symptoms is a safe and promising course of treatment.

During the slump test it is important to question the subject carefully about any pain which is produced. The slump position can be painful for asymptomatic subjects. As for any clinical examination procedure, for the slump to be diagnostic, the symptoms produced by the slump must be those of which the subject has complained.

THE SLUMP TEST IN EXAMINATION

A subjective report of aggravating activities which resemble the slump position is a good indicator for including the slump test in the objective examination. To clarify with a few common examples:

- cervical flexion while getting into or out of a car
- long sitting, e.g. in rowing
- prolonged thorocolumbar flexion in sport, e.g. hockey
- kicking a ball
- bending to pick up a ball.

The type and distribution of the symptoms are less reliable indicators for the need for slump examination. Symptoms reproduced by slump may be neural in origin or caused by neural movement against a neighbouring injured structure. Such symptoms have no uniquely identifiable qualities. They may be localized to an affected vertebral level, follow the distribution of a peripheral nerve or present as poorly localized and diffuse. They may be non-segmental and non-sclerotomal (Marks 1989). The authors have found, nevertheless, that the slump test is invaluable in the extended examination of all posterior thigh and persistent low back pain.

There is also no clear link between mechanism of injury and the subsequent value of slump testing during the objective examination. It is tempting to believe that injuries which occur during activities which mimic the neural tensioning of the slump test would be better investigated using the slump. Examples of such activites are bending forward and kicking a football, or lifting with straight knees and fully flexed hips and trunk. However, in clinical practice, the slump test can reproduce symptoms which began with activities like downhill running which do not mimic the slump position. The reason for this probably lies in the variety of ways in which free movement of neural structures can be compromised. Any structure or tissue through which neural tissue moves could potentially restrict the free glide of that neural tissue. Examples of such structures are muscle injured by swelling, spasm or local adhesions, intervertebral foraminal space reduced due to swelling of surrounding structures or deformity of the bony margins of the space, and fracture to bones adjacent to the spinal cord, nerves or nerve roots. Additionally, any intrusion into the spinal canal may limit spinal cord glide, as can adhesions between neural and adjacent structures due to direct injury.

In summary, the most useful indicator for slump testing which can be gained during the subjective examination is the description of the activity which now causes the symptoms.

TREATMENT CONSIDERATIONS

Precautions and contraindications for use of the slump test

Precautions
- irritability
- presence of neurological signs or symptoms
- reproduction of neurological symptoms

Contraindications
- worsening neurological signs or symptoms
- tethered cord syndrome
- cauda equina syndrome
- spinal instability in flexion

The clinician should consider using the slump as a treatment procedure when symptoms or lack of mobility are reproduced by the slump test and eased when a part of the slump position is released. When no sinister pathology or contraindications exist, whether to proceed with slump as treatment depends on the patient's response to the test. The method of incorporation of slump into patient management, like that of any other technique, depends in part on the irritability of the patient's condition. If a condition is non-irritable, symptoms which are provoked by the patient's activities or the clinician's examination will quickly settle to pre-provocation level. Irritable symptoms, once provoked, do not settle quickly and the longer they take to settle the more irritable they may be considered. The subjective examination should aim to clarify the activities-related irritability, which guides the clinician's objective examination. Whenever irritability is suspected, examination procedures should be limited or modified so that the patient's symptoms are minimally provoked. If the functional activity which reproduces the symptoms is reassessed immediately following the slump test and the range or pattern of movement is the same or better or the patient reports symptoms to be the same or lessened, it is safe to proceed with using the slump as treatment. If the functional activity is worse or the patient reports an increase in symptoms it is not wise to use the slump as treatment, and if the slump is used for reassessment later it should be modified to avoid aggravation of the problem. When the response both within and between treatment sessions is understood, the technique can be reduced or progressed as necessary. In addition, if the clinician is currently using a different treatment type which is significantly improving the symptoms, it is advisable to persist with the existing regime of treatment until the clinician is not satisfied with the progress before including the slump in treatment. Positive slump findings are commonly improved using spinal palpatory techniques. In the opinion of the authors, particular attention should be paid to the mobilization of the thoracolumbar and lumbosacral junctions when the slump test is positive. While it is not a hard and fast rule, it is a valuable clinical practice to determine the effect of joint mobilization on slump findings prior to using the slump as a treatment technique.

Whether or not the slump test is positive, the patient should be reassessed following the test to ascertain the test effect.

METHODS OF TREATMENT

There are several ways to use the slump as a treatment technique. Commonly the slump is used to apply a sustained stretch at the point of pain reproduction or movement limitation. How much pain is produced and how long the clinician sustains the stretch depends on the assessment and reassessment findings. Until the clinician is confident that the slump will not aggravate the problem, gentle stretches of short duration are recommended. Alternatively, the pain or restriction may be treated by intermittent stretch as might be applied through e.g. repeated knee flexion/extension or cervical flexion/extension. The rhythmical oscillations used may be large or small in amplitude. Again

the optimum amount and duration of such treatment can best be determined by observing the response.

Examination of hamstring pain

Several clinicians advocate a special role for the slump test in the differential diagnosis and treatment of pain in the posterior thigh (Bourke et al 1986, Kornberg 1985, Kornberg & Lew 1989, Lew 1988, Williamson 1987).

Posterior thigh pain and hamstring muscle weakness commonly lead to a diagnosis of hamstring injury. Most tests for hamstring injury, however, also challenge the low back and neural structures. Even local tenderness over the hamstring muscles does not ensure a correct diagnosis of hamstring injury. Palpable tenderness and localized muscle pain may be due to an injury to that muscle. It may also be caused by visceral disease (Kellgren 1939) or injury to the lumber spine (McCall et al 1979, Mooney & Robertson 1976), nerve roots and posterior dura (Kuslich et al 1991). McCall et al (1979) concluded that pain and palpable tenderness could be elicited in the referred area without palpable tenderness over the site of pathology. Therefore tenderness and pain in the hamstring muscle do not conclusively prove local hamstring pathology.

Pain produced in the posterior thigh by the slump test but relieved during the cervical extension component should not be due to hamstring pathology since altering cervical posture during the slump test should in no way affect the hamstring muscle (Maitland 1979). The slump test therefore provides an opportunity to differentiate and treat that posterior thigh pain which is not due to hamstring muscle pathology.

Kornberg (1985) investigated the frequency of positive slump test (when changing only the cervical posture during the slump test changed the hamstring pain) in a group of Australian Rules footballers, who were diagnosed as having hamstring strain. He found that compared to the control group (Australian Rules footballers with no hamstring or back pain) the incidence of positive slump was significantly higher (p < .001)

Kornberg and Lew (1989) studied footballers diagnosed as having a grade 1 hamstring strain with a positive slump test. The diagnosis of grade 1 hamstring strain was made if the player presented with posterior thigh pain without bruising, hamstring tenderness on palpation, limitation of SLR and pain with isometric hamstring contraction. They found that using the slump test as a stretching technique in combination with traditional treatment was superior to traditional treatment alone. Slump treated players recovered faster and only one player missed one game. In contrast, those who received traditional treatment alone each missed a minimum of two games (Table 33.1).

These studies suggest that posterior thigh pain in these footballers may originate from neural structures. If so, it

Table 33.1 Contingency table summarizing data from experimental and control groups of subjects

	0 games missed	1+ games missed
Experimental[1]	11 (4.71)[2]	1·(7.29)
Control[3]	0 (6.29)	16 (9.71)

($x^2 = 20.47$, df = 1, $p < 0.001$)

1 Traditional treatment with slump stretching technique
2 Numbers in parentheses, expected frequencies
3 Traditional treatment

may be why many so-called hamstring injuries are slower to heal and more recurrent than might be expected of a muscle injury.

Modifying the test and treatment

The slump test may be considered as a set of steps, each of which adds some tension to the dura/cord. Although the basic slump technique has been described above, it should be considered a guideline only. It is common in clinical practice to produce varying pain responses depending on the subject's position and the sequence of application of these slump components. The description of the activity which causes pain best indicates the sequence of slump which might be appropriate. To illustrate, consider the example of a patient who complained of occipital headache with prolonged sitting. The slump test was used when palpatory techniques failed to reproduce symptoms. In the sequence detailed above, no symptoms were produced. However, when the cervical spine was flexed after bilateral lower limb extension and the position sustained for 1 minute, the headache was reproduced. The problem was successfully treated by using this slump sequence and sustained stretch over three visits. Innovative adaptation of techniques are often required in the hunt for and treatment of elusive symptoms and the slump test should not be considered a rigid tool but a highly malleable one. The clinician may wish to add lateral trunk flexion or rotation, replace ankle dorsiflexion with plantar flexion/ inversion, slump stretch in side lying rather than sitting, or treat using repeated knee extension, cervical flexion or thoracic extension while the subject is held in the slump position, to make just a few of the many possible suggestions.

As was mentioned previously, whenever irritability is suspected, modified examination procedures should be used so that the patient's symptoms are minimally provoked.

Regardless of the order or method of application of the slump components, one important principle must be adhered to if differential diagnosis is desired. The stabilized part of the body must not move while the remote part of the body is moved, if neural structures are to be incriminated. In a subject with posterior thigh pain, if the knee is allowed to flex while the cervical spine is extended, it cannot be determined whether it was the cervical

extension or the knee flexion which eased the pain, leaving the clinician unsure of whether neural structures or the hamstrings are incriminated. In the slumped subject with occipital headache on full cervical flexion, if the cervical spine moves while the knees are flexed, a change in symptoms incriminates either cervical or neural structures. The part of the body in which the symptoms are felt must be held still while a remote section of the body is moved in order to incriminate a structure which moves between the two sites. If this principle of stabilization of one section of the body while a remote section is moved is clearly understood, the slump test becomes a flexible assessment tool with many useful variations. The clinician is advised to persist with the refinement of technique to ensure optimum stabilization.

Technique

As with the performance of any other technique, the more reliable the clinician's technique the more reliable is the information obtained. A few commonly observed technical weaknesses are worthy of comment.

When beginning the slump test, ensure that the subject sinks into full lumbar flexion. It is often necessary to spend some minutes teaching the pelvic rotation required to achieve this. It is not uncommon for people to be quite unaware of how to voluntarily flex their lumbar spines and it can demand considerable patience from the therapist to produce this apparently simple movement. There is a tendency for students to allow subjects to flex at the hip rather than bow the thoracic and lumbar spine.

Having achieved this, the next challenge is to the stabilization skills of the therapist. Thoracic and lumbar flexion must be firmly maintained by a secure downward compression through the shoulders. The tendency for the trunk to be dragged into lateral flexion towards the therapist should be avoided unless specifically desired. Since this overpressure should be maintained by the therapist's bodyweight rather than arms, the couch height should be adjustable to accommodate variations in subject size. When teaching friends or relatives of the person how to apply the slump as a home treatment, it is difficult to avoid the tendency for them to compress the spine thereby preventing thoracic and lumbar flexion. This can be prevented by positioning the subject in full flexion before applying the stabilizing pressure through the shoulders.

When the cervical spine is allowed to maximally flex, this position is securely overpressured from the back of the head using either the hand of the arm through which the shoulders are held, or the therapist's chin. Care should be taken to flex the cervical spine rather than apply a downward shearing force through the back of the head. If the person complains of cervicothoracic pain, immediately check the technique. This is the second most difficult thing to teach the relatives or friends helping with a home slump program. It is not uncommon for the patient to develop neck pain if the technique is performed badly. Maximal cervical flexion is limited by the front of the chest. There is no need to apply more overpressure than required to maintain this or the available end of range.

Students learning slump technique seem to find the next step the most awkward, although it is the simplest to learn well. If the therapist is not standing well towards the front of the subject, it will be difficult to reach the foot or ankle while maintaining the spinal stabilization. When the therapist begins the slump test, one foot should be in line with the subject's spine and the other stepped well forward to be in line with the place to which the therapist must move to in order to complete the test. It is the same principle as that required for safe lifting technique.

When removing the stabilization from the head in order to allow cervical extension, first allow extension to neutral, check for any change in pain, then allow full extension. It occasionally happens that the subject's pain is eased with extension to neutral but returns again at end of range cervical extension (Maitland 1991).

Progression of treatment

If the patient is responding to slump treatment it is usually unnecessary to alter the nature of treatment. If the subject initially responded but the response has plateaued before full recovery, slump can be progressed by increasing the pain provoked if the clinician deems this safe and appropriate, or by increasing the neural stretch by gradually adding in previously modified or deleted components of the slump.

Home routines

If it is desirable for the person to continue slump stretching at home and there is no reason why the stretch should not begin with knee extension, it is often easiest to teach the person to begin in long sitting with ankle dorsiflexion maintained by a wall. The person can then roll their lumbar, thoracic and cervical spines into flexion and get a partner to assist with overpressure.

NEUROLOGICAL EXAMINATION

If neurological signs or symptoms are complained of, a complete neurological examination mapping out the area of deficit is warranted prior to using the slump as a treatment technique and caution should be exercised when it is used for assessment. If neurological symptoms are provoked during a slump assessment the technique should be stopped at that point until the irritability of such symptoms is understood. At the next treatment session, the neurological examination should be repeated, comparing any deficit to that recorded on the previous visit. If the clinician suspects the slump test or treatment may be contributing to the amplification of signs or symptoms, and this continues to be the case despite attempts to modify the procedure, slump treatment should be abandoned.

The slump is important in the clinical examination and treatment of sporting injuries which result in low back or limb pain. It appears to aid in the differentiation of posterior thigh pain and to be useful for the treatment of subjects with posterior thigh pain and positive slump. When contraindications do not exist, it should be used as a routine test procedure for all sporting injuries resulting in low back and limb pain.

REFERENCES

Adams C B T, Logue V 1971 Studies in cervical spondylotic myelopathy. (1) Movement of the cervical roots, dura and cord and their relationship to the course of the extrathecal roots. Brain 94:557-568

Bourke A, Alchin C, Little K, Sargood J 1986 Hamstring symptoms and lumbar spine relationship in sports people: a pilot study. Proceedings of the Australian Physiotherapy Association, National Conference, Hobart, pp 309-321

Breig A 1960 Biomechanics of the central nervous system. Almquist & Wiksell, Stockholm

Breig A, Troup J D G 1979 Biomechanical considerations in the straight-leg-raising test. Spine 4(3):242-250

Goddard M P, Reid J D 1965 Movements induced by staight-leg-raising in the lumbo-sacral roots, nerves and plexus, and in the intrapelvic section of the sciatic nerve. Journal of Neurology, Neurosurgery and Psychiatry 28:12-18

Kellgren J H 1939 On the distribution of pain arising from deep somatic structures with charts of segmental pain areas. Clinical Science 4:35-46

Kornberg C 1985 Incidence of referred pain in Australian Rules football players with a diagnosis of grade one hamstring strain. Unpublished postgraduate diploma dissertation, Lincoln Institute of Health Sciences, School of Physiotherapy, Melbourne

Kornberg C, Lew P 1989 The effect of stretching neural structures on grade 1 hamstrings injuries. Journal of Orthopaedic and Sports Physical Therapy 10(12):481-489

Kuslich S D, Ulstrom C L, Michael C J 1991 The tissue origin of low back pain and sciatica: a report of pain response to tissue stimulation during operations on the lumbar spine using local anesthesia. Orthopaedic Clinics of North America 22(2):181-187

Lew P 1988 The slump test: a possible differentiation test. Proceedings of International Federation of Orthopaedic Manipulative Therapists Congress, Cambridge, pp 33-34

McCall E W, Park W M, O'Brien J P 1979 Induced pain referral from posterior lumbar elements in normal subjects. Spine 4(5):441-446

Maitland G D 1979 Negative disc exploration: positive canal signs. Australian Journal of Physiotherapy 25(3):129-134

Maitland G D 1985 The slump test: examination and treatment. Australian Journal of Physiotherapy 31(6):215-219

Maitland G D 1991 Personal communication

Marks R 1989 Distribution of pain provoked from lumbar facet joints and related structures during diagnostic spinal infiltration. Pain 39:37-40

Massey A 1982 The slump test. Unpublished postgraduate diploma dissertation, South Australian Institute of Technology, School of Physiotherapy, Adelaide

Mooney V, Robertson J 1976 The facet syndrome. Clinical Orthopaedics and Related Research 115:149-154

O'Connell J E A 1943 Sciatica and the mechanism of the production of the clinical syndrome in the protrusion of the lumbar intervertebral disc. British Journal of Surgery 30:315-327

O'Connell J E A 1946 The clinical signs of meningeal irritation. Brain 69:9-21

Phillips K, Lew P, Matyas T 1989 The inter-therapist test-retest reliability of the slump test. Australian Journal of Physiotherapy 35(2):89-94

Reid J D 1958 Ascending nerve roots and tightness of dura mater. New Zealand Medical Journal 57:16-26

Smith C G 1956 Changes in length and position of the segments of the spinal cord with changes in posture in the monkey. Radiology 66:259-266

Williamson A 1987 Recurrent hamstring lesions and lower limb tissue mobility. Proceedings of the Australian Sports Medicine Federation, National Scientific Conference, Adelaide 2:441-452

34. Special considerations for the female athlete

Melinda M. Cooper

BACK PAIN IN THE CHILDBEARING YEAR

When treating spinal problems in pregnant athletes assessment needs to be as detailed and comprehensive as in the non-pregnant athlete. There are additional concerns when dealing with pregnant athletes.

It is the author's opinion that spinal symptoms which present in pregnancy need to be assessed in their own right and not necessarily be attributed to the pregnancy. If thorough assessment and appropriate treatment does not improve the symptoms, it may then be feasible that the symptoms are intrinsic to the pregnancy and the therapist will need to advise the athlete that similar symptoms are likely in subsequent pregnancies. Implicit to this, is the need for the athlete to make a complete recovery prior to planning a future pregnancy and to give careful consideration to the number and spacing of pregnancies.

Subjective assessment

In addition to the usual history, it is useful to know if the athlete regularly had back pain premenstrually or during menstruation. It is possible that women who have 'hormonal' back pain differ from those with demonstrable musculoskeletal pathology and thus the prognosis would differ, with the former less likely to make a complete recovery with treatment.

It is necessary to learn at which stage during the pregnancy the symptoms began and whether it was present in the same site and to the same intensity in a previous pregnancy.

The athlete's parity and ages of other children are also important. Women who have children less than three years apart are involved in frequent and heavy lifting in the daily care of their toddlers. Also, women who have their children close together, i.e. less than three years apart may not have had sufficient time between respective pregnancies and lactations to have stabilized their hormonal levels or to have completely recovered from these experiences. It is the author's opinion that women who do not fully recover after each pregnancy are very likely to carry residual problems into future pregnancies and thus compound their symptoms.

Objective assessment

Examination procedures will need to be modified according to the gestational stage of the athlete. Lumbar and lower thoracic flexion will be limited by a large abdomen from the second trimester. Tests performed in supine should be minimized after 20 weeks.

Examination and treatment in prone on the plinth is both possible and often highly desirable and is effected by the judicious use of pillows and cushions. When assessing or treating in prone it is extremely important to frequently ask the woman how she is feeling, since her face is not observable.

Some women find this position uncomfortable and will therefore need to be treated either in modified prone on bean bags or side-lying on the plinth.

Frequent reassessments by getting the woman to replicate the aggravating movements after short bouts of treatment is not always advisable in pregnant patients in their third trimester. Often, they experience difficulty getting into positions and require a considerable amount of time to do so.

Treatment

Many treatment modalities used for non-pregnant athletes are also suitable for pregnant women.

Manual therapy techniques are very successful but care must be taken if manipulation is considered as a treatment option. All the joints of the pregnant body are affected by hormonal changes and the author has observed many women with symptoms of joint laxity in the first trimester, especially in the multiparous population. This joint laxity is usually a feature of later pregnancy and it is commonly accepted that the joints of the pelvis and lumbar spine are particularly affected. It is inadvisable to use manipulations

695

in this region. It is therefore important to ascertain the stage of pregnancy and to use more controlled and less vigorous treatment techniques later in pregnancy, while being aware that a number of women will display laxity early in their pregnancies.

Where there is obvious thoracic stiffness and/or kyphosis which is impeding postural corrective work, mid thoracic spine manipulations are indicated. When combined with effective remedial exercise, these are an excellent treatment modality.

Positioning the pregnant woman in supine is undesirable due to the compression of the maternal inferior vena cava by the gravid uterus which could compromise uterine blood flow. Pregnant women may also experience symptoms of supine hypotensive syndrome where they feel faint and dizzy and their blood pressure lowers (Beischer & Mackay 1976). Treatment techniques in supine should therefore be avoided from 20 weeks' gestation.

Orthotic pelvic and low back bracing can be useful in cases of demonstrable instability of lumbar, sacral or pubic joints in conjunction with dynamic abdominal bracing techniques. There are many types of braces available but none provide the one answer to all instability problems. Trochanter belts may be useful for some patients with pubic symphysis problems while other patients respond well to wide (15–20 cm) elasticized supports which cover the low lumbar and upper sacral levels and fasten under the abdomen with velcro across the pubic symphysis. Wide bandaging (15–20 cm) has also been found to be both effective in reducing symptoms while weightbearing. It is also inexpensive and simple for the woman to apply herself. The author frequently uses taping for postural correction especially in the thoracic region, which may often negate the need for pelvic/lumbar orthotics where the problem is both instability and postural in nature.

When considering electrotherapy as treatment, great care is warranted during pregnancy. Any electrotherapy which can permeate the pelvic or abdominal cavities is contraindicated during pregnancy. This includes ultrasound pulsed or continuous over the lumbar, sacral and pubic joints due to the risk of insonating placental tissues and the foetus at therapeutic doses where the sound waves are absorbed by the structures. Pregnant women over 20 weeks' gestation should not be receiving electrically driven traction because of the risks associated with being in supine.

Differential diagnoses

All orthopaedic presentations should be assessed subjectively and objectively, including movement assessment and palpation. This will ensure a more accurate understanding of the pathology. Many symptoms are dismissed as a particular pathology merely because of their site. An example of this is pubic symphysis pain. Pain in the central

groin area does not necessarily mean that the pubic symphysis is unstable. The author has treated a number of such presentations which may have been round ligament strain. The round ligament of the uterus inserts via a fatty digitation into the labia (Anderson 1978). At this point it certainly appears as pubic pain. However, accurate palpation usually reveals the symptoms to be worse unilaterally and centrally the symphysis is not symptomatic. Such presentations respond well to soft tissue mobilizations of the affected site.

Conversely, pubic symphysis strains are difficult to treat and usually require gentle mobilizations, dynamic abdominal bracing and orthotic use. Pectineal lesions may also appear at first glance to be pubic symphysis problems.

During pregnancy, there are enormous changes to all systems of the body. The author believes that many of the musculoskeletal symptoms encountered during pregnancy are as much due to changes in fascia as to the hormonal changes themselves. As a result, manual skills involving myofascial releases in addition to joint and soft tissue mobilizations and exercise should be considered by physiotherapists in their treatment regimen.

PELVIC FLOOR DYSFUNCTION

Symptoms associated with pelvic floor dysfunction can affect people of all ages and both sexes. The most commonly noted area of female pelvic floor dysfunction is incontinence. In Australia, it has been estimated that at least 700 000 people suffer urinary incontinence and of these less than 30% have sought assistance (Fonda & Wellings 1987). Simple stress urinary incontinence with coughing and sneezing has been reported to occur in 20% of women. The incidence rises to 36% in women between the ages of 45 and 59 years (Chiarelli 1987). Women are most likely to develop stress incontinence initially during pregnancy. Indeed, it has been stated that up to 64.5% of pregnant women experience incontinence (Beck & Hsu 1963).

The majority of stress urinary incontinence is mild and infrequent but these early symptoms have a strong tendency to worsen with pregnancy, childbirth, menopause and chronic coughing. Similarly, while women who develop incontinence in pregnancy may encounter a respite in their symptoms during the post-natal period, these women are more likely to develop the problem more severe degree during menopause.

Physiotherapists who are involved in continence management see many women complaining of urinary incontinence with weightbearing sports such as tennis, squash and aerobics but the author was unable to find current research linking sports, athletes and urinary incontinence. It is probable that female athletes suffer symptoms of pelvic floor dysfunction at a similar rate to their non-athletic counterparts.

Clinically, the author has observed a number of female athletes who have delayed seeking assistance for their symptoms, believing erroneously that their symptomatology is, to a certain degree, 'normal' for women or that nothing can be done for it. It is also possible that a number of these athletes will prematurely retire from their chosen sport because of this condition.

The soft tissues of the pelvic floor are particularly vulnerable in the childbearing year and after menopause. The author believes that as more female athletes continue to exercise and compete to some extent during pregnancy and return to their sports very soon after giving birth it is likely that these women will be subject to problems of incontinence and pelvic floor weakness. Similarly, many women are taking up sport and/or continuing sport into their menopausal years and beyond, where incontinence is very likely to be a problem.

Physiotherapists are in a position to be able to identify women at risk of developing or aggravating symptoms of incontinence and to educate, advise and/or treat as appropriate. All women should be educated about pelvic floor and sphincter weakness. Clinical experience suggests that particular attention should be given to women who are:

- pregnant
- parous, especially women who have had large babies, prolonged second stage of labour, operative vaginal delivery
- obese (in the sporting population this is usually not a problem unless the athlete is involved in weight sports such as weightlifting, discus or shotput)
- weightlifting
- chronically constipated
- peri-menopausal
- already symptomatic regardless of parity and degree of severity of symptoms
- known to have defective collagen disorders.

To this end, an understanding of pelvic floor anatomy and continence mechanisms is essential.

Applied anatomy

The pelvic floor is comprised of fascial, connective and muscular tissue and all components are important in maintaining function.

There are several layers of fascia and two layers of muscle (Fig. 34.1a).

Perineal group

This is made up of the bulbocavernosus, ischiocavernosus and transverse perineal muscles (Fig. 34.1b). The latter muscles serve to brace the perineum against downward pressure from the superior pelvic cavity. Innervation is by the pudendal nerve (S2, S3, S4).

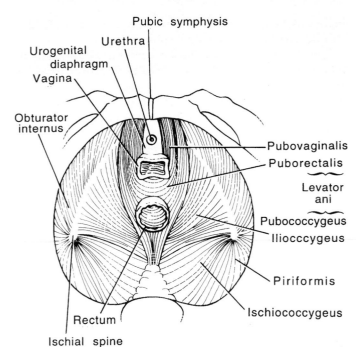

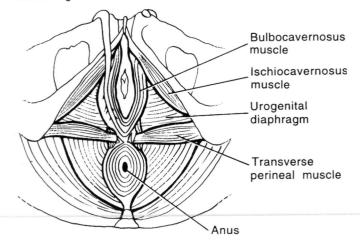

Fig. 34.1 Female pelvic diaphragm, (A) Superior view (B) Inferior view. Source: adapted from Wilder (1988)

The levator ani group

This is comprised of the deeper pelvic floor muscles of the pubococcygeus, puborectalis, iliococcygeus and ischiococcygeus. Innervation is by the pudendal nerve (S2, S3, S4). Pubococcygeus fibres pass posteriorly to partially insert into the lateral walls of the vagina and in part continue to insert onto the anterior surface of the coccyx. Innervation is from below by perineal branches of the pudendal nerve. The puborectalis, however, is innervated from direct motor branches of S3 and S4 to its pelvic surface.

It is a muscular loop which runs deep to the pubococcygeus around the recto-ano flexure, maintaining continence as a flap-valve mechanism. It is intimately blended with the striated external anal sphincter.

These muscles of the pelvic floor have more fascial tissue than contractile tissue which implies that with overstretching and constant straining (e.g. constipation, repetitive heavy lifting, childbirth) fascial damage can be permanent. If this occurs, then the dynamic function of the contractile elements of the pelvic floor becomes critically important in maintaining continence, support of pelvic structures and sexual function.

The bladder functions as a reservoir for urine until it fills to approximately 300–350 mL (Fonda & Wellings 1987). At that point a signal is sent to the brain which is recognized as the first sensation to void. This can usually be suppressed until full capacity is reached (average 500 mL). Urine does not normally leak out because of the well-supported bladder neck which acts like a valve. The bladder neck and proximal urethra are comprised of numerous elastic fibres in the urethral wall which suggest a passive occlusive role. The pelvic floor abuts the urethral length more distally and a pelvic floor contraction elevates the anterior vaginal wall moving the urethra towards the pubic symphysis (see Fig. 34.2).

The posterior pubo-urethral ligaments are fibromuscular bands that act as suspensory supports for the urethra. They contain contractile elements under neural control and functionally they prevent excessive posterior displacement of the urethra.

Pathology

Where bladder neck descent is due to poor pelvic floor support, the same increase in intra-abdominal pressure which normally occludes the bladder neck will in fact be a distracting force and the woman will lose urine (Fig. 34.2) (Chiarelli 1987). Prolapse may also occur where there is disruption to the pubo-urethral ligaments (Jones 1950).

Increases in intra-abdominal pressure occur commonly with coughing, sneezing and pregnancy. High impact activities of running, jumping and even racquet serves where there are strong abdominal contractions can cause incontinence and prolapse descent where the bladder neck is inadequately supported.

Assessment

During various other physiotherapy assessments performed on the female athlete, it is necessary to be alert to the impact of incontinence and take every opportunity to educate and thus assist in preventing the problem worsening. If the athlete does not present directly with an incontinence problem it is valuable nonetheless to inquire. For example, when the client is asked about coughing and its effect on back pain, it is also very useful to note if she suffers any incontinence at the same time.

The therapist may not intend to treat that symptom immediately but by being aware of it the physiotherapist can take the opportunity to give simple advice about pelvic floor exercises and perhaps return to the issue at a later date.

When the athlete presents overtly with pelvic floor symptoms, a detailed assessment is warranted. It is highly recommended to refer the patient to a physiotherapist working in the area of women's health, who has skills in assessing incontinence types and severity, prolapse and pelvic floor strength.

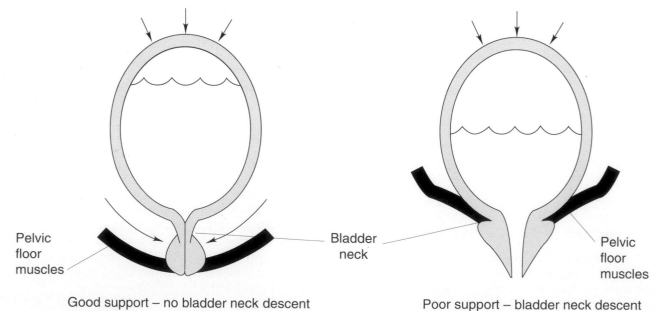

Good support – no bladder neck descent   Poor support – bladder neck descent

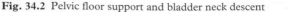

Fig. 34.2 Pelvic floor support and bladder neck descent

In assessing the various muscle contractions of the pubococcygeus, puborectalis and the superficial perineals most physiotherapists working in this field use a modified Oxford scale of grading 0–5 (Chiarelli 1989) whereby grade 0 represents no palpable contraction and grade 5 represents a strong squeeze, lift and hold and is readily repeatable. Usually, there is good occlusive power of the levator ani against the examiner's fingers. Clinical experience in treating women with incontinence suggests that both contractile strength and endurance are important. Female athletes who participate in long distance running or long sporting matches need very good endurance to keep them dry through the event.

It is the author's opinion that women who are participating in weightbearing competitive sports or weightbearing recreational activities should have grade 4 or better contractile strength and endurance of the levator ani when assessed during vaginal examination by an experienced women's health physiotherapist. The forces generated in weightbearing activities and rapidly changing directions such as running, squash and netball will be transmitted to the pelvic floor via ground reaction forces. If the pelvic floor strength is insufficient to meet these demands, the woman will develop urine leakage, lack of anal control or a dragging heavy feeling in the vagina (possibly, anterior vaginal wall descent or other prolapse). These symptoms will get worse with age and repetitive aggravating activities.

Treatment

Treatment will always consist of pelvic floor strengthening. If the woman's strength is less than grade 4 she will require a home program of daily pelvic floor exercises. All women should be instructed in pelvic floor bracing. Before each cough, sneeze or lifting manoeuvre the woman should tighten the pelvic floor. Female athletes who are participating in sports involving weights need to be particularly aware of this.

Perineometry can be a useful clinical tool to assist in pelvic floor strengthening. Intravaginal weighted cones can also be used by clients to continue their home program of strengthening. In women whose pelvic floor strength is grade 3 or less and not improving sufficiently rapidly with pelvic floor exercises alone, electrotherapy may also be of benefit. Interferential therapy using a two electrode approach over the perineum and/or anus and inferior to the pubic symphysis can be of benefit. Laycock and Green (1988) found that frequencies of 10–50 Hz were useful for genuine stress incontinence and 5–10 Hz for symptoms of urgency. Both applications are more comfortable using a carrier wave of 2 kHz and surged.

Female athletes will initially need advice concerning bladder voiding habits. Going to the toilet too frequently and deliberately reducing the fluid intake in the attempt to keep dry are pointless tasks that inevitably aggravate the situation. Restricting fluid intake is also potentially dangerous during exercise as it can cause dehydration.

The physiotherapist needs to encourage the client to drink 2 L or more (depending upon weather and exercise levels) of non-caffeinated fluid per day. She must drink before sport and preferably at frequent intervals during it.

Normal voiding occurs 3–5 times per day, 300–500 mL per void and at 3–5 hourly intervals. These are useful parameters and the woman should be encouraged to 'train' her bladder accordingly. It is commonly accepted that pelvic floor exercises are invaluable as a means of assisting to defer the urge to void during bladder retraining. Perineal support and distraction techniques are also useful although not always as practicable as pelvic floor exercises which can be done entirely privately and while engaged in other activities.

The author believes that specific pelvic floor training may also be required in women with very specific symptoms. For example, the woman who consistently loses a small amount of urine during her serve at squash may benefit from learning to deliberately contract the pelvic floor during isolated components of her serve until she can maintain control throughout the entire manoeuvre. The author has found that a monitored skipping program provides useful training.

The athlete contracts her pelvic floor and begins to skip initially using slow alternating leg patterns and gradually progresses to faster skips and then to double leg patterns. She notes the moment that her pelvic floor begins to feel heavy and reduces the amplitude and speed of skipping until she regains that sensation of control. This program can be extended as she develops more control.

Some athletes who still leak in spite of improving their pelvic floor strength and endurance can benefit from intravaginal devices which assist in supporting the bladder neck during sport.

One super or two average width tampons can be inserted side-by-side into the vagina to support the anterior vaginal wall. Various other products are on the market which can also be used intravaginally, such as the 'Femcare' sponge.

Female athletes with pelvic floor dysfunctional symptoms should be reviewed regularly even after active physiotherapy has ceased. If the woman is pregnant when she presented initially, she should be seen 4–6 weeks before delivery to ascertain that strength and function have been maintained. If she initially presented post-natally, she should be seen again after breastfeeding has ceased and/or there has been a resumption of her normal menstrual cycle. Athletes who have been deemed to be 'at risk' of pelvic floor dysfunction should be seen prior to or early in pregnancy. Similarly, the perimenopausal athlete should be seen at 3–6 monthly intervals.

Other women should be reviewed 6-monthly. These follow-up visits serve to remind patients of the importance of maintaining good pelvic floor function for life, and can assist in detecting early signs of deterioration. Assessment and treatment measures can then be promptly employed.

There do exist some women whose continence mechanisms are inherently inadequate. This may be due to inherited factors such as insufficient or defective connective tissue that predisposes these women to incontinence at an early age with or without the stresses of childbirth, ageing, menopause or increasing weight gain (Dwyer & Glenning 1990). Physiotherapists also need to be aware that female athletes with excessive joint mobility associated with loose connective tissue could be at risk of incontinence and should be encouraged to develop their pelvic floor strength as much as possible.

If pelvic floor strengthening is limited by inherent problems, and there is inadequate assistance from intravaginal devices during sport, surgery may need to be considered. Thorough examination and urodynamic assessment is recommended prior to surgery and the results of surgery have been found to be better in women who have undergone physiotherapy treatment pre-operatively (Klarskov et al 1991).

The author recommends that surgery be considered when all other conservative measures have been tried and proved to be insufficiently effective, and that the female athlete give serious consideration to changing her sport in an attempt to prevent the condition deteriorating and thus avoid the physical and emotional distress associated with pelvic floor dysfunction.

EXERCISE IN THE CHILDBEARING YEAR

To exercise or not while pregnant is an age-old question. Many recommendations have been made for pregnant women which are very similar to today's present guidelines (American College of Obstetricians and Gynaecologists 1985). O'Neill et al (1990) considered the historical perspective of exercise in pregnancy and concluded that much of the advice given to pregnant women has been based on social factors and society's attitudes towards women. The last decade, by contrast, has witnessed research into the acute foetal effects of exercise, and epidemiological studies evaluating the chronic foetal effects of repeated exercise in pregnancy. Such research serves to validate the contemporary guidelines on exercise in pregnancy published by the American College of Obstetricians and Gynaecologists in 1985.

The maternal benefits from exercise in pregnancy have yet to be clearly established. Some researchers have suggested that exercise in pregnancy is related to shorter labour duration, while others have found no such correlations (Collings et al 1983, Revelli 1992). Clapp (1990a) found that pregnant runners and 'aerobic dancers' had significantly fewer deliveries involving operative procedures such as forceps and ventouse (or vacuum extraction), episiotomies and caesarian sections.

He also found that babies born to female athletes who continued to exercise in pregnancy had significantly lower birth weights than babies born to athletes who had ceased exercise during pregnancy.

O'Neill et al (1992) found that exercising pregnant women consistently underestimated their actual heart rates when using the Borg system (Borg 1982) of determining heart rate from rates of perceived exertion. It is therefore wise to encourage the pregnant athlete to not rely on 'listening to her body' but to take her pulse regularly.

Issues concerning low foetal birth weight which may be an indicator that the well-being of the foetus and neonate is compromised, teratogenicity or the risk of foetal abnormalities due to raised maternal core temperature, increased cardiovascular strain on maternal systems and injury to the maternal musculoskeletal system require further research to put physiotherapist's minds at ease with respect to advising athletes exercising in pregnancy.

When considering exercise in pregnancy, it is helpful to differentiate between specific exercise for pregnancy and general/fitness exercise in pregnancy.

Specific exercise

It is commonly accepted among women's health workers that the following exercises are essential information for all pregnant women regardless of pre-pregnancy fitness levels:

- Pelvic floor exercises. These are the *most* important muscles affected by pregnancy and childbirth. A pamphlet such as the one produced by the Continence Foundation of Australia should be given to all women to explain these exercises and to reinforce what the physiotherapist has taught them.
- Backcare and effective lifting exercises
- Posture—this area needs to be brought to the attention of the athlete. The author has observed a number of pregnant athletes who have erroneously assumed that a high level of fitness is synonymous with good posture. The physiotherapist may need to prescribe corrective exercises for the individual athlete's needs.
- Abdominal strengthening. The author has found the following guide useful. In the first trimester, emphasis is on improving abdominal strength and teaching functional dynamic abdominal bracing. Pelvic rocking needs to be mastered in all positions at this stage before the abdomen becomes too large. All exercise positions are safe to use at this stage. In the second trimester, emphasis is on maintaining strength and positions will need to be modified by 20 weeks' gestation.
Ideally, no exercises should be performed in supine as the weight of the gravid uterus can compress the maternal inferior vena cava and precipitate maternal supine hypotensive syndrome (Beischer & Mackay 1976) where the mother feels faint and nauseated due to a drop in blood pressure. It is also possible that the supine position may compromise uterine blood and

How to do the exercises

- Sit upright or stand up, thighs slightly apart, close your back passage and front passages, and draw them up inside you. Hold this SQUEEZE AND LIFT feeling for five seconds, then let go slowly and rest for 10 seconds. Repeat five times. This completes the short exercise session.
- While doing this exercise, try not to use your seat or tummy muscles, or to hold your breath. Try to repeat it at one or two hourly intervals throughout the day.

If you have difficulty closing back and front passages at the same time, try closing them separately, like this:

- Sit on the toilet. Start to pass water, then try to stop the stream, and also close your vagina. Concentrate on the front muscles you are using. Repeat once more.
- Sit or stand upright, and draw in the back passage as though trying to control diarrhoea.

Practise these movements separately several times. This will help you to find out which muscles you are using. When you feel sure you are making the correct movements, try doing them together as described above.

Remember…

- Pelvic floor contractions are entirely private. You can do them at any time.
- The muscles will only become stronger if they are exercised accurately and strongly many times a day.
- It could take several months before you feel the benefit, so persistence is essential.

[Reprinted with permission from Health, Western Australia.]

thus have a negative effect on foetal well-being. In addition, the altered angle of pull of the rectus abdominus due to the enlarging abdomen implies that this muscle is working at a mechanical disadvantage and may predispose the pregnant woman to developing a diastasis of the rectus abdominus muscle. In the third trimester, emphasis is on protection of the more vulnerable musculoskeletal structures of the pelvic floor, pelvis, lower back and abdomen.

Female athletes who are pregnant need to be reminded to attend physiotherapy ante-natal classes to learn this information in detail in addition to their childbirth education.

General exercise/fitness

In the author's opinion, pregnant female athletes fall into one of two groups with respect to exercise in pregnancy.

Firstly, some pregnant female athletes wish to cease their regular exercise or sport during pregnancy but may wish to continue with some exercise program. These women are well advised to follow the ACOG guidelines (Table 34.1).

The second group of pregnant female athletes represents a dilemma to the advising health professional. These women wish to continue their sport or exercise throughout their gestation. For these athletes, the author has developed the guide to modification of exercise in pregnancy shown in the box on p. 655.

Modifications

The athlete needs to readjust her exercise philosophy and shift her focus from performance to the health and social benefits of exercise. She should cease competition as early into the pregnancy as possible.

Table 34.1 American College of Obstetricians and Gynecologists guidelines for exercise during pregnancy and pospartum

1 Regular exercise (at least three times per week) is preferable to intermittent activity. Competitive activities should be discouraged.
2 Vigorous exercise should not be performed in hot, humid weather or during a period of febrile illness.
3 Ballistic movements (jerky, bouncy motions) should be avoided. Exercise should be done on a wooden floor or a tightly carpeted surface to reduce shock and provide a sure footing.
4 Deep flexion or extension of joints should be avoided because of connective tissue laxity. Activities that require jumping, jarring motions, or rapid changes in direction should be avoided because of joint instability.
5 Vigorous exercise should be preceded by a five-minute period of muscle warm-up. This can be accomplished by slow walking or stationary cycling with low resistance.
6 Vigorous exercise should be followed by a period of gradually declining activity that includes gentle stationary stretching. Because connective tissue laxity increases the risk of joint injury, stretches should not be taken to the point of maximum resistance.
7 Heart rate should be measured at times of peak activity. Target heart rates and limits established in consultation with the physician should not be exceeded.
8 Care should be taken to gradually rise from the floor to avoid orthostatis hypotension. Some form of activity involving the legs should be continued for a brief period.
9 Liquids should be taken liberally before and after exercise to prevent dehydration. If necessary, activity should be interrupted to replenish fluids.
10 Women who have led sedentary lifestyles should begin with physical activity of very low intensity and advance activity levels very gradually.
11 Activity should be stopped and the physician consulted if any unusual symptoms appear.

Pregnancy only

1 Maternal heart rate should not exceed 140 beats/minute.
2 Strenuous activities should not exceed 15 minutes in duration.
3 No exercise should be performed in the supine position after the fourth month of gestation is completed.
4 Exercises that employ the Valsalva manoeuvre should be avoided.
5 Calorie intake should be adequate to meet not only the extra energy needs of pregnancy, but also of the exercise performed.
6 Maternal core temperature should not exceed 38°C.

Reprinted with permission from American College of Obstetricians and Gynecologists Exercise During Pregnancy and Postnatal period (ACG Home Exercise Programs). Washington DC, ACOG, 1985, p 4.

Sport in pregnancy

Jogging

- Do not commence in pregnancy.
- Do not continue if there is pelvic floor insufficiency or joint soreness.
- Take care with external environment, i.e. temperature, terrain.
- Consider alternating with non-weightbearing exercise.
- Shorten distance or increase time to complete the distance, or decrease the speed of jogging as pregnancy progresses.

Cycling

- Can initiate in pregnancy.
- Take care with posture.
- Change to stationary cycling from the second trimester.

Swimming

- Can initiate in pregnancy but with care. If not a competent swimmer, choose water aerobics approach.
- Use of the kickboard is a useful alternative for the less competent swimmer.
- Take care with breaststroke (pubic symphysis strain).
- Take care with temperature of water. Do not exercise in water with a temperature of 30°C or more.
- Respiratory changes may make swimming more difficult in late pregnancy. Use kickboard or take more time to swim each lap.

Scuba diving

- Scuba diving is contraindicated during pregnancy. If the need for decompression should arise, there is an increased risk of air embolism and nitrogen gas being pushed across the placenta. There is also evidence of an increased risk of miscarriage associated with this sport (Artal & Wiswell 1986, Hornsby 1989).

Water skiing

- Do not initiate in pregnancy.
- Must be very competent to continue for first trimester only.
- Snug fitting wetsuit pants are essential.
- Discontinue single ski and barefoot skiing as soon as possible.

Diving

- No high board diving and no diving competitions after first trimester.

Weightlifting

- Cease in pregnancy.

Contact sports

- Contact sports e.g. basketball, netball, hockey, football, volleyball, gymnastics, competition dance, horse-back riding, should not continue during pregnancy. They are not recommended due to the risk of abdominal and breast trauma (Revelli et al 1992, Artal & Wiswell 1986) Furthermore, in the event of injury the problem may be difficult to treat as there are many modalities that are contraindicated during pregnancy. e.g. nonsteroidal anti-inflammatories, some electrotherapy.

Racquet sports

- Considered safer than contact sports, but it is recommended that the athlete change from competition as soon as possible.
- Change from singles to doubles.
- Care with heat stress, especially if playing indoors and ventilation is limited.

Softball or baseball

- No sliding into bases or blocking bases.
- Change sports by second trimester.

Golf

- There is no need to cease during pregnancy but there will be a need to modify swing as abdomen grows.

Winter sports

- Do not initiate in pregnancy.
- Care with additional stress on cardiovascular system from cold.
- Ensure proper hydration.
- Competent participants only should continue in pregnancy.
- Participants must be fit prior to the season.
- Cross-country skiing is preferred to downhill skiing, or skating.

Activities often need to be modified to such an extent that it probably negates any benefits from participation. Therefore, it is recommended that the athlete seek alternatives to these activities early in the pregnancy so transition to another form of exercise is easier, in preference to doing no exercise.

Self-monitoring ideas

Heart rate. Take pulse, carotid/radial before exercise and immediately after 15 minutes of exercise at the higher intensity phase. Adjust activity accordingly. Remember, you cannot rely on listening to your body.

Talk test. Be able to talk (but not sing!) during exercise.

Dehydration. Urine should be pale or clear, with 250–500 mL per void. Drink 2 L or more of non-caffeinated fluid daily. Drink before, during and after exercise.

Overheating. Avoid weightbearing aerobic exercise forms in hot, humid or poorly ventilated conditions. If in doubt, take rectal temperature before and after exercise. A reasonable safe upper limit is 38.7°C (Clapp 1990b).

Weight gain. Ensure kilojoule intake is sufficient. This is especially important if maternal weight was low at conception. Ensure adequate calcium intake e.g. three serves of dairy products per day.

Check for fatigue and soreness. Especially low back pain, pubic symphysis pain, sacroiliac strain, calf cramps, pelvic floor strain or insufficiency. If these conditions are treated promptly the pregnant athlete may continue with exercise but will need to be closely monitored for symptoms while exercising.

Stop exercise if any of the following symptoms occur: any bleeding but especially vaginal, dizziness, shortness of breath, palpitations, faintness, tachycardia, abdominal pain, chest pain, nausea (increases). These symptoms should be reported to the doctor. Symptoms of back pain, pubic symphysis pain, exacerbations of old injuries and other pains directly related to the activity need to be reported to the physiotherapist.

Do not continue exercise if suffering from infections even if these infections seem minor, such as upper respiratory tract and urinary tract infections.

The pregnant athlete needs to remember that pregnancy is in itself aerobic, and therefore she does not need to achieve maximum heart rate to improve her cardiovascular fitness.

She will need to be encouraged to respond to her body's pregnant needs. For example, if she is nauseous and vomiting or unduly fatigued, rest is indicated.

A variety of exercise is preferred in pregnancy. If weightbearing exercise is preferred, non-weightbearing exercise such as swimming and cycling could be performed on alternate days. Repetitive weightbearing exercise is more demanding on the maternal cardiovascular system (Artal & Wiswell 1986, Revelli et al 1992). In the author's experience repetitive intense weightbearing exercise which may include jumping, hopping, skipping or use of trampolines can produce symptoms of pelvic floor dysfunction.

In addition to her regular exercise, the athlete should be encouraged to attend weekly ante-natal physiotherapy fitness classes for variety of exercise types, information, social networking and supervision.

The athlete who continues to exercise at moderate to high intensities needs to be advised on monitoring her response to exercise. The information in the box is useful as a hand-out for the athlete for home use.

After reviewing the literature (ACOG 1985, Artal et al 1986, Kulpa et al 1987, Revelli et al 1992, Clapp 1991, Wallace et al 1986, White 1992, Williams 1991) and from the author's clinical experience, the guidelines shown in the box on the opposite page have been found to be appropriate when discussing sport in pregnancy.

SUMMARY

All pregnant athletes should be assessed by their obstetrician for their medical and obstetric suitability concerning their exercise plans. They should be instructed by the physiotherapist in specific exercises for the pelvic floor, posture and abdominal musculature. They should be instructed to avoid exercises in the supine position, ballistic exercises and exercises at the extreme end of range as outlined by the ACOG guidelines.

The pregnant athlete who will continue to exercise unsupervised needs to be encouraged to cease competition as soon as possible and to decrease the intensity at which she was exercising pre-pregnancy. A variety of exercise types such as swimming, walking and stationary cycling are recommended. She should be instructed in self-monitoring techniques.

REFERENCES

American College of Obstetricians and Gynaecologists 1985 Home exercise program: exercise during pregnancy and the post-natal period. American College of Obstetricians and Gynaecologists, Washington D C

Anderson J 1978 Grant's atlas of anatomy. Williams & Wilkins, Baltimore, fig. 3–31

Artal R, Wiswell K (eds) 1986 Exercise in pregnancy. Williams & Wilkins, Baltimore

Beck R, Hsu N 1991 Pregnancy, childbirth and the menopause related to the development of stress incontinence. American Journal of Obstetrics and Gynaecology 91:820

Beischer N A, Mackay E V 1976 Obstetrics and the newborn for midwives and students. W B Saunders, Sydney, p 191

Borg G A V 1982 Psychophysical bases of perceived exertion. Medical Science in Sports and Exercise 14:377–381

Chiarelli P 1987 The physiotherapist's contribution to incontinence and other symptoms of pelvic floor dysfunction. In: Collins M (ed) Women's health through lifestages. Australian Physiotherapy Association (NSW Branch), Sydney

Chiarelli P 1989 The role of physiotherapy in treatment of urinary incontinence. Australian Family Physician 18:949–953

Clapp J F 1990a The course of labour after endurance exercise during pregnancy. American Journal of Obstetrics and Gynaecology 163(6):1799–1805

Clapp J F 1990b Exercise in pregnancy: a brief clinical review. Foetal Medicine Review 2:89–101

Clapp J F 1991 The changing thermal response to endurance exercise during pregnancy. American Journal of Obstetrics and Gynaecology 165(6):1684–1689

Collings C A, Curet L B, Mullin J P 1983 Maternal and fetal responses to a maternal aerobic exercise program. American Journal of Obstetrics and Gynaecology 145(6):702–707

Dwyer P L, Glenning P P 1990 Anatomy and neurology of the lower urinary tract. Current Opinion in Obstetrics and Gynaecology 2:573–579

Fonda D, Wellings C 1987. Urinary incontinence. AECD, Melbourne, p 1

Hornsby A (ed) 1989 Encyclopedia of recreational diving, PADI USA, Ch. 2, pp 54–55

Jones E 1950 Role of active exercise in pelvic muscle physiology. Western Journal of Surgery, Obstetrics and Gynaecology 58:1

Klarskov P, Nielsen K K, Kromann-Andersen R, Maegaard E 1991 Long-term results of pelvic floor training and surgery for female genuine stress incontinence. International Urogynaecological Journal 2:132–135

Kulpa P J, White B, Visscher R 1987 Aerobic exercise in pregnancy. American Journal of Obstetrics and Gynaecology 156(6):1395–1401

Laycock J, Green R J 1988 Interferential therapy in the treatment of incontinence. Physiotherapy April 74(4):161–168

O'Neill M E, Schnier A, Cooper K A, Boyce E S, Hunyor S N 1990 Historical perspective of exercise during pregnancy. Australian Physiotherapy Association Journal of National Women's Health Group 9(2):7–10

O'Neill M E, Cooper K A, Mills C M, Boyce E S, Hunyor S N 1992 Accuracy of Borg's ratings of perceived exertion in the prediction of heart rates during pregnancy. British Journal of Sports Medicine 26(2):121–124

Revelli A, Durando A, Massobrio M 1992 Exercise in pregnancy: a review of maternal and fetal effects. Obstetrics and Gynaecology Survey 47(6):355–367

Wallace A M, Boyer D B, Dan A, Holm K 1986 Aerobic exercise, maternal self-esteem and physical discomforts during pregnancy. Journal of Nurse-Midwifery 31(6):255–261

White J 1992 Exercising for two–what's safe for the active pregnant woman? Physician and Sports Medicine 20(5):179–186

Williams H 1991 Exercise and pregnancy—a G.P.'s perspective. Australian Physiotherapy Association Journal of National Women's Health Group 10(1):11–16

Considerations for the sports physiotherapist

35. Eating for peak performance

Louise M. Burke, Mark Hargreaves

As far back as the ancient Olympic competitions, athletes have eaten special diets or foods in the hope of improving their performance. Early interest in sports nutrition focused on the search for an ergogenic food or nutrient, particularly for use in the competition arena. However, since the 1960s there has been a dramatic change in the interest and understanding of nutrition for athletes, largely reflecting our increased knowledge of exercise science. The emphasis today is on matching nutritional goals directly to the physiological and biochemical effects of exercise, and to understanding the needs arising from training as well as competition.

THE PRINCIPLES OF THE TRAINING DIET

It is the training program that largely determines the nutritional needs of an athlete, since it is the predominant influence on both energy expenditure and life style. At the elite level at least, training is a daily commitment, with some athletes undertaking more than one session each day and some sessions lasting in excess of two hours. Such a training load not only affects the athlete's energy and nutrient requirements, but also has a large impact on social and life style factors (including dietary practices), thus influencing the athlete's in meeting nutritional goals.

The everyday nutritional goals of an athlete should encompass issues of general health as well as the specific needs of training. The following goals have been proposed (Burke & Read 1989):

- To provide basic nutrient requirements, including meeting any additional or increased needs that arise from a strenuous exercise program
- To incorporate nutritional practices that promote long-term health, and reduce the risk of the chronic disease patterns of affluent Western countries
- To achieve and maintain an appropriate body weight and level of body fat
- To promote recovery between training or competition and to support physiological adaptation by providing a suitable nutritional environment

- To experiment with intended competition practices so that beneficial strategies can be identified, and familiarization and habituation can occur.

In setting a base for everyday eating patterns, the athlete should adopt the concept of the 'healthy' or varied diet recommended for the general population. National dietary guidelines and nutrition policies have been established by many countries to embody nutrition messages for both short-term and long-term health (US Departments of Agriculture and Health and Human Services 1990, National Health and Medical Research Council 1992). Athletes, as part of the general community, might embrace these recommendations for their health advantages alone. However, it will be seen in the following discussion that population dietary guidelines (such as the guidelines for Australians summarized in Table 35.1) well encapsulate the special nutritional needs of athletes.

Inherent in the correct use of dietary guidelines is the recognition that the recommendations apply to a population, and that even when the average dietary intake of a population exceeds nutrient requirements, there will be subgroups within the population with specialized needs and

Table 35.1 Draft dietary guidelines for Australians

1 Enjoy a wide variety of nutritious foods.
2 Eat plenty of breads and cereals (preferably wholegrain), vegetables (including legumes) and fruits.
3 Eat a diet low in fat, in particular low in saturated fat.
4 Maintain a healthy body weight by balancing physical activity and food intake.
5 If you drink alcohol, limit your intake.
6 Eat only a moderate amount of sugar and foods containing added sugar.
7 Choose low salt foods and use salt sparingly.
8 Drink plenty of water.
9 Encourage and support breastfeeding.

Companion guidelines
10 Eat foods containing calcium. This is particularly important for girls and women.
11 Eat foods containing iron. This is partcularly important for girls, women, vegetarians and athletes.

Source: National Health and National Research Council (1992)

individuals who fail to achieve adequate nutrient intake. Athletes can be regarded as one such specialized subgroup (American Dietetic Association 1987), and even within their ranks individual needs must be recognized.

Energy intake

The energy intake of an athlete is an important starting point in the assessment of nutritional status, in that it underlies at least two of the goals of training nutrition proposed earlier. Energy intake influences body weight and body fat levels through its balance with energy expenditure, and also determines the potential for nutrient intake. A high energy intake, coupled with a varied selection of foods, should provide nutrient intakes well in excess of the levels considered adequate for the healthy population (American Dietetic Association 1987). Of course, not all athletes consume a high energy intake, and some athletes also restrict their dietary variety, often in the belief that performance will be enhanced by eliminating certain 'bad foods' (e.g. red meat) or by heavily emphasizing other 'good foods' (e.g. carbohydrate foods). Such athletes are at risk of inadequate nutrient intake.

The energy needs of individual athletes vary with age, sex, body mass and body composition, with the most important variable being the exercise (training) load. Sherman and Lamb (1988) found that an athlete undertaking strenuous training may have an energy expenditure 1.5 to 3 times greater than a sedentary counterpart, often with 30–40% of the day's energy expenditure occurring during two to four hours of intense training. Dietary surveys of athletes have shown that some individuals and groups report very high energy intakes, but also that there is a wide range in reported energy intakes within a group of athletes (Short & Short 1983). The highest energy consumers appear to be strength-training athletes with large body mass, and endurance athletes undertaking lengthy training sessions each day. When expressed per kg of body mass, these endurance athletes have been reported to consume over 0.21 MJ/kg/day (50 kcal/kg/day) (Brotherhood 1984). It is also noted that the requirements of growth in adolescent athletes also impose additional energy demands.

When energy requirements are large, it can be difficult for athletes to meet their needs from bulky high fibre and high carbohydrate foods. Access to food may also be limited by training, travelling and other life style commitments. In these circumstances, athletes may need counselling to make use of more compact carbohydrate and energy sources, and to adopt the pattern of frequent 'grazing' that is characteristic of high energy consumers (Kirsch & von Ameln 1981, Burke & Read 1987).

Body weight and body fat

Body mass and composition are functions of an athlete's genetics, diet and training (Brownell et al 1987) and will reflect the structural and functional characteristics that are specifically favourable for the sport involved. The physique of an athlete will be determined by the inherited characteristics that have been selective in determining athletic pursuits, and by the changes achieved through the conditioning effect of high-level training.

Brownell et al (1987) have suggested that there are three different patterns of body weight/body fat among sports. The first includes sports that are essentially passive and based largely on skill (eg. golf and archery), in which performance is largely independent of body fat levels. The second category involves sports with specific weight divisions for competition, and includes weightlifting, wrestling, boxing, lightweight rowing and horse racing. In these sports, athletes generally try to compete in weight divisions that are below their normal training weight, thus trying to gain an advantage over a lighter opponent. Short-term weight loss is often achieved over the days leading up to the event, using techniques such as dehydration, food restriction and the use of diuretics and laxatives (Steen & Brownell 1990). These practices may be deleterious to both health and performance particularly when the weight loss is extreme (greater than 5% of body weight) and repeated frequently (American College of Sports Medicine 1976, Brownell et al 1987).

The final category includes sports where low body mass and low body fat levels are considered necessary for optimal performance. The advantages of low body fat range from physical or mechanical (e.g. in distance running and triathlons) to values of aesthetics and appearance (e.g. gymnastics and ballet dancing).

It is possible to identify or describe a typical physical profile for various types of athletes, and even to distinguish between players in different positions in a team game, and athletes in different events in the same sport (Fleck 1983, Withers 1987a, 1987b). However, there is enough variation in body characteristics and body fat levels between elite athletes in the same sport to advise against the establishment of rigid body fat prescriptions for each sport. It is preferable to nominate a range of acceptable values for each sport, and then monitor the health and performance of individual athletes within this range.

Although some athletes easily achieve body composition suited to their sports, others may need to manipulate characteristics such as muscle mass or body fat levels, through changes in diet and training. It is important that these athletes can identify suitable and realistic goals, take appropriate measures to achieve the desired changes, and have a suitable means of measuring the results. For example, a gain in body mass should be achieved principally by the gain of muscle mass, while weight loss should be achieved by the loss of body fat. Nett changes in body weight (ie. use of scales) will not distinguish changes in individual body compartments. Thus techniques of measuring body composition and changes in body composition are required.

There are a number of methods available to estimate body composition and body fat levels, ranging from simple measurements of subcutaneous adipose tissue to more expensive and high-tech methods such as hydrostatic weighing, bioelectrical impedance, total body conductivity and near infra-red spectrophotometry (for review see Brodie 1988a, 1988b). While hydrostatic weighing ('underwater' weighing) is regarded as the criterion method of body density assessment, the measurement of skinfold fat ('pinch' test or caliper test) remains a practical, simple and inexpensive technique for the estimation of body fat levels. In Australia the common practice is to determine the sum of measurement of subcutaneous fat at 7–8 sites around the body. Errors incumbent in the use of predictive formulae to estimate percentage body fat are avoided by simply using the sum of these skinfold measurements to reflect adiposity (for a description of the sum of skinfold technique see review by Kerr 1994). As with all techniques of body composition assessment, care should be taken to maximize the validity and reliability of readings, and to interpret the results carefully in light of residual error.

Loss of body fat should be achieved by adjustment of energy intake and energy expenditure patterns, at a maximum rate of 1–1.5 kg/week to minimize the loss of muscle tissue (Yarrows 1988), and with a diet that still provides adequate nutrient intake. The potential for safe and healthy loss of body fat should always be assessed before weight loss goals are set. In general, a high level of training may allow the sum of skinfolds to be as low as 35–45 mm for males and 40–55 mm for females. However, individuals should be discouraged from achieving (or attempting to achieve) these very low levels of body fat unless definite advantages can be proven and disadvantages are minimal. As previously mentioned, individual history may reveal the health and training consequences of various body fat levels, thus allowing athletes to set their own 'optimum' or 'goal' body fat level.

While the present fashion among some athletic groups is the achievement of minimum body fat levels per se, athletes are warned about the possible lack of improvement from lowered body fat, as well as the potential for harmful side effects. The disadvantages of very low body fat remain mostly speculative, but reflect both direct consequences on the body (eg. loss of body warmth/ insulation) as well as the indirect consequences of the combination of chronic low energy/nutrient intake, excessive training and psychological factors that were successful in achieving the weight loss. Eating disorders are well documented among athletes (see review by Wilmore 1991).

Recent interest has focused on athletes whose goal body fat level seems not to be 'naturally' achieved. There has long been evidence both anecdotally and from dietary surveys that a significant number of athletes, particularly female, struggle to keep body fat levels low and report their energy intakes and requirements to be 'less than they deserve' (Clark et al 1988). Many dietary studies of female endurance athletes (Drinkwater et al 1984, Marcus et al 1985) have reported intakes that suggest an energy balance oddity—energy intake that seems too low to match energy expenditure from training. Although this has been explained by some as an artifact of poor dietary assessment methodology (Brotherhood 1984), others argue that the low intakes are so striking in some cases and seem so consistent across studies that some attention is merited (Brownell et al 1987).

In reviewing the weight control practices of athletes, Brownell et al (1987) discuss the set-point theory of body fat maintenance (Keesey 1986). They propose that athletes who reduce body fat below the natural level that their body wishes to defend, or lose body fat from critical sites, may induce some complex metabolic changes. They propose that a decrease in metabolic rate and/or an increase in food efficiency could result from the chronic restriction of food intake and the maintenance of body fat below the natural or regulated level. There may also be some implications for menstrual function. While this work remains somewhat speculative and offers no real cure for affected athletes other than to reassess their goals, the prevention of this problem would be best served by the safe and conservative methods of weight loss already proposed.

Protein and vitamins

Whether athletes have increased requirements for protein and vitamins and whether increased intakes of these nutrients will improve athletic performance continues to be a point of controversy. Comprehensive reviews of protein research (Lemon 1991a, 1991b, 1991c) have summarized the following major mechanisms by which protein requirements are increased by exercise:

- the contribution of protein catabolism to the fuel requirements of exercise (training and competition)
- a positive nitrogen balance during periods of heavy resistance training
- repair/recovery needs following muscle damage and efflux of muscle enzymes.

Although Lemon (1991a) cites some evidence to support beneficial effects of very high protein intakes in strength athletes, total protein requirements based on both estimates (Brotherhood 1984) and nitrogen balance studies (Tarnopolsky et al 1988) appear to be in the order of 1–1.5 g of protein per kg body mass per day for both endurance and strength training athletes, provided that both carbohydrate and energy requirements are also met. With high energy requirements and protein intake at the typical Western level of 12–15% of total energy intake, there would seem little problem for most athletes

Table 35.2 Ready reckoner of protein-rich foods

Approximately 10 g of protein is provided by the following foods:		
Low-fat animal foods	grilled fish	50 g (cooked weight)
	tuna or salmon	50 g
	lean beef or lamb	35 g (cooked weight)
	veal	35 g (cooked weight)
	turkey or chicken	40 g (cooked weight)
	game meat (rabbit, venison)	35 g (cooked weight)
	eggs	2 small
	cottage cheese	70 g
	reduced-fat cheese (11% fat slices)	30 g = 1.5 sl
	non-fat fruit yoghurt	200 g carton
	skim milk	300 mL
	liquid meal supplement (Sustagen or Exceed Sports Nutrition Supplement)	150 mL
Vegetable foods	wholemeal bread	4 sl (120 g)
	wheat flake cereal	3 cups (90g)
	untoasted muesli	1 cup (100g)
	cooked pasta or noodles	2 cups (300 g) cooked
	brown rice	2 cups (350 g)
	cooked lentils	3/4 cup (150 g)
	cooked kidney beans	3/4 cup (150 g)
	baked beans	4/5 cup (200 g)
	cooked soy beans or tofu	120 g
	nuts	60 g
	seeds (e.g. sesame)	60 g

Source: NUTTAB 1991, Australian Department of Community Services and Health

to meet these targets (see Table 35.2 for a ready reckoner of protein-rich foods).

Amino acid supplements, providing individual amino acids singly or in combinations, are currently enjoying wide interest (and use) among athletes. Amino acids supplements do not contribute greatly to total protein intake, but are proposed to enhance performance via specific metabolic effects. For example, it has been proposed that supplementation with ornithine/arginine or arginine/lysine combinations may stimulate growth hormone release, while the ingestion of the branched chain amino acids (valine, leucine and isoleucine) during endurance exercise has been suggested to reduce neurotransmitter-induced central fatigue. Investigation of the metabolic and performance effects of amino acid supplementation is preliminary and further work is required before any benefits can be clearly decided (for review see Burke 1992). In the meantime, athletes should also consider the considerable expense and the risks associated with consuming large doses of individual amino acids. Lemon (1991b) points out that the health consequences remain largely untested but include the potential for interference with amino acid absorption, metabolic imbalances and toxicity.

Indeed, indiscriminate use of large doses of L-tryptophan supplements was cited as the cause of numerous deaths and over 1500 cases of a rare blood disorder, eosinophilia-myalgia syndrome, during the 1980s (Teman & Hainline 1991).

The present consensus on vitamins is that studies have failed to show any beneficial effects of vitamin supplementation for athletic performance (see reviews by van der Beek 1985, Belko 1987, Williams 1985). With high energy intakes, the majority of athletes should be able to achieve vitamin intakes well in excess of the population recommended dietary intake levels, provided an adequately varied diet is chosen. Some athletes may benefit from dietary counselling to achieve their dietary potential, while problems remain for athletes who continue to be chronic low energy consumers. In such cases long-term broad range nutrient supplementation may be required.

Carbohydrate requirements for daily training

Daily training sessions, often intense and prolonged, have become a feature of many sports, and in most cases the resulting energy and carbohydrate requirements of training become more demanding than those of competition itself. The daily normalization or recovery of muscle and liver carbohydrate stores is considered a priority of the training diet of heavily training athletes.

Factors involved in the degree and rate of muscle glycogen resynthesis have been well reviewed (Ivy 1991, Robergs 1991), and include the extent of muscle trauma, the severity of muscle glycogen depletion and dietary carbohydrate intake.

Post-exercise glycogen synthesis is discussed in more detail later. The importance of a high carbohydrate diet for heavily training athletes has been illustrated in a number of studies (Costill & Miller 1980, Costill et al 1988, Jacobs et al 1982). These studies showed that athletes who failed to ingest sufficient carbohydrate to match the demands of their training commitments succumbed to chronic muscle glycogen depletion and fatigue.

The population dietary guidelines already recommend that carbohydrate intakes should be above the levels currently typical of the Western diet, and this should be achieved principally by increasing the consumption of complex carbohydrate and fibre-containing foods (National Health and Medical Research Council 1992). Several authorities have attempted to set guidelines for the needs of endurance athletes in order to maximize their capacity for daily glycogen restoration. Recommendations for carbohydrate intake have been set both on the basis of absolute intake (8–10 g of carbohydrate per kg body mass per day—Costill 1988) or as a percentage of the total diet (carbohydrates should provide 65–70% of total energy intake—American Dietetic Association 1987). The emphasis on nutritious carbohydrate foods will help the athlete to meet requirements (possibly elevated) for protein and micronutrients. Sugar and refined carbohydrate foods offer the advantages of being compact and pleasant to eat, and can be useful in providing a smaller contribution to the total carbohydrate intake without significantly disturbing the nutrient density of the diet. Table 35.3 provides a ready reckoner of carbohydrate-rich foods to help in the planning of high carbohydrate diets.

Iron status

Iron status is crucially involved in exercise performance through the role of iron in oxygen transport (myoglobin

Table 35.3 Ready reckoner of carbohydrate-rich foods

Approximately 50 g of carbohydrate is supplied by the following foods:

Cereals	bread	4 slices (120 g)
	bread roll	1 large or 2 small (120 g)
	muffin or crumpet	2 (130 g)
	breakfast cereal	= 2.5–3 cups (80 g) Weeties or 'light' cereal
		= 1–1.5 cups muesli flakes or 'heavier' cereal
		= 5 Weetbix
	rolled oats	90 g (1 cup)
	untoasted muesli	100 g (1 cup)
	porridge	600 g (2.5 cups)
	scones/pancakes	120 g (2 average size)
	wholemeal cake, low fat	120 g (1 large or 2 small slices)
	dry biscuit	90 g (16)
	rice cakes	50 g (3)
	plain muesli bar	2 bars
	sweet biscuit	75 g (8 plain, 4 cream)
	popcorn	100 g
	rice	170 g (1 cup)
	pasta/noodles	200 g (1.5 cups)
Vegetables	potatoes	360 g (1 large, 3 small)
		360 g mashed (1.5 cups)
	carrots/pumpkin/peas	800 g (4 cups)
	corn	300 g (1.5 cups)
Legumes	kidney, soy beans	300 g (1.5 cups)
	baked beans	500 g (2 cups)
	lentils	300 g (1.5 cups)
Fruit	fresh fruit	3 medium apples, oranges
	2 medium bananas	
	juice	500 mL sweetened
		700 mL unsweetened
	dried fruit	80 g (4 tbsp)
	canned/stewed fruit	400 g sweetened (2 cups)
		800 g unsweetened (4 cups)
	fruit salad, fresh	400 g (2 cups)
Dairy products	skim milk	1 L
	fruit non-fat yoghurt	400 g (2 cartons)
	plain non-fat yoghurt	800 g (4 cartons)
	low-fat icecream	250 g (2 cups)
Sugary foods	sugar	50 g (2 heaped tbsp)
	jam and honey	60 g (3 tbsp)
	plain lollies	50-60 g
Drinks	soft drinks and flavoured mineral water	500 mL
	cordial	800–1000 mL
	fruit juice	500–700 mL
	sports drinks	600–800 mL
	liquid meal drinks	250–350 mL
	carbo-loader drinks	200–250 mL
	low-fat milkshake/ fruit smoothie	350–500 mL

Source: NUTTAB 1991, Australian Department of Community Services and Health

and hemoglobin) and in aerobic metabolism (cytochromes and other ferroenzymes). Inadequate iron status will therefore impair exercise performance, and has gained the attention of sports scientists in recent years (Newhouse & Clement 1988, Haymes & Lamanca 1989). There is still a lack of consensus on many issues—for example, the hematological/biochemical parameters of 'optimum iron status', the level of iron deficiency that causes impairment of performance, and methods of distinguishing reduced iron status from exercise-mediated changes in iron metabolism. Nevertheless, it is agreed that at least some athletes are at risk of low iron status due to increased iron losses and, importantly, poor intake of bioavailable iron. The solution to this problem includes recognition of high risk athletic groups (including females, adolescents, vegetarians and endurance athletes, particularly a combination of these), and early detection and monitoring of iron depletion. Treatment may include iron supplementation, but a successful plan of management should also undertake to modify excessive iron losses and improve dietary intake. Iron-rich foods are summarized in Table 35.4.

Table 35.4 Iron-rich foods

Food	Serve	mg iron
Heme iron foods		
liver	100 g (cooked weight)	11.0 mg
liver pate	40 g (2 tbsp)	2-3 mg
lean steak	100 g (cooked weight)	4.0 mg
chicken (dark meat)	100 g (cooked weight)	1.2 mg
fish	100 g (cooked weight	0.6–1.4 mg
oysters	100 g	3.9 mg
salmon	100 g (small tin)	1.5 mg
Non-heme iron foods		
eggs	100 g (2)	2.0 mg
breakfast cereal (fortified)	30 g (1 cup)	2.5 mg
wholemeal bread	60 g (2 sl)	1.4 mg
spinach (cooked)	145 g (1 cup)	4.4 mg
lentils/kidney beans (cooked)	100 g (2/3 cup)	2.5 mg
tofu	100 g	1.9 mg
sultanas	50 g	0.9 mg
dried apricots	50 g	2.0 mg
almonds	50 g	2.1 mg

Source: NUTTAB 1991, Australian Department of Community Services and Health

Amenorrhea, bone density, calcium and stress fractures

Menstrual dysfunction in female athletes may include a number of problems (see review by Highet 1989), with most attention being focused on secondary amenorrhea. There is great variation in the reported incidence of secondary amenorrhea in groups of female athletes, due at least in part to differences in the definition of menstrual irregularities as well as in the calibre of the athletes studied (Highet 1989). However, it is agreed that young, intensively training females are at much greater risk of developing disturbances to the menstrual cycle than sedentary women, and that chronic exercise is either directly or indirectly responsible for this.

Numerous causes have been suggested for menstrual dysfunction in female athletes, including the type of exercise (eg. runners are at higher risk than swimmers), training intensity and training mileage. However, as reviewed by Loucks and Horvath (1985), studies have been unable to show a consistent factor across all sports.

The relationship between body weight or body fat levels and amenorrhea has received generous attention, with surveys noting an increased incidence of amenorrhea among groups of athletes who tend to be leaner and lighter, such as runners and dancers (Sanborn et al 1982). Again, numerous studies have failed to support that low body fat levels per se or 'critical body fat' levels are a universal cause of amenorrhea in athletes (Carlberg et al 1983, Linnell et al 1984, Sanborn et al 1987). Other suggested causes are rapid changes in body fat, or the depletion of specific body fat stores that are critical for the sustenance of pregnancy and lactation (Brownell et al 1987). There is some support for the theory proposed earlier that the body will try to defend some aspects of its body fat with metabolic adaptations (Brownell et al 1987). Some dietary surveys of runners have reported that amenorrheic subjects consumed significantly less energy per kg body mass that eumenorrheic controls, despite training similar or greater distances (Drinkwater et al 1984, Marcus et al 1985, Nelson et al 1986).

Other nutrient shortfalls, such as inadequate protein intake, have been noted in the diets of amenorrheic athletes, although it is possible to establish whether this is directly linked or simply associated with low energy intakes. Vegetarianism (Pirke et al 1986) and eating disorders (Gadpaille et al 1987) have both been suggested as primary risk factors.

Thus, at the moment, there seems to be no single theory that can adequately explain the cause of amenorrhea in athletes, but it is possible to identify a number of connected factors that may impose a threat in certain individuals. It is possible that individuals have personal thresholds to certain factors and that factors may act synergistically. Anecdotal evidence supports that some athletes can control whether they menstruate, by manipulating their training intensity or body fat levels.

Proof of a link between secondary amenorrhea and reduced bone density has strengthened in recent years (see review by Martin & Bailey 1987). Reduced bone mass in female athletes at first seems a paradoxical situation, since weightbearing exercise is known as a potent stimulus for bone formation (see review by Bailey et al 1986). However, in reviewing the results of 10 studies Martin and Bailey (1987) conclude that chronic hypoestrogenism, a feature of amenorrhea, is associated with a significant loss of calcium from trabecular bone, and that the bone-enhancing effects of exercise are not sufficient to compensate for this. While this condition was quickly dubbed 'sports osteoporosis' or 'athletic osteoporosis', osteopenia is probably a more accurate term, to distinguish it from the bone disease that afflicts the aged population.

While low estrogen levels are being implicated as the major cause of this bone loss in females, not all amenorrheic athletes develop low bone density and some normally menstruating athletes also have low bone density. Other factors contributing to negative calcium balance have been sought, including race, build, family history and, not surprisingly, calcium intake. In reviewing the role of dietary calcium and osteoporosis, Heaney (1987) offered the following summary:

- Calcium intake is positively related to calcium balance and bone mass, and negatively related to the rate of bone loss. A low calcium intake has a permissive role in the development of low bone density.
- Calcium operates as a threshold nutrient: above a certain intake further increases in intake produce no additional effect on bone.

Nutritional surveys of athletes (Marcus et al 1985, Berning et al 1985) frequently report calcium intakes that are below the recommended dietary intake levels. Thus it seems probable that some amenorrheic athletes contribute to their loss of bone mass by an inadequate calcium intake. Dietary risk factors include low total energy intake, poor food choice and variety, and the presence of eating behaviour problems. Across a number of countries, calcium intake is tied closely to the intake of dairy products (Nordin 1990).

It is speculated that reduced bone density may have both short-term and long-term consequences on health and athletic performance. Whether reduced bone density is directly related to stress fractures in athletes remains controversial. While bone strength is related to bone density, the incidence of stress fractures will also be influenced by the stress load or trauma experienced by the bones, making issues such as training load, biomechanical factors, training surfaces and equipment (eg. shoes) equally as important. Indeed, a study of elite Australian athletes has reported that the incidence of stress fractures was largely independent of bone mineral density (Carbon et al 1990). However, this and other studies (Marcus et al 1985, Lloyd et al 1986) have reported a significant correlation between stress fractures and amenorrhea among female athletes. The long term consequence of osteopenia in athletes is even more speculative in that its large-scale occurrence is too recent for any effect on old-age osteoporosis to be noted. However, it seems plausible that athletes who enter menopause with an already reduced bone density, would be expected to reach the bone's 'critical fracture threshold' earlier.

Stress fractures, reduced bone density and athletic amenorrhea must be viewed carefully, since they can occur as separate or interconnected problems in female athletes. The management and prevention of each must continue to be highly specific and individual, taking into account the mixed aetiology of each problem. However, it is likely that athletic amenorrhea will underlie many cases of reduced bone density, and the problem of negative calcium balance in this situation must be seen as one of estrogen deficiency rather than a primary calcium deficiency. The cornerstone of management is either the restoration of menses (sometimes made possible by alterations to diet, body fat or training load), or estrogen replacement therapy. Many females may benefit from dietary counselling to ensure adequate nutritional status to maintain both menstrual and bone integrity, including advice on correcting low energy intakes, suboptimal intake of nutrients including calcium, and disordered eating behaviour (good food sources of calcium are summarised in Table 35.5.) Preliminary work (Drinkwater et al 1986) reports that the restoration of menstrual function in amenorrheic runners can lead to an increase in bone density and that early intervention is important, since trabecular bone loss from untreated amenorrhea of long origin (as little as three years) may be irreversible (Cann et al 1988). Whether high dose calcium supplementation is useful as an adjunct to hormone therapy in treating or preventing bone loss remains speculative.

NUTRITION FOR COMPETITION

Besides the essential contribution of skill, success in sports performance may be determined by the capacity of the athlete to produce work or expend energy. An increased understanding of the metabolism of exercise has allowed scientists to identify some of the factors that limit performance or cause fatigue. These factors are impaired homeostasis (both at the cellular level and of the whole body) and depletion of fuel substrates. Training produces a number of physiological adaptations that allow athletes to produce more work and to delay the onset of fatigue. Even so, athletes should prepare for competition by understanding the factors limiting performance in their specific event, and by taking further steps to reduce the effects of their factors.

Some important goals of competition nutrition are (Burke & Read 1989):

- To ensure adequate carbohydrate fuel stores in the pre-competition phase
- During prolonged events, to promote maximum duration of fuel stores, and where appropriate supply additional carbohydrate during exercise.
- To promote the maintenance of homeostasis, particularly that of temperature regulation including the prevention of dehydration
- In weight-matched sports, to achieve the required body weight division without sacrificing fuel stores and hydration levels
- To avoid gastrointestinal discomfort during the event.
- To promote recovery after competition, particularly in sports involving repeated events over the same or successive days, or events in a weekly fixture.

Carbohydrate nutrition

In view of the importance of carbohydrates for exercise performance (Costill 1988, Hargreaves 1991), athletes should strive to optimize muscle and liver glycogen availability prior to competition, maintain a high rate of carbohydrate oxidation during the event and promote replenishment of the body carbohydrate reserves afterwards.

An exercise-diet regimen known as glycogen loading (or carbohydrate loading) has been used by endurance athletes in order to increase the availability of muscle and liver glycogen prior to exercise. The original protocol, as described by Scandinavian researchers in the late 1960s, used extremes of diet and exercise to achieve this goal. More recent work (Sherman et al 1981) has demonstrated that trained athletes need only reduce their training and increase dietary carbohydrate intake to 8–10 g per kg body mass per day, or 65–70% of total energy in order to achieve similar increases in muscle glycogen (see Table 35.6 for a sample diet). Since regular training involves day-to-day depletion and repletion of muscle glycogen and increases muscle glycogen synthase activity, the depletion phase of the 'classical' glycogen loading regime does not appear to be necessary in trained athletes. Although most studies examining the potential benefits of glycogen loading have focused on endurance sports, some researchers have suggested benefits during high intensity exercise (Greenhaff

Table 35.5 Calcium-rich foods

Food	Serving	mg calcium
Skim milk	200 ml (glass)	250 mg
Low fat (1–2%) milk	200 ml (glass) (Calcium added)	285 mg
Reduced-fat cheese	20 g (1 slice) (11% fat slices)	160 mg
Cottage cheese	100 g (1/2 cup)	80 mg
Non-fat fruit yoghurt	200 g (carton)	350 mg
Low-fat icecream	60 g (2 tbsp)	90 mg
Salmon (with bones)	100 g (small tin)	335 mg
Sardines (oil drained)	100 g (drained weight)	380 mg
Oysters	100 g	135 mg
Almonds	50 g	125 m
Tahini	20 g (tbsp)	190 mg
Spinach (cooked)	145 g (1 cup)	72 mg
Soy milk	200 ml (glass)	45 mg
Fortified soy milks	200 ml (glass) (e.g. So Good)	290 mg
Tofu	100 g	130 mg

Source   NUTTAB 1991, Australian Department of Community Services and Health

Table 35.6 A plan suitable for carbohydrate loading

These menu plans provide about 600 g of carbohydrate per day - providing the recommended carbohydrate intake of 8–10 g/kg body mass per day for a 60–65 kg athlete. They may need to be adapted for athletes outside this weight range. These menus are proposed for carbohydrate loading days only—while meeting carbohydrate intake goals, they do not meet all the nutrient requirements for everyday eating.

Day 1: (602 g CHO, 12 200 kJ – CHO = 80% of energy)

Breakfast	2 cups wheat flake cereal + 1 cup skim milk
	1 cup sweetened canned peaches
	250 mL sweetened fruit juice
Snack	2 thick slices toast + scrape marg + tbsp honey on each
	250 mL sports drink
Lunch	2 large bread rolls with light salad
	375 mL can of soft drink
Snack	large coffee scroll (unbuttered)
	250 mL sweetened fruit juice
Dinner	3 cups of boiled rice (made into 'stir fry' with small amount of lean ham, peas, corn and onion)
	250 mL sweetened fruit juice
Snack	2 crumpets + scrape marg + tbsp jam on each

Extra water during day

Day 2: (605 g CHO, 12 700 kJ – CHO = 77% of energy)

Breakfast	2 cups porridge + 1 cup skim milk
	1 banana
	250 mL sweetened fruit juice
Snack	2 muffins + scrape marg. + tbsp jam on each
Lunch	stack of three large pancakes + 60 mL maple syrup + small scoop icecream
	250 ml sweetened fruit juice
Snack	50 g jellybeans
Dinner	3 cups cooked pasta + 1 cup tomato pasta sauce
	2 slices bread
	250 mL sports drink
Snack	1 cup fresh fruit salad
	1/2 carton low fat fruit yoghurt
	Extra water during day

Day 3:

The athlete may like to switch to a low residue diet to reduce gastrointestinal contents and improve comfort during the event.
- Use menus for Day 1 or 2, switching to white bread, white cereals etc.
- From lunch onwards, replace some or all of solid food with 500 mL snacks of commercial carbo-loader or liquid meal supplements

et al 1987). It may also be relevant to athletes involved in intermittent activities such as basketball, football, and hockey. At the very least, athletes involved in high intensity activity should ensure their muscles contain adequate glycogen prior to competition; whether increased muscle glycogen availability increases performance remains to be fully clarified.

The pre-game meal should consist predominantly of carbohydrate (see Table 35.7) and be ingested 3–4 hours prior to exercise. Such a meal will alleviate hunger and ensure adequate availability of carbohydrate prior to exercise. Athletes who fast for 6–12 hours prior to exercise may suffer from reduced carbohydrate availability late in prolonged exercise, since liver glycogen is particularly susceptible to alterations in dietary carbohydrate intake. Furthermore, such feeding may promote an increase in muscle glycogen levels if these are less than optimal (Coyle

et al 1985). Ingestion of carbohydrate in the 3–4 hours prior to exercise will produce alterations in the metabolic response to exercise, including a slight fall in blood glucose during the first 30–60 min of exercise, despite normalization of the blood glucose and insulin levels prior to the commencement of exercise. Nevertheless, an increase in carbohydrate oxidation during exercise, following ingestion of approximately 300 g of carbohydrate 4 hours prior to exercise, results in an increase in endurance performance (Sherman et al 1989). The pre-event meal should also provide fluid to ensure full hydration, and avoid any foods known by the athlete to cause gastrointestinal discomfort during the following exercise bout. A meal low in fat, protein and fibre is often advised, and in cases where athletes experience difficulty in consuming solid foods prior to exercise, commercially available liquid meal supplements (e.g. Sustagen Sport or Exceed Sports meal) may be helpful.

Over the years it has been recommended that athletes avoid the ingestion of carbohydrate in the hour prior to strenuous exercise. This may be associated with lowered blood glucose levels with the onset of exercise and increased muscle glycogenolysis (Costill et al 1977, Hargreaves et al 1985) and impaired endurance performance (Foster et al 1979). These effects were attributed, in part, to the hyperinsulinemia resulting from carbohydrate ingestion which, together with the onset of muscle contraction, produced a rapid decline in blood glucose. In addition, the antilipolytic effect of insulin reduced the availability of free fatty acids, further enhancing the reliance on muscle glycogen. However, several recent studies have not shown these negative effects of pre-exercise carbohydrate ingestion on exercise performance and some have even observed enhanced performance (Gleeson et al 1986). Thus, it may be necessary to review the general recommendation that carbohydrates be avoided in the hour prior to exercise. In any event, since there are likely to be individual differences in the response to pre-exercise carbohydrate ingestion, it is suggested that athletes experiment with various pre-exercise feeding regimes during training to define their optimal strategy.

Table 35.7 Ideas for suitable pre-competition meals

Breakfast cereal with reduced fat milk and fruit
Muffins or crumpets with jam/honey
Pancakes with syrup
Baked beans on toast
Canned spaghetti on toast or muffins
Pasta with tomato/vegetarian sauce (low oil cooking)
Rice dish (low oil cooking), e.g. 'fried' rice in nonstick pan or 'creamed rice' made with low fat milk
Baked potato with low fat filling
Fruit salad with non fat fruit yoghurt
Liquid meal supplement (e.g. Sustagen sport or Exceed Sports meal)

NB: many athletes may need to choose low fibre versions (e.g. white bread or white rice rather than wholemeal varieties)

Table 35.8 General guidelines for fluid and carbohydrate requirements for athletes

Sports	Fluid needs	Cho needs	Comment
Weight-division sports (e.g. lightweight rowing, wrestling, and boxing)	Variable	Generally not needed	The athlete is encouraged to 'make weight' without resorting to severe dehydration and fasting. There may be some opportunity to top up fluid fuel levels after the weigh-in. If the athlete is still dehydrated, extra care should be taken with fluid intake needs/opportunities during the event.
Brief events (e.g. sprints, throwing events)	Not applicable	Not applicable	There is generally no need or opportunity to replace fluid and carbohydrate during an event. For multiple events spread over the day, the athlete is encouraged to rehydrate and refuel between events with appropriate fluids and foods.
Non-endurance events (e.g. 10 km run)	Variable (e.g. minimal 1 litre per hour)	Generally not needed	Sweat losses will vary with the length, intensity and environmental conditions of events. The athlete should use opportunities during the event to keep fluid deficits below a litre (approximately). Fluid replacement with water will generally be adequate, however sports drinks are also suitable. Fluid deficits should be replaced after the event, and rapid fuel recovery can be assisted by immediate intake of carbohydrate-rich foods and fluids.
Team events (e.g. basketball, soccer, football)	Variable (e.g. 500-1000mL per hour or more)	May be useful in some sports (e.g. 50g per hour)	Sweat losses will vary between players and sports, according to the length and intensity of individual play, and the environmental conditions. In tournament conditions there may be inadequate time for complete recovery of fluid and fuel needs between games. In this situation aggressive intake of a carbohydrate-rich fluid (e.g. sports drink) during the game will provide additional fuel.
Endurance events > 90 mins (e.g. marathon, 80 km cycle, Olympic distance triathlon)	500-1000mL per hour (more in extreme conditions)	Approximately 50 g per hour	Opportunities for regular intake of carbohydrate-rich fluids (e.g. sports drinks) should be encouraged in these sports—e.g. aid stations, breaks in play. Sweat losses will vary as above; carbohydrate needs will vary according to pre-existing glycogen stores, and the length and intensity of the event. The athlete is advised to keep pace with sweat losses as well as possible. Rehydrate fully and refuel after the event.
Ultra-endurance events—>4 hours (e.g. Ironman Triathlon)	500-1000mL per hour (or more in extreme conditions)	Approximately 50 g per hour	As for endurance events. The sodium in sports drinks may be useful in reducing the risk of hyponatremia in susceptible athletes. Solid forms of carbohydrate may be eaten to prevent/alleviate hunger as well as continue to supply additional fuel.

There is little question that carbohydrate ingestion is of benefit during endurance exercise, where the reliance on carbohydrate is high and fatigue is often associated with muscle glycogen depletion and hypoglycemia. Numerous studies have observed increased exercise time to exhaustion and work output with carbohydrate ingestion (Coyle et al 1983, 1986, Mitchell et al 1989a). Rather than slowing or sparing muscle glycogen oxidation, the beneficial effects of carbohydrate ingestion are related to its ability to maintain blood glucose levels and a high rate of carbohydrate oxidation when endogenous carbohydrate stores are low (Coyle et al 1986, Hargreaves & Briggs 1988). In addition, an attenuation of the counterregulatory hormonal response to exercise (Mitchell et al 1990) suggests a possible sparing of liver glycogen. Carbohydrate ingestion at the point of fatigue increases blood glucose and carbohydrate oxidation initially, but these effects are soon reversed as the rate of muscle glucose utilization exceeds the rate of carbohydrate absorption from the gut (Coggan & Coyle 1987). In contrast, carbohydrate ingestion late in exercise, but prior to the point of fatigue, is more effective in maintaining blood glucose levels and carbohydrate oxidation throughout exercise. Based on numerous studies, it appears that athletes need to ingest carbohydrate at a rate that will supply them with approximately 1 g of carbohydrate per minute. This can be achieved by the ingestion of 600–1000 mL/hr of solutions containing 5–10% carbohydrate; the typical concentration of commercially available carbohydrate-electrolyte replacement drinks ('sports drinks').

Important practical considerations in the choice of carbohydrate foods and fluids for consumption during prolonged exercise include the avoidance of gastrointestinal upset and the interplay between fluid and energy delivery (see next section). Carbohydrate-containing liquids are easier to ingest and better tolerated during most types of exercise than solid foods, and offer the advantage of simultaneous fluid replacement. The choice and concentration of the carbohydrate fluid will depend on the required rate of carbohydrate and fluid replacement. A highly concentrated carbohydrate solution (15–20%) has been shown to reduce the rate of gastric emptying and fluid delivery (Mitchell et al 1989b) but will increase the rate of delivery of carbohydrate from the stomach. Athletes are advised to experiment with various strategies during training to determine their optimal competition plan. The priority of fluid and carbohydrate needs will vary according to environmental conditions, and the length and intensity of the event. Table 35.8 provides a summary of the general needs for fluid and carbohydrate in various sports events.

In view of the importance of muscle glycogen for exercise performance, its resynthesis is an important metabolic process during recovery from strenuous exercise. Although exhaustive exercise will activate the metabolic pathways involved in glycogen resynthesis, full restoration of muscle glycogen levels is critically dependent upon adequate carbohydrate intake. Ingestion of this carbohydrate should occur as soon as possible after exercise in order to promote rapid glycogen resynthesis (Ivy et al 1988a). The optimal rate of carbohydrate ingestion is 50–100 g every two hours (Blom et al 1987, Ivy et al 1988b), aiming for a total intake of 600–800 g in 24 hours. The type of carbohydrate consumed influences the rate of glycogen synthesis, with glucose and sucrose resulting in faster rates of muscle glycogen resynthesis than fructose (Blom et al 1987); fructose may make a greater contribution to liver glycogen resynthesis. Studies comparing 'simple' and 'complex' carbohydrate foods have reported that they are equally effective in restoring muscle glycogen over 24 hours of recovery (Costill et al 1981). However, recent work which defines carbohydrate foods on a more physiological basis has reported that carbohydrate foods with a high glycemic index (high glycemic response) are associated with greater muscle glycogen synthesis during 24 hours of recovery than foods with a low glycemic index (Burke et al 1992, see review by Coyle 1991).

Muscle damage, often observed following strenuous exercise activity with a large eccentric component, is another factor to be considered in post-exercise recovery. Such muscle damage is associated with a reduced ability for glycogen resynthesis (Costill et al 1990, O'Reilly et al 1987, Sherman et al 1983), which is partially overcome by increasing carbohydrate intake (Costill et al 1990). Thus, athletes should be aware of the potential need for increased dietary carbohydrate intake following exercise that produces muscle damage and soreness.

Fluid balance during exercise

During exercise in air, evaporation of sweat from the skin is the major mechanism of heat loss. The sweating rate is determined by the thermal load, which in turn is influenced by the exercise intensity and environmental conditions (ambient temperature, relative humidity, wind direction and speed, sun:shade ratio). Water losses as a result of heavy sweating can be as high as 1.5-2 L/hr and the water lost is derived from all body fluid compartments, including the vascular space (Nose et al 1988a). The physiological responses to this dehydration include an increase in heart rate to maintain cardiac output, increases in resistance and capacitance in some vascular beds to displace blood volume centrally, and mobilization of water from the extravascular to the intravascular space. In the longer term, fluid replacement is a more effective way of minimizing the ill effects of dehydration. Infusion of saline during exercise, to simulate the ideal rate of fluid replacement, results in expansion of the plasma volume, lower heart rates, improved core-to-skin heat transfer and lower body temperatures at the end of exercise (Nose et al 1990). Fluid ingestion results in similar effects. Thus, athletes should be encouraged to drink during exercise, especially in hot environments when sweat losses may be large.

Over the years there has been much debate on the optimal volume and composition of rehydration beverages designed to enhance exercise performance. It has been difficult to examine the effects of fluid ingestion per se, since many beverages also contain carbohydrate which will minimize carbohydrate depletion. Recent results, however, have shown improved exercise performance with ingestion of fluids that contain relatively small amounts of substrate (Bethell et al 1990, Maughan et al 1989). The fluid volume requirement will be determined by the rate of fluid loss (ie. the sweating rate). It has been suggested, however, that athletes may have difficulty in ingesting much more than 500–1000 mL/hr (Noakes 1990), which will mean they are likely to incur a small water deficit. Although it is difficult for athletes to ingest large volumes of fluid, they should be encouraged to drink smaller volumes frequently in order to maintain a reasonable degree of gastric filling, an important determinant of gastric emptying (Noakes et al 1991, Mitchell & Voss 1991).

The bioavailability of ingested fluids is determined by gastric emptying and intestinal absorption, which are influenced by exercise intensity, ambient temperature, dehydration and fluid composition. An increase in the carbohydrate/electrolyte content to high levels (10–20%) is associated with impaired gastric emptying (Mitchell et al 1989b); glucose polymers may provide an advantage over glucose at higher concentrations (Sole & Noakes 1989), although this has not been observed in all studies. Inclusion of a smaller amount of carbohydrate/electrolyte (5–10%) may actually enhance fluid delivery, relative to water, by stimulating intestinal absorption, and has the added advantage of providing substrate.

Since sweat is hypotonic the emphasis should be on water replacement; however, the inclusion of sodium chloride in ingested fluid will enhance glucose and fluid absorption in the intestine and minimize the risk, in some individuals, of hyponatremia during ultraendurance exercise (Noakes 1990). The optimal sodium concentration remains to be determined. Although the body has well developed mechanisms for restoring fluid and electrolyte balance, drinking should be encouraged in the recovery period in order to facilitate restoration of body fluid levels. Recovery of lost volume is more rapid with ingestion of fluid containing small amounts of sodium and glucose, since ingestion of water alone will reduce fluid recovery by lowering plasma osmolality, removing dipsogenic drive and stimulating urine production (Nose et al 1988b).

Athletes participating in sports that have weight classifications often undergo acute dehydration in order to 'make weight' prior to competition. Since hypohydration results in decreased plasma and blood volumes, increased plasma osmolality, decreased skin blood flow and sweating, increased body temperature and increased heart rate during exercise, such practice should be discouraged for reasons of safety and exercise performance.

PUTTING THEORY INTO PRACTICE

Although our understanding of exercise physiology and sports nutrition has become sophisticated, it is uncertain whether athletes are fully utilizing this knowledge in the sports arena. Turning theory into practice requires awareness of the importance of nutrition, specialized dietary knowledge, adequate access to a suitable food supply, skills in food preparation, and general interest and motivation. Studies of the dietary patterns of athletes shows that some or all of these factors may be missing and that specialized nutrition education for various groups of athletes is warranted (Burke et al 1991). Many health professionals are involved in the various levels of dietary education and supervision, ranging from the initial detection of dietary problems to the organization of food plans for travelling and competing teams. A sports dietitian can provide special expertise to give advice or help manage the challenges in sports nutrition. Services may include group education sessions, preparation of nutrition education material, consultancy to teams or sporting organisations, and the assessment and counselling of individual athletes. A sports dietitian may be found at many sports medicine centres or clinics, at sports institutes, or by contacting the Dietitians Association.

REFERENCES

American College of Sports Medicine 1976 Position stand on weight loss in wrestlers. Medicine and Science in Sports and Exercise 8:xi–xiii

American Dietetic Association 1987 Position stand on nutrition for physical fitness and athletic performance for adults. Journal of the American Dietetic Association 87:933–939

Bailey D A, Martin A D, Houston C S, Howie J L 1986 Physical activity, nutrition, bone density and osteoporosis. Australian Journal of Science and Medicine in Sport 18(3):3–8

Belko A Z 1987 Vitamins and exercise—an update. Medicine and Science in Sports and Exercise 19 (Suppl 5):191–196

Berning J, Sanborn C F, Brooks S M, Wagner W W 1985 Caloric deficit in distance runners (abst). Medicine and Science in Sports and Exercise 17:242

Bethell L R, Leiper J B, Maughan R J 1990 Consumption of dilute glucose-electrolyte solutions improves exercise capacity in man. Journal of Physiology 429:60P

Blom P C S, Hostmark A T, Vaage O, Kardel K, Hermansen L 1987 Effect of different sugar diets on the rate of muscle glycogen synthesis. Medicine and Science in Sports and Exercise 19:491–496

Brodie D A 1988a Techniques of measurement of body composition Part 1. Sports Medicine 5:11–40

Brodie D A 1988b Techniques of measurement of body composition Part 2. Sports Medicine 5:74–98

Brotherhood J R 1984 Nutrition and sports performance. Sports Medicine 1:350–389

Brownell K D, Steen S N, Wilmore J 1987 Weight regulation in athletes: analysis of metabolic and health effects. Medicine and Science in Sports and Exercise 19:546–556

Burke L M 1992 Protein and amino acid needs of the athlete. State of the Art Review 28, Australian Sports Commission

Burke L M, Read R S D 1987 Diet patterns of elite Australian male triathletes. Physician and Sports Medicine 15(2):140–155

Burke L M, Read R S D 1989 Sports nutrition: approaching the nineties. Sports Medicine 8:80–100

Burke L M, Gollan R A, Read R S D 1991 Dietary intake and food use of groups of elite Australian male athletes. International Journal of Sport Nutrition 1:378–394

Burke L M, Collier G, Hargreaves M 1993 Muscle glycogen storage following prolonged exercise: effect of glycaemic index of carbohydrate feedings Journal of Applied Physiology 75:1019-23

Cann C E, Cavanaugh D J, Schnurpel K, Martin M C 1988 Menstrual history is the primary determinant of trabecular bone density in women runners (abst). Medicine and Science in Sports and Exercise 20(suppl.):59

Carbon R, Sambrook P N, Deakin V, Fricker P, Eisman J, Kelly P, Maguire K, Yeates M G 1990 Bone density of elite female athletes with stress fractures. Medical Journal of Australia 153:373–376

Carlberg K A, Buckman M T, Peake G T, Riesdesel M L 1983 Body composition of oligo/amenorrheic athletes. Medicine and Science in Sports and Exercise 15:215–217

Clark N, Nelson M, Evans W 1988 Nutrition education for elite female runners. Physician and Sportsmedicine 16(2):124–136

Coggan A R, Coyle E F 1987 Reversal of fatigue during prolonged exercise by carbohydrate infusion or ingestion. Journal of Applied Physiology 63:2388–2395

Coggan A R, Coyle E F 1989 Metabolism and performance following carbohydrate ingestion late in exercise. Medicine and Science in Sports and Exercise 21:59–65

Costill D L 1988 Carbohydrates for exercise: dietary demands for optimal performance. International Journal of Sports Medicine 9:1–18

Costill D L, Coyle E F, Dalsky G, Evans W, Fink W, Hoopes D 1977 Effects of elevated plasma FFA and insulin on muscle glycogen usage during exercise. Journal of Applied Physiology 43:695–699

Costill D L, Miller J M 1980 Nutrition for endurance sport: carbohydrate and fluid balance. International Journal of Sports Medicine 1:2–14

Costill D L, Sherman W M, Fink W J, Maresh C, Witten M, Miller J M 1981 The role of dietary carbohydrates in muscle glycogen resynthesis after strenuous running. American Journal of Clinical Nutrition 34:1831–1836

Costill D L, Flynn M G, Kirwan J P, Houmard J A, Mitchell J B, Thomas R T, Park S H 1988 Effects of repeated days of intensified training on muscle glycogen and swimming performance. Medicine and Science in Sports and Exercise 20:249–254

Costill D L, Pascoe D D, Fink W J, Robergs R A, Barr S I, Pearson D 1990 Impaired muscle glycogen resynthesis after eccentric exercise. Journal of Applied Physiology 69:46–50

Coyle E F, Hagberg J M, Hurley B F, Martin W H, Ehsani A A, Holloszy J O 1983 Carbohydrate feeding during prolonged strenuous exercise can delay fatigue. Journal of Applied Physiology 55:230–235

Coyle E F, Coggan A R, Hemmert M K, Lowe R C, Walters T J 1985 Substrate use during prolonged exercise following a pre-exercise meal. Journal of Applied Physiology 59:429–433

Coyle E F, Coggan A R, Hemmert M K, Ivy J L 1986 Muscle glycogen utilization during prolonged strenuous exercise when fed carbohydrate. Journal of Applied Physiology 61:165–172

Coyle E F 1991 Timing and method of increased carbohydrate intake to cope with heavy training, competition and recovery. Journal of Sports Sciences 9 (special issue) 29–52

Drinkwater B L, Nilson K, Chestnut C H, Bremner W J, Shainholtz S S 1984 Bone mineral content of amenorrheic and eumenorrheic athletes. New England Journal of Medicine 311:277–281

Drinkwater B L, Nilson K, Ott S, Chestnut C H 1986 Bone mineral density after resumption of menses in amenorrheic athletes. Journal of the American Medical Association 256:380–382

Fleck S J 1983 Body composition of elite American male athletes. American Journal of Sports Medicine 11:398–402

Foster C, Costill D L, Fink W J 1979 Effects of pre-exercise feedings on endurance performance. Medicine and Science in Sports and Exercise 11:1–5

Gadpaille W J, Sanborn C F, Wagner W W 1987 Athletic amenorrhea, major affective disorders and eating disorders. American Journal of Psychiatry 144:939–942

Gleeson M, Maughan R J, Greenhaff P L 1986 Comparison of the effects of pre-exercise feeding of glucose, glycerol and placebo on endurance and fuel homeostasis in man. European Journal of Applied Physiology 55:645–653

Greenhaff P L, Gleeson M, Maughan R J 1987 The effects of dietary manipulation on blood acid-base status and the performance of high intensity exercise. European Journal of Applied Physiology 56:331–337

Hargreaves M 1991 Carbohydrates and exercise. Journal of Sports Sciences 9(special issue):17–28

Hargreaves M, Costill D L, Katz A, Fink W J 1985 Effect of fructose ingestion on muscle glycogen usage during exercise. Medicine and Science in Sports and Exercise 17:360–363

Hargreaves M, Briggs C A 1988 Effect of carbohydrate ingestion on exercise metabolism. Journal of Applied Physiology 65:1553–1555

Haymes E M, Lamanca J F 1989 Iron loss in runners during exercise: implications and recommendations. Sports Medicine 7:277–285

Heaney R P 1987 The role of calcium in the prevention and treatment of osteoporosis. Physician and Sports Medicine 15(1):88–89

Highet R 1989 Athletic amenorrhea: an update on aetiology. Sports Medicine 7:82–108

Ivy J L 1991 Muscle glycogen synthesis before and after exercise. Sports Medicine 11:6–19

Ivy J L, Katz A L, Cutler C L, Sherman W M, Coyle E F 1988a Muscle glycogen synthesis after exercise: effect of time of carbohydrate ingestion. Journal of Applied Physiology 64:1480–1485

Ivy J L, Lee M C, Brozinick J T, Reed M J 1988b Muscle glycogen storage after different amounts of carbohydrate. Journal of Applied Physiology 65:2018–2023

Jacobs I, Westlin N, Karlsson J, Rasmussen M, Houghton B 1982 Muscle glycogen and diet in elite soccer players. European Journal of Applied Physiology 31:203–208

Keesey R E 1986 A set-point theory of obesity. In: Brownell K D, Foreyt P D (eds) Handbook of eating disorders: physiology and treatment of obesity, anorexia and bulimia. Basic Books, New York, pp 63–87

Kerr D 1994 Kinanthropometry. In: Burke L, Deakin V (eds) Clinical sports nutrition. McGraw Hill, Sydney

Kirsch K A, von Ameln H 1981 Feeding patterns of endurance athletes. European Journal of Applied Physiology 47:197–208

Lemon P W R 1991a Effect of exercise on protein requirements. Journal of Sports Sciences 9(special issue):53–70

Lemon P W R 1991b Protein and amino acid needs of the strength athlete. International Journal of Sport Nutrition 1:127–145

Lemon P W R 1991c Does exercise alter dietary protein requirements? In: Brouns F, Saris W, Newsholme E (eds) Advances in nutrition and top sport. Karger, Basel, pp 15–37

Linnell S L, Stager J M, Blue P W, Oyster N, Robertshaw D 1984 Bone mineral content and menstrual regularity in female runners. Medicine and Science in Sports and Exercise 16:343-348

Lloyd T, Triantafyllou S J, Baker E R Houts P S, Whiteside J A, Kalenak A, Stumpf P G 1986 Women athletes with menstrual irregularity have increased musculoskeletal injuries. Medicine and Science in Sports and Exercise 18:374–379

Loucks A B, Horvath S M 1985 Athletic amenorrhoea: a review. Medicine and Science in Sports and Exercise 17:56–72

Marcus R, Cann C, Madvig P, Minkoff J, Goddard M, Bayer M, Martin M, Gaudiani L, Haskell W 1985 Menstrual function and bone mass in elite women distance runners: endocrine and netabolic features. Annals of Internal Medicine 102:158–163

Martin A D, Bailey D 1987 Skeletal integrity in amenorrhoeic athletes. Australian Journal of Science and Medicine in Sport 19(1):3–7

Maughan R J, Fenn C E, Leiper J B 1989 Effects of fluid, electrolyte and substrate ingestion on endurance capacity. European Journal of Applied Physiology 58:481–486

Mitchell J B, Costill D L, Houmard J A, Fink W J, Pascoe D D, Pearson D R 1989a Influence of carbohydrate dosage on exercise performance and glycogen metabolism. Journal of Applied Physiology 67:1843–1849

Mitchell J B, Costill D L, Houmard J A, Fink W J, Robergs R A, Davis J A 1989b Gastric emptying: influence of prolonged exercise and carbohydrate concentration. Medicine and Science in Sports and Exercise 21:269–274

Mitchell J B, Costill D L, Houmard J A, Flynn M G, Fink W J, Beltz J D 1990 Influence of carbohydrate ingestion on counterregulatory hormones during prolonged exercise. International Journal of Sports Medicine 11:33–36

Mitchell J B, Voss K W 1991 The influence of volume on gastric emptying and fluid balance during prolonged exercise. Medicine and Science in Sports and Exercise 23:314–319

National Health and Medical Research Council 1992 Draft dietary guidelines for Australians. Australian Government Publishing Service, Canberra

Nelson M E, Fisher E C, Catsos P O, Meredith C N, Turksoy R N, Evans W J 1986 Diet and bone status in amenorrheic runners. American Journal of Clinical Nutrition 43:910-916

Newhouse I J, Clement D B 1988 Iron status: an update. Sports Medicine 5:337–52

Noakes T D 1990 The dehydration myth and carbohydrate replacement during prolonged exercise. Cycling Science 23–29

Noakes T D, Rehrer N J, Maughan R J 1991 The importance of volume in regulating gastric emptying. Medicine and Science in Sports and Exercise 23:307–313

Nordin B E C 1990 Calcium. In: Truswell A S (ed) Recommended nutrient intakes: Australia papers. Australian Professional Publications, Sydney, pp 201–206

Nose H, Mack G W, Shi X, Nadel E R 1988a Shift in body fluid compartments after dehydration in humans. Journal of Applied Physiology 65:318–324

Nose H, Mack G W, Shi X, Nadel E R 1988b Role of osmolality and plasma volume during rehydration in humans. Journal of Applied Physiology 65:325–331

Nose H, Mack G W, Shi X, Morimoto K, Nadel E R 1990 Effect of saline infusion during execise on thermal and circulatory regulations. Journal of Applied Physiology 69:609–616

O'Reilly K P, Warhol M J, Fielding R A, Frontera W, Meredith C N, Evans W J 1987 Eccentric exercise-induced muscle damage impairs muscle glycogen repletion. Journal of Applied Physiology 63:252–256

Pirke K M, Schweiger U, Laessle R, Dickhaut B, Schweiger M, Waechtler M 1986 Dieting influences the menstrual cycle: vegetarian versus nonvegetarian diet. Fertility and Sterility 46:1083–1088

Robergs R A 1991 Nutrition and exercise determinants of post-exercise glycogen synthesis. International Journal of Sport Nutrition 1:307–337

Sanborn C F, Albrecht B H, Wagner W W 1987 Athletic amenorrhea: lack of association with body fat. Medicine and Science in Sports and Exercise 19:207–212

Sanborn C F, Martin B J, Wagner W W 1982 Is athletic amenorrhea specific to runners? American Journal of Obstetrics and Gynecology 143:859–61

Sherman W M, Costill D L, Fink W J, Miller J M 1981 The effect of exercise and diet manipulation on muscle glycogen and its subsequent utilization during performance. International Journal of Sports Medicine 2:114–118

Sherman W M, Costill D L, Fink W J, Hagerman F C, Armstrong L E, Murray T F 1983 Effect of a 42,2 km footrace and subsequent rest or exercise on muscle glycogen and enzymes. Journal of Applied Physiology 55:1219–1224

Sherman W M, Lamb D R 1988 Nutrition and prolonged exercise. In: Lamb D R, Murray R (eds) Perspectives in exercise science and sports medicine Volume 1: Prolonged exercise. Benchmark Press, Indianapolis, pp 213–280

Sherman W M, Brodowicz G, Wright D A, Allen W K, Simonsen J, Dernbach A 1989 Effects of 4 h pre-exercise carbohydrate feedings on cycling performance. Medicine and Science in Sports and Exercise 21:598–604

Sole C C, Noakes T D 1989 Faster gastric emptying for glucose-polymer and fructose solutions than for glucose in humans. European Journal of Applied Physiology 58:605–612

Short S H, Short W R 1983 Four-year study of university athletes' dietary intake. Journal of the American Dietetic Association 82:632–645

Steen N S, Brownell K D 1990 Patterns of weight loss and regain in wrestlers: has the tradition changed? Medicine and Science in Sports and Exercise 22:762–768

Tarnopolsky M A, MacDougall J D, Atkinson S A 1988 Influence of protein intake and training status on nitrogen balance and lean body mass. Journal of Applied Physiology 64:187–193

Teman A J, Hainline B 1991 Eosinophilia-myalgia syndrome. Physician and Sports Medicine 19(2):81-86

US Departments of Agriculture and Health and Human Services 1990 Dietary guidelines for Americans. Home and Garden Bulletin 232

van der Beek E J 1985 Vitamins and endurance training: food for running or faddish claims? Sports Medicine 2:175–197

Williams M H 1985 Nutritional aspects of human physical and athletic performance, 2nd edn. Charles C Thomas, Springfield, ch 6

Wilmore J H 1991 Eating and weight disorders in the female athlete. International Journal of Sport Nutrition 1:104–117

Withers R T, Craig N P, Bourdon P C, Norton K I 1987a Relative body fat and anthropometric prediction of body density of male athletes. European Journal of Applied Physiology 56:191–200

Withers R T, Whittingham N O, Norton K I, Ellis M W, Cricket A 1987b Relative body fat and anthropometric prediction of body density of female athletes. European Journal of Applied Physiology 56:169–180

Yarrows S A 1988 Weight loss through dehydration in amateur wrestling. Journal of the American Dietetic Association 88:491–493

36. Touring with teams

Peter Duras

Tours with sporting teams have provided many physiotherapists with the highlights of their professional careers. Responsibilities are great, but the experience can be a uniquely rewarding one. The ability to convert the excitement of the initial appointment into the satisfaction of having served the team well depends on the ability to meet an array of challenges not usually encountered in the clinical or club setting. Care of athletes and officials requires the physiotherapist to assume a range of responsibilities which may include aspects of management, nutrition, stress reduction and recovery from fatigue.

Ideally all teams should be accompanied by at least a doctor, a physiotherapist, a masseur and a sports psychologist. In reality, limited funding leads many sporting organizations to select a physiotherapist as the team's sole medical official. It is assumed that the therapist will provide massage when required, and can manage most minor medical problems. For that reason, a number of the most commonly encountered medical hazards are outlined in this chapter. While the emphasis will be on the situations which are more likely to occur when travelling internationally with elite teams, many of these difficulties and principles apply while touring in one's own country, particularly when great distances are covered.

FUNCTIONS OF THE TOURING SPORTS PHYSIOTHERAPIST

Most physiotherapists working for amateur sporting associations do so without a formal contract or definition of roles. An English study (Hall 1989) showed that only one of 25 chartered physiotherapists operating with national teams in Olympic sports had a job description. Usually an invitation is issued and accepted, and the roles are assumed rather than specified. Though this allows the physiotherapist more flexibility, it also adds some uncertainty.

Typically the touring physiotherapist is expected to:

- Participate in pretour medical screening or obtain relevant medical details from team members using a questionnaire
- Advise athletes prior to departure of the steps which should be taken to prevent and minimize health and injury risks
- Protect team members from injury on tour by identifying areas of risk and encouraging effective preventive techniques
- Obtain the treatment equipment, kit and supplies appropriate to the size, nature and destination of the team and the time spent away
- Effectively assess and treat injuries in conjunction with other members of the medical team, in order to facilitate the athlete's safe and rapid return to sport
- Assist in the recovery from exercise and the reduction of stress and fatigue. This includes the provision of massage as required
- Provide first aid and be capable of managing minor medical problems if a team doctor is not available
- Refer to appropriate medical personnel or gain access to emergency care when required
- Advise athletes and coach on the safe return to training and competition after injury.
- Keep accurate records of injuries and treatment given throughout the tour
- Facilitate success and assist management with the smooth functioning of the team.

Special requirements

There are a number of skills and areas of specialized knowledge that will equip the clinically competent sports physiotherapist to cope with the many demands of the travelling team. These include knowledge of the sport, the ability to work with others and relate to the team members, adaptability, dedication and sound personal health.

A knowledge of the physical and psychological demands of the sport and the type of injuries that are likely to occur is essential. A familiarity with the nature of training, conditioning and competition is required to formulate prevention strategies, and determine aetiology, treatment and the readiness of an athlete to return to play after injury.

The physiotherapist who does not understand and appreciate all facets of the sport, its terminology and its importance to the athlete will have difficulty communicating and gaining the trust of athletes and officials.

The sports physiotherapist needs to be familiar with the relevant rules of the sport. These include regulations controlling access to injured players on the field, the use of tape and braces, drug testing procedures and the banned substances for that sport. When travelling with a team of disabled sportspeople the physiotherapist should have a working knowledge of the appropriate classification system.

The physiotherapist must have the ability to communicate and work closely with coaches, management and other health professionals in the team. Success depends on mutual respect and understanding of each other's role and expertise, as well as a knowledge of one's own limitations.

Confrontation, uncertainty and inaccurate or conflicting advice must be avoided in order to reduce the athlete's stress in the pressure-cooker situation of international competition. There is a variety of personalities on tour, each with its own peculiarities. The physiotherapist should have the ability to develop a rapport with members of the team, while remaining apolitical and professionally objective.

From the start of preparation for the tour to completion of the final report the organizational skills of the physiotherapist will be put to full use. Assessing team needs, making the necessary contacts, selecting and procuring equipment, and arranging for its transport and insurance are part of this process. So too is the keeping of adequate clinical records.

Adaptability and versatility are valuable assets on tour. Conditions are seldom ideal and can change dramatically on moving to a new location. Space, time, comfort, equipment and specialist support are usually limited. The ability to adapt and operate successfully under those conditions will earn respect and may set an example for athletes trying to cope with a difficult environment. Similarly, the dedicated physiotherapist will realize that the first priority must always be provision of care for the athlete. Unless the team is a small one on a brief tour, this will mean long hours working, travelling and servicing training and competition venues. The opportunities to relax, shop, tour and socialize will be limited by the need to be accessible to athletes and management. In order to meet these heavy demands, the physiotherapist should set aside time for rest, meals and exercise, and needs to possess good health and the ability to cope with stress.

Competence in first aid is required, and it is desirable that formal training and certification be obtained.

Proficiency in sports massage is now requested by many sports in order to enhance recovery after exercise, reduce fatigue, pain, tension and muscle spasm, facilitate relaxation and treat injuries.

Finally, there is no substitute for experience. Previous successful tours build confidence and establish the physiotherapist's ability to meet the requirements of team travel.

PREPARATION

The first stage of preparation involves gathering details of the nature and size of the team, composition of the medical squad, destinations and dates of travel and competition. Contact should be established with the manager and the medical personnel accompanying the team, in order to develop a working relationship at the preparatory stage. Information about the destinations can be obtained from acquaintances, athletes, sports officials and particularly colleagues who have visited the area. Embassies, tourist bureaux and guide books can supply further details. Investigation should focus on local health hazards, the safety of food and water, vaccinations required, and the range and extremes of climate conditions. Details of the voltages and plug types used in the countries on the tour are also required for any electrotherapy equipment carried.

The quality and ease of access to medical facilities at each destination should also be canvassed in advance. The host organization may provide a comprehensive polyclinic free of charge at major games. At most events, however, it is more difficult to obtain satisfactory medical specialist and emergency care. Contact with physiotherapists in the host country can be a great source of information and assistance.

Medical or team reports from previous tours can often be accessed. They are likely to provide a wealth of information on the number and type of injuries treated, equipment and supplies used, difficulties encountered, solutions to these problems and suggested improvements.

If possible, the physiotherapist should meet all members of the team in order to participate in their medical screening, individually assess their needs, and give advice on preventing or minimizing problems commonly encountered on tour. If this cannot be arranged, a circular should be sent to team members which incorporates a summary of this advice and a questionnaire seeking details of medical history, current injuries or illness, medication, allergies, vaccinations received, medical insurance held and any special dietary or other requirements. The circular should include a form authorizing any medical assistance considered necessary for the athlete, and another authorizing the team doctor or physiotherapist to discuss any relevant injury or illness with team management for the express purpose of determining the fitness of the athlete to participate. These forms and questionnaires should be completed and returned by the athlete. In the case of a minor it is essential that written permission be obtained from the parent or guardian (see Ch. 38).

Having collected this information, it should be possible to plan strategies and start acquiring the equipment and supplies needed to meet the team's requirements.

At least one meeting involving all team officials should be held well before departure, offering the opportunity to establish a working relationship, discuss the role of each person and disseminate information. Potential problems should be raised and management strategies designed. In particular, the importance of patient confidentiality and informed consent should be discussed and understood, and the appropriate lines of communication formulated between medical staff, athletes, coaches, selectors and management. Fitch (1989) points out that team personnel have a duty both to the athlete and to coaches and team management. It is essential that players understand this dual responsibility, and that they authorize the physiotherapist to release to the coach or administrator information relevant to their fitness to train or compete. Should a team member ask a physiotherapist not to report a significant injury, it is important that the physiotherapist convince the player that such a course of action is not in his or her best interests or those of the team. This approach is preferable to relying wholly on the written authorization.

Medical screening

Several weeks prior to departure a medical assessment should be carried out, preferably involving the team doctor and physiotherapist. The object of this screening is to identify potential problems and take the necessary steps to minimize their impact. Each athlete should be examined and a thorough history taken. Chronic and current injuries or illness need to be thoroughly assessed. Are there areas of pain, weakness or loss of flexibility that require attention? Is treatment being received, and is satisfactory progress being made? A letter may be requested from the athlete's practitioner or direct contact made so that treatment can be instigated, continued or modified if required. If there is doubt about the athlete's ability to recover or reach satisfactory performance standards, the athlete may be excluded from the team or advised to withdraw. Existing injuries frequently deteriorate further while on tour despite intensive treatment, and players may jeopordize their chances of future selection by performing poorly while on tour.

All athletes, particularly the inexperienced, should have warm-up, stretching, taping and other prevention protocols checked. Are there any medical problems such as asthma, diabetes or allergies to tape or medication? Any medication currently in use should be checked against the list of prohibited drugs in that sport. The athlete should take adequate medical supplies for the whole tour as it can be difficult to obtain the same or equivalent preparations abroad. If no medical officer is accompanying the team it may also be wise if the athlete's doctor prescribes appropriate sedatives and non-steroidal anti-inflammatories, to be used if necessary under the supervision of the physiotherapist.

The immunization status of each team member should be checked and suitably upgraded under the guidance of an experienced medical officer. Tetanus-diphtheria protection is usually required. Medical personnel and players of contact sports should have hepatitis B vaccination. Over 100 countries carry the risk of malaria and may require

chemoprophylaxis. The World Health Organization issues annual recommendations on the vaccinations required in different countries (Sando 1992).

The weight of each athlete should be recorded and monitored throughout the tour. Ideally, fitness tests and a dental examination should also be carried out. Team officials should also undertake the medical examination prior to departure, as they must be fit enough to cope with travel and working long hours under difficult conditions.

At the pre-departure medical screening or training camp, time should be set aside for the doctor or physiotherapist to brief the team on health related issues. If this is not possible the information should be included in the circular to team members. The following areas may be covered.

The composition of the medical team and arrangements for treatment must be included. Athletes should be encouraged to report injuries or illness immediately.

The relevance of prohibited substances in the sport is vital. Athletes must understand that many prescribed and 'over the counter' medications contain banned substances. Many nose drops and sprays, cough mixtures and influenza remedies contain prohibited substances such as pseudoephedrine. Some substances are permitted in one form but banned in others (e.g. salbutamol, a frequently used antiasthmatic, is permitted in aerosol form only). All medication must be cleared by the doctor or physiotherapist on tour, who should be familiar with the current list of prohibited substances in the sport. Drug testing procedures can be outlined (see Ch. 37).

Athletes should be warned of three common problems with diet. Traveller's diarrhoea may occur, usually caused by the ingestion of a strain of E. coli, with food or water. Water supplies can also be contaminated with flagellates, amoebae or other pathogenic bacteria. Careful washing of hands is essential before eating and after using the toilet. If water and food are a hazard, athletes should eat where recommended only, and avoid icecream, shellfish, salads, raw vegetables and unskinned fruit. Only bottled or boiled water should be used for drinking or brushing teeth. Ice for drinks should be made from purified water. The doctor or physiotherapist may need to supervise meal preparation and obtain uncontaminated drinks and ice for consumption. Naturally, drink bottles must not be shared. Players should have their own containers or marked cups to prevent the risk of cross-infection.

Athletes are often very particular about their food intake. The physiotherapist should intervene on the team's behalf when meals lack variety, freshness, quantity or quality, or differ unacceptably from the athlete's familiar diet. Not everyone views roast monkey brains as a delicacy.

Conversely, in a games village or hotel an unlimited supply of excellent food may be freely available, and it is easy to gain unwanted kilos, especially if bored or un-occupied. Regular weighing will help to monitor dietary problems. Physiotherapists should be aware that in some sports eating disorders such as anorexia nervosa are common in female athletes (Thornton 1990).

Athletes should be advised on methods of coping with lengthy periods of travel and jetlag, a topic covered later in this chapter.

Athletes have a personal responsibility to prevent the spread of infection within the team. Information needs to be provided on risk factors and prevention strategies for potential problems ranging from tinea to HIV/AIDS. The Australian Sports Medicine Federation's infectious diseases policy (1993) gives a number of recommendations, with a particular focus on the blood-borne infections, notably HIV and Hepatitis B. In broad terms, the risk of transmission of infectious diseases can be reduced by maintaining high standards of hygiene, not sharing baths, towels, razors or drink containers, reporting and treating open wounds immediately, and vaccination where appropriate. It is vital that athletes or officials with a significant bacterial or viral infection be isolated, to reduce the risk of spreading the infection to others (Bruckner & Khan 1993).

Equipment, supplies and treatment kit

The choice of equipment and supplies depends on the size of the team, length of the trip and the personal preferences of the physiotherapist. Despite the extra weight and bulk, the physiotherapist should aim to be as well equipped and as self-sufficient as possible. This means taking equipment rather than depending on hiring or acquiring while on tour. Physiotherapists can recount numerous stories of promised equipment which failed to materialize, vital parts broken or missing, huge hidden costs and unfamiliar models.

Battery operation and miniaturization, resulting from solid state and microprocessor technology, have produced a range of electromedical equipment which is smaller, lighter, more reliable and far more practical for the travelling physiotherapist. Laser and microstimulation units are available in pen sized models, TENS in pocket size, and interferential incorporated in multiple therapy units weighing under 2 kg. Ultrasound, the most popular modality, can be obtained in compact combinations with other equipment including high-voltage stimulation.

If the physiotherapist is not taking their own equipment, it is important to borrow or hire the items well in advance in order to become familiar with their operation, check their working order, arrange insurance, and package them for transport. Electromedical items may require special padded boxes and should be clearly marked as fragile. Small items of value such as portable lasers are best carried as hand luggage. Spare fuses, batteries and possibly a battery charger should be taken. Batteries should be removed from machines when in transit to avoid airport security problems and to prevent accidental discharge.

Power supplies can be a problem overseas, and voltages at each destination must be carefully checked. The majority of countries in Europe, the Middle East, Africa, South America, Oceania and much of mainland Asia supply power in the range 220–250 V, while the USA, Japan and a number of other countries vary from 100–117 volts. Use of a voltage significantly different from that of the equipment can interfere with output and operation, blow fuses, severely damage the unit and endanger the patient or operator. Some equipment comes with a voltage selector incorporated. If not, a transformer of sufficient V Amp rating should be used to obtain the correct output. International power supplies also vary from 50–60 cycles. These variations can cause overheating of equipment which must be checked frequently for temperature rises and switched off when not in use.

Plugs also vary greatly overseas. Sets of universal adaptors for travellers are easily purchased, but these often lack an earthing pin. It may be safer to fit a local pin to the equipment or to a power board with safety cut-outs which then provides multiple sockets of the home plug type. An extension cord is also desirable.

A portable treatment table is essential on most tours. The convenience more than compensates for the extra weight and bulk.

A list of equipment and supplies which should be considered can be found in Table 36.1. Examples of products available in Australia are given in brackets (no endorsement is implied). Keep an inventory of all supplies for Customs, and advise the team manager in advance how much excess weight you will take.

These supplies will be inaccessible at times, especially when in transit. It is prudent to carry Bandaids, throat lozenges, analgesics, safety pins, tape and scissors, plus motion sickness tablets on the plane.

If travelling with a team of wheelchair or amputee athletes add specialised skin dressings like Duoderm and additional 2nd Skin or silicon gel sheets for skin breakdown. Extra adhesive foam is handy for padding wheelchairs.

Physiotherapy treatment areas

Although team accommodation is usually limited, the physiotherapist should obtain a separate room for treatment, close to that of the doctor. This room usually becomes the team's social centre. Establish a waiting area and an appointments list. Set up the room to maximize lighting, privacy, comfort and function.

This is usually more difficult at training and competition venues. Areas allocated vary from the dark corner of a change room to the luxury of equipment and space in a polyclinic. Inspect the areas in advance where possible to locate the optimum working areas, plus access to ice, running water, power, telephones, medical facilities and the sports field. If no ice is available take your own. Request improvements if conditions are unsatisfactory.

DUTIES IN THE FIELD

The physiotherapist must establish the requirements of the team members, manager and coach, find out in advance whether he or she is allowed on the arena if an athlete or

Table 36.1 Equipment and supplies

Medical supplies
Lockable medical kit
Stethoscope
Emergency airway
Penlight torch
Scissors, personally identified
Tweezers, nail clippers
Air splints
Disposable gloves
Instant and reusable cold packs
Plastic bags for ice
Cold spray (Skefron)
Skin lubricants (Vaseline)
'Heat' creams (Metsal, Fanalgon)
Anti-inflammatory creams or gels (Movelat, Difflam)
Bruising dispersant (Lasonil, or Hirudoid)
Antihistamine cream
Anti-irritant for bites or rashes (Stingose)
Anti-fungal agent (Tinaderm, Canesten)
Nasal spray or drops (Spray Tish, Drixine)
Eye drops (Visine)
Motion sickness tablets (Dramamine)
Analgesics (Aspro Clear, Panadol)
Antihistamines (Fabahistin)
Antacids (Mylanta)
Burns cream (Butesin Picrate)
Antiseptic solution (Betadine)
Antiseptic spray or ointment (Savlon)
Cotton buds, alcohol swabs
Ultrasound and contact gel
Massage oil
Foam padding (Leukofoam)
Splinting and basic orthotic material
Thermometer

Bandages
Rigid Zinc Oxide (ZnO) strapping tapes 12 mm, 25 mm, 38 mm, 50 mm
Waterproof ZnO tape 25 mm
Elastic adhesive bandages, hypoallergenic and ZnO
Fixomull stretch or Hypafix tape 50 mm
Elastic compression bandages 50 mm, 75 mm, 100 mm
Tubular support bandage, (Flexigrip or equivalent)
Underwrap
Adhesive spray
Bandage clips
Bandaids
Triangular bandages
2nd Skin or silicon gel sheets
Sterile dressing kit
Assorted dressings
Steri strips and butterfly closures

General
Insect repellant
Sunscreen, lip balm
Small ice and drink containers
Electrolyte replacement
Condoms, tampons
Digital scales
Swiss army style pocket knife
Pocket sewing kit
Mouthguard
Record cards, pens and marker pen
Tissues, safety pins, rubber bands
Small gifts, badges
Disposable razors
Current list of permitted and prohibited medication

player is injured, know the location of medical facilities (including stretchers), and have a planned set of procedures in case of serious injuries.

The physiotherapist must also arrive early to set up the treatment area, liaise with medical personnel on site, obtain ice and assist with pre-event massage, taping amd warm-up routines, and as a member of the team, offer support and encouragement. The physiotherapist must be able to provide assessment and emergency care of injuries quickly, and be located easily by players or officials. In a team sport the obvious position is on the bench, ready to advise the coach on the injured player's ability to continue. In other sports it may well be in the warm-up or massage area. Any seriously ill or injured athlete requiring further medical attention or hospitalization must be accompanied by the physiotherapist, in order to facilitate and monitor optimal care. When in doubt aim for the largest teaching hospital.

At the end of each event all injuries must be assessed, immediate care and advice provided, and a time set for follow up treatment. Assist with post-event cool-down, stretches and massage if required.

PROBLEMS ENCOUNTERED ON TOUR

Murphy's Law applies to most travelling teams: whatever can go wrong probably will. Team members can be hit by cars, bitten by dogs or suffer virtually any known medical disorder. Many problems relate to stress or the high activity levels of athletes, and not all can be avoided. The following are some of the factors that may contribute to the physical and/or psychological problems.

Poor mattresses and pillows combined with the rigours of travel mean that there will probably be a number of neck and back conditions needing treatment.

Working with unfamiliar athletes, coaches and medical staff, each with their own methods and peculiarities, can be daunting. It should be seen as an opportunity to exchange ideas, learn more about the sport and increase knowledge.

Be wary of the press. An unofficial or misleading press release can be embarrassing and cause unnecessary alarm at home. The team manager is the correct person to talk to the press, and should be supplied with accurate information without abusing the player's right to confidentiality.

The physiotherapist should not condone any method which has been banned by the International Olympic Committee Medical Commission, which is not in accord with professional ethics or which might be harmful to the athlete (Sando 1992, Smith 1992). Physiotherapists in most countries do not have the right to supply prescription medication and should refrain from doing so. Unrestricted preparations, often incorporating lower dosages, can be used where appropriate.

Athletes who walk excess distances while shopping, touring or moving around a large games village may develop unnecessary leg soreness or low back pain, especially if hills are involved. Disabled athletes are even more prone to skin, spinal or limb problems if covering this extra territory.

If travelling with a team of young people, it must be remembered that children are more susceptible to heat stress, dehydration and hypothermia than adults, and that the immature musculoskeletal system is subject to a number of developmental, overuse and trauma associated problems. The physiotherapist should ensure that training, competition, diagnosis and treatment are appropriate to the growth and development of the child.

Athletes and officials on tour are subject to stress from a wide variety of sources. These may involve noise, extremes of climate, jetlag, poor food, accommodation or transport, constant shifting, loss of familiar routines, injury, illness, pressure to perform, size and standard of competition, interpersonal conflict and personal problems not associated with the sport. The physiotherapist must be aware of the stress affecting him or herself and other members of the team. In the treatment setting, team members may relax and discuss these problems, or may exhibit signs suggesting inability to cope. These include muscle tension, hypochondria, insomnia, aggression, agitation and loss of energy or concentration. Strategies which may be used to provide support in these situations include meditation, relaxation techniques, massage, positive imagery, personal counselling, social support and intervention to reduce or remove the source of stress. In many cases of anxiety the physiotherapist's contribution as a positive, sympathetic and sensitive contact may be all that is required (see Ch. 19).

OTHER DUTIES

Record keeping and physiotherapy report

Though sometimes difficult, it is vital that accurate records of assessment and treatment are kept for medico-legal reasons and to provide information for epidemiological studies, for the final report and for correspondence with the player's personal practitioner after the tour. A diary allows portability and privacy, and details can be transferred to patient cards later. Some countries, notably Canada, have developed a system where case notes are carried by athletes, providing greater continuity and detail. These should be updated and a record kept for the physiotherapist's own use.

A physiotherapy report should be sent to the team manager or parent sporting organisation following the tour. A summary of treatments and injuries encountered should be given, excluding information which would identify individual athletes. Detail the equipment and supplies used and any costs incurred. Outline significant problems encountered, recommend possible improvements and acknowledge assistance given.

Registration and insurance

Few countries require visiting physiotherapists to obtain registration when treating members of their own team (Sando 1992, Smith 1992). When demanded at major games, temporary registration is usually facilitated by the organizing body, free of charge. Several Australian State Registration Boards demand that physiotherapists accompanying teams from other states acquire temporary registration. Physiotherapists should limit treatment to team members and athletes.

The physiotherapist's professional indemnity or malpractice insurance policy should be carefully read to ensure that the countries being visited are not excluded. The insurance company should be informed of the destination and nature of your appointment, and any difficulties discussed in advance.

Comprehensive insurance, paid for by the sporting club or organization, is essential for all equipment taken on tour.

Team members should be advised to take out comprehensive health insurance. Medical care provided in other countries can be extremely expensive and is not usually covered by Australia's national health scheme. Insurance should also cover the cost of evacuation home by plane, often the best option if a person is seriously ill or injured overseas.

Air travel

Although extended jet travel has long been part of the athlete's life, it can still adversely affect performance. The principal problem is jetlag, a disruption of circadian rhythms experienced when flying across three or more time zones. The symptoms of psychological and physiological desynchronization include difficulty sleeping, fatigue, confusion, irritability, digestive disorders, stiffness, headaches and loss of sensory motor function (Loat & Rhodes 1989). The body clock takes approximately one day per time zone to adjust, and adjustment is more difficult when travelling eastward than east to west. Dehydration occurs due to dry air in the cabin and the consumption of drinks containing alcohol or caffeine. Low cabin pressures and exposure to cigarette smoke can combine to significantly reduce the oxygen carrying capacity of the blood, while venous congestion and lower limb oedema occur with tight clothing and prolonged sitting on the plane. Finally, upper respiratory tract infections are an extremely common problem amongst athletes following lengthy air travel especially when crossing several time zones (Bradshaw 1988).

These problems can be minimized by adopting the following guidelines (Ledoux 1988, Loat & Rhodes 1989, Bruckner & Khan 1993):

1. Watches should be set on the destination time and appropriate sleeping and eating patterns adopted as early as possible
2. Sufficient rest should be gained prior to departure
3. Total travel time between home and accommodation at the destination should be minimized. Lengthy train or bus travel and delays in terminals and stations add greatly to the stresses of air travel

4. Excess food, especially fats, should be avoided before and during the flight
5. Plenty of water, mineral water or fruit juice should be drunk on the plane
6. Alcohol, coffee, tea, cola, smoking and salt should be avoided
7. Light, loose fitting clothing should be worn, and athletes should stretch and move around the cabin regularly
8. If arriving during the day, time should be spent outdoors, having a light exercise session and attempting to settle into the local pattern of eating and sleeping times immediately.

Prolonged travel can pose particular problems for disabled athletes (Perriman 1992). Amputees may suffer stump irritation or swelling during long flights, making it difficult to fit prostheses on arrival. Ice, bandaging, elevation and the use of crutches or a wheelchair may be necessary for several days. Quadriplegic athletes susceptible to skin breakdown should lie down every two hours and travel with an airline cushion. Aisle chairs should be arranged in advance to aid movement around the plane.

SUMMARY

The demands placed on sporting bodies and governments to produce winning performances have led to an increasingly professional approach to sport. As a result, the number of touring teams has grown enormously. The knowledge, skill and versatility of the sports physiotherapist allow him or her to play a pivotal role in serving the varying needs of these groups. The level of professionalism and dedication displayed will determine whether that contribution is fully appreciated and of maximum value to athletes.

REFERENCES

Australian Sports Medicine Federation 1993 Infectious diseases policy, 3rd edn. ASMF, Canberra

Badewitz-Dodd L 1992 Drugs and sport, 2nd edn. MIMS Australia, Sydney

Bond J 1988 Minimising jet lag and jet stress: some thoughts for the travelling athlete. Sports Coach 12(1):56-57

Bottomley M 1990 Athletes at an overseas venue: the role of the team doctor. In: Payne S D W Medicine, sport and the law. Blackwell Scientific, ch 11

Bracker M D 1985 How I manage traveler's diarrhea. The Physician and Sportsmedicine 13(11):63-67

Bradshaw C 1988 Medical report on Australian junior athletic team's tour to the world junior championships. Sports Health 6 (4):18-22

Bruckner P, Khan K 1993 Clinical sports medicine. McGraw-Hill, Sydney, ch 45-47

Burke L, Read R 1989 Sports nutrition approaching the nineties. Sports Medicine 8(2):80-100

Campbell S The coach physiotherapist relationship. Physiotherapy in Sport 9(2):9-12

Donike M et al 1985 Screening procedure in doping control. In: Lungquist A, Peltokallio P, Tikkanen H (eds) Sports medicine in track and field. IAAF, Kuovola, Finland, pp 117-130

Dornan P 1990 The recognition of stress as a factor in athletic rehabilitation. Sports Health 8 (2):15-16

Eriksson B O et al 1990 Sports medicine: health and medication Guinness Publishing, Enfield, Middlesex, ch 41

Fallon K E 1990 The disabled athlete. In: Bloomfield J, Fricker P A, Fitch K D (eds) Textbook of science and medicine in sport. Blackwell Scientific, Melbourne, pp 488-511

Fitch K D 1989 Ethical guidelines of health care for sports medicine. Sports Health 7(2):27-28

Georgilopoulos P 1992 Personal communication

Gray B 1990 Exercise and the human immune system. Excel 6(3):12-14

Hall J 1989 The role of chartered physiotherapists in Olympic sports. Physiotherapy 75(12)686-690

Haynes S 1989 The permitted use of medicines in sport. National program on drugs in sport, Curtain, Canberra

Hillman R S, Smith R P 1991 Travel. In: Strauss R H (ed) Sports medicine 2nd edn. W B Saunders, Philadelphia, pp 273-281

Huckstep R L 1986 A simple guide to trauma, 4th edn. Churchill Livingstone, Edinburgh

International Olympic Committee Medical Commission 1990 List of doping classes and methods of doping. IOC, Lausanne

Kerr G, Fowler B 1988 The relationship between psychological factors and sports injuries. Sports Medicine 6:127-134

Ledoux M 1988 Planning your travel and overseas intake: the effects of jet lag. Canadian Physiotherapy Association Sports Physiotherapy Newsletter 13(2):15-18

Loat C E R, Rhodes E C 1989 Jet-lag and human performance. Sports Medicine 8(4):226-238

McDonald V 1992 Personal communication

Maguire K 1988 Dilemmas in sports medicine. Sport Health 6(1):12-14

Perriman D 1992 Personal communication

Peterson L, Renstrom P 1986 Sports injuries: their prevention and treatment. Methuen Australia, North Sydney, chs 4,7

Ray R, Feld F 1989 The team physician's medical bag. Clinics in Sports Medicine 8(1):139-145

Rund D 1986 Essentials of emergency medicine, 2nd edn. East Norwalk, Connecticut

Sando B G 1992 The team physician. In: Bloomfield J, Fricker P A, Fitch K D (eds) Textbook of science and medicine in sport. Blackwell Scientific, pp 422-436

Smith R B 1992 Personal communication

Thornton J S 1990 Feast or famine: eating disorders in athletes. Physician and Sportsmedicine 18(4)116-122

Wallner F D 1991 Care of the high performance athlete on tour. Proceedings of Australian Sports Medicine Federation's 1991 sports medicine workshop. ASMF, Canberra

37. Drugs in sport

Peter Brukner

Drugs are widely used by athletes both in the treatment of injury and to enhance performance. It is important that all professionals involved in the management of athletes have a basic knowledge of the types of drugs available, their clinical use and possible complications of their use.

THERAPEUTIC DRUGS

Analgesics

Analgesics or painkillers are widely used in our society. Aspirin, paracetamol and codeine are the most widely used analgesics, either by themselves or in combination with other analgesics. In the treatment of sporting injuries, analgesics are used in the acute phase immediately after injury to reduce pain. They may be used subsequently depending on the degree and duration of pain. They are also used to facilitate movement, which is essential for appropriate rehabilitation.

Aspirin has an analgesic effect at dosages of 250–300 mg. At higher dosages aspirin also has an anti-inflammatory effect, but this is associated with a higher incidence of side effects, particularly of the gastrointestinal system. Aspirin and paracetamol both have an anti-pyretic effect. Paracetamol has no influence on the inflammatory process.

Codeine is a more potent analgesic. It is a narcotic analgesic and therefore was previously in the International Olympic Committee (IOC) list of banned substances, along with morphine and pethidine. It was removed from this list in 1993.

Topical analgesics

Topical analgesics are used extensively by athletes and are known as 'sports rubs', 'heat rubs' and 'liniments'. Most commercially available topical analgesics contain a combination of substances such as menthol, methyl salicylate, camphor and eucalyptus oil.

The majority act as counter-irritants which inflame and irritate the skin. Most products contain two or more active ingredients that produce redness, dilate blood vessels, stimulate pain receptors and stimulate heat and cold receptors. The type and intensity of the effect depends on the particular ingredients, their concentration, how much is applied and how it is applied.

Although the exact mechanism of action of counter-irritants is unknown, it is possible that stimulation of nociceptors by a noxious stimulus such as a counter-irritant can inhibit the response of central neurones transmitting pain messages nearby. Rubbing topical agents into the skin may also suppress pain transmission by stimulating nerve fibres (Barone 1989).

Topical agents should not be used to replace a proper warm-up as there is likely to be no effect on muscles.

Topical agents may irritate the skin and occasionally cause blistering. Contact dermatitis also has been reported.

Topical anti-inflammatory agents

A number of topical anti-inflammatory products are available. These include indomethacin (Indospray), benzydamine (Difflam) and adrenocortical extract (Movelat). Topical indomethacin appears to be effective in reducing inflammation in superficial overuse injuries (Akemark & Forsskahl 1990).

NSAIDs

The non-steroidal anti-inflammatory drugs (NSAIDs) are widely used in the treatment of sporting injuries. The first drugs used were aspirin and the salicylates, while more recently other NSAIDs have been introduced. All these drugs have analgesic, anti-inflammatory and anti-pyretic properties. They are also widely used in the treatment of arthritis.

Mode of action

Inflammation occurs at the site of injury. A local soft tissue injury such as a ligament tear causes the release of

729

arachidonic acid from cell walls. The arachidonic acid is converted by a number of enzymes, in particular cyclo-oxygenase, to a variety of prostaglandins, thromboxane and prostacyclins. These substances act as mediators of the inflammatory response.

The NSAIDs have been shown to interfere with the conversion of arachidonic acid to prostaglandin by inhibiting the action of cyclo-oxygenase (Vane 1971). It is thought that NSAIDs also interfere elsewhere in the inflammatory response, but the exact mechanisms are uncertain.

Are NSAIDs effective?

In spite of the widespread use of NSAIDs, there is conflicting evidence on their effectiveness. There have been numerous clinical trials studying the effectiveness of NSAIDs in the management of acute soft tissue injuries. These have been reviewed by Clyman (1986), Weiler et al (1987) and Almekinders (1990). Most of the studies lacked a placebo group and compared one NSAID with another. Of the eight well designed studies which included a placebo and studied a single type of ligamentous injury, only four showed a significantly better outcome in the treatment group than in the placebo group (Almekinders 1990).

NSAIDs are commonly used in the treatment of overuse injuries such as tendonitis and bursitis, but there is no scientific evidence to support their use.

Animal studies have shown NSAIDs to have some beneficial effect (Vogel 1977, Dahners et al 1988, Almekinders & Gilbert 1986) and there may be valid reasons why the clinical trials do not reflect the popular view among clinicians that these drugs are effective in the management of acute injuries. One of the main methodological problems is the difficulty with the assessment of efficacy which in most studies relies mainly on subjective evaluation. Some workers consider that the effectiveness of NSAIDs in acute injuries is due to their analgesic effect, which allows earlier mobility.

More studies are needed to investigate the effectiveness of NSAIDs, particularly in the management of overuse injuries. In the meantime, the precise criteria for the use of NSAIDs in the management of sporting injuries remain a matter of debate.

Which NSAID?

There are a large number of NSAIDs currently available, as shown in Table 37.1.

The various clinical trials have failed to show that any one NSAID is consistently more effective than any other. Clinical experience tells us that there is some variation in individual response to different NSAIDs. However, in general, the choice of NSAID is not made on the grounds of efficacy alone, but on dosage schedule and side effect profile.

Table 37.1   Commonly used NSAIDs

Drug	Trade names	Usual dose (mg)	Times daily
Aspirin	Ecotrin, SRA, ASA	650	3–4
Diclofenac	Voltaren	25–50	2–3
Diflusinal	Dolobid	250–500	2
Ibuprofen	Brufen, Motrin, Rufen	400	3–4
Indomethacin	Indocid, Indocin	25–50	3
Ketoprofen	Orudis,	50–100	2–4
	Orudis-SR	100–200	1
Naproxen	Naprosyn, Anaprox	250–500	2
Piroxicam	Feldene	10–20	1–2
Sulindac	Clinoril	100–200	2
Tenoxicam	Tilcotil	20	1

Compliance is an important component of patient management and may be more so in the athlete. There are considerable differences in the dosage schedules of the various NSAIDs (Table 37.1).

Dosage schedules are dependent on the plasma half-life of the drug. Half-lives of NSAIDs vary from one hour to approximately 60 hours. Generally drugs with longer half-lives have a slower onset of action and require less frequent doses. Compounds such as piroxicam and tenoxicam have long plasma half-lives and can be given once every 24 hours. The NSAIDs with short half lives may be effective when given only two or three times a day, possibly due to the slow diffusion of NSAIDs into and out of the joint or synovial space.

Side effects

In general, the NSAIDs are safe drugs with minimal serious side effects, particularly in view of their widespread use. The most common side effects involve the gastrointestinal system, especially epigastric pain, nausea, indigestion and heartburn. The newer NSAIDs and enteric-coated forms of aspirin have a considerably lower incidence of dyspeptic symptoms than aspirin. There does not appear to be much difference in the incidence of gastrointestinal side effects among the different NSAIDs. As with the clinical efficacy, there appears to be considerable individual variation and another NSAID may be prescribed if the original choice causes side effects.

Dyspeptic side effects can be minimized by using the minimum effective dose, taking the drug with or immediately after food or milk, or by using antacids. Alcohol, cigarettes and coffee may aggravate the dyspepsia. Certain NSAIDs are available in suppository form which will reduce, but probably not eliminate, the gastric side effects. The incidence of peptic ulceration with the short term use of NSAIDs is rare. Gastric bleeding, in particular occult bleeding, does occur and may contribute to the high incidence of iron depletion seen in athletes. Clinicians should be wary of prescribing long term use of these drugs in iron-depleted athletes.

Other side effects occasionally seen with these drugs include asthma, allergic rhinitis, rashes, tinnitus, deafness, headache and confusion. These are all unusual. The occasional incidence of bone marrow suppression associated with the use of phenylbutazone has resulted in that drug being rarely prescribed.

The NSAIDs have a number of important drug interactions. Interactions have been reported with anti-coagulants, anti-hypertensives, diuretics and peripheral vasodilators.

Summary

NSAIDs are widely used in the treatment of many different types of sporting injuries, yet convincing evidence of their efficiency in the treatment of sprains and strains is lacking. The primary treatment of these conditions remains the early use of R.I.C.E. and subsequent physiotherapy. There may be a more clearcut role for the NSAIDs in the treatment of overuse injuries such as tendinitis and bursitis where inflammation is the primary pathology rather than a secondary factor.

There appear to be no great differences in the effectiveness of individual drugs. The choice should be made on the basis of patient tolerance and probable compliance, with preference being given to those which have a once or twice a day dosage schedule. Clinicians should be particularly concerned regarding the relationship of long term NSAID therapy, occult gastrointestinal bleeding and iron depletion.

Corticosteroids

Corticosteroids are the most potent anti-inflammatory drugs available to the medical practitioner. The presence of potentially harmful side effects prevents the use of long term systemic corticosteroids. The use of both short term systemic and local injection of corticosteroids remains controversial.

Local injection

Local injection of corticosteroid minimizes the risk of side effects associated with the systemic administration of the drug and allows the corticosteroid to be placed at the site of the injury. Local injection of corticosteroids has been used in the treatment of a number of inflammatory conditions, as shown in the box.

The effect of local corticosteroid injection in many of these conditions can be dramatic. Many athletes relate stories of their 'miraculous' cure and return to athletic activity and, as a result, desperate athletes may present to a medical practitioner demanding a 'cortisone injection' to enable them to return to their sporting activity.

As well as their potent anti-inflammatory action, the locally injected corticosteroid may have other effects.

> **Conditions in which local injection of corticosteroid may be used**
>
> Bursitis
> Paratendonitis
> Tenosynovitis
> Joint synovitis
> Osteoarthritis
> Chronic muscle strain
> Trigger points

Corticosteroids may have an inhibitory effect on collagen synthesis and thus interfere with the tissue repair process (Gray et al 1981). The rapid relief of symptoms after corticosteroid injection may mask the protective pain mechanism and result in overuse of a damaged joint. This may lead to increased degenerative changes. These changes appear to be dose-related and the use of repeated injections is discouraged (Leadbetter 1990).

The use of local corticosteroid injection is particularly effective in the treatment of bursitis. Conditions such as sub-acromial, olecranon, pre-patellar and retro-calcaneal bursitis may be resistant to alternative forms of treatment combined with NSAIDs, possibly due to poor blood supply. These bursitides often respond well to local injection. However, injections should only be used as part of the management program and the practitioner must continue to seek the cause of the problem, particularly in overuse injuries.

Intra-articular injections, particularly into weightbearing joints, are controversial. They should be performed with great care and reserved for those who develop a post-traumatic chronic synovitis which does not respond to non-steroidal anti-inflammatory drugs. Apophyseal joint injections can be effective in the management of patients whose back pain is primarily emanating from these joints and who have only short-lived response to manual therapy. Controversy surrounds the use of injectable corticosteroid into the epidural space.

Injections into tendons have also been a source of considerable controversy. A reported increased tendency to rupture after injection has led to this practice being virtually abandoned (Ford & De Bender 1979, Kelly et al 1984, Kleinman & Gross 1983). Some practitioners advocate the injection of tendon sheaths, while others advocate the 'bathing' of the tendon with corticosteroid by injection around, but not into, the tendon. The long term effects of these practices are unknown.

The use of injected corticosteroid in acute mono-articular exacerbations of osteoarthritis has been practised by rheumatologists for many years. An acute attack of gouty arthritis may also respond well to aspiration and corticosteroid injection.

Some clinicians recommend the injection of trigger points with corticosteroid, but others consider massage, dry needling or local anaesthetic injection to be just as effective (Travell & Simons 1983).

The main side effect of corticosteroid injection, apart from the possible damage to articular cartilage previously mentioned, is infection. This is a rare occurrence and should be prevented by strict aseptic techniques, particularly when performing intra-articular injections. The presence of an overlying skin infection is a contraindication to injection.

Corticosteroid injections commonly cause a short term exacerbation of symptoms, a phenomenon known as 'post-injection flare' which may commence soon after injection and usually subsides within 24–48 hours. This phenomenon is thought to be due to a crystalline synovitis. Patients should always be warned that it may occur.

Corticosteroid injections have a reputation of being a particularly painful procedure, but if local anaesthetic is added to the injection, the problem can be minimized. The abolition of pain after the local anaesthetic injection may be diagnostically significant.

There are a number of different forms of injectable corticosteroid available and there is no convincing evidence of difference in efficacy among them. They include hydrocortisone, betamethasone (Celestone), methylprednisolone (Depo-Medrol) and triamcinalone (Kenacort).

The use of local corticosteroid injections may produce dramatic amelioration of symptoms. However, their use should be restricted to conditions, such as bursitis, which have not responded to less interventional forms of therapy. It should only be considered to be part of the treatment management and may, by reducing pain and inflammation, allow other forms of therapy e.g. exercise therapy, to be initiated. Intra-articular injections, particularly in weight-bearing joints, should be approached with considerable caution because of possible long term damage to articular cartilage. Injection technique must be aseptic, the number of injections to any one site should be restricted to no more

Table 37.2 IOC list of doping classes and methods

Banned classes of drugs
Stimulants
Narcotics
Anabolic steroids
Beta blockers
Diuretics
Peptide hormones and analogues

Banned doping methods
Blood doping
Pharmacological, chemical and physical manipulation

Classes of drugs subject to certain restrictions
Alcohol
Marijuana
Local anaesthetics
Corticosteroids

---

than three (Leadbetter 1990) and injections should not be performed at less than 4-week intervals.

Systemic use

Corticosteroids are rarely used systemically in the treatment of sporting injuries because of the potential side effects (Behrens & Goodwin 1990). Occasionally, in chronic inflammatory conditions or acute exacerbation, a short course of prednisolone may be given using high doses over a period of a week. One condition reported to respond well to this regimen is osteitis pubis (Gonik & Stringer 1985). This form of treatment should only be considered when all other forms of treatment have failed.

DRUG ABUSE IN SPORT

Drug abuse in sport goes back almost as far as sport itself, with the first reported instance taking place during the Ancient Olympics where athletes consumed hallucinogenic brews of mushrooms and seeds to enhance their performance. In the last 30 or 40 years, however, drug problems have attracted considerable attention to the point where drugs are probably the major problem affecting sport today.

The use of amphetamines, anabolic steroids, growth hormone, testosterone, blood doping, erythropoietin and other substances by athletes in a large range of sports has forced sporting bodies to address this issue.

The International Olympic Committee (IOC), through its Medical Commission, has issued a list of banned substances which has been adopted in part or full by most sporting organisations. Many banned substances are found in commonly used medications.

Despite the existence of the list and the regular drug testing carried out at major international championships such as the Olympic Games and World Championships, the drug problem remains. However, with the publicity surrounding the disqualification of Canadian 100 metre gold medallist Ben Johnson at the 1988 Seoul Olympics, the authorities realized that competition testing alone is insufficient to control the problem. Since then, many countries have instituted random drug testing both in and out of season in a serious attempt to confront the problem. Random drug testing combined with stiff penalties for offenders represents the sporting world's best chance to combat this serious problem.

The IOC list of doping classes and methods is shown in Table 37.2, and a list of main classes, their clinical uses, effect on performance and side effects is found in Table 37.3.

Stimulants

Stimulants are a large group of substances that increase alertness and mask fatigue. There are a number of different

Table 37.3 Banned drugs and their effects

Type of drug	Examples	Medical usage	Effect on performance	Side effects
Stimulants Amphetamines	dexamphetamine dimethylamphetamine	narcolepsy childhood hyperkinetic syndrome	may delay fatigue, increase alertness	anxiety, insomnia, dizziness, euphoria, headache, nausea, vomiting, confusion, psychosis, hypertension, addiction
Adrenaline-like substances	adrenaline, ephedrine, pseudoephedrine, phenylpropanolamine	contained in most over-the-counter cold remedies	no convincing evidence of performance enhancement	anxiety, irritability, insomnia, headaches, hypertension
Caffeine	caffeine (limited use allowed)	tonics, diet pills, analgesics	possible effect on muscle contraction and fat metabolism	irritability, insomnia, palpitations, peptic ulceration
Cocaine	cocaine	nasal anaesthetic	increased alertness	impaired hand-eye co-ordination, aggression, cardiac and cerebral abnormalities
Narcotic analgesics	pethidine, morphine	moderate to severe pain	no evidence of improved performance, may be able to compete with injury	nausea, vomiting, dizziness, respiratory depression, addiction
Anabolic steroids	Oral: methandrostenolone (Dianabol) Injectable: Nandrolone (Deca-Durabolin)	hypogonadism, severe osteoporosis, breast carcinoma	increased muscle bulk, increased muscle strength, anti-catabolic effect possibly improving recovery	acne, baldness, gynaecomastia, decreased sperm production, testis size and sex drive, increased aggression, liver abnormalities, hypertension, hypercholesterolaemia
Beta blockers (certain sports only)	propranol (Inderal), atenolol (Tenormin), pindolol (Visken), metoprolol (Lopresor)	hypertension, angina, arrhythmias, tremor, migraine	reduce tremor in shooting and archery, adverse effects on aerobic and anaerobic capacity	insomnia, fatigue, depression, impaired sexual performance
Diuretics	frusemide (Lasix), hydrochlorthiazide (Dyazide, Moduretic, Hydrodiuril) chlorthiazide (Chlotride, Diuril)	hypertension, oedema, congestive cardiac failure	rapid weight loss, decreased concentration of drugs in urine	electrolyte imbalance, dehydration, muscle cramps
Peptide hormones	human chorionic gonadotrophin (HCG)	hypogonadism	may increase endogenous production of steroids	as in corticosteroids
	corticotrophin (ACTH) corticrophin	steroid-responsive conditions	euphoria	
	human growth hormone (HGH)	dwarfism	anecdotal evidence only	allergic reactions, diabetogenic effect, acromegaly
	erythropoietin (EPO)	chronic renal failure	increased endurance	increased blood viscosity, myocardial infarction

types of stimulants. These include the psychomotor stimulants such as the amphetamines and cocaine, and the sympathomimetic amines such as ephedrine and pseudo-ephedrine which are found in many over-the-counter cold remedies and central nervous system (CNS) stimulants such as high doses of caffeine.

Amphetamines were first used during World War 2 when it was noted that they increased alertness and enabled the troops in the trenches to stay awake. After the war, they were used by athletes, often with disastrous consequences, and a number of deaths occurred as a result of excessive use of amphetamines.

The sympathomimetic amines are widely used in cough and cold remedies. There is no convincing evidence of an effect on performance, but they remain on the banned list and athletes must take care to avoid accidental usage (Wadler & Hainline 1989).

Cocaine is an illegal drug, sometimes used socially for the euphoric sensation it produces. Its effect on sporting performance is uncertain, but most anecdotal reports describe a negative effect, particularly on vision and co-ordination. It is addictive and its widespread use in American colleges has resulted in the tragic deaths of some outstanding young athletes.

Caffeine is one of the most widely used substances in our society. It is found in coffee, tea, chocolate, cocoa and cola drinks as well as in a number of medications. In high doses caffeine is a CNS stimulant and may also have a ergogenic effect in endurance activities through its effect on fat metabolism. The use of high doses of caffeine has been banned and a urinary concentration of greater than 12 micrograms/L is defined as a positive test.

This urinary level is said to correspond to the ingestion of 500 mg of caffeine, the equivalent of 6–8 cups of coffee, 10 cans of cola or three family bars of chocolate consumed over a short time. However, athletes must take care when ingesting caffeine-containing products as urine levels produced from a particular dose of caffeine may vary considerably.

Narcotic analgesics

This group, which contains morphine and derivatives, is used in the management of moderate to severe pain. Codeine, a member of the group, is widely used in combination with other analgesics such as paracetamol and aspirin in the relief of moderate pain. It is also used clinically in the treatment of diarrhoea. Codeine was removed from the IOC list of banned substances in 1993.

Although there is no evidence that these drugs have any ergogenic effect, they are banned because of the possibility that their use may enable athletes with severe injuries to play without pain. It is also part of the general attempt to reduce the usage of these drugs, some of which are addictive.

Anabolic steroids

The anabolic steroids are derivatives of the male sex hormone testosterone. These drugs have been used by power athletes to increase muscle bulk and strength. Additional effects include psychological effects such as increased aggression and appetite, and a possible anti-catabolic effect which may enable improved recovery.

Anabolic steroids come in two forms: oral steroids such as methandrostenolone (Dianabol) and stanozolol (Winstrol), and injectable forms such as nandrolone (Deca-Durabolin). Despite evidence of potentially serious side effects, anabolic steroids have been widely used since the 1950s.

These side effects range from the primarily cosmetic effects such as acne, hair loss and gynaecomastia to more serious effects such as reduction in testicular size and sperm count, kidney and liver tumours, behavioural and psychiatric problems, hypertension and hypercholesterolaemia.

An additional effect in adolescents whose bones have not yet fused is premature closure of the epiphyseal growth plates, resulting in permanent shortening of the long bones.

Anabolic steroid use by females may result in the development of facial hair, increased body hair, deepening of the voice and enlargement of the clitoris. Some of these changes may be irreversible.

The side effects of anabolic steroids vary considerably among individual users and are not necessarily dose related. Despite widespread publicity concerning the dangers of anabolic steroid use, it still remains the number one drug problem in sport today.

Beta blockers

Beta blockers are pharmaceutical agents widely used in the treatment of hypertension, cardiac arrhythmias, angina and tremor. The reduction in tremor has resulted in the use of beta blockers in sports such as shooting and archery. The use of beta blockers is banned in the following sports: shooting, archery, bobsleigh, diving, luge, biathlon, modern pentathlon and ski jumping.

Diuretics

Diuretics, or fluid tablets as they are known, are used in medicine for the treatment of mild hypertension, cardiac failure and fluid retention. They have been used by athletes who need to lose weight quickly in sports where weight limits apply, and have also been used to dilute the concentration of other drugs in the urine. Side effects of these drugs include electrolyte imbalance and dehydration.

Peptide hormones

Human chorionic gonadotrophin (HCG) has been used by athletes in an attempt to increase endogenous production of steroids as well as to counteract the testicular atrophy caused by ingestion of anabolic steroids. Side effects include headaches, depression and fluid retention.

Human growth hormone (HGH) was, until recently, only available from human cadaver pituitary extracts and was thus in short supply and very expensive. With the use of genetic engineering, synthetic HGH is now available for the treatment of growth hormone deficiency or dwarfism.

The increased availability of synthetic human growth hormone, despite restrictions on its therapeutic use, has resulted in athletes experimenting with its use. There is no scientific evidence of any ergogenic effect and serious side effects include the development of acromegaly which involves excessive bony growth (particularly in the jaw), cardiac problems and an increased tendency to develop diabetes. At present, human growth hormone cannot be detected by the urinary drug test.

Blood doping and erythropoietin

Blood doping, in its usual form, involves the withdrawal of blood from the athlete followed by re-transfusion after a suitable period of time, usually four to eight weeks, during which time the number of red blood cells had increased to the pre-withdrawal level. The addition of the extra blood or red cells alone would then result in an increased number of red cells available to transport oxygen to the exercising muscles.

This practice has been used to improve endurance, but is potentially dangerous particularly if cross-matched blood is used rather than the athlete's own blood. Research is currently progressing on a suitable test to detect the use of blood doping.

Erythropoietin is a hormone involved in the regulation of red blood cell production and its synthetic form has proven valuable in the treatment of anaemia secondary to chronic renal failure. It is used by athletes for the same purpose as blood doping, i.e. to increase the haematocrit.

It does not have the risk involved with blood transfusion, but has the potential serious side effect of increasing blood viscosity by increasing the percentage of red blood cells in the blood. This may cause sluggish blood flow and has the potential, when combined with dehydration, to precipitate cerebral and coronary thrombosis. Deaths associated with its use have been reported (Cowart 1989).

Alcohol

Alcohol is not banned by the IOC, but breath or blood alcohol tests may be requested by an international sporting federation. Alcohol affects performance in a number of ways. It may impair reaction time, hand-eye co-ordination, accuracy, balance, gross motor skills, strength, body temperature regulation and hydration (Wadler & Hainline 1990).

Marijuana

Marijuana is not prohibited by the IOC, but as its use is illegal in many countries, a number of sports federations have included it on their list of banned substances. As with alcohol, marijuana use has a negative effect on sports performance. It impairs psychomotor skills, alters perception of time and impairs concentration. The well recognized 'amotivational syndrome' associated with long term marijuana use may be particularly damaging to a sporting career (Hollister 1986).

Local anaesthetics

The IOC has a number of restrictions on the use of injectable local anaesthetics. The use of cocaine as a local anaesthetic is prohibited. Only local or intra-articular injections may be used, and then only when medically justified. A physician using a local anaesthetic is required to submit details including diagnosis, dose and route of administration in writing to the IOC Medical Commission if under that body's jurisdiction.

Corticosteroids

The use of corticosteriods is banned by the IOC except for topical use, inhalational use and local or intra-articular injection. Under IOC rules, any physician wishing to administer corticosteroids intra-articularly or locally to a competitor must give written notification to the IOC Medical Commission.

DRUG TESTING

Drug testing has become so commonplace in both amateur and professional sport that it is essential for the sports medicine professional providing services to the team or individual to be familiar with the list of banned substances and the drug testing procedure itself. Often the practitioner will be expected to accompany the competitor to the drug testing area, and needs to be able to establish that the correct procedures have been carried out.

The criteria for deciding which athlete is tested varies from event to event. At some competitions, placegetters will be tested; at others, competitors are selected randomly; at other times, certain events may be targeted for testing.

A chaperone provided by the drug testing agency hands a written form to the competitor who signs the form acknowledging that he or she has been notified of selection for a drug test. The chaperone then remains with the competitor until the test is completed. From this point, the competitor is entitled to have a representative present, either a team official or member of the medical support team.

In the drug control room, the Drug Control Officer invites the athlete to select a sealed urine sample collection container, check the seal and open the package. From this moment on, the competitor is the only one allowed to handle the container until the sample bottles have been filled. The competitor moves to the toilet area and, in the presence and sight of the chaperone only, provides a urine sample. A sample of at least 80 mL is required. The chaperone must have a direct view of the passing of the urine and ensure that the urine sample remains uncontaminated until the security sealing process has commenced.

The competitor then returns to the drug control room where he or she is invited to select a set of 'Envopacs' (Fig. 37.1). Each set consists of two identically numbered Envopacs distinguished by the prefix A and B. Each Envopac is sealed with a coded red seal. The Drug Control Officer and the competitor must ensure that the Envopac

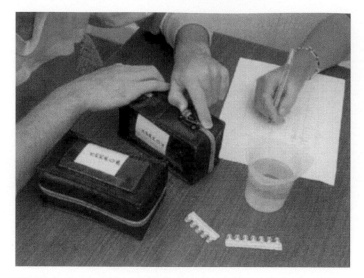

Fig. 37.1 A competitor breaks the envopac seals

numbers and the Envopac seal codes correspond with those on the master form.

The competitor must break the Envopac seals and unzip each Envopac, taking out the bottles. He or she must check the bottle number and prefix to ensure that it corresponds with the Envopac number and prefix. The competitor then dispenses 60 mL of urine into the A bottle and the remainder into the B bottle, leaving a few drops in the bottom of the sample collection container for measurement of urine pH and specific gravity.

The competitor then secures the bottle caps, checks for leakages, returns the bottles to the corresponding Envopacs and closes them. He or she then selects two coded blue Envopac seals and places a seal into each Envopac zipper clasp with the Envopac codes facing up.

The Drug Control Officer then completes the drug testing form, recording the Envopac numbers and Envopac seal numbers. The competitor is also asked to list all medications taken in the previous week, including over-the-counter medications, prescription drugs and any other substances taken by mouth, injection, inhalation or suppository. This medical declaration form should include all vitamins, amino acids and other supplements. It is vitally important that this list be completed accurately, as all substances taken in that period are likely to show up in the sample.

The competitor, his or her representative and the drug control officer then check all the written information and, if satisfied, sign the drug testing form. The competitor is given a copy of the form.

The samples are then sent in the sealed Envopacs to an accredited laboratory where the sample is analysed using gas chromatography and mass spectrometry. Initially only the A sample is analysed.

If the laboratory finds a possible positive test result in the sample in the A bottle, it informs the drug testing agency who then informs the competitor that a possible positive result has been recorded. The competitor, or a representative, is then entitled to be present at the unsealing and testing of the B sample.

If the B sample also proves positive, the relevant sporting organizations are informed. Most sporting bodies now have severe penalties in place for proven drug taking.

SUMMARY

Drug use is widespread in sport. The use in the management of musculoskeletal injuries is common, but in many cases evidence of any beneficial effect is lacking.

The use of performance enhancing drugs should be actively discouraged on both medical and ethical grounds. The therapist can play an important role in counselling athletes and providing other methods by which performance may be improved.

REFERENCES

Akemark C, Forsskahl B 1990 Topical indomethacin in overuse injuries in athletes. A randomised double-blind study comparing elemetacin with oral indomethacin and placebo. International Journal of Sports Medicine 11:393-396

Almekinders L 1990 The efficacy of nonsteroidal anti-inflammatory drugs in the treatment of ligament injuries. Sports Medicine 9(3):137-142

Almekinders L C, Gilbert G A 1986 Healing of experimental muscle strains and the effects of nonsteroidal anti-inflammatory medication. American Journal of Sports Medicine 14:303-308

ASDA 1990 Drug testing in sport. Australian Sports Drug Agency, Canberra

Barone J 1989 Topical analgesics: how effective are they? Physician and Sportsmedicine 17(2):162-168

Behrens T W, Goodwin J S 1990 Oral corticosteroids. In: Leadbetter W B, Buckwalter J A, Gordon S L (eds) Sports-induced inflammation. American Orthopaedic Society for Sports Medicine, Park Ridge

Clyman B 1986 Role of non-steroidal anti-inflammatory drugs in sports medicine. Sports Medicine 3:242-244

Cowart V S 1989 Erythropoietin: a dangerous new form of blood doping. Physician and Sportsmedicine 17(8):115-118

Dahners L E, Philips H O, Almekinders L C 1988 The effect of piroxicam on ligament healing in rats. Transaction of the Orthopaedic Research Society 11:77

Ford L T, De Bender J 1979 Tendon rupture after local steroid injection. South Medical Journal 72:827-830

Gonik B, Stringer C A 1985 Postpartum osteitis pubis. South African Medical Journal 78:213-214

Gray R G T, Tenbeaum J, Gottlieb N L 1981 Local corticosteroid injection treatment in rheumatic disorders. Seminars in Arthritis and Rheumatology 10:231-254

Hollister L 1986 Health aspects of cannabis. Pharmacology Review 38:1

Kelly D W, Carter V S, Jobe F W, Kerlan R K 1984 Patellar and quadriceps tendon ruptures: jumper's knee. American Journal of Sports Medicine 12:375-380

Kleinman M, Gross A E 1983 Achilles tendon rupture following steroid injection. Report of three cases. Journal of Bone and Joint Surgery 65A:1345-1347

Leadbetter W B 1990 Corticosteroid injection therapy in sports injuries. In: Sports-induced inflammation: clinical and basic science concepts. American Academy of Orthopaedic Surgeons, Park Ridge

Travell J G, Simons D G 1983 Myofascial pain and dysfunction. The trigger point manual. Williams & Wilkins, Baltimore

Vane J R 1971 Inhibition of prostaglandin synthesis as a mechanism of aspirin like drugs. Nature 231:232-235

Vogel H G 1977 Mechanical and chemical properties of various connective tissue organs in rats as influenced by non-steroid antirheumatic drugs. Connective Tissue Research 5:91-95

Wadler G I, Hainline B 1989 Drugs and the athlete. F A Davis, Philadelphia

Weiler J M, Albright J P, Buckwalter J A 1987 Non-steroidal anti-inflammatory drugs. In: Lewis A J, Furst D E (eds) Anti-inflammatory agents in sports medicine. Marcel Dekker, New York

38. Legal requirements

Hayden Opie

Sports physiotherapy is a diverse, if not idiosyncratic, occupation. Practices and knowledge vary according to sport, level of play, region and available resources. Idiosyncrasy is prominent in geographic limits to qualification to practise. Nevertheless, there are unifying elements and this book seeks to encompass both the diversity and the unity of sports physiotherapy.

Law displays similar unity and diversity; if anything, the geographic boundaries are more pronounced. Diversity exists in the many national and regional legal systems resting on different cultural, religious and social foundations, some over 1000 years old. Even though most English-speaking nations derive their legal systems from the English common law, differences exist among them. Unity is present because wherever human activity occurs it produces similar problems needing legal solutions.

Therefore, to produce a complete and detailed statement of the law as it affects sports physiotherapy is an overly demanding task for a chapter in this book. Furthermore, it is assumed that non-lawyer physiotherapists and students will prefer general rather than detailed discussion of the legal issues and their implications. These considerations have guided the preparation of this chapter. Aspects of sports physiotherapy having legal dimensions are identified and considered in general and non-technical terms, hopefully offering both a conceptual and practically useful guide for physiotherapist and student. This chapter is a point of first reference. The reader with a specific inquiry about the law in a particular place, or needing legal advice on some eventuality, would be wise to consult a legal professional practising locally.

SPORTS PHYSIOTHERAPY AND THE LAW

Sports physiotherapy

Physiotherapy is an established medical science. Even though sports physiotherapy is a relatively new discipline of physiotherapy, it has become an important field of practice. It is characterized by a quickly widening range and depth of knowledge and skill, as well as rapid growth in demand for that knowledge and skill as the sports world recognizes the medical basis of sport.

Not only are the traditional roles of the physiotherapist in injury management and rehabilitation important, but the sports physiotherapist can expect involvement with injury prevention and performance improvement or conditioning at both practical and theoretical levels. Attendance at a sports event or travel with a team will often necessitate proficiency in first aid and cardiopulmonary resuscitation. Matters can be complicated by the different grades at which sport is played and, therefore, the levels at which sports physiotherapy is practised. The pressures of elite sport are demanding and the need for rapid, if not immediate, return to competition, as well as potentially conflicting obligations to team athletes and management, raise unusual issues.

Sports physiotherapy is often practised by someone whose primary focus is in the area. On the other hand, a general practitioner may encounter injured athletes from time to time. The latter practitioner must not be too proud and should refer the athlete to the 'specialist' physiotherapist. Grayson (1992) suggests that the days are long past when it was sufficient to say to a patient, 'You had best give up your sport.' Sport can be a serious and important activity like work and it behoves the physiotherapist to search for solutions to injury problems, not circumvent them.

The delivery of sports physiotherapy to an athlete may be part of a wider sports medicine effort. Particularly in professional and elite sports, the physiotherapist will work with a range of health professionals including doctors, nutritionists, masseurs and trainers. The relationships between them have legal and ethical dimensions which will be considered later.

Different terminology occurs within the English speaking world. In the USA and Canada, the term 'trainer' often refers to a group delivering first aid and rehabilitative care, including but not limited to physiotherapists. In Australia and New Zealand, it is unusual to describe sports physiotherapists as trainers. Similarly, in the USA 'physician' is commonly used to describe doctors. In this chapter, the terms 'doctor', 'physiotherapist' and 'trainer' will be used and are mutually exclusive.

Law

In common law countries or regions, there are two principal kinds of law: statute law and common law.

Statute law is made by Parliaments (or legislatures) and their delegates. Laws made by Parliaments are usually referred to as Acts. Laws made by their delegates have many names, including by-laws, ordinances, regulations and rules. The delegates may be local councils, statutory authorities, professional associations or the executive arm of government such as the President (USA) or Cabinet (Australia). Some countries have more than one legislature. In Australia, Canada and the USA, there is a federal legislature with power to make statute law for the whole country, and regional legislatures (states in Australia and USA, provinces in Canada) with power for that region only. The laws which govern the sharing of responsibility for making statute law between federal and regional legislatures are usually called constitutions.

The common law is made by courts. They apply legal principles originating in the customs of England prior to the Norman conquest and developed over subsequent centuries to meet the changing needs of society. Common law courts use the doctrine of precedent, which means that a court in a region is obliged to adhere to the statements of legal principle made by superior courts having authority over the same region. These statements are contained in the written judgements of courts and may be explained or criticized in academic literature. Not all judgements are used for this purpose. Only those which are considered important are published for future use in developing and stating legal principles. Very occasionally unreported judgements whose existence is otherwise well known will be used as precedents.

Each country or region has its own hierarchy of courts. Thus, the territory for which a hierarchy is responsible will correspond to the territory for which a legislature is responsible. For example, in the USA there is a hierarchy of federal courts and a separate hierarchy of courts in each state. One court will have ultimate authority; in the USA that is the Supreme Court. When there is no precedent for deciding a particular case within its territory, a court may have regard to statements of principle made by courts in other common law countries and regions. It is not unusual for English courts to seek guidance from decisions of Australian and Canadian courts, and vice versa. Aided by modern computer database and communications technology, such cross-referencing is increasing. Also, courts will only decide the issue in dispute before them as presented by the parties to the case. They will avoid broad statements of principle and usually do not decide theoretical or hypothetical issues. Only when an issue comes before the court as a dispute between parties will it be resolved.

Most court judgements do not involve argument over the principles of law necessary to reach a decision. These cases turn on their facts. As such, they do not create precedents of legal principle for future cases; they only apply existing principles. This case-by-case decision-making process arguably achieves an acceptable consistency of outcome. However, there is significant scope for variance; for example, different judges and juries may perceive the facts of similar cases in differing ways.

Most legal proceedings do not involve any formal judgement by a court. These cases are settled before a trial is held, usually on confidential terms. Often cases are settled by a defendant (even though he or she had some confidence in succeeding) because the cost of proving the point (taking into account the chance of failure), is greater than paying a portion of the plaintiff's claim. This tends to happen most frequently where the defendant is insured and the insurance company, which controls the defence, will give greater weight to financial considerations than personal feelings (such as a desire to protect one's professional prestige) in making a decision to settle.

Thus, cases which are not reported, turn on their facts or are settled out of court, are of little importance in the development of legal principle.

Interaction of sports physiotherapy and the law

Legislation

Legislation may affect sports physiotherapy in various ways. In most places it controls the practice of physiotherapy generally. Typically, a registering authority is established to fix qualifications for the practice of the profession and to provide for the certification of those people who qualify to practise. Penalties will be set for unauthorized practice, in particular the use of modalities for treatment by ultrasound and microwave, for example. Thus, it may be unlawful for trainers to use those modalities.

The registering authority may be a delegate of the legislature empowered to make detailed rules for governing the profession. Sometimes the authority will double as the professional association for physiotherapists. The rules made by the authority may provide for the recognition of and qualification for specialist disciplines within the profession, including sports physiotherapy.

Legislation can be relevant in other ways. It will regulate pharmaceutical preparations which are available only on a doctor's prescription. In some parts of Canada and the USA, physiotherapists who voluntarily render emergency first aid to injured athletes are protected by Good Samaritan statutes from liability for causing or aggravating injuries.

Common law

Common law is probably more important to sports physiotherapy than legislation because the physiotherapist/patient relationship is almost exclusively regulated by common law. Three features of that relationship receive substantial consideration in this chapter. They are the circumstances when the relationship arises and how it is defined, the standard of professional performance required of the physiotherapist, and confidentiality. In various ways, the three are connected.

One consequence of the relatively recent emergence of sports physiotherapy as a recognized discipline is that there are few reported court cases involving the practice of sports physiotherapy. This comment can be applied to sports medicine professionals generally. Hence, it is necessary to envisage how general principles of law might be applied in the context of sport. This can be supplemented by considering specific principles developed for analogous problems in other fields of health care.

SPORTS PHYSIOTHERAPIST/ ATHLETE RELATIONSHIP

Creation

Among professional relationships, that between doctor and patient is one of the oldest. The law developed to regulate it can be applied to the emerging sports physiotherapist/athlete relationship.

That relationship will occur when the sports physiotherapist undertakes the care of the athlete. The occasion for doing so may exist because the athlete consults or is referred to the physiotherapist's practice, a sports team requests the physiotherapist to render physiotherapy and related health care services to its players, or the physiotherapist may fortuitously be present when emergency assistance is needed at a sports event. Normally very little, if anything, is said between the athlete and physiotherapist about the relationship.

The legal dimensions of the sports physiotherapist/athlete relationship are influenced by the circumstances in which the care is undertaken. The physiotherapist may be working as an independent contractor (in the sense of being in practice alone or in partnership), or as an employee of a team, school or clinic or other health care organization. The care may be paid or voluntary, planned or unplanned, rendered in an emergency or not.

Implications

The development of the sports physiotherapist/athlete relationship generates various rights and obligations.

Authority to practise

The physiotherapist is authorized to administer physiotherapy and related lawful health care to the athlete. There are three aspects to this proposition. As a threshold matter, the physiotherapist must possess current authority to practise physiotherapy in the place where the care is provided. This may be of special significance to physiotherapists accompanying touring teams (see below). Secondly, the health care practised must be physiotherapy and not a form of care which may be the restricted preserve of other health professionals, for example doctors and dentists. Thirdly, the athlete must consent to the administration of physiotherapy (see below).

A definition of physiotherapy is important. Legislation which regulates the practice of physiotherapy often provides one. This may be a more or less comprehensive statement, or a partial one listing the modalities which may be used by a qualified physiotherapist. A court called on to interpret or amplify any such definition is likely to follow the views of the profession.

Skill and care

Legal rules govern the standard of care delivered to the athlete. When there is a contract, usually where the athlete pays for the care (e.g. the athlete has initiated a consultation at the physiotherapist's clinic), the standard will be that which the contract specifies. Rarely is anything expressly indicated and, in that absence, the law will set a standard which reflects appropriate professional skill. The terminology varies, but 'due care and skill' is often used by the courts. Independently of the contract, the law will often recognize a duty to exercise professional skill. In common law countries this duty falls under the ambit of the law of torts (civil wrongs) and is known as the tort of negligence. Because of the sports physiotherapist/athlete relationship the law requires that the physiotherapist avoid negligence by exercising 'reasonable care' or 'ordinary care and skill'. Again, various terms are used.

'Due care and skill' and 'reasonable care' are based on professional standards and as such they are regarded as having more or less the same content. This means that whether or not the patient has a contract with the physiotherapist (for instance, there will be no contract between them if the service is paid for by a parent or the physiotherapist is engaged by a team) or whether the service is paid or voluntary, the standard of professional skill to be exercised must be the same. Charitable care does not justify 'cheap' or deficient care. Occasionally, a contract will specify a higher or lower standard which might override both the due care and skill and the reasonable care standards. This will depend on a complex array of factors, especially if the standard is lower (see below).

Confidence and trust

Physiotherapy's ethics require information about the athlete which is received in the course of the sports physiotherapist/ athlete relationship to be kept in confidence. This will extend beyond information received direct from the athlete to that received from professional colleagues. Among the ethical principles adopted by the World Confederation for Physical Therapy is one which requires physiotherapists to ' hold in confidence all personal information entrusted to them and...not [to] discuss a patient's affairs with other than those responsible for the patient's care' (World 1982). Similar ethical rules have been adopted by local professional associations. A failure to abide by the relevant confidentiality rule usually amounts to professional misconduct and involves the risk of disciplinary action by the local authorities.

Ethical rules of associations will not usually be directly enforceable by athletes. Confidentiality may be imposed indirectly: a court can imply a term to that effect in the contract between the athlete and physiotherapist; an action in negligence may be available for injury sustained if the confidence is broken; or the general law of breach of confidence will protect against disclosures whether or not there is a contract (Skene 1990).

The obligation of confidence is not absolute. There are many exceptions, including the following. The athlete may authorize disclosure. This might occur expressly, such as when the athlete requests that a health report be given to the manager of a professional team interested in employing the athlete. The authority may be given impliedly where, say, the physiotherapist must prepare instructions for the manufacture and fitting of a prosthetic device, or must refer the athlete to a colleague and provide a copy of the treatment history. Legislation may authorize disclosure, for example where certain injuries or illnesses must be reported to public health authorities. The common law justifies (and may even require) disclosure where it is in the athlete's or the public's interest. Just when that is so is controversial.

Obviously, the athlete will not trust the physiotherapist if the athlete believes that information made available will be passed to others improperly. However, the sports physiotherapist/athlete relationship necessitates trust in another important way. The physiotherapist must be frank and honest with the athlete. There must be sufficient information made available for the athlete to make choices about health care options and to receive adequate care from others. For example, to discover an injury and not inform the patient would in almost all cases be a dereliction of duty. Again, the duty is not absolute. A therapeutic privilege is widely recognized as entitling the withholding of information if its revelation would be medically counterproductive in a significant way. Also, the common law does not usually permit the patient to have access to the physiotherapist's records. Those belong to the physiotherapist. Legislation in various regions may modify this access rule, for example the *Access to Health Records Act 1990* (UK) requires disclosure of health records (subject to some exceptions) when requested by the patient and certain other people, such as parents of a child patient.

These rules have the important objective of encouraging the free and open flow of information between athlete and physiotherapist. Unless information about the athlete's health is readily available the task of treatment is inhibited. On the other hand, circumstances may warrant withholding information from the athlete or divulging it to third parties. As shall be seen, the law does not always provide a clear definition of the boundary between these conflicting influences, because practices and problems in sports physiotherapy have run ahead of the law and specific precedents are yet to emerge.

LIABILITY OR MALPRACTICE LITIGATION

Since the sports physiotherapist has duties to the athlete arising from the relationship between them, there may be occasions when a breach of one or more of those duties occurs or is alleged. This is the field of liability or malpractice litigation. This section of the chapter will cover a range of topics connected with liability. The previous background and statements of principle will be applied to circumstances involving an absence of consent to treatment, unskilful care and breach of confidence. Other topics concerning sharing responsibility for liability and risk management will be considered in the following section.

Before doing so, it may be helpful to place the problem in context and to say something about the litigation process. Emphasis will be on liability for physical injuries.

The scope and nature of the problem

Of all legal issues, liability litigation generates the greatest interest, or concern, among sports physiotherapists. The words 'negligence' and 'malpractice' figure prominently when 'talking law' with health professionals. The reason may stem from some personal involvement as a defendant or witness in a court action, the dramatisation of litigation in the media and in gossip, or because premiums for professional indemnity insurance have risen markedly.

Inherent in participation in sport is the risk of accidentally sustaining severe injury: the dangers of death, paralysis and other disablement are present in varying degrees. Fortunately, such outcomes are rare compared with the levels of participation, and are usually justified by the overall health and recreational benefits to be gained for the community. It is impossible to eliminate risk from life.

However, being the victim of a physiotherapist's negligence is not one of the inherent risks of sports participation. Just because an athlete is prepared to risk life and limb in meeting the physical demands of a sport does not mean that he or she is entitled to anything less than the standards of physiotherapy to be expected in other circumstances.

If an athlete accuses a physiotherapist of being responsible for some injury from which the athlete is suffering, it will most likely be because one of four things has occurred as a result of allegedly inappropriate care.

1. An injury suffered in participation has been aggravated, for example moving a person who has sustained a broken spine thereby causing paralysis (*Welch v. Dunsmuir Joint Union High School District 1958*).
2. An injury or condition is not identified and subsequent participation in sport exposes the athlete to injury inflicted by opponents or caused by the demands of participation, for example not detecting a neck injury which is converted into major paralysis by an opponent's legitimate tackle (*Robitaille v. Vancouver Hockey Club Ltd 1981*).
3. There may be an unduly long recovery period or failure to make normal recovery, for example something as simple as where incorrect or inadequate application of ice delays recovery from soft tissue injuries (Murphy 1992).
4. An injury may occur in the course of treatment, for example a burn.

It is quite easy to generate a high level of alarm—if not a 'siege mentality'—over the prospect of being sued for such events. Factors which contribute to this include the following. There is a widely held view that society, particularly in the USA, displays a growing propensity to use litigation to settle disputes—the 'sue syndrome' (Graham 1986). Related to this is the perception that if someone suffers misfortune it must be another's fault and that person must therefore pay compensation. Doctors and, to a lesser extent, physiotherapists are regarded as fair targets for compensation demands because they are considered to be relatively wealthy and probably insured (and what is wrong with taking money from an insurer?). There are ever higher public expectations of successful recovery from injury due to spectacular gains in the knowledge and skills of medical science. These fuel the belief that if an athlete fails to recover from injury it must be the fault of the medical personnel. Changes in the way that health care is delivered— especially the move to clinics—have tended to depersonalize the patient's experience. The deliverer of care is no longer a close family friend. The consequence is that a strong social disincentive to litigation—not wishing to make a fuss over how well a friend helped you—is markedly diminished.

However, the prospect of being sued can be overstated. The limited empirical evidence available indicates that athletes are not lining up to sue sports physiotherapists. A survey of all reported cases in the USA from federal and state courts from 1960 to July 1989 found only nine cases which called into question the standard of care delivered by athletic trainers (Leverenz & Helms 1990). The published results do not reveal how many, if any, of these athletic trainers were physiotherapists but it has been said that there are no reported cases in the USA discussing the liability of physiotherapists (Mitten 1994). A 20% sample of actions commenced in the Supreme and County Courts of Victoria, Australia, in 1979–1990 found no litigation by athletes against medical personnel (Opie 1992).

While this evidence may go some way to allaying the fears which give rise to the siege mentality, it should not be taken as a basis for disregarding the prospect of liability litigation or of not seeking to understand the role of law in the practice of sports physiotherapy. The findings of Leverenz & Helms disclose that 66% of the identified cases had occurred since 1979. This suggests that litigation against trainers is a recent and growing phenomenon and is consistent with the relatively recent emergence of sports medicine as a field of health care. It must also be recognized that a sports physiotherapist may become involved in litigation, even though she or he may not be found liable (Walker et al 1984). Some lawyers adopt the 'shotgun' approach and take action against almost anyone who is potentially involved, and let matters sort themselves out as the litigation proceeds. There is always a chance of becoming a witness, and an understanding of legal processes will aid that role. Finally, as will be demonstrated below, the law can become a very helpful tool of practice management: obtaining an understanding of it may lead to a better and more rewarding professional relationship with athletes.

It is important to appreciate the differing perspectives on liability litigation held by physiotherapists and lawyers. Mention has been made of the alarm over litigation which is often expressed in sports medicine circles. On the other hand, a plaintiff's lawyer sometimes feels that he or she is representing the weak against the strong and is the person of last resort to whom the athlete turns. The truth lies in between. Since little is achieved in a climate of confrontation, a few moments taken to focus on the respective roles of sports physiotherapist and lawyer may prove instructive.

The endeavours of sports physiotherapists in caring for athletes will be aimed at preventing injury, producing or restoring physical well being, maximizing performance and promoting pleasure from participation in sport. From the viewpoint of the physiotherapist, the athlete and the community, these endeavours are very worthy.

In contrast, in the present context, when the sports physiotherapist's work encounters that of the lawyer representing an athlete, it is because something has gone wrong—the athlete has been seriously hurt. In these circumstances the lawyer's role is to assist the injured athlete in exercising any legal right to compensation which may exist. Compensation can be very important to the athlete because he or she may be unable to work and will face loss of income either temporarily or permanently. For the elite athlete, there may loss of endorsement and related income. Medical and other expenses will also need to be met.

The present structure of the legal system in most common law countries and regions requires that the athlete prove the injury was sustained as a result of the fault of somebody else. New Zealand is an important exception where compensation benefits are available to victims of medical misadventure under its universal no-fault accident compensation scheme and the right to sue is abrogated. In some jurisdictions workers' compensation laws may prevent or limit professional athletes from bringing malpractice actions against physiotherapists. To prove fault someone must be shown to be legally to blame because that person wrongfully performed an act which caused the injury or did not take action to prevent it. The organization which has employed the physiotherapist or upon whose behalf he or she has acted may be liable as well.

To decide whether legal liability exists, the legal system adopts an adversarial approach under which the athlete's arguments and lawyers are matched against those of the sports physiotherapist. This approach places the defendant physiotherapist in the 'firing line'. It is bad enough that an athlete in care has been seriously injured; matters are only made worse for the physiotherapist by being accused of having caused or aggravated the injury and having to defend an expensive and reputation threatening lawsuit.

It is, therefore, not surprising that bad feelings toward lawyers have been generated. Some lawyers have been perceived as 'ambulance chasers' or 'creative litigators' in their efforts to drum up new business. Indeed, there may be a feeling in some circles that lawyers are having 'sport' at the expense of medical professionals in order to make money.

From the perspective of people involved in sport the foregoing depicts a negative side to the role of law and lawyers. However, there is another and important aspect, concerning encouraging safe administration and practice in sport. In addition to seeking to compensate the injured athlete, the law aims to encourage safety by deterring a repetition of injury by imposing legal liability upon those who could have prevented the injury occurring. This serves as an example to others and assists in fixing appropriate community standards for future safe activity. Another objective of the law, which is of less importance in the present context, is that the imposition of liability acts as a form of retribution and can assuage feelings of revenge.

In one Australian court case (*Watson v. Haines* 1987), the athlete became a quadriplegic while playing the position of hooker in school rugby league. This was despite briefings given by medical researchers to senior Education Department officials that people with the anatomical characteristics of the plaintiff (a relatively long, thin neck) should not play in that position. The A\$2 187 460.81 awarded against the state of New South Wales and the consequent publicity resulted in greater awareness by the sport's authorities of the need for safety measures and arguably saved a number of young players from a similar fate.

Consent

One of the implications of the sports physiotherapist/athlete relationship discussed above is that the physiotherapist must have authority to practise.

An absence of authority, in the sense of not being licensed to practise in the territory or of exercising skills which are the preserve of others, may be important in two ways. First, it may be used to support an allegation of unskilful treatment which has caused injury, for example undertaking a procedure beyond the scope of physiotherapy and within the expertise of a doctor. Second, where the 'physiotherapist' is not licensed, the permission which the athlete has given to receive treatment may be regarded as obtained fraudulently because, by offering or providing services as a physiotherapist, there is a representation that the person is lawfully entitled to do so. If harm is caused by the fraud there will be legal liability. A separate matter is whether, due to the fraud, the athlete's consent is invalidated and, thus, any touching of the athlete for the purposes of examination or treatment constitutes battery. The answer can be controversial and local advice should be sought. One view is that this is a fraud as to a surrounding circumstance, not to the nature of the act, and therefore the consent is not affected. On the other hand, to hold liability in battery is a desirable deterrent and punishment for such behaviour.

As a general rule, the athlete's consent to undergo examination or to receive treatment is necessary to avoid battery. Touching without consent (battery) or threatened touching without consent (assault) is unlawful. In the event of assault or battery, a sum of money, known as 'damages', may be awarded to the athlete as compensation. A criminal offence might be committed as well.

Consent may be given expressly, orally or in writing. Before medical operations or other major treatment programs, it is common practice to seek written consent. The athlete must be aware that he or she is giving consent (signing a form thought to be a receipt is not consent) and possess sufficient knowledge of the proposed procedure to make the consent valid. For instance, agreeing to ultrasound is not consent to traction. There has been much debate over what is sufficient knowledge. Current thinking in much of the common law world is that as long as the basic nature of the therapy is disclosed, the consent is valid. Thus, actions for battery will succeed only where there has been no consent at all (in the sense that the basic nature of the treatment has not been made known and agreed to) or the treatment has exceeded the consent given. An allegation that the athlete was not given sufficiently detailed information on the procedure for administration of the treatment, success rates and risks in order to make an informed choice about treatment is regarded as falling within the ambit of the physiotherapist's duty to exercise reasonable care (see below). Failure to sufficiently inform does not invalidate the consent (Fleming 1992, Keeton 1984, *Reibl v. Hughes* 1980, *Rogers v. Whitaker* 1992).

Once given, consent may be withdrawn. Treatment should cease at that point. Difficulties arise when the treatment is life-sustaining but this will rarely be an issue in sports physiotherapy.

The delivery of emergency care is not regarded as battery even in the absence of any prior consent from the athlete. It is uncertain whether this is because the common law regards such conduct as justified or because it implies consent. In either event, the result is the same. Even so, it has been recommended that health professionals caring for sports teams have athletes sign consent forms in contemplation of the administration of emergency care (Savastano 1968). Usually, the athlete will indicate a desire for the physiotherapist to proceed even though this may be given abruptly or hardly at all if he or she is distressed by pain. The definition of emergency care assumes more importance when the athlete is not in a position to give consent, for example is unconscious. Legal terminology defining an emergency varies between regions and reflects subtle differences. Legislation may be relevant. Anything that is life-threatening or, maybe, a serious risk to health is an emergency. It is apparent that the views of health professionals will be of great importance in providing the content of this definition. Steps taken to stabilize an injury pending arrival of superior medical services will most probably be regarded as within the scope of emergency care not requiring further consent.

To acquiesce in minor treatment such as bandaging or application of antiseptic or ice amounts to implied consent.

Administering treatment to children raises special and complex issues. Children do not reach full legal capacity until they attain the age of majority. This age varies between regions, but is commonly 18–21 years.

The first issue is whether a child can consent to physiotherapy and, if so, at what age. It is well recognized that children possess certain legal capacities, especially in regard to making contracts for 'essentials', such as food and clothing. That principle can be extended to health care. However, the concern is that a child, because of his or her immaturity, may make important decisions which are not in the child's best long-term interests. Recently, English courts have emphasized that the child's intellectual and emotional development should be examined to determine whether the child is sufficiently mature or competent to make a decision about medical treatment (*Gillick v. West Norfolk and Wisbech Area Health Authority* 1986). The age at which this competency is reached will vary according to the child and the nature of the decision, but 15 years may be indicative. The implication is that the decision of such a competent child to have or refuse physiotherapy will prevail over the opposing views of a person having legal responsibility for the child—a parent or guardian. In the USA, the general position is that a child may not consent to medical treatment involving a risk of serious injury or death, but lesser treatments may be consented to provided the child has the capacity of the average person to weigh the risks and benefits (Keeton 1984).

A cautious approach when dealing with apparently mature children would entail obtaining the consent of both the child and a parent or legal guardian. If this is not forthcoming, advice should be sought from local lawyers and ethical committees.

When treating immature children, the consent of a parent or guardian should always be obtained.

Emergency care is delivered to children according to the principles outlined above, but may be complicated where a parent refuses permission, perhaps on religious grounds. While this will be extremely rare in relation to the type of care likely to be provided by physiotherapists, common law and legislation often make provision for the delivery of emergency care in the face of parental opposition and reference should be made to local laws.

Unskilful care: contracts

Mention has been made of the duty to exercise due care and skill which is implied in a contract between an athlete and a sports physiotherapist for the provision of physiotherapy. 'Due care and skill' is the normal contractual standard of skill to be expected. This standard is essentially the same as the standard of reasonable care imposed by the tort of negligence. For that reason the two standards will be considered below in connection with negligence.

Before treatment is commenced, the physiotherapist may say something indicating that a particular result will be achieved from the therapy. This will be interpreted by a court as a contractual promise or guarantee of outcome—it need not be in writing. Should it not be fulfilled, the physiotherapist will be in breach of the contract even though due care and skill has been exercised. For that reason, it is generally regarded as rash to offer estimates of recovery in such a way as to permit their being interpreted as promises. Quite apart from possible legal consequences, it is unfair to build inflated expectations.

As a means of protection from legal liability, some practitioners seek to exempt themselves from the obligation to exercise due care and skill. This is attempted by an exclusion clause in the contract. Whether this can achieve its aim is considered below under the heading 'Risk management'.

Unskilful care: negligence

For purposes of analysis, it is common practice to divide the tort of negligence into three parts: duty, breach and damage.

Duty is concerned with whether the alleged wrongdoer was obliged to take care for the injured person's safety. Usually, the existence of the sports physiotherapist/athlete relationship imposes on the sports physiotherapist a duty to take reasonable care not to injure an athlete in his or her charge. The duty covers both action and inaction.

Breach is the most important issue for present (and most) purposes and will be considered in detail below. It is concerned with whether the care taken by the sports physiotherapist has conformed to the standard of reasonable care expected of a person in similar circumstances.

The third part examines whether the breach of the duty of care caused damage or harm which is not remote. This terminology is favoured in Australia, England and New Zealand, whereas Canadian and United States courts prefer 'proximate cause'. There are variations in approach, but they are not particularly significant in this context. The issue of damage can be important in circumstances where it is alleged by an athlete that, for example incorrect procedures for stabilizing a spinal injury caused or aggravated paralysis, whereas the physiotherapist may contend that the paralysis occurred contemporaneously with the spinal injury. A different causation issue arises in cases where the alleged breach of duty is a failure to disclose the risks of treatment. Here the athlete must show that he or she (or a reasonable person in the same position) would not have undergone the treatment if informed of the risks. This issue will be touched on below.

Other important elements of an athlete's claim in the tort of negligence will be whether any defences are available to the physiotherapist, and the calculation of damages payable. Defences will be considered below, in 'Shared resposibility for injury' and 'Risk management'. Damages are the monetary compensation for harms suffered, including lost income, health care expenses, physical and mental disability, and pain and suffering.

Negligence: breach of the duty of care

Physiotherapy is a skilled profession. The relevant skills are not possessed by ordinary people. The performance of any physiotherapist must be judged by the standards of the profession, not those of ordinary people. An often-quoted statement of this principle is from a judgement of McNair J (*Bolam v. Friern Hospital Management Committee* 1957):

…where you get a situation which involves the use of some special skill or competence…The test is the standard of the ordinary skilled man exercising and professing to have that special skill. A man need not possess the highest expert skill; it is well-established law that it is sufficient if he exercises the ordinary skill of an ordinary competent man exercising that particular art.

Other descriptors such as the 'prudent' or 'reasonable' person have been used. Their meanings do not differ markedly in the common law world. The attention of the court is not only on the possession of a skill but on its exercise. The exercise of the skill will contain aspects connected with technique as well as judgement. McNair J's reference to special skill is not to a 'specialty' as widely used in the health professions. It is intended to distinguish the physiotherapist's skills from those of ordinary people.

The remainder of this section will consider four issues arising from this principle.

1. What is meant by an ordinary competent sports physiotherapist?
2. What is meant by reasonable care in connection with the exercise of a special skill?
3. How does a court go about deciding whether reasonable care has been exercised and how does this relate to professional practices?
4. What practical guidance may be drawn from the cases and literature on steps to be taken to comply with the legal standard of care?

The ordinary competent sports physiotherapist

The common law recognizes that within professions there may be specialties. Designation of specialties has probably reached its peak in the professional arrangements for doctors. Legally, this means that the orthopedic surgeon will not be judged by the standard of the ordinary competent doctor (general practitioner), but by the standard of the ordinary competent orthopedic surgeon.

In contrast, a person may specialize in an area of practice, in the sense of that is where most of his or her work is to be found. This may be for reasons of economics, interest or demographics. For instance, a doctor's clinic which is located in an area where a large proportion of children reside will tend to concentrate on pediatrics. However, that doctor is not judged by the standard of the pediatrician, but by the knowledge and skill in pediatrics expected of the ordinary competent doctor practising as a general practitioner.

The significance of this for the sports physiotherapist will depend upon whether sports physiotherapy is a recognized specialty within the profession of physiotherapy. This will usually be a local matter.

If specialization has not been recognized, the standard of care expected in most circumstances will be that of the ordinary competent physiotherapist. Complications occur when the physiotherapist either gains a post-graduate qualification in sports physiotherapy or adopts the title 'sports physiotherapist' or 'sports physiotherapy specialist'. The former might be regarded in law as conferring a specialized skill while the latter is arguably a representation that the person concerned possesses some higher level of skill not found among ordinary physiotherapists. In both cases the courts will probably judge the physiotherapist's performance against a higher or specialized standard relevant to the circumstances. However, this may vary between regions and there could be difficulties in establishing the content of that standard. Local advice should be sought on this issue.

Where there is a recognized sports physiotherapy specialization, the standard of care required will be set according to the knowledge and skill to be expected of the specialist sports physiotherapist. This standard may be found in the prerequisites to formal recognition as a specialist established by the relevant authorities. For instance, in Australia, a specialist sports physiotherapist is one who has completed the process of specialisation in sports physiotherapy available through the Australian College of Physiotherapists.

There has been a tendency, most frequently in the USA, to determine standards by reference to physiotherapists practising in the same locality. However, the advent of conference travel, modern communications and database technologies has tended to nationalize, if not internationalize, the practice of physiotherapy. The emphasis placed on geographically based standards has declined correspondingly (Mitten 1994).

Reasonable care

The court's task is twofold: to set the standard of reasonable care required by the tort of negligence by reference to what the ordinary competent physiotherapist would have done in the circumstances of the case; and to find the actual conduct of the physiotherapist in question. If the latter falls short of the former, the duty is breached.

Whether breach has occurred is an issue of fact judged in the circumstances of the particular case. Infinite and subtle variation of circumstances mean that court decisions cannot be predicted with certainty. Partially for that reason, a court's decision in a case is not a precedent for another even though it may have similar facts. At best it is a guide. Thus, lawyers are reluctant to provide unqualified answers to hypothetical questions about breach of duty, as well as to questions based on actual facts.

Further theoretical explanation of the standard of reasonable care is complicated by the factual emphasis of the inquiry. Nevertheless, legal principles provide a framework for what amounts to reasonable care. The standard of care expected of the ordinary competent physiotherapist is an objective or externally fixed standard. It is not correct to inquire whether the particular physiotherapist accused of negligence performed as well as usual or even exercised all the skill and knowledge which he or she possessed (that is, did his or her best). That would be subjective. The notion of reasonable care requires comparison with an external standard.

Accordingly, no allowance is made for the absence of skill or the inexperience of the novice (*Gillespie v. Southern Utah State College* 1983). The standard required is that of the ordinary competent physiotherapist.

Notwithstanding the assertion of McNair J that possession of the highest expert skill is not expected, courts have tended to set progressively higher standards. Advances in science and corresponding increases in community expectations partly account for this. So does insurance, especially in relation to motor vehicle accidents, where courts and juries know that the defendant driver is insured. Although they are not meant to take that into account, they have set higher standards of driver safety in their desire to see the victim compensated. This sentiment has carried over into medical liability litigation. While 'reasonable' suggests something which is average or 'fair enough', the standard in practice may be more demanding. Nevertheless, the physiotherapist is not regarded as a guarantor of recovery. The courts carefully point out that failure to make full recovery does not of itself indicate that there has been negligent medical care (*Gillespie v, Southern Utah State College* 1983).

One aspect of determining what the ordinary competent physiotherapist would have done involves the courts in examining how he or she would respond to foreseeable risks of harm to the athlete. Foreseeable risks are those which are not fanciful or far fetched. To determine that response, the courts use a risk analysis. It is often expressed as an algebraic formula, although a computation is rarely made. The use of the formula may be intangible. Liability is said to occur if:

$$B < P.L$$

where

B is the burden of adequate precautions
P is the probability of injury occurring
L is the gravity of the injury (the amount of the loss).

Breach of the duty of care is determined in accordance with the knowledge reasonably available when the alleged breach occurred. Occasionally an injury or a medical advance must occur before it is realized that a danger exists or means are discovered to avoid it. In those circumstances, no liability will be incurred if the physiotherapist acted in accordance with current knowledge and skill. Liability is not to be judged with the benefit of hindsight.

Reference has been made to a court case involving an athlete who had broken his neck playing rugby league (*Watson v. Haines* 1987). That case illustrates the operation of the risk analysis principles. The gravity of the foreseeable injury—quadriplegia (L)—was great if it materialized and, given that the athlete possessed the relevant anatomical characteristic (a relatively long thin neck), there was a small but significant probability (P) that the injury would occur if he played as hooker. Weighed against those factors, the cost and difficulty (B) of steps to inform school coaches of the risks identified by the research and of establishing a program to screen those boys who were at risk were much smaller. Indeed, the boys could continue playing rugby—they only needed to avoid playing positions involving the risk. The court was able to conclude that B < P.L and held the state liable. The court said that had the coaches been sued they would not have been liable because as ordinary coaches knowledge of the risk was something which could not be reasonably expected to be within their expertise at the time. Given the publicity which the case attracted, a coach would not avoid liability on that basis now.

Establishing the reasonable care standard and the relevance of professional practices

It will be apparent that the content of the variables central to the application of the risk analysis will be largely set by scientific evidence. The knowledge of risks, appropriate avoidance measures and level of skill to be displayed will be set by the educational programs, conferences, research, publications and professional practices and standards of sports physiotherapy. They will be proven to the court by evidence from experts who have appropriate experience and knowledge. Thus, to the extent that there are concerns that issues of liability are out of the hands of the sports physiotherapy profession, they may be allayed. Overall, there is correspondence among legal outcomes and professional standards (Weistart 1985).

It is not uncommon for differing bodies of opinion to evolve among sports physiotherapists concerning the appropriate measures to be adopted for a particular contingency. Rather than decide which opinion is to amount in law to reasonable behaviour, the traditional approach of the courts has been to regard the physiotherapist as acting reasonably if his or her conduct corresponded to a responsible body of professional opinion. McNair J has said (*Bolam V. Friern Hospital Management Committee 1957*):

[A doctor] is not guilty of negligence if he has acted in accordance with a practice accepted as proper by a responsible body of medical men skilled in that particular art...Putting it the other way round, a man is not negligent, if he is acting in accordance with such a practice, merely because there is a body of opinion...[that takes]...a contrary view. At the same time, that does not mean that a medical man can obstinately and pigheadedly carry on with some old technique if it has been proved

to be contrary to what is really substantially the whole of informed medical opinion.

This approach is regarded by some as conferring a privileged position on the medical professions. In contrast, a sport administrator is not absolved of liability because one body of opinion allows play to continue in what another regards as dangerous conditions. Here, the court would choose between the competing views.

The willingness of courts to automatically defer to a common or recognized medical practice when setting the standard of reasonable care is subject to strong criticism. In some quarters it is viewed as conceding to the medical professions the court's right to decide when a breach of the duty of care has occurred.

Medical care may be depicted as having three phases: (1) diagnosis; (2) providing information and advice on treatment options; and (3) delivery of treatment. In regard to phases (1) and (3), courts appear more willing to accept compliance with a common practice as constituting reasonable conduct. Even if not willing to do so automatically, courts will place great importance on such compliance (*Rogers v. Whitaker* 1992).

However, in connection with phase (2), an athlete may maintain that the information or advice was inadequate. As mentioned earlier, this will be linked to a further allegation related to causation; namely, that the athlete would not have undergone the treatment if better informed and would not have suffered some undesired outcome. (There is debate over whether this should be judged by what the particular athlete or a reasonable athlete would have done.) Thus, an action of this kind may succeed notwithstanding that the treatment is rendered with all possible skill and care. In these situations the courts display much less willingness to regard the physiotherapist's actions in relation to provision of advice and information as reasonable just because they accord with a responsible body of medical opinion, or even the whole of informed opinion. There is in many quarters a retreat from the theory of 'doctor knows best'. This is closely linked to the notion of patient autonomy or self-determination: the right of a patient to decide what is to happen to his or her body, life and welfare. From this perspective the athlete would wish to receive understandable information relevant to his or her circumstances (e.g. age and overall health status) about the diagnosis, contemplated treatment, material risks of failure and complications, prospects of success, prognosis if treatment is delayed or not received, and alternative methods of treatment (Willis 1972). The greater the patient's desire for information, the greater the duty to provide it. There are significant differences between common law countries on this information and advice issue and uncertainty cloaks the legal principles in some of them. English courts (*Sidaway v. Bethlem Royal Hospital* 1985) have exhibited reluctance to depart from the traditional position whereas United States courts (*Canterbury v. Spence* 1972) and, to a lesser extent, Australian (*Rogers v. Whitaker* 1992) and Canadian (*Reibl v. Hughes* 1980) courts, have emphasised the patient's right to receive information. Thus, the test for determining how much information the patient is legally entitled to receive varies. There is a range: (1) what the reasonable doctor would provide based on medical disclosure practices which may or may not account for the athlete's needs for information; (2) what the reasonable athlete in the position of the patient/athlete would wish to know; and (3) what the particular athlete would wish to know on whether the information is reasonably required or not. Legal doctrine and debate covers this range. Risks which are immaterial or already known to the athlete do not have to be disclosed.

Some regions accept the existence of a therapeutic privilege, although there are variations in its scope. The privilege may justify 'withholding information…when…[the physiotherapist]…judges on reasonable grounds that the patient's health, physical or mental, might be seriously harmed by the information' (*F v. R* 1983). It may apply also where the patient's temperament or emotional state precludes using the information as the basis of a rational decision. In Ontario, the existence of a therapeutic privilege has been rejected (*Meyer Estate v. Rogers* 1991), and in England it does not become an issue because the only information and advice which has to be provided is that which a responsible body of opinion would regard as necessary.

The quantity and nature of information and advice which an athlete is entitled to expect from a sports physiotherapist and the extent of the right of the physiotherapist to withhold information depend on local law which is subject to the variations mentioned. However, it is suggested that an appropriate ethical standard ought to encompass high regard to equipping the athlete with information to make informed decisions. There will need to be appropriate liaison with other health professionals who may be treating the athlete. Such an approach is most likely to fulfil any legal obligations.

Guidance from the cases and literature concerning compliance with the standard of care

The variable factual nature of whether the standard of care required of the sports physiotherapist has been broken means that previous court decisions and the views of commentators should be approached with caution when seeking to establish guidelines for non-negligent behaviour.

However, there are recurrent issues and themes. These will be addressed below. Many concern attendance at sports events and training sessions. The list is indicative, not exhaustive. It should become readily apparent that the matters listed will, if implemented, make it easier for the physiotherapist to fulfil his or her role in a proper and rewarding manner. Further guidance on appropriate standards of care may be found in other chapters of this book.

Much will depend on the circumstances of the physiotherapist's engagement. For instance, it is not uncommon for teams to appoint a physiotherapist but not a doctor, perhaps because a doctor is not available or a physiotherapist is considered a more economical all-round option. Thus, the physiotherapist might be looked to for first aid or supervision of medical facilities at a venue in circumstances where primary responsibility might otherwise rest with a doctor. While these may be tasks which either a doctor or a physiotherapist can undertake lawfully, the physiotherapist must resist any pressure to act beyond the bounds of his or her professional competence.

There are many matters which can only be dealt with in advance of attendance at a sports event or training session. They include:

1. Keeping abreast of advances in knowledge and technique and being well practised in them (Drowatzky 1985), particularly, training and refresher courses in first aid and cardiopulmonary resuscitation. This might be expected to include how to recognize and stabilize acute trauma, especially head, spine and extremity injuries (Walker et al 1984).
2. Planning with care personal first aid and physiotherapy kits and ensuring their good order (Murphy 1992).
3. Checking the first aid and physiotherapy facilities provided at a venue and drawing attention to deficiencies and requesting that they be rectified. Deficiencies will be judged according to factors such as foreseeable volumes of use and minimum standards recognized by the profession.
4. Ensuring that arrangements are in place for access to superior emergency care (Drowatzky 1985). For example, where is the nearest telephone? Is there road access for an ambulance? Who has the key to the locked gate on the driveway leading from the street? This may involve detailing another person to make the necessary arrangements and inquiries.
5. If appointed to a club or school team for a season, the physiotherapist should be involved in or receive reports on pre-participation examinations and become familiar with each player's history and physical condition (Drowatzky 1986, Walker 1984).
6. If appointed to a national or regional team consisting of athletes with whose histories and existing injuries the physiotherapist is unfamiliar, the details should be discovered and, if necessary, each player's personal doctor or physiotherapist contacted (Murphy 1992). One objective of doing so is to ensure that the injured

athlete is not subjected to conflicting treatment philosophies (Murphy 1992).

7. Before accepting appointment as a team or venue physiotherapist, it should be ascertained whether there will exist channels of communication with relevant decision-makers so that the physiotherapist's recommendations on improved emergency and treatment facilities will be received and implemented. Authority should be obtained to decide on a player's fitness to participate, and to refer him or her to further medical care should the occasion warrant. It is unsatisfactory if medically unqualified coaches or managers can override the physiotherapist's judgement and require players to return to play when it is unsafe to do so. Should a physiotherapist fail in these respects in isolation, it is unlikely that he or she would be legally liable. However, if these suggestions are implemented successfully, the delivery of care will be superior and incidents which might develop legal complications will be less likely to occur.

8. Mental and physical preparation for events should not be overlooked. This will include rehearsal and planning of expected tasks, such as pre-game massage, taping, questions for players with injuries, setting out equipment and organizing assistants, and making sure of the availability and suitability of personal equipment for likely conditions, such as weather (Murphy 1992).

In summary, these points relate to preparation for emergency care, equipment and facilities, management structures impinging on health care delivery, medical histories and the physiotherapist's personal preparedness to fulfil the role. A failure to take reasonable care in relation to any of these points risks legal liability.

Once at the venue but before an event or training session commences there are further matters including:

1. Checking equipment and facilities to ensure that they comply with specifications.
2. The planned pre-event treatment and questions (see above) should be dealt with.
3. A physiotherapist might be expected to supervise or assist with appropriate warm-up exercises. Correct warming-up reduces the risk of injury, especially muscle pulls (Murphy 1992). Whether it is the physiotherapist's duty to become involved with warm-ups will depend on the job description. One who is in attendance only to assist with first aid will probably have no such duty. However, the team physiotherapist will quite likely be responsible for warming-up, especially if the team lacks a fitness trainer.

Most legal liability claims concerning medical care arise out of the treatment (or absence of it) delivered immediately following an injury. Thus, events and training periods warrant special attention. (This is not to suggest that attention should be focused entirely on these periods. The reason for liability is often found in a failure to take care in regard to matters pertaining to the time preceding the event or training session, such as those listed above.) The following matters concern skills, management structures and the deployment of facilities under the conditions of an event or training session.

1. The physiotherapist should honour arrangements to be in attendance or ensure there is a replacement.
2. Recognized safety standards and precautions should be implemented, such as 'head-bin' (removal of concussed players from further participation) and 'blood-bin' (removal of bleeding players until the wound is sealed). If the physiotherapist's preparation is thorough (see above), these precautions will have been established as policies and clear authority will have been obtained to enforce them (perhaps in conjunction with other medical personnel). Thus, the only issue is whether reasonable care is taken to implement the safety standard on any particular occasion.
3. Provision of emergency care has a high-profile because of the potentially grave implications resulting from lack of due skill in execution. Resuscitation (Grayson 1992, Murphy 1992) and movement of players with severe head and spinal injuries (Drowatzky 1985, *Welch v. Dunsmuir Joint Union High School District* 1958) are obvious potential problem areas.
4. Participation in a sport notwithstanding the presence of an injury or health risk is another major area for concern over potential litigation. There are a number of dimensions to this concern.
   (a) An athlete injured during participation may wish to re-enter the event. The legal risk is that the physiotherapist's diagnosis may fail to detect the injury or understate its severity, with the result that the player re-enters and aggravates the original injury. If the diagnosis has not been undertaken with reasonable care, there will be liability for the aggravation. It has been advocated that any doubt should mean the athlete cannot re-enter (Walker 1984).
   (b) There is perhaps a greater risk of liability in circumstances where pressure to re-enter immediately is absent. There have been cases where a failure in diagnosis caused aggravation of the injury over time (*Walton v. Portland Trail Blazers* 1978, *Price v. Milawski* 1978) or at a subsequent event (*Robitaille v. Vancouver Hockey Club Ltd* 1981).
   (c) Participation may be contra-indicated because of injury or health condition, but the athlete insists on participation. This is a difficult problem and will be considered below under 'Specific situations'.

(d) The administration of pain killing injections to enable an athlete to participate is fraught with legal danger. It is 'inexcusable practice…to inject any sprained ligament with local anaesthetic and let…[the athlete]…carry on playing' (Crane 1990). There have been cases in which athletes alleged that injuries were aggravated because they continued to play while pain killers masked the warning signs of serious injury (*Ridge v. San Diego Chargers* 1980). This dimension cannot be dismissed as irrelevant to physiotherapists just because the administration of pain killing injections is outside the proper scope of the practice of physiotherapy. Quite apart from the chance that a physiotherapist may transgress the limits of the discipline, it is not beyond the bounds of possibility that he or she may become implicated if administration occurs with the physiotherapist's knowledge and tacit approval.

The need for compliance with the standard of care does not conclude with the treatment rendered at an event. Subsequent rehabilitative treatment and exercise come under its umbrella. Matters for consideration include the following.

1. A sports physiotherapist is not expected to force an athlete to follow the rehabilitation program or to attend for treatments. However, reasonable care is required in relation to the design of the program, explaining its nature and risks, administering treatment, monitoring progress to assess whether the program is achieving its objectives, supervising the athlete in performing exercises in a proper manner, informing the athlete of the consequences if he or she does not follow the program to its planned conclusion and, perhaps, making some effort to follow-up if the athlete inexplicably terminates treatment.

2. Where the athlete is to self-administer treatment by, say, modalities employing heat or cold, instruction in the modalities' proper and safe use, pointing out usual and other material dangers, will be required.

Further matters of general application include the following.

1. Maintenance of adequate records can often be overlooked in the hurly-burly of change-room routine. Records are important for future reference for the physiotherapist and other medical personnel. In that way they facilitate good care. They may also prove useful for research on injury prevention and improved care techniques. It must be acknowledged that, for legal proceedings, records are a two-edged sword because, as evidence of the treatment, they can suggest liability. However, inadequate records are indicative of poor care and that should be sufficient incentive to maintain good ones.

2. The team physiotherapist may have responsibilities in regard to less qualified medical personnel such as trainers. These responsibilities need to be defined carefully. Depending on the circumstances, they may include selection and training of personnel, as well as devising appropriate systems for supervision and reporting injuries. A common misconception is that if a person being supervised is negligent, the supervisor is liable. Unless the trainer is the physiotherapist's employee (in which case vicarious liability may apply) it will be unusual for the physiotherapist to be liable merely because the trainer commits an isolated negligent act. Rather, liability will arise where the system is negligently devised or implemented negligently overall.

Imperfections in the legal system

The outcome of legal claims is not always in accord with that which might be expected from recognized medical practices. A variety of other factors have a role in influencing outcomes. These include the skill of the lawyers involved, sympathy which judge and jury feel for the claimant, impressiveness of witnesses and financial considerations prompting settlement. While a physiotherapist may be 'right' in relation to particular conduct, the legal outcome can be different because of the cost and difficulty of so proving. There is continuing and inconclusive debate on how to rid the legal system of these imperfections.

SPECIFIC SITUATIONS

Emergencies

It has been recognized that the prospect of incurring legal liability may deter people from voluntarily rendering emergency aid at the scene of accidents. Those who might render aid are said to be reluctant to do so for fear of being accused of, and being held legally liable for, making matters worse or, at least, not making them better. The response of Parliaments in some places (mainly Canada and the USA) has been to enact Good Samaritan laws which offer protection from liability. These laws differ markedly according to who delivers the emergency care (some laws apply only to doctors), the location of delivery (care at hospitals is normally excluded), the definition of emergency care (what is an emergency and its duration) and the conduct of the carer. In regard to the last variable, protection may apply no matter how defective the care has been, only in the absence of gross negligence, or only if the injured person's condition is not worsened (Todaro 1986). A volunteer is usually one who acts for no charge or prospect of financial reward. An arrangement whereby expenses are reimbursed may disqualify a person from volunteer status. This is another issue where advice should be sought as to the precise terms of the local law.

Participation in the face of medical risks

Recreational, elite and other competitive athletes challenge their respective physical capabilities when participating. That is one of the characteristics of sport. In doing so there are health benefits measured in terms of physical fitness and mental diversion and relaxation. There are, however, health risks such as cardiac arrest, arthritis and injury. The worth to the community in health terms of any particular class of sporting activity must be assessed by an overall weighing up of benefits and risks. Sport governing bodies are increasingly aware of the need to modify game rules to make sports safer without necessarily detracting from the nature of the game. Physiotherapists have an important role to play in discovering and publicising the nature of injury risks and suggesting ways in which sports may be made safer. The extent of the legal obligations of sport governing bodies and scientific personnel in this regard has not received sustained attention in the courts. It is possible that in the future this will change although it is speculation to say just when and how.

Of immediate concern are cases where an athlete participates notwithstanding that a health condition or injury indicates that participation should be deferred or avoided altogether. These situations can occur where there is loss of a paired organ, certain musculoskeletal problems or simply a knee that requires further rest after reconstruction. This has become an increasingly controversial issue, especially in the USA where a number of well known athletes have died from pre-existing health conditions (Greenberg 1993). Legal concerns arise when the physiotherapist, acting alone or in conjunction with other medical personnel, approves participation only to see activation or worsening of an injury or condition. For instance, a young man with a relatively long thin neck ought not to be approved to play in the front row of rugby scrum (*Watson v. Haines* 1987). The first issue is whether the injury or condition was known or ought to have been detected. If so, the next is whether approval should have been given. The answers will depend on what is required by the standard of reasonable care, as explained above.

Occasionally a determined, foolishly enthusiastic or impatient athlete will wish to participate notwithstanding medical advice to the contrary. Normally, a physiotherapist does not have power to restrain such an individual from participating. (That is why it can be valuable to have the team's authority to decide who may play, although any decision against the athlete playing must not contravene laws against discrimination (Greenberg 1993, Manno 1991).) Even so, medical personnel are obliged to provide advice and information so that the decision to participate is an informed decision with knowledge of the risks and knowledge that participation is contrary to medical advice. In potentially troublesome cases, it may be desirable to have the advice-giving process witnessed, the athlete sign a release (but see below under, 'Risk management') (Greenberg 1993, Manno 1991) and the physiotherapist put his or her opposition and reasons in writing. Where the athlete is a child or mentally incompetent special problems are encountered because of concern that the athlete is not fit to make important decisions. In such cases, the physiotherapist should clearly indicate his or her opposition to participation to whoever has responsibility for the athlete's welfare. If that fails, local legal and ethical advice ought to be sought and, in extreme cases, it may be a matter for local welfare agencies. A release will be ineffective because such athletes lack legal capacity.

A different approach can be appropriate for elite athletes. Here the physiotherapist's function may be to have the athlete in playing condition as soon as possible. This function derives from the circumstances that the athlete may be without income while sidelined or be at risk of losing a sponsor, ranking, a place in a team or the chance to participate in an Olympic Games. These matters may justify adopting less conservative treatment practices than would be the case for a weekend recreational player. Furthermore, the elite athlete may not wish to miss the opportunity to play in a special event even though an injury has not fully healed. In such cases, the physiotherapist should proceed as discussed above in regard to providing advice and information so that the athlete may make an informed decision.

Fan syndrome

A physiotherapist may come to identify closely with the performances of elite athletes. He or she may assume the status of a confidant and become among the most enthusiastic of fans. At this stage there is a strong prospect of falling victim to 'fan syndrome'. The syndrome distorts appropriate clinical judgement. Athletes will be told what they wish to hear. Unrealistic recovery periods will be mentioned, poor performances will be credited to a combination of unfortunate circumstances (not the result of injury-diminished ability) and retirement will be depicted as far away when medical prudence might dictate otherwise.

The especially dangerous aspect of fan syndrome is that the victim-physiotherapist will rarely be aware of having contracted it.

Often it will seem as if having fan syndrome does not matter because athlete and physiotherapist are as one. However, almost inevitably the athlete will learn that care has not been what it ought to have been and the athlete's pleasure over being told comforting news will turn to accusation.

When working with elite athletes it is difficult to avoid becoming bonded to the pursuit of their goals. However, it must not be forgotten that the physiotherapist has an overriding professional function to perform. If fan syndrome obscures proper clinical judgement there is the risk of legal liability. Indeed, the misguided physiotherapist-fan does not assist the athlete's interests.

TEAM PHYSIOTHERAPISTS

The sports physiotherapist/athlete relationship is usually bipartite where the athlete has consulted or been referred to the physiotherapist's practice or the physiotherapist has rendered emergency care. This means the obligations relating to the exercise of care and skill and to trust and confidence are defined in the context of two parties—the physiotherapist and the athlete.

In contrast, the sports physiotherapist/athlete relationship may arise because a third party has engaged the services of the physiotherapist to care for the athlete. The relationship is then tripartite. The third party may be a professional sports team which employs the athlete. It may be a national or regional sports association charged with fielding a representative team, and the athlete has been selected for that team. This section will investigate the effect the tripartite relationship has upon the obligations pertaining to the exercise of care and skill and to trust and confidence. It will also seek to identify areas where the physiotherapist's responsibilities to athlete and team may conflict.

Skill and care

Since the physiotherapist has been engaged by or appointed to the team, he or she owes a duty to the team to exercise the requisite level of skill in examining or testing prospective athletes as well as caring for the team's existing players. Determining what that level is and whether it has been satisfied will be in accordance with the principles set out earlier in this chapter—but, as shall be shown, not exclusively so. It is increasingly common for the terms of engagement or appointment to stipulate that the physiotherapist must be available to attend certain events, training sessions and tours.

The breach of any such duty or stipulation will render the physiotherapist liable to the team, in addition to any liability for loss sustained by the athlete. Depending on the circumstances, this may warrant dismissal as team physiotherapist and the payment of damages for loss suffered by the team. A team's financial loss can be difficult to prove, but could, for example, be constituted by salary payments to an injured star player who would have returned to competition sooner had appropriate care been provided.

The team employs the physiotherapist with the objective of treating athletes so that they are fit to play. Insofar as the athlete wishes to return from injury as soon as practicable, the athlete and team hold a common objective. However, that may not always be the case. A star player's contract may provide for him or her to continue to be paid when disabled by injury. Faced with a choice between a conservative medical approach to recovery and declaration of fitness, compared with one which is more adventurous or speculative, the athlete might be expected to opt for the former—better to wait a few extra weeks and be certain of not aggravating the injury. However, to the club, that star player at 90% fitness may be superior to the replacement. Accordingly, the physiotherapist might be pressured directly or indirectly to adopt the adventurous practice.

How is this dilemma, occasioned by conflicting interests of team and athlete, to be resolved? First, the athlete should be given sufficient information to make an informed decision on whether to participate. If the athlete remains disinclined to take the risk, there may be a term of his or her contract with the team providing for a dispute or grievance resolution procedure whereby a decision on fitness for play is made by independent medical personnel. Otherwise, the weight of legal principle and commentary favours the view that the physiotherapist's duty is principally to the athlete as an individual patient and that his or her health and welfare must be the primary considerations in case of conflict between team and athlete (Drowatzsky 1985, Grayson 1992).

Fan syndrome is a dangerous complicating factor in these cases. The syndrome may induce the physiotherapist who has become an enthusiastic team supporter to side with team management against an athlete. Some court cases have been reported in the literature where this has been alleged to occur (Drowatzky 1985). Perhaps the most alarming case involved doctors who were influenced by management's view that a Canadian professional ice hockey player was a malingerer. The doctors negligently failed to treat him when he was suffering from a spinal injury. This injury was subsequently aggravated during normal play with catastrophic results and the doctors were found in breach of their legal obligations to the player (*Robitaille v. Vancouver Hockey Club Ltd* 1981).

Confidence and trust

The team will expect reports from the physiotherapist on the health and fitness of the athlete. Such information would normally be subject to the restrictions of confidentiality found in the bipartite physiotherapist/athlete relationship. Confidential information may be disclosed to third parties by the physiotherapist with the consent of the athlete. It is quite common for athletes to expressly give consent when they join the team or enter into professional employment contracts. Otherwise, it is widely accepted that some form of consent is to be implied from the circumstances of team membership and that health care is arranged by the team. Selection and training programs would be seriously inhibited if team medical personnel were not at liberty to pass on information about athletes' health and fitness. The terms of the express or implied consent will vary on a case-by-case basis: the two key variables are the nature of the information and the class of people to whom disclosure is permitted. The usual scope of consent will be to authorize disclosure of information relevant to athletic performance to team management and other members of the team's medical staff. It is desirable that such arrangements be clearly defined and agreed to by the athlete and, preferably, be recorded in writing.

The tripartite relationship will also mean that the team's management may become involved in decisions about appropriate treatment for the athlete. The nature and timing of treatment may have important implications for team planning which the athlete may wish to take into account. However, in the final analysis decisions about treatment are for the athlete taking into account his or her own overall situation.

The physiotherapist may obtain information that an athlete is not fully fit to play but be requested by the athlete not to inform the coach or selectors. The athlete's motives might range from not wishing to miss a final or major event through to needing a match payment which would otherwise be lost. This presents a dilemma. For the physiotherapist to properly advise and treat the athlete, there must be trust between them such that the athlete is confident to make full and frank disclosure of the existence and extent of injuries knowing that, when requested, the physiotherapist will not pass on 'sensitive' health information. On the other hand, the physiotherapist has obligations to the team. The legal niceties of the physiotherapist providing information to team management when requested not to do so by the athlete, especially where the information is volunteered by the athlete rather than discovered by medical observation, have not received much legal analysis in the courts.

Information discovered by the physiotherapist should be passed on. If the athlete announces that he or she will only inform the physiotherapist of the injury or condition if the information is not passed on, the legal position is probably that the physiotherapist should state that he or she is bound to inform the team. It is unlikely that an athlete could restrain the physiotherapist from revealing the information. In reaching this conclusion relevant supporting factors are that the athlete is usually under a personal obligation to the team to reveal performance-relevant health information and would be unlikely to receive a court's assistance to force the physiotherapist not to honour the physiotherapist's obligations to the team. However, this is another issue on which local legal advice should be taken.

A further issue merits brief mention. Early in this chapter it was stated that the sports physiotherapist must be frank and honest with the athlete concerning his or her health and injuries. One complaint about team medical personnel which receives mention in United States' literature is that players, mainly in American football, have been permitted to continue participating in their sport without being told they were injured or without knowledge of the full extent of the injury (Berry & Wong 1993, *Krueger v. San Francisco Forty Niners* 1987). This may even extend to an allegation that non-disclosure has been dishonest or fraudulent (*Krueger v. San Francisco Forty Niners* 1987). Subject to the exceptional situation of therapeutic privilege discussed above, athletes must be given sufficient details of their injuries to make informed decisions about continued participation, as well as to avoid aggravating them and to receive treatment for complications in later life. The duty to be frank and honest with the athlete will override any perceived responsibility to the team.

CONFIDENTIALITY

Relevant principles applicable to confidentiality have been considered above under the headings 'Sports Physiotherapist/Athlete Relationship' and 'Team Physiotherapists'. This section concerns some additional points.

The first is research. Competing interests are at stake: patients' privacy as protected by confidentiality, and benefits for future generations to be gained by improved medical science coming from research dependent on access to otherwise confidential information. As a preliminary it should be noted that general statements of a physiotherapist's experience over the years in treating people recovering from certain kinds of injury would not normally involve any disclosure of confidential information.

Typically, the issue of competing interests arises in one of two circumstances. First, a physiotherapist may wish to use information which he or she has gathered about the medical histories of individuals or groups of athletes for the purposes of publishable research. Second, specialist researchers may request a clinic or team to grant access to their medical histories as a means of primary data collection for epidemiological research.

Ideally, the consent of athletes should be obtained prior to medical information about them being made available to others either in published form or through inspection of histories by researchers. An example of this approach is to be found in the practice whereby team membership agreements contain a clause granting consent to the use of information about athletes for scientific research, provided their identities remain confidential.

Sometimes it is not practicable or desirable to obtain consent because the athlete can no longer be found or because knowledge that the athlete is the subject of an epidemiological study may cause undue alarm. It is usual for local medical research authorities to develop guidelines to deal with such situations, incorporating various safeguards to protect privacy. These typically include anonymity of the athlete in published research, disclosure of such information to researchers only where it is strictly necessary to the project (if practicable, names and other identifying data to be withheld) and access only for qualified researchers. Provided these safeguards are met, the public interest in promoting research will most likely be regarded as outweighing the privacy interests of the athlete, and disclosure will not breach confidentiality. This is, however, a somewhat murky area and may depend on the value and nature of the research. Local advice should be taken.

A team physiotherapist may participate in a medical examination of a prospective player with whom there is no other connection. The information gained from the examination may be passed to the team, as that is the purpose of the examination. Otherwise, it is confidential. This applies even though the athlete may prove unfit for employment and no further relationship ensues. A related matter is that according to some United States legal authorities, the physiotherapist who examines such prospective players must at least inform them of serious health problems which he or she discovers so the athlete may have them treated (*Betesh v. United States* 1974). This duty arguably extends to exercising reasonable care in conducting examinations so as to detect at least, serious health defects (King 1981).

SHARED RESPONSIBILITY FOR INJURY

Notwithstanding that the physiotherapist may have acted wrongfully, he or she may not be liable for all the harm which the athlete has suffered. The relevant laws are technical and subject to local differences. Consequently, they will be described in general terms only and local legal advice should be sought.

Causation

Usually, the allegation is one of aggravating an existing injury. Since the original injury is not caused by the physiotherapist's act, there is liability only to the extent that the athlete is harmed beyond the consequences of the original injury had the injury received proper care.

Multiple wrongdoers and contribution

Liability may be shared with others who have been responsible for the athlete's care, such as doctors, radiologists and trainers. This is particularly the case where the athlete complains that an injury remained undetected or improperly diagnosed over a period of time during which he or she was treated by a number of medical personnel. Most regions have legislation which prescribe rules for sharing liability in these circumstances. This area of law is known as contribution. A common, but not the only, formula is for liability to be borne according to what a court considers just and equitable having regard to each person's responsibility for the harm. This permits a flexible approach for dealing with widely varying fact situations. However, significant debate has occurred over the correct approach to be taken in applying that rule.

Contributory negligence

Contributory negligence is a defence to an action in negligence. In some places it is a defence to an action in contract. It occurs where an athlete fails to take reasonable care for his or her own safety and this contributes to causing the injury. The principles for deciding whether there has been such a failure are analogous to those considered under the heading 'Negligence: breach of the duty of care' above. For example, a delay in recovery may be a combination of poor medical treatment and failure by the athlete to follow instructions for proper care of the injury. Reasonable care for one's safety may even require seeking alternative advice when it is apparent that proper care is not being received (*Robitaille v. Vancouver Hockey Club Ltd* 1981). At common law, contributory negligence acted to defeat a person's claim completely and this remains the case in a few places. However, most places have legislation which permits a court to apportion or share responsibility between the various wrongdoers and the contributorily negligent injured athlete. Thus, after establishing his or her case against the wrongdoers and proving the value of the loss, the athlete will have the damages reduced according to what a court considers just and equitable, having regard to the athlete's share in responsibility for the harm. This is a common formula, but by no means the only one, especially in the USA. In the USA contributory negligence is called comparative negligence when apportionment is permitted.

Vicarious liability

The most common form of vicarious liability occurs in the relationship between an employer and employee. The employer will be liable for most wrongful acts committed by the employee in the course of his or her employment notwithstanding that the employer may not have been personally at fault, for example, the partners in a clinic will be vicariously liable for burns caused negligently by a non-partner physiotherapist who is their employee. One rationale for this rule is that employers profit from their employees' work and should be responsible for the losses as well. Another is that employers are more likely to be insured and able to pay the injured person's damages.

It is often misunderstood that the employer's vicarious liability does not relieve the employee of liability. The athlete can sue either or both, but cannot recover damages twice over.

In cases where the employer is sued, the law in some places permits the employer to recover the damages paid to the athlete from the employee whose wrongful conduct produced the vicarious liability.

Whether or not a worker is an employee can be a complex issue, and legal tests vary between regions. A physiotherapist working for a hospital or full-time for a team is an employee, whereas one who is in practice on his or her own or as a partner in a clinic is an independent contractor. The significance of the difference between an employee and an independent contractor for present purposes is that while a person who engages an employee is open to vicarious liability, someone who engages an independent contractor is not usually vicariously liable for the contractor's wrongful conduct. If an insurance company sends a potential life insurance client to a medical clinic for a check-up and pays the doctor's bill, the doctor is an independent contractor. Hence, if that doctor negligently injures the patient during the examination, the insurance company will not be vicariously liable. While this rule will often apply to team physiotherapists who are in private practice, that will not always be the case. Such a physiotherapist may become part of the team's organization and be subject to its control, even if only in a general way and on a part-time basis, so that he or she will be regarded as an employee in connection with the delivery of physiotherapy services related to athletes' involvement with the team (*Barry and Wong Robitaille v. Vancouver Hockey Club Ltd* 1981) but not private health matters (*Wilson v. Vancouver Hockey Club Ltd* 1985). Whether or not this occurs may be a matter of circumstance and degree.

Practical implications of this include the following. An employee physiotherapist should discover whether the insurance policy taken by the employer insures the employee against his or her own liability to athletes as well as the employer's vicarious liability. It is often possible to have such insurance. As part of the employment agreement, the employer may be requested to indemnify the employee against liability to athletes which he or she may incur in the course of employment, or at least agree not to seek indemnity from the employee should the employer be held vicariously liable. On the other hand, employer physiotherapists may wish to resist such requests for commercial reasons. They should also have insurance which protects them against vicarious liability for the wrongful conduct of their employees.

Supervision of other sports medicine staff

The team sports physiotherapist may often be called upon to supervise or help train other members of the sports medicine staff. Typically, these people will be appointed by the team, and apart from being work colleagues, they will have no other connection with the physiotherapist.

Accordingly, the physiotherapist will not be vicariously liable for their wrongful behaviour in the sense that an employer is liable.

However, the physiotherapist does owe a duty to the athlete to take reasonable care in relation to the supervision and training. Should the physiotherapist expressly or impliedly direct the other staff member to perform some action which is wrongful or provide unsuitable training, there will be personal (as opposed to vicarious) liability to the injured athlete. This does not mean there is liability for each wrongful act of the supervised staff member. Provided the physiotherapist has designed and implements a proper system of supervision, isolated acts of negligence by supervised staff members do not place the physiotherapist in breach his or her own duty to the athlete.

RISK MANAGEMENT

There are many dimensions to managing the risks of litigation. The first encompasses measures to avoid the occurrence of events which might involve the physiotherapist in legal liability. The precautions discussed above under the heading 'Negligence: breach of the duty of care' are especially relevant. Prevention is better than cure. It is important to think carefully and methodically about risk management. That should involve identifying the risks, evaluating their nature and gravity and developing a safety plan which can be implemented to systematically eliminate or minimize risks. Particularly when working for a team or venue, an essential element of risk management is obtaining a clear definition of the expected role and responsibilities, as well as the relationship to other health professionals. The best time for doing so is when the agreement of appointment or renewal is negotiated.

Naturally, this kind of risk management might be taken to extremes so that resources and energy are claimed to be directed away from the delivery of health care. The unflattering term 'defensive medicine' has been used to describe these situations. However, it should be remembered that most steps which have been identified for managing risks are likely to lift the standard of care provided. That is a desirable objective, quite apart from any incidental reduction of exposure to legal liability.

The second dimension of risk management encompasses measures to avoid the occurrence of legal liability. These involve legal steps such as having athletes complete consent forms or agree to exclude liability.

The reasons for obtaining an athlete's consent before administering physiotherapy are considered above under the heading 'Consent'. (Remember, consent once given can be withdrawn, in some emergency circumstances explicit consent is not necessary, and the consent of a parent or legal guardian may be required for treatment given to children.) Sometimes it is convenient or desirable to obtain consent in writing because it is a better record than an oral consent. However, a consent form is usually regarded only as evidence of a state of affairs, namely, that consent was given. An athlete may be able to prove that there was no consent and the written document is not an accurate record of his or her state of mind. Usually, strong evidence will be necessary to do so because the indication of consent supplied by the signed form must be negated.

Sometimes a consent form can record (at least in general terms) what an athlete has been told in regard to proposed treatment. This may be appropriate where major or complicated treatment is planned and will provide some evidence in connection with the physiotherapist's information and advice-giving duties.

It is desirable to have standard forms of consent drafted and checked regularly by a lawyer.

An exclusion clause, as its name suggests, is intended to provide relief from legal liability which would normally apply but for the presence of the clause. They are sometimes called exemption clauses or, in the USA, releases or waivers. A variant is the limitation clause, which does not entirely exclude liability but imposes a monetary ceiling. These clauses constitute agreements between athlete and physiotherapist and contemplate that certain kinds of incident may occur for which the physiotherapist is not to be legally liable. Since the clauses seek to modify the balance between the contracting parties which the law considers 'normal', they often receive a hostile reception in the courts and from Parliaments. While waivers prepared expertly may succeed, they are, among other things (Manno 1991), they are frequently illegal, are interpreted narrowly by courts in favour of the person who appears disadvantaged and are rarely of any effect against children. Parents and legal guardians are widely regarded as not being entitled to agree to exclusion clauses on children's behalf. However, an alternative is to seek an indemnity from the parent or guardian which requires payment by the parent or guardian to the physiotherapist of an amount equal to any damages which the latter is ordered to pay to the child athlete.

Notwithstanding the limits and reservations which have been mentioned above, exclusions can achieve their purposes in some situations, but this requires local advice and careful and skilled legal drafting.

The third dimension is insurance. Insurance is important. Very simply, it is usually a contract whereby, in exchange for a payment called a premium, the insurer agrees to indemnify the insured (the physiotherapist) in respect of awards of damages and associated legal costs which the insured is liable to pay in certain circumstances defined in the policy. Thus, if all other risk management measures have failed to avoid liability arising, the insurer rather than the physiotherapist will pay.

Most physiotherapists will hold legal liability insurance cover of some kind. This insurance can go by different names according to locality and insurance company. It is often arranged by professional associations as part of a compulsory or voluntary uniform scheme. A prime consideration is whether the existing insurance covers the sports physiotherapy activity to be engaged in. For instance, the policy may cover a physiotherapy practice during 'normal' hours and activity, but not protect voluntary work at a weekend mass participation marathon or with a touring team in a foreign country. Thus, an extension may be necessary to cover the 'unusual' activity. Another important point to note is the insurance policy's requirements for the physiotherapist to report the happening of incidents which might give rise to liability—failure to do so may invalidate the cover for that incident. The maximum limit of cover for any one incident must be noted. If liability exceeds the maximum cover, the physiotherapist will have to the pay the excess. At the very least these issues should be investigated and reviewed from time to time with an adviser.

When working for a team or venue, it may be possible to have the team's or venue's insurance extended to protect the physiotherapist, or it may do so already. This can avoid a surcharge on the physiotherapist's normal private practice policy premium.

Reference should also be made to the insurance position of employees discussed above under the heading 'Vicarious liability'.

The fourth and final dimension is not normally within the control of individual physiotherapists but warrants brief mention. Parliaments have enacted laws which regulate the circumstances in which legal proceedings may be taken. Some are specific to health care professions, others are of general application. Statutes of limitation fix time periods within which legal proceedings may be commenced. These periods vary from place to place. It is common for them not to commence to run against children until they reach the age of full legal capacity. In some states of the USA, shorter than usual periods may apply to sectors of the health care professions. This has been a legislative response to concern about growth in medical malpractice litigation. A related development in the USA is to be found in special notification and procedural arrangements for health care litigation. Local advice should be taken on these matters.

PERFORMANCE-ENHANCING DRUG CONTROL

Not only do the International Olympic Committee, major international sports federations and some national laws prohibit the use of certain performance-enhancing substances and techniques by athletes, they have created offences aimed at those who may in various ways assist or encourage athletes to break the anti-doping rules. In part this is a response to disclosures during the Ben Johnson affair of the pivotal role in doping practices played by medically and scientifically qualified people.

The anti-doping rules of sport have undergone dramatic expansion in complexity and reach in recent years and it is not practical to analyse the rules here. It will suffice to identify the following implications and issues for a physiotherapist who renders prohibited assistance or incites breaking the rules (or engages in related prohibited activity):

1. Banishment from official association with the sport concerned and denial of access to government-funded facilities and programs in certain countries;
2. Disciplinary action by the local physiotherapy regulatory authority for professional misconduct (*State Medical Board of Ohio v. Murray* 1993, Mitten 1994);
3. Legal action by athletes alleging physical harm suffered through using dangerous prohibited substances or techniques
4. Drug trafficking or customs offences in some countries.

Occasionally, athletes will seek advice on which substances and practices are banned so as to avoid breaking the rules. Information is usually obtained from doctors or, in some countries, services provided by sport or government. However, if a physiotherapist does provide advice, he or she will be under a duty to take reasonable care to ensure that the advice is accurate. The potential for rendering inaccurate advice was highlighted during 1992 when controversy arose over the status of clenbuterol as a prohibited anabolic steroid and stimulant.

REGISTRATION

Consideration was given above (under the headings 'Legislation' and Authority to practise') to the regulatory bodies for physiotherapy and to the need for physiotherapists to be licensed to practise. These regulatory arrangements apply to physiotherapy generally, are technical and vary between regions, especially in the USA (Baker & Rode 1975). Accordingly, it is not proposed to consider them further in the context of sports physiotherapy other than to focus on two specific issues.

The physiotherapist must possess current authority to practise physiotherapy in the legal region where care is provided. This means that a physiotherapist who is travelling with a team in a foreign country, or even in another state or province of his or her own country, should obtain local registration in the region visited before treating team athletes while on tour. Most local laws allow for temporary registration and it should be obtainable without too much trouble, given that the physiotherapist will be only treating members of his or her own team. However, in practice it is almost routine for local registration to be overlooked. Indeed, regulatory bodies rarely concern themselves with the issue, although there have been notable exceptions such as when visiting team physiotherapists were required to register in New Zealand in connection with the 1990 Auckland Commonwealth Games. In most places, the unregistered physiotherapist risks criminal prosecution. The absence of registration would be an embarrassing (but not necessarily crucial) disclosure in any action by an athlete concerning injury alleged to have been caused by the physiotherapist during the tour.

Especially in team sports, physiotherapists will often work alongside and supervise trainers as fellow members of the sports medicine staff. Trainers will not be qualified to practise physiotherapy in their own right. To determine the permissible limits of the trainer's role vis-à-vis the physiotherapist's role, reference will have to be made to the definition of physiotherapy found in the relevant regulatory legislation. In some places a comprehensive definition is provided by the legislation. In others the approach has been to leave physiotherapy undefined but at the same time restrict the use of certain modalities and techniques (such as microwave and ultrasound). Under this approach a court would have to decide on the basis of expert evidence whether any particular activity was physiotherapy.

Obviously, public safety is the main motive for such control. Unauthorised use is often punishable by the criminal law which may impose a fine or even imprisonment.

It may come to the attention of the physiotherapist that a trainer is practising restricted physiotherapy techniques or using restricted modalities, or is highly likely to do so. The physiotherapist may be tempted to instruct the trainer in the proper methods on the basis that, once trained, the risk of the trainer injuring an athlete is significantly reduced. However, the physiotherapist risks being held to be an accomplice to any breach by the trainer of the criminal provisions of physiotherapy laws, disciplinary action for unprofessional conduct, and liability in negligence to an athlete injured by the trainer. Also, teams and venues which own restricted modalities could risk liability if they take insufficient steps to ensure that unqualified employees do not use the modalities. In a limited number of places, it may be lawful for a trainer to use some restricted modalities under supervision of a physiotherapist or, in some states of the USA, in his or her own right under legislation regulating athletic trainers.

REFERENCES

Books and articles

Baker B B, Rode C A 1975 Legal implications concerning the use of physical therapy modalities by athletic trainers. Athletic Training 10(4):208-211

Berry R C, Wong G M 1993 Law and business of the sports industries 2nd edn. Auburn House Publishing, Dover, Massachusetts, vol II

Crane J 1990 Association football: the team doctor. In: Payne S D W (ed) Medicine, sport and the law. Blackwell Scientific Publications, Oxford

Drowatzky J N 1985 Legal duties and liability in athletic training. Athletic Training 20(1):10-13

Fleming J G 1992 The law of torts, 8th edn. Law Book Company, Sydney, p 81

Graham L S 1986 Avoiding the 'sue syndrome'. The Physician and Sportsmedicine 14(2):66

Grayson E 1992 Sports medicine and the law. In: Payne S D W (ed) Medico-legal hazards of rugby union. Blackwell Special Projects, Oxford

Greenberg M J 1993 To play or not to play. The sports Lawyer XI Sept/Oct: 1,3,7,10

Keeton W P (ed) 1984 Prosser and Keeton on torts, 5th edn. West Publishing, St Paul, pp.114-121

King J H 1981 The duty and standard of care for team physicians. Houston Law Review 18:657-705

Leverenz L J, Helms L B 1990 Suing athletic trainers: part I. Athletic Training 25(3):212-218

Manno A 1991 A high price to compete: the feasibility and effect of waivers used to protect schools from liability for injuries to athletes with high medical risks. Kentucky Law Journal 79:867-881

Mitten M J 1994 Liability of sports medicine providers and related entities. In: Uberstine G A (ed) Law of professional and amateur sports. Clark Boardman Callaghan, Deerfield Illinois

Murphy K 1992 The role of the physiotherapist in club and international rugby football. In: Payne S D W (ed) Medico-legal hazards of rugby union, Blackwell Special Projects, Oxford

Opie H 1992 Nature and incidence of personal injury litigation in sport and recreation. Unpublished

Savastano A A 1968 The team physician and the law. Rhode Island Medical Journal 51:558-565

Skene L 1990 You, your doctor and the law. Oxford University Press, Melbourne

Todaro G J 1986 The volunteer team physician: when are you exempt from civil liability? The Physician and Sportsmedicine 14(2):147-153

Walker E J, Bianco E A, Hartmann P M 1984 Legal aspects of sports medicine. In: Birrer R B (ed) Sports medicine for the primary care physician. Appleton-Century-Crofts, Norwalk

Weistart J C 1985 Legal consequences of standard setting for competitive athletes with cardiovascular abnormalities. Journal of American College of Cardiology 6:1191-1197

Willis G C 1972 The legal responsibilities of the team physician. The Journal of Sports Medicine Sept/Oct:28-29

World Confederation for Physical Therapy 1982 Ethical principles for physical therapists 8

Cases

Betesh v. United States (1977) 400 Fed Supp 238 (Dist of Columbia)

Bolam v. Friern Hospital Management Committee [1957] 1 WLR 582 (Queen's Bench, England)

Canterbury v. Spence (1972) 464 Fed Rep, 2d Series 772 (CA Dist of Columbia)

F. v. R. (1983) 33 SASR 189 (SC SA)

Gillespie v. Southern Utah State College (1983) 669 Pac Rep, 2d Series 861 (SC Utah)

Gillick v. West Norfolk and Wisbech Area Health Authority [1986] AC 112 (House of Lords)

Krueger v. San Francisco Forty Niners (1987) 234 Cal Rep 579 (CA Calif)

Meyer Estate v. Rogers (1991) 6 Can Cases on the Law of Torts 2nd Series 102 (Ontario)

Price v. Milawski (1978) 82 DLR 3rd Series 130 (CA Ontario)

Reibl v. Hughes [1980] 2 SCR 880 (SC Canada)

Ridge v. San Diego Chargers. In: Pitt M B 1980 Malpractice on the sidelines: developing a standard of care for team sports physicians. COMM/ENT 2:579-598

Robitaille v. Vancouver Hockey Club Ltd (1981) 124 DLRReports 3d Series 228 (CA British Columbia)

Rogers v. Whitaker (1992) L 175 CLR 479 (High Couurt of Australia)

Sidaway v. Bethlem Royal Hospital [1985] AC 871 (House of Lords)

State Medical Board of Ohio v. Murray (1993) 613 NE 2nd series 636 (sc Ohio)

Walton v. Portland Trail Blazers 1978. In: Berry R C, Wong G M 1986 Law and business of the sports industries, 2nd edn. Auburn House Publishing, Dover, Massachusetts, vol II

Watson v. Haines (1987) Aust Torts Rep ¶80-094 (SC NSW)

Welch v. Dunsmuir Joint Union High School District (1958) 326 Pac Rep, 2d Series 633 (CA California)

Wilson v. Vancouver Hockey Club Ltd (1985) 22 DLR, 4th Series 516 (CA British Columbia)

Index